Acquisitions Editor: Emily Lupash
Product Manager: Andrea M. Klingler
Marketing Manager: Christen Murphy
Designer: Joan Wendt
Art by: Dragonfly Media Group
Compositor: Aptara, Inc.

KT-528-314

Fourth Edition

Copyright © 2011 Lippincott Williams & Wilkins, a Wolters Kluwer business

351 West Camden Street   Two Commerce Square, 2001 Market Street
Baltimore, MD 21201   Philadelphia, PA 19103

Printed in The People's Republic of China

Not authorized for Sale in North America or the Caribbean

First Edition, 1994
Second Edition, 2000
Third Edition, 2006

Unless otherwise indicated, all photographs are Copyright © Fitness Technologies Press, Frank I. Katch, and Victor L. Katch, 5043 Via Lara Lane, Santa Barbara, CA, 93111. This material is protected by copyright. No photograph may be reproduced in any form or by any means without permission from the copyright holders.

Appendix B Copyright © 1991, 1999, 2010 by Fitness Technologies, Inc. 5043 Via Lara Lane, Santa Barbara, CA, 93111. This material is protected by copyright. No part of it may be reproduced in any manner or by any means without written permission from the copyright holder.

Appendices C and D Copyright © 1991, 1999, 2010 by William D. McArdle, Frank L. Katch, Victor L. Katch and Fitness Technologies, Inc. This material is protected by copyright. No part of it may be reproduced in any manner or by any means without written permission from the copyright holder.

All rights reserved. This book is protected by copyright. No part of this book may be reproduced in any form or by any means, including photocopying, or utilized by any information storage and retrieval system without written permission from the copyright owner.

The publisher is not responsible (as a matter of product liability, negligence, or otherwise) for any injury resulting from any material contained herein. This publication contains information relating to general principles of medical care that should not be construed as specific instructions for individual patients. Manufacturers' product information and package inserts should be reviewed for current information, including contraindications, dosages, and precautions.

Library of Congress Cataloging-in-Publication Data

Katch, Victor L.
    Essentials of exercise physiology / Victor L. Katch, William D. McArdle, Frank I. Katch.— 4th ed.
        p. ; cm.
    William D. McArdle is first named author on previous edition.
    Abridgement of: Exercise physiology / William D. McArdle, Frank I. Katch, Victor L. Katch. 7th ed. c2010.
    Includes bibliographical references and index.
    Summary: "This is a textbook for undergraduate Exercise Physiology courses"—Provided by publisher.
    Summary: "The fourth edition of Essentials of Exercise Physiology represents a compact version of the seventh edition of Exercise Physiology: Nutrition, Energy, and Human Performance, ideally suited for an undergraduate l introductory course in exercise physiology"—Provided by publisher.
    ISBN 978-1-60831-267-2 (alk. paper)
    1. Exercise—Physiological aspects.   I. McArdle, William D.   II. Katch, Frank I.   III. McArdle, William D. Exercise physiology.
IV. Title.
    [DNLM: 1. Exercise—physiology.   2. Physical Fitness—physiology.   3. Sports Medicine.   QT 260]
    QP301.M1149 2011
    612'.044—dc22

                                                                    2010031304

The publishers have made every effort to trace the copyright holders for borrowed material. If they have inadvertently overlooked any, they will be pleased to make the necessary arrangements at the first opportunity.

To purchase additional copies of this book, call our customer service department at **(800) 638-3030** or fax orders to **(301) 223-2320.** International customers should call **(301) 223-2300.**

Visit Lippincott Williams & Wilkins on the Internet: http://www.lww.com. Lippincott Williams & Wilkins customer service representatives are available from 8:30 am to 6:00 pm, EST.

Essentials of Exercise Physiology

FOURTH EDITION

Victor L. Katch (Ann Arbor, MI)
Professor, Department of Movement Science
School of Kinesiology

Associate Professor, Pediatrics
School of Medicine
University of Michigan
Ann Arbor, Michigan

William D. McArdle (Sound Beach, NY)
Professor Emeritus, Department of Family, Nutrition, and Exercise Science
Queens College of the City University of New York
Flushing, New York

Frank I. Katch (Santa Barbara, CA)
International Research Scholar, Faculty of Health and Sport
Agder University College
Kristiansand, Norway

Instructor and Board Member
Certificate Program in Fitness Instruction
UCLA Extension, Los Angeles, CA

Former Professor and Chair of Exercise Science
University of Massachusetts
Amherst, Massachusetts

055572

Wilkins

THE HENLEY COLLEGE LIBRARY

DEDICATION

To Heather, Erika, Leslie, Jesse, Ryan, and Cameron: you light up my life.
— Victor L. Katch

To my grandchildren, Liam, Aiden, Quinn, Dylan, Kelly Rose, Owen, Henry, Kathleen (Kate), Grace, Elizabeth, Claire, and Elise. Keep your eye on the ball, your skis together, and go for the gold. All my love, Grandpa; and to Guido F. Foglia, my mentor, my "brother," and my unbelievably good and loyal friend.
— Bill McArdle

To my beautiful wife Kerry, who has been there for me from the beginning, and our great children, David, Kevin, and Ellen.
— Frank I. Katch

Preface

The fourth edition of *Essentials of Exercise Physiology* represents an updated, compact version of the seventh edition of *Exercise Physiology: Nutrition, Energy, and Human Performance*, ideally suited for an undergraduate introductory course in exercise physiology or health-related science. *Essentials of Exercise Physiology* maintains many of the features that have made *Exercise Physiology: Nutrition, Energy, and Human Performance*, a leading textbook in the field since 1981 and the First Prize winner in medicine of the British Medical Association's 2002 Medical Book Competition. This *Essentials* text continues the same strong pedagogy, writing style, and graphics and flow charts of prior editions, with considerable added materials.

In preparing this edition, we incorporated feedback from students and faculty from a wide range of interests and disciplines. We are encouraged that all reviewers continue to embrace the major theme of the book: "**understanding interrelationships among energy intake, energy transfer during exercise, and the physiologic systems that support that energy transfer.**"

ORGANIZATION

We have rearranged material within and among chapters to make the information flow more logically. To improve readability, we have combined topic headings, incorporated common materials, and rearranged other materials necessary for an essentials text. This restructuring now makes it easier to cover most of the chapters in a one-semester course and adapt materials to diverse disciplines.

Section I, "Introduction to Exercise Physiology," introduces the historical roots of exercise physiology and discusses professional aspects of exercise physiology and the interrelationship between exercise physiology and sports medicine.

Section II, "Nutrition and Energy," consists of three chapters and emphasizes the interrelationship between food energy and optimal nutrition for exercise. A critical discussion includes the alleged benefits of commonly promoted nutritional (and pharmacologic) aids to enhance performance.

Section III, "Energy Transfer," has four chapters that focus on energy metabolism and how energy transfers from stored nutrients to muscle cells to produce movement during rest and various physical activities. We also include a discussion of the measurement and evaluation of the different capacities for human energy transfer.

Section IV, "The Physiologic Support Systems," contains four chapters that deal with the major physiologic systems (pulmonary, cardiovascular, neuromuscular, and endocrine) that interact to support the body's response to acute and chronic physical activity and exercise.

Section V, "Exercise Training and Adaptations," includes three chapters that describe application of the scientific principles of exercise training, including the highly specific functional and structural adaptation responses to chronic exercise overload. We discuss the body's response to resistance training and the effects of different environmental challenges on energy transfer and exercise performance. We also critique the purported performance-enhancing effects of various "physiologic" agents.

Section VI, "Optimizing Body Composition, Successful Aging, and Health-Related Physical Activity Benefits," contains three chapters that feature health-related aspects of regular physical activity. We include a discussion of body composition assessment; the important role physical activity plays in weight control, successful aging, and disease prevention; and clinical aspects of exercise physiology.

WORKBOOK FORMAT

The Questions & Notes workbook sections remain integrated into each chapter. This pedagogical element encourages students to answer different questions about what they read. This concurrent active reading/learning element enhances student understanding of text material to a greater extent than simply reading and underlining the content on the page.

Highlights of New and Expanded Content

The following points highlight new and expanded content of the fourth edition of *Essentials of Exercise Physiology*:

- Each section has undergone a major revision, incorporating the most recent research and information about the topic.
- We have included new emerging topics within each chapter based on current research.
- We include updated selected references at the end of every chapter.
- Where applicable, we include relevant Internet websites related to exercise physiology.
- We include additional *For Your Information* boxes and have added new and updated material to the *Close Up boxes*.
- The full-color art program continues to be a stellar feature of the textbook. We have updated and expanded the art program and tables to maintain consistent with the 2010 seventh edition of *Exercise Physiology: Nutrition, Energy, and Human Performance.*

Special Features

- **Close Up Boxes.** This popular feature focuses on timely and important exercise, sport, and clinical topics in exercise physiology that relate to chapter content. Many of the boxes present practical applications to related topics of interest. This material, often showcased in a step-by-step, illustrated format, provides relevance to the practice of exercise physiology. Some Close Up boxes contain self-assessment or laboratory-type activities.
- **For Your Information Boxes.** These boxes throughout the text highlight key information about different exercise physiology areas. We designed these boxes to help bring topics to life and make them relevant to student learning.
- **Thought Questions.** Thought Questions at the end of each chapter section summary encourage integrative, critical thinking to help students apply information from the chapter. The instructor can use these questions to stimulate class discussion about chapter content and application of material to practical situations.

- **Questions & Notes.** This feature facilitates student learning by focusing on specific questions related to important material presented in the text.
- **Appendices.** Useful current information is at the student's fingertips:

  Appendix A: The Metric System and Conversion Constants in Exercise Physiology

  Appendix B: Metabolic Computations in Open-Circuit Spirometry

  Appendix C: Evaluation of Body Composition—Girth Method

  Appendix D: Evaluation of Body Composition—Skinfold Method

User's Guide

Essentials of Exercise Physiology, 4th edition, was created and developed as a compact version of the popular *Exercise Physiology: Nutrition, Energy, and Human Performance*, 7th edition. This comprehensive package integrates the basic concepts and relevant scientific information to understand nutrition, energy transfer, and exercise training. Please take a few moments to look through this User's Guide, which will introduce you to the tools and features that will enhance your learning experience.

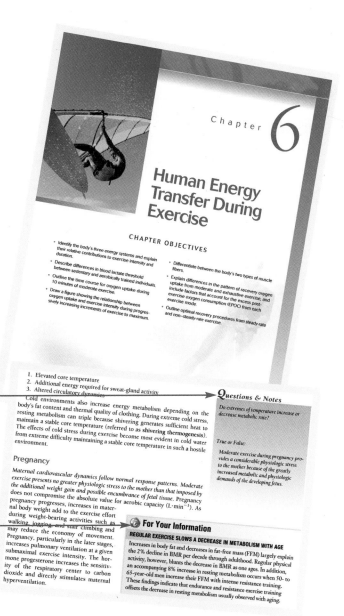

Chapter Objectives open each chapter and present learning goals to help you focus on and retain the crucial topics discussed in each chapter.

Questions & Notes, located in the margin of the odd-numbered pages, enhance your understanding of text material by using an integrated workbook format that presents questions to help drive home key topics and provide a place to take notes and jot down questions.

For Your Information Boxes highlight key information about different exercise physiology areas and help bring topics to life, making them exciting and relevant for all readers.

Beautiful Illustrations throughout the text help to draw attention to important concepts in a visually stimulating and intriguing manner. Detailed, full-color drawings and photographs amplify and clarify the text and are particularly helpful for visual learners.

Close Up Boxes explore real-life cases and practical applications of exercise physiology applied to elite athletes and average people.

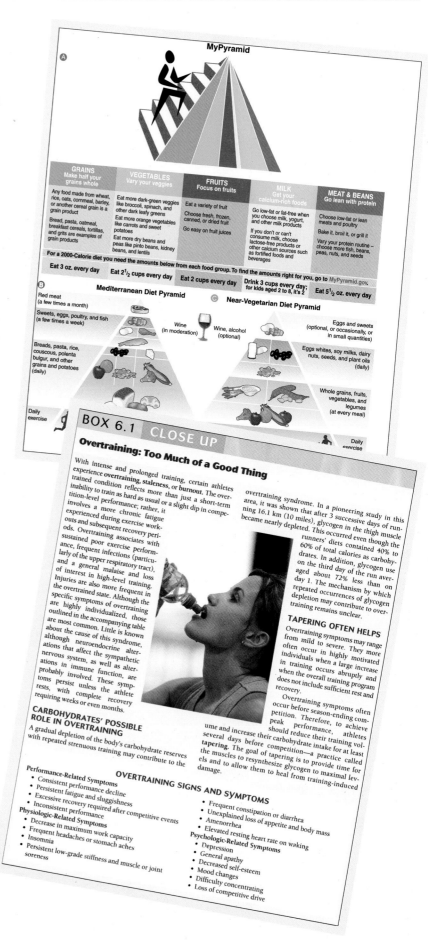

BOX 6.1 CLOSE UP

Overtraining: Too Much of a Good Thing

With intense and prolonged training, certain athletes experience **overtraining, staleness,** or **burnout.** The overtrained condition reflects more than just a short-term inability to train as hard as usual or a slight dip in competition-level performance; rather, it involves a more chronic fatigue experienced during exercise workouts and subsequent recovery periods. Overtraining associates with sustained poor exercise performance, frequent infections (particularly of the upper respiratory tract), and a general malaise and loss of interest in high-level training. Injuries are also more frequent in the overtrained state. Although the specific symptoms of overtraining are highly individualized, those outlined in the accompanying table are most common. Little is known about the cause of this syndrome, although neuroendocrine alterations that affect the sympathetic nervous system, as well as alterations in immune function, are probably involved. These symptoms persist unless the athlete rests, with complete recovery requiring weeks or even months.

CARBOHYDRATES' POSSIBLE ROLE IN OVERTRAINING

A gradual depletion of the body's carbohydrate reserves with repeated strenuous training may contribute to the

overtraining syndrome. In a pioneering study in this area, it was shown that after 3 successive days of running 16.1 km (10 miles), glycogen in the thigh muscle became nearly depleted. This occurred even though the runners' diets contained 40% to 60% of total calories as carbohydrates. In addition, glycogen use on the third day of the run averaged about 72% less than on day 1. The mechanism by which repeated occurrences of glycogen depletion may contribute to overtraining remains unclear.

TAPERING OFTEN HELPS

Overtraining symptoms may range from mild to severe. They more often occur in highly motivated individuals when a large increase in training occurs abruptly and when the overall training program does not include sufficient rest and recovery.

Overtraining symptoms often occur before season-ending competition. Therefore, to achieve peak performance, athletes should reduce their training volume and increase their carbohydrate intake for at least several days before competition—a practice called **tapering.** The goal of tapering is to provide time for the muscles to resynthesize glycogen to maximal levels and to allow them to heal from training-induced damage.

OVERTRAINING SIGNS AND SYMPTOMS

Performance-Related Symptoms
• Consistent performance decline
• Persistent fatigue and sluggishness
• Excessive recovery required after competitive events
• Inconsistent performance

Physiologic-Related Symptoms
• Decrease in maximum work capacity
• Frequent headaches or stomach aches
• Insomnia
• Persistent low-grade stiffness and muscle or joint soreness

• Frequent constipation or diarrhea
• Unexplained loss of appetite and body mass
• Amenorrhea
• Elevated resting heart rate on waking

Psychologic-Related Symptoms
• Depression
• General apathy
• Decreased self-esteem
• Mood changes
• Difficulty concentrating
• Loss of competitive drive

Thought Questions, located at the conclusion of each chapter part, encourage critical thinking and problem-solving skills to help students use and apply information learned throughout each chapter in a practical manner.

THOUGHT QUESTIONS

1. How does aerobic and anaerobic energy metabolism affect optimal energy transfer capacity for a (1) 100-m sprinter, (2) 400-m hurdler, and (3) marathon runner?

2. How can elite marathoners run 26.2 miles at a pace of 5 minutes per mile, yet very few can run just 1 mile in 4 minutes?

3. In prolonged aerobic exercise such as marathon running, explain why exercise capacity diminishes when

glycogen reserves deplete even though stored fat contains more than adequate energy reserves.

4. Is it important for weight lifters and sprinters to have a high capacity to consume oxygen? Explain.

5. From an exercise perspective, what are some advantages of having diverse sources of potential energy for synthesizing the cells' energy currency ATP?

Summaries at the end of each chapter provide a numbered list of the need-to-know facts and important information to help you review and remember what you have learned.

SUMMARY

1. The major energy pathway for ATP production differs depending on exercise intensity and duration. Intense exercise of short duration (100-m dash, weight lifting) derives energy primarily from the intramuscular phosphagens ATP and PCr (immediate energy system). Intense exercise of longer duration (1–2 min) requires energy mainly from the reactions of anaerobic glycolysis (short-term energy system). The long-term aerobic system predominates as exercise progresses beyond several minutes in duration.

2. The steady-rate oxygen uptake represents a balance between exercise energy requirements and aerobic ATP resynthesis.

3. The oxygen deficit represents the difference between the exercise oxygen requirement and the actual oxygen consumed.

4. The maximum oxygen uptake, or VO$_{2max}$, represents quantitatively the maximum capacity for aerobic ATP resynthesis.

5. Humans possess different types of muscle fibers, each with unique metabolic and contractile properties. The two major fiber types include low glycolytic, high oxidative, slow-twitch fibers and low oxidative, high glycolytic, fast-twitch fibers.

6. Understanding the energy spectrum of exercise forms a sound basis for creating optimal training regimens.

7. Bodily processes do not immediately return to resting levels after exercise ceases. The difference in recovery from light and strenuous exercise relates largely to the specific metabolic and physiologic processes in each exercise.

STUDENT RESOURCES

Inside the front cover of your textbook you will find your personal access code. Use it to log on to *thePoint.lww.com/Essentials4e*, the companion website for this textbook. On the website you can access various supplemental materials available to help enhance and further your learning. These assets include animations, a quiz bank, and the fully searchable online text.

Acknowledgments

The fourth edition of *Essentials of Exercise Physiology* represents a team effort. We are pleased to thank the many dedicated professionals at Lippincott Williams & Wilkins, particularly the outstanding efforts of our Product Manager Andrea Klingler, who spearheaded this effort with her sense of good judgment and tireless attention to detail. Other publishing team members include the expert talents of the following individuals: Jennifer Clements, Art Director; Emily Lupash, Acquisitions Editor; Amy Rowland, Editorial Assistant; and Loftin Paul Montgomery, Permissions Department. We also thank the many reviewers, colleagues, and adopters of the first three editions for their insightful comments and helpful suggestions.

VICTOR L. KATCH
WILLIAM D. MCARDLE
FRANK I. KATCH

Contents

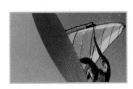
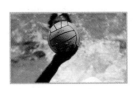
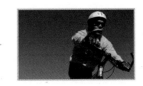

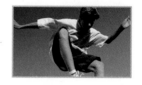
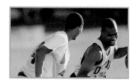
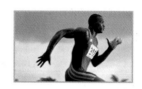

Introduction to Exercise Physiology

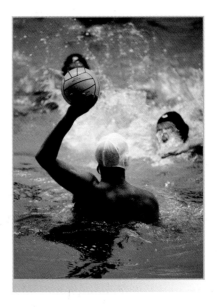

Exercise physiology enjoys a rich historical past filled with engaging stories about important discoveries in anatomy, physiology, and medicine. Fascinating people and unique events have shaped our field. The ancient Greek physician Galen (131–201 AD) wrote 87 detailed essays about improving health (proper nutrition), aerobic fitness (walking), and strengthening muscles (rope climbing and weight training). From 776 BC to 393 AD, the ancient Greek "sports nutritionists" planned the training regimens and diets for Olympic competitors, which included high-protein meat diets believed to improve strength and overall fitness. New ideas about body functioning emerged during the Renaissance as anatomists and physicians exploded every notion inherited from antiquity. Gutenberg's printing press in the 15th century disseminated both classic and newly acquired knowledge. Consequently, the typical person gained access to local and world events, and education became more accessible to the masses as universities developed and flourished throughout Europe.

The new anatomists went beyond simplistic notions of the early Greek scholar Empedocles' (ca. 500–430 BC) four "bodily humors" and elucidated the complexities of the circulatory, respiratory, and digestive systems. Although the supernatural still influenced discussions of physical phenomena, many people turned from dogma and superstition to experimentation as their primary source of knowledge. By the middle of the 19th century, fledgling medical schools in the United States began to graduate their students, many who assumed positions of leadership in academia and allied medical sciences. The pioneer physicians taught in medical schools, conducted research, and wrote textbooks. Some became affiliated with departments of physical education and hygiene, where they oversaw programs of physical training for students and athletes. These early efforts to infuse biology and physiology into the school curriculum helped to shape the origin of modern exercise physiology.

Part 1 Chapter 1 chronicles the achievements of several of the early American physician-scientists. The writing and research efforts (begun in 1860) by a college president and his physician son at Amherst College, MA, gave birth to exercise physiology as we know it today. Our history in the United States also includes the first exercise physiology laboratory at Harvard University begun in 1891 and

He who does not know what he is looking for will not lay hold of what he has found when he gets it.

— Claude Bernard,
Introduction à l'étude de la medecine expérimentale
(*The Introduction to the Study of Experimental Medicine.* 1865. Translated by H.C. Greene; Henry Schuman, Inc., New York, 1927)

the rigorous course of study for students in the Department of Anatomy, Physiology, and Physical Training. The chapter also highlights scientific contributions of current American and Nordic researchers who have impacted the field of exercise physiology.

The study of exercise physiology pioneers and their 2 millennia of contributions in chemistry, nutrition, metabolism, physiology, and physical fitness helps us to more clearly understand our historical underpinnings. It also places in proper perspective the state and direction of our field today.

Part 2 of Chapter 1 discusses the various roles of an exercise physiologist in the workplace and includes certification and education requirements necessary to achieve professional status.

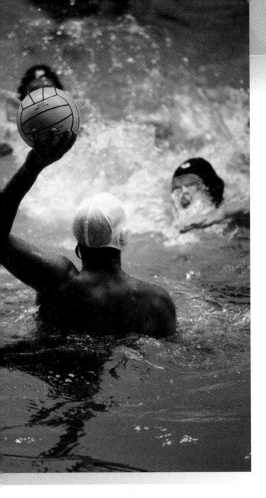

Origins of Exercise Physiology: Foundations for the Field of Study

CHAPTER OBJECTIVES

- Briefly outline Galen's contributions to health and scientific hygiene.

- Discuss the beginnings of the development of exercise physiology in the United States.

- Discuss the contributions of George Wells Fitz to the evolution of the academic field of exercise physiology.

- List contributions of Nordic scientists to the field of exercise physiology.

- Outline the course of study for the first academic 4-year program in the United States from the Department of Anatomy, Physiology, and Physical Training at Harvard University.

- Describe the creation of the Harvard Fatigue Laboratory, its major scientists, and its contributions to the field of exercise physiology.

- Describe the different jobs of an exercise physiologist.

- Discuss the roles of social networking and how they relate to exercise physiologists.

- List two of the most prominent exercise physiology professional organizations.

INTRODUCTION

The ability to impact the environment depends on our capacity for physical activity. Movement represents more than just a convenience; it is fundamental to human evolutionary development—no less important than the complexities of intellect and emotion.

In this century, scientists have amassed considerable new knowledge about physical activity so that exercise physiology is now a separate academic field of study within the biological sciences. Exercise physiology as an academic discipline consists of three distinct components (**Fig. 1.1**):

1. Body of knowledge built on facts and theories derived from research
2. Formal course of study in institutions of higher learning
3. Professional preparation of practitioners and future investigators and leaders in the field

The current academic discipline of exercise physiology emerged from the influences of several traditional fields—primarily anatomy, physiology, and medicine. Each of these disciplines uniquely contributes to our understanding human structure and function in health and disease. Human physiology integrates aspects of chemistry, biology, nutrition, and physics to explain biological events and their sites of occurrence. Physiologists grapple with questions such as, "What factors regulate body functions?" and "What sequence of events occurs between the stimulus and the response in the regulatory process?" The discipline of physiology compartmentalizes into subdisciplines, usually based on either a systems approach (e.g., pulmonary, cardiovascular, renal, endocrine, neuromuscular) or a broad area of study (e.g., cell, invertebrate, vertebrate, comparative, human).

Part 1 of this chapter briefly outlines the genesis from antiquity to the present state of exercise physiology worldwide. We emphasize the growth of formal research laboratories and the publication of textbooks in the field. The roots of exercise physiology have many common links to antiquity, with the knowledge explosion of the late 1950s greatly increasing the number of citations in the research literature. Consider the terms *exercise* and *exertion*. In 1946, a hand search of resource manuals yielded only 12 citations in five journals. By 1962, the number increased to 128 citations in 51 journals, and by 1981, 655 citations appeared in 224 journals. These increases, however, have been dwarfed by the exponential increase in new scientific knowledge in the exercise physiology-related fields during the past decade. Eleven years ago in early October, more than 6000 citation listings for *exercise* and *exertion* appeared in more than 1400 journals. On October 13, 2010, the number of citations for the single term *exercise* returned 180,066 citations, and adding the term *exertion* yielded 54,451 more entries! It is not a stretch to say that exercise physiology indeed represents a mature field of study.

The historical underpinnings of exercise physiology form an important base for students pursuing a graduate degree. Many students complete course work, internships, and research experiences that provide sufficient preparation for continued education to become an exercise physiologist. In part 2 of this chapter we introduce various roles that the modern-day exercise physiologist will assume in different clinical and professional settings. We also review different academic and professional certifications offered by different professional organizations.

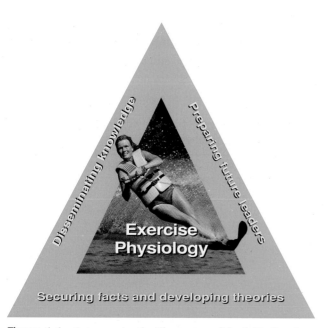

Figure 1.1 Science triangle. Three parts of the field of study of exercise physiology: (1) the body of knowledge evidenced by experimental and field research engaged in the enterprise of securing facts and developing theories, (2) the formal course of study in institutions of higher learning for the purpose of disseminating knowledge, and (3) preparation of future leaders in the field. (Adapted from Tipton, C.M.: Contemporary exercise physiology: Fifty years after the closure of the Harvard Fatigue Laboratory. *Exerc. Sport Sci. Rev.,* 26:315, 1998.)

Part 1 Origins of Exercise Physiology: From Ancient Greece to the United States

The origins of exercise physiology begin with the influential Greek physicians of antiquity. Scholars in the United States and Nordic countries fostered the scientific assessment of sport and exercise as a respectable field of inquiry.

EARLIEST DEVELOPMENT

The first real focus on the physiology of exercise probably began in early Greece and Asia Minor. Exercise, sports, games, and health concerned even earlier civilizations, including the Minoan and Mycenaean cultures, the great biblical empires of David and Solomon, Assyria, Babylonia, Media, and Persia, and the empires of Alexander. The ancient civilizations of Syria, Egypt, Greece, Arabia, Mesopotamia, Persia, India, and China also recorded references to sports, games, and health practices that included personal hygiene, exercise, and training. The doctrines and teachings of Susruta (Sushruta, an Indian physician) promoted the influence of different modes of exercise on human health and disease. For example, Susruta considered obesity a disease caused by an increase in the humor *vayu* (from increases in lymph chyle) and believed that a sedentary lifestyle contributed to obesity. The greatest influence on Western Civilization, however, came from the early Greek physicians Herodicus (ca. 480 BC), Hippocrates (460–377 BC), and Claudius Galenus or Galen (131–201 AD). Herodicus, a physician and athlete, strongly advocated proper diet in physical training. His early writings and devoted followers influenced Hippocrates, the famous physician and "father of preventive medicine" who contributed 87 treatises on medicine, including several on health and hygiene.

Five centuries after Hippocrates, during the early decline of the Roman Empire, Galen became the most well-known and influential physician who ever lived. Galen began studying medicine at about 16 years of age. During the next 50 years, he enhanced current thinking about health and scientific hygiene, an area some might consider applied exercise physiology. Throughout his life, Galen taught and practiced the seven "laws of health" that comprised breathing fresh air, eating proper foods, drinking the right beverages, exercising, getting adequate sleep, having a daily bowel movement, and controlling one's emotions (sound familiar as modern dogma?). Galen scribed at least 80 treatises and about 500 essays related to human anatomy and physiology, nutrition, growth and development, the benefits of exercise and deleterious consequences of sedentary living, and diverse diseases and their treatment. Among his notable contributions, Galen introduced the concept of *polisarkia* (too much food intake, too little exercise) now known as morbid obesity. One of the first laboratory-oriented physiologist–physicians, Galen conducted original experiments in physiology, comparative anatomy, and medicine; he dissected animals (e.g., goats, pigs, cows, horses, and elephants). As physician to the gladiators (most likely the first "sports medicine" physician), Galen treated torn tendons and muscles using surgical procedures that he invented and recommended rehabilitation therapies and exercise regimens. For example, for lower-back discomfort, subjects were suspended upside down in a vertical position to relieve pressure in the lumbar region. Galen followed the Hippocratic school of medicine that believed in logical science grounded in observation and experimentation, not superstition or deity dictates. Galen wrote detailed descriptions about the forms, kinds, and varieties of "swift" vigorous exercises, including their proper quantity and duration. Galen's writings about exercise and its effects might be considered the first formal "how to" manuals about such topics, which remained influential for the next 15 centuries. The beginnings of "modern day" exercise physiology include the periods of Renaissance, Enlightenment, and Scientific Discovery in Europe. During this time, Galen's ideas continued to influence the writings of the early physiologists, physicians, and teachers of hygiene and health. For example, in Venice in 1539, the Italian physician Hieronymus Mercurialis (1530–1606) published *De Arte Gymnastica Apud Ancientes* (*The Art of Gymnastics Among the Ancients*). This text, influenced by Galen and other Greek and Latin authors, profoundly affected subsequent writings about gymnastics (physical training and exercise) and health (hygiene) in Europe and 19th century America. The panel in **Figure 1.2**, redrawn from *De Arte Gymnastica*, acknowledges the early Greek influence of one of Galen's well-known essays, "Exercise with the Small Ball." This depiction illustrates his regimen of specific strengthening exercises featuring discus throwing and rope climbing.

Questions & Notes

Name the most famous of the Greek physicians.

What does the term polisarkia *mean?*

State one important tenet of the Hippocrates School of Medicine.

List 3 contributions of Galen to the study of exercise physiology.

1.

2.

3.

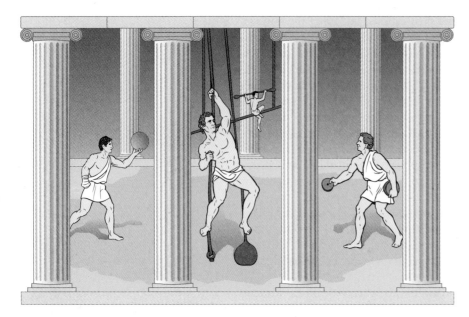

Figure 1.2 The early Greek influence of Galen's famous essay, "Exercise with the Small Ball" clearly appears in Mercurialis' *De Arte Gymnastica*, a treatise about the many uses of exercise for preventive and therapeutic medical and health benefits. The three panels represent the exercises as they might have been performed during Galen's time.

EARLY UNITED STATES EXPERIENCE

By the early 1800s in the United States, European science-oriented physicians and experimental anatomists and physiologists strongly promoted ideas about health and hygiene. Before 1800, only 39 first-edition American-authored medical books had been published; several medical schools were founded (e.g., Harvard Medical School, 1782–1783); seven medical societies existed (the first was the New Jersey State Medical Society in 1766); and only one medical journal existed (*Medical Repository*, initially published on July 26, 1797). Outside the United States, 176 medical journals were published, mostly from Britain (e.g., *Foreign Medical Review*, *London Medical Journal*, *Physical Journal of London*), France (e.g., *Le Journal de Medicine, Chirurgie et Pharmacie, Gazette Medical de Paris*), Germany (*Deliciae Medicae et Chirurgicae, Natur and Medizin Kunst und Literature Geschichte, Acta Medicorum Berolinen, Chirurgisch*), and Italy (*Giornale per Servire alla Storia Ragionata della Medicina di questo Secole*). By 1850, the number of indigenous medical journals published in the United States increased to 117. Interestingly, the first medical publication in America in 1677 by Thomas Thatcher, a minister, "A Brief Guide in The Small Pox and Measles" appeared more than 100 years before the founding of Harvard Medical School. The famous classic first edition of *Gray's Anatomy, Descriptive and Surgical* (now known simply as *Gray's Anatomy*) was first published in 1858 in the United Kingdom (3 years before British anatomist Henry Gray's death at age 34 years from smallpox) and in the United States in 1859. Medical journal publications in the United States increased tremendously during the first half of the 19th century. Steady growth in the number of scientific contributions from France and Germany influenced the thinking and practice of American medicine. An explosion of information reached the American public through books, magazines, newspapers, and traveling "health salesmen" who sold an endless variety of tonics and elixirs, promising to optimize health and cure disease. Many health reformers and physicians from 1800 to 1850 used "strange" procedures to treat disease and bodily discomforts. To a large extent, scientific knowledge about health and disease was in its infancy. Lack of knowledge and factual information spawned a new generation of "healers," who fostered quackery and primitive practices on a public that was all too eager to experiment with almost anything that seemed to work. If a salesman could offer a "cure" to combat gluttony (digestive upset) and other physical ailments, the product or procedure would become the common remedy.

The "hot topics" of the early 19th century (alas, still true today) included nutrition and dieting (slimming), general information about exercise, how to best develop overall fitness, training (gymnastic) exercises for recreation and preparation for sports, and personal health and hygiene. Although many health faddists practiced "medicine" without a license, some enrolled in newly created medical schools (without entrance requirements), obtaining MD degrees in as little as 16 weeks. During the time of the early British American colonies, approximately 3500 medical practitioners provided medical services, yet only about 400 had received "degrees" in medicine. By the mid-19th century, medical school graduates began to assume positions of leadership in academia and allied medical sciences. Physicians either taught in medical school and conducted research (and wrote textbooks) or were affiliated with departments of physical education and hygiene, where they would oversee programs of physical training for students and athletes.

Austin Flint, Jr., MD: Important American Physician–Physiologist

Austin Flint, Jr., MD (1836–1915), a pioneer American physician–physiologist, contributed significantly to the

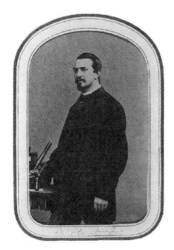

Figure 1.3   Austin Flint, Jr., MD American physician–physiologist, taught that muscular exercise should be taught from a strong foundation of science and laboratory experimentation.

Questions & Notes

Name the first medical school in the United States.

Describe Austin Flint's major contribution to the field of exercise physiology.

burgeoning literature in physiology (**Fig. 1.3**). A respected physician, physiologist, and successful textbook author, he fostered the belief among 19th century American physical education teachers that muscular exercise should be taught from a strong foundation of science and experimentation. Flint, professor of physiology and microscopic anatomy in the Bellevue Hospital Medical College of New York (founded in 1736, the oldest public hospital in the United States), chaired the Department of Physiology and Microbiology from 1861 to 1897 and also served as New York State's first Surgeon General. In 1866, he published a series of five classic textbooks, the first titled *The Physiology of Man; Designed to Represent the Existing State of Physiological Science as Applied to the Functions of the Human Body* (the cloth edition of this 500-page text first sold for $4.50). Eleven years later, Flint published *The Principles and Practice of Medicine*, a synthesis of his first five textbooks consisting of 987 pages of meticulously organized sections with supporting documentation. This tome included illustrations of equipment used to record physiological phenomena, including the Frenchman Etienne-Jules Marey's (1830–1904) early cardiograph for registering the wave form and frequency of the pulse and a refinement of his sphygmograph instrument for making pulse measurements—the forerunner of modern cardiovascular instrumentation (**Fig. 1.4**).

Dr. Flint, well trained in the scientific method, received the American Medical Association's prize for basic research on the heart in 1858. He published his medical school thesis, "The Phenomena of Capillary Circulation," in an 1878 issue of the *American Journal of the Medical Sciences*. His 1877 textbook included many exercise-related details about the influence of posture and exercise on pulse rate, the influence of muscular activity on respiration, and the influence of exercise on nitrogen elimination. Flint also published a well-known monograph in 1871 that influenced future work in the early science of exercise, "On the Physiological

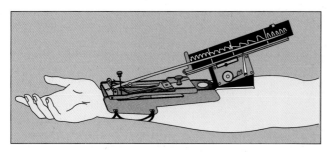

Figure 1.4   Etienne-Jules Marey's advanced sphygmograph.

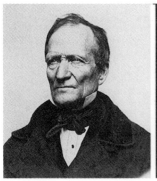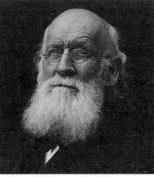

Figure 1.5 Drs. Edward Hitchcock (1793–1864) (*left*) and Edward Hitchcock, Jr. (1828–1911) (*right*), father and son educators, authors, and scientists who pioneered the sports science movement in the USA.

Effects of Severe and Protracted Muscular Exercise, with Special Reference to its Influence Upon the Excretion of Nitrogen." Flint was well aware of scientific experimentation in France and England and cited the experimental works of leading European physiologists and physicians, including the incomparable François Magendie (1783–1855) and Claude Bernard (1813–1878) and the influential German physiologists Justis von Liebig (1803–1873), Edward Pflüger (1829–1910), and Carl von Voit (1831–1908). Flint also discussed the important contributions to metabolism of Antoine Lavoisier (1743–1784) and to digestive physiology from pioneer American physician–physiologist William Beaumont (1785–1853).

Through his textbooks Flint influenced Edward Hitchcock, Jr., MD, the first medically trained and science-oriented professor of physical education (see next section). Hitchcock quoted Flint about the muscular system in his syllabus of *Health Lectures*, which became required reading for all students enrolled at Amherst College between 1861 and 1905.

Amherst College Connection

Two physicians, father and son, pioneered the American sports science movement (**Fig. 1.5**). Edward Hitchcock, DD, LL.D. (1793–1864), served as professor of chemistry and natural history at Amherst College and as president of the College from 1845 to 1854. He convinced the college president in 1861 to allow his son Edward (1828–1911), an Amherst graduate (1849) with a Harvard medical degree (1853) to assume the duties of his anatomy course. On August 15, 1861, **Edward Hitchcock, Jr.**, became Professor of Hygiene and Physical Education with full academic rank in the Department of Physical Culture at an annual salary of $1000—a position he held almost continuously until 1911. Hitchcock's professorship became the second such appointment in physical education in an American college. The first, to John D. Hooker 1 year earlier at Amherst College in 1860, was short lived because of Hooker's poor health. Hooker resigned in 1861, and Hitchcock (Jr.) was appointed in his place.

The original idea of a Department of Physical Education with a professorship had been proposed in 1854 by William Augustus Stearns, DD, the fourth president of Amherst College. Stearns considered physical education instruction essential for the health of students and useful to prepare them physically, spiritually, and intellectually. In 1860, the Barrett Gymnasium at Amherst College was completed and served as the training facility where all students were required to perform systematic exercises for 30 minutes daily, 4 days a week (**Fig. 1.6**). A unique

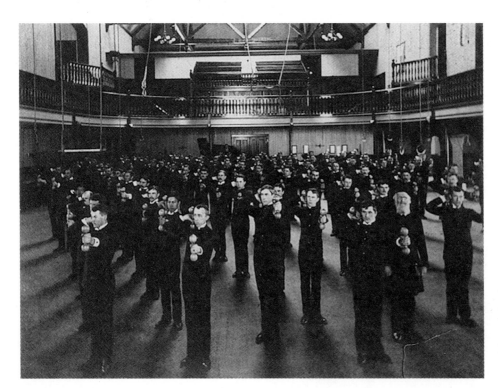

Figure 1.6 Dr. Edward Hitchcock, Jr. (second from right, with beard) with the entire class of students perform regimented barbell exercises at Amherst College in the 1890s. (Photo courtesy of Amherst College Archives, and by permission of the Trustees of Amherst College, 1995.)

feature of the gymnasium was Hitchcock's scientific laboratory that included strength and anthropometric equipment and a spirometer to measure lung function, which he used to measure the vital statistics of all Amherst students. Dr. Hitchcock was the first to statistically record basic data on a large group of subjects on a yearly basis. These measurements provided solid information for his counseling duties concerning health, hygiene, and exercise training.

In 1860, the Hitchcocks coauthored an anatomy and physiology textbook geared to college physical education (Hitchcock E, Hitchcock E, Jr: *Elementary Anatomy and Physiology for Colleges, Academies, and Other Schools.* New York: Ivison, Phinney & Co., 1860); 29 years earlier, the father had published a science-oriented hygiene textbook. Interestingly, the anatomy and physiology book predated Flint's similar text by 6 years. This illustrated that an American-trained physician, with an allegiance to the implementation of health and hygiene in the curriculum, helped set the stage for the study of exercise and training well before the medical establishment focused on this aspect of the discipline. A pedagogical aspect of the Hitchcocks' text included questions at the bottom of each page about topics under consideration. In essence, the textbook also served as a "study guide" or "workbook." **Figure 1.7** shows sample pages from the 1860 book on muscle structure and function.

Questions & Notes

Name the first "professor" of physical education in the United States.

Name the father–son team who started the first physical education program in the United States.

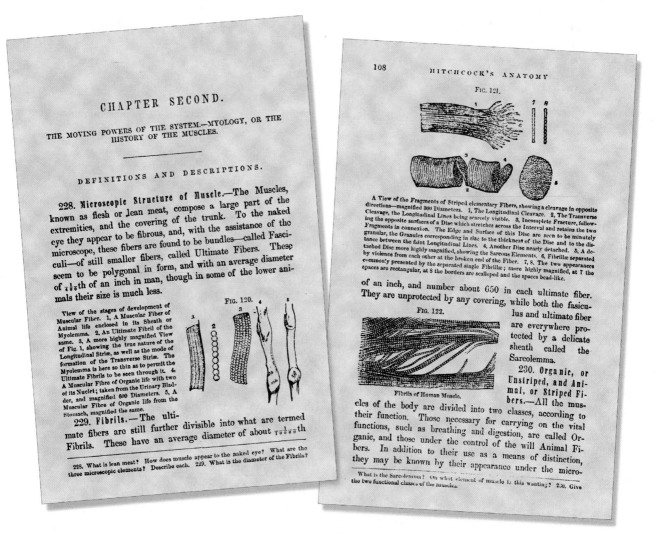

Figure 1.7   Examples from the Hitchcocks' text on muscle structure and function. Note that study questions appear at the bottom of each page, the forerunner of modern workbooks (Reproduced from Hitchcock, E., and Hitchcock, E., Jr.: (1860). *Elementary Anatomy and Physiology for Colleges, Academies, and Other Schools.* New York: Ivison, Phinney & Co., 1860: pp., 132, 137. (Materials courtesy of Amherst College Archives, and permission of the Trustees of Amherst College, 1995.)

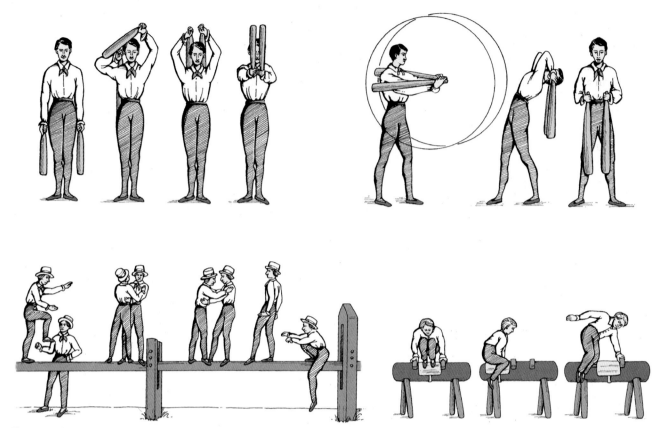

Figure 1.8 Exercise with Indian clubs (*top*). Exercise on a balance beam and pommel horse (*bottom*). These kinds of exercises were performed routinely in physical activity classes at Amherst College from 1860 to 1920. Changes in girth anthropometric measurements showed significant improvements in body dimensions (primarily upper arm and chest) from the workouts.

An 1880 reprint of the book contained 373 woodcut drawings about the body's physiological systems, including detailed drawings of exercise apparatus (bars, ladders, ropes, swings) and different exercises performed with Indian clubs or "scepters," one held in each hand. **Figure 1.8** shows examples of exercises with Indian clubs and those performed on a balance beam and pommel horse by Amherst College students from 1860 to the early 1890s.

Anthropometric Assessment of Body Build

From 1861 to 1888, Hitchcock, Jr. became interested in the influence of bodily measurements on overall health. He measured all students enrolled at Amherst College for six measures of segmental height, 23 girths, six breadths, eight lengths, and eight indices of muscular strength, lung capacity, and pilosity (amount of hair on the body). In 1889, Hitchcock, Jr., and Hiram H. Seelye, MD, his colleague who also served as college physician from 1884 to 1896 in the Department of Physical Education and Hygiene, published a 37-page anthropometric manual that included five tables of anthropometric statistics based on measurements of students from 1861 to 1891. Hitchcock's measurement methods undoubtedly influenced European-trained anthropometrists in France and England in the early 1890s, notably the French biometrician Alphonese Bertillon (1853–1914), who developed a formal criminal identification system based on physical measurements.

Hitchcock, Jr., performed pioneering anthropometric studies at the college level, and the military made the first detailed anthropometric, spirometric, and muscular strength measurements on Civil War soldiers in the early 1860s. Trained military anthropometrists (practitioners with a specialty in taking body measurements according to strict standards) used a unique device, the andrometer (**Fig. 1.9**), to secure the physical dimensions of soldiers for purposes of fitting uniforms. The andrometer, originally devised in 1855 by a tailor in Edinburgh, Scotland, determined the proper clothing size for British soldiers. Special "sliders" measured total height; breadth of the neck, shoulders, and pelvis; and length of the legs and height to the knees and crotch. Most current university exercise physiology research laboratories and numerous medical school, military, and ergonomic and exercise research laboratories include quantitative assessment procedures to routinely assess aspects of muscular strength, anthropometry, and body composition.

George Wells Fitz, MD: A Key Exercise Physiology Pioneer

George Wells Fitz, MD (1860–1934), physician and pioneer exercise physiology researcher (**Fig. 1.10**), helped establish the Department of Anatomy, Physiology, and Physical Training at Harvard University in 1891, shortly after he

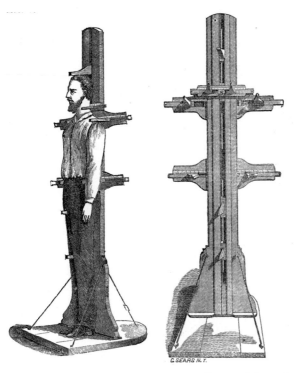

Describe possible practical uses of anthropometric data.

Discuss why George Wells Fitz is considered an important exercise physiology pioneer.

Where was the first exercise physiology laboratory located?

Figure 1.9 The United States Sanitary Commission first used the andrometer at numerous military installations along the Atlantic seaboard during the early 1860s to properly size soldiers for their military uniforms.

received his MD degree from Harvard Medical School in 1891. One year later, Fitz developed the first formal exercise physiology laboratory, where students investigated the effects of exercise on cardiorespiratory function, including muscular fatigue, metabolism, and nervous system functions. Fitz, uniquely qualified to teach this course based on his sound experimental training at Harvard's Medical School under the tutelage of well-known physiologists, also designed new recording and measuring devices. Fitz published his research in the prestigious *Boston Medical and Surgical Journal*, including studies on muscle cramping, the efficacy of protective clothing, spinal curvature, respiratory function, carbon dioxide measurement, and speed and accuracy of simple and complex movements. He also wrote a textbook (*Principles of Physiology and Hygiene* [New York: Holt, 1908] and revised physiologist HN Martin's *The Human Body. Textbook of Anatomy, Physiology and Hygiene; with Practical Exercises* [Holt, 1911]). Well-known researchers in the new program included distinguished Harvard Medical School physiologists Henry Pickering Bowditch (1840–1911), whose research produced the "all or none principle" of cardiac contraction and "treppe" (staircase

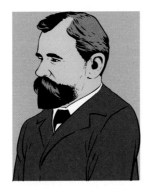

Figure 1.10 George Wells Fitz, MD, physician and pioneer exercise physiology researcher.

BOX 1.1 CLOSE UP

Course of Study: Department of Anatomy, Physiology, and Physical Training, Lawrence Scientific School, Harvard University, 1893

Few of today's undergraduate physical education major programs could match the strong science core required at Harvard in 1893. The accompanying table lists the 4-year course of study of the department's fourth-year requirements listed in the 1893 course catalog. Along with core courses, Professor Fitz established an exercise physiology laboratory. The following describes the laboratory's objectives:

"A well-equipped laboratory has been organized for the experimental study of the physiology of exercise. The object of this work is to exemplify the hygiene of the muscles, the conditions under which they act, the relation of their action to the body as a whole affecting blood supply and general hygienic conditions, and the effects of various exercises on muscular growth and general health."

First Year

Experimental Physics
Elementary Zoology
Morphology of Animals
Morphology of Plants
Elementary Physiology and Hygiene (taught by Fitz[1])
General Descriptive Chemistry
Rhetoric and English Composition
Elementary German
Elementary French
Gymnastics and Athletics (taught by Sargent and Lathrop)

Second Year

Comparative Anatomy of Vertebrates
Geology
Physical Geography and Meteorology
Experimental Physics
General Descriptive Physics
Qualitative Analysis
English Composition
Gymnastics and Athletics (taught by Sargent and Lathrop)

Third Year (at Harvard Medical School)

General Anatomy and Dissection
General Physiology (taught by Bowditch and Porter)
Histology (taught by Minot and Quincy)
Hygiene
Foods and Cooking [Nutrition] (at Boston Cooking School)
Medical Chemistry
Auscultation and Percussion
Gymnastics and Athletics (taught by Sargent and Lathrop)

Fourth Year

Psychology (taught by James)
Anthropometry (Sargent[2])
Applied Anatomy and Animal Mechanics [Kinesiology] (taught by Sargent[3])
Physiology of Exercise (taught by Fitz[4])
Remedial Exercise (taught by Fitz[5])
History of Physical Education (taught by Sargent and Fitz[6])
Forensics
Gymnastics and Athletics (Sargent and Lathrop[7])

COURSE EXPLANATION

[1]The Elementary Physiology of and Hygiene of Common Life, Personal Hygiene, Emergencies. Half-course. One lecture and one laboratory hour each week throughout the year (or three times a week, first half-year). Dr. G.W. Fitz. This is a general introductory course intended to give the knowledge of human anatomy, physiology, and hygiene, which should be possessed by every student; it is suitable also for those not intending to study medicine or physical training.

[2]Anthropometry. Measurements and Tests of the Human Body, Effects of Age, Nurture and Physical Training. Lectures and practical exercises. Half-course. Three times a week (first half-year). Dr. Sargent. This course affords systematic training in making measurements and tests of persons for the purpose of determining individual strength and health deficiencies. Practice is also given in classifying measurements, forming typical groups, etc., and in determining the relation of the individual to such groups. This course must be preceded by the course in General Anatomy at the Medical School, or its equivalent.

[3]Applied Anatomy and Animal Mechanics. Action of Muscles in Different Exercises. Lectures and Demonstrations. Half-course. Three times a week (second half-year). Dr. Sargent. The muscles taking part in the different exercises and the mechanical conditions under which they work are studied. The body is considered as a machine. The development of force, its utilization and the adaptation of the different parts to these ends are made prominent in the work. This course must be preceded by the course in General Anatomy at the Medical School, or its equivalent.

[4]Physiology of Exercise. Experimental work, original work and thesis. Laboratory work six hours a week. Dr. G.W. Fitz. This course is intended to introduce the student to the fundamental problems of physical education and to give him the training in use of apparatus for investigation and in the methods in such work. This course is preceded by the course in General Physiology at the Medical School, or its equivalent.

[5] Remedial Exercises. The Correction of Abnormal Conditions and Positions. Lectures and Demonstrations. Half-course. Twice a week (second half-year). Dr. G.W. Fitz. Deformities such as spinal curvature are studied and the corrective effects of different exercises observed. The students are trained in the selection and application of proper exercises, and in the diagnosis of cases when exercise is unsuitable.

[6] History of Physical Education. Half-course. Lecture once a week and a large amount of reading. Drs. Sargent and G.W. Fitz. The student is made acquainted with the literature of physical training; the history of the various sports is traced and the artistic records (statuary, etc.) studied.

[7] Gymnastics and Athletics. Dr. Sargent and Mr. J.G. Lathrop. Systematic instruction is given throughout the four years in these subjects. The students attend the regular afternoon class in gymnastics conducted by Dr. Sargent, work with the developing appliances to remedy up their own deficiencies and take part in the preliminary training for the various athletic exercises under Mr. Lathrop's direction. Much work is also done with the regular apparatus of the gymnasium.

phenomenon of muscle contraction), and William T. Porter (1862–1949), internationally recognized experimental physiologist who founded Harvard Apparatus, Inc., in 1901). Charles S. Minot (1852–1914), a Massachusetts Institute of Technology–educated chemist with European training in physiology, taught the histology course, and acclaimed Harvard psychologist and philosopher, trained as a physician, William James (brother of novelist Henry James, 1842–1910) offered the fourth year psychology course. The new 4-year course of study, well grounded in the basic sciences even by today's standards, provided students with a rigorous, challenging curriculum in what Fitz hoped would be a new science of physical education. The third year of study was taken at the medical school (see the table in the Close Up Box 1.1 on page 12).

Prelude to Exercise Science: Harvard's Department of Anatomy, Physiology, and Physical Training (BS Degree, 1891–1898)

Harvard's new physical education major and exercise physiology research laboratory focused on three objectives:

1. Prepare students, with or without subsequent training in medicine, to become directors of gymnasia or instructors in physical training.
2. Provide general knowledge about the science of exercise, including systematic training to maintain health and fitness.
3. Provide suitable academic preparation to enter medical school.

Physical education students took general anatomy and physiology courses in the medical school; after 4 years of study, graduates could enroll as second-year medical students and graduate in 3 years with an MD degree. Dr. Fitz taught the physiology of exercise course; thus, he deserves recognition as the first person to formally teach such a course. The new degree included experimental investigation and original work and a thesis, including 6 hours a week of laboratory study. The prerequisite for Fitz's physiology of exercise course included general physiology or its equivalent taken at the medical school. The Physiology of Exercise course introduced students to the fundamentals of physical education and provided training in experimental methods related to exercise physiology. In addition to the course in remedial exercise, students took a required course in applied anatomy and animal mechanics. This thrice-weekly course, taught by Dr. Dudley Sargent (1849–1924), was the forerunner of modern biomechanics courses. Its prerequisite was general anatomy or its equivalent taken at the medical school.

Before its dismantling in 1900, nine men graduated with BS degrees from the Department of Anatomy, Physiology, and Physical Training. The first graduate, James Francis Jones (1893), became instructor in Physiology and Hygiene and director of Gymnasium at Marietta College, Marietta, Ohio. One year after Fitz's untimely resignation from Harvard in 1899, the department changed its

*Q**uestions & Notes**

Describe and detail similarities between Harvard's exercise physiology academic requirements and the requirements for your major.

curricular emphasis to anatomy and physiology (dropping the term *physical training* from the department title). This terminated (at least temporarily) a unique experiment in higher education. For almost a decade before the turn of the century, the field of physical education was moving forward on a strong scientific foundation similar to other more developed disciplines. Unfortunately, this occasion to nurture the next generation of students in exercise physiology (and physical education) was momentarily stymied. Twenty years would pass before Fitz' visionary efforts to "study the physiological and psychological effects of exercise" and establish exercise physiology as a bona fide field of investigation would be revived, but outside of a formal physical education curriculum.

One of the legacies of the Fitz-directed "Harvard experience" between 1891 and 1899 was the mentoring it provided specialists who began their careers with a strong scientific basis in exercise and training and its relationship to health. They were taught that experimentation and the discovery of new knowledge about exercise and training furthered the development of a science-based curriculum. Unfortunately, it would take another 60 years before the next generation of science-oriented educators led by physiologists such as A.V. Hill (1886–1977) and D.B. Dill (1891–1986), who were not trained educators would again exert strong influence on the physical education curriculum and propel exercise physiology to the forefront of scientific investigation. By 1927, 135 institutions in the United States offered bachelor's degree programs in Physical Education with coursework in the basic sciences; this included four master's degree programs and two doctoral programs (Teachers College, Columbia University and New York University). Since then, programs of study with differing emphasis in exercise physiology have proliferated. Currently, more than 170 programs in the United States and 53 in Canada offer masters or doctoral degrees with specialization in a topic related to Kinesiology and Exercise Science with course work in exercise physiology.

Exercise Studies in Research Journals

In 1898, three articles on physical activity appeared in the first volume of the *American Journal of Physiology*. Other articles and reviews subsequently appeared in prestigious journals, including the first published review in *Physiological Reviews* (2:310, 1922) on the mechanisms of muscular contraction by Nobel laureate A.V. Hill. The German applied physiology publication *Internationale Zeitschrift für angewandte Physiologie einschliesslich Arbeitsphysiologie* (1929–1940; now *European Journal of Applied Physiology and Occupational Physiology; www.springerlink.com/content/108306/*) became a significant journal for research about exercise physiology-related topics. The *Journal of Applied Physiology*, first published in 1948, contained the classic paper by British growth and development researcher J.M. Tanner (1920–2010) on ratio expressions of physiological data with reference to body size and function (a "must read" for exercise physiologists). The official journal of the American College of Sports Medicine (*www.acsm.org/*), *Medicine and Science in Sports*, first appeared in 1969. It aimed to integrate both medical and physiological aspects of the emerging fields of sports medicine and exercise science. The official name of this journal changed in 1980 to *Medicine and Science in Sports and Exercise*.

First Textbook in Exercise Physiology

Debate exists over the question: "What was the first textbook in exercise physiology?" Several textbook authors give the distinction of being "first" to the English translation of Fernand Lagrange's *The Physiology of Bodily Exercise*, originally published in French in 1888. We disagree. To deserve such historical recognition, a textbook should meet the following three criteria:

1. Provide sound scientific rationale for major concepts.
2. Provide summary information (based on experimentation) about important prior research in a particular topic area (e.g., contain scientific references to research in the area).
3. Provide sufficient "factual" information about a topic area to give it academic legitimacy.

The Lagrange book represents a popular book about health and exercise with a "scientific" title. Based on the aforementioned criteria, the book does not exemplify a bona fide exercise physiology text; it contains fewer than 20 reference citations (based on observations of friends performing exercise). By disqualifying the Lagrange book, what text qualifies as the first exercise physiology text? Possible candidates for "first" include these four choices published between 1843 and 1896:

1. Combe's 1843 text, *The Principles of Physiology Applied to the Preservation of Health, and to the Improvement of Physical and Mental Education.* New York: Harper & Brothers.
2. Hitchcock and Hitchcock's 1860 book, *Elementary Anatomy and Physiology for Colleges, Academies, and Other Schools.* New York: Ivison, Phinney & Co.
3. Kolb's insightful 1893 book, *Physiology of Sport.* London: Krohne and Sesemann.
4. Martin's 1896 text, *The Human Body. An Account of its Structure and Activities and the Conditions of its Healthy Working.* New York: Holt & Co.

CONTRIBUTIONS OF THE HARVARD FATIGUE LABORATORY (1927–1946)

The real impact of laboratory research in exercise physiology (along with many other research specialties) occurred in 1927, again at Harvard University, 27 years after Harvard closed the first exercise physiology laboratory in the United States. The 800-square-foot Harvard Fatigue Laboratory in the basement of Morgan Hall of Harvard University's Business School legitimized exercise physiology as an important area of research and study.

BOX 1.2   CLOSE UP

What's in a Name?

A lack of unanimity exists for the name of the departments offering degrees (or even coursework) in exercise physiology. This box lists examples of 49 names of departments in the United States that offer essentially the same area of study. Each provides some undergraduate or graduate emphasis in exercise physiology (e.g., one or several courses, internships, work-study programs, laboratory rotations, or inservice programs).

Allied Health Sciences
Exercise and Movement Science
Exercise and Sport Science
Exercise and Sport Studies
Exercise Science
Exercise Science and Human Movement
Exercise Science and Physical Therapy
Health and Human Performance
Health and Physical Education
Health, Physical Education, Recreation and Dance
Human Biodynamics
Human Kinetics
Human Kinetics and Health
Human Movement
Human Movement Sciences
Human Movement Studies
Human Movement Studies and Physical Education
Human Performance
Human Performance and Health Promotion
Human Performance and Leisure Studies
Human Performance and Sport Science
Interdisciplinary Health Studies
Integrative Biology
Kinesiology
Kinesiology and Exercise Science

Movement and Exercise Science
Movement Studies
Nutrition and Exercise Science
Nutritional and Health Sciences
Performance and Sport Science
Physical Culture
Physical Education
Physical Education and Exercise Science
Physical Education and Human Movement
Physical Education and Sport Programs
Physical Education and Sport Science
Physical Therapy
Recreation
Recreation and Wellness Programs
Science of Human Movement
Sport and Exercise Science
Sport Management
Sport, Exercise, and Leisure Science
Sports Science
Sport Science and Leisure Studies
Sport Science and Movement Education
Sport Studies
Wellness and Fitness
Wellness Education

Many of 20th century's great scientists with an interest in exercise affiliated with the Fatigue Laboratory. Renowned Harvard chemist and professor of biochemistry Lawrence J. Henderson, MD (1878–1942) established the laboratory. David Bruce Dill (1891–1986; **Fig. 1.11**), a Stanford PhD in physical chemistry, became the first and only scientific director of the laboratory. While at Harvard, Dill refocused his

Questions & Notes

Describe the significance of the Harvard Fatigue Laboratory to the development of exercise physiology.

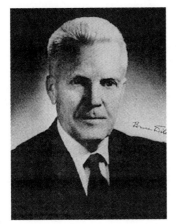

Figure 1.11   David Bruce Dill (1891–1986), prolific experimental exercise physiologist, helped to establish the highly acclaimed Harvard Fatigue Laboratory.

efforts from biochemistry to experimental physiology and became the driving force behind the laboratory's numerous scientific accomplishments. His early academic association with physician Arlie Bock (a student of famous high-altitude physiologist Sir Joseph F. Barcroft (1872–1947) at Cambridge, England, and Dill's closest friend for 59 years), and contact with 1922 Nobel laureate Archibald Vivian Hill provided Dill with the confidence to successfully coordinate the research efforts of dozens of scholars from 15 different countries. Hill convinced Bock to write a third edition of Bainbridge's text, *Physiology of Muscular Activity*, and Bock invited Dill to coauthor this 1931 book.

Similar to the legacy of the first exercise physiology laboratory established in 1891 at Harvard's Lawrence Scientific School 31 years earlier, the Harvard Fatigue Laboratory demanded excellence in research and scholarship. Cooperation among scientists from around the world fostered lasting collaborations. Many of its charter scientists influenced a new generation of exercise physiologists worldwide.

OTHER EARLY EXERCISE PHYSIOLOGY RESEARCH LABORATORIES

Other notable research laboratories helped exercise physiology become an established field of study at colleges and universities. The Nutrition Laboratory at the Carnegie Institute in Washington, DC (established 1904) initiated experiments in nutrition and energy metabolism. The first research laboratories established in a department of physical education in the United States originated at George Williams College in 1923 (founded by the YMCA Training School in Chicago, Illinois, now merged with Aurora College, Aurora, Illinois); University of Illinois (1925), Springfield College, Massachusetts (1927); and Laboratory of Physiological Hygiene at the University of California, Berkeley (1934). In 1936, Franklin M. Henry (**Fig. 1.12**)

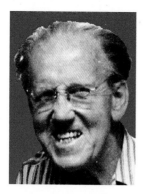

Figure 1.12 F.M. Henry (1904–1993), University of California, Berkeley, psychologist, physical educator, and researcher who first proposed physical education as an academic discipline. He conducted basic experiments in oxygen uptake kinetics during exercise and recovery, muscular strength, and cardiorespiratory variability during steady-rate exercise, determinants of heavy-work endurance exercise, and neural control factors related to human motor performance.

assumed responsibility for the laboratory; shortly thereafter, his research appeared in various physiology and motor performance-oriented journals (120 articles in peer-reviewed journals; 1975 ACSM Honor Award).

NORDIC CONNECTION (DENMARK, SWEDEN, NORWAY, AND FINLAND)

Denmark and Sweden also pioneered the field of exercise physiology. In 1800, Denmark became the first European country to require physical training (military-style gymnastics) in the school curriculum. Since then, Danish and Swedish scientists have continued to contribute significant research in both traditional physiology and the latest subdisciplines in exercise physiology and adaptations to physical training.

Danish Influence

In 1909, the University of Copenhagen endowed the equivalent of a Chair in Anatomy, Physiology, and Theory of Gymnastics. The first Docent, Johannes Lindhard, MD (1870–1947), later teamed with August Krogh, PhD (1874–1949), an eminent scientist who specialized in physiological chemistry and research instrument design and construction, to conduct many of the classic experiments in exercise physiology (**Fig. 1.13**). For example, Professors Lindhard and Krogh investigated gas exchange in the lungs, pioneered studies of the relative contribution of fat and carbohydrate oxidation during exercise, measured blood flow redistribution during different exercise intensities, and quantified cardiorespiratory dynamics in exercise.

By 1910, Krogh and his wife Marie (**Fig. 1.14**), a physician, had proven through a series of ingenious, decisive

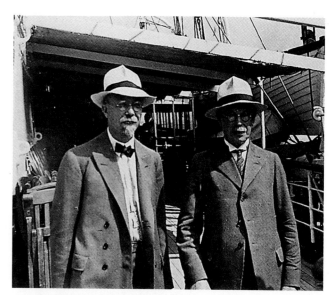

Figure 1.13 Professors August Krogh and Johannes Lindhard, early 1930s, pioneering exercise physiology experimental scientists.

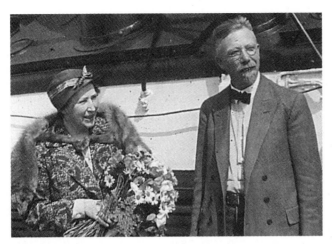

Figure 1.14 Marie Krogh (a physician and researcher) and August Krogh, Nobel Prize achievement in Physiology or Medicine in 1920 that explained capillary control of blood flow in resting and exercising muscle. Dr. Krogh published more than 300 scientific papers in scientific journals on many topics in exercise physiology.

experiments that diffusion governs pulmonary gas exchange during exercise and altitude exposure, not oxygen secretion from lung tissue into the blood as postulated by British physiologists Sir John Scott Haldane and James Priestley. Krogh published a series of experiments (three appearing in the 1919 *Journal of Physiology*) concerning the mechanism of oxygen diffusion and transport in skeletal muscles. He won the Nobel Prize in physiology or medicine in 1920 for discovering the mechanism for capillary control of blood flow in resting and exercising muscle. In recognition of the achievements of this renowned scientist, an institute to honor this cradle for exercise physiology research in Copenhagen bears his name (August Krogh Institute; *www1.bio.ku.dk/English*).

Three other Danish researchers—physiologists Erling Asmussen (1907–1991; ACSM Citation Award, 1976 and ACSM Honor Award, 1979), Erik Hohwü–Christensen (1904–1996; ACSM Honor Award, 1981), and Marius Nielsen (b. 1903)—conducted significant exercise physiology studies (**Fig. 1.15**). These "three musketeers," as Krogh called them, published voluminously during the 1930s to 1970s. Asmussen, initially an assistant in Lindhard's laboratory, became a prolific researcher, specializing in muscle fiber architecture and mechanics. He also published papers with Nielsen and Christensen on many applied topics, including muscular strength and performance, ventilatory and cardiovascular response to changes in posture and exercise intensity, maximum

Questions & Notes

Name 8 non-American notable exercise scientists and their country of origin.

1.

2.

3.

4.

5.

6.

7.

8.

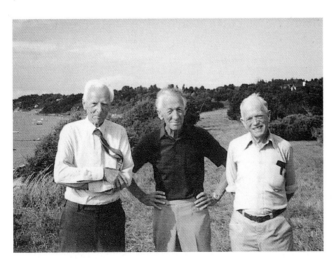

Figure 1.15 Drs. Erling Asmussen (*left*), Erik Hohwü-Christensen (*center*), and Marius Nielson (*right*), 1988, acclaimed exercise physiology researchers.

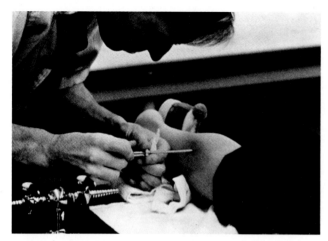

Figure 1.16 Swedish researcher Dr. Bengt Saltin taking a muscle biopsy of gastrocnemius muscle after an endurance training program. (Photo courtesy of Dr. David Costill.)

working capacity during arm and leg exercise, changes in oxidative response of muscle during exercise, comparisons of positive and negative work, hormonal and core temperature response during different intensities of exercise, and respiratory function in response to decreased ambient oxygen levels.

Christensen became Lindhard's student in Copenhagen in 1925. In his 1931 doctoral thesis, Christensen reported studies of cardiac output, body temperature, and blood sugar concentration during intense exercise on a cycle ergometer, compared arm versus leg exercise, and quantified the effects of training. Together with Krogh and Lindhard, Christensen published an important 1936 review article describing physiological dynamics during maximal exercise. With J.W. Hansen, he used oxygen uptake and the respiratory quotient to describe how diet, state of training, and exercise intensity and duration affected carbohydrate and fat utilization. Discovery of the concept of "carbohydrate loading" actually occurred in 1939. Experiments by physician Olé Bang in 1936, inspired by his mentor Ejar Lundsgaard, described the fate of blood lactate during exercise of different intensities and durations. The research of Christensen, Asmussen, Nielsen, and Hansen took place at the Laboratory for the Theory of Gymnastics at the University of Copenhagen. Today, the August Krogh Institute continues the tradition of basic and applied research in exercise physiology. Since 1973, Swedish-trained scientist Bengt Saltin (**Fig. 1.16**) (the only Nordic researcher besides Erling Asmussen to receive the ACSM Citation Award [1980] and ACSM Honor Award [1990]; former student of Per-Olof Åstrand, discussed in the next section) continues his noteworthy scientific studies at the Muscle Research Institute in Copenhagen.

Swedish Influence

Modern exercise physiology in Sweden can be traced to Per Henrik Ling (1776–1839), who in 1813 became the first director of Stockholm's Royal Central Institute of Gymnas-

tics (RCIG). Ling, in addition to his expertise in exercise and movement and as a fencing master, developed a system of "medical gymnastics" that incorporated his studies of anatomy and physiology, which became integral to Sweden's school curriculum in 1820. Ling's son, Hjalmar Ling (1820–1886), published an important textbook about the "kinesiology of body movements" in 1866 (from a translation in Swedish: *The First Notions of Movement Science. Outline Regarding the Teaching at RCIG and an Introduction with References to the Elementary Principles of Mechanics and Joint-Science*). As a result of Per Henrik and his son Hjalmar's philosophy and pioneering influences, physical education graduates from the RCIG were extremely well schooled in the basic biological sciences in addition to proficiency in many sports and games. The RCIG graduates were all men until 1864 when women were first admitted. Ling's early teachings and curriculum advances consisted of four branches of his System of Gymnastics—the most influential and long lasting being medical gymnastics that has evolved into the discipline of physiotherapy. Course work included anatomy and physiology, pathology with dissections, and basic study in movement science (*Rörelselära* in Swedish). One of Ling's lasting legacies was his steadfast insistence that RCIG graduates have a strong science background. This was carried out by Ling's disciples, who assumed positions of leadership in predominantly Germany, France, Denmark, Belgium, and England, with the influence extending to the United States beginning in the 1830s. Founded in 1813, the Gymnastik-Och Idrottshögskolan or Swedish School of Sport and Health Sciences (GIH) has the distinction as the oldest University College in the world within its field. GIH along with the Department of Physiology in the Karolinska Institute Medical School in Stockholm, the Royal Institute of Technology, Stockholm University, and Örebro University conduct research in exercise physiology and musculoskeletal health and disease.

Per-Olof Åstrand, MD, PhD (b. 1922; **Fig. 1.17**) is the most famous graduate of the College of Physical Education (1946); in 1952, he presented his doctoral thesis at the Karolinska Institute Medical School. Åstrand taught in the Department of Physiology in the College of Physical Education from 1946 to 1977; it then became a department at

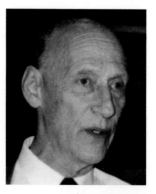

Figure 1.17 Dr. Per-Olof Åstrand, Department of Physiology, Karolinska Institute, Stockholm, was instrumental in charting the modern course of exercise physiology research.

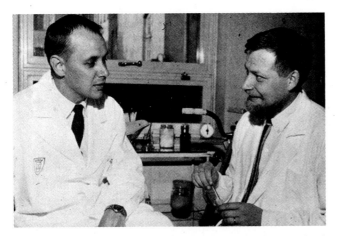

Figure 1.18   Drs. Jonas Bergström (*left*) and Eric Hultman (*right*), Karolinska Institute, Stockholm, pioneered needle biopsy techniques to assess the ultrastructural architecture of muscle fibers and their biochemical functions.

the Karolinska Institute, where he served as professor and department head from 1977 to 1987. Christensen, Åstrand's mentor, supervised his thesis, which evaluated physical working capacity of men and women ages 4 to 33 years. This important study, among others, established a line of research that propelled Åstrand to the forefront of experimental exercise physiology for which he achieved worldwide fame. Four of his papers, published in 1960 with Christensen as coauthor, stimulated further studies on the physiological responses to intermittent exercise. Åstrand has mentored an impressive group of exercise physiologists, including "superstar" Dr. Bengt Saltin.

Two Swedish scientists from the Karolinska Institute, Drs. Jonas Bergström and Erik Hultman (**Fig. 1.18**), conducted important needle biopsy experiments in the mid 1960s. With this procedure, muscle could be studied under various conditions of exercise, training, and nutritional status. Collaborative work with other Scandinavian researchers (Saltin and Hultman from Sweden and Hermansen from Norway) and researchers in the United States (e.g., Gollnick [d. 1994], Washington State University) provided new vistas from which to view the physiology of exercise.

Norwegian and Finnish Influence

The new generation of exercise physiologists trained in the late 1940s analyzed respiratory gases with a highly accurate sampling apparatus that measured minute quantities of carbon dioxide and oxygen in expired air. Norwegian scientist Per Scholander (1905–1980) developed the method of analysis (and analyzer that bears his name) in 1947.

Another prominent Norwegian researcher, **Lars A. Hermansen** (1933–1984: **Fig. 1.19**; ACSM Citation Award, 1985), from the Institute of Work Physiology

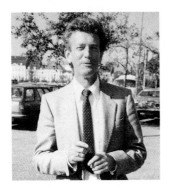

Figure 1.19   Lars A. Hermansen (1933–1984), Institute of Work Physiology, Oslo.

Questions & Notes

Who was Per Henrik Ling and why is he an important historical figure?

Name 2 famous Danish exercise physiologists.

  1.

  2.

Name 2 famous Swedish exercise physiologist.

  1.

  2.

Name a famous Norwegian exercise physiologist.

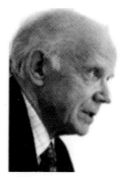

Figure 1.20 Dr. Paavo Komi, Finland's pioneer researcher in biomechanics and exercise work physiology.

made many contributions, including a classic 1969 article titled "Anaerobic Energy Release," which appeared in the initial volume of *Medicine and Science in Sports*.

In Finland, Martti Karvonen, MD, PhD (ACSM Honor Award, 1991) from the Physiology Department of the Institute of Occupational Health, Helsinki, achieved notoriety for a method to predict optimal exercise training heart rate, now called the "Karvonen formula" (see Chapter 14). Paavo Komi (**Fig. 1.20**), Department of Biology of Physical Activity, University of Jyväskylä, has been Finland's most

prolific researcher with numerous experiments published in the combined areas of exercise physiology and sport biomechanics.

OTHER CONTRIBUTORS TO EXERCISE PHYSIOLOGY

In addition to the American and Nordic scientists who achieved distinction as exercise scientists, many other "giants" in the fields of physiology and experimental science made monumental contributions that indirectly contributed to the knowledge base in exercise physiology. These include the physiologists shown in **Figure 1.21**: Antoine Laurent Lavoisier (1743–1794; fuel combustion); Sir Joseph Barcroft (1872–1947; altitude); Christian Bohr (1855–1911; oxygen–hemoglobin dissociation curve); John Scott Haldane (1860–1936; respiration); Otto Myerhoff (1884–1951; Nobel Prize, cellular metabolic pathways); Nathan Zuntz (1847–1920; portable metabolism apparatus); Carl von Voit (1831–1908) and his student, Max Rubner (1854–1932; direct and indirect calorimetry, and specific dynamic action of food); Max von Pettenkofer (1818–1901; nutrient metabolism); and Eduard F.W. Pflüger (1829–1910; tissue oxidation).

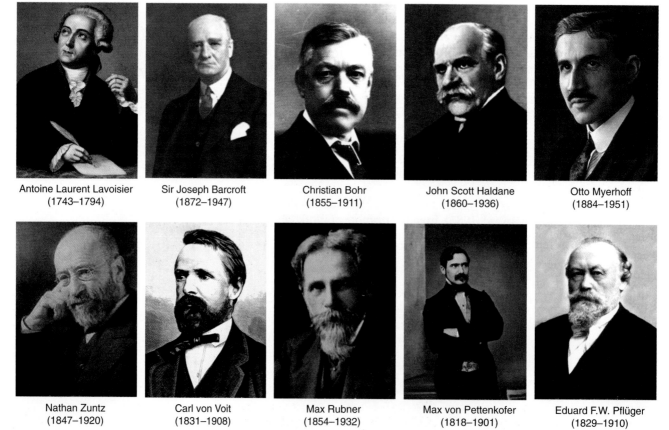

Antoine Laurent Lavoisier
(1743–1794)

Sir Joseph Barcroft
(1872–1947)

Christian Bohr
(1855–1911)

John Scott Haldane
(1860–1936)

Otto Myerhoff
(1884–1951)

Nathan Zuntz
(1847–1920)

Carl von Voit
(1831–1908)

Max Rubner
(1854–1932)

Max von Pettenkofer
(1818–1901)

Eduard F.W. Pflüger
(1829–1910)

Figure 1.21 Ten prominent scientist–researchers who paved the way in the development of modern exercise physiology.

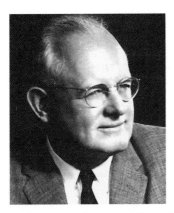

Figure 1.22   Dr. Thomas Kirk Cureton (1901–1993), prolific researcher and author, helped to establish the influential graduate program at the University of Illinois that mentored many leading exercise physiologists.

Questions & Notes

Name a famous Finnish exercise physiologist.

Name the pioneering physical fitness researcher from the University of Illinois.

Perform an internet search using the term exercise performance. *How many "hits" do you find?*

The field of exercise physiology also owes a debt of gratitude to the pioneers of the physical fitness movement in the United States, notably Thomas K. Cureton (1901–1993; ACSM charter member, 1969 ACSM Honor Award; **Fig. 1.22**) at the University of Illinois, Champaign. Cureton, a prolific and innovative physical educator and pioneer researcher, trained four generations of students beginning in 1941 who later established quality research programs and influenced many leading exercise physiologists. These early physical education graduates with an exercise physiology specialty soon assumed leadership positions as professors of physical education with teaching and research responsibilities in exercise physiology at numerous colleges, universities, and military establishments in the United States and throughout the world. Dr. Cureton was author or coauthor of 50 textbooks about exercise, health, sport-specific training and physical fitness and served on the President's Council on Physical Fitness and Sports (*www.fitness.gov*) under five presidents. Cureton, a champion masters swimmer, established 14 age-group world records, also tutored Sir Roger Bannister (b. 1929), who first shattered the sub 4-minute mile barrier on May 6, 1954.

CONTEMPORARY DEVELOPMENTS

Exercise Physiology, the Internet, and Online Social Networking

Since publication of the third edition of this textbook in 2006, topics related to exercise physiology on the Internet have expanded tremendously. Information about almost every topic area, no matter how seemingly remote, can quickly be obtained through the popular search engines Google (*www.google.com*) and Yahoo! (*www.yahoo.com*) and others such as AltaVista, Ask Jeeves, Inktomi, LookSmart, Teoma, Bing Walhello, and Open Directory. On June 29, 2010, there were 1,880,000 hits for the term *exercise physiology* (Google search); and 17,800,102 "hits" via Yahoo! Adding the word *muscle* to that search narrowed the selection to *only* 755,000 entries, with a further reduction to 60,100 links when adding *DNA*. At this point, if we still wanted to pinpoint the search further because of an interest about *DNA*, *muscle*, and *twins*, the search returned 7900 entries, still a sizable number. Going still further, adding *Greenland* returned 2000 entries, with further restriction to 207 entries by adding *pygmies*. The point becomes clear—the Internet provides a wonderful repository of useful information to target a focus of inquiry—no matter how specific. When you reach this point, you must make qualitative decisions about how to sift through the information to determine what is pertinent (and reliable) to your needs.

An Example from This Section Consider an example discussed in this section for Galen, one of the most influential Greek physicians of antiquity. Entering the term Galen into a June 29, 2010 Google search yields an overwhelming 5,600,000 entries! But do not be overwhelmed by this unbelievable number of Web sites that deal in some way with topics related to Galen. Check out the first entry (*en.wikipedia.org/wiki/Galen*); that single search by itself provides a goldmine of useful information about Galen. The blue hyperlinks (words highlighted in blue) will lead to further details about his life and times. Clicking on the first term in blue, *Pergamon* (*en.wikipedia.org/wiki/Pergamum*), provides much useful information about this ancient Greek city (with continuing details about the location of the city during the Greek "ancient" period). Along the way, you can discover information about the Greek Bronze Age and about ancient Greece, including the development of early public school education and how boys were trained in athletics to prepare for military service (*en.wikipedia.org/wiki/Ancient_Greece#Education*). At this point, you may want to know more specific details about Galen and sports medicine. By adding the term *Galen sports medicine* to the search yields 35,400 Web URLs (Universal Record Locator or specific pages of information). The fifth entry titled "the father of sports medicine (Galen)" looks like it might provide useful information (*www.ncbi.nlm.nih.gov/pubmed/350061*). This entry links to one of the largest research databases in the world (PubMed) sponsored by the U.S. National Library of Medicine and the National Institutes of Health (*www.ncbi.nlm.nih.gov/pubmed/*). The following presents information from that link that identifies an article by GA Snook in the *American Journal of Sports Medicine* in 1978 regarding Galen:

> **Snook GA. The father of sports medicine (Galen).**
> *Am. J. Sports Med.,* 6(3):128–131, 1978.
>
>   Although there were many physicians who treated athletes before Galen, I believe that he was the first to devote a major portion of his time to this field of endeavor. Furthermore, his systematic observations, his aggressive pursuit of newer and better ways of treatment, his teaching, and his publishing of his observations make him a kindred soul to the team physician and practitioners of sports medicine of today. It is for these reasons that I believe that he can justly be called the "Father of Sports Medicine."

Online Social Networking Online Social Networking refers to the common grouping of individuals into more specific groups. The four most popular social networking sites as of October 2009 (based on inbound links and complete monthly visitors) include Facebook (*www.facebook.com*), MySpace (*www.myspace.com*), Twitter (*www.twitter.com*), and LinkedIn (*www.linkedin.com*). Other popular sites include Classmates.com (*www.classmates.com*), and Ning (*www.ning.com*). Such sites allow Internet users to gather and share information or experiences about specific topics (from Galen the ancient physician to genetics related to molecular biology in exercise physiology)

and develop friendships and continue professional relationships. Numerous electronic discussion groups exist in exercise physiology and related areas, many with thousands of subscribers. New bulletin boards with specific areas of interest (e.g., pediatric exercise immunology, molecular biology and exercise) enable subscribers to receive and reply to the same inquiry. Many of the field's top scientists routinely participate in discussion groups, which makes "lurking" (computer slang for following the interchanges but rarely participating) a productive pastime. Anyone with an Internet connection and e-mail address can participate in a discussion group of interest. Appendix E lists frequently cited journals in exercise physiology. Entering the journal name in one of the Internet search engines directs you to that site.

CONTEMPORARY PROFESSIONAL EXERCISE PHYSIOLOGY ORGANIZATIONS

Just as knowledge dissemination via publications in research and professional journals signals expansion of a field of study, development of professional organizations to certify and monitor professional activities becomes critical to continued growth. The American Association for the Advancement of Physical Education (AAAPE), formed in 1885, represented the first professional organization in the United States to include topics related to exercise physiology. This association predated the current American Alliance for Health, Physical Education, Recreation, and Dance (AAHPERD; *www.aahperd.org/*).

Until the early 1950s, the AAHPERD represented the predominant professional organization for exercise physiologists. As the field expanded and diversified its focus, a separate professional organization was needed to more fully respond to professional needs. In 1954, Joseph Wolffe, MD, and 11 other physicians, physiologists, and physical educators founded the American College of Sports Medicine (ACSM; *www.acsm.org*). Presently, the ACSM has more than 20,000 members in 75 countries, including 15,000 ACSM Certified Professionals and 6500 conference attendees (as of October 2009). The ACSM now represents the largest professional organization in the world for exercise physiology (including allied medical and health areas). The ACSM's mission "promotes and integrates scientific research, education, and practical applications of sports medicine and exercise science to maintain and enhance physical performance, fitness, health, and quality of life." The ACSM publishes the quality and well-cited research journal *Medicine and Science in Sport and Exercise* and other resource publications, including the *Health & Fitness Journal, Exercise and Sport Science Reviews,* the 2010 *Guidelines for Exercise Testing and Prescription* (8th edition), *ACSM's Resource Manual for Clinical Exercise Physiology* (2nd edition), *ACSM's Resource Manual for Guidelines for Exercise Testing and Prescription* (6th edition), and *ACSM's Certification Review* (3rd edition).

BOX 1.3   CLOSE UP

How to Discern Reliable Historical Research

The purpose of historical research has changed through the ages. The earliest writers of history focused on literary rather than scientific objectives; they preserved beloved folktales, created epics to entertain or inspire, defended and promoted numerous causes, zealously protected the privilege of a class, and glorified the state and exalted the church. In contrast, ancient Greek scholars envisioned history as a search for the truth—the application of exacting methods to select, verify, and classify facts according to specific standards that endure the test of critical examination and preserve an accurate record of past events. Historical research enlarges our world of experience and provides deeper insights into what has been successfully and unsuccessfully tried.

Historical scholars collect and validate source materials to formulate and verify hypotheses. Unlike experimental research, their methods feature observations and insights that cannot be repeated under conventional laboratory conditions.

COLLECTING SOURCE MATERIAL

Historians' initial and most important problem-solving task seeks to obtain the best available data. Historians must distinguish between primary and secondary source materials.

PRIMARY SOURCES

Primary sources comprise the basic materials of historical research. This prized form of "data" derives from:

1. Testimony from reliable eyewitnesses and earwitnesses to past events.
2. Direct examination of actual "objects" used in the past.

A historian collects evidence from the closest witness to the past event or condition. Primary source materials include records preserved with the conscious intent of transmitting information. For example, a newspaper account of what transpired at a meeting has less intrinsic historical value than the meeting's official minutes. Records of past ideas, conditions, and events exist in written form (e.g., official records or executive documents, health records, licenses, annual reports, catalogs, and personal records—diaries, autobiographies, letters, wills, deeds, contracts, lecture notes, original drafts of speeches, articles, and books), visual (pictorial) form (photographs, movies, microfilms, drawings, paintings, etchings, coins,

sculpture), mechanical form (tape recordings, phonograph records, dictations), electronic form (digital "memory" on disc or tape), and sometimes oral form (myths, folktales, family stories, dances, games, ceremonies, reminiscences by eyewitnesses to events).

SECONDARY SOURCES

Secondary sources include information provided by a person who did not directly observe the event, object, or condition. The original publication of a research report in a scientific journal represents a primary source (often used by modern researchers to provide context to their experiments), summaries in encyclopedias, newspapers, periodicals, the Internet, and other references qualify as secondary materials. The more interpretations that separate a past event from the reader, the less trustworthy the evidence becomes; the transition often distorts and changes the facts. For this reason, secondary sources are less reliable. However, secondary sources acquaint a neophyte historian with major theoretical issues and suggest locations for uncovering primary source materials.

CRITICIZING SOURCE MATERIAL

Historians critically examine the trustworthiness of their source material. Through external criticism, the historian checks the authenticity and textual integrity of the "data" (time, place, and authorship) to determine its admissibility as reliable evidence. Enterprising and exacting investigation becomes part of external criticism—tracking down anonymous and undated documents, ferreting out forgeries, discovering plagiarism, uncovering incorrectly identified items, and restoring documents to their original forms.

After completing external criticism, the historian engages in internal criticism to establish the meaning and trustworthiness of a document's contents. Internal criticism determines the following:

1. Conditions that produced the document
2. Validity of the writer's intellectual premises
3. Competency, credibility, and possible author bias
4. Correctness of data interpretation

Careful historical research provides insight about how past facts influence current events. Whether an accurate record of the past predicts and influences future circumstances remains a hotly debated topic among historians.

Other important professional organizations related to exercise physiology include the International Council of Sport Science and Physical Education (ICSSPE; *www.icsspe.org/*), founded in 1958 in Paris, France, originally under the name the International Council of Sport and Physical Education. The ICSSPE serves as an international umbrella organization concerned with promoting and disseminating results and findings in the field of sport science. Its main professional publication, *Sport Science Review*, deals with thematic overviews of sport sciences research. The Federation Internationale de Medicine Sportive (FIMS; *www.fims.org*), composed of the national sports medicine associations of more than 100 countries, originated in 1928 during a meeting of Olympic medical doctors in Switzerland. The FIMS promotes the study and development of sports medicine throughout the world and hosts major international conferences in sports medicine every 3 years; it also produces position statements on topics related to health, physical activity, and sports medicine. A joint position statement with the World Health Organization (WHO; *www.who.int*) titled "Physical Activity and Health" denotes one of the FIMS's best-known documents. Other organizations representing exercise physiologists include the European College of Sport Science (ECSS; *www.ecss.de*), British Association of Sport and Exercise Sciences (BASES; *www.bases.org.uk*), and American Society of Exercise Physiology (ASEP; *www.asep.org*).

A COMMON LINK

One theme unites the 2300-year history of exercise physiology—the value of mentoring by visionaries who spent an extraordinary amount of time "infecting" students with a passion for science. These demanding but inspiring relationships developed researchers who nurtured the next generation of productive scholars. This nurturing process from mentor to student remains fundamental to the continued academic enhancement of exercise physiology. The connection between mentor and student remains the hallmark of most fields of inquiry—from antiquity to the present. The mentoring process includes a love of discovery through the scientific method. In Part 2, we explore the fundamentals of the scientific process. The pioneers in our field (and contemporary researchers) incorporated these principles in their quest toward new discoveries.

 SUMMARY

1. Exercise physiology as an academic field of study consists of three distinct components: (1) a body of knowledge built on facts and theories derived from research, (2) a formal course of study at institutions of higher learning, and (3) professional preparation of practitioners and future leaders in the field.

2. Exercise physiology has developed as a field separate from physiology because of its unique focus on the study of the functional dynamics and adaptations to human movement and associated physiological responses.

3. Galen, one of the first "sports medicine" physicians, wrote prolifically, producing at least 80 treatises and perhaps 500 essays on topics related to human anatomy and physiology, nutrition, growth and development, the benefits of exercise and deleterious consequences of sedentary living, and diseases and their treatment.

4. Austin Flint, Jr., MD (1836–1915), one of the first American pioneer physician–scientists, incorporated studies about physiological responses to exercise in his influential medical physiology textbooks.

5. Edward Hitchcock, Jr., (1828–1911), Amherst College Professor of Hygiene and Physical Education, devoted his academic career to the scientific study of physical exercise and training and body size and shape. His 1860 text on anatomy and physiology, coauthored with his father, significantly influenced the sports science movement in the United States after 1860. Hitchcock's insistence on the need for science applied to physical education undoubtedly influenced Harvard's commitment to create an academic Department of Anatomy, Physiology, and Physical Training in 1891.

6. George Wells Fitz, MD (1860–1934) created the first departmental major in Anatomy, Physiology, and Physical Training at Harvard University in 1891; the following year, he started the first formal exercise physiology laboratory in the United States. Fitz was probably first to teach an exercise physiology course at the university level.

7. The real impact of laboratory research in exercise physiology (along with many other research specialties) occurred in 1927 with the creation of the Harvard Fatigue Laboratory at Harvard University's business school. Two decades of outstanding work by this laboratory legitimized exercise physiology as a key area of research and study.

8. The Nordic countries (particularly Denmark and Sweden) played an important historical role in developing the field of exercise physiology. Danish physiologist August Krogh (1874–1949) won the 1920 Nobel Prize in physiology or medicine for discovering the mechanism that controlled capillary blood flow in resting or active muscle; Krogh's basic experiments led him to conduct other experiments with exercise scientists worldwide. His pioneering work in exercise physiology continues to inspire exercise physiology studies in many areas, including oxygen uptake kinetics and metabolism, muscle physiology, and nutritional biochemistry.

9. Publications of applied and basic exercise physiology research have increased as the field expands into different areas. The Internet and online social networking offer unique growth potential for information dissemination in this area.

10. The ACSM, with more than 20,000 members from North America and 75 other countries, represents the largest professional organization in the world for exercise physiology (including allied medical and health areas).

11. One theme unites the 2300-year history of exercise physiology—the value of mentoring by professors who spent an extraordinary amount of time "infecting" students with a passion for science.

Part 2	The Exercise Physiologist

Many individuals view exercise physiology as an undergraduate or graduate academic major (or concentration) completed at an accredited college or university. In this regard, only those who complete this academic major have the "right" to be called an "exercise physiologist." However, many individuals complete undergraduate and graduate degrees in related fields with considerable coursework and practical experience in exercise physiology or related areas. Consequently, the title "exercise physiologist" could also apply so long as a person's academic preparation is adequate. Resolution of this dilemma becomes difficult because no national consensus exists as to what constitutes an acceptable (or minimal) academic program of course work in exercise physiology. In addition, there are no universal standards for hands-on laboratory experiences (anatomy, kinesiology, biomechanics, and exercise physiology), demonstrated level of competency, and internship hours that would stand the test of national certification or licensure. Moreover, because areas of concentration within the field are so broad, consensus certification testing becomes challenging. No national accreditation or licensure exists to certify exercise physiologists.

WHAT DO EXERCISE PHYSIOLOGISTS DO?

Exercise physiologists assume diverse careers. Some use their research skills primarily in colleges, universities, and private industry settings. Others are employed in health, fitness, and rehabilitation centers, and others serve as educators, personal trainers, managers, and entrepreneurs in the health and fitness industry.

Exercise physiologists also own health and fitness companies or are hands-on practitioners who teach and service the community, including corporate, industrial, and governmental agencies. Some specialize in other types of professional work such as massage therapy, and others go on to pursue professional degrees in physical therapy, occupational therapy, nursing, nutrition, medicine, and chiropractic.

Table 1.1 presents a partial list of different employment descriptions for a qualified exercise physiologist in one of six major areas.

EXERCISE PHYSIOLOGISTS AND HEALTH AND FITNESS PROFESSIONALS IN THE CLINICAL SETTING

The well-documented health benefits of regular physical activity have enhanced exercise physiologists' role beyond traditional lines. A clinical exercise physiologist becomes part of the health and fitness professional team. This team

Questions & Notes

What is the ACSM? Summarize its mission.

List 3 possible job opportunities for exercise physiology graduates.

1.

2.

3.

Table 1.1	Partial List of Employment Opportunities for Qualified Exercise Physiologists

SPORTS	COLLEGE UNIVERSITY	COMMUNITY	CLINICAL	GOVERNMENT MILITARY	BUSINESS	PRIVATE
Sports director	Professor	Manage/direct health/wellness programs	Test/supervise cardiopulmonary patients	Fitness director/ manager	Sports management	Personal health/ fitness consultant
Strength/ conditioning coach	Researcher	Community education	Evaluate/supervise special populations (diabetes, obesity, arthritis, dyslipidemia, cystic fibrosis, cancer, hypertension, children, low pregnancy)	Health fitness director in correctional institutions	Health/ fitness promotion	Own business
Director, manager of state/national teams	Administrator	Occupational rehabilitation	Exercise technologist in cardiology practice	Sports nutrition programs	Sport psychologist	
Consultant	Teacher		Researcher		Health/ fitness club instructor	
	Instructor					

approach to preventive and rehabilitative services requires different personnel depending on the program mission, population served, location, number of participants, space availability, and funding level. A comprehensive clinical program may include the following personnel in addition to an exercise physiologist:

- Physicians
- Certified personnel (exercise leaders, health and fitness instructors, directors, exercise test technologists, preventive and rehabilitative exercise specialists, preventive and rehabilitative exercise directors)
- Dietitians
- Nurses
- Physical therapists
- Occupational therapists
- Social workers
- Respiratory therapists
- Psychologists
- Health educators

Sports Medicine and Exercise Physiology: A Vital Link

The traditional view of **sports medicine** involves rehabilitating athletes from sports-related injuries. *A more contemporary view relates sports medicine to the scientific and medical (preventive and rehabilitative) aspects of physical activity, physical fitness, and exercise and sports performance.* A close

link ties sports medicine to clinical exercise physiology. Sports medicine professionals and exercise physiologists work hand in hand with similar populations. These include, at one extreme, sedentary people who need only a modest amount of regular exercise to reduce risk of degenerative diseases, and at the other extreme, able-bodied and disabled athletes who strive to further enhance their performance.

Carefully prescribed physical activity significantly contributes to overall health and quality of life. In conjunction with sports medicine professionals, clinical exercise physiologists test, treat, and rehabilitate individuals with diverse diseases and physical disabilities. In addition, prescription of physical activity and athletic competition for physically challenged individuals plays an important role in sports medicine and exercise physiology, providing unique opportunities for research, clinical practice, and professional advancement.

TRAINING AND CERTIFICATION BY PROFESSIONAL ORGANIZATIONS

To properly accomplish responsibilities in the exercise setting, health and fitness professionals must integrate unique knowledge, skills, and abilities related to exercise, physical fitness, and health. Different professional organizations provide leadership in training and certifying health and fitness professionals at different levels. Table 1.2 lists organizations offering training and certification programs with diverse emphases and specializations. The ACSM has

Table 1.2 Organizations Offering Training or Certification Programs Related to Physical Activity	
ORGANIZATION	**AREAS OF SPECIALIZATION AND CERTIFICATION**
Aerobics and Fitness Association of America (AFAA) 15250 Ventura Blvd., Suite 200 Sherman Oaks, CA 91403	AFP Fitness Practitioner, Primary Aerobics Instructor, Personal Trainer & Fitness Counselor, Step Reebok Certification, Weight Room/Resistance Training Certification, Emergency Response Certification
American College of Sports Medicine (ACSM) 401 West Michigan St. Indianapolis, IN 46202	Exercise Leader, Health/Fitness Instructor, Exercise Test Technologist, Health/Fitness Director, Exercise Specialist, Program Director
American Council on Exercise (ACE) 5820 Oberlin Dr., Suite 102 San Diego, CA 92121	Group Fitness Instructor, Personal Trainer, Lifestyle & Weight Management Consultant
Canadian Aerobics Instructors Network (CAIN) 2441 Lakeshore Rd. West, PO Box 70009 Oakville, ON L6L 6M9 Canada	CIAI Instructor, Certified Personal Trainer
Canadian Personal Trainers Network (CPTN) Ontario Fitness Council (OFC) 1185 Eglington Ave. East, Suite 407 North York, ON M3C 3C6 Canada	CPTN/OFC Certified Personal Trainer, CPTN Certified Specialty Personal Trainer, CPTN/OFC Assessor of Personal Trainers, CPTN/OFC Course Conductor for Personal Trainers
Canadian Society for Exercise Physiology 1600 James Naismith Dr., Suite 311 Gloucester, ON K1B 5N4	CFC (Certified Fitness Consultant), PFLC (Professional Fitness & Lifestyle Consultant), AFAC (Accredited Fitness Appraisal Center)
The Cooper Institute for Aerobics Research 12330 Preston Rd. Dallas, TX 75230	PFS (Physical Fitness Specialists; Personal Trainer), GEL (Group Exercise Leadership; Aerobic Instructor), ADV.PFS (Advanced Physical Fitness specialist, Biomechanics of Strength Training, Health Promotion Director)
Disabled Sports USA 451 Hungerford Dr., Suite 100 Rockville, MD 20850	Adapted Fitness Instructor
National Academy of Sports Medicine (NASM) 5845 E. Still Creek, Circle Suite 206 Mesa, AZ 85206	(CPT) Certified Personal Trainer
Jazzercise 2808 Roosevelt Blvd. Carlsbad, CA 92008	Certified Jazzercise Instructor
International Society of Sports Nutrition 600 Pembrook Dr. Woodland Park, CO 80863	Sports Nutrition Certification Body Composition Certification
National Strength & Conditioning Association (NSCA) P.O. Box 38909 Colorado Springs, CO 80937	Certified Strength & Conditioning Specialist, Certified Personal Trainer
YMCA of the USA 101 North Wacker Dr. Chicago, IL 60606	Certified Fitness Leader (Stage I—Theory, II—Applied Theory, III—Practical), Certified Specialty Leader, Trainer of Fitness Leaders, Trainer of Trainers

emerged as the preeminent academic organization offering comprehensive programs in areas related to the health and fitness profession. ACSM certifications encompass cognitive and practical competencies that are evaluated by written and practical examinations. The candidate must successfully complete each of these components (scored separately) to receive the world-recognized ACSM certification. The ACSM offers a wide variety of certification programs throughout the United States and in other countries (*www.acsm.org*).

ACSM QUALIFICATIONS AND CERTIFICATIONS

Health and fitness professionals should be knowledgeable and competent in different areas, including first-aid and CPR certification, depending on personal

Questions & Notes

Go on-line and search ACSM.org for their various certification programs in your geographic area.

Table 1.3	Major Knowledge and Competency Areas Required for Individuals Interested in ACSM Certifications

Exercise physiology and related exercise science
Pathophysiology and risk factors
Health appraisal, fitness, and clinical testing
Electrocardiography and diagnostic techniques
Patient management and medications
Medical and surgical management
Exercise prescription and programming
Nutrition and weight management
Human behavior and counseling
Safety, injury prevention, and emergency procedures
Program administration, quality assurance, and outcome
   assessment
Clinical and medical considerations (ACSM Certified Personal
   Trainer only)

From American College of Sports Medicine. (2010). *ACSM's Guidelines for Exercise Testing and Prescription* (8th Ed.). Baltimore: Lippincott Williams & Wilkins.

interest. Table 1.3 presents content areas for different ACSM certifications. Each has general and specific learning objectives.

Health and Fitness Track

The **Health and Fitness Track** encompasses the Exercise Leader, Health/Fitness Instructor, and Health/Fitness Director categories.

Exercise Leader

An **Exercise Leader** must know about physical fitness (including basic motivation and counseling techniques) for healthy individuals and those with cardiovascular and pulmonary diseases. This category requires at least 250 hours of hands-on leadership experience or an academic background in an appropriate allied health field. Examples of general objectives for an Exercise Leader in exercise physiology include:

1. Define *aerobic* and *anaerobic metabolism*.
2. Describe the role of carbohydrates, fats, and proteins as fuel for aerobic and anaerobic exercise performance.
3. Define the relationship of METs (multiples of resting metabolism) and kilocalories with levels of physical activity.

Health/Fitness Instructor

An undergraduate degree in exercise science, kinesiology, physical education, or appropriate allied health field represents the minimum education prerequisite for a **Health/Fitness Instructor**. These individuals must demonstrate competency in physical fitness testing, designing and executing exercise programs, leading exercise, and organizing and operating fitness facilities. The Health/Fitness Instructor has added responsibility for (1) training or supervising exercise leaders during an exercise program and (2) serving as an exercise leader. Health/Fitness Instructors also function as health counselors to offer multiple intervention strategies for lifestyle change.

Health/Fitness Director

The minimum educational prerequisite for **Health/Fitness Director** certification requires a postgraduate degree in an appropriate allied health field. Health/Fitness Directors must acquire a Health/Fitness Instructor or Exercise Specialist certification. This level requires supervision by a certified program director and physician during an approved internship or at least 1 year of practical experience. Health/Fitness Directors require leadership qualities that ensure competency in training and supervising personnel and proficiency in oral presentations.

Clinical Track

The **clinical track** indicates that certified personnel in these areas provide leadership in health and fitness or clinical programs. These professionals possess added clinical skills and knowledge that allow them to work with higher risk, symptomatic populations.

Exercise Test Technologist

Exercise Test Technologists administer exercise tests to individuals in good health and various states of illness. They need to demonstrate appropriate knowledge of functional anatomy, exercise physiology, pathophysiology, electrocardiography, and psychology. They must know how to recognize contraindications to testing during preliminary screening, administer tests, record data, implement emergency procedures, summarize test data, and communicate test results to other health professionals. Certification as an Exercise Test Technologist does *not* require prerequisite experience or special level of education.

Preventive/Rehabilitative Exercise Specialist

Unique competencies for the category include the ability to lead exercises for persons with medical limitations (particularly cardiorespiratory and related diseases) and healthy populations. The position requires a bachelor's or graduate degree in an appropriate allied health field and an internship of 6 months or more (800 hours), largely with cardiopulmonary disease patients in a rehabilitative setting. The **Preventive/Rehabilitative Exercise Specialist** conducts and administers exercise tests; evaluates and interprets clinical data and formulates exercise prescriptions; conducts exercise sessions; and demonstrates leadership, enthusiasm, and creativity. This person can respond appropriately to complications during exercise testing and training and can modify exercise prescriptions for patients with specific needs.

Preventive/Rehabilitative Program Director

A **Preventive/Rehabilitative Program Director** holds an advanced degree in an appropriate allied health-related area. The certification requires an internship or practical experience of at least 2 years. This health professional works with cardiopulmonary disease patients in a rehabilitative setting, conducts and administers exercise tests, evaluates and interprets clinical data, formulates exercise prescriptions, conducts exercise sessions, responds appropriately to complications during exercise testing and training, modifies exercise prescriptions for patients with specific limitations, and makes administrative decisions regarding all aspects of a specific program.

SUMMARY

1. A close link ties sports medicine to clinical exercise physiology. Sports medicine professionals and exercise physiologists work side by side with similar populations. These include, at one extreme, sedentary people who need only a modest amount of regular exercise to reduce their risk of degenerative diseases and patients recovering from surgery or requiring regular exercise to combat a decline in functional capacity brought on by serious illness. At the other extreme are able-bodied and disabled athletes who strive to enhance their sports performance.

2. In their clinical role, exercise physiologists alongside sports medicine professionals test, treat, and rehabilitate individuals with diverse diseases and physical disabilities.

3. The ACSM has emerged as the preeminent academic organization offering comprehensive certification programs in several areas related to the health and fitness profession. ACSM certifications encompass cognitive and practical competencies that are evaluated by written and practical examinations.

THOUGHT QUESTIONS

1. Discuss advantages for personal trainers to become trained in exercise physiology and related areas or obtain a special certification from a recognized organization. Why can't a person just have practical experience and learn to apply it to others?

2. How would you account for the differences that exist in quality of certification requirements of different organizations?

3. Discuss whether professionals in the field should be required by their certifying organization to take continuing education courses and subscribe to professional research journals.

SELECTED REFERENCES

American Association for Health, Physical Education, and Recreation. *Research Methods Applied to Health, Physical Education, and Recreation.* Washington, DC: American Association for Health, Physical Education, and Recreation, 1949.

Asmussen, E.: Muscular exercise. In: *Handbook of Respiration.* Section 3. Respiration. Vol. II. Fenn, W.O. and Rahn, H. (eds.). Washington, DC: American Physiological Society, 1965.

Åstrand, P.O.: Influence of Scandinavian scientists in exercise physiology. *Scand. J. Med. Sci. Sports.*, 1:3, 1991.

Bang, O., et al.: Contributions to the physiology of severe muscular work. *Skand. Arch. Physiol.*, 74(Suppl):1, 1936.

Barcroft, J.: *The Respiratory Function of the Blood. Part 1. Lesson from High Altitude.* Cambridge: Cambridge University Press, 1925.

Berryman, J.W.: The tradition of the "six things nonnatural": Exercise and medicine from Hippocrates through antebellum America. *Exerc. Sport Sci. Rev.*, 17:515, 1989.

Berryman, J.W.: The rise and development of the American College of Sports Medicine. *Med. Sci. Sports Exerc.*, 25:885.

Berryman, J.W.: *Out of Many, One. A History of the American College of Sports Medicine.* Champaign, IL: Human Kinetics, 1995.

Berryman, J.W., Thomas K. Cureton, Jr.: pioneer researcher, proselytizer, and proponent for physical fitness. *Res. Q. Exerc. Sport.*, 67:1, 1996.

Buskirk, E.R.: From Harvard to Minnesota: keys to our history. *Exerc. Sport Sci. Rev.,* 20:1, 1992.

Buskirk, E.R.: Early history of exercise physiology in the United States. Part 1. A contemporary historical perspective. In: *History of Exercise and Sport Science.* Messengale, J.D., and Swanson, R.A. (eds.). Champaign, IL: Human Kinetics, 1997.

Christensen, E.H., et al.: Contributions to the physiology of heavy muscular work. *Skand. Arch. Physiol. Suppl.*, 10, 1936.

Consolazio, C.F.: *Physiological Measurements of Metabolic Functions in Man.* New York: McGraw-Hill Book Co., 1961.

Cureton, T.K., Jr.: *Physical Fitness of Champion Athletes.* Urbana, IL: University of Illinois Press, 1951.

Dill, D.B.: *Life, Heat, and Altitude: Physiological Effects of Hot Climates and Great Heights.* Cambridge, MA: Harvard University Press, 1938.

Dill, D.B.: The Harvard Fatigue Laboratory: Its development, contributions, and demise. *Circ. Res.,* 20(suppl I):161, 1967.

Dill, D.B.: Arlie V. Bock, pioneer in sports medicine. December 30, 1888–August 11, 1984. *Med. Sci. Sports Exerc.,* 17:401, 1985.

Gerber, E.W.: *Innovators and Institutions in Physical Education.* Philadelphia: Lea & Febiger, 1971.

Green, R.M.: *A Translation of Galen's Hygiene.* IL: Charles C. Thomas, Springfield, MA 1951.

Henry, F.M.: Aerobic oxygen consumption and alactic debt in muscular work. *J. Appl. Physiol.,* 3:427:1951.

Henry, F.M.: Lactic and alactic oxygen consumption in moderate exercise of graded intensity. *J. Appl. Physiol.,* 8:608, 1956.

Henry, F.M. Physical education: an academic discipline. *JOHPER,* 35:32, 1964.

Hermansen, L.: Anaerobic energy release. *Med. Sci. Sports,* 1:32, 1969.

Hermansen, L., Andersen, K.L.: Aerobic work capacity in young Norwegian men and women. *J. Appl. Physiol.,* 20:425, 1965.

Hoberman, J.M.: The early development of sports medicine in Germany. In: *Sport and Exercise Science.* Berryman, J.W., and Park, R.J. (eds.). Urbana, IL: University of Illinois Press, 1992.

Horvath, S.M., Horvath, E.C.: *The Harvard Fatigue Laboratory: Its History and Contributions.* Englewood Cliffs, CA: Prentice-Hall, 1973.

Johnson, R.E., et al.: *Laboratory Manual of Field Methods for the Biochemical Assessment of Metabolic and Nutrition Conditions.* Boston: Harvard Fatigue Laboratory, 1946.

Katch, V.L.: The burden of disproof. *Med. Sci. Sports Exerc.* 18:593, 1986.

Kerlinger, F.N.: *Foundations of Behavioral Research,* 2nd Ed. New York: Holt, Rinehart, and Winston, 1973.

Krogh, A.: *The Composition of the Atmosphere; An Account of Preliminary Investigations and a Programme.* Kobenhavn: A.F. Host, 1919.

Kroll, W.: *Perspectives in Physical Education.* New York: Academic Press, 1971.

Leonard, F.G.: *A Guide to the History of Physical Education.* Philadelphia: Lea & Febiger.

Lusk, G.: *The Elements of the Science of Nutrition.* 2nd Ed. Philadelphia: W.B. Saunders, 1909.

Park, R.J.: Concern for health and exercise as expressed in the writings of 18th century physicians and informed laymen (England, France, Switzerland). *Res. Q.,* 47:756, 1976.

Park, R.J.: The attitudes of leading New England transcendentalists toward healthful exercise, active recreation and proper care of the body: 1830–1860. *J. Sport Hist.,* 4:34, 1977.

Park, R.J.: The research quarterly and its antecedents. *Res. Q. Exerc. Sport.,* 51:1, 1980.

Park, R.J.: The emergence of the academic discipline of physical education in the United States. In: *Perspectives on the Academic Discipline of Physical Education.* Brooks, G.A. (ed.). Champaign, IL: Human Kinetics, 1981.

Park, R.J.: Edward M. Hartwell and physical training at the Johns Hopkins University, 1879–1890. *J. Sport Hist.,* 14:108, 1987.

Park, R.J.: Physiologists, physicians, and physical educators: Nineteenth century biology and exercise, hygienic and educative. *J. Sport Hist.,* 14:28, 1987.

Park, R.J.: The rise and demise of Harvard's B.S. program in Anatomy, Physiology, and Physical Training. *Res. Q. Exerc. Sport,* 63:246, 1992.

Park, R.J.: Human energy expenditure from *Australopithecus afarensis* to the 4-minute mile: Exemplars and case studies. *Exerc. Sport Sci. Rev.,* 20:185, 1992.

Park, R.J.: A long and productive career: Franklin M. Henry—Scientist, mentor, pioneer. *Res. Q. Exerc. Sports,* 65:295, 1994.

Park, R.J.: High-protein diets, "damaged hearts," and rowing men: antecedents of modern sports medicine and exercise science, 1867–1928. *Exerc. Sport. Sci. Rev.,* 25:137, 1997.

Payne, J.F.: *Harvey and Galen. The Harveyan Oration, Oct. 19, 1896.* London: Frowde, 1897.

Schmidt-Nielsen, B.: August and Marie Krogh and respiratory physiology. *J. Appl. Physiol.,* 57:293, 1984.

Scholander, P.F.: Analyzer for accurate estimation of respiratory gases in one-half cubic centimeter samples. *J. Biol. Chem.,* 167:235, 1947.

Shaffel, N.: The evaluation of American medical literature. In: *History of American Medicine.* Martilbanez, F. (ed.). New York: MD Publications, 1958.

Tipton, C.M.: Exercise physiology, part II: A contemporary historical perspective. In: *The History of Exercise and Sports Science.* Messengale, J.D., and Swanson, R.A. (eds.). Champaign, IL: Human Kinetics, 1997.

Tipton, C.M.: Contemporary exercise physiology: Fifty years after the closure of the Harvard Fatigue Laboratory. *Exerc. Sport Sci. Rev.,* 26:315, 1998.

Tipton, C.M.: Historical perspective: The antiquity of exercise, exercise physiology and the exercise prescription for health. *World Rev. Nutr. Diet.,* 98:198, 2008.

Tipton, C.M.: Susruta of India, an unrecognized contributor to the history of exercise physiology. *J. Appl. Physiol.,* 104:1553, 2008.

Nutrition and Energy

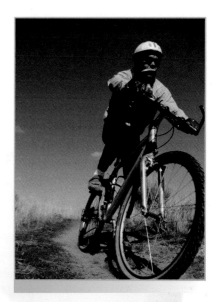

Proper nutrition forms the foundation for physical performance. The foods we consume provide fuel for biologic work and chemicals for extracting and using potential energy within this fuel. Food also provides essential elements to synthesize new tissue and repair existing cells. Individuals often train for optimum exercise performance, only to fall short from inadequate, counterproductive, and sometimes harmful nutritional practices based on "junk" science vigorously promoted on the Internet and in popular fitness magazines.

Chapter 2 reviews the six broad categories of nutrients: carbohydrates, lipids, proteins, vitamins, minerals, and water. Understanding each nutrient's role in energy metabolism and tissue synthesis clarifies one's knowledge of the interaction between food intake and storage and exercise performance. No nutritional "magic bullets" exist per se, yet the quantity and blend of nutrients in the daily diet profoundly affect exercise capacity, training responsiveness, and the potential to achieve positive health outcomes. **Chapter 3** presents key information about food as an energy source and what constitutes an optimum diet for exercise and good health. **Chapter 4** concludes with a discussion of nutritional and pharmacologic supplements and their possible role as ergogenic aids to physical performance.

What is a scientist after all? It is a curious man looking through a keyhole, the keyhole of nature, trying to know what's going on.

— Jacques Yves Cousteau

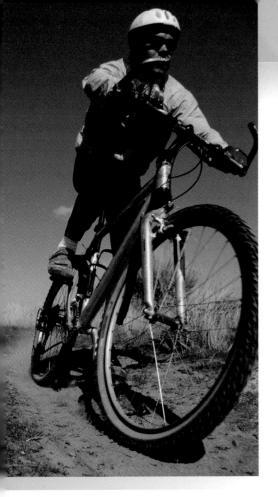

Chapter

2

Macronutrients and Micronutrients

CHAPTER OBJECTIVES

- Distinguish differences among monosaccharides, disaccharides, and polysaccharides.

- Discuss carbohydrates' role as an energy source, protein sparer, metabolic primer, and central nervous system fuel.

- Define and give an example of a triacylglycerol, saturated fatty acid, polyunsaturated fatty acid, monounsaturated fatty acid, and trans-fatty acid.

- List major characteristics of high- and low-density lipoprotein cholesterol and discuss the role of each in coronary heart disease.

- List four important functions of fat in the body.

- Define essential and non-essential amino acids and give food sources for each.

- List one function for each fat- and water-soluble vitamin and explain the potential risks of consuming these micronutrients in excess.

- Outline three broad roles of minerals in the body.

- Define *osteoporosis*, *exercise-induced anemia*, and *sodium-induced hypertension*.

- Describe how regular physical activity affects bone mass and the body's iron stores.

- Outline factors related to the female athlete triad.

- List the functions of water in the body.

- Define *heat cramps*, *heat exhaustion*, and *heat stroke*.

- Explain factors that affect gastric emptying and fluid replacement.

- List five predisposing factors to hyponatremia with prolonged exercise.

The carbohydrate, lipid, and protein **macronutrients** consumed daily supply the energy to maintain bodily functions during rest and diverse physical activities. The macronutrients help to maintain and enhance the organism's structural and functional integrity with exercise training. **Part 1** discusses each macronutrient's general structure, function, and source in the diet and emphasizes their importance in sustaining physiologic function during physical activity.

CARBOHYDRATES

All living cells contain **carbohydrates**. With the exception of lactose and a small amount of glycogen obtained in animal tissues, plant sources provide all of the dietary carbohydrate. Atoms of carbon, hydrogen, and oxygen combine to form a carbohydrate or sugar molecule, always in a ratio of 1 atom of carbon and 2 atoms of hydrogen for each oxygen atom. The general formula $(CH_2O)n$ represents a simple carbohydrate, where *n* equals from 3 to 7 carbon atoms.

Monosaccharides

*The **monosaccharide** molecule forms the basic unit of carbohydrates.* The molecule's number of carbon atoms determines its category. The Greek name for this number, ending with "ose," indicates sugars. For example, 3-carbon monosaccharides are **trioses**, 4-carbon sugars are **tetroses**, 5-carbon sugars are **pentoses**, 6-carbon sugars are **hexoses**, and 7-carbon sugars are **heptoses**. The hexose sugars,

glucose, fructose, and galactose, represent the nutritionally important monosaccharides.

Glucose, also called *dextrose* or *blood sugar*, consists of 6 carbon, 12 hydrogen, and 6 oxygen atoms ($C_6H_{12}O_6$; **Fig. 2.1**). This sugar forms when energy from sunlight interacts with water, carbon dioxide, and the green pigment cholorophyl. It occurs naturally in food or is produced through the digestion (**hydrolysis**) of more complex carbohydrates. After absorption by the small intestine, glucose can function in one of these four ways:

1. Used directly by the cell for energy
2. Stored as glycogen in the muscles and liver
3. Converted to fats for energy storage
4. Provide carbon skeletons to synthesize non-essential amino acids

Fruits and honey provide the main source of **fructose** (also called *levulose* or *fruit sugar*), the sweetest of the monosaccharides. The small intestine absorbs some fructose directly into the blood, and the liver converts it to glucose. **Galactose** does not exist freely in nature; rather, it forms milk sugar (**lactose**) in the mammary glands of lactating animals. In the body, galactose freely converts to glucose for energy metabolism.

Disaccharides

Combining two monosaccharide molecules forms a **disaccharide** or double sugar. The monosaccharides and disaccharides collectively make up the **simple sugars**.

Each of the disaccharides contains glucose as a principal component. The three disaccharides of nutritional importance include:

1. **Sucrose:** Glucose + fructose; the most common dietary disaccharide; composed of 12 atoms of carbon, 22 atoms of hydrogen, and 11 atoms of oxygen ($C_{12}H_{22}O_{11}$). It occurs naturally in most foods that

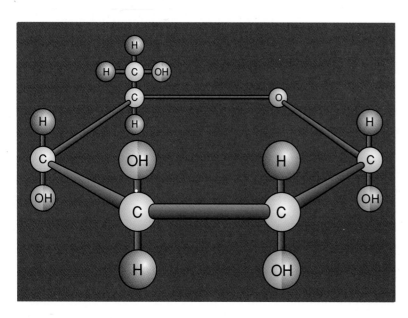

Figure 2.1 The three-dimensional ring structure of the simple glucose molecule resembles a hexagonal plate to which H and O atoms form during photosynthesis. The sugar forms when energy from sunlight interacts with water, carbon dioxide, and the green pigment cholorophyl.

contain carbohydrate, particularly beet sugar, cane sugar, brown sugar, maple syrup, and honey

2. **Lactose:** Glucose + galactose; found in natural form only in milk and often called *milk sugar*
3. **Maltose:** Glucose + glucose; occurs in beer, cereals, and germinating seeds

Polysaccharides

Polysaccharides include plant and animal categories.

Plant Polysaccharides
Starch and fiber represent the two most common forms of plant polysaccharides.

Starch   **Starch,** the storage form of plant polysaccharide, forms from hundreds of individual sugar molecules joined together. It appears as large granules in seed and corn cells and in grains that make bread, cereal, spaghetti, and pastries. Large amounts also exist in peas, beans, potatoes, and roots, in which starch stores energy for the plant's future needs. The term **complex carbohydrates** refers to dietary starch.

Fiber   **Fiber,** classified as a non-starch, structural polysaccharide, includes cellulose, the most abundant organic molecule on earth. Fibrous materials resist hydrolysis by human digestive enzymes. Plants exclusively contain fiber, which constitutes the structure of leaves, stems, roots, seeds, and fruit coverings. Fibers differ in physical and chemical characteristics and physiologic action; they occur primarily within the cell wall as cellulose, gums, hemicellulose, pectin, and noncarbohydrate lignins. Other fibers—mucilage and the gums—serve as integral components of the plant cell itself.

Animal Polysaccharides
During the process of **glucogenesis,** a few hundred to thousands of glucose molecules combine to form **glycogen,** the large storage polysaccharide in mammalian muscle and liver. **Figure 2.2** illustrates that a well-nourished 80-kg person stores approximately 500 g of

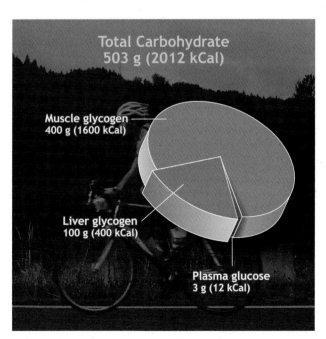

Figure 2.2   Distribution of carbohydrate energy in a typical 80-kg person.

*Q*uestions *& Notes*

List the 3 types of carbohydrates.

1.

2.

3.

List the 2 types of polysaccharides.

1.

2.

Give the recommended fiber intake for men and women up to age 50 years.

Men:

Women:

Write the chemical formula for glucose.

Give 2 examples of a simple sugar.

1.

2.

List the 2 most common plant polysaccharides.

1.

2.

Give an example of a food with a high fiber content.

BOX 2.1 CLOSE UP

Health Implications of Dietary Fiber

Americans typically consume about 12 to 15 g of fiber daily, far short of the recommendations of the Food and Nutrition Board of the National Academy of Sciences (*www.iom.edu/About-IOM/Leadership-Staff/Boards/Food-and-Nutrition-Board.aspx*) of 38 g for men and 25 g for women up to age 50 years and 30 g for men and 21 g for women older than age 50 years.

Fibers hold considerable water and give "bulk" to the food residues in the intestines, often increasing stool weight and volume by 40% to 100%. This bulking-up action may aid gastrointestinal functioning and reduce the chances of contracting colon cancer and other gastrointestinal diseases later in life. Increased fiber intake, partcularly **water-soluble fibers,** may modestly reduce serum cholesterol. These include pectin and guar gum present in oats (rolled oats, oat bran, oat flour), legumes, barley, brown rice, peas, carrots, and diverse fruits.

For men with elevated blood lipids, adding 100 g of oat bran to their daily diets reduced serum cholesterol levels by 13% and lowered the low-density lipoprotein (LDL) component of the cholesterol profile. In contrast, the **water-insoluble fibers**—cellulose; hemicellulose; lignin; and cellulose-rich products, such as wheat bran—did not reduce cholesterol levels.

Current nutritional wisdom maintains that a dietary fiber intake of between about 20 to 40 g per day depending on age and gender (ratio of 3:1 for water-insoluble to soluble fiber) plays an important part of a well-structured diet. Persons with marginal levels of nutrition should not consume excessive fiber because increased fiber intake decreases the absorption of calcium, iron, magnesium, phosphorus, and trace minerals. The figure below highlights the fiber content of common foods listed by overall fiber content. Note that 1 cup of Fiber One Bran Cereal (General Mills) provides 100% of the recommended daily value for dietary fiber for women up to age 50 years.

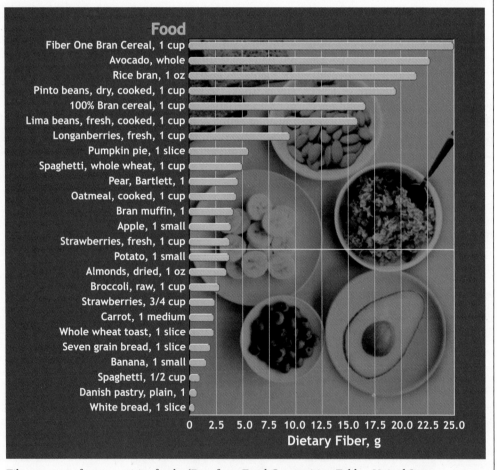

Fiber content of representative foods. (Data from Food Composition Tables, United States Department of Agriculture.) *www.nal.usda.gov/fnic/foodcomp/search*

carbohydrate. Of this, approximately 400 g exists as muscle glycogen (largest reserve) and 90 to 110 g exists as liver glycogen (highest concentration representing between 3% to 7% of the liver's weight), but only about 2 to 3 g exists as blood glucose. Each gram of carbohydrate (glycogen or glucose) contains about 4 kCal of energy (see Chapter 3), with the average-size individual storing between 1500 and 2000 kCal as carbohydrate, enough total energy to power a 20-mile run.

Muscle glycogen serves as the major source of carbohydrate energy for active muscles during exercise. In contrast to muscle glycogen, liver glycogen reconverts to glucose for transport in the blood to the working muscles. **Glycogenolysis** describes this reconversion process (glycogen → glucose); it provides a rapid extramuscular glucose supply. Unlike liver, muscle cells do not contain the enzyme to remake glucose from stored glycogen. Thus, glucose (or glycogen) within a muscle cell cannot supply the carbohydrate needs of surrounding cells. Depleting liver and muscle glycogen through dietary restriction or intense exercise stimulates glucose synthesis from structural components of the other macronutrients (principally protein's amino acids) through the process of **gluconeogenesis** (glucose formation from non-glucose sources).

Hormones regulate liver and muscle glycogen stores by controlling the level of circulating blood sugar. Elevated blood sugar cause the pancreas' beta (β) cells to secrete additional **insulin** that facilitates the muscles' uptake of the glucose excess, inhibiting further insulin secretion. This *feedback regulation* maintains blood glucose at an appropriate physiologic concentration. In contrast, if blood sugar decreases below normal (**hypoglycemia**), the pancreas' alpha (α) cells immediately secrete **glucagon** to increase glucose availability and normalize the blood sugar level. Known as the **insulin antagonist** hormone, blood glucose increases when glucagon stimulates liver glycogenolysis and gluconeogenesis.

Diet Affects Glycogen Stores

The body stores comparatively little glycogen so dietary intake can considerably affect its quantity. For example, a 24-hour fast or a low-carbohydrate, normal-calorie (isocaloric) diet dramatically reduces glycogen reserves. In contrast, maintaining a carbohydrate-rich isocaloric diet for several days doubles the body's carbohydrate stores compared with a normal, well-balanced diet. The body's upper limit for glycogen storage equals about 15 g per kilogram (kg) of body mass, which is equivalent to 1050 g for the average 70-kg man or 840 g for a typical 56-kg woman. To estimate your body's maximum glycogen storage capacity (in grams), multiply your body weight in kilograms (lb ÷ 2.205 = kg) by 15.

Carbohydrates' Role in the Body

Carbohydrates serve three primary functions related to energy metabolism and exercise performance:

1. **Energy source.** Energy from bloodborne glucose and muscle glycogen breakdown ultimately powers muscle action (particularly high-intensity exercise) and other more "silent" forms of biologic work. For physically active people, adequate daily carbohydrate intake maintains the body's limited glycogen stores. However, more is not necessarily better; if dietary carbohydrate intake exceeds the cells' capacity to store glycogen, the carbohydrate excess readily converts to fat, thus triggering an increase in the body's total fat content.
2. **Protein sparer.** Adequate carbohydrate intake preserves tissue proteins. Normally, protein contributes to tissue maintenance, repair, and growth and as a minor nutrient energy source. With reduced glycogen reserves, gluconeogenesis synthesizes glucose from protein (amino acids) and the glycerol portion of the fat molecule (triacylglycerol). This metabolic process increases carbohydrate availability and maintains plasma glucose levels under three conditions:
   a. Dietary restriction
   b. Prolonged exercise
   c. Repeated bouts of intense training
3. **Metabolic primer.** Byproducts of carbohydrate breakdown serve as a "primer" to facilitate the body's use of fat for energy, particularly in the liver. Insufficient carbohydrate metabolism (either through limitations in glucose transport into the cell, as occurs in diabetes, or glycogen

*Q*uestions *&* Notes

Define hypoglycemia.

List 3 important functions of carbohydrates in the body.

1.

2.

3.

Describe the role of insulin in the body.

🛈 For Your Information

IMPORTANT CARBOHYDRATE CONVERSIONS

Glucogenesis—Glycogen synthesis from glucose (glucose → glycogen)

Gluconeogenesis—Glucose synthesis largely from structural components of noncarbohydrate nutrients (protein → glucose)

Glycogenolysis—Glucose formation from glycogen (glycogen → glucose)

depletion through inadequate diet or prolonged exercise) increases dependence on fat utilization for energy. When this happens, the body cannot generate a sustained high level of aerobic energy transfer from fat-only metabolism. This consequence reduces an individual's maximum exercise intensity.

Fuel for the Central Nervous System   The central nervous system requires carbohydrate for proper functioning. Under normal conditions, the brain uses blood glucose almost exclusively for fuel without maintaining a backup supply of this nutrient. In poorly regulated diabetes, during starvation, or with a low carbohydrate intake, the brain adapts metabolically after about 8 days to use relatively large amounts of fat (in the form of ketones) as an alternative to glucose as the primary fuel source.

At rest and during exercise, the liver serves as the main source to maintain normal blood glucose levels. In prolonged intense exercise, blood glucose eventually decreases below normal levels because of liver glycogen depletion and active muscles' continual use of available blood glucose. Symptoms of a modest hypoglycemia include feelings of weakness, hunger, and dizziness. This ultimately impacts exercise performance and may partially explain "central" or neurologic fatigue associated with prolonged exercise or starvation.

Recommended Carbohydrate Intake

Figure 2.3 illustrates the carbohydrate content of selected foods. Rich carbohydrate sources include cereals, cookies, candies, breads, and cakes. Fruits and vegetables appear as

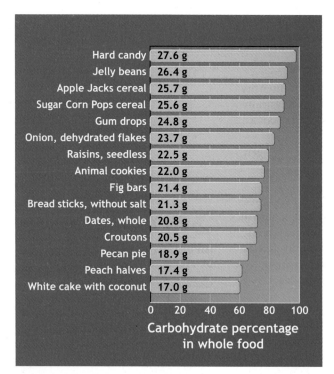

	Carbohydrate percentage in whole food
Hard candy	27.6 g
Jelly beans	26.4 g
Apple Jacks cereal	25.7 g
Sugar Corn Pops cereal	25.6 g
Gum drops	24.8 g
Onion, dehydrated flakes	23.7 g
Raisins, seedless	22.5 g
Animal cookies	22.0 g
Fig bars	21.4 g
Bread sticks, without salt	21.3 g
Dates, whole	20.8 g
Croutons	20.5 g
Pecan pie	18.9 g
Peach halves	17.4 g
White cake with coconut	17.0 g

Figure 2.3   Percentage of carbohydrates in commonly served foods. The insert in each bar displays the number of grams of carbohydrate per ounce (28.4 g) of food.

less valuable sources of carbohydrates because the food's total weight (including water content) determines a food's carbohydrate percentage. The dried portions of fruits and vegetables exist as almost pure carbohydrate. For this reason, hikers and ultraendurance athletes rely on dried apricots, pears, apples, bananas, and tomatoes to provide ready but relatively lightweight carbohydrate sources.

Carbohydrates account for between 40% and 55% of the total calories in the typical American diet. For a sedentary 70-kg person, this translates to a daily carbohydrate intake of about 300 g. Average Americans consume about half of their carbohydrate as simple sugars, predominantly as sucrose and high-fructose corn syrup. This amount of simple sugar intake represents the yearly intake equivalent to 60 pounds of table sugar (16 teaspoons of sucrose a day) and 46 pounds of corn syrup!

For more physically active people and those involved in exercise training, carbohydrates should equal about 60% of daily calories or 400 to 600 g, predominantly as unrefined, fiber-rich fruits, grains, and vegetables. During periods of intense exercise training, we recommend that carbohydrate intake increase to 70% of total calories consumed (8 to 10 g per kg of body mass).

Carbohydrate Confusion

Frequent and excessive consumption of more rapidly absorbed forms of carbohydrate (i.e., those with a high glycemic index; see page 39) may alter the metabolic profile and possibly increase disease risk for obesity, type 2 diabetes, abnormal blood lipids, and coronary heart disease, particularly for individuals with excess body fat. For example, eating a high-carbohydrate, low-fat meal reduces fat breakdown and increases fat synthesis more in overweight men than lean men. Dietary patterns of women over a 6-year period showed that those who ate a starchy diet of potatoes and low-fiber, higher glycemic processed white rice, pasta, and white bread along with non-diet soft drinks experienced 2.5 times the rate of type 2 diabetes than women who ate less of those foods and more fiber-containing unrefined whole-grain cereals, fruits, and vegetables.

All Carbohydrates are Not Physiologically Equal   Digestion and absorption rates of different carbohydrate-containing foods might explain the carbohydrate intake–diabetes link. Whereas low-fiber processed starches and simple sugars in soft drinks digest quickly and enter the blood at a relatively rapid rate (i.e., have a high glycemic index), slow-release forms of high-fiber, unrefined complex carbohydrates and carbohydrate foods rich in lipids slow digestion to minimize surges in blood glucose. The rapid increase in blood glucose that accompanies refined processed starch and simple sugar intake increases insulin demand, stimulates the pancrease to overproduce insulin which accentuates hyperinsulinemia, increases plasma triacylglycerol concentrations, and augments fat synthesis. Consistently eating such foods can reduce the body's sensitivity to insulin (i.e., the body resists insulin's effects), thus requiring progressively greater insulin output to control blood sugar levels. *Type 2 diabetes results when the pancreas cannot produce sufficient insulin to regulate blood glucose or becomes insensitive to the effects of insulin, causing it to rise.* In contrast, diets with fiber-rich, low-glycemic carbohydrates tend to lower blood glucose and the insulin response after eating, improve blood lipid profiles, and increase insulin sensitivity.

A Role in Obesity?   About 25% of the adult population produces excessive insulin in response to a "challenge" of rapidly absorbed carbohydrates (adminstering a set quantity of glucose to track the insulin outcome). These insulin-resistant individuals (i.e., require more insulin to regulate blood glucose) increase their risk for obesity by consistently consuming such a diet. Weight gain occurs because excessive insulin facilitates glucose oxidation at the expense of fatty acid oxidation; it also stimulates fat storage in adipose tissue.

The insulin surge in response to high-glycemic carbohydrate intake often abnormally decreases blood glucose. This "rebound hypoglycemia" sets off hunger signals that may trigger overeating. A repetitive scenario of high blood sugar followed by low blood sugar exerts the most profound effect on sedentary obese individuals who show the greatest insulin resistance and an exaggerated insulin response to a blood glucose challenge. Regularly engaging in low to moderate physical activity produces the following three beneficial effects:

1. Improves insulin sensitivity to reduce the insulin requirement for a given glucose uptake.
2. Stimulates plasma-derived fatty acid oxidation to decrease fatty acid availability to the liver, thereby depressing any increase in plasma very low-density lipoprotein (VLDL) cholesterol and triacylglycerol concentration.
3. Exerts a potent positive influence for weight control.

Glycemic Index

The glycemic index serves as a relative (qualitative) indicator of carbohydrates' ability to increase blood glucose levels. Blood sugar increase, termed the *glycemic response*, is quantified after ingesting a food containing 50 g of a carbohydrate or carbohydrate-containing food and comparing it over a 2-hour period with a "standard" for carbohydrate, usually white bread or glucose, with an assigned value of 100. The glycemic index expresses the percentage of total area under the blood glucose response curve for a "specific food" compared with only glucose. Thus, a food with a glycemic index of 45 indicates that ingesting 50 g of the food increases blood glucose concentrations to levels that reach 45% compared with 50 g of glucose. The glycemic index provides a more useful physiologic concept than simply classifying a carbohydrate based on its chemical configuration as simple or complex, as sugars or starches, or as available or unavailable. A high glycemic index rating does not necessarily indicate poor nutritional quality because carrots, brown rice, and corn, with their rich quantities of health-protective micronutrients, phytochemicals, and dietary fiber, have relatively high indices.

The revised glycemic index listing also includes the **glycemic load** associated with consuming specified serving sizes of different foods. Whereas the glycemic index compares equal quantities of a carbohydrate-containing food, the glycemic load quantifies the overall glycemic effect of a typical portion of food. This represents the amount of available carbohydrate in that serving and the glycemic index of the food. A high glycemic load reflects a greater expected elevation in blood glucose and a greater insulin response (release) to that food. Consuming a diet with a high glycemic load on a regular basis is associated with an increased risk for type 2 diabetes and coronary heart disease.

Figure 2.4 lists the glycemic index for common items in various food groupings. For easy identification, foods are placed into high, medium, and low categories. Interestingly, a food's index rating does not depend simply on its

Questions & Notes

Name the carbohydrate type that when consumed in excess contributes to type 2 diabetes.

Explain the difference between the glycemic index and glycemic load.

Give 3 beneficial effects of regular exercise for obese individuals.

1.

2.

3.

Give the typical carbohydrate intake for a sedentary 70-kg person.

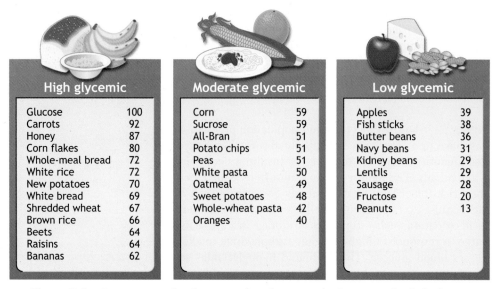

Figure 2.4 Categorization for glycemic index of common food sources of carbohydrates.

classification as a "simple" (mono- and disaccharides) or "complex" (starch and fiber) carbohydrate. This is because the plant starch in white rice and potatoes has a higher glycemic index than the simple sugar fructose in apples and peaches. A food's fiber content slows digestion rate, so many fiber-containing vegetables such as peas, beans, and other legumes have low glycemic indexes. Ingesting lipids and proteins also tends to slow the passage of food into the small intestine, reducing the glycemic load of the meal's carbohydrate content.

Carbohydrate Use During Exercise

The fuel mixture used during exercise depends on the intensity and duration of effort, including the exerciser's fitness and nutritional status.

Intense Exercise Stored muscle glycogen and bloodborne glucose primarily contribute to the total energy required during intense exercise and in the early minutes of exercise when oxygen supply fails to meet aerobic metabolism demands.

Figure 2.5 shows that early during intense exercise, the muscles' uptake of circulating blood glucose increases sharply and continues to increase as exercise progresses. After 40 minutes, glucose uptake increases 7 to 20 times the uptake at rest, with the highest use occurring in the most intense exercise. Carbohydrates' large energy contribution occurs because they are the only macronutrient that provides energy without oxygen (i.e., anaerobically). During intense aerobic exercise, intramuscular glycogen becomes the preferential energy fuel. This provides an advantage because glycogen supplies energy for exercise twice as rapidly than fat and protein (see Chapter 8).

Moderate and Prolonged Exercise During the transition from rest to submaximal exercise, almost all

energy comes from glycogen stored in active muscles. Over the next 20 minutes, liver and muscle glycogen provide about 40% to 50% of the energy requirement, with the remainder from fat breakdown with minimal amounts from blood glucose. As exercise continues and glycogen stores deplete, fat catabolism increases its percentage contribution to the total energy for muscular activity. Additionally, bloodborne glucose becomes the major source of the limited carbohydrate energy. Eventually, liver glucose output does not keep pace with its use, and blood glucose concentration declines toward hypoglycemic levels.

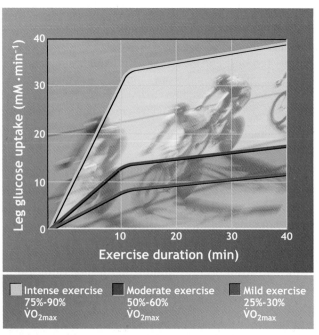

Figure 2.5 Generalized response for blood glucose uptake of the leg muscles during cycling in relation to exercise duration and intensity. Exercise intensity is expressed as a percentage of $\dot{V}O_2$max (maximal oxygen consumption).

An inability to maintain a desired level of performance (often referred to as **fatigue**) can occur if exercise progresses to the point where liver and muscle glycogen decrease severely, even with sufficient oxygen available to the muscles and almost unlimited potential energy from stored fat. Endurance athletes commonly refer to fatigue under these conditions as **bonking** or **hitting the wall**. Research does not fully explain why carbohydrate depletion coincides with the onset of fatigue in prolonged submaximal exercise. The answer may relate to one or more of the following three reasons:

1. Key role of blood glucose in central nervous system function.
2. Muscle glycogen's role as a "primer" in fat breakdown.
3. Relatively slow rate of energy release from fat compared with carbohydrate breakdown.

LIPIDS (OILS, FATS, AND WAXES)

A lipid (from the Greek *lipos*, meaning fat) molecule has the same structural elements as carbohydrate except that it differs in its atomic linkages. Specifically, the lipid's ratio of hydrogen-to-oxygen considerably exceeds that of carbohydrate. For example, the formula $C_{57}H_{110}O_6$ describes the common lipid stearin with an H-to-O ratio of 18.3:1; for carbohydrate the ratio equals 2:1. Lipid, a general term, refers to a heterogeneous group of compounds that includes oils, fats, and waxes and related compounds. Oils remain liquid at room temperature, whereas fats remain solid. Approximately 98% of dietary lipid exists as triacylglycerols (see next section). Lipids can be placed into one of three main groups: **simple lipids**, **compound lipids**, and **derived lipids**.

Simple Lipids

The simple lipids or "neutral fats" consist primarily of **triacylglycerols**. They constitute the major storage form of fat; more than 90% of body fat exists as triacylglycerol, predominantly in adipose cells. This molecule consists of two different atom clusters. A glycerol component has a 3-carbon molecule that itself does not qualify as a lipid because of its high water solubility. The other component consists of three clusters of carbon-chained atoms termed fatty acids that attach to the glycerol molecule. Fatty acids contain straight hydrocarbon chains with as few as 4 carbon atoms or more than 20, although chain lengths of 16 and 18 carbons are most prevalent.

Figure 2.6 illustrates the basic structure of saturated and unsaturated fatty acid molecules. All lipid-containing foods contain mixtures of different proportions of saturated and unsaturated fatty acids.

Saturated Fatty Acids
Saturated fatty acids contain only single bonds between carbon atoms, with the remaining bonds attaching to hydrogen. A saturated the fatty acid holds as many hydrogen atoms as chemically possible (i.e., saturated relative to hydrogen).

Saturated fatty acids occur plentifully in beef, lamb, pork, chicken, and egg yolk and in dairy fats of cream, milk, butter, and cheese. Saturated fatty acids from plants include coconut and palm oil, vegetable shortening, and hydrogenated margarine; commercially prepared cakes, pies, and cookies rely heavily on saturated fatty acids.

Unsaturated Fatty Acids
Unsaturated fatty acids contain one or more double bonds along the main carbon chain. Each double bond in the carbon chain reduces the number of potential hydrogen-binding sites; therefore, the molecule remains unsaturated relative to hydrogen. Monounsaturated fatty acids contain one double bond along the main carbon chain; examples include

Questions & Notes

List 2 factors that determine the fuel mixture used during exercise.

1.

2.

Name 2 low glycemic foods.

1.

2.

Give one possible exercise-related outcome of low muscle glycogen levels.

Give the major differences between a saturated and an unsaturated fatty acid.

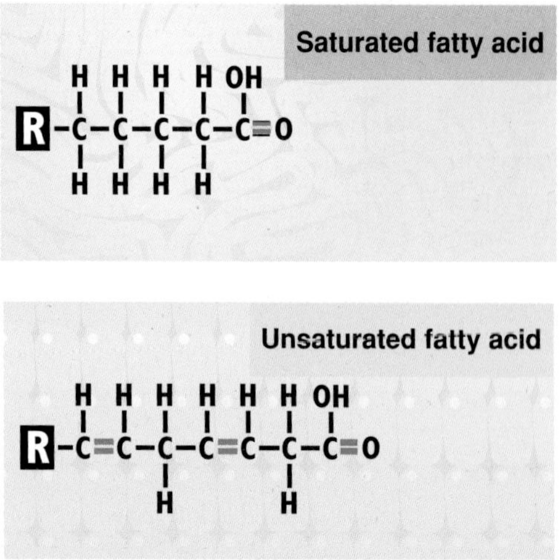

Figure 2.6 The presence or absence of double bonds between the carbon atoms constitutes the major structural difference between saturated and unsaturated fatty acids. *R* represents the glycerol portion of the triacylglycerol molecule.

canola oil; olive oil; peanut oil; and oil in almonds, pecans, and avocados. Polyunsaturated fatty acids contain two or more double bonds along the main carbon chain; examples include safflower, sunflower, soybean, and corn oils.

Fatty acids from plant sources are typically unsaturated and liquefy at room temperature. Lipids with more carbons in the fatty acid chain and containing more saturated fatty acids remain firmer at room temperature.

Fatty Acids in the Diet

The average person in the United States consumes about 15% of their total calories as saturated fats (equivalent to more than 50 pounds per year). This contrasts with the Tarahumara Indians of Mexico, whose diet typically contains only 2% of total calories as saturated fat (high in complex, unrefined carbohydrate). The strong relationship between saturated fatty acid intake and coronary heart disease risk has prompted health professionals to recommend replacing at least a portion of dietary saturated fatty acids with unsaturated fatty acids. Monounsaturated fatty acids lower coronary risk even below average levels. Recommendations include no more than 10% of total energy intake as saturated fatty acids, with the remainder distributed in equal amounts among saturated, polyunsaturated, and monounsaturated fatty acids.

Compound Lipids

Compound lipids consist of neutral fat combined with phosphorus (**phospholipids**) and glucose (**glucolipids**). Another group of compound fats contains the **lipoproteins**, which are formed primarily in the liver from the union of triacylglycerols, phospholipids, or cholesterol with protein. *Lipoproteins serve important functions because they constitute the main form for lipid transport in the blood.* If blood lipids did not bind to protein, they literally would float to the top like cream in non-homogenized milk.

High- and Low-Density Lipoprotein Cholesterol

Four types of lipoproteins exist according to their gravitational densities: chylomicrons, high density, low density, and very low density. Chylomicrons form after emulsified lipid droplets leave the small intestine and enter the lymphatic vasculature. Normally, the liver takes up chylomicrons, metabolizes them, and delivers them to adipose tissue for storage.

The liver and small intestine produce **high-density lipoprotein (HDL)**. Of the lipoproteins, HDLs contain the greatest percentage of protein and the least total lipid and cholesterol. Degradation of a **very-low density lipoprotein (VLDL)** produces a **low-density lipoprotein (LDL)**. The VLDL contains the greatest percentage of lipid. VLDLs transport triacylglycerols (formed in the liver from fats, carbohydrates, alcohol, and cholesterol) to muscle and adipose tissue. The enzyme **lipoprotein lipase** acts on VLDL to transform it to a denser LDL molecule with less lipid. LDL and VLDL contain the greatest lipid and least protein content.

"Bad" Cholesterol (Low-Density Lipoprotein) Among the lipoproteins, LDLs, which normally carry between 60% and 80% of the total serum cholesterol, have the greatest affinity for cells located in the arterial wall. LDL delivers cholesterol to arterial tissue where the LDL oxidizes to ultimately participate in the proliferation of smooth muscle cells and other unfavorable changes that damage and narrow arteries. These three factors influence serum LDL concentration:

1. Regular exercise
2. Visceral fat accumulation
3. Diet composition

"Good" Cholesterol (High-Density Lipoprotein) Unlike LDL, HDL operates as so-called "good" cholesterol to protect against heart disease. HDL acts as a scavenger in the **reverse transport of cholesterol** by removing it from the arterial wall and transporting it to the liver, where it joins in bile formation for excretion from the intestinal tract.

The amounts of LDL and HDL cholesterol and their specific ratios (e.g., HDL/total cholesterol) and subfractions provide more meaningful indicators of coronary artery disease risk than just total cholesterol in blood. Regular aerobic exercise and abstinence from cigarette smoking increase HDLs and favorably affect the LDL/HDL ratio. The role of exercise on the blood lipid profile is discussed more fully in Chapter 17.

Derived Lipids

Derived lipids include substances formed from simple and compound lipids. **Cholesterol**, the most widely known derived lipid, exists only in animal tissue. Cholesterol does not contain fatty acids but shares some of the physical and chemical characteristics of lipids. From a dietary viewpoint, cholesterol is considered a lipid. Cholesterol is widespread in the plasma membrane of all animal cells and is obtained either through food intake (**exogenous cholesterol**) or synthesis within the body (**endogenous cholesterol**). Even if an individual maintains a "cholesterol-free" diet (which is difficult to achieve), endogenous cholesterol synthesis usually varies between 0.5 to 2.0 g (500–2000 mg·d^{-1}) daily. *The body forms more cholesterol with a diet high in saturated fatty acids because saturated fat facilitates the liver's cholesterol synthesis.* The rate of endogenous synthesis usually meets the body's needs; hence, severely reducing cholesterol intake, except in pregnant women and in infants (who require exogeneous cholesterol), causes little harm.

Cholesterol participates in many complex bodily processes, including the following five functions:

1. Builds plasma membranes
2. Precursor in synthesizing vitamin D
3. Synthesizes adrenal gland hormones, including estrogen, androgen, and progesterone
4. Serves as a component for bile (emulsifies lipids during digestion)
5. Helps tissues, organs, and body structures form during fetal development

Five rich sources of cholesterol include:

1. Egg yolk
2. Red meats
3. Organ meats (liver, kidney, and brains)
4. Shellfish (shrimp, lobster, crab, scallops, clams, oysters, mussels)
5. Dairy products (ice cream, cream cheese, butter, and whole milk)

Foods of plant origin contain no cholesterol.

Trans-Fatty Acids: The Unwanted Fat

Trans-fatty acids derive from the hydrogenation of unsaturated corn, soybean, or sunflower oil. This fatty acid forms when one of the hydrogen atoms along the restructured carbon chain moves from its naturally occurring position (*cis* position) to the opposite side of the double bond that separates two carbon atoms (*trans* position). The richest trans-fat sources include vegetable shortenings, some margarines, crackers, candies, cookies, snack foods, fried foods, baked goods, salad dressings, and other processed foods made with partially hydrogenated vegetable oils.

Health concern about trans-fatty acids center on their possible detrimental effects on serum lipoproteins. A diet high in margarine and commercial baked goods like cookies, cakes, doughnuts, pies and deep-fried foods prepared with hydrogenated vegetable oils increases LDL cholesterol concentration by a similar amount as a diet high in saturated fatty acids. Unlike saturated fats, hydrogenated oils also decrease the concentration of beneficial HDL cholesterol. In light of the strong evidence that trans-fatty acids place individuals at increased risk for heart disease, the Food and Drug Administration (FDA) has mandated that food processors include the amount of trans-fatty acids on nutrition labels. The FDA estimates the average American consumes approximately 2.2 kg of trans-fats yearly. In Dec, 2006, New York City became the nation's first city to enforce a ban on essentially all trans-fats in foods prepared in the City's 24,000 eateries—from fast foods and delicatessens to five-star restaurants. A full statewide California ban on trans fat became law on January 1, 2010. Calgary, Canada, was the first city in Canada to ban *trans* fat.

Fish Oils (and Fish) Are Healthful

Greenland Eskimos who consume large quantities of lipids from fish, seal, and whale have a low incidence of coronary heart disease. Their health profiles indicate the potential for two long-chain polyunsaturated fatty acids, eicosapentaenoic acid (EHA) and docosahexaenoic acid (DHA), to confer health benefits.

*Q*uestions & Notes

Describe the major differences between exogenous and endogenous cholesterol.

List the 4 types of lipoproteins.

1.

2.

3.

4.

Describe the major function of lipoproteins.

List the 3 factors that influence LDL concentrations in the body.

1.

2.

3.

Do foods of plant origin contain cholesterol?

These oils belong to an omega-3 fatty acid family found primarily in the oils of shellfish and cold-water herring, salmon, sardines, bluefish, mackerel, and sea mammals. **Omega-3 fatty acids** may prove beneficial in the treatment of diverse psychological disorders in addition to decreasing overall heart disease risk and mortality rate (chance of ventricular fibrillation and sudden death), inflammatory disease risk, and for smokers the risk of contracting chronic obstructive pulmonary disease.

Several mechanisms explain how eating fish possibly protects against heart disease. Fish oil may serve as an antithrombogenic agent to prevent blood clot formation on arterial walls. It may also inhibit the growth of atherosclerotic plaques, reduce pulse pressure and total vascular resistance (increase arterial compliance), and stimulate endothelial-derived nitric oxide (see Chapter 10) to facilitate myocardial perfusion. The oil's lowering effect on triacylglycerol provides additional heart disease protection.

Lipids in Food

Figure 2.7 shows the approximate percentage contribution of common food groups to the total lipid content of the typical American diet. Plant sources contribute about 34% to the daily lipid intake, and the remaining 66% comes from lipids of animal origin.

Lipid's Role in the Body

Four important functions of lipids in the body include:

1. Energy reserve
2. Protection of vital organs and thermal insulation
3. Transport medium for fat-soluble vitamins
4. Hunger suppressor

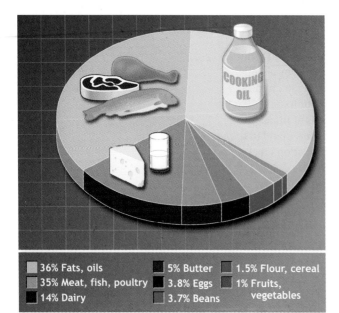

36% Fats, oils   5% Butter   1.5% Flour, cereal
35% Meat, fish, poultry   3.8% Eggs   1% Fruits, vegetables
14% Dairy   3.7% Beans

Figure 2.7 Contribution from the major food groups to the lipid content of the typical American diet.

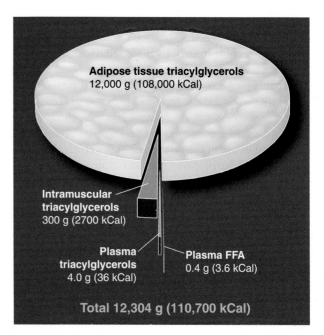

Adipose tissue triacylglycerols
12,000 g (108,000 kCal)

Intramuscular
triacylglycerols
300 g (2700 kCal)

Plasma
triacylglycerols
4.0 g (36 kCal)

Plasma FFA
0.4 g (3.6 kCal)

Total 12,304 g (110,700 kCal)

Figure 2.8 Distribution of fat energy within a typical 80-kg man.

Energy Reserve Fat constitutes the ideal cellular fuel for three reasons: Each molecule (1) carries large quantities of energy per unit weight, (2) transports and stores easily, and (3) provides a ready energy source. At rest in well-nourished individuals, fat provides as much as 80% to 90% of the body's energy requirements. One g of pure lipid contains about 9 kCal of energy, more than twice the energy available in 1 g of carbohydrate or protein from lipid's greater number of hydrogen.

Approximately 15% of the body mass for men and 25% for women consists of fat. **Figure 2.8** illustrates the total mass (and energy content) of fat from various sources in an 80-kg young adult man. The amount of fat in adipose tissue triacylglycerol translates to about 108,000 kCal. Most of this energy remains available for exercise and would supply enough energy for a person to run four round trips nonstop between Santa Barbara, California, and San Francisco, California (or Ann Arbor, Michigan, to Green Bay, Wisconsin) or three round trips between Queens, New York, and Pittsburgh, Pennsylvania. These runs assume a theoretical energy expenditure of about 100 kCal per mile. Contrast this with the limited 2000 kCal reserve of stored glycogen that would provide only enough energy for a 20-mile run. Viewed from a different perspective, the body's energy reserves from carbohydrate could power intense running for only about 1.6 hours, but the fat reserves would last 75 times longer, or about 120 hours! As was the case for carbohydrates, fat as a fuel "spares" protein to carry out two of its three main functions of tissue synthesis and repair.

Protection and Insulation Up to 4% of the body's fat protects against trauma to the vital organs, the heart, lungs, liver, kidneys, spleen, brain, and spinal cord. Fats stored just below the skin in the subcutaneous fat layer provide insulation, determining one's ability to tolerate extremes of cold exposure. This insulatory layer of fat probably affords little protection except to deep-sea divers, ocean or channel swimmers, or Arctic inhabitants or others exposed to cold-related environments. In contrast, excess body fat hinders temperature regulation during thermal stress, most notably during sustained exercise in air, when the body's heat production can increase 20 times above resting levels. In this case, the barrier of insulation from subcutaneous fat retards the flow of heat from the body.

Vitamin Carrier and Hunger Suppressor Dietary lipid serves as a carrier and transport medium for the fat-soluble A, D, E, and K vitamins, which require an intake of about 20 g of dietary fat daily. Thus, voluntarily reducing lipid intake concomitantly depresses the body's level of these vitamins and may ultimately lead to vitamin deficiency. In addition, dietary lipid delays the onset of "hunger pangs" and contributes to satiety after meals because emptying lipid from the stomach takes about 3.5 hours after its ingestion. This explains why weight-loss diets that contain some lipid sometimes prove initially successful in blunting the urge to eat more than the heavily advertised extreme so-called "fat-free" diets.

Recommended Lipid Intake

In the United States, dietary lipid represents between 34% and 38% of total calorie intake. Most health professionals recommend that lipids should not exceed 30% of the diet's total energy content. Unsaturated fatty acids should supply at least 70% of total lipid intake.

For dietary cholesterol, the American Heart Association (*www.aha.org*) recommends no more than 300 mg (0.01 oz) of cholesterol consumed daily, an intake equivalent to about 100 mg per 1000 kCal of food ingested. Three hundred mg of cholesterol almost equals the amount in the yolk of one large egg and just about one-half of the daily cholesterol consumed by the average American man.

Consume Lipids in Moderation In the quest to achieve good health and optimal exercise performance, prudent practice entails cooking with and consuming lipids derived primarily from vegetable sources. This approach may be too simplistic, however, because total saturated and unsaturated fatty acid intake constitutes more than a minimal risk for diabetes and heart disease. If so, then one should reduce the intake of all lipids, particularly those high in saturated and trans-fatty acids. Concerns also exist over the association of high-fat diets with ovarian, colon, endometrium, and other cancers. Another beneficial effect of reducing the diet's total lipid content relates to weight control. The energy requirements of various metabolic pathways make the body particularly efficient in converting excess calories from dietary lipid to stored fat.

Table 2.1 lists the saturated, monounsaturated, and polyunsaturated fatty acid content of various sources of dietary lipids. All fats contain a mix of each fatty acid type, yet different fatty acids predominate in certain foods. Several polyunsaturated fatty acids, most prominently linoleic acid (present in cooking and salad oils), must be consumed because they serve as precursors of *essential fatty acids* the body cannot synthesize. Humans require about 1% to 2% of total energy intake from linoleic acid (an omega-6 fatty acid). The best sources for alpha-linolenic acid or one of its related omega-3 fatty acids, EPA and DHA, include cold-water fatty fish (salmon, tuna, or sardines) and oils such as canola, soybean, safflower, sunflower, sesame, and flax.

Questions & Notes

Give the 4 major functions of lipids in the body.

1.

2.

3.

4.

State the recommended lipid intake as a percentage of the daily total kCal intake.

State the recommended cholesterol intake in mg per 1000 kCal of food ingested.

List 3 reasons why lipid represents the ideal cellular fuel.

1.

2.

3.

List 2 examples of high saturated fatty acid foods.

1.

2.

List 2 examples of high polyunsaturated foods.

1.

2.

Table 2.1	Examples of Foods High and Low in Saturated Fatty Acids, Foods High in Monounsaturated and Polyunsaturated Fatty Acids, and the Polyunsaturated to Saturated Fatty Acid (P/S) Ratio of Common Fats and Oils					

HIGH SATURATED	%	HIGH MONOSATURATED	%	FATS AND OILS	P/S RATIO
Coconut oil	91	Olives, black	80	Coconut oil	0.2/1.0
Palm kernel oil	82	Olive oil	75	Palm oil	0.2/1.0
Butter	68	Almond oil	70	Butter	0.1/1.0
Cream cheese	57	Canola oil	61	Olive oil	0.6/1.0
Coconut	56	Almonds, dry	52	Lard	0.3/1.0
Hollandaise sauce	54	Avocados	51	Canola oil	5.3/1.0
Palm oil	51	Peanut oil	48	Peanut oil	1.9/1.0
Half & half	45	Cashews, dry roasted	42	Soybean oil	2.5/1.0
Cheese, Velveeta	43	Peanut butter	39	Sesame oil	3.0/1.0
Cheese, mozzarella	41	Bologna	39	Margarine, 100% corn oil	2.5/1.0
Ice cream, vanilla	38	Beef, cooked	33	Cottonseed oil	2.0/1.0
Cheesecake	32	Lamb, roasted	32	Mayonnaise	3.7/1.0
Chocolate almond bar	29	Veal, roasted	26	Safflower oil	13.3/1.0
LOW SATURATED	**%**	**HIGH POLYUNSATURATED**	**%**		
Popcorn	0	Safflower oil	77		
Hard candy	0	Sunflower oil	70		
Yogurt, nonfat	2	Corn oil	58		
Crackerjacks	3	Walnuts, dry	51		
Milk, skim	4	Sunflower seeds	47		
Cookies, fig bars	4	Margarine, corn oil	45		
Graham crackers	5	Canola oil	32		
Chicken breast, roasted	6	Sesame seeds	31		
Pancakes	8	Pumpkin seeds	31		
Cottage cheese, 1%	8	Tofu	27		
Milk, chocolate, 1%	9	Lard	11		
Beef, dried	9	Butter	6		
Chocolate, mints	10	Coconut oil	2		

Data from the Science and Education Administration. (1985, 1986). *Home and Garden Bulletin 72, Nutritive value of foods.* Washington, DC: US Government Printing Office; Agricultural Research Service, United States Department of Agriculture. (1975). *Nutritive value of American foods in common units. Agricultural Handbook no. 456.* Washington, DC: US Government Printing Office.

Contribution of Fat in Exercise

The contribution of fat to the energy requirements of exercise depends on two factors:

1. Fatty acid release from triacylglycerols in the fat storage sites.
2. Delivery in the circulation to muscle tissue as free fatty acids (FFA) bound to blood albumin.

Triacylglycerols stored within the muscle cell also contribute to exercise energy metabolism. **Figure 2.9** shows that FFA uptake by active muscle increases during hours 1 and 4 of moderate exercise. In the first hour, fat (including intramuscular fat) supplies about 50% of the energy; by the third hour, fat contributes up to 70% of the total energy requirement. *With greater dependence on fat catabolism (e.g., with carbohydrate depletion), exercise intensity decreases to a level governed by the body's capacity to mobilize and oxidize fat.*

PROTEINS

A normal-size adult contains between 10 and 12 kg of protein, primarily located within skeletal muscle. The caloric equivalent for this mass of protein ranges between 18,160 and 21,792 kCal (1 kg = 454 g; 1 g protein = 4 kCal. Thus, $454 \times 4 = 1816$ kCal $\times 10$ kg = 18,160 kCal). Structurally, proteins resemble carbohydrates and lipids because they contain carbon, oxygen, and hydrogen. They differ because they also contain nitrogen (~16% of the molecule) along with sulfur and occasionally phosphorus, cobalt, and iron.

Amino Acids

Just as glycogen forms from the linkage of many simple glucose subunits, protein forms from amino acid "building-block" linkages. Peptide bonds join amino acids in chains representing diverse forms and chemical combinations; combining two amino acids produces a dipeptide, and three amino acids linked together form a tripeptide. A linear configuration of up to as many as 1000 amino acids produces a polypeptide; combining more than 50 amino acids forms a polypeptide protein of which humans can synthesize about 80,000 different kinds. Whereas single cells contain thousands of different protein molecules, the body contains approximately 50,000 different protein-containing compounds. The biochemical functions and properties of each protein depend on the sequencing of its specific amino acids.

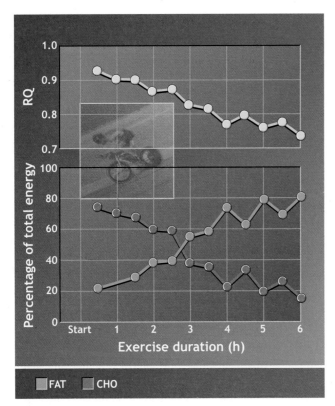

Figure 2.9 Generalized percentage contribution of macronutrient catabolism in relation to oxygen consumption of the leg muscles during prolonged exercise.

*Q*uestions & *Notes*

State the percentage of nitrogen contained in most protein molecules.

Describe the general chemical structure of an amino acid.

State the major difference between an essential and a nonessential amino acid.

State one example of an essential amino acid.

State one example of a nonessential amino acid.

Figure 2.10 shows the four common features that constitute the general structure of all amino acids. Of the 20 different amino acids required by the body, each contains a positively charged amine group at one end and a negatively charged organic acid group at the opposite end. The amine group consists of 2 hydrogen atoms attached to nitrogen (NH_2), and the organic acid group (technically termed a carboxylic acid group) joins 1 carbon atom, 2 oxygen atoms, and 1 atom of hydrogen symbolized chemically as COOH. The remainder of the amino acid molecule contains a side chain, which may take several different forms. *The specific structure of the side chain dictates the amino acid's particular characteristics.* **Figure 2.11** illustrates the structure of the non-essential amino acid alanine found in a wide variety of animal and vegetable foods, particularly meats. This amino acid plays an important role in the glucose–alanine cycle in the liver to synthesize glucose.

Essential and Non-essential Amino Acids   The body requires 20 different amino acids, although tens of thousands of the same amino acids may combine in a single protein compound. Of the different amino acids, eight (nine in infants) cannot be synthesized in the body at a sufficient rate to prevent impairment of normal cellular function. These make up the indispensable or **essential amino acids** because they must be ingested preformed in foods. The body manufactures the remaining 12 **non-essential amino acids**. This does not mean they are unimportant; rather, they form from compounds already existing in the body at a rate that meets demands for normal growth and tissue repair.

Animals and plants manufacture proteins that contain essential amino acids. *No health or physiological advantage comes from an amino acid derived from an animal compared with the same amino acid derived from vegetable origin.* Plants synthesize protein (and thus amino acids) by incorporating nitrogen from the soil (along with carbon, oxygen, and hydrogen from air and water). In contrast,

ⓘ For Your Information

THE NINE ESSENTIAL AMINO ACIDS

1. Histidine (infants)
2. Leucine
3. Lysine
4. Isoleucine
5. Methionine
6. Phenylalanine
7. Threonine
8. Tryptophan
9. Valine

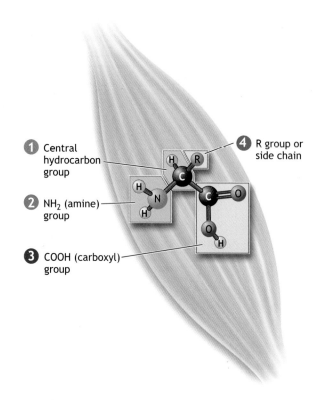

Figure 2.10   Four common features of amino acids.

animals do not possess a broad capability for protein synthesis; they obtain much of their protein from ingested sources.

Constructing a body protein requires specific amino acid availability at the time of protein synthesis. **Complete proteins** or higher quality proteins come from foods with all of the essential amino acids in their correct ratio. This maintains protein balance and allows tissue growth and repair. An **incomplete protein** or lower quality protein lacks one or more of the essential amino acids. Diets that contain mostly incomplete protein eventually produce protein malnutrition despite the food source's adequacy for energy and protein quantity.

Sources of Proteins

The two protein sources include those in the diet and those synthesized in the body.

Dietary Sources   Complete proteins are found in eggs, milk, meat, fish, and poultry. Eggs provide the optimal mixture of essential amino acids among food sources; hence, eggs receive the highest quality rating compared with other foods. Presently, almost two-thirds of dietary protein in the United States comes from animal sources, whereas 90 years ago, protein consumption occurred equally from plants and animals. Reliance on animal sources for dietary protein accounts for a relatively high current intake of cholesterol and saturated fatty acids.

The "**biologic value**" or protein rating of food refers to its completeness for supplying essential amino acids. Animal sources contribute high-quality protein, whereas vegetables (lentils, dried beans and peas, nuts, and cereals) remain incomplete in one or more of the essential amino acids; thus, these rate lower in biologic value. Eating a variety of plant foods (grains, fruits, and vegetables), each providing a different quality and quantity of amino acids, contributes all of the required essential amino acids. **Table 2.2** lists examples of common food sources of protein and their relative protein rating.

Synthesis in the Body   Enzymes in muscle facilitate nitrogen removal from certain amino acids and subsequently pass nitrogen to other compounds in the biochemical reactions of **transamination** illustrated in **Figure 2.12**. An amine group shifts from a donor amino acid to an acceptor acid, and the acceptor thus becomes a new amino acid. *This allows amino acids to form from non–nitrogen-carrying organic compounds generated in metabolism.*

Deamination represents the opposite process to transamination. It involves removal of an amine group from the amino acid molecule, with the remaining carbon skeleton converting to a carbohydrate or lipid or being used for energy. The cleaved amine group forms urea in the liver for excretion by the kidneys. Urea must dissolve in water, so

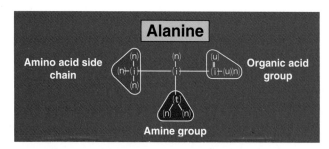

Figure 2.11   Chemical structure of the common, non-essential amino acid alanine. Animal sources of this amino acid include meat, seafood, caseinate, dairy products, eggs, fish, and gelatin. Vegetarian sources include beans, nuts, seeds, soy, whey, brewer's yeast, brown rice bran, corn, legumes, and whole grains.

Table 2.2	Rating of Common Sources of Dietary Protein
FOOD	**PROTEIN RATING**
Eggs	100
Fish	70
Lean beef	69
Cow's milk	60
Brown rice	57
White rice	56
Soybeans	47
Brewer's hash	45
Whole-grain wheat	44
Peanuts	43
Dry beans	34
White potato	34

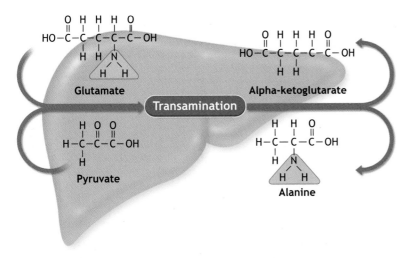

Figure 2.12 The biochemical process of transamination provides for the intramuscular synthesis of amino acids from nonprotein sources. An amine group from a donor group transfers to an acceptor, non–nitrogen-containing acid to form a new amino acid.

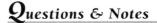

excessive protein catabolism (involving increased deamination) promotes fluid loss.

For deamination and transamination, the remaining carbon skeleton of the non-nitrogenous amino acid residue further degrades during energy metabolism. In well-nourished individuals at rest, protein breakdown (**catabolism**) contributes between 2% to 5% of the body's total energy requirement. During its **catabolism**, protein first degrades into its amino acid components. The liver then strips the nitrogen from the amino acid molecule (via deamination) to form urea (H_2NCONH_2) for excretion.

Protein's Role in the Body

No body "reservoirs" of protein exist; all protein contributes to tissue structures or exists as constituents of metabolic, transport, and hormonal systems. Protein constitutes between 12% and 15% of the body mass, but its content in different cells varies considerably. A brain cell, for example, contains only about 10% protein, but protein represents up to 20% of the mass of red blood cells and muscle cells. The systematic application of resistance training increases the protein content of skeletal muscle, which represents about 65% of the body's total protein.

Amino acids provide the building blocks to synthesize RNA and DNA, the heme components of the oxygen-binding hemoglobin and myoglobin compounds, the catecholamine hormones epinephrine and norepinephrine, and the neurotransmitter serotonin. Amino acids activate vitamins that play a key role in metabolic and physiologic regulation.

Tissue synthesis (**anabolism**) accounts for more than one-third of the protein intake during rapid growth in infancy and childhood. As growth rate declines, so does the percentage of protein retained for anabolic processes. Continual turnover of tissue protein occurs when a person attains optimal body size and growth stabilizes. Adequate protein intake replaces the amino acids continually degraded in the turnover process.

Proteins serve as primary constituents for plasma membranes and internal cellular material. Proteins within cell nuclei called nucleoproteins "supervise" cellular protein synthesis and transmit hereditary characteristics. Structural proteins are the key components in hair, skin, nails, bones, tendons, and ligaments, and globular proteins comprise the nearly 2000 different enzymes that dramatically accelerate chemical reactions and regulate the catabolism of fats,

Questions & Notes

Describe a complete protein.

Describe transamination.

Describe deamination.

ⓘ For Your Information

FATE OF AMINO ACIDS AFTER NITROGEN REMOVAL

After deamination, the remaining carbon skeletons of the α-keto acids pyruvate, oxaloacetate, or α-ketoglutarate follow one of three distinct biochemical routes:

1. *Gluconeogenesis*—18 of the 20 amino acids serve as a source for glucose synthesis.
2. *Energy source*—The carbon skeletons oxidize for energy because they form intermediates in citric acid cycle metabolism or related molecules.
3. *Fat synthesis*—All amino acids provide a potential source of acetyl-CoA to furnish substrate to synthesize fatty acids.

carbohydrates, and proteins during energy release. Proteins also regulate the acid–base quality of the body fluids, which contributes to neutralizing (buffering) excess acid metabolites formed during vigorous exercise.

Vegetarian Approach to Sound Nutrition

True vegetarians (**vegans**) consume nutrients from only two sources—plants and dietary supplements. Vegans represent fewer than 1% of the U.S. population, although nearly 10% of Americans consider themselves "almost" vegetarians.

An increasing number of competitive and champion athletes consume diets consisting predominately of nutrients from varied plant sources, including some dairy and meat products. Considering the time required for training and competition, athletes often encounter difficulty in planning, selecting, and preparing nutritious meals from predominantly plant sources without relying on supplementation. The fact remains that two-thirds of the world's population subsists on largely vegetarian diets with little reliance on animal protein. Well-balanced vegetarian and vegetarian-type diets provide abundant carbohydrates, which is crucial when training intensely. *Vegetarian-type diets have the following characteristics: usually low or devoid of cholesterol, high in fiber, low in saturated and high in unsaturated fatty acids, and rich in fruit and vegetable sources of antioxidant vitamins and phytochemicals.*

Obtaining ample high-quality protein becomes the vegetarian's main nutritional concern. A **lactovegetarian** diet includes milk and related products such as ice cream, cheese, and yogurt. The lactovegetarian approach minimizes the problem of acquiring sufficient high-quality protein and increases the intake of calcium, phosphorus, and vitamin B_{12} (produced by bacteria in the digestive tract of animals). Good meatless sources of iron include fortified ready-to-eat cereals, soybeans, and cooked farina (fine flour or meal made from cereal grains or starch), and cereals and wheat germ contain a relatively high concentration of zinc. Adding eggs to the diet ensures an ample intake of high-quality protein (**ovolactovegetarian diet**).

Figure 2.13 displays the contribution of various food groups to the protein content of the American diet. By far, the greatest protein intake comes from animal sources, with only about 30% from plant sources.

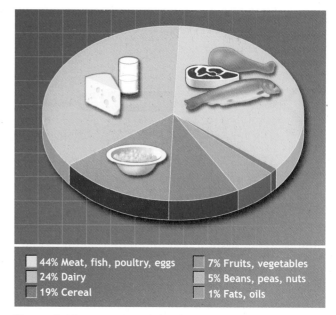

☐ 44% Meat, fish, poultry, eggs   ☐ 7% Fruits, vegetables
☐ 24% Dairy   ☐ 5% Beans, peas, nuts
☐ 19% Cereal   ☐ 1% Fats, oils

Figure 2.13 Contribution from the major food sources to the protein content of the typical American diet.

Recommended Protein Intake

Protein intake that exceeds three times the recommended level does not enhance exercise capacity during intensive training or subsequent sports performance. *For athletes, muscle mass does not increase simply by eating high-protein foods.* If lean tissue synthesis resulted from all the extra protein intake consumed by the typical athlete, then muscle mass would increase tremendously. For example, eating an extra 100 g (400 kCal) of protein daily would translate to a daily 500-g (1.1-lb) increase in muscle mass. This obviously does not happen. Additional dietary protein, after deamination, provides for energy or recycles as components of other molecules, including stored fat in subcutaneous depots. Dietary protein intake substantially above recommended values can prove harmful because excessive protein breakdown strains liver and kidney function from the production and elimination of urea and other solutes.

Table 2.3 lists the recommended protein requirements for adolescent and adult men and women. On average, 0.83 g protein per kg body mass represents the recommended daily intake. To determine the protein requirement for

	MEN		WOMEN	
RECOMMENDED AMOUNT	**ADOLESCENT**	**ADULT**	**ADOLESCENT**	**ADULT**
Grams of protein per kg of body weight	0.9	0.8	0.9	0.8
Grams of protein per day based on average weight[a]	59.0	56.0	50.0	44.0

Table 2.3 Recommended Protein Intake for Adolescent and Adult Men and Women

[a]Average weight is based on a "reference" man and woman. For adolescents (ages 14–18 years), the average weight equals 65.8 kg (145 lb) for young men and 55.7 kg (123 lb) for young women. For adult men, the average weight equals 70 kg (154 lb); for adult women, the average weight equals 56.8 kg (125 lb).

men and women ages 18 to 65 years, multiply body mass in kg by 0.83. Thus, for a 90-kg man, the total protein requirement equals 75 g (90 × 0.83). The protein requirement holds even for overweight people; it includes a reserve of about 25% to account for individual differences in protein requirements for about 98% of the population. Generally, the protein requirement (and the quantity of the required essential amino acids) decreases with age. In contrast, the protein required for infants and growing children equals 2.0 to 4.0 g per kg body mass to facilitate growth and development. Pregnant women should increase their daily protein intake by 20 g·d^{-1}, and nursing mothers should increase intake by 10 g·d^{-1}. *A 10% increase in the calculated protein requirement, particularly for a vegetarian-type diet, accounts for dietary fiber's effect in reducing the digestibility of many plant-based protein sources.* Stress, disease, and injury usually increase protein requirements.

Protein Requirements for Physically Active People

Any discussion of protein requirements must include the assumption of adequate energy intake to match the added needs of exercise. *If energy intake falls below the total energy expended during intense training, even augmented protein intake may fail to maintain nitrogen balance.* This occurs because a disproportionate quantity of dietary protein catabolizes to balance an energy deficit rather than augment tissue maintenance and muscle development.

The common practice among weight lifters, body builders, and other power athletes who consume liquids, powders, or pills made of predigested protein represents a waste of money and may actually be counterproductive for producing the intended outcome. For example, many preparations contain proteins predigested to simple amino acids through chemical action in the laboratory. Available evidence does not support the notion that simple amino acids absorb more easily or facilitate muscle growth. In fact, the small intestine absorbs amino acids rapidly when they are part of more complex di- and tripeptide molecules. The intestinal tract handles proteins effectively in their more complex form. In contrast, a concentrated amino acid solution draws water into the small intestine, which can cause irritation, cramping, and diarrhea in susceptible individuals.

Researchers have questioned the necessity of advocating a larger protein requirement for these three groups of athletes:

1. Growing adolescent athletes.
2. Athletes involved in resistance training (to enhance muscle growth) and endurance training programs (to counter increased protein breakdown for energy).
3. Wrestlers and football players subjected to recurring muscle trauma.

Inadequate protein intake can reduce body protein, particularly from muscle, with a concomitant impairment in performance. If athletes do require additional protein, then more than likely their increased food intake will compensate for training's increased energy expenditure. Nonetheless, this may not occur in athletes with poor nutritional habits or who voluntarily diet and reduce their energy intake to hopefully gain a competitive advantage.

Do Athletes Require More Protein? Much of the current understanding of protein dynamics and exercise comes from studies that have expanded the classic method of determining protein breakdown through urea excretion. For example, the output of "labeled" CO_2 from amino acids (either injected or ingested) increases during exercise in proportion to the metabolic rate. As exercise progresses, the concentration of plasma urea also increases, coupled with a dramatic increase in nitrogen excretion in sweat (often occurring without changing urinary nitrogen excretion). The sweat mechanism helps to excrete nitrogen produced from protein breakdown during exercise. Furthermore, oxidation of plasma and intracellular amino acids increases

$\mathcal{Q}$**uestions & Notes**

Describe a "vegan" diet.

Give the RDA for protein for an adult male and female.

Male:

Female:

Do athletes require more protein? Discuss.

For Your Information

FOOD DIVERSITY: CRUCIAL FOR VEGETARIANS

A vegan diet provides all of the essential amino acids if the Recommended Daily Allowance for protein includes 60% of protein from grain products, 35% from legumes, and the remaining 5% from green leafy vegetables. A 70-kg person who requires about 56 g of protein can obtain the essential amino acids by consuming approximately 1¼ cups of beans; ¼ cup of seeds or nuts; about 4 slices of whole-grain bread; 2 cups of vegetables (half being green leafy); and 2½ cups of diverse grain sources such as brown rice, oatmeal, and cracked wheat.

significantly during moderate exercise independent of changes in urea production. Protein use for energy reached its highest level when subjects exercised in the glycogen-depleted state. This emphasizes the important role of carbohydrate as a protein sparer, meaning that carbohydrate availability impacts the demand on protein "reserves" in exercise. Protein breakdown and accompanying gluconeogenesis (glucose synthesis from protein) undoubtedly become important factors in endurance exercise and frequent intense training when glycogen reserves diminish. Eating a high-carbohydrate diet with adequate energy intake preserves muscle protein in athletes who train hard and for protracted durations.

We *recommend that athletes who train intensely for 2 to 6 hours daily consume between 1.2 and 1.8 g of protein per kg of body mass daily.* This protein intake falls within the range typically consumed by physically active men and women, thus obviating the need to consume supplementary protein. With adequate protein intake, consuming animal sources of protein does not facilitate muscle strength or size gains with resistance training compared with protein intake from plant sources.

SUMMARY

1. Carbon, hydrogen, oxygen, and nitrogen represent the primary structural units for most of the body's biologically active substances.

2. Whereas specific combinations of carbon with oxygen and hydrogen form carbohydrates and lipids, proteins consist of combinations of carbon, oxygen, and hydrogen, including nitrogen and minerals.

3. Simple sugars consist of chains of from 3 to 7 carbon atoms with hydrogen and oxygen in the ratio of 2 to 1. Glucose, the most common simple sugar, contains a 6-carbon chain, $C_6H_{12}O_6$.

4. Three classifications commonly define carbohydrates: monosaccharides (glucose and fructose); disaccharides (two monosaccharides as in sucrose, lactose, and maltose); and polysaccharides, which contain three or more simple sugars to form plant starch and fiber and the large animal polysaccharide glycogen.

5. Whereas glycogenolysis reconverts glycogen to glucose, gluconeogenesis synthesizes glucose largely from the carbon skeletons of amino acids.

6. Fiber, a non-starch, structural plant polysaccharide, offers considerable resistance to human digestive enzymes. Technically not a nutrient, water-soluble and water-insoluble dietary fibers still confer health benefits for gastrointestinal functioning and cardiovascular disease.

7. Americans typically consume 40% to 50% of their total calories as carbohydrates, with about half in the form of simple sugars, predominantly sucrose and high-fructose corn syrup.

8. Carbohydrates, stored in limited quantity in liver and muscle, serve four important functions: major source of energy, spares protein breakdown, metabolic primer for fat metabolism, and fuel for the central nervous system.

9. Muscle glycogen and blood glucose become the primary fuels for intense exercise. The body's glycogen stores also provide energy in sustained, intense aerobic exercise such as marathon running, triathlon-type events, long-distance cycling, and endurance swimming.

10. A carbohydrate-deficient diet rapidly depletes muscle and liver glycogen, profoundly affecting capacity for both intense anaerobic exercise and long-duration aerobic exercise. Individuals who exercise regularly should consume at least 60% of their daily calories as carbohydrates (400–600 g), predominantly in unrefined, fiber-rich complex form.

11. Similar to carbohydrates, lipids contain carbon, hydrogen, and oxygen atoms but with a higher ratio of hydrogen to oxygen. Lipid molecules consist of one glycerol molecule and three fatty acid molecules.

12. Plants and animals synthesize lipids into one of three groups: simple lipids, compound lipids, and derived lipids.

13. Saturated fatty acids contain as many hydrogen atoms as chemically possible; thus, the molecule is considered saturated relative to hydrogen. High saturated fatty acid intake elevates blood cholesterol and promotes coronary heart disease.

14. Unsaturated fatty acids contain fewer hydrogen atoms attached to the carbon chain. These fatty acids exist as either monounsaturated or polyunsaturated with respect to hydrogen.

15. Dietary lipid represents between 34% to 38% of the typical person's total caloric intake. Prudent recommendations suggest a 30% level or lower, of which 70% to 80% should be unsaturated fatty acids.

16. Lipids provide the largest nutrient store of potential energy for biologic work. They protect vital organs, provide insulation from cold, transport fat-soluble vitamins, and depress hunger.

17. During light and moderate exercise, fat contributes about 50% of the energy requirement. As exercise

continues, fat becomes more important, supplying more than 70% of the body's energy needs.

18. Proteins differ chemically from lipids and carbohydrates because they contain nitrogen in addition to sulfur, phosphorus, and iron.

19. Subunits called amino acids form proteins. The body requires 20 different amino acids.

20. The body cannot synthesize 8 (9 in children) of the 20 amino acids; they must be consumed in the diet and thus comprise the essential amino acids.

21. All animal and plant cells contain protein. Complete (higher quality) proteins contain all the essential amino acids; the other protein type represents incomplete or lower quality proteins. Proteins from the animal kingdom are of higher quality.

22. Consuming a variety of plant foods provides all the essential amino acids because each food source contains a different quality and quantity of amino acids.

23. For adults, the recommended protein intake equals 0.83 g per kg of body mass.

24. Protein breakdown above the resting level occurs during endurance and resistance training exercise to a degree greater than previously thought. Athletes in intense training (2–6 h·d^{-1}) should consume between 1.2 and 1.8 g of protein per kg of body mass daily.

25. Reduced carbohydrate reserves from either diet or exercise increase protein catabolism, making it imperative to maintain optimal levels of glycogen during strenuous training.

THOUGHT QUESTIONS

1. Outline a presentation to a high school class about how to eat "well" for a physically active, healthy lifestyle.

2. Many college students do not eat well-balanced meals. Give your recommendations concerning macronutrient intake to ensure proper energy reserves for moderate and intense physical activities. Are supplements of these macronutrients necessarily required for physically active individuals?

3. Explain the importance of regular carbohydrate intake when maintaining a high level of daily physical activity. Additionally, what are some "non-exercise" health benefits for a diet rich in food sources containing unrefined, complex carbohydrates?

4. Discuss a rationale for recommending adequate carbohydrate intake, rather than excess protein, for a person who wants to increase muscle mass through resistance training.

Part 2 Micronutrients: Facilitators of Energy Transfer and Tissue Synthesis

VITAMINS

The Nature of Vitamins

The formal discovery of vitamins revealed that the body requires these essential organic substances in minute amounts to perform highly specific metabolic functions. Vitamins, often considered accessory nutrients, do *not* perform these three commonly assumed functions:

1. Supply energy.
2. Serve as basic building units for other compounds.
3. Contribute substantially to the body's mass.

A prolonged inadequate intake of a particular vitamin can trigger symptoms of vitamin deficiency and lead to severe medical complications. For example,

 For Your Information

NATURAL VERSUS LABORATORY-MADE VITAMINS

No difference exists between a vitamin obtained naturally from food and a vitamin produced synthetically. Manufacturers gain huge profits in advertising vitamins as "natural" or "organically isolated," yet such vitamins are chemically identical to those synthesized in the laboratory.

symptoms of thiamin deficiency occur after only 2 weeks on a thiamin-free diet, and symptoms of vitamin C deficiency appear after 3 or 4 weeks. At the other extreme, consuming the fat-soluble vitamins A, D, E, and K in excess can produce a toxic overdose manifested by hair loss, irregularities in bone formation, fetal malformation, hemorrhage, bone fractures, abnormal liver function, and ultimately death.

Classification of Vitamins

Thirteen different vitamins have been isolated, analyzed, classified, and synthesized and have had their recommended intake levels established. Vitamins are classified as either **fat-soluble** (vitamins A, D, E, and K) or **water-soluble** (vitamin C and the B-complex vitamins: vitamin B_6 [pyridoxine], vitamin B_1 [thiamin], vitamin B_2 [riboflavin], niacin [nicotinic acid], pantothenic acid, biotin, folic acid, and vitamin B_{12} [cobalamin]).

Fat-Soluble Vitamins   Fat-soluble vitamins dissolve and store in the body's fatty tissues and do not require daily intake. In fact, symptoms of a fat-soluble vitamin insufficiency may not appear for years. Dietary lipid provides the source of fat-soluble vitamins. Whereas the liver stores vitamins A, D, and K, vitamin E distributes throughout the body's fatty tissues. Prolonged intake of a "fat-free" diet accelerates a fat-soluble vitamin insufficiency. Table 2.4 lists the major bodily functions, dietary sources, and symp-

toms of a deficiency or excess for the fat-soluble vitamins for men and women ages 19 to 50 years. Chapter 3 discusses the dietary reference intakes (DRIs), including tolerable upper intake levels for all vitamins (and minerals) for different life-stage groups.

Water-Soluble Vitamins   Vitamin C (ascorbic acid) and the B-complex group constitute the nine water-soluble vitamins. They act largely as **coenzymes**—small molecules that combine with a larger protein compound (apoenzyme) to form an active enzyme that accelerates interconversion of chemical compounds. Coenzymes participate directly in chemical reactions; when the reaction runs its course, coenzymes remain intact and participate in further reactions. Water-soluble vitamins play an essential role as part of coenzymes in the cells' energy-generating reactions.

Because of their solubility in water, water-soluble vitamins disperse in the body fluids without appreciable storage, with the excess voided in urine. If the diet regularly contains less than 50% of the recommended values for water-soluble vitamins, marginal deficiencies may develop within 4 weeks. Table 2.5 summarizes food sources, major bodily functions, and symptoms from an excess and deficiency of water-soluble vitamins. The B-complex vitamins serve as coenzymes in energy-yielding reactions during carbohydrate, fat, and protein breakdown. They also contribute to hemoglobin synthesis and red blood cell formation.

Table 2.4	Food Sources, Major Bodily Functions, and Symptoms of Deficiency or Excess of the Fat-Soluble Vitamins for Healthy Adults (Ages 19–50 Years)[a]			
VITAMIN	**DIETARY SOURCES**	**MAJOR BODILY FUNCTIONS**	**DEFICIENCY**	**EXCESS**
Vitamin A (retinol)	Provitamin A (beta–carotene) widely distributed in green vegetables; retinol present in milk, butter, cheese, fortified margarine	Constituent of rhodopsin (visual pigment); maintenance of epithelial tissues; role in mucopolysaccharide synthesis	Xeropthalmia (keratinization of ocular tissue), night blindness, permanent blindness	Headache, vomiting, peeling of skin, anorexia, swelling of long bones
Vitamin D	Cod-liver oil, eggs, dairy products, fortified milk, and margarine	Promotes growth and mineralization of bones; increases absorption of calcium	Rickets (bone deformities) in children; osteomalacia in adults	Vomiting, diarrhea, weight loss, kidney damage
Vitamin E (tocopherol)	Seeds, green leafy vegetables, margarines, shortenings	Functions as an antioxidant to prevent cell damage	Possibly anemia	Relatively nontoxic
Vitamin K (phylloquinone)	Green leafy vegetables, small amount in cereals, fruits, and meats	Important in blood clotting (helps form active prothrombin)	Conditioned deficiencies associated with severe bleeding, internal hemorrhages	Relatively nontoxic; synthetic forms at high doses may cause jaundice

[a]Food and Nutrition Board, National Academy of Sciences. (2009). Available at *http://www.nal.usda.gov/fnic/etext/000105.html*. This website provides interactive dietary reference intakes for health professionals.

Table 2.5	Food Sources, Major Bodily Functions, and Symptoms of Deficiency or Excess of the Water-Soluble Vitamins for Healthy Adults (Ages 19–50 Years)[a]			
VITAMIN	**DIETARY SOURCES**	**MAJOR BODILY FUNCTIONS**	**DEFICIENCY**	**EXCESS**
Vitamin B$_1$ (thiamin)	Pork, organ meats, whole grains, legumes	Coenzyme (thiamin prophosphate) in reactions involving removal of carbon dioxide	Beriberi (peripheral nerve changes, edema, heart failure)	None reported
Vitamin B$_2$ (riboflavin)	Widely distributed in foods	Constituent of two flavin nucleotide coenzymes involved in energy metabolism (FAD and FMN)	Reddened lips, cracks at mouth corner (cheilosis), eye lesions	None reported
Vitamin B$_3$ (niacin-nicotinic acid)	Liver, lean meats, grains, legumes (can be formed from tryptophan)	Constituent of two coenzymes in oxidation-reduction reactions (NAD$^+$ and NADP)	Pellagra (skin and gastrointestinal lesions, nervous mental disorders)	Flushing, burning and tingling around neck, face, and hands
Vitamin B$_5$ (pantothenic acid)	Widely distributed in foods	Constituent of coenzyme A, which plays a central role in energy metabolism	Fatigue, sleep disturbances, impaired coordination, nausea	None reported
Vitamin B$_6$ (pyridoxine)	Meats, vegetables, whole-grain cereals	Coenzyme (pyridoxal phosphate) involved in amino acid and glycogen metabolism	Irritability, convulsions, muscular twitching, dermatitis, kidney stones	None reported
Folate	Legumes, green vegetables, whole-wheat products	Coenzyme (reduced form) involved in transfer of single-carbon units in nucleic acid and amino acid metabolism	Anemia, gastrointestinal disturbances, diarrhea, red tongue	None reported
Vitamin B$_7$ (biotin)	Legumes, vegetables, meats	Coenzymes required for fat synthesis, amino acid metabolism, and glycogen (animal starch) formation	Fatigue, depression, nausea, dermatitis, muscular pains	None reported
Vitamin B$_{12}$ (cobalamin)	Muscle meats, eggs, dairy products, (absent in plant foods)	Coenzyme involved in transfer of single-carbon units in nucleic acid metabolism	Pernicious anemia, neurologic disorders	None reported
Vitamin C (ascorbic acid)	Citrus fruits, tomatoes, green peppers, salad greens	Maintains intercellular matrix of cartilage, bone, and dentine, important in collagen synthesis	Scurvy (degeneration of skin, teeth, blood vessels, epithelial hemorrhages)	Relatively nontoxic; possibility of kidney stones

[a]Food and Nutrition Board, National Academy of Sciences. (2009). Available at *http://www.nal.usda.gov/fnic/etext/000105.html*

Vitamin C serves these four functions:

1. Cofactor in enzymatic reactions.
2. Scavenger of free radicals in antioxidative processes.
3. Collagen synthesis.
4. Maintain intracellular matrix of bone and cartilage.

Vitamin Toxicity Excess vitamins function as potentially harmful chemicals once enzyme systems catalyzed by specific vitamins saturate. A higher probability exists for overdosing with fat-soluble than water-soluble vitamins.

Fat-soluble vitamins should not be consumed in excess without medical supervision. Adverse reactions from excessive fat-soluble vitamin intake occur at a lower level than with water-soluble vitamins. Women who consume excess vitamin A (as retinol but not in the provitamin carotene form) early in pregnancy increase the risk of birth defects in their infants. Excessive vitamin A accumulation (called **hypervitaminosis A**) causes irritability; swelling of bones; weight loss; and dry, itchy skin in young children. In adults, symptoms include nausea, headache, drowsiness, loss of hair, diarrhea, and bone brittleness from calcium loss. Discontinuing excessive vitamin A consumption reverses these symptoms. A regular excess of vitamin D can damage the kidneys. An "overdose" from vitamins E and K rarely occurs, but intakes above the recommended level provide *no* health or fitness benefits.

Vitamins' Role in the Body

Vitamins contain no useful energy for the body; instead, they link and regulate the sequence of metabolic reactions that release energy within food molecules. They also play an intimate role in tissue synthesis and other biologic processes. A vitamin participates repeatedly in metabolic reactions regardless of the person's physical activity level. This means that the vitamin needs of athletes do not exceed those of sedentary counterparts. **Figure 2.14** summarizes the important biologic functions of vitamins in the body.

Individuals who expend considerable energy exercising need not consume special foods or supplements that increase the diet's vitamin content above established requirements. Also, at high levels of daily physical activity, food intake usually increases to sustain the added energy requirements of exercise. Additional food consumed through a variety of nutritious meals proportionately increases vitamin and mineral intake. This general rule has several possible exceptions. First, vitamin C and folic acid exist in foods that usually comprise only a small part of most Americans' total caloric intake; the availability of these foods also varies by season. Second, some athletic groups consume relatively low amounts of vitamins B_1 and

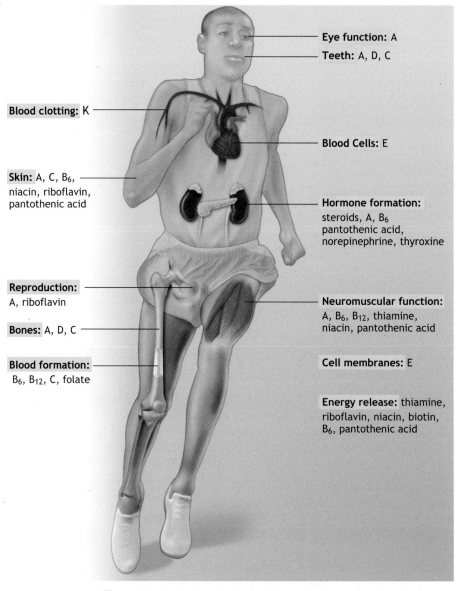

Figure 2.14 Biologic functions of vitamins.

B$_6$. An adequate intake of these two vitamins occurs if the daily diet contains fresh fruit, grains, and uncooked or steamed vegetables. Individuals on meatless diets should consume a small amount of milk, milk products, or eggs (or a vitamin supplement) because only foods of animal origin contain vitamin B$_{12}$.

Free Radical Production and Antioxidant Role of Specific Vitamins

Most of the oxygen consumed in the mitochondria during energy metabolism combines with hydrogen to produce water. Normally, about 2% to 5% of oxygen forms the oxygen-containing free radicals superoxide (O$_2^-$), hydrogen peroxide (H$_2$O$_2$), and hydroxyl (OH$^-$) from electron "leakage" along the electron transport chain (see Chapter 5). A **free radical** represents a chemically reactive molecule or molecular fragment with at least one unpaired electron in its outer orbital or valence shell. These are the same free radicals produced by heat and ionizing radiation and carried in cigarette smoke, environmental pollutants, and even some medications.

A buildup of free radicals increases the potential for cellular damage or **oxidative stress** to biologically important substances (see Close up Box 2.2: *Increased Metabolism During Exercise and Free Radical Production*, on page 58). Oxygen radicals exhibit strong affinity for the polyunsaturated fatty acids in the lipid bilayer of cell membranes. During oxidative stress, deterioration occurs in the plasma membrane's fatty acids. Membrane damage occurs through a series of chain reactions termed **lipid peroxidation**. These reactions, which incorporate oxygen into lipids, increase the vulnerability of the cell and its constituents. Free radicals also facilitate LDL cholesterol oxidation and thus accelerate the atherosclerotic process. Oxidative stress ultimately increases the likelihood of cellular deterioration associated with advanced aging, cancer, diabetes, coronary artery disease, and a general decline in central nervous system and immune function.

Vitamins Behave as Chemicals The most recent nationally representative data available on dietary supplement use showed that an estimated 175 million Americans use supplements, spending in excess of $30 billion annually. Of this total, vitamin–mineral pills and powders, often at potentially toxic dosages, represent the most common form of supplement used by the general public, accounting for approximately 70% of the total annual supplement sales. Particularly susceptible marketing targets include exercise enthusiasts, competitive athletes, and coaches and personal trainers who assist individuals achieve peak performance. More than 50% of competitive athletes in some sports consume supplements on a regular basis, either to ensure adequate micronutrient intake or to achieve an excess with the hope of enhancing exercise performance and training responsiveness. *More than 55 years of research data do not provide evidence that consuming vitamin (and mineral) supplements improves exercise performance, the hormonal and metabolic responses to exercise, or the ability to train arduously and recover from such training in healthy persons with nutritionally adequate diets.* When vitamin–mineral deficiencies appear in physically active people, they often occur among these three groups:

1. Vegetarians or groups with low energy intake such as dancers, gymnasts, and weight-class sport athletes who strive to maintain or reduce body weight.
2. Individuals who eliminate one or more food groups from their diet.
3. Individuals (e.g., endurance athletes) who consume large amounts of processed foods and simple sugars with low micronutrient density.

Questions & Notes

Describe what generally happens to the excess intake of the B-complex vitamins.

Describe a free radical.

Name the 3 most important antioxidant vitamins.

1.

2.

3.

🛈 For Your Information

RICH DIETARY SOURCES OF ANTIOXIDANT VITAMINS

- β-carotene (best known of the pigmented compounds or carotenoids give color to yellow, orange, and green leafy vegetables and fruits): Carrots; dark-green leafy vegetables such as spinach, broccoli, turnips, beet, and collard greens; sweet potatoes; winter squash; and apricots, cantaloupe, mangos, and papaya
- Vitamin C: Citrus fruits and juices; cabbage, broccoli, and turnip greens; cantaloupe; green and red sweet peppers; and berries
- Vitamin E: Poultry, seafood, vegetable oils, wheat germ, fish liver oils, whole-grain breads and fortified cereals, nuts and seeds, dried beans, green leafy vegetables, and eggs

BOX 2.2 CLOSE UP

Increased Metabolism During Exercise and Free Radical Production

Exercise produces reactive oxygen in at least two ways. The first occurs via an electron leak in the mitochondria, probably at the cytochrome level, to produce superoxide radicals. The second occurs during alterations in blood flow and oxygen supply—underperfusion during intense exercise followed by substantial reperfusion in recovery—which trigger excessive free radical generation. The reintroduction of molecular oxygen in recovery also produces reactive oxygen species that cause oxidative stress. Some argue that the potential for free radical damage increases during trauma, stress, and muscle damage and from environmental pollutants, including smog.

The risk of oxidative stress increases with intense exercise. Exhaustive endurance exercise by untrained persons produces oxidative damage in the active muscles. Intense resistance exercise also increases free radical production, indirectly measured by malondialdehyde, the lipid peroxidation byproduct. Variations in estrogen levels during the menstrual cycle do not affect the mild oxidative stress that accompanies moderate-intensity exercise. The accompanying figure illustrates how regular aerobic exercise affects oxidative response and the potential for tissue damage including protective adaptive responses.

Nothing can stop oxygen reduction and free radical production, but an elaborate natural defense exists within the cell and extracellular space against its damaging effects. This defense includes enzymatic and non-enzymatic mechanisms that work in concert to immediately counter potential oxidative damage. Three major antioxidant enzymes include **superoxide dismutase**, **catalase**, and **glutathione peroxidase**. The nutritive-reducing vitamins A, C, and E and the vitamin A precursor β-carotene also serve

important protective functions. These antioxidant vitamins protect the plasma membrane by reacting with and removing free radicals to squelch the chain reaction.

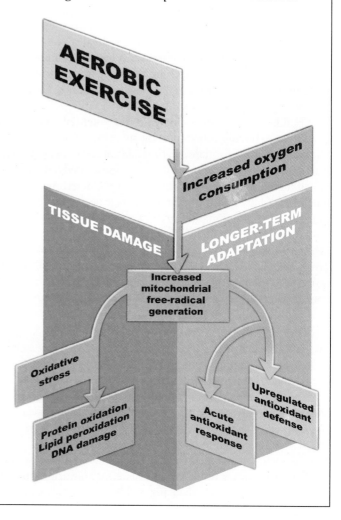

Any significant excess of vitamins function as chemicals or essentially drugs in the body. For example, a megadose of water-soluble vitamin C increases serum uric acid levels, which precipitates gout in people predisposed to this disease. At intakes greater than 1000 mg daily, urinary excretion of oxalate (a breakdown product of vitamin C) increases, accelerating kidney stone formation in susceptible individuals. In iron-deficient individuals, megadoses of vitamin C may destroy significant amounts of vitamin B_{12}. In healthy people, vitamin C supplements frequently irritate the bowel and cause diarrhea.

Excess vitamin B_6 may induce liver and nerve damage. Excessive riboflavin (B_2) intake can impair vision, and a megadose of nicotinic acid (niacin) serves as a potent

vasodilator and inhibits fatty acid mobilization during exercise, rapidly depleting muscle glycogen. Folic acid concentrated in supplement form can trigger an allergic response, producing hives, lightheadedness, and breathing difficulties. Megadoses of vitamin A can induce toxicity to the nervous system, and excess vitamin D intake can damage kidneys.

Vitamins and Exercise Performance

Figure 2.15 illustrates that the water-soluable B-complex vitamins play key roles as coenzymes to regulate energy-yielding reactions during carbohydrate, fat, and protein catabolism. They also contribute to hemoglobin synthesis and red blood cell production. The belief that "if a little is good, more must be better" has led many coaches, athletes, fitness enthusiasts, and even some scientists to advocate using vitamin supplements above recommended levels. The facts do not support such advice for individuals who consume an adequate diet.

Supplementing with vitamin B_6, an essential cofactor in glycogen and amino acid metabolism, did not benefit the metabolic mixture metabolized by women during intense aerobic exercise. In general, athletes' status for this vitamin equals reference standards for the population and does not decrease with strenuous exercise to a level warranting supplementation. For endurance-trained men, 9 days of vitamin B_6 supplementation (20 mg per day) provided no ergogenic effect on cycling to exhaustion performed at 70% of aerobic capacity.

Chronic high-potency, multivitamin–mineral supplementation for well-nourished, healthy individuals does not augment aerobic fitness, muscular strength, neuromuscular performance after prolonged running, and general athletic performance. In addition to the B-complex group, no exercise benefits exist for excess vitamins C and E on stamina, circulatory function, or energy metabolism. Short-term daily supplementation with 400 IU of vitamin E produced no effect on normal neuroendocrine and metabolic responses to strenuous exercise or performance time to exhaustion. Vitamin C status in trained athletes, assessed by serum concentrations and urinary ascorbate levels, does not differ from untrained individuals despite large differences in daily physical activity level. Active persons typically increase their daily energy intake to match their increased energy requirement; thus, a proportionate increase occurs in micronutrient intake, often in amounts that exceed recommended levels.

Briefly describe the function of minerals in the body.

ⓘ For Your Information

HOW ANTIOXIDANT VITAMINS SERVE TO NEUTRALIZE FREE RADICALS

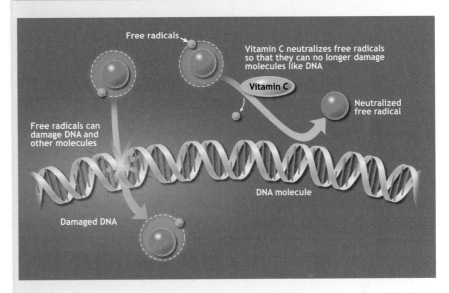

Free radicals

Vitamin C neutralizes free radicals so that they can no longer damage molecules like DNA

Vitamin C

Neutralized free radical

Free radicals can damage DNA and other molecules

DNA molecule

Damaged DNA

MINERALS

The Nature of Minerals

Approximately 4% of the body's mass (~2 kg for a 50-kg woman) consists of 22 mostly metallic elements collectively called **minerals**. Minerals serve as constituents of enzymes, hormones, and vitamins; they combine with other chemicals (e.g., calcium phosphate in bone and iron in the heme of hemoglobin) or exist singularly (e.g., free calcium in body fluids). In the body, **trace minerals** are those required in amounts 100 mg a day or below, and **major minerals** are required in amounts 100 mg daily or above. Excess minerals serve no useful physiologic purpose and can produce toxic effects.

Kinds, Sources, and Functions of Minerals

Most major and trace minerals occur freely in nature, mainly in the waters of rivers, lakes, and oceans; in topsoil; and beneath the earth's surface. Minerals exist in the root systems of plants and in the body structure of animals that consume plants and water containing minerals. **Table 2.6** lists the major bodily

ⓘ For Your Information

NOT WHAT MOST PEOPLE THINK

Think again if you are counting on your daily multivitamin pill to ward off the killer chronic diseases cancer or heart disease. The largest study to date of multivitamin use in 161,808 postmenopausal women published in the February 2009 *Archives of Internal Medicine* reported that vitamin supplementation did *not affect* the risk of cancer, heart disease, or overall mortality—and it made no difference how long the supplements were taken. This is unfortunate because Americans spend about $23 billion annually on these supplements. The study's lead author offers this advice: "Get nutrients from food. Whole foods are better than dietary supplements."

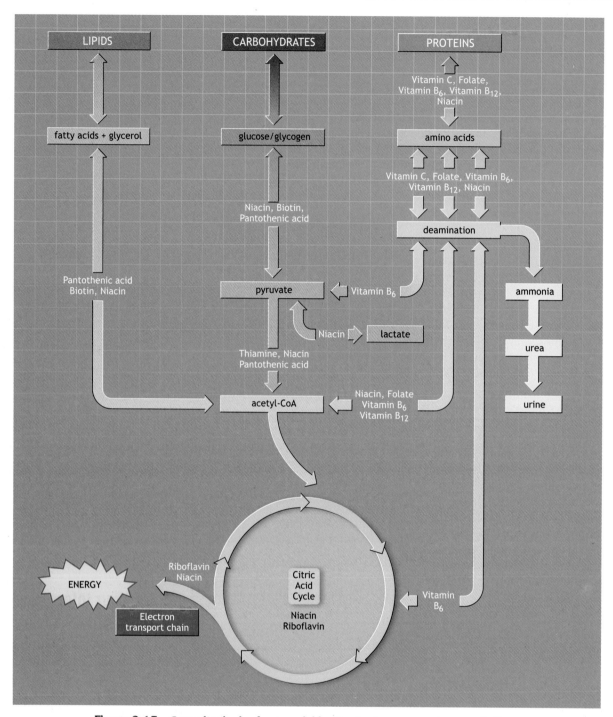

Figure 2.15 Generalized role of water-soluble vitamins in macronutrient metabolism.

functions, dietary sources, and symptoms of a deficiency and excess for important major and trace minerals.

Minerals often become part of the body's structures, and existing chemicals and serve three broad roles:

1. Provide structure in forming bones and teeth.
2. Help to maintain normal heart rhythm, muscle contractility, neural conductivity, and acid–base balance.
3. Help to regulate cellular metabolism by becoming part of enzymes and hormones that modulate cellular activity.

Figure 2.16 lists minerals that participate in catabolic and anabolic cellular processes. Minerals activate numerous reactions, releasing energy during carbohydrate, fat, and protein catabolism. Minerals help to synthesize biologic nutrients—glycogen from glucose, triacylglycerols from fatty acids and glycerol, and proteins from amino acids. Without the essential minerals, the fine balance would be disrupted between catabolism and anabolism. Minerals also form important constituents of hormones. An inadequate thyroxine production from iodine deficiency, for example,

Table 2.6	Important Major and Trace Minerals for Healthy Adults (Ages 19–50 Years): Their Food Sources, Functions, and Effects of Deficiencies and Excesses[a]			
MINERAL	**DIETARY SOURCES**	**MAJOR BODILY FUNCTIONS**	**DEFICIENCY**	**EXCESS**
Major				
Calcium	Milk, cheese, dark green vegetables, dried legumes	Bone and tooth formation; blood clotting; nerve transmission	Stunted growth; rickets, osteoporosis; convulsions	Not reported in humans
Phosphorus	Milk, cheese, yogurt, meat, poultry, grains, fish	Bone and tooth formation; acid-base balance	Weakness, demineralization of bone; loss of calcium	Erosion of jaw (phossy jaw)
Potassium	Leafy vegetables, cantaloupe, lima beans, potatoes, bananas, milk, meats, coffee, tea	Fluid balance; nerve transmission; acid-base balance	Muscle cramps; irregular cardiac rhythm; mental confusion; loss of appetite; can be life-threatening	None if kidneys function normally; poor kidney function causes potassium buildup and cardiac arrhythmias
Sulfur	Obtained as part of dietary protein, and present in food preservatives	Acid-based balance; liver function	Unlikely to occur with adequate dietary intake	Unknown
Sodium	Common salt	Acid-based balance; body water balance; nerve function	Muscle cramps; mental apathy; reduced appetite	High blood pressure
Chlorine (chloride)	Part of salt-containing food; some vegetables and fruits	Important part of extracellular fluids	Unlikely to occur with adequately dietary intake	With sodium, contributes to high blood pressure
Magnesium	Whole grains, green leafy vegetables	Activates enzymes in protein synthesis	Growth failure; behavioral disturbances; weakness, spasms	Diarrhea
Trace				
Iron	Eggs, lean meats, legumes, whole grains, green leafy vegetables	Constituent of hemoglobin and enzymes involved in energy metabolism	Iron deficiency anemia (weakness, reduced resistance to infection)	Siderosis; cirrhosis of liver
Fluorine	Drinking water, tea, seafood	May be important to maintain bone structure	Higher frequency of tooth decay	Mottling of teeth; increased bone density; neurologic disturbances
Zinc	Widely distributed in foods	Constituent of digestive enzymes	Growth failure; small sex glands	Fever, nausea, vomiting, diarrhea
Copper	Meats, drinking water	Constituent of enzymes associated with iron metabolism	Anemia, bone changes (rare in humans)	Rare metabolic condition (Wilson's disease)
Selenium	Seafood, meat, grains	Functions in close association with vitamin E	Anemia (rare)	Gastrointestinal disorders; lung irritation
Iodine (iodide)	Marine fish and shellfish, dairy products, vegetables, iodized salt	Constituent of thyroid hormones	Goiter (enlarged thyroid)	Very high intakes depress thyroid activity
Chromium	Legumes, cereals, organ meats, fats, vegetable oils, meats, whole grains	Constituent of some enzymes; involved in glucose and energy metabolism	Rarely reported in humans; impaired glucose metabolism	Inhibition of enzymes; occupational exposures; skin and kidney damage

[a]Food and Nutrition Board, National Academy of Sciences. (2009). *http://www.nal.usda.gov/fnic/etext/000105.html.*

slows resting metabolism. In extreme cases, this predisposes a person to obesity. The synthesis of insulin, the hormone that facilitates cellular glucose uptake, requires zinc as do approximately 100 enzymes, and the mineral chlorine forms the digestive acid hydrochloric acid.

Minerals and Physical Activity

Food sources in a well-balanced diet readily provide the minerals required by the body. The next sections describe specific functions for important minerals related to physical activity.

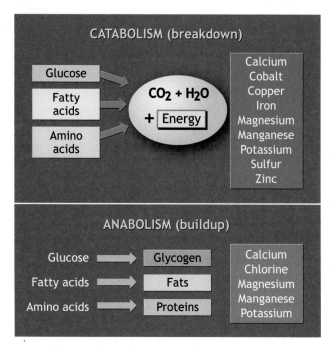

Figure 2.16 Minerals contribute to macronutrient catabolism (breakdown) and anabolism (buildup).

Calcium

Calcium, the most abundant mineral in the body, combines with phosphorus to form bones and teeth. These two minerals represent about 75% of the body's total mineral content of about 2.5% of body mass. In ionized form (~1% of the body's 1200 mg of cal-

cium), calcium is involved in these six important functions:

1. Muscle action
2. Blood clotting
3. Nerve impulse transmission
4. Activation of several enzymes, (e.g., tissue transglutaminase, mitochondrial glycerol phosphate dehydrogenase [mGPD])
5. Synthesis of calciferol (active form of vitamin D)
6. Fluid transport across cell membranes

Osteoporosis: Calcium Intake, and Exercise   The skeleton contains more than 99% of the body's total calcium. With calcium deficiency, the body draws on its calcium reserves in bone to replace the deficit. With prolonged negative imbalance, **osteoporosis** (literally meaning "porous bones") eventually develops as the bones lose calcium mass (mineral content) and calcium concentration (mineral density) and progressively become porous and brittle. **Figure 2.17** illustrates two opposing processes: (1) the buildup of calcium by its efficient transport from the small intestine for storage in the bone matrix (note that the blue arrowhead points into the bone) and (2) inadequate calcium intake or the ineffective absorption of calcium by the intestinal mucosa, where calcium travels in the opposite direction from the bone into bodily fluids, called *calcium resorption*. Leaching of calcium from the bones remains a destructive process that leaves bones hollow and fenestrated. The end result, osteoporosis, negatively impacts males and females of all ages.

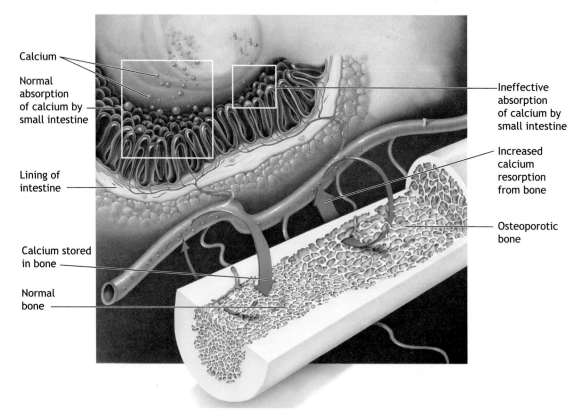

Figure 2.17   (1) Calcium buildup by its efficient transport from the small intestines for storage in the bone matrix (note that the large *blue arrowhead* points into the bone) and (2) the opposing process of ineffective calcium intestinal absorption, where calcium leaches from the bones (large *blue arrowhead* points into blood stream), leaving them brittle and likely to fracture.

Osteoporosis currently affects 44 million Americans, or 55% of people 50 years of age and older, with 68% women. Today in the United States, approximately 10 million individuals already live with the disease, and almost 34 million more are estimated to have low bone mass (**osteopenia**). Fifty percent of all women eventually develop osteoporosis, primarily from their relatively low calcium intake and the loss of the calcium-conserving hormone estrogen at menopause. Men are not immune; men with osteoporosis totalled 2 million in 2009. This number is expected to exceed 20 million in 2020 (*www.nof.org/*). Osteoporosis, a silent disease that sometimes goes undetected for years until a bone fracture occurs. It accounts for more than 1.6 million fractures yearly, including about 700,000 spinal fractures, 250,000 wrist fractures, 300,000 hip fractures, and 300,000 fractures at other sites. Among women older than age 60 years, osteoporosis has reached near-epidemic proportions. On average, 24% of hip fracture patients older than 50 years of age die in the year following their fracture.

Dietary Calcium Crucial.   As a general guideline, adolescent boys and girls (ages 9–13 years of age) and young adult men and women (14–18 years of age) require 1300 mg of calcium daily or about as much calcium in six 8-oz glasses of milk. For adults between the ages of 19 and 50 years, the daily requirement decreases to 1000 mg. Although growing children require more calcium per unit body mass on a daily basis than adults, many adults remain deficient in calcium intake. For example, the typical adult's daily calcium intake ranges between 500 and 700 mg. More than 75% of adults consume less than the recommended amount, and about 25% of women in the United States consume less than 300 mg of calcium daily. Athletes, female dancers, gymnasts, and endurance competitors are the most prone to calcium dietary insufficiency.

Exercise Helps.   *Regular exercise slows the rate of skeletal aging.* Regardless of age or gender, young children and adults who maintain physically active lifestyles achieve greater bone mass compared with sedentary counterparts. For men and women who remain physically active, even at ages 70 and 80 years, bone mass exceeds that of sedentary individuals of similar age. The decline in vigorous exercise as one ages closely parallels the age-related loss of bone mass.

Exercise of moderate intensity provides a safe and potent stimulus to maintain and even increase bone mass. **Weight-bearing exercise** represents a particularly desirable form of exercise; examples include walking, running, dancing, and rope skipping. Resistance training, which generates considerable muscular force against the body's long bones, also proves beneficial. Exercise benefits depend on adequate calcium availability for the bone-forming process.

Female Athlete Triad: An Unexpected Problem for Women Who Train Intensely

A paradox exists between exercise and bone dynamics for athletic premenopausal women. Women who train intensely and emphasize weight loss often engage in **disordered eating behaviors,** which in the extreme, cause life-threatening complications (see *How to Recognize Warning Signs of Disordered Eating* in

 For Your Information

FIFTEEN RISK FACTORS FOR OSTEOPOROSIS

1. Advancing age
2. History of fracture as an adult, independent of cause
3. History of fracture in a parent or sibling
4. Cigarette smoking
5. Slight build or tendency toward being underweight
6. White or Asian female
7. Sedentary lifestyle
8. Early menopause
9. Eating disorder
10. High protein intake (particularly animal protein)
11. Excess sodium intake
12. Alcohol abuse
13. Calcium-deficient diet before and after menopause
14. High caffeine intake (equivocal)
15. Vitamin D deficiency (prevalent in ~40% of adults)

 For Your Information

BONE HEALTH DIAGNOSTIC CRITERIA BASED ON VARIATION (STANDARD DEVIATION [SD]) OF OBSERVED BONE DENSITY VALUES COMPARED WITH VALUES FOR A GENDER-MATCHED YOUNG ADULT POPULATION

Normal	<1.0 SD below mean
Osteopenia	1.0 to 2.5 SD below mean
Osteoporosis	>2.5 SD below mean
Severe osteoporosis	> 2.5 SD below mean plus one or more fragility fractures

 For Your Information

REGULAR EXERCISE AND INCREASED MUSCLE STRENGTH SLOW SKELETAL AGING

Moderate- to high-intensity aerobic exercise (weight bearing) performed 3 days per week for 50 to 60 minutes each builds bone and retards its rate of loss. Muscle-strengthening exercises also benefit bone mass. Individuals with greater back strength and those who train regularly with resistance exercise have a greater spinal bone mineral content than weaker and untrained individuals.

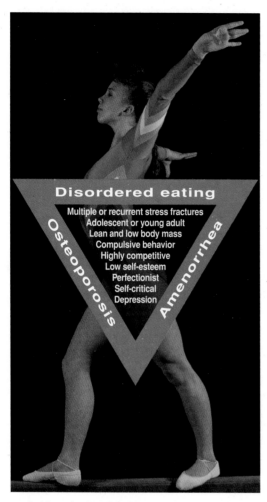

Figure 2.18 The female athlete triad: disordered eating, amenorrhea, and osteoporosis.

Chapter 16). Disordered eating decreases energy availability. This has the effect of reducing body mass and body fat to a point where the menstrual cycle becomes irregular (**oligomenorrhea**) or ceases (**secondary amenorrhea**). The tightly integrated continuum illustrated in **Figure 2.18** that begins with disordered eating and ends with energy drain, amenorrhea, and eventual osteoporosis reflects the clinical entity labeled the **female athlete triad**.

Many girls and young women who participate in sports have at least one of the triad's disorders, particularly disordered eating behavior. Many female athletes of the 1970s and 1980s believed the loss of normal menstruation reflected hard training and the inevitable consequence of athletic success. Whereas the prevalence of amenorrhea among female athletes in body weight-related sports (distance running, gymnastics, ballet, cheerleading, figure skating, and body building) probably ranges between 25% and 65%, no more than 5% of the general population suffer from this condition.

Sodium, Potassium, and Chlorine

The minerals sodium, potassium, and chlorine, collectively termed **electrolytes**, dissolve in the body as electrically charged ion particles. Sodium and chlorine represent the chief minerals contained in blood plasma and extracellular fluid. Electrolytes modulate fluid movement within the body's various fluid compartments. This allows for a constant, well-regulated exchange of nutrients and waste products between the cell and its external fluid environment. Potassium represents the chief intracellular mineral.

Establishing proper electrical gradients across cell membranes represents the most important function of sodium and potassium ions. A difference in electrical balance between the cell's interior and exterior allows nerve impulse transmission, muscle stimulation and contraction, and proper gland functioning. Electrolytes maintain plasma membrane permeability and regulate the acid and base qualities of body fluids, particularly blood.

Sodium: How Much Is Enough? The wide distribution of sodium in foods makes it easy to obtain the daily requirement without adding salt to foods. In the United States, sodium intake regularly exceeds the daily level recommended for adults of 2400 mg or the amount of one heaping teaspoon of table salt (sodium makes up about 40% of salt). The typical Western diet contains about 4500 mg of sodium (8–12 g of salt) each day. This represents 10 times the 500 mg of sodium the body actually needs. Reliance on table salt in processing, curing, cooking, seasoning, and preserving common foods accounts for the large sodium intake. Aside from table salt, common sodium-rich dietary sources include monosodium glutamate (MSG), soy sauce, condiments, canned foods, baking soda, and baking powder.

A normal sodium balance in the body usually occurs throughout a range of dietary intakes. For some individuals, excessive sodium intake becomes inadequately regulated. A chronic excess of dietary sodium can increase fluid volume and possibly increase peripheral vascular resistance; both factors could elevate blood pressure to levels that pose a health risk. **Sodium-induced hypertension** occurs in about one-third of hypertensive individuals in the United States.

For decades, the first line of defense in treating high blood pressure attempted to minimize excess sodium from the diet. Conventional wisdom maintains that by reducing sodium intake, perhaps the body's sodium and fluid levels would be reduced, thereby lowering blood pressure. Sodium restriction per se, however, does not lower blood pressure in people with normal blood pressure. Certain individuals, however, remain "**salt sensitive**"—reducing dietary sodium decreases their blood pressure and thus provides a prudent, nonpharmacologic first line of defense.

Iron

The body normally contains between 3 to 5 g (about one-sixth oz) of iron. Of this amount, approximately 80% exists in functionally active compounds, predominantly combined with hemoglobin in red blood cells. This iron–protein compound increases the oxygen-carrying capacity of blood approximately 65 times. Iron also serves

Table 2.7	Recommended Dietary Allowances for Iron[a]	
	AGE (y)	IRON (mg/d)
Children	1–3	7
	4–8	10
Men	9–13	8
	14–18	11
	19–70	8
Women	9–13	8
	14–18	15
	19–50	18
	51–70	8
Pregnant	<19	27
	≥19	27
Lactating	<19	10
	≥19	9

[a]Food and Nutrition Board, Institute of Medicine. (2002). *Dietary Reference Intakes: Recommended Intakes for Individuals.* Washington, DC: National Academy Press. Available at *www.iom.edu.*

*Q*uestions & Notes

Briefly describe the female athlete triad.

as a structural component of myoglobin (~5% of total iron), a compound similar to hemoglobin that stores oxygen for release within muscle cells. Small amounts of iron exist in cytochromes, the specialized substances that transfer cellular energy.

Iron Stores About 20% of the body's iron does not combine in functionally active compounds. **Hemosiderin** and **ferritin** constitute the iron stores in the liver, spleen, and bone marrow. These stores replenish iron lost from the functional compounds and provide the iron reserve during periods of insufficient dietary iron intake. A plasma protein, **transferrin**, transports iron from ingested food and damaged red blood cells to tissues in need. Plasma levels of transferrin often reflect the adequacy of the current iron intake.

Athletes should include normal amounts of iron-rich foods in their daily diets. People with inadequate iron intake or with limited rates of iron absorption or high rates of iron loss often develop a reduced concentration of hemoglobin in the red blood cells. This extreme condition of iron insufficiency, commonly called **iron deficiency anemia**, produces general sluggishness, loss of appetite, and reduced capacity to sustain even mild exercise. "Iron therapy" normalizes the hemoglobin content of the blood and exercise capacity. Table 2.7 lists recommendations for iron intake for children and adults.

For Your Information

SIX PRINCIPLES TO PROMOTE BONE HEALTH

1. *Specificity:* Exercise provides a local osteogenic effect.
2. *Overload:* Progressively increasing exercise intensity promotes continued improvement.
3. *Initial values:* Individuals with the smallest total bone mass have the greatest potential for improvement.
4. *Diminishing returns:* As one approaches the biologic ceiling for bone density, further gains require greater effort.
5. *More not necessarily better:* Bone cells become desensitized in response to prolonged mechanical-loading sessions.
6. *Reversibility:* Discontinuing exercise overload reverses the positive osteogenic effects of exercise.

For Your Information

LESS MAY BE EVEN MORE BENEFICIAL

The Centers for Disease Control and Prevention (*www.cdc.gov*) says that nearly 70% of adult Americans should follow a low-salt diet that cuts recommended daily sodium intake of 2300 mg to 1500 mg, about that found in two-thirds of a teaspoon of salt. The three groups at special risk for sodium sensitivity include (1) people with existing hypertension (30.5% of the adult population), (2) those age 40 years and older without hypertension (34.4%), and (3) African Americans ages 20 to 39 years without hypertension (4.2%). And reducing sodium intake may have health benefits beyond lowering blood pressure; it may improve flow-mediated dilatation, the measure of a blood vessel's healthy ability to relax.

BOX 2.3   CLOSE UP

Lowering High Blood Pressure with Dietary Intervention: The DASH Diet

Nearly 50 million Americans have hypertension, a condition that, if left untreated, increases the risk of stroke, heart attack, and kidney failure. Fifty percent of people with hypertension seek treatment; only about half of these individuals achieve long-term success. One reason for the lack of compliance concerns possible side effects of readily available antihypertensive medication. For example, fatigue and impotence often discourage patients from maintaining a chronic medication schedule required by pharmacologic treatment of hypertension.

THE DASH APPROACH

Research using DASH (Dietary Approaches to Stop Hypertension; *www.nhlbi.nih.gov/health/public/heart/hbp/dash/new_dash.pdf*) shows that this diet lowers blood pressure in some individuals to the same extent as pharmacologic therapy and often more than other lifestyle changes. Two months of the diet reduced systolic pressure by an average of 11.4 mm Hg; diastolic pressure decreased by 5.5 mm Hg. Every 2 mm Hg reduction in systolic pressure lowers heart disease risk by 5% and stroke risk by 8%. Further good news emerges from recent research indicating that the standard DASH diet combined with a daily dietary salt intake of 1500 mg produces even greater blood pressure reductions than achieved with the DASH diet only.

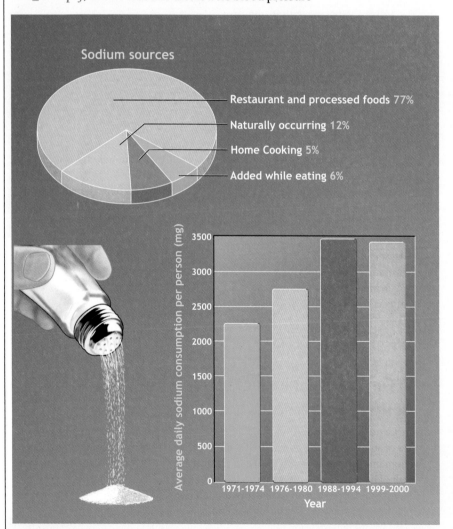

Sodium sources

Restaurant and processed foods 77%

Naturally occurring 12%

Home Cooking 5%

Added while eating 6%

Consumer groups and the American Medical Association (*www.ama.org*) urge the limitation of salt in foods to combat high blood pressure, prevalent in about 40% of the U.S. population. Adults now consume 4000 mg of sodium daily, almost double the 2400 mg (1 tsp of salt) recommended. Much of this excess comes from restaurant and processed foods.

Table 1 shows the general goals and nature of the DASH diet for a 2100-calorie (kCal) eating plan with its high content of fruits, vegetables, and dairy products and low-fat composition. In addition, a 24-year follow-up of women whose diets most closely resembled the DASH plan were 24% less likely to develop heart disease and 18% less likely to have a stroke.

Table 1	Daily Nutrient Goals Used in the DASH Studies for a 2100-Calorie Eating Plan

Total fat	27% of calories	Sodium	2300 mg[a]
Saturated fat	6% of calories	Potassium	4700 mg
Protein	18% of calories	Calcium	1250 mg
Carbohydrate	55% of calories	Magnesium	500 mg
Cholesterol	150 mg	Fiber	30 g

FOOD GROUP	DAILY SERVINGS	SERVING SIZES
Grains[b]	6–8	1 slice bread 1 oz dry cereal[c] ½ cup cooked rice, pasta, or cereal
Vegetables	4–5	1 cup raw, leafy vegetable ½ cup cut-up raw or cooked vegetable ½ cup vegetable juice
Fruits	4–5	1 medium fruit ¼ cup dried fruit ½ cup fresh, frozen, or canned fruit ½ cup fruit juice
Fat-free or low-fat milk and mild products	2–3	1 cup milk or yogurt 1½ oz cheese
Lean meats, poultry, and fish	≤6	1 oz cooked meats, poultry, or fish 1 egg
Nuts, seeds, and legumes	4–5 per week	⅓ cup or 1½ oz nuts 2 tbsp peanut butter 2 tbsp or ½ oz seeds ½ cup cooked legumes (dry beans and peas)
Fats and oils	2–3	1 tsp soft margarine 1 tsp vegetable oil 1 tbsp mayonnaise 2 tbsp salad dressing
Sweets and added sugars	≤5 per week	1 tbsp sugar 1 tbsp jelly or jam ½ cup sorbet, gelatin 1 cup lemonade

[a]1500 mg sodium was a lower goal tested and found to be even better for lowering blood pressure. It was particularly effective for middle-aged and older individuals, African Americans, and those who already had high blood pressure.
[b]Whole grains are recommended for most grain servings as a good source of fiber and nutrients.
[c]Serving sizes vary between ½ cup and 1¼ cups, depending on cereal type. Check the product's Nutrition Facts label.
DASH, Dietary Approaches to Stop Hypertension. From US Department of Health and Human Services, National Institutes of Health, National Heart, Lung, and Blood Institute (2006). *Your Guide to Lowering Your Blood Pressure with DASH*. Available at *www.nhlbi.nih.gov/health/public/ heart/hbp/dash/new_dash.pdf*.

Sample DASH Diet

Table 2 shows a sample DASH diet (including recommended substitutions to reduce sodium to 1500 mg daily) consisting of approximately 2100 kCal. This level of energy intake provides a stable body weight for a typical 70-kg person. More physically active and heavier individuals should boost their portion size or the number of individual items to maintain their weight. Individuals desiring to lose weight or who are lighter or sedentary should eat less but not less than the minimum number of servings for each food group shown on page 68.

(continued)

BOX 2.3 CLOSE UP

Lowering High Blood Pressure with Dietary Intervention: The DASH Diet (Continued)

Table 2 Sample DASH Diet (Including Recommended Substitutions to Reduce Sodium to 1500 mg Daily) Consisting of Approximately 2100 kCal

2300 mg SODIUM MENU	SODIUM (mg)	SUBSTITUTION TO REDUCE SODIUM TO 1500 mg	SODIUM (mg)
Breakfast			
¾ cup bran flakes cereal:	220	3/4 cup shredded wheat cereal	1
1 medium banana	1		
1 cup low-fat milk	107		
1 slice whole wheat bread:	149		
1 tsp soft (tub) margarine	26	1 tsp unsalted soft (tub) margarine	0
1 cup orange juice	5		
Lunch			
¾ cup chicken salad:[a]	179	Remove salt from the recipe[a]	120
2 slices whole wheat bread	299		
1 tbsp Dijon mustard	373	1 tbsp regular mustard	175
Salad:			
½ cup fresh cucumber slices	1		
½ cup tomato wedges	5		
1 tbsp sunflower seeds	0		
1 tsp Italian dressing, low calorie	43		
½ cup fruit cocktail, juice pack	5		
Dinner			
3 oz beef, eye of the round:	35		
2 tbsp beef gravy, fat free	165		
1 cup green beans, sautéed with:	12		
½ tsp canola oil	0		
1 small baked potato:	14		
1 tbsp sour cream, fat free	21		
1 tbsp grated natural cheddar cheese, reduced fat	67	1 tbsp natural cheddar cheese, reduced fat, low sodium	1
1 small whole-wheat roll:	148		
1 tsp soft (tub) margarine	26	1 tsp unsalted soft (tub) margarine	0
1 small apple	1		
1 cup low-fat milk	107		
Snacks			
⅓ cup almonds, unsalted	0		
¼ cup raisins	4		
½ cup fruit yogurt, fat-free, no sugar added	86		
Totals	2101		1507

[a]1500 mg sodium was a lower goal tested and found to be even better for lowering blood pressure. It was particularly effective for middle-aged and older individuals, African Americans, and those who already had high blood pressure.
DASH, Dietary Approaches to Stop Hypertension. From US Department of Health and Human Services, National Institutes of Health, National Heart, Lung, and Blood Institute (2006). *Your Guide to Lowering Your Blood Pressure with DASH.* Available at *www.nhlbi.nih.gov/health/public/heart/hbp/dash/new_dash.pdf.*

REFERENCES

Calton J.B.: Prevalence of micronutrient deficiency in popular diet plans. *J. Int. Soc. Sports Nutr.,* 10:24, 2010.

Smith P.J., et al.: Effects of the dietary approaches to stop hypertension diet, exercise, and caloric restriction on neurocognition in overweight adults with high blood pressure. *Hypertension,* 55:1331, 2010.

Troyer J.L., et al.: The effect of home-delivered Dietary Approach to Stop Hypertension (DASH) meals on the diets of older adults with cardiovascular disease. *Am. J. Clin. Nutr.,* 91:1204, 2010.

Of Concern to Vegetarians   *The relatively low bioavailability of non-heme iron places women on vegetarian-type diets at risk for developing iron insufficiency.* Female vegetarian runners have a poorer iron status than their counterparts who consume the same quantity of iron from predominantly animal sources. Including vitamin C–rich food in the diet enhances dietary iron bioavailability. This occurs because ascorbic acid increases the solubility of non-heme iron, making it available for absorption at the alkaline pH of the small intestine. The ascorbic acid in one glass of orange juice, for example, stimulates a threefold increase in non-heme iron absorption from a breakfast meal.

Females: A Population at Risk   Inadequate iron intake frequently occurs among young children, teenagers, and females of childbearing age, including physically active women.

Iron loss during a menstrual cycle ranges between 5 and 45 mg. This produces an additional 5-mg dietary iron requirement daily for premenopausal females, increasing the average monthly dietary iron intake need by about 150 mg. The small intestine absorbs only about 15% of ingested iron. This depends on one's current iron status, form of iron ingested, and meal composition. An additional 20 to 25 mg of iron becomes available each month (from the additional 150-mg monthly dietary requirement) for synthesizing red blood cells lost during menstruation. Not surprisingly, 30% to 50% of American women experience dietary iron insufficiencies from menstrual blood loss, including their limited dietary iron intake.

Athletes and Iron Supplements   *If an individual's diet contains the recommended iron intake, supplementing with iron does not increase hemoglobin, hematocrit, or other measures of iron status.* Any increase in iron loss with exercise training coupled with poor dietary habits in adolescent and premenopausal women could strain an already limited iron reserve. This does not mean that individuals involved in strenuous training should take supplementary iron or that indicators of sports anemia result from dietary iron deficiency or exercise-induced iron loss. Iron overconsumption or overabsorption could potentially cause harm. Over-the-counter supplements containing high levels of iron should not be used indiscriminately; excessive iron can accumulate to toxic levels and contribute to diabetes, liver disease, and heart and joint damage. Iron excess may even facilitate growth of latent cancers and infectious organisms. Athletes' iron status should be monitored by periodic evaluation of hematologic characteristics and iron reserves.

Minerals and Exercise Performance

Consuming mineral supplements above recommended levels on an acute or chronic basis does not benefit exercise performance or enhance training responsiveness. However, loss of water and the mineral salts sodium chloride and potassium chloride in sweat does pose an important challenge in prolonged, hot weather exercise. Excessive water and electrolyte loss impairs heat tolerance and exercise performance and can trigger heat cramps, heat exhaustion, or heat stroke. The yearly number of heat-related deaths during spring and summer football practice provides a tragic illustration of the importance of replacing fluids and electrolytes. During practice or competition, an athlete may sweat up to 5 kg of water. This corresponds to about 8.0 g of salt depletion because each kilogram (1 L) of sweat contains about 1.5 g of salt (of which 40% represents sodium). Immediate replacement of water lost through sweating should become the overriding consideration.

Defense Against Mineral Loss in Exercise   Vigorous exercise
triggers a rapid and coordinated release of the hormones **vasopressin** and **aldosterone** and the enzyme **renin** to minimize sodium and water loss

Questions & Notes

Give the recommended iron intake for a college-aged male and female.

Describe the term sports anemia *and those most susceptible.*

 For Your Information

FUNCTIONAL ANEMIA; NORMAL HEMOGLOBIN BUT LOW IRON RESERVES

A relatively high prevalence of non-anemic iron depletion exists among athletes in diverse sports as well as in recreationally active women and men. Low values for hemoglobin within the "normal" range often reflect **functional anemia** or **marginal iron deficiency.** Depleted iron reserves and reduced iron-dependent protein production (e.g., oxidative enzymes) with a relatively normal hemoglobin concentration (non-anemic) characterize this condition. The ergogenic effects of iron supplementation on aerobic exercise performance and training responsiveness benefit these iron-deficient athletes.

Current recommendations support iron supplementation for non-anemic physically active women with low serum ferritin (measure of iron reserves) levels. Supplementation in this case exerts little effect on hemoglobin concentration and red blood cell volume. Any improved exercise capacity likely occurs from increased muscle oxidative capacity, not the blood's increased oxygen transport capacity.

BOX 2.4 CLOSE UP

Exercise-Induced Anemia: Fact or Fiction?

Research has focused on the influence of vigorous training on the body's iron status, primarily because of interest in endurance sports and increased participation of women in such activities. The term "sports anemia" frequently describes reduced hemoglobin levels approaching **clinical anemia** (12 g per 100 mL of blood for women and 14 g per 100 mL for men) attributable to intense training. Some researchers maintain that exercise training creates an added demand for iron that often exceeds its intake. This taxes iron reserves, which eventually slows hemoglobin synthesis or reduces iron-containing compounds within the cell's energy transfer system. Individuals susceptible to an "iron drain" could experience reduced exercise capacity because of iron's crucial role in oxygen transport and utilization.

Heavy training could theoretically create an augmented iron demand (facilitating development of clinical anemia). This loss of iron could come from iron loss in sweat and hemoglobin loss in urine caused by red blood cell destruction with increased temperature, spleen activity, and circulation rates and from mechanical trauma (**foot-strike hemolysis**) from the feet repetitively pounding the running surface. Gastrointestinal bleeding may also occur with long-distance running. Such iron loss, regardless of the cause, stresses the body's iron reserves for synthesizing 260 billion new red blood cells daily in the bone marrow of the skull, upper arm, sternum, ribs, spine, pelvis, and upper legs. Iron losses pose an additional burden to women because they have the greatest iron requirement yet lowest iron intake.

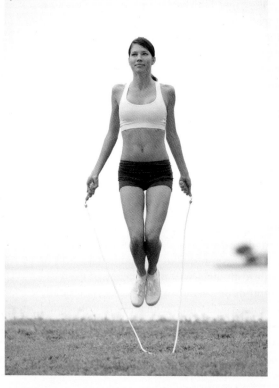

Suboptimal hemoglobin concentrations and hematocrits occur frequently among endurance athletes, thus supporting the possibility of an exercise-induced anemia. On closer scrutiny, however, transient reductions in hemoglobin concentration occur in the early phase of training and then return toward pretraining values.

A decrease in hemoglobin concentration with training parallels the disproportionately large expansion in plasma volume compared with total hemoglobin. Thus, total hemoglobin (an important factor in endurance performance) remains the same or increases somewhat with training, yet hemoglobin concentration (expressed in mg per 100 mL blood) decreases in the expanding plasma volume.

Aerobic capacity and exercise performance normally improve with training despite the apparent dilution of hemoglobin. Although vigorous exercise may induce some mechanical destruction of red blood cells (including minimal iron loss in sweat), these factors do not appear to strain an athlete's iron reserves to precipitate clinical anemia as long as iron intake remains within the normal range. Applying stringent criteria for what constitutes anemia and insufficiency of iron reserves makes "true" sports anemia much less prevalent among highly trained athletes than believed. For male collegiate runners and swimmers, large changes in training volume and intensity during various phases of the competitive season did not reveal the early stages of anemia. Data from female athletes also confirm that the prevalence of iron deficiency anemia did *not* differ in comparison with specific athletic groups or with nonathletic controls.

through the kidneys and sweat. An increase in sodium conservation by the kidneys occurs even under extreme marathon running in warm, humid weather during which sweat output often reaches 2 L per hour. Adding a slight amount of salt to fluid ingested or food consumed

usually replenishes electrolytes lost in sweat. For runners during a 20-day road race in Hawaii, plasma minerals remained normal when the athletes consumed an unrestricted diet *without* mineral supplements. This finding (and the findings of others) indicates that ingesting "athletic drinks" provides no special benefit in replacing the minerals lost through sweating compared with ingesting the same minerals in a well-balanced diet. Taking extra salt may prove beneficial for prolonged exercise in the heat when fluid loss exceeds 4 or 5 kg. This can be achieved by drinking a 0.1% to 0.2% salt solution (adding 0.3 tsp of table salt per L of water). Intense exercise during heat stress can produce a mild potassium deficiency. A diet that contains the recommended amount of this mineral corrects any deficiencies. Drinking an 8-oz glass of orange or tomato juice replaces the calcium, potassium, and magnesium lost in 3 L (7 lb) of sweat, a sweat loss not likely to occur if an individual performs less than 60 minutes of vigorous exercise. Older age Master's athletes and other older recreational enthusiasts who take blood pressure medications should remain vigilant against dehydration symptoms (dizziness, lightheadedness, nausea) during exercise from the medication's effect to lower the blood pressure coupled with water and fluid losses from the environmental and exercise effects.

Give the amount of salt needed per liter of water to make a "homemade" fluid replacement drink.

SUMMARY

1. Vitamins neither supply energy nor contribute to body mass. These organic substances serve crucial functions in almost all bodily processes and must be obtained from food or dietary supplementation.

2. Thirteen known vitamins are classified as either water soluble or fat soluble. Vitamins A, D, E, and K comprise the fat-soluble vitamins; vitamin C and the B-complex vitamins constitute the water-soluble vitamins.

3. Excess fat-soluble vitamins can accumulate in body tissues and increase to toxic concentrations. Except in relatively rare instances, excess water-soluble vitamins remain nontoxic and eventually pass in the urine.

4. Vitamins regulate metabolism, facilitate energy release, and serve important functions in bone formation and tissue synthesis.

5. Vitamins C and E and β-carotene serve key protective antioxidant functions. A diet with appropriate levels of these micronutrients reduces the potential for free radical damage (oxidative stress) and may protect against heart disease and cancer.

6. Excess vitamin supplementation does not improve exercise performance or the potential for sustaining hard, physical training. Serious illness can occur from regularly consuming excess fat-soluble and, in some cases, water-soluble vitamins.

7. Approximately 4% of body mass consists of 22 elements called minerals. They distribute in all body tissues and fluids.

8. Minerals occur freely in nature; in the waters of rivers, lakes, oceans; and in soil. The root system of plants absorbs minerals; minerals eventually incorporate into the tissues of animals that consume plants.

9. Minerals function primarily in metabolism as important parts of enzymes. Minerals provide structure to bones and teeth and in synthesizing glycogen, fat, and protein.

10. A balanced diet provides adequate mineral intake except in geographic locations with inadequate iodine in the soil.

11. Osteoporosis has reached epidemic proportions among older individuals, especially women. Adequate calcium intake and regular weight-bearing exercise or resistance training can protect against bone loss at any age.

12. Women who train vigorously often do not match energy intake to energy output. Reduced body weight and body fat can adversely affect menstruation and cause advanced bone loss at an early age. Restoration of normal menses does not necessarily restore bone mass.

13. About 40% of American women of childbearing age have dietary iron insufficiency. This could lead to iron-deficiency anemia, which negatively affects aerobic exercise performance and the ability to perform heavy training.

14. For women on vegetarian-type diets, the relatively low bioavailability of non-heme iron increases risk for iron insufficiency. Vitamin C (in food or supplement form) increases intestinal non-heme iron absorption.

15. Excessive sweating during exercise produces losses of body water and related minerals; these should be replaced during and after exercise. Sweat loss during exercise usually does not increase mineral requirements above recommended values.

THOUGHT QUESTIONS

1. Discuss specific conditions that justify vitamin and mineral supplementation.

2. Discuss factors that may contribute to gender-specific recommendations for vitamin and mineral intakes.

3. Outline the dynamics of bone loss and give suggestions to high school females regarding protection against future osteoporosis.

Part 3   Water

WATER IN THE BODY

Age, gender, and body composition influence an individual's body water content, which can range from 40% to 70% of total body mass. Water constitutes 72% of muscle weight and approximately 50% of the weight of body fat (adipose tissue). Thus, differences among individuals in relative percentage of total body water largely result from variations in body composition (i.e., differences in fat-free versus fat tissue).

The body contains two fluid "compartments." The first, the **intracellular** compartment, refers to fluid inside cells; the second **extracellular** compartment includes (1) blood plasma (~20% of total extracellular fluid) and (2) interstitial fluids, which primarily comprise fluid flowing in the microscopic spaces between cells. Six sources of interstitial fluid include:

1. Lymph
2. Saliva
3. Fluids in the eyes
4. Fluids secreted by glands and the digestive tract
5. Fluids that bathe the nerves of the spinal cord
6. Fluids excreted from the skin and kidneys

Much of the fluid lost through sweating comes from extracellular fluid, predominantly blood plasma.

Functions of Body Water

Water serves six important functions:

1. Provides the body's transport and reactive medium.
2. Diffusion of gases occurs across moist body surfaces.
3. Waste products leave the body through the water in urine and feces.
4. Absorbs considerable heat with only minimal changes in temperature from its heat-stabilizing qualities.
5. Watery fluids lubricate joints, keeping bony surfaces from grinding against each other.
6. Being noncompressible, water provides structure and form through the turgor it imparts to the body's tissues.

Water Balance: Intake Versus Output

The water content of the body remains relatively stable over time. Appropriate fluid intake rapidly restores any imbalance. **Figure 2.19** displays the sources of water intake and water loss (output). The bottom panel illustrates that fluid balance can change dramatically during exercise, especially in a hot, humid environment.

Water Intake   In a normal environment, a sedentary adult requires about 2.5 L of water daily. For an active person in a warm environment, the water requirement often increases to between 5 and 10 L daily. Three sources provide this water:

1. Liquids
2. Foods
3. Metabolic processes

The average individual living in a generally thermoneutral environment normally consumes about 1200 mL or 41 oz of water daily. Fluid intake can increase five or six times above normal during exercise and thermal stress. A decline in body weight of 2 lb in exercise represents a fluid loss of approximately 1 qt of fluid. At the extreme, an individual lost 13.6 kg (30 lb) of water weight during a 2-day, 17-hour, 55-mile run across the desert in Death Valley, California. Proper fluid ingestion with salt supplements kept the body weight loss to only 1.4 kg. In this example, fluid loss and replenishment represented between 3.5 and 4 gal of liquid!

Most fruits and vegetables contain considerable water—more than 90% (e.g., lettuce, celery, cucumber, red and green tomatoes, spinach, zucchini, watermelon, cantaloupe, eggplant, sweet peppers, cabbage and broccoli); in contrast, butter, oils, dried meats, and chocolate, cookies, and cakes contain relatively little water (<20%).

Metabolizing food molecules for energy forms carbon dioxide and water. For a sedentary person, **metabolic water** provides about 25% of the daily water requirement. This includes 55 g of water from the complete breakdown of 100 g of carbohydrate, 100 g of water from 100 g of protein breakdown, and 107 g of water from 100 g of fat catabolism. Additionally, each gram of glycogen joins with 2.7 g of water as the glucose units link together thus making glycogen a

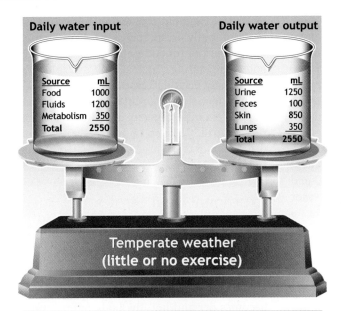

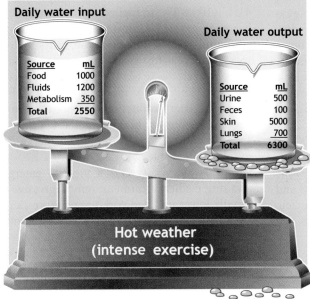

Figure 2.19 Water balance in the body. *Top.* Little or no exercise in normal ambient temperature and humidity. *Bottom.* Moderate to intense exercise in a hot, humid environment.

heavy energy fuel. Glycogen subsequently releases this water during its catabolism for energy. For runners and other endurance athletes who consume additional carbohydrates to "overstock" their muscles' glycogen content, this practice provides a double-edged sword. On the one hand, additional glycogen is essential for elite performance, yet the additional water storage decreases exercise economy because the extra body mass increases energy expenditure.

Water Output   The body loses water in four ways:

1. In urine
2. Through the skin
3. As water vapor in expired air
4. In feces

The kidneys normally reabsorb about 99% of the 140 to 160 L of filtrate formed each day, leaving from 1000 to 1500 mL or about 1.5 qt of urine for excretion daily. Every gram of solute (e.g., the urea end-product of protein

Questions & Notes

Name the 2 fluid compartments of the body.

1.

2.

List 4 ways water is lost from the body.

1.

2.

3.

4.

ⓘ For Your Information

HYDRATION TERMINOLOGY

- *Euhydration:* Normal daily water variation
- *Hyperhydration:* New steady-state condition of increased water content
- *Hypohydration:* New steady-state condition of decreased water content
- *Rehydration:* Process of gaining water from hypohydrated state toward euhydration

ⓘ For Your Information

DON'T RELY ON ORAL TEMPERATURE

Oral temperature does not usually provide an accurate measure of deep body temperature after strenuous exercise. Large and consistent differences occurred between oral and rectal temperatures; for example, the average rectal temperature of 103.5°F after a 14-mile race in a tropical climate differed from a "normal" 98°F when temperature was assessed orally. This 5.5°F discrepancy partly results from evaporative cooling of the mouth and airways during relatively high ventilatory volumes immediately after heavy exercise.

breakdown) eliminated by the kidneys requires about 15 mL of water. From a practical standpoint, consuming large quantities of protein for energy via a high-protein diet *accelerates* dehydration during exercise.

A small amount of water, perhaps 350 mL, termed **insensible perspiration**, continually seeps from the deeper tissues through the skin to the body's surface. Subcutaneous sweat glands also produce water loss through the skin. Evaporation of sweat's water component provides the refrigeration mechanism to cool the body. The daily sweat rate under most conditions amounts to between 500 and 700 mL. This by no means reflects sweating capacity; for example, a well-trained, acclimatized person produces up to 12 L of sweat (equivalent of 12 kg) at a rate of 1 L per hour during prolonged exercise in a hot environment.

Insensible water loss of 250 to 350 mL per day occurs through small water droplets in exhaled air. The complete moistening of all inspired air passing down the pulmonary airways accounts for this loss. Exercise affects this source of water loss. For physically active individuals, the respiratory passages release 2 to 5 mL of water each minute during strenuous exercise, depending on climatic conditions. Ventilatory water loss happens least in hot, humid weather and most in cold temperatures (inspired air contains little moisture). At altitude, the less dense inspired air volumes, which require humidification, also increase fluid loss compared with sea-level conditions.

Intestinal elimination produces between 100 and 200 mL of water loss because water constitutes approximately 70% of fecal matter. The remainder comprises nondigestible material, including bacteria from the digestive process and the residues of digestive juices from the intestine, stomach, and pancreas. With diarrhea or vomiting, water loss can increase to between 1500 and 5000 mL.

WATER REQUIREMENT DURING EXERCISE

The loss of body water represents the most serious consequence of profuse sweating. Three factors determine water loss through sweating:

1. Severity of physical activity
2. Environmental temperature
3. Humidity

The major physiologic defense against overheating comes from evaporation of sweat from the skin's surface. The evaporative loss of 1 L of sweat releases about 600 kCal of heat energy from the body to the environment. **Relative humidity**, which refers to the water content of the ambient air, impacts the efficiency of the sweating mechanism in temperature regulation. At 100% relative humidity, the ambient air is completely saturated with water vapor. This blocks evaporation of fluid from the skin surface to the air, thus minimizing this important avenue for body cooling. When this happens, sweat beads on the skin and eventually rolls off without generating a cooling effect.

Dry air can hold considerable moisture, so fluid evaporates rapidly from the skin. This enables the sweat mechanism to function at optimal efficiency to regulate body temperature. Interestingly, sweat loss equal to 2% to 3% of body mass decreases plasma volume. This amount of fluid loss strains circulatory functions and ultimately impairs exercise capacity and diminishes thermoregulatory control. Chapter 15 presents a more comprehensive discussion of thermoregulatory dynamics during exercise in hot climates.

Exertional Heat Stroke

Heat stroke, the most serious and complex heat stress malady, requires immediate medical attention. Heat stroke syndrome reflects a failure of heat-regulating mechanisms triggered by excessively high body temperatures. With thermoregulatory failure, sweating usually ceases, the skin becomes dry and hot, the body temperature increases to 41°C (105.8°F) or higher, and the circulatory system becomes strained. Unfortunately, subtle symptoms often confound the complexity of exertional hyperthermia. Instead of ceasing, sweating can occur during intense aerobic exercise (e.g., 10-km running race) in young, hydrated, and highly motivated individuals. With high metabolic heat production, the body's heat gain greatly exceeds avenues for heat loss. If left untreated, circulatory collapse and damage to the central nervous system and other organs will lead to death.

Heat stroke represents a medical emergency. While awaiting medical treatment, only aggressive treatment to rapidly lower elevated core temperature can avert death; the magnitude and duration of hyperthermia determine organ damage and mortality. Immediate treatment includes alcohol rubs and application of ice packs. Whole-body cold- or ice-water immersion remains the *most effective* treatment for a collapsed hyperthermic athlete.

Practical Recommendations for Fluid Replacement in Exercise

Depending on environmental conditions, total sweat loss during a marathon run in elite athletes at world record pace averages about 5.3 L (12 lb). The fluid loss corresponds to an overall reduction of 6% to 8% of body mass. *Fluids must be consumed regularly during physical activity to avoid dehydration and its life-threatening consequences.*

Fluid replacement maintains plasma volume to optimize the circulatory and sweating response. Ingesting "extra" water before exercising in the heat provides some thermoregulatory protection. Pre-exercise hyperhydration (1) delays dehydration, (2) increases sweating during exercise, and (3) blunts the increase in body temperature compared with exercising without prior fluids. As a practical step, a person should consume 400 to 600 mL (13–20 oz) of cold water 10 to 20 minutes before exercising. This

BOX 2.5   CLOSE UP

How to Distinguish Among Heat Cramps, Heat Exhaustion, and Heat Stroke

Human heat dissipation occurs by (1) redistribution of blood from deeper tissues to the periphery and (2) activation of the refrigeration mechanism provided by evaporation of sweat from the surface of the skin and respiratory passages. During heat stress, cardiac output increases, vasoconstriction and vasodilation move central blood volume toward the skin, and thousands of previously dormant capillaries threading through the upper skin layer open to accommodate blood flow. Conduction of heat away from warm blood at the skin's cooled surface provides about 75% of the body's heat-dissipating functions. Heat production during physical activity often strains heat-dissipating mechanisms, especially under high ambient temperature and humidity. This triggers a broad array of physical signs and symptoms collectively termed *heat illness*, ranging in severity from mild to life threatening.

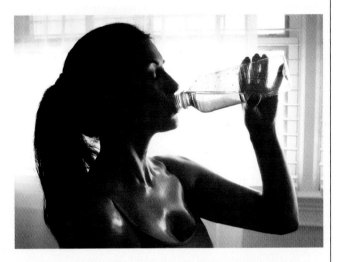

CONDITION	CAUSES	SIGNS AND SYMPTOMS	PREVENTION
Heat Cramps	Intense, prolonged exercise in the heat; negative Na^+ balance	Tightening cramps, involuntary spasms of active muscles; low serum Na^+	Replenish salt loss; ensure acclimatization
Heat Syncope	Peripheral vasodilation and pooling of venous blood; hypotension; hypohydration	Giddiness; syncope, mostly in upright position during rest or exercise; pallor; high rectal temperature	Ensure acclimatization and fluid replenishment; reduce exertion on hot days; avoid standing
Heat Exhaustion	Cumulative negative water balance	Exhaustion; hypohydration, flushed skin; reduced sweating in extreme dehydration; syncope; high rectal temperature	Proper hydration before exercise and adequate replenishment during exercise; ensure acclimatization
Heat Stroke	Extreme hyperthermia leading to thermoregulatory failure; aggravated by dehydration	Acute medical emergency; includes hyperpyrexia (rectal temp > 41°C), lack of sweating, and neurologic deficit (disorientation, twitching, seizures, coma)	Ensure acclimatization; identify and exclude individuals at risk; adapt activities to climatic constraints

prudent practice should be combined with continual fluid replacement during exercise.

Gastric Emptying

The small intestine absorbs fluids after they pass from the stomach. The following seven factors influence gastric emptying:

1. **Fluid temperature.** Cold fluids (5°C or 41°F) empty from the stomach at a faster rate than fluids at body temperature.
2. **Fluid volume.** Keeping fluid volume in the stomach at a relatively high level speeds gastric emptying and may compensate for any inhibitory effects of the beverage's carbohydrate or electrolyte content. Optimizing the effect of stomach volume on gastric emptying occurs by consuming

Questions & Notes

Give the major physiologic defense against overheating.

400 to 600 mL of fluid immediately before exercise. Then regularly ingesting 150 to 250 mL of fluid (at 15-minute intervals) throughout exercise continually replenishes the fluid passed into the intestine and maintains a large gastric volume during exercise.

3. **Caloric content.** Increased energy content decreases the gastric emptying rate.

4. **Fluid osmolarity.** Gastric emptying slows when the ingested fluid contains concentrated electrolytes or simple sugars, whether as glucose, fructose, or sucrose. For example, a 40% sugar solution empties from the stomach at a rate 20% slower than plain water. *As a general rule, between a 5% and 8% carbohydrate–electrolyte beverage consumed during exercise in the heat contributes to temperature regulation and fluid balance as effectively as plain water.* As an added bonus, this drink maintains glucose metabolism and glycogen reserves in prolonged exercise.

5. **Exercise intensity.** Exercise up to an intensity of about 75% of maximum does not negatively affect gastric emptying, at which point the stomach's emptying rate becomes restricted.

6. **pH.** Marked deviations from 7.0 decrease the emptying rate.

7. **Hydration level.** Dehydration decreases gastric emptying and increases the risk of gastrointestinal distress.

The tradeoff between ingested fluid composition and the gastric emptying rate must be evaluated based on environmental stress and energy demands. Exercise in a cold environment does not stimulate much fluid loss from sweating. In this case, reduced gastric emptying and subsequent water absorption are tolerated, and a more concentrated sugar solution (15–20 g per 100 mL of water) may prove beneficial. *For survival, the primary concern during prolonged exercise in the heat becomes fluid replacement.* Chapter 4 addresses the desirable composition of "sports drinks" and their effects on fluid replacement.

Adequacy of Rehydration

Preventing dehydration and its consequences, especially a dangerously elevated body temperature (**hyperthermia**), requires adherence to an adequate water replacement schedule. This often becomes "easier said than done" because some individuals believe ingesting water hinders exercise performance. For some athletes, chronic dehydration remains a way of life during the competitive season. Competitors intentionally lose considerable fluid so they can compete in a lower weight class—often with fatal outcomes if dehydration becomes severe enough to precipitate cardiovascular abnormalities from electrolyte imbalances. Chronic dehydration also occurs in ballet, in which dancers focus on body weight to appear thin. Many individuals on weight loss programs incorrectly believe that restricting fluid intake in some way accelerates body

fat loss. At the extreme, some fanatics and new-age, self-help gurus advocate abstinence of food and fluids for several days while participating in spiritual ceremonies and other so-called "mind and body cleansing" activities while enclosed in sealed heat chambers (essentially saunas covered with plastic tarps called sweat lodges) that exceed 115°F. In a recent tragedy (October 2009), three people died as part of a group crowded into a homemade structure without air circulation for purposes of "cleansing their bodies of toxins!"

Monitoring changes in body weight provide a convenient method to assess (1) fluid loss during exercise or heat stress and (2) adequacy of rehydration in recovery. In addition to having athletes "weigh in" before and after practice, coaches can minimize weight loss by providing scheduled water breaks during practice or training sessions and unrestricted access to water during competition. Each 0.45 kg (1 lb) of body weight loss corresponds to 450 mL (15 oz) of dehydration. After exercising, the thirst mechanism provides an imprecise guide to water needs. If rehydration depended entirely on a person's thirst, it could take several days to reestablish fluid balance after severe dehydration.

Hyponatremia: Water Intoxication

Under normal conditions, one can consume a maximum of about 9.5 L (10 qt) of water daily without unduly straining the kidneys or diluting chemical concentrations of body fluids. Consuming more than 9.5 L can produce **hyponatremia** or water intoxication, a condition related to dilution of the body's normal sodium concentration. In general, mild hyponatremia exists when serum sodium concentration decreases below 135 $mEq \cdot L^{-1}$; serum sodium below 125 $mEq \cdot L^{-1}$ triggers severe symptoms.

A sustained low plasma sodium concentration creates an osmotic imbalance across the blood–brain barrier that forces rapid water influx into the brain. The swelling of brain tissue leads to a cascade of symptoms that range from mild (headache, confusion malaise, nausea, and cramping) to severe (seizures, coma, pulmonary edema, cardiac arrest, and death). The five most important predisposing factors to hyponatremia include:

1. Prolonged intense exercise in hot weather.
2. Poorly conditioned individuals who experience excessive sweat loss with high sodium concentration.
3. Physical activity performed in a sodium-depleted state because of a "salt-free" or "low-sodium" diet.
4. Use of diuretic medication for hypertension.
5. Frequent intake of large quantities of sodium-free fluid during prolonged exercise.

Hyponatremia results from extreme sodium loss through prolonged sweating coupled with dilution of existing extracellular sodium and accompanying reduced osmolality from consuming fluids with low or no sodium. Hyponatremia can occur in experienced athletes. The likely scenario includes intense, ultramarathon-type, continuous exercise lasting 6 to 8 hours, although it can occur in only 4 hours. Nearly 30% of athletes who competed in an Ironman Triathlon experienced symptoms of hyponatremia; these occurred most frequently late in the race or in the recovery after competition. In a large study of more than 18,000 ultra-endurance athletes (including triathletes), approximately 9% of collapsed athletes during or after competition presented with symptoms of hyponatremia. An experienced ultramarathoner required hospitalization after consuming nearly 20 L of fluid during a continuous 62-mile, 8.5-hour run.

ⓘ For Your Information

SIX STEPS TO REDUCE OVERHYDRATION AND HYPONATREMIA RISK DURING PROLONGED EXERCISE

1. Drink 400 to 600 mL (14–22 oz) of fluid 2 to 3 hours before exercise.
2. Drink 150 to 300 mL (5–10 oz) of fluid about 30 minutes before exercise.
3. Drink no more than 1000 mL·h^{-1} (33 oz) of plain water spread over 15-minute intervals during or after exercise.
4. Add approximately 1/4 to 1/2 tsp of salt per 32 oz of ingested fluid.
5. Do not restrict salt in the diet.
6. Adding 5 to 8% glucose to the rehydration drink facilitates intestinal water uptake via the glucose–sodium transport mechanism.

 ## SUMMARY

1. Water constitutes 40% to 70% of an individual's total body mass. Muscle contains 72% water by weight, and water represents only about 50% of the weight of body fat.

2. Approximately 62% of total body water occurs intracellularly (inside the cells), and 38% occurs extracellularly in the plasma, lymph, and other fluids outside the cell.

3. Aqueous solutions supply food and oxygen to cells, and waste products always leave via a watery medium. Water gives structure and form to the body and regulates body temperature.

4. The normal average daily water intake of 2.5 L comes from liquid intake (1.2 L), food (1.0 L), and metabolic water produced during energy-yielding reactions (0.3 L).

5. Daily water loss occurs through urine (1.0–1.5 L), through the skin as insensible perspiration (0.35 L) and sweat (500–700 mL), as water vapor in expired air (0.25–0.35 L), and in feces (0.10 L).

6. Hot weather exercise greatly increases the body's water requirement because of fluid loss via sweating. In extreme thermal conditions, fluid needs increase five or six times above normal.

7. Heat cramps, heat exhaustion, and heat stroke comprise the major forms of heat illness. Heat stroke represents the most serious and complex of these maladies.

8. Several factors affect the rate of gastric emptying: keeping fluid volume in the stomach at a relatively high level speeds gastric emptying, concentrated sugar solutions impair gastric emptying and fluid replacement, and cold fluids empty from the stomach more rapidly than fluids at body temperature.

9. Maintaining plasma volume (so circulation and sweating progress optimally) represents the primary aim of fluid replacement. For the ideal replacement schedule during exercise, fluid intake should match fluid loss. Monitoring change in body weight during and after workouts indicates the effectiveness of fluid replacement.

10. Optimal gastric volume for fluid replacement occurs by consuming 400 to 600 mL of fluid immediately before exercise followed by regular ingestion of 250 mL of fluid every 15 minutes during exercise.

11. Drinking concentrated sugar-containing beverages slows the rate of gastric emptying; this could disrupt fluid balance in exercise, especially during heat stress.

12. The ideal oral rehydration solution contains between 5% and 8% carbohydrates. This beverage concentration replenishes carbohydrate without adversely affecting fluid balance and thermoregulation.

13. Excessive sweating and ingesting large volumes of plain water during prolonged exercise decrease extracellular sodium concentration and sets the stage for hyponatremia (water intoxication), a potentially dangerous malady.

 ## THOUGHT QUESTIONS

1. What specific approaches might a coach establish for athletes to guard against dehydration and possible heat injury? Include factors that optimize fluid replenishment.

2. Describe the ideal fluid (in terms of content and quantity) to consume before, during, and after exhausting exercise.

SELECTED REFERENCES

Adams-Hillard, P.J., Deitch, H.R.: Menstrual disorders in the college age female. *Pediatr. Clin. North Am.*, 52:179, 2005.

American Dietetic Association; Dietitians of Canada; American College of Sports Medicine: American College of Sports Medicine position stand. Nutrition and athletic performance. *Med. Sci. Sports Exerc.*, 2009;41:709, 2009. Review.

American College of Sports Medicine, American Dietetic Association and Dietitians of Canada: Joint Position Statement. Nutrition and athletic performance. *Med. Sci. Sports Exerc.*, 32:2130, 2000.

American College of Sports Medicine: American College of Sports Medicine Position Stand. Osteoporosis and exercise. *Med. Sci. Sports Exerc.*, 27:i, 1995.

American College of Sports Medicine: Position stand on physical activity and bone health. *Med. Sci. Sports Exerc.*, 36:1985, 2004.

Aoi, W.: Exercise and food factors. *Forum Nutr.*, 61:147, 2009.

Barberger-Gateau, P., et al.: Dietary patterns and risk of dementia: the Three-City cohort study. *Neurology.*, 69:1921, 2007.

Bartali, B., et al.: Serum micronutrient concentrations and decline in physical function among older persons. *JAMA.*, 299:3208, 2008.

Bartoszewska, M., et al.: Vitamin D, muscle function, and exercise performance. *Pediatr. Clin. North Am.*, 57:849, 2010.

Boon, H., et al.: Substrate source use in older, trained males after decades of endurance training. *Med. Sci. Sports Exerc.*, 39:2160, 2007.

Cases, N., et al.: Differential response of plasma and immune cell's vitamin E levels to physical activity and antioxidant vitamin supplementation. *Eur. J. Clin. Nutr.*, 59:781, 2005.

Coyle, E.F.: Improved muscular efficiency displayed as Tour de France champion matures. *J. Appl. Physiol.*, 98:2191, 2005.

Cox, G.R., et al.: Daily training with high carbohydrate availability increases exogenous carbohydrate oxidation during endurance cycling. *J. Appl. Physiol.*, 109:126, 2010.

Davies, J.H., et al.: Bone mass acquisition in healthy children. *Arch. Dis. Child.*, 90:373, 2005.

Davis, J.K., Green, J.M.: Caffeine and anaerobic performance: ergogenic value and mechanisms of action. *Sports Med.*, 39:813, 2009.

Demark-Wahnefried, W., et al.: Lifestyle intervention development study to improve physical function in older adults with cancer: outcomes from Project LEAD. *J. Clin. Oncol.*, 24:3465, 2006.

Donsmark, M., et al.: Hormone-sensitive lipase as mediator of lipolysis in contracting skeletal muscle. *Exerc. Sport Sci. Rev.*, 33:127, 2005.

Erdman, K.A., et al.: Influence of performance level on dietary supplementation in elite Canadian athletes. *Med. Sci. Sports Exerc.*, 38:349, 2006.

Fairey A.S., et al.: Randomized controlled trial of exercise and blood immune function in postmenopausal breast cancer survivors. *J. Appl. Physiol.*, 98:1534, 2005.

Feiereisen, P., et al.: Is strength training the more efficient training modality in chronic heart failure? *Med. Sci. Sports Exerc.*, 39:1910, 2007.

Food and Nutrition Board, Institute of Medicine: *Dietary Reference Intakes for Energy, Carbohydrates, Fiber, Fat, Protein and Amino Acids*. Washington, D.C.: National Academy Press, 2002.

Foskett, A., et al.: Carbohydrate availability and muscle energy metabolism during intermittent running. *Med. Sci. Sports Exerc.*, 401:96, 2008.

Gaine, P.C., et al.: Postexercise whole-body protein turnover response to three levels of protein intake. *Med. Sci. Sports Exerc.*, 39:480, 2007.

Ganio, M.S., et al.: Effect of various carbohydrate-electrolyte fluids on cycling performance and maximal voluntary contraction. *Int. J. Sport Nutr. Exerc. Metab.*, 20:104, 2010.

Geleijnse, J.M., et al.: Effect of low doses of n-3 fatty acids on cardiovascular diseases in 4,837 post-myocardial infarction patients: design and baseline characteristics of the Alpha Omega Trial. *Am. Heart J.*, 159:539, 2010.

Godek, S.F., et al.: Sweat rate and fluid turnover in American football players compared with runners in a hot and humid environment. *Br. J. Sports Med.*, 39:205, 2005.

Green, H.J., et al.: Mechanical and metabolic responses with exercise and dietary carbohydrate manipulation. *Med. Sci. Sports Exerc.*, 391:139, 2007.

Greydanus, D.E., et al.: The adolescent female athlete: current concepts and conundrums. *Pediatr. Clin. North Am.*, 57:697, 2010.

Gropper S.S., et al.: Iron status of female collegiate athletes involved in different sorts. *Biol. Trace Elem. Res.*, 109:1, 2006.

Guadalupe-Grau, A., et al.: Exercise and bone mass in adults. *Sports Med.*, 39:439, 2009.

Hamilton, K.L.: Antioxidants and cardioprotection. *Med. Sci. Sports Exerc.*, 39:1544, 2007.

Irwin, M.L.: Randomized controlled trials of physical activity and breast cancer prevention. *Exerc. Sport Sci. Rev.*, 34:182, 2006.

Jentjens, R.L., Jeukendrup, A.E.: High rates of exogenous carbohydrate oxidation from a mixture of glucose and fructose ingested during prolonged cycling exercise. *Br. J. Nutr.*, 93:485, 2005.

Jeukendrup, A.E., et al.: Nutritional considerations in triathlon. *Sports Med.*, 35:163, 2005.

Jeukendrup, A.E., Wallis, G.A.: Measurement of substrate oxidation during exercise by means of gas exchange measurements. *Int. J. Sports Med.*, 26 Suppl 1:S28, 2005.

Jeukendrup, A.E.: Carbohydrate intake during exercise and performance. *Nutrition*, 20:669, 2004.

Jeukendrup, A.E.: Carbohydrate and exercise performance: the role of multiple transportable carbohydrates. *Curr. Opin. Clin. Nutr. Metab. Care*, 13:452, 2010.

Klungland Torstveit, M., Sundgot-Borgen, J.: The female athlete triad: are elite athletes at increased risk. *Med. Sci. Sports Exerc.*, 37:184, 2005.

Kobayashi, I.H., et al.: Intake of fish and omega-3 fatty acids and risk of coronary heart disease among Japanese: The Japan Public Health Center-Based (JPHC) Study Cohort 1. *Circulation,* 113:195, 2006.

Lanou, A.J., et al.: Calcium, dairy products, and bone health in children and young adults: a reevaluation of the evidence. *Pediatrics,* 115:736, 2005.

Lecarpentier, Y.: Physiological role of free radicals in skeletal muscles. *J. Appl. Physiol.,* 103:1917, 2007.

Li, W.C., et al.: Effects of exercise programs on quality of life in osteoporotic and osteopenic postmenopausal women: a systematic review and meta-analysis. *Clin. Rehabil.,* 23(10):888, 2009.

Lindsey, C., et al.: Association of physical performance measures with bone mineral density in postmenopausal women. *Arch. Phys. Med. Rehabil.,* 86:1102, 2005.

Liu, J.F., et al.: Blood lipid peroxides and muscle damage increased following intensive resistance training of female weightlifters. *Ann. N. Y. Acad. Sci.,* 1042:255, 2005.

Lonn, E., et al.: Effects of long-term vitamin E supplementation on cardiovascular events and cancer: a randomized controlled trial. *JAMA,* 293:1338, 2005.

Loucks, A.B.: New animal model opens opportunities for research on the female athlete triad. *J. Appl. Physiol.,* 103:1467, 2007.

Lukaski, H.C.: Vitamin and mineral status: effects on physical performance. *Nutrition,* 20:632, 2004.

Ma, Y., et al.: Dietary quality 1 year after diagnosis of coronary heart disease. *J. Am. Diet. Assoc.,* 108:240, 2008.

Maughan, R.J., Shirreffs, S.M.: Development of individual hydration strategies for athletes. *Int. J. Sport Nutr. Exerc. Metab.,* 18:457, 2008.

Myint, P.K., et al.: Plasma vitamin C concentrations predict risk of incident stroke over 10 y in 20649 participants of the European Prospective Investigation into Cancer Norfolk prospective population study. *Am. J. Clin. Nutr.,* 87:64, 2008.

Pikosky, M.A., et al.: Increased protein maintains nitrogen balance during exercise-induced energy deficit. *Med. Sci. Sports Exerc.,* 40:505, 2008.

Popp, K.L., et al.: Bone geometry, strength, and muscle size in runners with a history of stress fracture. *Med. Sci. Sports Exerc.,* 41: 2145, 2009.

Qi, L., et al.: Whole grain, bran, and cereal fiber intakes and markers of systemic inflammation in diabetic women. *Diabetes Care,* 29:207, 2006.

Reinking, M.F., Alexander, L.E.: Prevalence of disordered-eating behaviors in undergraduate female collegiate athletes and nonathletes. *J. Athl. Train.,* 40:47, 2005.

Rosner, MH.: Exercise-associated hyponatremia. *Semin. Nephrol.* 29:271, 2009.

Roth, E.M., Harris, W.S.: Fish oil for primary and secondary prevention of coronary heart disease. *Curr. Atheroscler Rep.,* 12:66, 2010.

Siu, P.M., et al.: Effect of frequency of carbohydrate feedings on recovery and subsequent endurance run. *Med. Sci. Sports Exerc.,* 36:315, 2004.

Simopoulos, A.P.: Genetic variants in the metabolism of omega-6 and omega-3 fatty acids: their role in the determination of nutritional requirements and chronic disease risk. *Exp. Biol. Med.,* 235:785, 2010.

Slentz, C.A., et al.: Inactivity, exercise training and detraining, and plasma lipoproteins. STRRIDE: a randomized, controlled study of exercise intensity and amount. *J. Appl. Physiol.,* 103:432, 2007.

Starnes, J.W., Taylor, R.P.: Exercise-induced cardioprotection: Endogenous mechanisms. *Med. Sci. Sports Exerc.,* 39:1537, 2007.

Stewart, K.J., et al.: Exercise effects on bone mineral density relationships to changes in fitness and fatness. *Am. J. Prev. Med.,* 28:453, 2005.

Suh, S.W., et al. Hypoglycemia, brain energetics, and hypoglycemic neuronal death. *Glia.,* 55:1280, 2007.

Thomas-John, M., et al.: Risk factors for the development of osteoporosis and osteoporotic fractures among older men. *J. Rheumatol.* 36:1947, 2009.

Torstveit, M.K., Sundgot-Borgen, J.: Low bone mineral density is two to three times more prevalent in non-athletic premenopausal women than in elite athletes: a comprehensive controlled study. *Br. J. Sports Med.,* 39:282, 2005.

Torstveit, M.K., Sundgot-Borgen, J.: The female athlete triad: are elite athletes at increased risk? *Med. Sci. Sports Exerc.,* 37:184, 2005.

Venables, M.C., Jeukendrup, A.E.: Endurance training and obesity: Effect on substrate metabolism and insulin sensitivity. *Med. Sci. Sports Exerc.,* 40:495, 2008.

Wallis, G.A., et al.: Oxidation of combined ingestion of maltodextrins and fructose during exercise. *Med. Sci. Sports Exerc.,* 37:426, 2005.

Westerlind, K.C., Williams, N.I.: Effect of energy deficiency on estrogen metabolism in premenopausal women. *Med. Sci. Sports Exerc.,* 39:1090, 2007.

Williams, PT.: Reduced diabetic, hypertensive, and cholesterol medication use with walking. *Med. Sci. Sports Exerc.,* 40:433, 2008.

NOTES

Food Energy and Optimum Nutrition for Exercise

CHAPTER OBJECTIVES

- Define *heat of combustion*, *digestive efficiency*, and *Atwater general factors*.

- Compute the energy content of a meal from its macronutrient composition.

- Compare the nutrient and energy intakes of physically active men and women with sedentary counterparts.

- Outline the MyPyramid recommendations.

- Describe the timing and composition of the pre-event (precompetition) meal, including reasons for limiting lipid and protein intake.

- Summarize effects of low, normal, and high carbohydrate intake on glycogen reserves and subsequent endurance performance.

- For endurance athletes, describe the potential negative effects of consuming a concentrated sugar drink 30 minutes before competition and the ideal composition of a "sports drink."

- Discuss possible reasons why consuming high-glycemic carbohydrates during intense aerobic exercise enhances endurance performance.

- Define *glucose polymer* and give the rationale for adding these compounds to a sports drink.

- Make a general recommendation concerning carbohydrate intake for athletes in intense training.

- Describe the most effective way to replenish glycogen reserves after an intense bout of training or competition.

- Compare classic carbohydrate loading with the modified procedure.

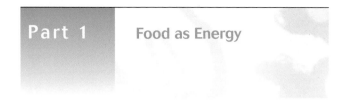

Part 1   Food as Energy

CALORIE—A MEASUREMENT OF FOOD ENERGY

One kilogram–calorie (kilocalorie [kCal], or simply calorie) expresses the quantity of heat necessary to raise the temperature of 1 kg (1 L) of water 1°C (from 14.5° to 15.5°C). For example, if a particular food contains 300 kCal, then releasing the potential energy trapped within this food's chemical structure increases the temperature of 300 L of water by 1°C. Different foods contain different amounts of potential energy. For example, one Triple Whopper hamburger with medium French fries and a CocaCola from Burger King (*www.bk.com*) contains 1930 kCal (about 60% of fat kCal from the burger and fries). The equivalent heat energy increases the temperature of 1930 L of water by 1°C.

Gross Energy Value of Foods

Laboratories use **bomb calorimeters**, similar to the one illustrated in **Figure 3.1**, to measure the total or gross energy

value of various food macronutrients. Bomb calorimeters operate on the principle of **direct calorimetry**, measuring the heat liberated as the food burns completely. The bomb calorimeter works as follows:

- A small, insulated chamber filled with oxygen under pressure contains a weighed portion of food.
- The food literally explodes and burns when an electric current ignites an electric fuse within the chamber.
- A surrounding water bath absorbs the heat released as the food burns (termed the *heat of combustion*). An insulating water jacket surrounding the bomb prevents heat loss to the outside.
- A sensitive thermometer measures the heat absorbed by the water. For example, the complete combustion of one beef, skinless, 20oz hot dog and a 1.4-oz bun with mustard and small French fries (2.4 oz) liberates 512 kCal of heat energy. This would raise 5.12 kg (11.3 lb) of ice water to the boiling point.

Heat of Combustion The heat liberated by the burning or oxidation of food in a bomb calorimeter represents its **heat of combustion** (total energy value of the food). *Burning 1 g of pure carbohydrate yields a heat of combustion of 4.20 kCal, 1 g of pure protein releases 5.65 kCal, and 1 g of pure lipid yields 9.45 kCal.* Because most foods in the diet consist of various proportions of these three macronutrients, the caloric value of a given food reflects the sum of the heats of combustion for these three macronutrients. This value demonstrates that complete lipid oxidation in the bomb calorimeter liberates about 65% more energy per gram than protein oxidation and 120% more energy than carbohydrate oxidation.

Net Energy Value of Foods

Differences exist in the energy value of foods when comparing the heat of combustion (gross energy value) determined by direct calorimetry with the *net* energy available to the body. This pertains particularly to protein because its nitrogen component does not oxidize. In the body, nitrogen atoms combine with hydrogen to form urea, which excretes in urine. Elimination of hydrogen in this manner represents a loss of approximately 19% of protein's potential energy. The hydrogen loss reduces protein's heat of combustion in the body to about 4.6 kCal per gram instead of 5.65 kCal per gram in the bomb calorimeter. In contrast, identical physiologic fuel values exist for carbohydrates and lipids (neither contains nitrogen) compared with their heats of combustion in the bomb calorimeter.

Digestive Efficiency

The ingested macronutrient availability to the body determines their ultimate caloric yield. *Availability* refers to

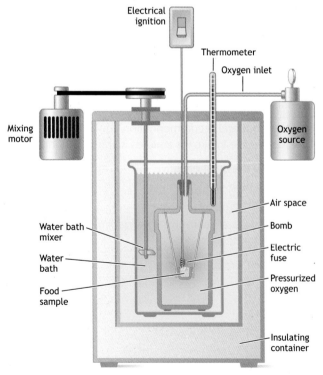

Figure 3.1 Bomb calorimetry directly measures the energy value of food.

completeness of digestion and absorption. Normally, about 97% of carbohydrates, 95% of lipids, and 92% of proteins become digested, absorbed, and available for energy conversion. Large variation exists in the digestive efficiency of protein, ranging from a high of 97% for animal protein to a low of 78% for dried peas and beans. Furthermore, less energy becomes available from a meal with a high-fiber content.

Considering average digestive efficiencies, the **net kCal value** per gram available to the body equals 4.0 for carbohydrates, 9.0 for lipids, and 4.0 for proteins. These corrected heats of combustion, known as the **Atwater general factors**, were named after Wilbur Olin Atwater (1844–1907), the scientist who first described energy release in the calorimeter (*www.sportsci.org/news/history/atwater/atwater.html*).

Energy Value of a Meal

The caloric content of any food can be determined from Atwater values if one knows its composition and weight. For example, how could we determine the kCal value for 1/2 cup (3.5 oz or about 100 g) of creamed chicken? Based on laboratory analysis of a standard recipe, the macronutrient composition of l g of creamed chicken contains 0.2 g of protein, 0.12 g of lipid, and 0.06 g of carbohydrate. Using the Atwater net kCal values, 0.2 g of protein contains 0.8 kCal (0.20 × 4.0), 0.12 g of lipid equals 1.08 kCal (0.12 × 9.0), and 0.06 g of carbohydrate yields 0.24 kCal (0.06 × 4.0). Therefore, the total caloric value of 1 g of creamed chicken equals 2.12 kCal (0.80 + 1.08 + 0.24). Consequently, a 100-g serving contains 100 times as much or 212 kCal. **Table 3.1** presents another example of kCal calculations for 3/4 cup or 100 g of vanilla ice cream.

Fortunately, the need seldom exists to compute kCal values because the United States Department of Agriculture has already made these determinations for almost all foods (*www.nal.usda.gov/fnic/foodcomp/search/*). Food-calorie guides available on the Internet make analyzing kCal values of food a relatively easy task (*www.nat.uiuc.edu/nat_welcome.html*).

(i) For Your Information

SPORTS THAT PROMOTE MARGINAL NUTRITION

Gymnasts; ballet dancers; ice dancers; and weight-class athletes in boxing, wrestling, rowing, and judo engage in arduous training. Owing to the nature of their sport, these athletes continually strive to maintain a lean, light body mass dictated by either esthetic or weight-class considerations. Energy intake often intentionally falls short of energy expenditure, and a relative state of malnutrition develops. Nutritional supplementation for these athletes may prove beneficial.

Questions & Notes

Give the heat of combustion for 1 g each of:

Carbohydrate:

Protein:

Lipid:

Give the Atwater factors for:

Carbohydrate:

Protein:

Lipid:

Of the 3 macronutrients, which one has the highest digestive efficiency?

Table 3.1	Method of Calculating the Caloric Value of a Food from Its Composition of Macronutrients

Food: Ice cream (vanilla)
Weight: 3/4 cup = 100 g

	COMPOSITION		
	PROTEIN	LIPID	CARBOHYDRATE
Percentage	4	13	21
Total grams	4	13	21
In 1 gram	0.04	0.13	0.21
Calories per gram	0.16	1.17	0.84
	(0.04 × 4.0 kCal)	(0.13 × 9.0 kCal)	(0.21 × 4.0 kCal)

Total calories per gram: 0.16 + 1.17 + 0.84 = 2.17 kCal
Total calories per 100 grams: 2.17 × 100 = 217 kCal

BOX 3.1   CLOSE UP

How to Read a Food Label

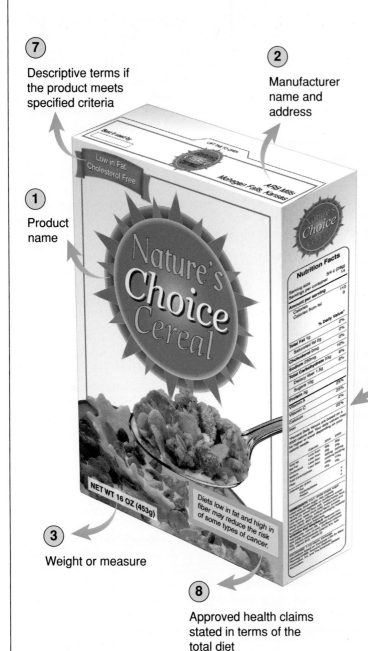

7 Descriptive terms if the product meets specified criteria

2 Manufacturer name and address

1 Product name

3 Weight or measure

8 Approved health claims stated in terms of the total diet

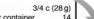

Nutrition Facts

| Serving size | 3/4 c (28 g) |
| Servings per container | 14 |

Amount per serving

| Calories | 110 |
| Calories from fat | 9 |

	% Daily Value*
Total Fat 1 g	2%
Saturated fat 0 g	0%
Trans fat 0 g	0%
Cholesterol 0 mg	0%
Sodium 250 mg	10%
Total Carbohydrate 23 g	8%
Dietary fiber 1.5 g	6%
Sugars 10 g	
Protein 3 g	
Vitamin A	25%
Vitamin C	25%
Calcium	2%
Iron	25%

*Percent Daily Values are based on a 2000 calorie diet. Your daily values may be higher or lower depending on your calorie needs.

	Calories	2000	2500
Total fat	Less than	65 g	80 g
Sat Fat	Less than	20 g	25 g
Cholesterol	Less than	300 mg	300 mg
Sodium	Less than	2400 mg	2400 mg
Total Carbohydrate		300 g	375 g
Fiber		25 g	30 g

Calories per gram:	
Fat	9
Carbohydrates	4
Protein	4

INGREDIENTS: Corn, whole wheat, sugar, rolled oats, brown sugar, rice, partially hydrogenated vegetable oil (sunflower and/or canola oil), wheat flour, salt, malted barley flour, corn syrup, whey (from milk), malted corn and barley syrup, honey, artificial flavor, annatto etract (color), BHT added to packaging material to preserve product freshness.
VITAMINS AND MINERALS: Reduced iron, niacinamide, vitamin B6, Vitamin A palmitate zinc oxide (source of zinc), riboflavin (vitamin B2), thiamin mononitrate (vitamin B1), folic acid, vitamin B12, vitamin D.

EXCHANGE: 1-1/2 starch, exchange calculations based on *Exchange Lists for Meal Planning* ©1995, American Diabetes Association, Inc. and The American Dietetic Association.

5 Serving size, number of servings per container, and calorie information

6 Nutrition information panel provides quantities of nutrients per serving, in both actual amounts and as "% Daily Values" based on a 2000-calorie energy intake

4 Ingredients in descending order of predominance by weight

In 1990, the United States Congress passed the **Nutrition Labeling and Education Act**, which brought sweeping changes for food labeling. All foods, except those containing only a few nutrients such as plain coffee, tea, and spices, now provide consistent nutrition information. The food label must display the following information prominently and in words an average person can understand (numbers in the figure relate to the numbered information below):

1. Product's common or usual name.
2. Name and address of manufacturer, packer, or distributor.
3. Net contents for weight, measure, or count.
4. All ingredients listed in descending order of predominance by weight.
5. Serving size, number of servings per container, and calorie information.
6. Quantities of specified nutrients and food constituents, including total food energy in calories; total fat (g); saturated fat (g); cholesterol (mg); sodium (mg); total carbohydrate, including starch, sugar, and fiber (g); and protein (g). As of 2006, the quantity of trans fat must be included as well.

7. Descriptive terms of content.
8. Approved health claims stated in terms of the total diet.

TERMS ON FOOD LABELS

Common terms and what they mean:

Free: Nutritionally trivial and unlikely to have physiologic consequences; synonyms include "without," "no," and "zero".

High: Twenty percent or more of the Daily Value (DV) for a given nutrient per serving; synonyms include "rich in" or "excellent in".

Less: At least 25% less of a given nutrient or calories than the comparison food.

Low: An amount that allows frequent consumption of the food without exceeding the nutrient's DV.

Good source: Product provides between 10% and 19% of a given nutrient's DV per serving.

Cholesterol Terms

Cholesterol free: Less than 2 mg per serving and 2 g or less of saturated fat per serving.

Low cholesterol: Twenty mg or less of cholesterol per serving and 2 g or less of saturated fat per serving.

Less cholesterol: Twenty-five percent or less of cholesterol per serving and 2 g or less of saturated fat per serving.

Fat Terms

Extra lean: Less than 5 g of fat, 2 g of saturated fat, and 95 mg of cholesterol per serving and per 100 g of meat, poultry, or seafood.

Fat free: Less than 0.5 g of fat per serving (no added fat or oil).

Lean: Less than 10 g of fat, 4.5 g of saturated fat, and 95 mg of cholesterol per serving and per 100 g of meat, poultry, or seafood.

Less fat: Twenty-five percent or less fat than the comparison food.

Low fat: Three grams or less of fat per serving.

Light: Fifty percent or less fat than the comparison food (e.g., "50% less fat than our regular cookies").

Less saturated fat: Twenty-five percent or less saturated fat than the comparison food.

Energy Terms

Calorie free: Fewer than 5 calories per serving.

Light: One-third fewer calories than the comparison food.

Low calorie: Forty calories or less per serving.

Reduced calorie: At least 25% fewer calories per serving than the comparison food.

Fiber Term

High fiber: Five g or more of fiber per serving.

Sodium Terms

Sodium free and *salt free:* Less than 5 mg of sodium per serving.

Low sodium: One hundred forty mg or less of sodium per serving.

Light: Low-calorie food with 50% sodium reduction.

Light in sodium: No more than 50% of the sodium of the comparison food.

Very low sodium: Thirty-five mg or less of sodium per serving.

REFERENCES

Nutritional Labeling and Education Act (NLEA) Requirements (8/94-2/95): *www.fda.gov/ICECI/InspectionGuides/ucm074948.htm*

U.S. Food and Drug Administration. Available at *www.fda.gov/Food/LabelingNutrition/Consumerinformation/ucm078889.htm twoparts* panel (This website provides complete description of the new food label and relevant terms and materials related to the label.)

Calories Equal Calories

Consider the following five common foods: raw celery, cooked cabbage, cooked asparagus spears, mayonnaise, and salad oil. To consume 100 kCal of each of these foods, one must eat 20 stalks of celery, 4 cups of cabbage, 30 asparagus spears, but only 1 Tbsp of mayonnaise or 4/5 tsp of salad oil. Thus, a small serving of some foods contains the equivalent energy value as a large quantity of other foods. Viewed from a different perspective, to meet daily energy needs, a sedentary young adult woman would have to consume more than 420 stalks of celery, 84 cups of cabbage, or 630 asparagus spears yet only 1.5 cups of mayonnaise or about 8 oz of salad oil. What is the major difference among these foods? Recall that high-fat foods contain more energy with little water, and foods low in fat or high in water tend to contain little energy.

 For Your Information

MORE LIPID EQUALS MORE CALORIES

Lipid-rich foods contain a higher energy content than foods that are relatively fat free. One glass of whole milk, for example, contains 160 kCal; the same quantity of skim milk contains only 90 kCal. If a person who normally consumes 1 qt of whole milk each day switches to skim milk, the total calories ingested each year would be reduced by the equivalent calories in 25 lb of body fat. Thus, following this switch for just 3 years theoretically represents the equivalent energy in 75 lb of body fat.

A calorie reflects food energy regardless of the food source. From an energy standpoint, 100 calories from mayonnaise equals the same 100 calories in 20 celery stalks, 100 calories of Ben and Jerry's Triple Carmel Chunk ice cream, or 30 asparagus spears! The more food consumed, the more calories consumed. An individual's caloric intake equals the sum of *all* energy consumed from either small or large quantities of foods. Celery and asparagus spears would become "fattening" foods if consumed in excess.

SUMMARY

1. A calorie or kilocalorie (kCal) represents a measure of heat that expresses the energy value of food.

2. Burning food in a bomb calorimeter permits direct quantification of the food's energy content.

3. The heat of combustion represents the amount of heat liberated in a food's complete oxidation. Average gross energy values equal 4.2 kCal per gram for carbohydrates, 9.4 kCal per gram for lipids, and 5.65 kCal per gram for proteins.

4. The coefficient of digestibility represents the proportion of food consumed digested *and* absorbed by the body. Coefficients of digestibility average approximately 97% for carbohydrates, 95% for lipids, and 92% for proteins.

5. The net energy values equal 4 kCal per gram of carbohydrates, 9 kCal per gram of lipids, and 4 kCal per gram of proteins. These Atwater general factors provide an estimate of the net energy value of foods in a diet and allow one to compute the caloric content of any meal from its carbohydrate, lipid, and protein composition.

6. A calorie represents a unit of heat energy regardless of food source. From an energy standpoint, 500 kCal of chocolate cheesecake topped with homemade whipped cream is no more fattening than 500 kCal of a carrot and lettuce salad; 500 kCal of onion and pepperoni pizza; or 500 kCal of a bagel with Coho salmon, red onions, and sour cream.

THOUGHT QUESTIONS

1. What factors other than the energy value of one's diet should you consider when formulating a healthful approach to weight control?

2. Explain the importance of considering food type in planning a weight loss diet.

Part 2	Optimal Nutrition for Exercise and Sports

From a nutritional and energy balance perspective, optimal food consumption must supply required nutrients for tissue maintenance, repair, and growth without excessive energy intake. Reasonable estimates have been made of specific nutrient needs for individuals of different ages and body sizes, with considerations for individual differences in digestion, storage capacity, nutrient metabolism, and daily energy expenditure. Establishing dietary recommendations for physically active men and women remains complicated by the specific energy requirements and training demands of particular sports and by individual dietary preferences. Sound nutritional guidelines form the framework for planning and evaluating food intake for individuals who exercise regularly. Part 2 describes nutrient requirements of sedentary and active individuals, including optimal nutrition guidelines for intense physical activity.

NUTRIENT CONSUMPTION OF THE SEDENTARY AND PHYSICALLY ACTIVE

Many coaches make dietary recommendations based on their "feelings" and past experiences rather than sound research evidence. The fact that athletes often obtain inadequate or incorrect information concerning dietary practices and the role of specific nutrients in exercise exacerbates the problem. Considering the total body of scientific evidence, physically active people and athletes do *not* require additional nutrients beyond those obtained in a balanced diet. *Physically fit Americans, including those involved in increased physical activity, consume diets that more closely approach dietary recommendations than less active peers of lower fitness levels.*

Inconsistencies exist among studies that relate diet quality to physical activity level or physical fitness. Relatively crude and imprecise self-reported measures of physical activity, unreliable dietary assessments, or small sample size help to explain part of the discrepancy. Table 3.2 contrasts the nutrient and energy intakes with national dietary recommendations of a large population-based cohort of nearly 7959 men and 2453 women classified as low, moderate, and high for cardiorespiratory fitness. The most significant four findings indicate the following:

1. A progressively lower body mass index with increasing levels of physical fitness for both men and women.
2. Remarkably small differences in energy intake related to physical fitness classification for women (≤94 kCal per day) and men (≤82 kCal per day); the moderate fitness group in both genders consumed the least calories.
3. A progressively higher dietary fiber intake and lower cholesterol intake across fitness categories.
4. Men and women with higher fitness levels generally consumed diets that more closely approached dietary recommendations (with respect to dietary fiber, percent of energy from total fat, percent of energy from saturated fat, and dietary cholesterol) than peers of lower levels of fitness.

Attention to proper diet does not mean athletes must join the ranks of the more than 40% of Americans who take nutritional supplements (spending more than $10 billion yearly) to micromanage their nutrient intake. *In essence, sound human nutrition represents sound nutrition for athletes.*

DIETARY REFERENCE INTAKES

Controversy surrounding use of the Recommended Dietary Allowances (RDAs) over the past 15 years caused the Food and Nutrition Board and scientific nutrition community to reexamine the usefulness of the RDAs. This process, which began in 1997, led the National Academies' Institute of Medicine in cooperation with Canadian scientists to develop the **Dietary Reference Intakes** (DRIs; *www.fnic.nal.usda.gov/interactiveDRI/*), a radically new and more comprehensive approach to nutritional recommendations for individuals. Think of the DRIs as the umbrella term for an array of new standards—the **RDAs, Estimated Average Requirements (EARs), Adequate Intakes (AIs),** and the **Tolerable Upper Intake Levels (ULs)**—for nutrient recommendations to plan and assess diets for healthy people.

The final nutrient recommendations included population data from Canada and the United States because of both countries' similar dietary patterns. Nutrient recommendations encompass daily intakes intended for health maintenance and upper-intake levels that reduce the likelihood of harm from excess nutrient intake. The DRIs differ from their predecessor RDAs by focusing more on promoting health maintenance and risk reduction for nutrient-dependent diseases (e.g., heart disease, diabetes, hypertension, osteoporosis, various cancers, and age-related macular degeneration) rather than preventing the deficiency diseases scurvy (vitamin C deficiency) or beriberi (vitamin B_1 deficiency). The DRIs also provide values for macronutrients and food components of nutritional importance for compounds believed to have health-protecting qualities (e.g., phytochemicals).

The DRI value also includes recommendations that apply to gender and life stages of growth and development based on age including pregnancy and lactation (*www.nap.edu*; search for Dietary Reference Intakes).

The following provides four different sets of values for the intake of nutrients and food components in the DRIs (**Fig. 3.2**):

1. **EAR:** Average level of daily nutrient intake to meet the requirement of half of the healthy individuals in a particular life stage and gender group. In addition to assessing nutritional adequacy of intakes of

*Q*uestions & Notes

In general, do athletes require different nutrients in different quantities than non-athletes? Discuss.

 For Your Information

EAT MORE YET WEIGH LESS

Physically active individuals generally consume more calories per kg of body mass than their sedentary counterparts. The extra energy required for exercise accounts for the larger caloric intake. Paradoxically, the most physically active men and women, who eat more on a daily basis, weigh less than those who exercise at a lower total caloric expenditure. Regular exercise allows a person to "eat more yet weigh less" while maintaining a lower percentage of body fat despite the age-related tendency toward weight gain that begins at about age 21 years and continues at about one pound of weight gained for the next 40 years! Physically active persons maintain a lighter and leaner body and a healthier heart disease risk profile despite their increased food intake.

Table 3.2 Mean (±SD) Nutrient Intake Based on 3-Day Diet Records By Level of Cardiorespiratory Fitness in 7959 Men and 2453 Women

VARIABLE	MALES LOW FITNESS (N = 786)	FEMALES LOW FITNESS (N = 233)	MALES MODERATE FITNESS (N = 2457)	FEMALES MODERATE FITNESS (N = 730)	MALES HIGH FITNESS (N = 4716)	FEMALES HIGH FITNESS (N = 1490)
Demographic and health data						
Age (y)	47.3 ± 11.1[a,b]	47.5 ± 11.2[b]	47.3 ± 10.3[c]	46.7 ± 11.6	48.1 ± 10.5	46.5 ± 11.0
Apparently healthy (%)	51.5[a,b]	55.4[a,b]	69.1[c]	71.1[c]	77.0	79.3
Current smokers (%)	23.4[a,b]	12.0[a,b]	15.8[c]	9.0[c]	7.8	4.2
BMI (kg · m^{-2})	30.7 ± 5.5[a,b]	27.3 ± 6.7[a,b]	27.4 ± 3.7[c]	24.3 ± 4.9[c]	25.1 ± 2.7	22.1 ± 3.0
Nutrient data						
Energy (kCal)	2378.6 ± 718.6[a]	1887.4 ± 607.5[a]	2296.9 ± 661.9[c]	1793.0 ± 508.2[c]	2348.1 ± 664.3	1859.7 ± 514.7
kCal · kg^{-1}	25.0 ± 8.1[a]	27.1 ± 9.4[a]	26.7 ± 8.4[c]	28.1 ± 8.8[c]	29.7 ± 9.2	31.7 ± 9.8
Carbohydrate (% kCal)	43.2 ± 9.4[b]	47.7 ± 9.6[b]	44.6 ± 9.1[c]	48.2 ± 9.0[c]	48.1 ±9.7	51.1 ± 9.4
Protein (% kCal)	18.6 ± 3.8	17.6 ± 3.7[a]	18.5 ± 3.8	18.1 ± 3.9	18.1 ± 3.8	17.7 ± 3.9
Total fat (% kCal)	36.7 ± 7.2[b]	34.8 ± 7.6[b]	35.4 ± 7.1[c]	33.7 ± 6.8[c]	32.6 ± 7.5	31.3 ± 7.5
SFA (% kCal)	11.8 ± 3.2[b]	11.1 ± 3.3	11.3 ± 3.2[c]	10.6 ± 3.2[c]	10.0 ± 3.2	9.6 ± 3.1
MUFA (% kCal)	14.5 ± 3.2[a,b]	13.4 ± 3.4[a,b]	13.8 ± 3.1[c]	12.8 ± 3.0[c]	12.6 ± 3.3	11.9 ± 3.2
PUFA (% kCal)	7.4 ± 2.2[a,b]	7.5 ± 2.2	7.5 ± 2.2	7.5 ± 2.2	7.4 ± 2.3	7.4 ± 2.4
Cholesterol (mg)	349.5 ± 173.2[b]	244.7 ± 132.8[b]	314.5 ± 147.5[c]	224.6 ± 115.6[c]	277.8 ± 138.5	204.1 ± 103.6
Fiber (g)	21.0 ± 9.5[b]	18.9 ± 8.2[a,b]	22.0 ± 9.7[c]	20.0 ± 8.3[c]	26.2 ± 11.9	23.2 ± 10.7
Calcium (mg)	849.1 ± 371.8[a,b]	765.2 ± 361.8[a,b]	860.2 ± 360.2[c]	774.6 ± 342.8[c]	924.4 ± 386.8	828.3 ± 372.1
Sodium (mg)	4317.4 ± 1365.7	3350.8 ± 980.8	4143.0 ± 1202.3	3256.7 ± 927.7	4133.2 ± 1189.4	3314.4 ± 952.7
Folate (mcg)	336.4 ± 165.2[b]	301.8 ± 157.6[a,b]	359.5 ± 197.0[c]	319.7 ± 196.2	428.0 ± 272.0	356.2 ± 232.5
Vitamin B$_6$ (mg)	2.4 ± 0.9[b]	2.0 ± 0.8[b]	2.4 ± 0.9[c]	2.0 ± 0.8[c]	2.8 ± 1.1	2.2 ± 0.9
Vitamin B$_{12}$ (mcg)	6.6 ± 5.5[a]	4.7 ± 4.2	6.8 ± 6.0	4.9 ± 4.2	6.6 ± 5.8	5.0 ± 4.2
Vitamin A (RE)	1372.7 ± 1007.3[a,b]	1421.9 ± 1135.3[b]	1530.5 ± 1170.4[c]	1475.1 ± 1132.9[c]	1766.3 ± 1476.0	1699.0 ± 1346.9
Vitamin C (mg)	117.3 ± 80.4[b]	116.7 ± 7.5[b]	129.2 ± 108.9[c]	131.5 ± 140.0	166.0 ± 173.2	153.5 ± 161.1
Vitamin E (AE)	11.5 ± 9.1[b]	10.8 ± 7.5	12.1 ± 8.6[c]	10.3 ± 6.5[c]	13.7 ± 11.4	11.5 ± 8.1

BMI, body mass index; SFA, saturated fatty acid; PUFA, polyunsaturated fatty acid; MUFA, monounsaturated fatty acid; RE, retinol equivalents; AE, alpha-tocopherol units.

[a]Significant difference between low and moderate fit, $P < 0.05$.

[b]Significant difference between low and high fit, $P < 0.05$.

[c]Significant difference between moderate and high fit, $P < 0.05$.

From: Brodney, S., et al.: Nutrient intake of physically active fit and unfit men and women. *Med. Sci. Sports Exerc.* 33:459, 2001.

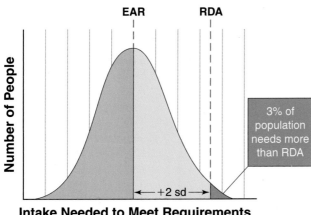

Figure 3.2   Theoretical distribution of the number of people adequately nourished by a given nutrient intake. For example, the number of people receiving adequate nutrition with 50 units of the nutrient is greater than those receiving only 15 units or who require 75 units. The Recommended Dietary Allowance (RDA) is set at an intake level that would meet the nutrient needs of 97% to 98% of the population (2 standard deviations [SD] above the mean). The Estimated Average Requirement (EAR) represents a nutrient intake value estimated to meet the requirement of 50% of the healthy individuals in a gender and life stage group.

population groups, the EAR provides a useful value for determining the prevalence of inadequate nutrient intake by the proportion of the population with intakes below this value.

2. **RDA:** The average daily nutrient intake level sufficient to meet the requirement of nearly 97% to 98% of healthy individuals in a particular life stage and gender group. For most nutrients, this value represents the EAR plus two standard deviations of the requirement.

3. **AI:** The AI provides a nutritional goal when no RDA exists. It represents a recommended average daily nutrient intake level based on observed or experimentally determined approximations or estimates of nutrient intake by a group (or groups) of apparently healthy people that are assumed as adequate; the AI is used when an RDA cannot be determined. The risk is low when intake is at or above the AI level.

4. **UL:** The highest average daily nutrient intake level likely to pose no risk of adverse health effects to almost all individuals in the specified gender and life stage group of the general population. The potential risk of adverse effects increases as intake increases above the UL.

The DRI report reveals that fruits and vegetables yield about one-half as much vitamin A as previously believed. This means that individuals who do not eat vitamin A–rich, animal-derived foods should upgrade their intake of carotene-rich fruits and vegetables. The report also sets a daily maximum intake level for vitamin A in addition to boron, copper, iodine, iron, manganese, molybdenum, nickel, vanadium, and zinc. Specific recommended intakes are provided for vitamins A and K, chromium, copper, iodine, manganese, molybdenum, and zinc. The report concludes that one can meet the daily requirement for the nutrients examined without supplementation. The exception is iron intake for which most pregnant women need supplements to meet their increased daily requirements.

Table 3.3 presents the RDIs for the vitamins for different life stage groups. Well-balanced meals provide an adequate quantity of all vitamins, regardless of a person's age and physical activity level. Similarly, mineral supplements generally confer little benefit because the required minerals occur readily in food and water. Individuals who expend considerable energy exercising generally do *not* need to consume special foods or supplements that increase their micronutrient intake above recommended levels. Also, at high levels of daily physical activity,

Questions & Notes

Briefly explain how the DRIs differ from the RDAs.

Name the 4 different parts of the DRIs.

1.

2.

3.

4.

Explain the difference between "RDA" and "EAR."

For Your Information

HEART-DIET LINKS

Research published in the *Archives of Internal Medicine* based on analysis of more than 200 studies involving millions of people indicates that vegetables, nuts, and the Mediterranean diet (rich in vegetables, nuts, whole grains, fish, and olive oil) make the list of "good" heart-healthy foods. Foods on the "bad" list include starchy carbohydrates such as white bread, and the trans fats in many cookies and French fries. Insufficient evidence exists to conclude that meat, eggs, and milk are either good or bad for the heart.

Table 3.3 Dietary Reference Intakes (DRIs): Recommended Intakes for Individuals: Vitamins

LIFE STAGE GROUP	VITAMIN A (µg/d)[a]	VITAMIN C (mg/d)	VITAMIN D (µg/d)[b,c]	VITAMIN E (mg/d)[d]	VITAMIN K (µg/d)	THIAMIN (mg/d)	RIBOFLAVIN (mg/d)	NIACIN (mg/d)[a]	VITAMIN B6 (mg/d)	FOLATE (µg/d)[f]	VITAMIN B12 (mg/d)	PANTOTHENIC ACID (mg/d)	BIOTIN (µg/d)	CHOLINE (mg/d)[a]
Infants														
0–6 mo	400*	40*	5*	4*	2.0*	0.2*	0.3*	2*	0.1*	65*	0.4*	1.7*	5*	125*
7–12 mo	500*	50*	5*	5*	2.5*	0.3*	0.4*	4*	0.3*	80*	0.5*	1.8*	6*	150*
Children														
1–3 y	300	15	5*	6	30*	0.5	0.5	6	0.5	150	0.9	2*	8*	200*
4–8 y	400	25	5*	7	55*	0.6	0.6	8	0.6	200	1.2	3*	12*	250*
Males														
9–13 y	600	45	5*	11	60*	0.9	0.9	12	1.0	300	1.8	4*	20*	375*
14–18 y	900	75	5*	15	75*	1.2	1.3	16	1.3	400	2.4	5*	25*	550*
19–30 y	900	90	5*	15	120*	1.2	1.3	16	1.3	400	2.4	5*	30*	550*
31–50 y	900	90	5*	15	120*	1.2	1.3	16	1.3	400	2.4	5*	30*	550*
51–70 y	900	90	10*	15	120*	1.2	1.3	16	1.3	400	2.4[h]	5*	30*	550*
>70 y	900	90	15*	15	120*	1.2	1.3	16	1.3	400	2.4[h]	5*	30*	550*
Females														
9–13 y	600	45	5*	11	60*	0.9	0.9	12	1.0	300	1.8	4*	20*	375*
14–18 y	700	65	5*	15	75*	1.0	1.0	14	1.2	400[f]	2.4	5*	25*	400*
19–30 y	700	75	5*	15	90*	1.1	1.1	14	1.3	400[f]	2.4	5*	30*	425*
31–50 y	700	75	5*	15	90*	1.1	1.1	14	1.3	400[f]	2.4	5*	30*	425*
50–70 y	700	75	10*	15	90*	1.1	1.1	14	1.5	400	2.4[h]	5*	30*	425*
>70 y	700	75	15*	15	90*	1.1	1.1	14	1.5	400	2.4[h]	5*	30*	425*
Pregnancy														
≤18 y	750	80	5*	15	75*	1.4	1.4	18	1.9	600[f]	2.6	6*	30*	450*
19–30 y	770	85	5*	15	90*	1.4	1.4	18	1.9	600[f]	2.6	6*	30*	450*
31–50 y	770	85	5*	15	90*	1.4	1.4	18	1.9	600[f]	2.6	6*	30*	450*
Lactation														
≤18 y	1200	115	5*	19	75*	1.4	1.6	17	2.0	500	2.8	7*	35*	550*
19–30 y	1300	120	5*	19	90*	1.4	1.6	17	2.0	500	2.8	7*	35*	550*
31–50 y	1300	120	5*	19	90*	1.4	1.6	17	2.0	500	2.8	7*	35*	550*

Note: This table (taken from the DRI reports, see *http://www.nap.edu/catalog.php?record_id=11537*) presents Recommended Dietary Allowances (RDAs) in **bold type** and Adequate Intakes (AIs) in ordinary type followed by an asterisk (*). RDAs and AIs may both be used as goals for individual intake. RDAs are set to meet the needs of almost all (97 to 98 percent) individuals in a group. For healthy breastfed infants, the AI is the mean intake. The AI for other life stage and gender groups is believed to cover needs of all individuals in the group, but lack of data or uncertainty in the data prevent being able to specify with confidence the percentage of individuals covered by this intake.

[a]As retinol activity equivalents (RAEs). 1 RAE = 1 mg retinol, 12 mg β-carotene, 24 mg α-carotene, or 24 mg β-cryptoxanthin. To calculate RAEs from REs of provitamin A carotenoids in foods, divide the REs by 2. For preformed vitamin A in foods or supplements and for provitamin A carotenoids in supplements, 1 RE = 1 RAE.

[b]Calciferol. 1 µg calciferol = 40 IU vitamin D.

[c]In the absence of adequate exposure to sunlight.

[d]As α-Tocopherol. α-Tocopherol includes *RRR*-α-tocopherol, the only form of α-tocopherol that occurs naturally in foods, and the 2*R*-stereoisometric forms of α-tocopherol (*RRR*-, *RSR*-, *RRS*, and *RSS*-α-tocopherol) that occur in fortified foods and supplements. It does not include the 2*S*-stereoisometric forms of α-tocopherol (*SRR*-, *SSR*-, *SR*-, and *SSS*-α-tocopherol), also found in fortified foods and supplements.

[e]As niacin equivalents (NE). 1 mg of niacin = 60 mg of tryptophan; 0–6 months = preformed niacin (not NE).

[f]As dietary folate equivalents (DFE). 1 DFE = 1 µg food folate = 0.6 µg of folic acid from fortified food or as a supplement consumed with food = 0.5 µg of a supplement taken on an empty stomach.

[g]Although AIs have been set for choice, there are few data to assess whether a dietary supply of choline is needed at all stages of the life cycle and it may be that the choline requirement can be met by endogenous synthesis at some of these stages.

[h]Because 10 to 30 percent of older people may malabsorb food-bound B₁₂, it is advisable for those older than 50 years to meet their RDA mainly by consuming foods fortified with B₁₂ or a supplement containing B₁₂.

[i]In view of evidence linking folate intake with neural tube defects in the fetus, it is recommended that all women capable of becoming pregnant consume 400 µg from supplements or fortified foods in addition to intake of food folate from a varied diet.

[j]It is assumed that women will continue consuming 400 mg from supplements or fortified food until their pregnancy is confirmed and they enter prenatal care, which ordinarily occurs after the end of the periconceptional period—the critical time for formation of the neural tube.

Sources: Dietary Reference Intakes for Calcium, Phosphorous, Magnesium, Vitamin D, and Fluoride (1997); Dietary Reference Intakes for Thiamin, Riboflavin, Niacin, Vitamin B₆, Folate, Vitamin B₁₂, Pantothenic Acid, Biotin, and Choline (1998); Dietary Reference Intakes for Vitamin C, Vitamin E, Selenium, and Carotenoids (2000); and Dietary Reference Intakes for Vitamin A, Vitamin K, Arsenic, Boron, Chromium, Copper, Iodine, Iron, Manganese, Molybdenum, Nickel, Silicon, Vanadium, and Zinc (2001).

food intake generally increases to sustain the added energy requirements of exercise. Additional food through a variety of nutritious meals proportionately increases vitamin and mineral intakes. Table 3.4 presents similar data for minerals for different life stage groups.

MYPYRAMID: THE ESSENTIALS OF GOOD NUTRITION

Key principles of good eating include *variety*, *balance*, and *moderation*. The typical pattern of food intake in the United States increases the risk for obesity, marginal micronutrient intakes, low high-density lipoprotein (HDL) and high low-density lipoprotein (LDL) cholesterol, type 2 diabetes, and elevated levels of homocysteine.

In April 2005, the U.S. government unveiled its latest attempt to personalize the approach of Americans to choose a healthier lifestyle that balances nutrition and exercise. The new color-coded food pyramid, termed **MyPyramid** (**Fig. 3.3**), offers a fresh look and a complementary Web site (*www.mypyramid.gov*) to provide personalized and supplementary materials on food intake guidance (e.g., the recommended number of cups of vegetables) based on age, gender, and level of daily exercise. The pyramid is based on the 2005 *Dietary Guidelines for Americans* published by the Department of Health and Human Services and the Department of Agriculture (*www.healthierus.gov/dietaryguidelines*). It provides a series of vertical color bands of varying widths with the combined bands for fruits (red band) and vegetables (green band) occupying the greatest width followed by grains, with the narrowest bands occupied by fats, oils, meats, and sugars. A personalized pyramid is obtained by logging on to the website. Note the addition of a figure walking up the left side of the pyramid to emphasize at least 30 minutes of moderate to vigorous daily physical activity. The *Guidelines*, formulated for the general population, also provide a sound framework for meal planning for physically active individuals. The principal message advises consuming a varied but balanced diet. Importance is placed on a diet rich in fruits and vegetables, cereals and whole grains, nonfat and low-fat dairy products, legumes, nuts, fish, poultry, and lean meats.

Figures 3.3B and **3.3C** present modifications of the basic pyramid. These apply to individuals whose diet consists largely of foods from the plant kingdom (**Near-Vegetarian Diet Pyramid**), or fruits, nuts, vegetables, fish, beans, and all manner of grains, with dietary fat composed mostly of monounsaturated fatty acids with mild ethanol consumption (**Mediterranean Diet Pyramid**). A Mediterranean-style diet protects individuals at high risk of death from heart disease. Its high content of monounsaturated fatty acids (generally olive oil with its associated phytochemicals) helps delay age-related memory loss, cancer, and overall mortality rate in healthy, elderly people. The dietary focus of all three pyramids also reduces risk for ischemic stroke and enhances the benefits of cholesterol-lowering drugs.

AN EXPANDING EMPHASIS ON HEALTHFUL EATING AND REGULAR PHYSICAL ACTIVITY

Scientists have responded to the rapidly rising number of overweight and obese adults and children and the increasing incidence of comorbidities associated with the overweight condition. The Institute of Medicine, the medical division of the National Academies, issued the *Guidelines* as part of its DRIs. The *Guidelines*, updated every 5 years, are currently under development for 2010 (*www.cnpp.usda.gov/dietaryguidelines.htm*). Recommendations emphasize that Americans (including children) spend at least 1 *hour* (not 30 minutes as previously recommended—about 400 to 500 kCal expended) over the course of

Questions & Notes

List 3 foods considered "good" for the heart.

1.

2.

3.

List the 3 principles of good eating.

1.

2.

3.

Describe the basis for the MyPyramid.

🛈 For Your Information

RECOMMENDED MEAL COMPOSITION

Suggested composition of a 2500-kCal diet based on recommendations of an expert panel of the Institute of Medicine, National Academies.

	Carbohydrate	Lipid	Protein
Percentage	60	15	25
Kilocalories	150	375	625
Grams	375	94	69
Ounces	13.2	3.3	2.4

Table 3.4 Dietary Reference Intakes (DRIs): Recommended Intakes for Individuals: Minerals

LIFE STAGE GROUP	CALCIUM (mg/d)	CHROMIUM (µg/d)	COPPER (µg/d)	FLUORIDE (mg/d)	IODINE (µg/d)	IRON (mg/d)	MAGNESIUM (mg/d)	MANGANESE (mg/d)	MOLYBDENUM (µg/d)	PHOSPHORUS (mg/d)	SELENIUM (µg/d)	ZINC (mg/d)
Infants												
0–6 mo	210*	0.2*	200*	0.01*	110*	0.27*	30*	0.003*	2*	100*	15*	2*
7–12 mo	270*	5.5*	220*	0.5*	130*	11*	75*	0.6*	3*	275*	20*	3
Children												
1–3 y	500*	11*	340	0.7*	90	7	80	1.2*	17	460	20	3
4–8 y	800*	15*	440	1	90	10	130	1.5*	22	500	30	5
Males												
9–13 y	1,300*	25*	700	2*	120	8	240	1.9*	34	1,250	40	8
14–18 y	1,300*	35*	890	3*	150	11	410	2.2*	43	1,250	55	11
19–30 y	1,000*	35*	900	4*	150	8	420	2.3*	45	700	55	11
31–50 y	1,000*	35*	900	4*	150	8	420	2.3*	45	700	55	11
51–70 y	1,200*	30*	900	4*	150	8	420	2.3*	45	700	55	11
>70 y	1,200*	30*	900	4*	150	8	420	2.3*	45	700	55	11
Females												
9–13 y	1,300*	21*	700	2*	120	8	240	1.6*	34	1,250	40	8
14–18 y	1,300*	24*	890	3*	150	15	360	1.6*	43	1,250	55	9
19–30 y	1,000*	25*	900	3*	150	18	310	1.8*	45	700	55	8
31–50 y	1,000*	25*	900	3*	150	18	320	1.8*	45	700	55	8
50–70 y	1,200*	20*	900	3*	150	8	320	1.8*	45	700	55	8
>70 y	1,200*	20*	900	3*	150	8	320	1.8*	45	700	55	8
Pregnancy												
≤18 y	1,300*	29*	1,000	3*	220	27	400	2.0*	50	1,250	60	13
19–30 y	1,000*	30*	1,000	3*	220	27	350	2.0*	50	700	60	11
31–50 y	1,000*	30*	1,000	3*	220	27	360	2.0*	50	700	60	11
Lactation												
≤18 y	1,300*	44*	1,300	3*	290	10	360	2.6*	50	1,250	70	14
19–30 y	1,000*	45*	1,300	3*	290	9	310	2.6*	50	700	70	12
31–50 y	1,000*	45*	1,300	3*	290	9	320	2.6*	50	700	70	12

Note: This table presents Recommended Dietary Allowances (RDAs) in **bold type** and Adequate Intakes (AIs) in ordinary type followed by an asterisk (*). RDAs are set to meet the needs of almost all (97 to 98 percent) individuals in a group. For healthy breastfed infants, the AI is the mean intake. The AI for other life stage and gender groups is believed to cover needs of all individuals in the group, but lack of data or uncertainty in the data prevent being able to specify with confidence the percentage of individuals covered by this intake.

Sources: Dietary Reference Intakes for Calcium, Phosphorous, Magnesium, Vitamin D and Fluoride (1997); Dietary Reference Intakes for Thiamin, Riboflavin, Niacin, Vitamin B₆, Folate, Vitamin B₁₂, Pantothenic Acid, Biotin, and Choline, (1998); Dietary Reference Intakes for Vitamin C, Vitamin E, Selenium, and Carotenoids (2000); and Dietary Reference Intakes for Vitamin A, Vitamin K, Arsenic, Boron, Chromium, Copper, Iodine, Iron, Manganese, Molybdenum, Nickel, Silicon, Vanadium, and Zinc (2001). These reports may be accessed via *http://www.nap.edu/catalog.php?record_id=11537.* Copyright 2006 by the National Academy of Sciences. Reprinted with permission.

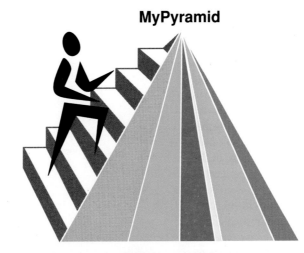

MyPyramid

GRAINS Make half your grains whole	VEGETABLES Vary your veggies	FRUITS Focus on fruits	MILK Get your calcium-rich foods	MEAT & BEANS Go lean with protein
Any food made from wheat, rice, oats, cornmeal, barley, or another cereal grain is a grain product Bread, pasta, oatmeal, breakfast cereals, tortillas, and grits are examples of grain products	Eat more dark-green veggies like broccoli, spinach, and other dark leafy greens Eat more orange vegetables like carrots and sweet potatoes Eat more dry beans and peas like pinto beans, kidney beans, and lentils	Eat a variety of fruit Choose fresh, frozen, canned, or dried fruit Go easy on fruit juices	Go low-fat or fat-free when you choose milk, yogurt, and other milk products If you don't or can't consume milk, choose lactose-free products or other calcium sources such as fortified foods and beverages	Choose low-fat or lean meats and poultry Bake it, broil it, or grill it Vary your protein routine – choose more fish, beans, peas, nuts, and seeds
For a 2000-Calorie diet you need the amounts below from each food group. To find the amounts right for you, go to MyPyramid.gov.				
Eat 3 oz. every day	Eat 2½ cups every day	Eat 2 cups every day	Drink 3 cups every day; for kids aged 2 to 8, it's 2	Eat 5½ oz. every day

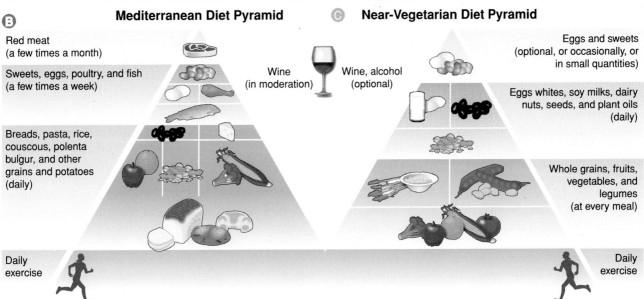

Mediterranean Diet Pyramid

Red meat (a few times a month)

Sweets, eggs, poultry, and fish (a few times a week)

Wine (in moderation)

Wine, alcohol (optional)

Breads, pasta, rice, couscous, polenta bulgur, and other grains and potatoes (daily)

Daily exercise

Near-Vegetarian Diet Pyramid

Eggs and sweets (optional, or occasionally, or in small quantities)

Eggs whites, soy milks, dairy nuts, seeds, and plant oils (daily)

Whole grains, fruits, vegetables, and legumes (at every meal)

Daily exercise

Figure 3.3   **A.** MyPyramid: A more comprehensive and personalized guide to sound nutrition. **B.** Mediterranean Diet Pyramid application to individuals whose diet consists largely of foods from the plant kingdom, or fruits; nuts; vegetables; all manner of grains; and protein derived from fish, beans, and chicken, with dietary fat composed mostly of monounsaturated fatty acids and with mild alcohol consumption. **C.** Near-Vegetarian Diet Pyramid without meat or dairy products consumed. The focus of the two pyramids in B and C on fruits and vegetables, particularly cruciferous and green leafy vegetables and citrus fruit and juice, also reduces risk for ischemic stroke and may potentiate the beneficial effects of cholesterol-lowering drugs.

each day in moderately intense physical activity (e.g., brisk walking; jogging; swimming; bicycling; lawn, garden, and house work) to maintain health and a normal body weight. This amount of regular physical activity, which was based on an assessment of the amount of exercise healthy people engage in each day, is twice that previously recommended in 1996 in a report from the United States Surgeon General. The advice represents a bold increase in exercise duration considering that 30 minutes of similar type exercise on most days significantly decreases disease risk; unfortunately, more than 60% of the U.S. population fails to incorporate even a moderate level of exercise into their lives, and shamefully, 25% do no exercise at all. In 2007, the American College of Sports Medicine in cooperation with the American Heart Association published guidelines presented in Chapter 13 for optimum exercise type and duration for people up to age 65 years and older than age 65 years (*www.acsm.org*).

The team of 21 experts also recommended for the first time a range for macronutrient intake plus how much dietary fiber to include in one's daily diet (previous reports over the past 60 years have dealt only with micronutrient recommendations). To meet daily energy and nutrient needs while minimizing the risk for chronic diseases, adults should consume between 45% and 65% of their total calories from carbohydrates. The maximum intake of added sugars (i.e., the caloric sweeteners added to manufactured foods and beverages such as soda, candy, fruit drinks, cakes, cookies, and ice cream) was placed at 25% of total calories. The range of acceptable lipid intake was placed at 20% to 35% of caloric intake, which is a range lower at the lower end of most recommendations and higher at the upper end of the 30% limit set by the American Heart Association, American Cancer Society, and National Institutes of Health. The panel also recommended that adult men age 50 years and younger consume 38 g of fiber daily and adult women consume 21 g a day, values considerably greater than the 12 to 15 g currently consumed.

Clearly, no single food or meal provides optimal nutrition and associated health-related benefits.

Diet Quality Index The Diet Quality Index (DQI-I), developed by the National Research Council Committee on Diet and Health, appraises the general "healthfulness" of one's diet. The index presented in Table 3.5 offers a simple scoring schema based on a risk gradient associated with diet and major diet-related chronic diseases. Respondents who meet a given dietary goal receive a score of 0; a score of 1 applies to an intake within 30% of a dietary goal; the score becomes 2 when intake fails to fall within 30% of the goal. The final score equals the total for all eight categories. The index ranges from 0 to 16, with a lower score representing a higher quality diet. A score of 4 or less reflects a more healthful diet; an index of 10 or higher indicates a less healthful diet that needs improvement.

EXERCISE AND FOOD INTAKE

Figure 3.4 illustrates the average energy intakes for males and females in the U.S. population grouped by age category. Mean energy intakes peak between ages 16 to 29 years and

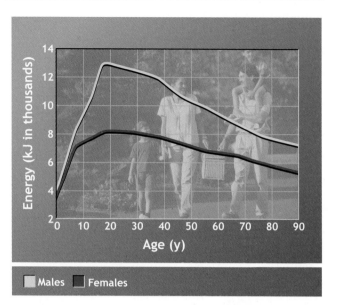

Figure 3.4 Average daily energy intake for males and females by age in the U.S. population during the years 1988 to 1991. (From Briefel, R.R., et al.: Total energy intake of the U.S. population: The Third National Health and Nutrition Examination Survey, 1988–1991. *Am. J. Clin. Nutr.*, 62(suppl):10725, 1995; and Troiano, R.P. Energy and fat intake of children and adolescents in the United States: Data from the National Health and Nutrition Survey. *Am. J. Clin. Nutr.*, 72:134, 2000.)

decline thereafter. A similar pattern occurs for males and females, although males reported higher daily energy intakes than females at all ages. Between ages 20 to 29 years, women consumed 35% fewer kCal than men on a daily basis (3025 kCal vs. 1957 kCal). With aging, the gender difference in energy intake decreased; at age 70 years, women consumed 25% fewer kCal than men.

Physical Activity Makes a Difference

For individuals who regularly engage in moderate to intense physical activities, food intake balances easily with daily energy expenditure. Lumber workers, for example, who typically expend nearly 4500 kCal daily, unconsciously adjust their energy intake to balance their energy output. For them, body weight remains stable despite an extremely large food intake. The balancing of food intake to meet a new level of energy output takes 1 to 2 days to attain new energy equilibrium. The fine balance between energy expenditure and food intake does not occur in sedentary people, in whom caloric intake chronically exceeds their relatively low daily energy expenditure. Lack of precision in regulating food intake at the low end of the physical activity spectrum contributes to "creeping obesity" in highly mechanized and technologically advanced societies.

Figure 3.5 presents data on energy intake from a large sample of elite male and female endurance, strength, and team sport athletes in the Netherlands. For men, daily energy intake ranged between 2900 and 5900 kCal; female competitors consumed 1600 to 3200 kCal. Except for the high-energy intake of athletes at extremes of performance and training, daily energy intake did not exceed 4000 kCal for men or 3000 kCal for women.

Extreme Energy Intake and Expenditure: The Tour de France During competition or periods of intense training, some sport activities require extreme energy output (sometimes in excess of 1000 kCal·h^{-1} in elite marathoners and professional cyclists) and a correspondingly high energy intake. For example, the daily energy requirements of elite cross-country skiers during 1 week of training averages 3740 to 4860 kCal for women and 6120 to 8570 kCal for men. **Figure 3.6** shows the variation in daily energy expenditure for a male competitor during the Tour de France professional cycling race. Energy expenditure averaged 6500 kCal daily for nearly 3 weeks during this event. Large daily variation occurred depending on the activity level for a particular day; the daily energy expenditure decreased to 3000 kCal on a "rest" day and increased to approximately 9000 kCal when the athlete was cycling over a mountain pass. By combining liquid nutrition with normal meals, the cyclist nearly matched daily energy expenditure with energy intake.

For Your Information

NUTRITIONAL GUIDELINES FOR THE GENERAL POPULATION

Population Goals	Major Guidelines
Overall healthy eating pattern	Consume a varied diet that includes foods from each of the major food groups with an emphasis on fruits, vegetables, whole grains, low-fat or nonfat dairy products, fish, legumes, poultry, and lean meats. Monitor portion size and number to ensure adequate not excess, intake.
Appropriate body weight (BMI = 25[a])	Match energy intake to energy needs. When weight loss is desirable, make appropriate changes to energy intake and expenditure (PA). Limit foods with a high sugar content and those with a high caloric density.
Desirable cholesterol profile	Limit foods high in saturated fat, *trans* fat, and cholesterol. Substitute unsaturated fat from vegetables, fish, legumes, and nuts.
Desirable blood pressure (systolic <140 mm Hg; diastolic <90 mm Hg)	Maintain a healthy body weight. Consume a varied diet with an emphasis on vegetables, fruits, and low-fat or nonfat dairy products. Limit sodium intake. Limit alcohol intake.

Modified from Krauss RM, et al. AHA dietary guidelines revision 2000: a statement for healthcare professionals from the Nutrition Committee of the American Heart Association. Circulation 102:2284, 2000.
[a]BMI, body mass index (kg·m^{-2}); PA, Physical Activity.

The Precompetition Meal

Athletes often compete in the morning after an overnight fast. Considerable depletion occurs in the body's carbohydrate reserves over 8 to 12 hours without eating (see Chapter 2); thus, precompetition nutrition takes on considerable importance even if the person follows appropriate dietary recommendations. *The precompetition meal provides the athlete with adequate carbohydrate energy and ensures optimal hydration.* Fasting before competition or intense training makes no sense physiologically because it rapidly depletes liver and muscle glycogen and ultimately impairs exercise performance. Consider the following three factors when individualizing an athlete's meal plans:

1. Food preference
2. Psychologic set
3. Food digestibility

As a general rule, foods high in lipid and protein should not be consumed on competition days. These foods digest slowly and remain in the digestive tract longer than carbohydrate foods containing similar calories. The timing of the precompetition meal also deserves consideration. Increased emotional stress and tension depress intestinal absorption because of a decrease in blood flow to the digestive tract. *Generally, 3 hours provides sufficient time to digest and absorb a carbohydrate-rich precompetition meal.*

High Protein: Not the Best Choice Many athletes become accustomed to and even depend on the classic "steak and eggs" precompetition meal. This meal may satisfy the athlete, coach, and restaurateur, but its benefits to exercise performance can actually hinder optimal performance.

Daily Energy Expenditure (kCal)

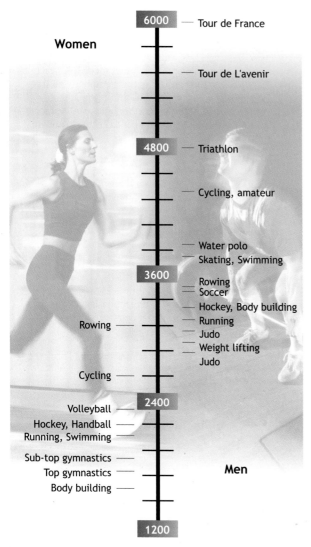

Figure 3.5 Daily energy intake in kilocalories per day in elite male and female endurance, strength, and team sport athletes. (From van Erp-Baart, A.M.J., et al.: Nationwide survey on nutritional habits in elite athletes. *Int. J. Sports Med.,* 10:53, 1989.)

High-protein precompetition meals should be modified or even abolished in favor of one high in carbohydrates for the following five reasons:

1. Dietary carbohydrates, not protein, replenish liver and muscle glycogen previously depleted from an overnight fast.
2. Carbohydrates digest and become absorbed more rapidly than proteins or lipids; thus, carbohydrates provide energy faster and reduce the feeling of fullness.
3. High-protein meals elevate resting metabolism more than high-carbohydrate meals because of greater energy requirements for protein's digestion, absorption, and assimilation. Additional metabolic heat places demands on the body's heat-dissipating mechanisms, which impairs exercise performance in hot weather.
4. Protein catabolism for energy facilitates dehydration during exercise because the byproducts of amino

acid breakdown require water for urinary excretion. Approximately 50 mL of water "accompanies" the excretion of each gram of urea in urine.
5. Carbohydrate provides the main energy nutrient for short-duration anaerobic exercise and prolonged, intense endurance activities.

Ideal Precompetition Meal   *The ideal precompetition meal maximizes muscle and liver glycogen storage and provides glucose for intestinal absorption during exercise.* The meal should accomplish these two goals:

1. Contain 150 to 300 g of carbohydrate (3–5 g per kg of body mass) in either solid or liquid form.
2. Be consumed within 3 to 4 hours before exercising.

The benefit of a precompetition meal depends on the athlete maintaining a nutritionally sound diet throughout training. Pre-exercise food cannot correct existing nutritional deficiencies or inadequate nutrient intake during the weeks before competition.

Liquid Meals   Commercially prepared **liquid meals** offer an alternative to the precompetition meal. Five benefits include the following:

1. Enhance energy and nutrient intake in training, particularly if daily energy output exceeds energy intake because of the athlete's lack of interest in food or nutrition mismanagement.
2. Provide a high glycemic carbohydrate for glycogen replenishment.
3. Contain some lipid and protein to contribute to satiety.
4. Supply fluid because these meals exist in liquid form.
5. Digest rapidly, essentially omitting residue in the intestinal tract.

Liquid meals prove particularly effective during daylong swimming and track meets or tennis, ice hockey, soccer, field hockey, martial arts, wrestling, volleyball, and basketball tournaments. During tournament competition, the athlete usually has little time for or interest in food. Athletes also can benefit from liquid meals if they experience difficulty maintaining a relatively large body mass and as a ready source of calories to gain weight.

Carbohydrate Intake Before, During, and After Intense Exercise

Whereas intense aerobic exercise continued for 1 hour decreases liver glycogen by about 55%, a 2-hour strenuous workout almost depletes the glycogen in the liver and specifically targeted exercised muscle fibers. Even maximal, repetitive, 1- to 5-minute bouts of exercise interspersed with brief rest intervals dramatically lowers liver and muscle glycogen levels (e.g., soccer, ice hockey, field hockey, European handball, and tennis). Carbohydrate supplementation improves prolonged exercise capacity and intermittent, high-intensity exercise performance. The "vulnerability" of the body's glycogen stores during intense exercise has focused research on the potential high performance benefits of carbohydrate intake just before and during exercise. Current research also continues to

Table 3.5	**The Diet Quality Index**		
RECOMMENDATION		**SCORE**	**INTAKE**
Reduce total lipid intake to 30% or less of total energy		☐ 0 ☐ 1 ☐ 2	<30% >30–40% >40%
Reduce saturated fatty acid intake to less than 10% of total energy		☐ 0 ☐ 1 ☐ 2	<10% 10–13% >13%
Reduce cholesterol intake to less than 300 mg daily		☐ 0 ☐ 1 ☐ 2	<300 mg 300–400 mg >400 mg
Eat 5 or more servings daily of vegetables and fruits		☐ 0 ☐ 1 ☐ 2	≥5 servings 3–4 servings 0–2 servings
Increase intake of starches and other complex carbohydrates by eating 6 or more servings daily of breads, cereals, and legumes		☐ 0 ☐ 1 ☐ 2	≥6 servings 4–5 servings 0–3 servings
Maintain protein intake at moderate levels		☐ 0 ☐ 1 ☐ 2	100% RDA 100–150% RDA >150% RDA
Limit total daily sodium intake to 2400 mg or less		☐ 0 ☐ 1 ☐ 2	≤2400 mg 2400–3400 mg >3400 mg
Maintain adequate calcium intake (approximately the RDA)		☐ 0 ☐ 1 ☐ 2	≥100% RDA 67–99% RDA <67% RDA

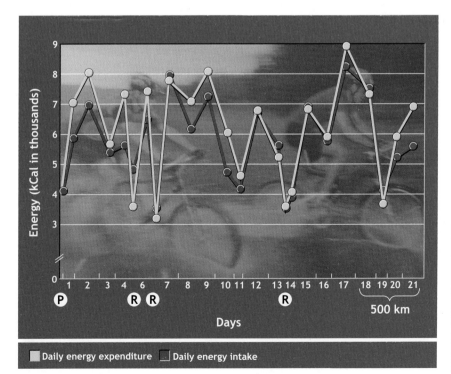

Figure 3.6 Variation in daily energy expenditure (*purple squares*) and energy intake (*yellow circles*) for a cyclist during the Tour de France competition. Note the extremely high energy expenditure values and the ability to achieve energy balance with liquid nutrition plus normal meals. P, stage; R, rest day. (Modified from the chapter *Adequacy of Vitamin Supply under Maximal Sustained Workloads: The Tour de France* by Wim H.M. Saris, Jaap Schrijver, Marie-Agnes v. Erp Baart, & Fred Brouns, published on pp. 205–212 in *Elevated Dosages of Vitamins* by Paul Walter et al., ISBN 0-920887-29-5 and ISBN 3-456-81679-0 ©1989 Hans Huber Publishers.)

Daily energy expenditure ☐ *Daily energy intake*

Energy (kCal in thousands)

Days

500 km

---

*Q*uestions & Notes

Give the average daily energy intake for males and females between ages 16 and 29 years.

Males:

Females:

Give the estimated daily energy expenditure for participants in the Tour de France.

List 2 food types that should NOT be consumed during days of athletic competition.

1.

2.

Give 3 reasons the precompetition meal should be higher in carbohydrate than in protein.

1.

2.

3.

i For Your Information

GLUCOSE POLYMERS

If a drink contains a glucose polymer (e.g., maltodextrin) rather than simple sugars, it minimizes the negative effects of concentrated sugar molecules on gastric emptying and maintains plasma volume. Short-chain polymers (3 to 20 glucose units) derived from cornstarch breakdown reduce the number of particles in solution (osmolality); this facilitates water movement from the stomach into the small intestine for absorption.

illustrate how to optimize carbohydrate replenishment during the postexercise recovery period.

Before Exercise

The potential endurance benefits of consuming simple sugars before exercise remain equivocal. One line of research contends that ingesting rapidly absorbed, high-glycemic carbohydrates within 1 hour before exercising accelerates glycogen depletion and negatively affects endurance performance by (1) causing an overshoot in insulin release, thus creating low blood sugar termed **rebound hypoglycemia** (that impairs central nervous system function during exercise) and (2) facilitating glucose influx into muscle (through a large insulin release) to increase carbohydrate use as fuel during exercise. Concurrently, high insulin levels inhibit lipolysis to reduce free fatty acid mobilization from adipose tissue. Greater carbohydrate breakdown and blunted fat mobilization contribute to premature glycogen depletion and early fatigue.

Recent research indicates that consuming glucose before exercise increases muscle glucose uptake but reduces liver glucose output during exercise to a degree that actually *conserves* liver glycogen reserves. From a practical standpoint, one way to eliminate any potential for negative effects from pre-exercise simple sugars necessitates ingesting them at least 60 minutes before exercise. This allows sufficient time to reestablish hormonal balance before exercise.

Pre-exercise Fructose Intake

The small intestine absorbs fructose more slowly than glucose with only a minimal insulin response without a decline in blood glucose. These observations have stimulated debate about whether fructose might provide a beneficial pre-exercise, exogenous carbohydrate fuel source for prolonged exercise. The theoretical rationale for fructose appears plausible, but its exercise benefits remain inconclusive. From a practical standpoint, consuming a high-fructose beverage often produces gastrointestinal distress (cramping, vomiting, and diarrhea), which should negatively impact exercise performance. *After it has been absorbed by the small intestine, fructose must also be converted to glucose in the liver. This time delay further limits fructose availability for energy.*

Glycemic Index and Pre-exercise Food Intake

The glycemic index helps to formulate the composition of the immediate pre-exercise meal. The basic idea is to make glucose available to maintain blood sugar and muscle metabolism without requiring an excess insulin release. The objective, to spare glycogen reserves, requires stabilizing blood glucose and optimizing fat mobilization and catabolism. Consuming low-glycemic index foods less than 30 minutes before exercise allows for a relatively slow rate of glucose absorption into the blood during exercise. This eliminates an insulin surge yet also provides a steady

supply of "slow-release" glucose from the digestive tract as exercise progresses. This effect theoretically should benefit long-term, intense exercise.

During Exercise

Consuming about 60 g of liquid or solid carbohydrates each hour during exercise benefits long-duration intense exercise and repetitive, short bouts of near-maximal effort. Sustained exercise below 50% of maximum intensity relies primarily on fat oxidation, with only a relatively small demand on carbohydrate breakdown. As such, consuming carbohydrate offers little benefit during such activity. In contrast, carbohydrate intake provides supplementary glucose during intense, aerobic exercise when glycogen utilization increases greatly. Exogenous carbohydrate accomplishes one or both of the following two goals:

1. Spares muscle glycogen because the ingested glucose powers the exercise.
2. Helps to stabilize blood glucose, which prevents headache, lightheadedness, nausea, and other symptoms of central nervous system distress.

Maintaining an optimal blood glucose level also supplies muscles with glucose during the later stages of prolonged exercise when glycogen reserves deplete. Consuming carbohydrates while exercising at 60% to 80% $\dot{V}O_{2max}$ (maximal oxygen consumption) postpones fatigue by 15 to 30 minutes. This effect offers potential for marathon runners who often experience muscle fatigue within 90 minutes of running. **Figure 3.7** shows that a single, concentrated carbohydrate intake almost 2 hours into exercise when blood

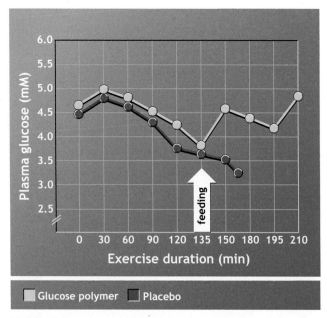

Figure 3.7 Average plasma glucose concentration during prolonged, high-intensity aerobic exercise when subjects consumed a placebo (*red*) or glucose polymer (*gold*; 3 g per kg body mass in a 50% solution). (Modified from Coggan, A.R., Coyle, E.F. Metabolism and performance following carbohydrate ingestion late in exercise. *Med. Sci. Sports Exerc.*, 21:59, 1989.)

glucose and glycogen reserves near depletion restores blood glucose levels; this strategy increases carbohydrate availability and delays fatigue because higher blood glucose levels sustain the muscles' energy needs.

Post-exercise Carbohydrate Intake

To speed glycogen replenishment after a hard bout of training or competition, one should immediately consume carbohydrate-rich, high-glycemic foods. Specifically, consume 50 to 75 g (2 to 3 oz) of moderate- to high-glycemic carbohydrates every 2 hours for a total of 500 g (7–10 g per kg body mass) or until consuming a large high-carbohydrate meal. If consuming carbohydrate immediately after exercise is impractical, meals containing 2.5 g of high-glycemic carbohydrates per kg of body mass consumed at 2, 4, 6, 8, and 22 hours after exercise rapidly restores muscle glycogen. For a 70-kg runner, for example, this would amount to a little more than 6 oz (2.5 g × 70 ÷ 28.4 g per oz = 6 oz).

To rapidly replenish glycogen reserves, avoid legumes, fructose, and milk products because of their slow rates of intestinal absorption. More rapid glycogen resynthesis occurs by remaining physically inactive during recovery. *Under optimal carbohydrate intake conditions, glycogen replenishes at a rate of about 5% per hour. Even under the best of circumstances, it would still require at least 20 hours to reestablish glycogen stores with glycogen depletion.*

GLUCOSE INTAKE, ELECTROLYTES, AND WATER UPTAKE

Adding carbohydrates to the oral rehydration beverage provides additional glucose energy for exercise when the body's glycogen reserves deplete. Determining the optimal fluid/carbohydrate mixture and volume to consume during exercise takes on importance when the objectives attempt to reduce fatigue and prevent dehydration. Consuming a large, dilute fluid volume may lessen carbohydrate uptake, and concentrated sugar solutions diminish fluid replacement.

The rate of stomach emptying greatly affects the small intestine's fluid and nutrient absorption. Exercise up to an intensity of about 75% $\dot{V}O_{2max}$ minimally (if at all) impacts gastric emptying and an exercise intensity greater than 75% $\dot{V}O_{2max}$ slows the emptying rate. Gastric volume greatly influences gastric emptying; its rate decreases as stomach volume decreases. It makes sense to maintain a relatively large stomach fluid volume to speed gastric emptying.

Consider Fluid Concentration

A key question concerns the possible negative effects of sugar drinks on water absorption from the digestive tract. Gastric emptying slows when ingested fluids contain an excessive concentration of particles in solution (increased osmolality) or possess high caloric content. Any factor that impairs fluid uptake negatively impacts prolonged exercise in hot weather, when adequate water intake and absorption play prime roles in the participant's health and safety. Ingesting up to an 8% glucose–sodium oral rehydration beverage causes little negative effect on

Questions & Notes

Give the major purpose of the precompetition meal.

Give 2 benefits of a precompetition liquid meal.

1.

2.

 ## For Your Information

FLUID INTAKE: PRACTICAL RECOMMENDATIONS

1. Monitor dehydration rate from changes in body weight (have athlete urinate before postexercise body weight determination to account for water lost in urine). Each pound of weight loss corresponds to about 450 mL (15 fluid oz) of dehydration.
2. Drink fluids at the same rate as their estimated rate of depletion. This means drinking at a rate close to 80% of sweating rate during prolonged exercise that produces cardiovascular stress, excessive heat, and dehydration.
3. Drink between 625 and 1250 mL each hour (250 mL every 15 min) of a 4% to 8% carbohydrate beverage to meet carbohydrate (30 to 60 g·h^{-1}) and fluid requirements.
4. Consuming 400 to 600 mL of fluid immediately before exercise optimizes the beneficial effect of increased stomach volume on fluid and nutrient passage into the intestine.
5. Fluid temperature per se probably does not play a major role in replenishing fluid during exercise.
6. Avoid beverages containing alcohol or caffeine because both compounds induce a diuretic effect (alcohol most pronounced) that facilitates water loss.

BOX 3.2   CLOSE UP

Recommended Oral Rehydration Beverage

The ideal oral rehydration beverage has these five qualities:

1. Tastes good.
2. Absorbs rapidly.
3. Causes little or no gastrointestinal distress.
4. Helps maintain extracellular fluid volume and osmolality.
5. Offers the potential to enhance exercise performance.

Consuming a 5% to 8% carbohydrate-electrolyte beverage during exercise in the heat contributes to temperature regulation and fluid balance as effectively as plain water. The drink also maintains glucose metabolism and glycogen reserves in prolonged exercise.

To determine a drink's carbohydrate percentage, divide its carbohydrate content (in grams) by the fluid volume (in milliliters) and multiply by 100. For example, 80 g of carbohydrate in 1000 mL (1 L) of water represents an 8% solution. Of course, various environmental and exercise conditions interact to influence the optimal composition of the rehydration solution. With relatively short-duration (30–60 minutes), intense aerobic effort, and high thermal stress, fluid replenishment takes on importance for health and safety; ingesting a more dilute carbohydrate–electrolyte solution (<5% carbohydrate) is advisable under such conditions. In cool weather, with less likelihood of significant dehydration, a more concentrated beverage of 15% carbohydrate suffices. Essentially, no differences exist among liquids containing glucose, sucrose, or starch as the preferred exogenous carbohydrate fuel source during exercise.

The optimal carbohydrate replacement rate ranges between 30 and 60 g (1–2 oz) per hour.

The accompanying figure illustrates the major factors that affect gastric emptying from the stomach and fluid absorption for the small intestine. A major factor to speed gastric emptying involves maintaining a relatively high fluid volume in the stomach.

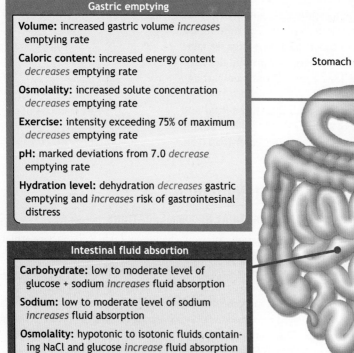

Gastric emptying

Volume: increased gastric volume *increases* emptying rate

Caloric content: increased energy content *decreases* emptying rate

Osmolality: increased solute concentration *decreases* emptying rate

Exercise: intensity exceeding 75% of maximum *decreases* emptying rate

pH: marked deviations from 7.0 *decrease* emptying rate

Hydration level: dehydration *decreases* gastric emptying and *increases* risk of gastrointesinal distress

Intestinal fluid absortion

Carbohydrate: low to moderate level of glucose + sodium *increases* fluid absorption

Sodium: low to moderate level of sodium *increases* fluid absorption

Osmolality: hypotonic to isotonic fluids containing NaCl and glucose *increase* fluid absorption

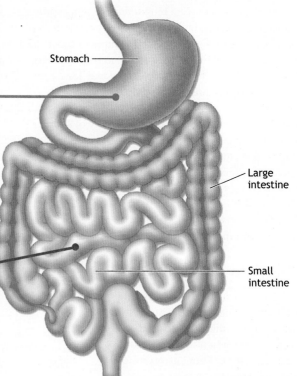

Stomach

Large intestine

Small intestine

gastric emptying. This beverage facilitates fluid uptake by the intestinal lumen because active cotransport of glucose and sodium across the intestinal mucosa stimulates water's passive uptake by osmotic action. Water replenishes effectively, and additional glucose uptake contributes to blood glucose maintenance. This glucose can then spare muscle and liver glycogen or provide for blood glucose reserves during the later stage of exercise.

Sodium's Potential Benefit

Adding a moderate amount of sodium to ingested fluid maintains plasma sodium concentration. The American College of Sports Medicine recommends that sports drinks contain 0.5 to 0.7 g of sodium per liter of fluid consumed during exercise lasting more than 1 hour. This benefits ultraendurance athletes at risk for hyponatremia (see Chapter 2), which results from significant sweat-induced sodium loss coupled with an unusually large intake of plain water. A beverage that tastes good to the individual contributes to voluntary rehydration during exercise and recovery. Adding a small amount of sodium to the rehydration beverage does the following to promote continued fluid intake and fluid retention during recovery from exercise:

1. Maintains plasma osmolality.
2. Reduces urine output.
3. Sustains the drive to drink.

CARBOHYDRATE NEEDS DURING INTENSE TRAINING

Repeated days of strenuous endurance workouts for distance running, swimming, cross-country skiing, and cycling can induce general fatigue that makes training progressively more difficult. Often referred to as "**staleness**," the gradual depletion of glycogen reserves probably triggers this physiologic state. In one experiment, in which athletes ran 16.1 km (10 miles) a day for 3 successive days, glycogen in the thigh muscles was nearly depleted, although the athletes' diets contained about 50% carbohydrate. By the third day, glycogen usage during the run was less than on the first day, and fat breakdown supplied the predominant fuel to power exercise. No further glycogen depletion occurred when daily dietary carbohydrate increased to 600 g (70% of caloric intake), further demonstrating the importance of maintaining adequate carbohydrate intake during training.

Diet, Glycogen Stores, and Endurance Capacity

In the late 1960s, scientists observed that endurance performance improved simply by consuming a carbohydrate-rich diet for 3 days before exercising. Conversely, endurance deteriorated if the diet consisted principally of lipids. In one series of classic experiments, subjects consumed one of three diets. The first maintained normal energy intake but supplied the majority of calories from lipids, with only 5% from carbohydrates. The second provided the normal allotment for calories with the typical percentages of the three macronutrients. The third provided 80% of calories as carbohydrates.

The results from this innovative study illustrated in **Figure 3.8** show that the glycogen content of leg muscles, expressed as grams of glycogen per 100 g of muscle,

Questions & Notes

Describe the advantage of adding a small amount of sodium to fluid ingested.

Describes what happens with gradual glycogen depletion.

For Your Information

MUSCLE GLYCOGEN SUPERCOMPENSATION ENHANCED BY PRIOR CREATINE SUPPLEMENTATION

A synergy exists between glycogen storage and creatine supplementation. For example, preceding a glycogen loading protocol with a creatine loading protocol (20 g per day for 5 days) produces a 10% greater glycogen packing in the vastus lateralis muscle compared with muscle glycogen levels achieved with only glycogen loading. It appears that increases in creatine and cellular volume with creatine supplementation facilitate subsequent storage of muscle glycogen.

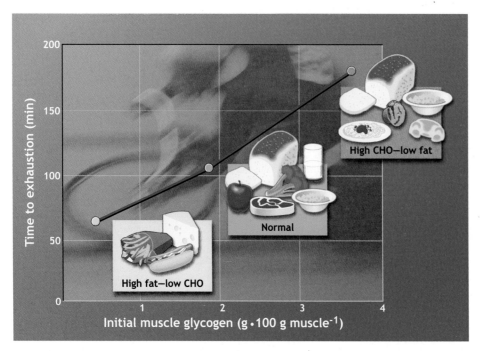

Figure 3.8 Classic experiment on the effects of a low-carbohydrate diet, mixed diet, and high-carbohydrate diet on glycogen content of the quadriceps femoris muscle and the duration of endurance exercise on a bicycle ergometer. With a high-carbohydrate diet, endurance time tripled compared with a diet low in carbohydrates. (Adapted from Bergstrom, J., et al.: Diet, muscle glycogen and physical performance. *Acta. Physiol. Scand.* 71:140, 1967.)

averaged 0.6 for subjects who consumed the low-carbohydrate diet, 1.75 for subjects who consumed the typical diet, and 3.75 for subjects who consumed the high-carbohydrate diet. Furthermore, the subjects' endurance capacity varied greatly depending on their pre-exercise diet. When subjects consumed the high-carbohydrate diet, endurance more than tripled compared with those consuming the low-carbohydrate diet!

These findings highlight the important role nutrition plays in establishing appropriate energy reserves for exercise. A diet deficient in carbohydrates rapidly depletes muscle and liver glycogen. Glycogen depletion subsequently affects performance in maximal, short-term anaerobic exercise and prolonged, intense aerobic effort. In addition to athletes, these observations also are germain to moderately active people who eat less than the recommended quantity of carbohydrates.

Enhanced Glycogen Storage: Carbohydrate Loading

A particular combination of diet plus exercise produces a significant "packing" of muscle glycogen, a procedure termed **carbohydrate loading** or **glycogen supercompensation**. The technique increases muscle glycogen levels more than levels achieved by simply maintaining a high-carbohydrate diet. Glycogen loading packs up to 5 g of glycogen into each 100 g of muscle in contrast to the normal value of 1.7 g. For athletes who follow the classic glycogen-loading procedure (see Close Up Box 3.3, *Strategies for Carbohydrate Loading, page 104*), enhanced muscle glycogen levels are maintained in a resting, nonexercising individual for at least 3 days if the diet contains about 60% of total calories as carbohydrate during the maintenance phase.

Exercise facilitates both the rate and magnitude of glycogen replenishment. For sports competition and exercise training, a diet containing between 60% and 70% of calories as carbohydrates should adequately maintain muscle and liver glycogen reserves. This diet ensures about twice the level of muscle glycogen compared with sedentary counterparts who consume a lower carbohydrate diet of 50%–60% carbohydrates. For well-nourished physically active individuals, the supercompensation effect remains relatively small. During intense training, individuals who do not upgrade daily caloric and carbohydrate intakes to meet increased energy demands may experience chronic muscle fatigue and staleness.

Individuals should learn all they can about carbohydrate loading before trying to manipulate their diet and exercise habits to achieve a supercompensation effect. If a person decides to supercompensate after weighing the pros and cons (see page 103), the new food regimen should be tried in stages during training and not for the first time before competition. For example, a runner should start with a long run followed by a high-carbohydrate diet. The athlete should maintain a detailed log of how the dietary manipulation affects performance. Subjective feelings should be noted during exercise depletion and replenishment phases. With positive results, the person should then try the complete series of depletion, low-carbohydrate diet and a high-carbohydrate diet but maintain the low-carbohydrate diet for only 1 day. If no adverse effects appear, the low-carbohydrate diet should be gradually extended to a maximum of 4 days.

Modified Loading Procedure

The less-stringent, modified dietary protocol removes many of the negative aspects of the classic glycogen-loading sequence. This 6-day protocol does not require prior exercise to deplete glycogen. The athlete trains at about 75% of $\dot{V}O_{2max}$ (85% HR_{max}) for 1.5 hours and then gradually reduces or tapers exercise duration on successive days. Carbohydrates represent approximately 50% of total caloric intake during the first 3 days. Three days before competition, the diet's carbohydrate content then increases to 70% of energy intake, replenishing glycogen reserves to about the same point achieved with the classic loading protocol.

Rapid Loading Procedure: A One-Day Requirement

The 2 to 6 days required to achieve supranormal muscle glycogen levels represents a limitation of typical carbohydrate loading procedures. Research has evaluated whether a shortened time period that combines a relatively brief bout of intense exercise with only 1 day of high-carbohydrate intake achieves the desired loading effect. Endurance-trained athletes cycled for 150 seconds at 130% of $\dot{V}O_{2max}$, followed by 30 seconds of all-out cycling. In the recovery period, the men consumed 10.3 $g \cdot kg$ body mass^{-1} of high-glycemic carbohydrate foods. Biopsy data presented in **Figure 3.9** indicated that carbohydrate levels increased 82% in all fiber types of the vastus lateralis muscle after only 24 hours. The increased glycogen storage equaled or exceeded values reported by others using a 2- to 6-day regimen. The short-duration loading procedure benefits individuals who do not wish to disrupt normal training with the time required and potential negative aspects of other nutrient loading protocols.

Limited Applicability and Negative Aspects

The potential benefits from carbohydrate loading apply only to intense and prolonged aerobic activities. *Unless the athlete begins competing in a state of depletion, exercising for less than 60 minutes requires only normal carbohydrate intake and glycogen reserves.* Carbohydrate loading and associated high levels of muscle and liver glycogen did not benefit athletes in a 20.9-km (13-mile) run compared with a run after a low-carbohydrate diet. Also, a single, maximal anaerobic exercise for 75 seconds did not improve by increasing muscle glycogen availability above normal through dietary manipulation before exercise.

In most sport competition and exercise training, a daily diet of 60% to 70% of total calories as carbohydrates provides for adequate muscle and liver glycogen reserves. This diet ensures about twice the level of muscle glycogen compared with the 45% to 50% carbohydrate amount of the typical American diet. For

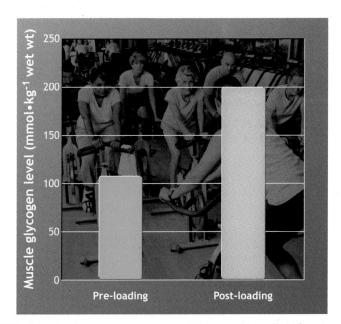

Figure 3.9 Muscle glycogen concentration of the vastus lateralis before (pre-loading) and after 180 seconds of near-maximal intensity cycling exercise followed by 1 day of high-carbohydrate intake (post-loading). (From Fairchild, T. J., et al.: Rapid carbohydrate loading after short bout of near maximal-intensity exercise. *Med. Sci. Sports Exerc.,* 34:980, 2002.)

*Q*uestions & Notes

Discuss potential benefits of carbohydrate loading.

 For Your Information

ADJUST CARBOHYDRATE INTAKE TO ENERGY EXPENDITURE AND BODY WEIGHT

Athletes who train arduously should consume 10 g of carbohydrates per kg of body mass daily. A 100-lb (45-kg) athlete who expends 2800 kCal daily requires approximately 450 g of carbohydrate, or 1800 kCal. An athlete who weighs 150 pounds (68 kg) and expends 4200 kCal per day should consume about 680 g of carbohydrates (2720 kCal). In both examples, carbohydrate intake equals 64% of total energy intake.

 For Your Information

KEEP THEM UNREFINED, COMPLEX, AND LOW GLYCEMIC

Little health risk exists in subsisting chiefly on a variety of fiber-rich complex carbohydrates if intake also supplies essential amino acids, fatty acids, minerals, and vitamins. The most desirable complex carbohydrates exhibit slow digestion and absorption rates. Such moderate- to low-glycemic types include whole-grain breads, cereals, pastas, legumes, most fruits, and milk and milk products.

BOX 3.3 CLOSE UP

Strategies for Carbohydrate Loading

The importance of muscle glycogen levels to enhance exercise performance remains unequivocal; time to exhaustion during intense aerobic exercise directly relates to the initial glycogen content of the liver and active musculature. In one series of experiments, muscle glycogen content increased sixfold, and endurance capacity tripled for subjects fed a high-carbohydrate diet compared with feeding the same subjects a low-carbohydrate (high-fat) diet of similar energy content. Carbohydrate loading provides a strategy to increase initial muscle and liver glycogen levels before prolonged endurance performance.

CLASSIC CARBOHYDRATE LOADING PROCEDURE

Classic carbohydrate loading involves a two-stage procedure.

Stage 1—Depletion

Day 1: Perform exhaustive exercise to deplete muscle glycogen in specific muscles.

Days 2, 3, and 4: Maintain low-carbohydrate food intake (high percentage of protein and lipid in the daily diet).

Stage 2—Carbohydrate Loading

Days 5, 6, and 7: Maintain high-carbohydrate food intake (normal percentage of protein in the daily diet).

Competition Day

Follow high-carbohydrate precompetition meal recommendation.

SPECIFICS OF PRECOMPETITION DIET-EXERCISE PLAN TO ENHANCE GLYCOGEN STORAGE

1. Use high-intensity, aerobic exercise for 90 minutes about 6 days before competition to reduce muscle and liver glycogen stores. Because glycogen loading occurs only in the specific muscles depleted by exercise, athletes must engage the major muscles involved in their sport.

2. Maintain a low-carbohydrate diet (60–100 g per day) for 3 days while training at moderate intensity to further deplete glycogen stores.

3. Switch to a high-carbohydrate diet (400–700 g per day) at least 3 days before competition and maintain this intake up to and as part of the precompetition meal.

Sample Meal Plans for Carbohydrate Depletion (Stage 1) and Carbohydrate Loading (Stage 2) Preceding an Endurance Event

MEAL	STAGE 1	STAGE 2
Breakfast	1/2 cup fruit juice 2 eggs 1 slice whole-wheat toast 1 glass whole milk	1 cup fruit juice 1 bowl hot or cold cereal 1 to 2 muffins 1 Tbsp butter coffee (cream and sugar)
Lunch	6 oz hamburger 2 slices bread 1 serving salad 1 Tbsp mayonnaise and salad dressing 1 glass whole milk	2–3 oz hamburger with bun 1 cup juice 1 orange 1 Tbsp mayonnaise 1 serving pie or cake
Snack	1 cup yogurt	1 cup yogurt, fruit, or cookies
Dinner	2 to 3 pieces chicken, fried 1 baked potato with sour cream 1/2 cup vegetables 2 Tbsp butter iced tea (no sugar)	1–1 1/2 pieces chicken, baked 1 baked potato with sour cream 1 cup vegetables 1/2 cup sweetened pineapple iced tea (sugar) 1 Tbsp butter
Snack	1 glass whole milk	1 glass chocolate milk with 4 cookies

Carbohydrate intake averages approximately 100 g or 400 kCal during Stage 1; Stage 2 carbohydrate intake increases to 400 to 700 g or about 1600 to 2800 kCal.

BOX 3.4 CLOSE UP

International Society of Sports Nutrition Position Stand: Nutrient Timing[a]

The following represents the position of the International Society of Sports Nutrition published in 2008 regarding nutrient timing and the intake of carbohydrates, proteins, and fats in reference to healthy, exercising individuals. The Society, composed of experts in the field of sports nutrition and exercise physiology (*www.sportsnutritionsociety.org*), makes the following eight points:

1. Maximal endogenous glycogen stores are best promoted by following a high-glycemic, high-carbohydrate (CHO) diet (600 to 1000 g CHO or ~8 to 10 g $CHO \cdot kg^{-1} \cdot d^{-1}$), and ingestion of free amino acids and protein (PRO) alone or in combination with CHO before resistance exercise can maximally stimulate protein synthesis.

2. During exercise, CHO should be consumed at a rate of 30 to 60 g of CHO/h in a 6% to 8% CHO solution (8 to 16 fluid oz) every 10 to 15 minutes. Adding protein (PRO) to create a CHO:PRO ratio of 3 to 4:1 may increase endurance performance and maximally promotes glycogen resynthesis during acute and subsequent bouts of endurance exercise.

3. Ingesting CHO alone or in combination with PRO during resistance exercise increases muscle glycogen, offsets muscle damage, and facilitates greater training adaptations after either acute or prolonged periods of supplementation with resistance training.

4. Postexercise (within 30 minutes) consumption of CHO at high dosages (8–10 g $CHO \cdot kg^{-1} \cdot d^{-1}$) have stimulate muscle glycogen resynthesis; adding PRO (0.2–0.5 g $PRO \cdot kg^{-1} \cdot d^{-1}$) to CHO at a ratio of 3 to 4:1 (CHO:PRO) may further enhance glycogen resynthesis.

5. Postexercise ingestion (immediately to 3 hours after exercise) of amino acids, primarily essential amino acids, stimulates robust increases in muscle protein synthesis; the addition of CHO may stimulate even greater levels of protein synthesis. Additionally, pre-exercise consumption of a CHO + PRO supplement may produce peak levels of protein synthesis.

6. During consistent, prolonged resistance training, postexercise consumption of varying doses of CHO + PRO supplements in varying dosages stimulate improvements in strength and body composition compared with control or placebo conditions.

7. The addition of creatine (Cr) (0.1 g $Cr \cdot kg^{-1} \cdot d^{-1}$) to a CHO + PRO supplement may facilitate even greater adaptations to resistance training.

8. Nutrient timing incorporates the use of methodical planning and eating of whole foods, nutrients extracted from food, and other sources. The timing of the energy intake and the ratio of certain ingested macronutrients are likely the attributes to allow for enhanced recovery and tissue repair after high-volume exercise, augmented muscle protein synthesis, and improved mood states when compared with unplanned or traditional strategies of nutrient intake.

[a]Kerksick C, et al.: International Society of Sports Nutrition position stand: nutrient timing. *J. Int. Soc. Sports Nutr.*, 3;5:17, 2008.

well-nourished athletes, any supercompensation effect from carbohydrate loading remains relatively small.

The addition of 2.7 g of water stored with each gram of glycogen makes this a heavy fuel compared with equivalent energy as stored fat. A higher body mass because of water retention often makes the athlete feel heavy, "bloated," and uncomfortable; any extra load also directly adds to the energy cost of weight-bearing running, racewalking, climbing activities, and cross-country skiing. The added energy cost may actually negate the potential benefits from increased glycogen storage. On the positive side, the water liberated during glycogen breakdown aids in temperature regulation to benefit exercise in hot environments.

The classic model for supercompensation is ill advised for individuals with certain health problems. A dietary carbohydrate overload, interspersed with periods of high lipid or protein intake, may increase blood cholesterol and urea nitrogen levels. This could pose problems to those predisposed to type 2 diabetes and heart disease and those with muscle enzyme deficiencies or renal disease. Failure to eat a balanced diet can produce deficiencies of some minerals and vitamins, particularly water-soluble vitamins; these deficiencies may require dietary

Questions & Notes

Under what condition would glycogen super-compensation be ill-advised?

supplementation. The glycogen-depleted state during the first phase of the glycogen-loading procedure certainly reduces one's capability to engage in intense training, possibly producing a detraining effect during the loading interval. Dramatically reducing dietary carbohydrate for 3 or 4 days could also set the stage for lean tissue loss because muscle protein serves as gluconeogenic substrate to maintain blood-glucose levels with low glycogen reserves.

SUMMARY

1. Within rather broad limits, a balanced diet from regular food intake provides the nutrient requirements of athletes and others engaged in exercise training and sports competition.

2. MyPyramid represents a model for good nutrition for most individuals, and includes regular physical activity. The guidelines emphasize diverse grains, vegetables, and fruits as major calorie sources, downplaying foods high in animal proteins, lipids, and dairy products.

3. For physically active individuals, consuming 400 to 600 g of carbohydrates particularly unrefined, low-glycemic polysaccharides should supply 60% to 70% of daily caloric intake.

4. The volume of daily physical activity largely determines energy intake requirements. Under most circumstances, daily energy requirements for physically active individuals probably do not exceed 4000 kCal for men and 3000 kCal for women. Under extremes of training and competition, these values approach 5000 kCal for women and 9000 kCal for men.

5. The relatively high caloric intakes of physically active men and women usually increase protein, vitamin, and mineral intake above recommended values.

6. The ideal precompetition meal maximizes muscle and liver glycogen storage and enhances glucose for intestinal absorption during exercise. High-carbohydrate and relatively low-lipid and low-protein meals generally fill this requirement. A carbohydrate-rich pre-event meal requires about 3 hours for digestion and absorption.

7. Commercially prepared liquid meals offer a practical approach to precompetition nutrition and energy supplementation because they balance nutritive value, contribute to fluid needs, and absorb rapidly.

8. Consuming low-glycemic index foods immediately before exercise allows for a relatively slow rate of glucose absorption into the blood. This should eliminate an insulin surge while providing a steady supply of "slow-release" glucose from the digestive tract during exercise.

9. Fluid volume within the stomach exerts the greatest effect on the rate of gastric emptying. One should consume 400 to 600 mL of fluid immediately before exercise with subsequent regular ingestion of 250 mL at 15-minute intervals throughout exercise.

10. Consuming a 5% to 8% carbohydrate-electrolyte beverage during exercise in the heat contributes to temperature regulation and fluid balance as effectively as plain water.

11. Following a bout of intense physical training or competition, a person should consume 50 to 75 g of moderate- to high-glycemic carbohydrates every 2 hours for a total of 500 g to speed glycogen replenishment.

12. It takes at least 20 hours (5% per hour) to fully re-establish pre-exercise glycogen stores.

13. Successive days of intense training gradually deplete glycogen reserves even with the typical pattern of carbohydrate intake.

14. A diet deficient in carbohydrate rapidly depletes muscle and liver glycogen to profoundly impair performance in maximal, short-term anaerobic exercise and prolonged, intense aerobic effort.

15. Carbohydrate loading can augment endurance performance. Athletes should become well informed about this procedure because of potential negative side effects.

16. Modifying the classic carbohydrate loading procedure augments glycogen storage without dramatically altering diet and exercise regimens.

THOUGHT QUESTIONS

1. Under what circumstances might an athlete require nutritional supplementation?

2. An athletic team has three matches scheduled on consecutive days. What should the athletes consume after each day's competition and why?

3. What advice would you give to a sprint athlete (runner or swimmer) who plans to carbohydrate load for competition?

4. Among physically active men and women, how can individuals who consume the greatest number of calories weigh less than those who consume fewer calories?

SELECTED REFERENCES

Achten, J., et al.: Higher dietary carbohydrate content during interspersed running training results in a better maintenance of performance and mood state. *J. Appl. Physiol.*, 96:1331, 2004.

Akabas, S.R., Dolins, K.R.: Micronutrient requirements of physically active women: what can we learn from iron? *Am. J. Clin. Nutr.*, 81(suppl):1246S, 2005.

Barnett, C., et al.: Muscle metabolism during sprint exercise in man: influence of sprint training. *J. Sci. Med. Sport*, 7:314, 2004.

Baty, J.J., et al.: The effect of a carbohydrate and protein supplement on resistance exercise performance, hormonal response, and muscle damage. *J. Strength Cond. Res.*, 21:321, 2007.

Berardi, J.M., et al.: Postexercise muscle glycogen recovery enhanced with a carbohydrate-protein supplement. *Med. Sci. Sports Exerc.*, 38:1106, 2006.

Billaut, F., Bishop, D.: Muscle fatigue in males and females during multiple-sprint exercise. *Sports Med.*, 39:257, 2009.

Blacker, S.D., et al.: Carbohydrate vs protein supplementation for recovery of neuromuscular function following prolonged load carriage. *J. Int. Soc. Sports Nutr.*, 7:2, 2010.

Bosch, A.N., Noakes, T.D.: Carbohydrate ingestion during exercise and endurance performance. *Indian J. Med. Res.*, 121:634, 2005.

Burgomaster, K.A., et al.: Six sessions of sprint interval training increases muscle oxidative potential and cycle endurance capacity in humans. *J. Appl. Physiol.*, 98:1985, 2005.

Burke, L.M., et al.: Energy and carbohydrate for training and recovery. *J. Sports Sci.*, 24:675, 2006.

Burke, L.M.: Nutrition for distance events. *J. Sports Sci.*, 25 (Suppl 1):S29, 2007. Review. Erratum in: *J. Sports Sci.*, 27 667, 2009.

Burns, S.F., et al.: A single session of resistance exercise does not reduce postprandial lipaemia. *J. Sports Sci.*, 23:251, 2005.

Cases, N., et al.: Differential response of plasma and immune cell's vitamin E levels to physical activity and antioxidant vitamin supplementation. *Eur. J. Clin. Nutr.*, 59:781, 2005.

Castell, L.M., et al.: BJSM reviews: A-Z of nutritional supplements: dietary supplements, sports nutrition foods and ergogenic aids for health and performance. Part 8. *Br. J. Sports Med.*, 44:468, 2010.

Castellani, J.W., et al.: Energy expenditure in men and women during 54h of exercise and caloric deprivation. *Med. Sci. Sports Exerc.*, 38:894, 2006.

Cochran, A.J., et al.: Carbohydrate feeding during recovery alters the skeletal muscle metabolic response to repeated sessions of high-intensity interval exercise in humans. *J. Appl. Physiol.*, 108:628, 2010.

Coggan, A.R., Coyle, E.F.: Carbohydrate ingestion during prolonged exercise: Effects on metabolism and performance. In: *Exercise and Sport Science Reviews*, Vol. 19. Holloszy, J.O. (ed.). Baltimore: Williams & Wilkins, 1991.

Cordain, L., et al.: Origins and evolutions of the Western diet: health implications for the 21st century. *Am. J. Clin. Nutr.*, 81:341, 2005.

Coyle, E.F.: Fluid and fuel intake during exercise. *J. Sports Sci.*, 22:39, 2004.

Currell, K., and Jeukendrup, A.E.: Superior endurance performance with ingestion of multiple transportable carbohydrates. *Med. Sci. Sports Exerc.*, 40:275, 2008.

Donaldson, C.M., et al.: Glycemic index and endurance performance. *Int. J. Sport Nutr. Exerc. Metab.*, 20:154. Review, 2010.

Erlenbusch, M., et al.: Effect of high-fat or high-carbohydrate diets on endurance exercise: a meta-analysis. *Int. J. Sport Nutr. Exerc. Metab.*, 15:1, 2005.

Fiala, K.A., et al.: Rehydration with a caffeinated beverage during the nonexercise periods of 3 consecutive days of 2-a-day practices. *Int. J. Sport Nutr. Exerc. Metab.*, 14:419, 2004.

Food and Nutrition Board, Institute of Medicine.: *Dietary Reference Intakes for Energy, Carbohydrates, Fiber, Fat, Protein and Amino Acids.* Washington, D.C.: National Academy Press, 2002.

Helge, J.W., et al.: Impact of a fat-rich diet on endurance in man: role of the dietary period. *Med. Sci. Sports Exerc.*, 30:456, 1998.

Hoffman, J.R., et al.: Effect of low-dose, short-duration creatine supplementation on anaerobic exercise performance. *J. Strength Cond. Res.*, 19:260, 2005.

Hoffman, J.R., et al.: Effects of beta-hydroxy beta-methylbutyrate on power performance and indices of muscle damage and stress during high-intensity training. *J. Strength Cond. Res.*, 18:747, 2004.

Horowitz, J.F., et al.: Energy deficit without reducing dietary carbohydrate alters resting carbohydrate oxidation and fatty acid availability. *J. Appl. Physiol.*, 98:1612, 2005.

Horowitz, J.F., et al.: Substrate metabolism when subjects are fed carbohydrates during exercise. *Am. J. Physiol.*, 276(5 Pt): E828, 1999.

Horowitz, J.F.: Fatty acid mobilization from adipose tissue during exercise. *Trends Endocrinol. Metab.*, 14:386, 2003.

Hulston, C.J., Jeukendrup, A.E.: No placebo effect from carbohydrate intake during prolonged exercise. *Int. J. Sport Nutr. Exerc. Metab.*, 19:275, 2009.

Iaia, F. M., et al.: Four weeks of speed endurance training reduces energy expenditure during exercise and maintains muscle oxidative capacity despite a reduction in training volume. *J. Appl. Physiol.*, 106:73, 2009.

Ivy, J.L., et al.: Effect of a carbohydrate-protein supplement on endurance performance during exercise of varying intensity. *Int. J. Sport Nutr. Exerc. Metab.*, 13:388, 2003.

Jeacocke, N.A., Burke, L.M.: Methods to standardize dietary intake before performance testing. *Int. J. Sport Nutr. Exerc. Metab.* 20:87. Review, 2010.

Jenkins, D. J., et al.: Glycemic index: an overview of implications in health and disease. *Am. J. Clin. Nutr.*, 76(suppl):266S, 2002.

Jentjens, R. L., et al.: Oxidation of combined ingestion of glucose and fructose during exercise. *J. Appl. Physiol.*, 96:1277, 2004.

Jentjens, R.L., Jeukendrup, A.E.: High rates of exogenous carbohydrate oxidation from a mixture of glucose and fructose ingested during prolonged cycling exercise. *Br. J. Nutr.*, 93:485, 2005.

Jeukendrup, A.E., Wallis, G.A.: Measurement of substrate oxidation during exercise by means of gas exchange measurements. *Int. J. Sports Med.*, 26(suppl 1):S28, 2005.

Kammer, L, et al.: Cereal and nonfat milk support muscle recovery following exercise. *J. Int. Soc. Sports Nutr.*, 6:11. 2009.

Kerksick, C., et al.: International Society of Sports Nutrition position stand: Nutrient timing. *J. Int. Soc. Sports Nutr.*, 3;5:17. 2008. Erratum in: *J. Int. Soc. Sports Nutr.*, 5:18, 2008.

Khanna, G.L., Manna, I.: Supplementary effect of carbohydrate-electrolyte drink on sports performance, lactate removal and cardiovascular response of athletes. *Indian J. Med. Res.*, 121:665, 2005.

Kirwin, J.P., et al.: A moderate glycemic meal before endurance exercise can enhance performance. *J. Appl. Physiol.*, 84:53, 1998.

Lambert, C.P., et al.: Macronutrient considerations for the sport of bodybuilding. *Sports Med.*, 34:317, 2004.

Lasheras, C., et al.: Mediterranean diet and age with respect to overall survival in institutionalized, nonsmoking elderly people. *Am. J. Clin. Nutr.*, 71:987, 2000.

Leiper, J.B., et al.: The effect of intermittent high-intensity running on gastric emptying of fluids in man. *Med. Sci. Sports Exerc.*, 37:240, 2005.

Liu, S., et al.: A prospective study of dietary glycemic load, carbohydrate intake, and risk of coronary heart disease in US women. *Am. J. Clin. Nutr.*, 71:1455, 2000.

McArdle, W.D., et al.: *Sports and Exercise Nutrition*, 3rd Ed. Baltimore: Lippincott Williams & Wilkins, 2009.

Morifuji, M., et al.: Dietary whey protein increases liver and skeletal muscle glycogen levels in exercise-trained rats. *Br. J. Nutr.*, 93:439, 2005.

Morrison, P.J., et al.: Adding protein to a carbohydrate supplement provided after endurance exercise enhances 4E-BP1 and RPS6 signaling in skeletal muscle. *J. Appl. Physiol.*, 104:1029, 2008.

Nick J.J., et al.: Carbohydrate feedings during team sport exercise preserve physical and CNS function. *Med. Sci. Sports Exerc.*; 37:306, 2005.

Nybo, L.: CNS fatigue and prolonged exercise: effect of glucose supplementation. *Med. Sci. Sports Exerc.*, 35:589, 2003.

Pelly, F., et al.: Catering for the athletes village at the Sydney 2000 Olympic Games: The role of sports dietitians. *Int. J. Sport Nutr. Exerc. Metab.*, 19:340, 2009.

Pi-Sunyer, X.: Glycemic index and disease. *Am. J. Clin. Nutr.*, 76(suppl): 290S, 2002.

Riddell, M.C., et al.: (2001). Substrate utilization during exercise with glucose and glucose plus fructose ingestion in boys ages 10–14 yr. *J. Appl. Physiol.*, 90:903, 2001.

Rodriguez, N.R., et al.: Position of the American Dietetic Association, Dietitians of Canada, and the American College of Sports Medicine: Nutrition and athletic performance. American Dietetic Association; Dietetians of Canada; American College of Sports Medicine. *J. Am. Diet. Assoc.*, 109:509, 2009.

Roy, L.B., et al.: Oxidation of exogenous glucose, sucrose, and maltose during prolonged cycling exercise. *J. Appl. Physiol.*, 96:1285, 2004.

Saunders, M.J., et al.: Effects of a carbohydrate-protein beverage on cycling endurance and muscle damage. *Med. Sci. Sports Exerc.*, 36:1233, 2004.

Sawka, M.N., et al.: Hydration effects on temperature regulation. *Int. J. Sports Med.*, 19(suppl 2):S108, 1998.

Shannon, K.A., et al.: Resistance exercise and postprandial lipemia: The dose effect of differing volumes of acute resistance exercise bouts. *Metabolism*, 54:756, 2005.

Shirreffs, S.M., et al.: Fluid and electrolyte needs for preparation and recovery from training and competition. *J. Sports Sci.*, 22:57, 2004.

Snyder, A.C.: Overtraining and glycogen depletion hypothesis. *Med. Sci. Sports Exerc.*, 30:1146, 1998.

Sparks, M.J., et al.: Pre-exercise carbohydrate ingestion: Effect of the glycemic index on endurance exercise performance. *Med. Sci. Sports Exerc.*, 30:844, 1998.

Stepto, N. K., et al.: Effect of short-term fat adaptation on high-intensity training. *Med. Sci. Sports Exerc.*, 34:449, 2002.

Stewart, R.D., et al.: Protection of muscle membrane excitability during prolonged cycle exercise with glucose supplementation. *J. Appl. Physiol.*; 103:331, 2007.

Tharion, W. J., et al.: Energy requirements of military personnel. *Appetite*, 44:47, 2005.

Theodorou, A.S.: Effects of acute creatine loading with or without carbohydrate on repeated bouts of maximal swimming in high-performance swimmers. *J. Strength Cond. Res.*, 19:265, 2005.

Trichopoulou, A., et al.: Adherence to a Mediterranean diet and survival in a Greek population. *N. Engl. J. Med.*, 348:2599, 2003.

Vogt, M., et al.: Effects of dietary fat on muscle substrates, metabolism, and performance in athletes. *Med. Sci. Sports Exerc.*, 35:952, 2003.

Von Duvillard, S.P., et al.: Fluids and hydration in prolonged endurance performance. *Nutrition*, 20:651, 2004.

Wakshlag, J.J., et al.: Biochemical and metabolic changes due to exercise in sprint-racing sled dogs: implications for postexercise carbohydrate supplements and hydration management. *Vet. Ther.*, 5:52, 2004.

Welsh, R. S., et al.: Carbohydrates and physical/mental performance during intermittent exercise to fatigue. *Med. Sci. Sports Exerc.*, 34;723, 2002.

Williams, M.H.: *Nutrition for Health, Fitness, and Sport*, 7th Ed. New York: McGraw-Hill. 2009.

Wismann, J., Willoughby, D.: Gender differences in carbohydrate metabolism and carbohydrate loading. *J. Int. Soc. Sports Nutr.*, 5:3:28, 2006.

Yeo, W.K., et al.: Fat adaptation followed by carbohydrate restoration increases AMPK activity in skeletal muscle from trained humans. *J. Appl. Physiol.*, 1051:519, 2008.

Zaryski, C., Smith, D. J.: (2005). Training principles and issues for ultra-endurance athletes. *Curr. Sports Med. Rep.*, 4:165, 2005.

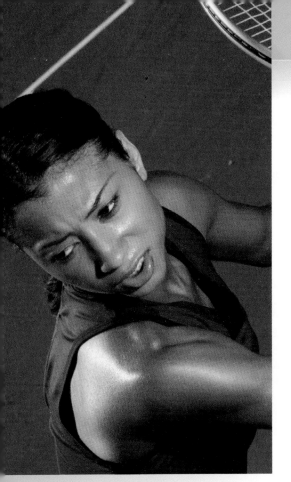

Chapter 4

Nutritional and Pharmacologic Aids to Performance

CHAPTER OBJECTIVES

- List four examples of substances alleged to provide ergogenic benefits.

- Summarize research concerning caffeine's potential as an ergogenic aid.

- Discuss the physiologic and psychologic effects of alcohol and how alcohol affects exercise performance.

- Explain how glutamine and phosphatidylserine affect exercise performance and the training response.

- Describe any positive and negative ergogenic effects of creatine supplementation.

- Explain how postexercise carbohydrate–protein–creatine supplementation augments responses to resistance training.

- Give the rationale for medium-chain triacylglycerol supplementation as an ergogenic aid.

- Discuss the possible ergogenic benefits and risks of clenbuterol, amphetamines, chromium picolinate, β-hydroxy-β-methylbutyrate, and buffering solutions.

- Discuss the positive and negative effects of anabolic steroids use as an ergogenic aid.

- Discuss the positive and negative effects of androstenedione use as an ergogenic aid.

- Describe the medical use of human growth hormone, including its potential dangers when used by healthy individuals.

- Describe the rationale for DHEA (dehydroepiandros-terone) as an ergogenic aid.

Ergogenic aids include substances and procedures believed to improve exercise capacity, physiologic function, or athletic performance. This chapter discusses the possible ergogenic role of selected commonly used nutritional and pharmacologic agents. Chapter 15 presents the use of physiologic manipulations and agents to enhance exercise performance.

Considerable literature concerns the effects of different nutritional and pharmacologic aids on exercise performance and training responsiveness. Product promotional materials often include testimonials and endorsements for untested products from sports professionals and organizations, media publicity, television infomercials, and websites. Frequently touted articles quote potential performance benefits from steroids (and steroid substitutes), alcohol, amphetamines, hormones, carbohydrates, amino acids (either consumed singularly or in combination), fatty acids, caffeine, buffering compounds, wheat-germ oil, vitamins, minerals, catecholamine agonists, and even marijuana and cocaine. Athletes routinely use many of these substances, believing their use can enhance mental and physical functions or the effects of training for sports performance.

Five mechanisms explain how ergogenic agents exert their effects:

1. By acting as a central or peripheral stimulant to the nervous system (e.g., caffeine, choline, amphetamines, alcohol).
2. By increasing the storage or availability (or both) of a limiting substrate (e.g., carbohydrate, creatine, carnitine, chromium).
3. By acting as a supplemental fuel source (e.g., glucose, medium-chain triacylglycerols).
4. By reducing or neutralizing performance-inhibiting metabolic byproducts (e.g., sodium bicarbonate, citrate, pangamic acid, phosphate).
5. By facilitating recovery from strenuous exercise (e.g., high-glycemic carbohydrates, water).

The indiscriminate use of ergogenic substances often increases the likelihood of adverse side effects that range from benign physical discomfort to life-threatening episodes. Many compounds also fail to conform to labeling requirements to correctly identify the strength of the product's ingredients and contaminents.

USED SINCE ANTIQUITY

Ancient athletes of Greece reportedly used hallucinogenic mushrooms for ergogenic purposes, and Roman gladiators ingested the equivalent of "speed" to enhance performance in the Circus Maximus (chariot racing stadium and mass entertainment venue in Rome beginning in 50 BC). Athletes of the Victorian era between 1840 to 1900 routinely used chemicals such as caffeine, alcohol, nitroglycerine, heroin, cocaine, and even strychnine (rat poison) for a competitive edge. Present-day athletes go to great lengths to promote all aspects of their health. They train hard; eat well-balanced meals; consume the latest sports drink with megadoses of vitamins, minerals, and amino acids; and seek and receive

medical advice for various injuries (no matter how minor). Yet ironically, they ingest synthetic agents, many of which precipitate adverse effects ranging from nausea, hair loss, itching, and nervous irritability to severe consequences of sterility, liver disease, drug addiction, psychotic episodes, and even death from liver and blood cancer.

Ergogenic aids, including illlgal drugs, to improve exercise performance in almost all sports have been making headlines since the 1950s. Improvements in doping control standards have apparently had a major impact on sports performance reflected by the lack of improvement in new world records, mainly in track and field. Perhaps the drug-tainted past has temporarily been put on hold. Particularly impressive is the decline in men and women's performances in the shotput, discus, javelin, and long jump.

Highly celebrated and idolized but now disgraced Olympians were required by the International Olympic Committee (IOC; *www.olympic.org*) to return their medals for illegal doping during the 2000 Sydney Olympic Games. Track star Marion Jones, who won five medals (gold in the 100-m and 200-m and 1600-m relay and bronze in the long jump and 40-m relay), pleaded guilty in 2007 to two counts of lying to investigators after vigorously denying steroid abuse over many years. Jones was sentenced to federal prison for 6 months, including 2 years' probation and community service.

FUNCTIONAL FOODS

An increasing belief in the potential for selected foods to promote health has led to the coined term **functional food.** Beyond meeting the three basic nutrition needs for survival, hunger satisfaction, and preventing adverse effects, functional foods and their bioactive components (e.g., olive oil, soy products, omega-3 fatty acids) promote well-being, health, and optimal bodily function and reduce disease risk (**Fig. 4.1**). Primary physiologic targets for this expanding branch of food science include gastrointestinal functions, antioxidant systems, and macronutrient metabolism. Enormous pressure exists to understand nutrition's role in optimizing an individual's genetic potential, susceptibility to disease, and overall performance. Unfortunately, the science base generated by research in this field of human nutrition often falls prey to nutritional hucksters and scam artists.

DOUBLE-BLIND, PLACEBO-CONTROLLED EXPERIMENT: THE PROPER MEANS TO EVALUATE ERGOGENIC CLAIMS

For today's exercise enthusiast and competitive athlete, dietary supplements usually consist of nonprescription plant extracts, vitamins, minerals, enzymes, and hormonal products. For a positive impact, these supplements must provide a nutrient that is undersupplied in the diet or exerts a drug-like influence on cellular function.

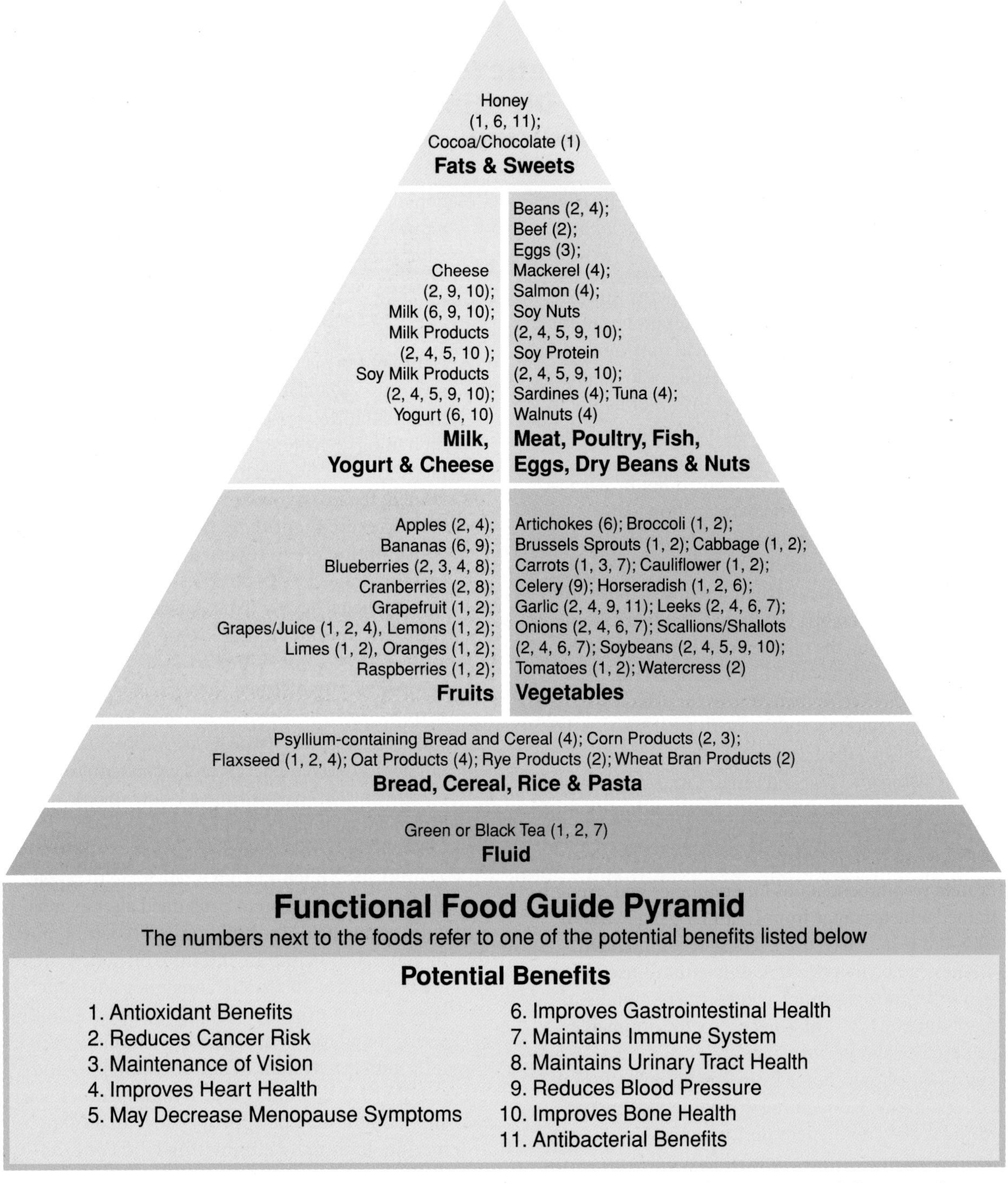

Honey
(1, 6, 11);
Cocoa/Chocolate (1)
Fats & Sweets

Cheese
(2, 9, 10);
Milk (6, 9, 10);
Milk Products
(2, 4, 5, 10);
Soy Milk Products
(2, 4, 5, 9, 10);
Yogurt (6, 10)

Beans (2, 4);
Beef (2);
Eggs (3);
Mackerel (4);
Salmon (4);
Soy Nuts
(2, 4, 5, 9, 10);
Soy Protein
(2, 4, 5, 9, 10);
Sardines (4); Tuna (4);
Walnuts (4)

**Milk,
Yogurt & Cheese**

**Meat, Poultry, Fish,
Eggs, Dry Beans & Nuts**

Apples (2, 4);
Bananas (6, 9);
Blueberries (2, 3, 4, 8);
Cranberries (2, 8);
Grapefruit (1, 2);
Grapes/Juice (1, 2, 4), Lemons (1, 2);
Limes (1, 2), Oranges (1, 2);
Raspberries (1, 2);

Artichokes (6); Broccoli (1, 2);
Brussels Sprouts (1, 2); Cabbage (1, 2);
Carrots (1, 3, 7); Cauliflower (1, 2);
Celery (9); Horseradish (1, 2, 6);
Garlic (2, 4, 9, 11); Leeks (2, 4, 6, 7);
Onions (2, 4, 6, 7); Scallions/Shallots
(2, 4, 6, 7); Soybeans (2, 4, 5, 9, 10);
Tomatoes (1, 2); Watercress (2)

Fruits **Vegetables**

Psyllium-containing Bread and Cereal (4); Corn Products (2, 3);
Flaxseed (1, 2, 4); Oat Products (4); Rye Products (2); Wheat Bran Products (2)

Bread, Cereal, Rice & Pasta

Green or Black Tea (1, 2, 7)
Fluid

Functional Food Guide Pyramid
The numbers next to the foods refer to one of the potential benefits listed below

Potential Benefits

1. Antioxidant Benefits
2. Reduces Cancer Risk
3. Maintenance of Vision
4. Improves Heart Health
5. May Decrease Menopause Symptoms

6. Improves Gastrointestinal Health
7. Maintains Immune System
8. Maintains Urinary Tract Health
9. Reduces Blood Pressure
10. Improves Bone Health
11. Antibacterial Benefits

Figure 4.1 Functional food guide pyramid. Different foods provide different benefits. (From University of Illinois at Chicago and the University of Illinois at Urbana-Champaign. *Functional Foods for Health*.) *www.Nutriwatch.org/04Foods/ff.html*

 For Your Information

BANNED SUBSTANCES

The World Anti-Doping Agency (WADA; *www.wada-ama.org/en/prohibitedlist.ch2*) currently bans the following nine categories of substances:

1. Anabolic androgenic steroids
2. Hormones and related substances
3. β_2 agonists
4. Hormone antagonists and modulators
5. Diuretics and other masking agents

6. Stimulants
7. Narcotics
8. Cannabinoids
9. Glucocorticosteroids

BOX 4.1 CLOSE UP

Key Points on Nutrition and Athletic Performance From the American Dietetic Association, Dietitians of Canada, and American College of Sports Medicine

The following key points summarize the current energy, nutrient, and fluid recommendations for active adults and competitive athletes.

1. Athletes need to consume adequate energy during periods of high-intensity and long-duration training to maintain body weight and health and maximize training effects. Low energy intakes results in loss of muscle mass; menstrual dysfunction; loss of or failure to gain bone density; an increased risk of fatigue, injury and illness; and a prolonged recovery process.

2. Body weight and composition should **not** be used as the sole criterion for sports participation, daily weigh-ins are discouraged. Optimal body fat levels depend on sex, gender, and heredity of the athlete. Body fat assessment techniques have inherent variability and limitations. Preferably, weight loss (fat loss) should take place during the off season or begin before the competitive season with a qualified sports dietitian.

3. Carbohydrate recommendations for athletes range from 6 to 10 $g \cdot kg^{-1}$ BW·d^{-1} (2.7–4.5 $g \cdot lb^{-1}$ BW·d^{-1}). Carbohydrates maintain blood glucose levels during exercise and replace muscle glycogen. The amount required depends on the athlete's total daily energy expenditure, type of sport, gender, and environmental conditions.

4. Protein recommendations for endurance and strength-trained athletes range from 1.2 to 1.7 $g \cdot kg^{-1}$ BW·d^{-1} (0.5–0.8 $g \cdot lb^{-1}$ BW·d^{-1}). These recommended intakes can be met through diet without use of protein or amino acid supplements. Energy intake to maintain body weight is necessary for optimal protein use and performance.

5. Fat intake should range from 20% to 35% of total energy intake. Consuming 20% or less of energy from fat does not benefit performance. Fat, fat-soluble vitamins, and essential fatty acids are important in the athletes diet. High-fat diets are not recommended for athletes.

6. Athletes who restrict energy intake or use severe weight loss practices, eliminate one or more food groups or consume high- or low-carbohydrate diets of low micronutrient density are at greatest risk of micronutrient deficiencies. Athletes should consume diets that provide at least the Recommended Dietary Allowance for all micronutrients.

7. Dehydration (water deficit in excess of 2%–3% body mass) decreases exercise performance; thus, adequate fluid intake before, during, and after exercise is important for optimal performance. Drinking prevents dehydration from occurring during exercise, and individuals should **not** drink in excess of sweating rate. After exercise, individuals should drink approximately 16 to 24 oz (450–675 mL) of fluid for every pound (0.5 kg) of body weight lost during exercise.

8. Before exercise, a meal or snack should provide sufficient fluid to maintain hydration and should be relatively low in fat and fiber to facilitate gastric emptying and minimize gastrointestinal distress, relatively high in carbohydrates to maximize maintenance of blood glucose, moderate in protein, composed of familiar foods, and well tolerated by the athlete.

9. During exercise, primary goals for nutrient consumption are to replace fluid losses and provide carbohydrates (~30–60 $g \cdot h^{-1}$) for maintenance of blood glucose levels. This is especially important for endurance events lasting longer than 1 h when the athlete has not consumed adequate food or fluid before exercise or when the athlete is exercising in extreme environments (heat, cold, or high altitude).

10. After exercise, dietary goals are to provide adequate fluids, electrolytes, energy, and carbohydrates to replace muscle glycogen and ensure rapid recovery. A carbohydrate intake of approximately 1.0 to 1.5 $g \cdot kg^{-1}$ BW (0.5–0.7 $g \cdot lb^{-1}$) during the first 30 min and again every 2 h for 4 to 6 h is adequate to replace glycogen stores. Protein consumed after exercise provides amino acids for building and repair of muscle.

11. In general, no vitamin and mineral supplements are required if an athlete consumes adequate energy from a variety of foods. Supplementation recommendations unrelated to exercise, such as folic acid for women of childbearing potential, should be followed. A multivitamin/mineral supplement may be appropriate if an athlete is dieting, habitually eliminating foods or food groups, is ill or recovering from injury, or has a specific micronutrient deficiency. Single-nutrient supplements may be appropriate for a specific medical or nutritional reason (e.g., iron supplements to correct iron-deficiency anemia).

12. Athletes should be counseled regarding the appropriate use of ergogenic aids to ensure safety, efficacy, potency, and legality.

13. Vegetarian athletes may be at risk for low intakes of energy, protein, fat, and key micronutrients such as iron, calcium, vitamin D, riboflavin, zinc, and vitamin B_{12}. Consultation with a sports dietitian is recommended to avoid these nutrition problems.

Nutrition and Athletic Performance. Joint position statement from the American Dietetic Association, Dietitians of Canada, and the American College of Sports Medicine. *Med. Sci. Sports Exerc.*, 41:709, 2009.

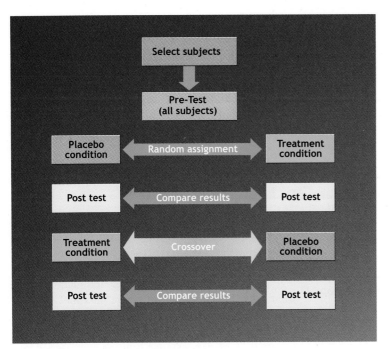

Figure 4.2 Example of a randomized, double-blind, placebo-controlled, cross-over study. After appropriate subject selection, participants are pre-tested and then randomly assigned to either the experimental or control (placebo) group. After treatment, a posttest is administered. Participants then cross over into the opposite group for the same time period as in the first condition. A second post-test follows. Comparisons of the post-tests determine the extent of a "treatment effect."

The ideal experiment to evaluate the performance-enhancing effects of an exogenous supplement requires that randomly assigned experimental and control subjects remain unaware or "blinded" to the substance administered. To achieve this goal, subjects receive a similar quantity or form of the proposed aid. The experimental subjects receive the alleged aid, and the control group subjects receive an inert compound or placebo. The placebo treatment evaluates the possibility of subjects performing well or responding better simply because they receive a substance they believe should benefit them (psychological or placebo effect). To further reduce experimental bias from influencing the outcome, those administering the treatment and recording the response must not know which subjects receive the treatment or placebo. In such a **double-blinded** experiment, both the investigators and the subjects remain unaware of the treatment condition. **Figure 4.2** illustrates the design of a double-blind, placebo-controlled study with an accompanying *crossover* with treatment and placebo conditions reversed.

Part 1   Nutritional Ergogenic Aids

BUFFERING SOLUTIONS

Dramatic alterations take place in the chemical balance of intracellular and extracellular fluids during all-out exercise durations of between 30 and 120 seconds. This occurs because muscle fibers rely predominantly on anaerobic energy transfer, which increases lactate formation with decreased intracellular pH. Increases in acidity inhibit the energy transfer and contractile qualities of

Questions & Notes

State the recommended protein intake for endurance and strength-trained athletes.

 For Your Information

URINE TESTING: THE METHOD OF CHOICE

Testing of urine samples provides the primary method for drug detection. Chemicals are added to the urine sample, which is then heated and vaporized in testing. The vapor passes through an absorbent column and an electric or magnetic field (gas chromatography and mass spectrometry). The pattern made by the molecules deflected by the field is compared with patterns made by known chemicals.

active muscle fibers. In the blood, increased concentrations of H^+ and lactate produce acidosis.

The bicarbonate aspect of the body's buffering system defends against an increase in intracellular H^+ concentration (see Chapter 9). Maintaining high levels of extracellular bicarbonate causes rapid H^+ efflux from cells and reduces intracellular acidosis. This fact has fueled speculation that increasing the body's bicarbonate (alkaline) reserve or pre-exercise alkalosis might enhance subsequent anaerobic exercise performance by delaying the decrease in intracellular pH. Research has produced conflicting results in this area from variations in pre-exercise doses of sodium bicarbonate and type of exercise to evaluate the ergogenic effects.

One study evaluated the effects of acute induced metabolic alkalosis on short-term fatiguing exercise that generated lactate accumulation. Six trained middle-distance runners consumed a **sodium bicarbonate** solution (300 mg per kg body mass) or a similar quantity of calcium carbonate placebo before running an 800-m race or under control conditions without an exogenous substance. Ingesting the alkaline drink increased pH and standard bicarbonate levels before exercise (Table 4.1). Study subjects ran an average of 2.9 sec faster under alkalosis and achieved higher post-exercise blood lactate, pH, and extracellular H^+ concentrations compared with the placebo or control subjects. Similar ergogenic effects of induced alkalosis also occur in short-term anaerobic performance with the alkalinizing agent exogenous **sodium citrate**.

The ergogenic effect of pre-exercise alkalosis (not banned by the World Anti-Doping Agency WADA; *www.wada-a.org*), either with sodium bicarbonate or sodium citrate before intense, short-term exercise, probably occurs from an increase in anaerobic energy transfer during exercise. Increases in extracellular buffering provided by exogenous buffers may facilitate coupled transport of lactate and H^+ across muscle cell membranes into extracellular fluid during fatiguing exercise. This delays decreases in intracellular pH and its subsequent negative effects on muscle function. A 2.9-second faster 800-m race time represents a dramatic improvement; it transposes to about 19 m at race pace, bringing a last place finisher to first place in most 800-m races.

Effects Relate to Dosage and Degree of Exercise Anaerobiosis

The interaction between bicarbonate dosage and the cumulative anaerobic nature of exercise influences potential ergogenic effects of pre-exercise bicarbonate loading. *For men and women, doses of at least 0.3 g per kg body mass ingested 1 to 2 hours before competition facilitate H^+ efflux from cells.* This enhances a single maximal effort of 1 to 2 minutes or longer term arm or leg exercise that lead to exhaustion within 6 to 8 minutes. No ergogenic effect occurs for typical resistance training exercises (e.g., squat, bench press). All-out effort lasting less than 1 minute may improve only for repetitive exercise bouts.

PHOSPHATE LOADING

The rationale concerning pre-exercise phosphate supplementation (**phosphate loading**) focuses on increasing extracellular and intracellular phosphate levels can produce three effects:

1. Increase adenosine triphosphate (ATP) phosphorylation.
2. Increase aerobic exercise performance and myocardial functional capacity.

Table 4.1	Performance Time and Acid–Base Profiles for Subjects Under Control, Placebo, and Induced Pre-exercise Alkalosis Conditions Before and Following an 800-m Race			
VARIABLE	**CONDITION**	**PRE-TREATMENT**	**PRE-EXERCISE**	**POST-EXERCISE**
pH	Control	7.40	7.39	7.07
	Placebo	7.39	7.40	7.09
	Alkalosis	7.40	7.49[b]	7.18[a]
Lactate (mmol·L^{-1})	Control	1.21	1.15	12.62
	Placebo	1.38	1.23	13.62
	Alkalosis	1.29	1.31	14.29[a]
Standard HCO_3^{-1} (mEq·L^{-1})	Control	25.8	24.5	9.90
	Placebo	25.6	26.2	11.0
	Alkalosis	25.2	33.5[b]	14.30[a]

	Control	Placebo	Alkalosis
Performance time (min:s)	2:05.8	2:05.1	2:02.9[c]

[a]Alkalosis values were significantly higher than placebo and control values post exercise.
[b]Pre-exercise values were significantly higher than pre-treatment values.
[c]Alkalosis time was significantly faster than control and placebo times.
From Wilkes, D., et al.: Effects of induced metabolic alkalosis on 800-m racing time. *Med. Sci. Sports Exerc.*, 15:277, 1983.

3. Augment peripheral oxygen extraction in muscle tissue by stimulating red blood cell glycolysis and subsequent elevation of erythrocyte 2,3-diphosphoglycerate (2,3-DPG).

The compound 2,3-DPG, produced within the red blood cells during anaerobic glycolytic reactions, binds loosely with hemoglobin subunits, reducing its affinity for oxygen. This releases additional oxygen to the tissues for a given decrease in cellular oxygen pressure.

Despite the proposed theoretical rationale for ergogenic effects with phosphate loading, benefits are not consistently observed. Some studies show improvement in $\dot{V}O_{2max}$ (maximal oxygen consumption) and arteriovenous oxygen difference after phosphate loading, but other studies report no effects on aerobic capacity and cardiovascular performance.

One reason for inconsistencies in findings concerns variations in exercise mode and intensity, dosage, and duration of supplementation; standardization of pretesting diets; and subjects' fitness level. *Presently, little reliable scientific evidence exists to recommend exogenous phosphate as an ergogenic aid.* On the negative side, excess plasma phosphate stimulates secretion of parathormone, the parathyroid hormone. Excessive parathormone production accelerates the kidneys' excretion of phosphate and facilitates resorption of calcium salts from the bones to decrease bone mass. Research has not determined whether short-term phosphate supplementation can negatively impact normal bone dynamics.

ANTI-CORTISOL–PRODUCING COMPOUNDS

The anterior pituitary gland secretes adrenocorticotropic hormone (ACTH), which induces adrenal cortex release of the glucocorticoid hormone **cortisol** (hydrocortisone) (see Chapter 12). Cortisol decreases the transport of amino acid into cells to depress anabolism and stimulate protein breakdown to its building block amino acids in all cells except the liver. The liberated amino acids circulate to the liver for glucose synthesis (gluconeogenesis) for energy. Cortisol serves as an insulin antagonist by inhibiting cellular glucose uptake and oxidation.

Prolonged, elevated serum concentration of cortisol from exogenous intake ultimately leads to excessive protein breakdown, tissue wasting, and negative nitrogen balance. The potential catabolic effect of exogenous cortisol has convinced body builders and others to use supplements in the hope that they inhibit the body's normal cortisol release. Some believe that depressing cortisol's normal increase after exercise augments muscular development with resistance training because muscle tissue synthesis progresses unimpeded in recovery. Athletes use the supplements glutamine and phosphatidylserine to produce an anticortisol effect.

Glutamine

Glutamine, a non-essential amino acid, exhibits many regulatory functions in the body, one of which provides an anticatabolic effect to enhance protein synthesis. The rationale for glutamine's use as an ergogenic aid comes from findings that glutamine supplementation effectively counteracts protein breakdown and muscle wasting from repeated use of exogenous glucocorticoids. In one study with female rats, infusing a glutamine supplement for 7 days countered the normal depressed protein synthesis and atrophy in skeletal muscle with chronic glucocorticoid administration. However, no research exists concerning the efficacy of excess glutamine in altering the normal hormonal milieu and training responsiveness in healthy men and women. For example, the potential anticatabolic and glycogen synthesizing

Questions & Notes

Briefly describe the ergogenic role of sodium bicarbonate.

Briefly describe the ergogenic role of phosphate loading.

Briefly describe the theoretical benefits of using anti-cortisol agents.

For Your Information

SOME POTENTIAL NEGATIVE SIDE EFFECTS

Individuals who bicarbonate load often experience abdominal cramps and diarrhea about 1 hour after ingestion. This adverse effect would surely minimize any potential ergogenic effect. Substituting sodium citrate (0.4–0.5 g per kg body mass) for sodium bicarbonate reduces or eliminates adverse gastrointestinal effects while still providing ergogenic benefits.

effects of exogenous glutamine have promoted speculation that supplementation might benefit resistance training effects. Daily glutamine supplementation (0.9 g per kg lean tissue mass) during 6 weeks of resistance training in healthy young adults did not affect muscle performance, body composition, or muscle protein degradation compared with a placebo. Any objective decision about glutamine supplements for ergogenic purposes must await supportive research studies, which presently are lacking.

Phosphatidylserine

Phosphatidylserine (PS) represents a glycerophospholipid typical of a class of natural lipids that comprise the structural components of biological membranes, particularly the internal layer of the plasma membrane that surrounds all cells. Speculation exists that PS, through its potential for modulating functional events in cell membranes (e.g., number and affinity of membrane receptor sites), modifies the body's neuroendocrine response to stress.

In one study, nine healthy men received 800 mg of PS derived from bovine cerebral cortex in oral form daily for 10 days. Three 6-minute intervals of cycle ergometer exercise of increasing intensity induced physical stress. Compared with the placebo condition, the PS treatment diminished ACTH and cortisol release without affecting growth hormone (GH) release. These results confirmed earlier findings by the same researchers that a single intravenous PS injection counteracted hypothalamic–pituitary–adrenal axis activation with exercise. Soybean lecithin provides the majority of PS supplementation by athletes, yet the research showing physiologic effects has used *bovine-derived* PS. Subtle differences in the chemical structure of these two forms of PS may create differences in physiologic action, including the potential ergogenic effects of this compound.

β-HYDROXY-β-METHYLBUTYRATE

β-Hydroxy-β-methylbutyrate (HMB), a bioactive metabolite generated in the breakdown of the essential branched-chain amino acid leucine, decreases protein loss during stress by inhibiting protein catabolism. In rats and chicks, less protein breakdown and a slight increase in protein synthesis occurred in muscle tissue (in vitro) exposed to HMB. An HMB-induced increase occurred in fatty acid oxidation in mammalian muscle cells exposed to HMB. Depending on the quantity of HMB in food (relatively rich sources include catfish, grapefruit, and breast milk), humans synthesize between 0.3 and 1.0 g of HMB daily, with about 5% from dietary leucine catabolism. HMB supplements are taken because of their potential nitrogen-retaining effects to prevent or slow muscle damage and inhibit muscle breakdown (proteolysis) with intense physical effort.

Research has studied the effects of exogenous HMB on skeletal muscle response to resistance training. In part one of a two-part study (**Fig. 4.3**), young men participated in two randomized trials. In the first study, 41 subjects received either 0, 1.5, or 3.0 g of HMB daily at two protein levels, either 117 g or 175 g daily, for 3 weeks. The men resistance trained during this time for 1.5 hours, 3 days a week. In the second study, 28 subjects consumed either 0 or 3.0 g of HMB daily and resistance trained for 2 to 3 hours, 6 days a week, for 7 weeks. In the first study, HMB supplementation depressed the exercise-induced increase in muscle proteolysis reflected by urinary 3-methylhistidine and plasma creatine phosphokinase [CPK] levels during the first 2 weeks of training. These biochemical indices of muscle damage were 20% to 60% lower in the HMB-supplemented group. In addition, the supplemented

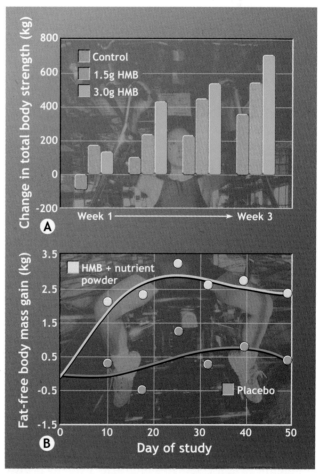

Figure 4.3 **A.** Change in muscle strength (total weight lifted in upper- and lower-body exercises) during study 1 (week 1–week 3) in subjects who supplemented with β-hydroxy-β-methylbutyrate (HMB). Each *group of bars* represents one complete set of upper- and lower-body workouts. **B.** Total-body electrical conductivity-assessed change in fat-free mass (FFM) during study 2 for a control group that received a carbohydrate drink (*placebo*) and a group that received 3 g of Ca-HMB each day mixed in a nutrient powder (*HMB + nutrient powder*). (From Nissen, S., et al.: Effect of leucine metabolite β-hydroxy–β-methylbutyrate on muscle metabolism during resistance-exercise training. *J. Appl. Physiol.*, 81:2095, 1996.)

group lifted more total weight during each training week (see **Fig. 4.3A**), with the greatest effect in the group receiving the largest HMB supplement. Muscular strength increased 8% in the unsupplemented group and more in the HMB-supplemented groups (13% for the 1.5-g group and 18.4% for the 3.0-g group). Added protein (not indicated in the graph) did not affect any of the measurements; one should view this lack of effect in proper context—the "lower" protein quantity ($115 \text{ g} \cdot \text{d}^{-1}$) equaled twice the RDA.

In the second study, individuals who received HMB supplementation had higher fat-free mass (FFM) than the unsupplemented group at 2 and 4 to 6 weeks of training (see **Fig. 4.3B**). At the last measurement during training, however, the difference between groups decreased and failed to differ from the difference between pretraining baseline values.

The mechanism for any HMB effect on muscle metabolism, strength improvement, and body composition remains unknown. Perhaps this metabolite inhibits normal proteolytic processes that accompany intense muscular overload. Although the results demonstrate an ergogenic effect for HMB supplementation, it remains unclear just what component of the FFM (protein, bone, water) HMB affects. Furthermore, the data in **Figure 4.3B** indicate potentially transient body composition benefits of supplementation that tend to revert toward the unsupplemented state as training progresses.

Not all research shows beneficial effects of HMB supplementation with resistance training. One study evaluated the effects of variations in HMB supplementation (approximately $3 \text{ g} \cdot \text{d}^{-1}$ vs. $6 \text{ g} \cdot \text{d}^{-1}$) on muscular strength during 8 weeks of whole-body resistance training in untrained young men. The study's primary finding indicated that HMB supplementation, regardless of dosage, produced *no difference* in most of the strength data (including 1-repetition maximum [1-RM] strength) compared with the placebo group. Additional studies must assess the long-term effects of HMB supplements on body composition, training response, and overall health and safety.

CHROMIUM

The trace mineral **chromium** serves as a cofactor for potentiating insulin function, although its precise mechanism of action remains unclear. Chronic chromium deficiency may trigger an increase in blood cholesterol and decrease the body's sensitivity to insulin, thus increasing the risk of type 2 diabetes. In all likelihood, some adult Americans consume less than the 50 to 200 mg of chromium, which is considered by the National Research Council Food and Nutrition Board's the Estimated Safe and Adequate Daily Dietary Intake (ESADDI). This occurs largely because chromium-rich foods such as brewer's yeast, broccoli, wheat germ, nuts, liver, prunes, egg yolks, apples with skins, asparagus, mushrooms, wine, and cheese do not usually constitute part of the regular daily diet. Food processing removes chromium from foods in natural form, and strenuous exercise and associated high carbohydrate intake also promote urinary chromium losses to increase the potential for chromium deficiency. For athletes with documented chromium-deficient diets, dietary modifications or use of chromium supplements to increase chromium intake seem prudent.

Chromium's Alleged Benefits

Chromium, touted as a "fat burner" and "muscle builder," represents one of the largest selling mineral supplements in the United States, second only to calcium. Supplement intake of chromium, usually as **chromium picolinate**, often achieves 600 μg daily. This picolinic acid combination supposedly improves chromium absorption compared with the inorganic salt chromium chloride.

Questions & Notes

Briefly describe the ergogenic benefits of HMB ingestion.

 For Your Information

POTENTIAL RISKS OF CHROMIUM EXCESS

Concerning the bioavailability of trace minerals in the diet, excessive dietary chromium inhibits zinc and iron absorption. At the extreme, this could induce iron-deficiency anemia, blunt the ability to train intensely, and negatively affect exercise performance requiring high-level aerobic metabolism.

Further potential bad news emerges from studies in which human tissue cultures that received extreme doses of chromium picolinate showed eventual chromosomal damage. Critics contend that such high laboratory dosages would not occur with supplement use in humans. Nonetheless, one could argue that cells continually exposed to excessive chromium (e.g., long-term supplementation) accumulate this mineral and retain it for years.

Generally, studies that suggest beneficial effects of chromium supplements on body fat and muscle mass incorrectly infer body composition changes from changes in body weight (or anthropometric measurements) instead of the more appropriate assessment methods discussed in Chapter 16. One study observed that supplementing daily with 200 μg (3.85 mmol) of chromium picolinate for 40 days produced a small increase in FFM and a decrease in body fat in young men who resistance trained for 6 weeks. No data were presented to document increases in muscular strength.

Another study reported increases in body mass without a change in strength or body composition in previously untrained female college students (no change in males) who received daily a 200-μg chromium supplement during a 12-week resistance training program compared with unsupplemented control subjects. When collegiate football players received daily supplements of 200 μg of chromium picolinate for 9 weeks, no changes occurred in body composition and muscular strength from intense weight-lifting training compared with a control group receiving a placebo. Among obese personnel enrolled in the U.S. Navy's mandatory remedial physical conditioning program, consuming 400 μg of additional chromium picolinate daily caused no greater loss in body weight or percentage of body fat and no increase in FFM compared with a group receiving a placebo.

A double-blind research design studied the effects of a daily chromium supplement (3.3–3.5 mmol either as chromium chloride or chromium picolinate) or a placebo for 8 weeks during resistance training in 36 young men. For each group, dietary intakes of protein, magnesium, zinc, copper, and iron equaled or exceeded recommended levels during training; subjects also had adequate baseline dietary chromium intakes. Chromium supplementation increased serum chromium concentration and urinary chromium excretion equally, regardless of its ingested form. Table 4.2 shows that compared with a placebo treatment, chromium supplementation did *not* affect training-related changes in muscular strength, physique, FFM, or muscle mass.

CREATINE

Meat, poultry, and fish provide rich sources of **creatine**; they contain approximately 4 to 5 g per kg of food weight. The body synthesizes only about 1 to 2 g of this nitrogen-containing organic compound daily, primarily in the kidneys, liver, and pancreas, from the amino acids arginine, glycine, and methionine. Thus, adequate dietary creatine becomes important for obtaining required amounts. Because the animal kingdom contains the richest creatine-containing foods, vegetarians experience a distinct disadvantage in obtaining ready sources of exogenous creatine. Skeletal muscle contains approximately 95% of the body's total 120 to 150 g of creatine.

Creatine supplements sold as creatine monohydrate (CrH_2O) come as a powder, tablet, capsule, and stabilized liquid (under such names as Rejuvinix, Cell Tech Hardcore, Muscle Marketing, and NOZ). A person can purchase creatine over the counter or via mail order as a nutritional supplement (without guarantee of purity). Ingesting a

Table 4.2	Effects of Two Different Forms of Chromium Supplementation on Average Values for Anthropometric, Bone, and Soft Tissue Composition Measurements Before and After Resistance Training					
	PLACEBO		CHROMIUM CHLORIDE		CHROMIUM PICOLINATE	
	PRE	POST	PRE	POST	PRE	POST
Age (y)	21.1	21.5	23.3	23.5	22.3	22.5
Stature (cm)	179.3	179.2	177.3	177.3	178.0	178.2
Weight (kg)	79.9	80.5[a]	79.3	81.1[a]	79.2	80.5
Σ4 skinfold thickness (mm)[b]	42.0	41.5	42.6	42.2	43.3	43.1
Upper arm (cm)	30.9	31.6[a]	31.3	32.0[a]	31.1	31.4[a]
Lower leg (cm)	38.2	37.9	37.4	37.5	37.1	37.0
Endomorphy	3.68	3.73	3.58	3.54	3.71	3.72
Mesomorphy	4.09	4.36[a]	4.25	4.42[a]	4.21	4.33[a]
Ectomorphy	2.09	1.94[a]	1.79	1.63[a]	2.00	1.88[a]
FFMFM (kg)[c]	62.9	64.3[a]	61.1	63.1[a]	61.3	62.7[a]
Bone mineral (g)	2952	2968	2860	2878	2918	2940
Fat-free body mass (kg)	65.9	67.3[a]	64.0	65.9[a]	64.2	66.1[a]
Fat (kg)	13.4	13.1	14.7	15.1	14.7	14.5
Body fat (%)	16.4	15.7	18.4	18.2	18.4	17.9

From Lukaski, H.C., et al.: Chromium supplementation and resistance training: Effects on body composition, strength, and trace element status of men. *Am. J. Clin. Nutr.*, 63:954, 1996.
[a]Significantly different from pretraining value.
[b]Measured at biceps, triceps, subscapular, and suprailiac sites.
[c]Fat-free, mineral-free mass.

liquid suspension of creatine monohydrate at the relatively high daily dose of 20 to 30 g for up to 2 weeks increases intramuscular concentrations of free creatine and PCr by 30%. These levels remain high for weeks after only a few days of supplementation. Sports governing bodies have not declared creatine an illegal substance.

Important Component of High-Energy Phosphates

The precise physiologic mechanisms underlying the potential ergogenic effectiveness of supplemental creatine remain poorly understood. Creatine passes through the digestive tract unaltered for absorption in the bloodstream from the intestinal mucosa. Just about all ingested creatine becomes incorporated within skeletal muscle (average concentration, 125 mM per kg dry muscle; range, 90–160 mM) via insulin-mediated active transport. About 40% of the total exists as free creatine; the remainder combines readily with phosphate to form PCr. Type II, fast-twitch muscle fibers store about four to six times more PCr than ATP. PCr serves as the cells' "energy reservoir" to provide rapid phosphate-bond energy to resynthesize ATP (refer to Chapter 5). This becomes important in all-out effort lasting up to 10 seconds. Because of limited amounts of intramuscular PCr, it seems plausible that any increase in PCr availability should accomplish the following three ergogenic effects:

1. Improve repetitive performance in muscular strength and short-term power activities.
2. Augment short bursts of muscular endurance.
3. Provide for greater muscular overload to enhance resistance training effectiveness.

Documented Benefits Under Certain Exercise Conditions

No serious adverse effects from creatine supplementation for up to 4 years have been reported. However, anecdotes indicate a possible association between creatine supplementation and cramping in multiple muscle areas during competition or lengthy practice in football players. This effect may occur from (1) altered intracellular dynamics from increased free creatine and PCr levels or (2) an osmotically induced enlarged muscle cell volume (greater cellular hydration) caused by increased creatine content. Gastrointestinal tract nausea, indigestion, and difficulty absorbing food have been linked to exogenous creatine ingestion.

Figure 4.4 illustrates the ergogenic effects of creatine loading on total work accomplished during repetitive sprint cycling performance. Active but untrained men performed sets of maximal 6-second bicycle sprints interspersed with various recovery periods (24, 54, or 84 s) between sprints to simulate sports conditions. Performance evaluations took place under creatine-loaded (20 g per day for 5 days) or placebo conditions. Supplementation increased muscle creatine (48.9%) and PCr (12.5%) levels compared with the placebo levels. Increased intramuscular creatine produced a 6% increase in total work accomplished (251.7 kJ before supplement vs. 266.9 kJ after creatine loaded) compared with the group that consumed the placebo (254.0 kJ before test vs. 252.3 kJ after placebo). Creatine supplements have benefited an on-court "ghosting" routine that involves simulated positional play of competitive squash players. It also augmented repeated sprint cycle performance after 30 minutes of constant load, submaximal exercise in the heat without disrupting thermoregulatory dynamics. Creatine's benefits to muscular performance also occur in normally active older men.

Figure 4.5 outlines mechanisms of how elevating intramuscular free creatine and PCr with creatine supplementation might enhance exercise

Questions & Notes

Name one product known to augment the effects of creatine loading.

Briefly describe the ergogenic benefits of creatine ingestion.

ⓘ For Your Information

CARBOHYDRATE INGESTION AUGMENTS CREATINE LOADING

Research supports the common belief among athletes that consuming creatine with a sugar-containing drink increases creatine uptake and storage in skeletal muscle. For 5 days, subjects received either 5 g of creatine four times daily or a 5-g supplement followed 30 minutes later by 93 g of a high-glycemic simple sugar four times daily. For the creatine-only supplement group, increases occurred for muscle phosphocreatine (PCr) (7.2%), free creatine (13.5%), and total creatine (20.7%). Larger increases took place for the creatine plus sugar-supplemented group (14.7% increase in muscle PCr, 18.1% increase in free creatine, and 33.0% increase in total creatine).

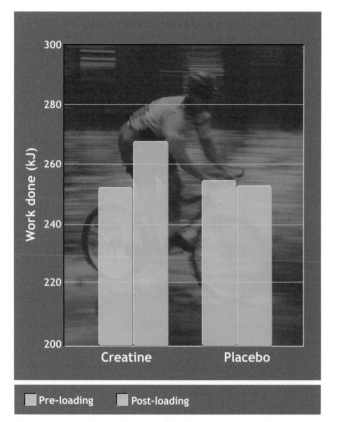

Figure 4.4 Effects of creatine loading versus placebo on total work accomplished during long-term (80-min) repetitive sprint-cycling performance. (From Preen, C.D., et al.: Effect of creatine loading on long-term sprint exercise performance and metabolism. *Med. Sci. Sports Exerc.*, 33:814, 2001.)

performance and training responses. Besides benefiting weight lifting and body building, improved immediate anaerobic power output capacity benefits sprint running; cycling; swimming; jumping; and all-out, repetitive rapid movements in football and volleyball. Increased intramuscular PCr concentrations should also enable individuals to increase training intensity in strength and power activities.

Oral supplements of creatine monohydrate (20–25 g per day) increase muscle creatine and performance in high-intensity exercise, particularly repeated intense muscular effort. The ergogenic effect does not vary between vegetarians and meat eaters. Even daily low doses of 6 g for 5 days improve repeated power performance. For Division I football players, creatine supplementation during resistance training increased body mass, lean body mass, cellular hydration, and muscular strength and performance. Similarly, supplementation augmented muscular strength and size increases during 12 weeks of resistance training.

Taking a high dose of creatine helps replenish muscle creatine levels after intense exercise. Such metabolic "reloading" should facilitate recovery of muscle contractile capacity, thus enabling athletes to sustain repeated efforts of intense exercise. Also, only limited information exists about long-term high doses of creatine supplemen-

tation in healthy individuals, particularly the effects on cardiac muscle and kidney function (creatine degrades to creatinine before excretion in urine). Short-term use (e.g., 20 g per day for 5 consecutive days) in healthy men does not detrimentally impact blood pressure, plasma creatine, plasma creatine kinase (CK) activity, or renal responses assessed by glomerular filtration rate and rates of total protein and albumin excretion. For healthy subjects, no differences emerged in plasma content and urine excretion rate for creatinine, urea, and albumin between control subjects and those consuming creatine for between 10 months and 5 years.

Creatine supplementation does *not* improve exercise performance that requires high levels of aerobic energy transfer or cardiovascular and metabolic responses. It also exerts little effect on isometric muscular strength or dynamic muscle force during a single movement.

Effects on Body Mass and Body Composition

Body mass increases of between 0.5 and 2.4 kg often accompany creatine supplementation independent of short-term changes in testosterone or cortisol concentrations. It remains unclear how much of the weight gain occurs from anabolic effects of creatine on muscle tissue

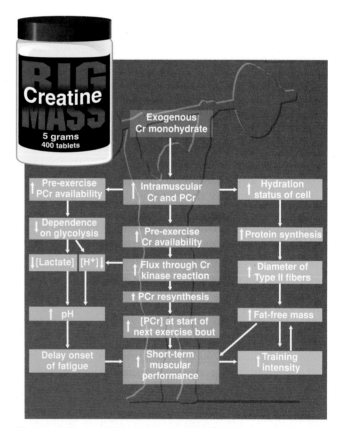

Figure 4.5 Possible mechanisms for how elevating intracellular creatine (Cr) and phosphocreatine (PCr) might enhance intense, short-term exercise performance and the exercise training response. (Modified from Volek, J.S., Kraemer, W.J.: Creatine supplementation: Its effect on human muscular performance and body composition. *J. Strength Cond. Res.*, 10:200, 1996.)

synthesis or osmotic retention of intracellular water from increased creatine stores.

Creatine Loading

Creatine Loading Many creatine users pursue a "loading" phase by ingesting 20 to 30 g of creatine daily for 5 to 7 days (usually as a tablet or powder added to liquid). A maintenance phase occurs after the loading phase, during which the person supplements with as little as 2 to 5 g of creatine daily. Individuals who consume vegetarian-type diets show the greatest increase in muscle creatine because of the low creatine content of their diets. Large increases also characterize "responders," that is, individuals with normally low basal levels of intramuscular creatine.

Three practical questions for those desiring to elevate intramuscular creatine with supplementation concern:

1. The magnitude and time course of intramuscular creatine increase.
2. The dosage necessary to maintain a creatine increase.
3. The rate of creatine loss or "washout" after cessation of supplementation.

To provide insight into these questions, researchers studied two groups of men. In one experiment, subjects ingested 20 g of creatine monohydrate ($\sim$0.3 g$\cdot$kg^{-1}) for 6 consecutive days, at which time supplementation ceased. Muscle biopsies were taken before supplement ingestion and at days 7, 21, and 35. Similarly, another group consumed 20 g of creatine monohydrate daily for 6 consecutive days. But instead of discontinuing supplementation, they reduced dosage to 2 g daily ($\sim$0.03 g$\cdot$kg^{-1}) for an additional 28 days. **Figure 4.6A** illustrates that muscle creatine concentration increased by approximately 20% after 6 days. Without continued supplementation, muscle creatine content gradually declined to baseline in 35 days. The group that continued to supplement with reduced creatine intake for an additional 28 days maintained muscle creatine at the increased level (**Fig. 4.6B**).

For both groups, the increase in total muscle creatine content during the initial 6-day supplement period averaged about 23 mmol per kg of dry muscle, which represented about 20 g (17%) of the total creatine ingested. Interestingly, a similar 20% increase in total muscle creatine concentration occurred with only a 3-g daily supplement. This increase occurred more gradually and required 28 days in contrast to only 6 days with the 6-g supplement.

Questions & Notes

Briefly explain the effects of creatine supplementation on exercise performance.

Discuss important factors to consider when trying to elevate intramuscular creatine.

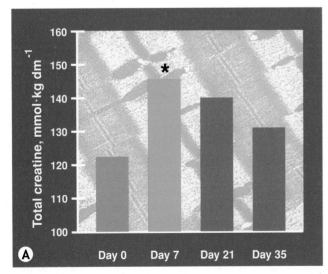 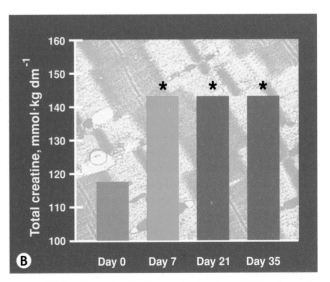

Figure 4.6 **A.** Muscle total creatine concentration in six men who ingested 20 g of creatine for 6 consecutive days. **B.** Muscle total creatine concentration in nine men who ingested 20 g of creatine for 6 consecutive days and thereafter ingested 2 g of creatine per day for the next 28 days. In both *A* and *B*, muscle biopsy samples were taken before ingestion (day 0) and on days 7, 21, and 35. Values refer to averages per kg dry muscle mass (dm). *Significantly different from day 0. (From Hultman, E., et al.: Muscle creatine loading in men. *J. Appl. Physiol.*, 81:232, 1996.)

A rapid and effective way to "creatine load" skeletal muscle requires ingesting 20 g of creatine monohydrate daily for 6 days and then switching to $2 \, g \cdot d^{-1}$. This keeps levels elevated for up to 28 days. If rapidity of "loading" is not a consideration, supplementing 3 g daily for 28 days achieves approximately the same high levels.

RIBOSE: AN ALTERNATIVE TO CREATINE ON THE SUPPLEMENT SCENE

Ribose has emerged as a competitor supplement to creatine to increase power and replenish high-energy compounds after intense exercise. The body readily synthesizes ribose, and the diet provides small amounts in ripe fruits and vegetables. Metabolically, the 5-carbon ribose sugar serves as an energy substrate for ATP resynthesis. Consuming exogenous ribose has been touted to quickly restore depleted ATP. To maintain optimal ATP levels and thus provide its ergogenic effect, recommended ribose doses range from 10 to 20 g per day. A compound that either increases ATP levels or facilitates its resynthesis could certainly benefit short-term, high-power output physical activities, yet only limited data have assessed this potential. A double-blind randomized experiment evaluated the effects of four doses of oral ribose daily at 4 g per dose on repeated bouts of maximal exercise and ATP replenishment after intermittent maximal muscle contractions. No difference in intermittent isokinetic knee extension force, blood lactate, or plasma ammonia concentration emerged between ribose and placebo trials. The exercise decreased intramuscular ATP and total adenine nucleotide content immediately after exercise and 24 hours later, yet oral ribose administration proved ineffective to facilitate recovery of these compounds.

GINSENG AND EPHEDRINE

The popularity of herbal and botanical remedies has soared as possible ways to improve health, control body weight, and improve exercise performance. **Ginseng** and **ephedrine** are marketed as nutritional supplements to "reduce stress," "revitalize," and "optimize mental and physical performance," particularly during times of fatigue and stress. Ginseng also is touted to play a role as an alternative therapy to treat diabetes, stimulate immune function, and improve male fertility. Clinically, 1 to 3 g of ginseng administered 40 minutes before an oral glucose challenge reduces postprandial glycemia in subjects without diabetes. As with caffeine, ephedrine and ginseng occur naturally and, for decades, have been used in folk medicine to enhance "energy."

Ginseng

Used in Asian medicine to prolong life, strengthen and restore sexual functions, and invigorate the body, the ginseng root (often sold as Panax or Chinese or Korean ginseng), serves no recognized medical use in the United States except as a soothing agent in skin ointments. Commercial ginseng root preparations usually take the form of powder, liquid, tablets, or capsules. Widely marketed foods and beverages also contain various types and amounts of ginsenosides. Because dietary supplements need not meet the same quality control for purity and potency as pharmaceuticals, considerable variation exists in the concentrations of marker compounds for ginseng, including levels of potentially harmful impurities, toxic pesticides, and heavy metal contamination like lead, cadmium, mercury, arsenic. Neither the Food and Drug Administration (FDA; *www.fda.gov*) nor state or federal agencies routinely test ginseng-containing products or other supplements for quality.

Reports of ginsing's ergogenic possibilities often appear in the lay literature, but a review of the research provides little evidence to support its effectiveness for these purposes. For example, volunteers consumed either 200 or 400 mg of the standardized ginseng concentrate every day for 8 weeks in a double-blind research protocol. Neither treatment affected submaximal or maximal exercise performance, ratings of perceived exertion, heart rate, oxygen consumption, or blood lactate concentrations. Similarly, no ergogenic effects emerged on diverse physiologic and performance variables after a 1-week treatment with a ginseng saponin extract administered in two doses of either 8 or 16 mg per kg of body mass. When effectiveness has been demonstrated, the research has failed to use adequate controls, placebos, or double-blind testing protocols. *At present, no compelling scientific evidence exists that ginseng supplementation offers any ergogenic benefit for physiologic function or exercise performance.*

Ephedrine

Unlike ginseng, Western medicine had recognized the potent amphetamine-like compound ephedrine (with sympathomimetic physiologic effects) found in several species of the plant ephedra (dried plant stem called ma huang [ma wong, ephedra sinica]). The ephedra plant contains ephedrine and pseudoephedrine, the two major active components first isolated by a Japanese researcher in 1928. The medicinal role of this herb has included treating asthma, symptoms of the common cold, hypotension, and urinary incontinence and as a central stimulant to treat depression. Physicians in the United States discontinued ephedrine's use as a decongestant and asthma treatment in the 1930s in favor of safer medications.

Ephedrine exerts both central and peripheral effects, with the latter reflected in increased heart rate, cardiac output, and blood pressure. Because of its β-adrenergic effect, ephedrine causes bronchodilation in the lungs. High ephedrine dosages can produce hypertension, insomnia, hyperthermia, and cardiac arrhythmias. Other possible side effects include dizziness, restlessness, anxiety, irritability, personality changes, gastrointestinal symptoms, and difficulty concentrating.

The potent physiologic effects of ephedrine have led researchers to investigate its potential as an ergogenic aid. No effect of a 40-mg dose of ephedrine occurred on indirect indicators of exercise performance or ratings of perceived exertion (RPE; see Chapter 13). The less concentrated pseudoephedrine also produced no effect on $\dot{V}O_{2max}$, RPE, aerobic cycling efficiency, anaerobic power output (Wingate test), time to exhaustion on a bicycle and a 40-km cycling trial, or physiologic and performance measures during 20 minutes of running at 70% of $\dot{V}O_{2max}$ followed by a 5000-m time trial.

FDA Bans Ephedrine   In early 2004, the United States federal government announced a ban on the sale of ephedra, the latest chapter in a long story that gained national prominence after the deaths of two football players (a professional National Football League [NFL] all-pro player and a university athlete) were linked to ephedra use in 2001. A little more than 1 month after the death of one of its players, the NFL was the first sports governing body to ban ephedra. In February 2003, the FDA announced a series of measures that included strong enforcement actions against firms making unsubstantiated claims for their ephedra-containing products. In early 2004, the ban on ephedrine took effect (*www.fda.gov/ola/2003/dietarysupplements1028.html* and *www.cfsan.fda.gov/~dms/ds-ephed.html*). A Utah judge then countered and blocked the FDA's action against Nutraceutical Corporation (a Utah-based corporation), and the banned herbal compound ephedra could again be marketed and sold to the general public. Nutraceutical had argued that ephedra was "safe" at recommended doses and accused the FDA of failing to adequately assess ephedra's effects at lower dosage levels. Finally, the U.S. Supreme Court in 2007 issued a "certiorari denied" without comment in the case, rejecting the lower court's challenge to the FDA's ban of ephedra. This final decision should once and for all curtail this product from being sold to an eager public looking for an "edge" in health and fitness.

AMINO ACID SUPPLEMENTS AND OTHER DIETARY MODIFICATIONS FOR AN ANABOLIC EFFECT

Many athletes and the lay public regularly consume **amino acid supplements** believing they boost testosterone, GH, insulin, and insulin-like growth factor I (IGF-I) to improve muscle size and strength and decrease body fat. The rationale for trying such nutritional ergogenic stimulants comes from the clinical use of amino acid infusion or ingestion in deficient patients to regulate anabolic hormones.

Research on healthy subjects does not provide convincing evidence for an ergogenic effect of the generalized use of amino acid supplements on hormone secretion, responsiveness to workouts, or exercise performance. In studies with appropriate design and statistical analysis, supplements of arginine, lysine, ornithine, tyrosine, and other amino acids, either singularly or in combination, produced *no* effect on GH levels or insulin secretion or on diverse measures of anaerobic power and all-out running performance at $\dot{V}O_{2max}$. Furthermore, elite junior weight lifers who supplemented with all 20 amino acids did not improve their physical performance or resting or exercise-induced responses of testosterone, cortisol, or GH. The indiscriminate use of amino acid supplements at dosages considered pharmacologic rather than nutritional increases risk of direct toxic effects or creation of an amino acid imbalance.

Prudent Means to Possibly Augment an Anabolic Effect

With resistance training, muscle hypertrophy occurs from a shift in the body's normal dynamic state of protein synthesis and degradation to greater tissue synthesis.

The normal hormonal milieu (e.g., insulin and GH levels) in the period following resistance exercise stimulates the muscle fiber's anabolic processes while inhibiting muscle protein degradation. Dietary modifications that increase amino acid transport into muscle, raise energy availability, or increase anabolic hormone levels would theoretically augment the training effect by increasing the rate of anabolism, depressing catabolism, or both. Either effect should create a positive body protein balance to improve muscular growth and strength (see Close Up Box 3.4: *International Society of Sports Nutrition Position Stand: Nutrient Timing,* on page 105).

Specific Timing of Carbohydrate–Protein-Creatine Supplementation Augments Response to Resistance Exercise

Studies of hormonal dynamics and protein anabolism indicate a transient but potential fourfold increase in protein synthesis with carbohydrate or protein supplements (or both) consumed *immediately after* resistance exercise workouts. This effect of supplementation in the immediate postexercise period of resistance exercise may also prove effective for tissue repair and synthesis of muscle proteins after aerobic exercise.

Drug-free male weightlifters with at least 2 years of resistance training experience consumed carbohydrate and protein supplements immediately after a standard resistance training workout. Treatment included one of the following: (1) a placebo of pure water, (2) a supplement of carbohydrate (1.5 g per kg body mass), (3) protein (1.38 g per kg body mass), or (4) carbohydrate and protein (1.06 g carbohydrate plus 0.41 g protein per kg body mass) consumed immediately after and then 2 hours after the training session. Compared with the placebo, each nutritive supplement produced a hormonal environment (elevated plasma concentrations of insulin and GH) in recovery conducive to protein synthesis and muscle tissue growth. Such data provide indirect evidence for a possible training benefit of increasing carbohydrate or protein intake (or both) immediately after resistance training workouts.

A recent study compared the effects of the strategic consumption of glucose, protein, and creatine (1) before, (2) after, or (3) before and after each resistance-training workout compared with supplementation in the hours not close to the workout (i.e., supplement timing) on muscle fiber hypertrophy, muscular strength, and body composition. Resistance-trained men matched for strength were placed in one of two groups; one group consumed a supplement (1 g per kg body weight) of glucose, protein, and creatine immediately before and after resistance training, and the other group received the same supplement dose in the morning and late evening of the workout day. Measurements of body composition by dual energy x-ray aborptiometry (DXA; see Chapter 16), strength (1-RM), muscle fiber type, cross-sectional area, contractile protein, creatine, and glycogen content from vastus lateralis muscle biopsies took place the week before and immediately after a 10-week training program. Supplementa-

tion in the immediate pre-postexercise period produced a greater increase in lean body mass and 1-RM strength in two of three measures (**Fig. 4.7**). Body composition changes were accompanied by greater increases in muscle cross-sectional

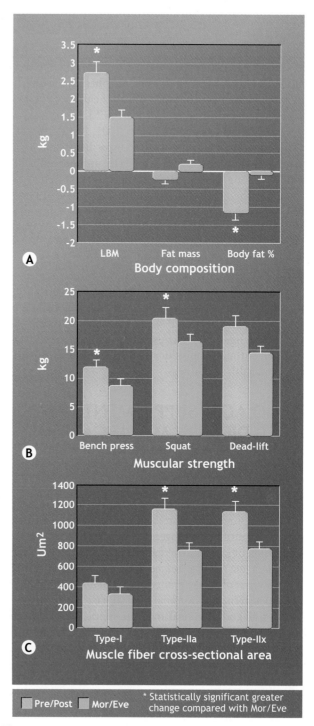

Figure 4.7 Effects of receiving a supplement (1 g per kg of body weight) or protein, glucose, and creatine immediately before (PRE) and after (POST) resistance exercise training or in the early morning (MOR) or late evening (EVE) of the training day on changes in body composition (**A**), 1-RM strength (**B**), and muscle cross-sectional area (**C**). *Statistically significant greater change compared with MOR-EVE. (From Cribb, P.J., Hayes, A.: Effects of supplement timing and resistance exercise on skeletal muscle hypertrophy. *Med. Sci. Sports Exerc.,* 38:1918, 2006.)

area of the type II muscle fibers and contractile protein content. These findings revealed that supplement timing provides a simple but effective strategy to enhance the desired adaptations from resistance training.

COENZYME Q-10 (UBIQUINONE)

Coenzyme Q-10 (CoQ_{10}; ubiquinone in oxidized form and ubiquinol when reduced), found primarily in meats, peanuts, and soybean oil, functions as an integral part of the mitochondrion's electron transport system of oxidative phosphorylation. This lipid-soluble natural component of all cells exists in high concentrations within myocardial tissue. CoQ_{10} has been used therapeutically to treat individuals with cardiovascular disease because of its role in oxidative metabolism and its antioxidant properties that promote scavenging of free radicals that damage cellular components. Because of its positive effect on oxygen uptake and exercise performance in cardiac patients, some consider CoQ_{10} a potential ergogenic nutrient for endurance performance. Based on the belief that supplementation could increase the flux of electrons through the respiratory chain and thus augment aerobic resynthesis of ATP, the popular literature touts CoQ_{10} supplements as a means to improve "stamina" and enhance cardiovascular function. However, no research data support such claims.

CoQ_{10} supplementation increases serum CoQ_{10} levels, but it does *not* improve a healthy person's aerobic capacity, endurance performance, plasma glucose or lactate levels at submaximal workloads, or cardiovascular dynamics compared with a placebo. One study evaluated oral supplements of CoQ_{10} on the exercise tolerance and peripheral muscle function of healthy, middle-aged men. Measurements included $\dot{V}O_{2max}$, lactate threshold, heart rate response, and upper extremity exercise blood flow and metabolism. For 2 months, subjects received either CoQ_{10} (150 mg per day) or a placebo. Blood levels of CoQ_{10} increased during the treatment period and remained unchanged in the control subjects. No differences occurred between groups for any of the physiologic or metabolic variables. Similarly, for trained young and older men, CoQ_{10} supplementation of 120 mg per day for 6 weeks did not benefit aerobic capacity or lipid peroxidation, a marker of oxidative stress. Recent data indicate that CoQ_{10} supplements (60 mg daily combined with vitamins E and C) did not affect lipid peroxidation during exercise in endurance athletes.

LIPID SUPPLEMENTATION WITH MEDIUM-CHAIN TRIACYLGLYCEROLS

Do high-fat foods or supplements elevate plasma lipid levels to make more energy available during prolonged aerobic exercise? To answer this question, one must consider these factors. First, consuming triacylglycerols composed of predominantly 12 to 18 carbon long-chain fatty acids *delays* gastric emptying. This negatively affects the rapidity of exogenous fat availability and slows fluid and carbohydrate replenishment, both crucial in intense endurance exercise. Second, after digestion and intestinal absorption (normally a 3- to 4-h process), long-chain triacylglycerols reassemble with phospholipids, fatty acids, and a cholesterol shell to form

Questions & Notes

Name 3 herbs and their purported ergogenic effects.

  Herb: Effect:

  1.

  2.

  3.

Give the formal names for the following herbs:

  CoQ10:

  MCT:

  HCA:

Describe the function of coenzyme Q-10.

 For Your Information

POSTEXERCISE GLUCOSE AUGMENTS PROTEIN BALANCE AFTER RESISTANCE TRAINING WORKOUTS

Healthy men familiar with resistance training performed eight sets of 10 repetitions of knee extensor exercise at 85% of maximum strength. Immediately after the exercise session and 1 hour later, they received either a glucose supplement (1.0 g per kg body mass) or a placebo of NutraSweet. Glucose supplementation reduced myofibrillar protein breakdown as reflected by decreased excretion of 3-methylhistidine and urinary nitrogen. Although not statistically significant, glucose supplementation also increased the rate of the amino acid leucine's incorporation into the vastus lateralis over the 10-hour post-exercise period. These alterations indicated that the supplemented condition produced a more positive body protein balance after exercise. The beneficial effect of a post-exercise high-glycemic glucose supplementation most likely occurred from increased insulin release with glucose intake, which should enhance muscle protein balance in recovery.

fatty droplets called chylomicrons that travel relatively slowly to the systemic circulation via the lymphatic system. In the bloodstream, the tissues remove the triacylglycerols bound to chylomicrons. The relatively slow rate of digestion, absorption, and oxidation of long-chain fatty acids make this energy source undesirable as a supplement to augment energy metabolism in active muscle during exercise.

Medium-chain triacylglycerols (MCTs) provide a more rapid source of fatty acid fuel. MCTs are processed oils, frequently produced for patients with intestinal malabsorption and other tissue-wasting diseases. Marketing for the sports enthusiast hypes MCTs as a "fat burner," "energy source," "glycogen sparer," and "muscle builder." Unlike longer chain triacylglycerols, MCTs contain saturated fatty acids with 8- to 10-carbon atoms along the fatty acid chain. During digestion, they hydrolyze by lipase action in the mouth, stomach, and intestinal duodenum to glycerol and medium-chain fatty acids (MCFAs). The water solubility of MCFAs enables them to move rapidly across the intestinal mucosa directly into the bloodstream via the portal vein without necessity of slow chylomicron transport by the lymphatic system as required for long-chain triacylglycerols. In the tissues, MCFAs move through the plasma membrane and diffuse across the inner mitochondrial membrane for oxidation. They pass into the mitochondria largely independent of the carnitine-acyl-CoA transferase system; this contrasts with the slower transfer and mitochondrial oxidation rate of long-chain fatty acids. MCTs do not usually store as body fat because of their relative ease of oxidation. Because ingesting MCTs elevates plasma free fatty acids (FFAs) rapidly, some speculate that supplementing with these lipids might spare liver and muscle glycogen during intense aerobic exercise.

Inconclusive Exercise Benefits

Consuming MCTs does not inhibit gastric emptying, but conflicting research exists about their use in exercise. Ingesting 30 g of MCTs (an estimated maximal amount tolerated in the gastrointestinal tract) before exercising contributed only between 3% and 7% of the total exercise energy cost.

Consuming about 3 oz (86 g) of MCT provides interesting results. Endurance-trained cyclists rode for 2 hours at 60% $\dot{V}O_{2peak}$; they then immediately performed a simulated 40-km cycling time trial. During each of three rides, they drank 2 L of beverages containing either 10% glucose, a 4.3% MCT emulsion, or 10% glucose plus a 4.3% MCT emulsion. **Figure 4.8** shows the effects of the beverages on average speed in the 40-km trials. Replacing the carbohydrate beverage with only the MCT emulsion impaired exercise performance by approximately 8%. The combined carbohydrate plus MCT solution consumed repeatedly during exercise significantly improved cycling speed by 2.5%. This small ergogenic effect occurred with (1) reduced total carbohydrate oxidation at a given level of oxygen uptake, (2) higher final circulating FFA and

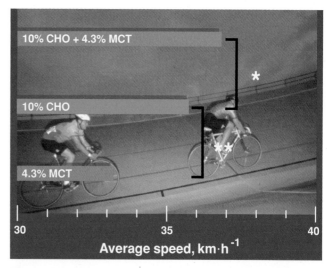

Figure 4.8 Effects of carbohydrate (CHO; 10% solution), medium-chain triacylglycerol (MCT; 4.3% emulsion), and carbohydrate + MCT ingestion during exercise on a simulated 40-km time-trial cycling speeds after 2 hours of exercise at 60% of peak oxygen uptake. *Significantly faster than 10% CHO trials; **significantly faster than 4.3% MCT trials. (From Van Zyl, C.G., et al.: Effects of medium-chain triacylglycerol ingestion on fuel metabolism and cycling performance. *J. Appl. Physiol.*, 80:2217, 1996.)

ketone levels, and (3) lower final glucose and lactate concentrations.

The small endurance performance enhancement with MCT supplementation probably occurred because this exogenous fatty acid source contributed to the total exercise energy expenditure including total fat oxidation in exercise. Consuming MCTs does not stimulate the release of bile, the fat-emulsifying agent from the gall bladder. Thus, cramping and diarrhea often accompany an excess intake of this lipid form. In general, the relatively small alterations in substrate availability and substrate oxidation by increasing the FFA availability during moderately intense aerobic exercise have only a small ergogenic effect on exercise capacity.

(–)-HYDROXYCITRATE: A POTENTIAL FAT BURNER?

(—)-Hydroxycitrate (HCA), a principal constituent of the rind of the fruit of Garcinia cambogia used in Asian cuisine, is the latest compound promoted as a "natural fat burner" to facilitate weight loss and enhance endurance performance. Metabolically, HCA operates as a competitive inhibitor of an enzyme that catalyzes the breakdown of citrate to oxaloacetate and acetyl-CoA in the cytosol, which limits the pool of 2-carbon acetyl compounds and reduces cellular ability to synthesize fat. Inhibition of citrate catabolism also slows carbohydrate breakdown. Thus, HCA supplementation should provide a way to conserve glycogen and increase lipolysis during endurance exercise. Research has shown that increasing plasma HCA availability with supplementation exerts *no effect* on skeletal muscle fat oxidation during rest or exercise, at least in endurance-trained humans. This casts serious doubt on the usefulness of large quantities of HCA as an anti-obesity agent or ergogenic aid.

PYRUVATE

Ergogenic effects have been extolled for **pyruvate**, the 3-carbon end product of the cytoplasmic breakdown of glucose in glycolysis. As a partial replacement for dietary carbohydrate, advocates say that consuming pyruvate enhances endurance performance and promotes fat loss. Pyruvic acid, a relatively unstable chemical, causes intestinal distress. Consequently, various forms of the salt of this acid (sodium, potassium, calcium, or magnesium pyruvate) are produced in capsule, tablet, or powder form. Supplement manufacturers recommend taking 2 to 4 capsules daily (a total of 2 and 5 g of pyruvate spread throughout the day and taken with meals). One capsule usually contains 600 mg of pyruvate. The calcium form of pyruvate contains approximately 80 mg of calcium with 600 mg of pyruvate. Some advertisements recommend doses of one capsule per 20 pounds of body weight. Manufacturers also combine creatine monohydrate and pyruvate; 1 g of creatine pyruvate provides about 80 mg of creatine and 400 mg of pyruvate. Recommended pyruvate doses range from 5 to 20 g per day. Pyruvate content in the normal diet ranges between 100 to 2000 mg daily. The largest dietary amounts occur in fruits and vegetables, particularly red apples (500 mg each), with smaller quantities in dark beer (80 mg per 12 oz) and red wine (75 mg per 6 oz).

Effects on Endurance Performance

Two double-blind, cross-over studies by the same laboratory showed that 7 days of daily supplementation of a 100-g mixture of pyruvate (25 g) plus dihydroxyacetone (DHA; 75 g, another 3-carbon compound of glycolysis), increased upper- and lower-body aerobic endurance by 20% compared with exercise with a 100-g supplement of an isocaloric glucose polymer. The pyruvate–DHA mixture increased cycle ergometer time to exhaustion of the legs by 13 minutes (66 min vs. 79 min); upper-body arm-cranking exercise time increased by 27 minutes (133 min vs. 160 min). A reduction also occurred for local muscle and overall body ratings of perceived exertion when subjects exercised with the pyruvate–DHA mixture compared with the placebo. Dosage recommendations range between 2 and 5 g of pyruvate spread throughout the day and consumed with meals.

Proponents of pyruvate supplementation maintain that elevations in extracellular pyruvate augment glucose transport into active muscle. Enhanced "glucose extraction" from blood provides the important carbohydrate energy source to sustain intense aerobic exercise while also conserving intramuscular glycogen stores. When the individual's diet contains 55% of total calories as carbohydrate, pyruvate supplementation also increases pre-exercise muscle glycogen levels. Both of these effects (higher pre-exercise glycogen levels and facilitated glucose uptake and oxidation by active muscle) benefit high-intensity endurance exercise similar to how pre-exercise carbohydrate loading and glucose feedings during exercise exert ergogenic effects.

Body Fat Loss Some research indicates that exogenous pyruvate intake augments body fat loss when accompanied by a low-energy diet. The precise role of pyruvate in facilitating weight loss remains unknown. Consuming pyruvate may stimulate small increases in futile metabolic activity (metabolism not coupled to ATP production) with a subsequent wasting of energy. Unfortunately, adverse side effects of a 30- to 100-g daily pyruvate intake include

Questions & Notes

Give one reason that long-chain fatty acids are undesirable as a supplement to augment energy metabolism.

Briefly describe how medium-chain triacylglycerols may act as an ergogenic supplement.

Give one negative effect of consuming medium-chain triacylglycerols.

Briefly describe how pyruvate supposedly acts as an ergogenic supplement.

ⓘ For Your Information

SKIP THE CARNITINE

Vital to normal metabolism, carnitine facilitates influx of long-chain fatty acids into the mitochondrial matrix, where they enter β-oxidation during energy metabolism. Patients with progressive muscle weakness benefit from carnitine administration, but healthy adults do not require carnitine supplements above that contained in a balanced diet. No research supports ergogenic benefits, positive metabolic alterations (aerobic or anaerobic), or body fat–reducing effects from carnitine supplementation.

diarrhea and some gastrointestinal gurgling and discomfort. *Until additional studies from independent laboratories reproduce existing findings for exercise performance and body fat loss, one should view with caution conclusions about the effectiveness of pyruvate supplementation.*

GLYCEROL

Glycerol is a component of the triacylglycerol molecule, a gluconeogenic substrate, an important constituent of the cells' phospholipid plasma membrane, and an osmotically active natural metabolite. The 2-carbon glycerol molecule achieved clinical notoriety (along with mannitol, sorbitol, and urea) for its role in producing an osmotic diuresis. This capacity for influencing water movement within the body makes glycerol effective in reducing excess accumulation of fluid (edema) in the brain and eye. Glycerol's effect on water movement occurs because extracellular glycerol enters the tissues of the brain, cerebrospinal fluid, and eye's aqueous humor at a relatively slow rate to create an osmotic effect that draws fluid from these tissues.

Ingesting a concentrated mixture of glycerol plus water increases the body's fluid volume and glycerol concentrations in plasma and interstitial fluid compartments. This sets the stage for fluid excretion from an increase in renal filtrate and urine flow. Because proximal and distal tubules reabsorb much of this glycerol, a large fluid portion of renal filtrate also becomes reabsorbed to avert a marked diuresis. When consumed with 1 to 2 L of water, glycerol facilitates water absorption from the intestine to cause extracellular fluid retention mainly in the plasma fluid compartment. The hyperhydration effect of glycerol supplementation reduces overall heat stress during exercise reflected by increased sweating rate; this lowers the heart rate and body temperature during exercise and enhances endurance performance during heat stress. Reducing heat stress with hyperhydration using glycerol plus water supplementation before exercise increases safety for the exercise participant. The typically recommended pre-exercise glycerol dosage of 1 g of glycerol per kg of body mass in 1 to 2 L of water lasts up to 6 hours.

Not all research demonstrates meaningful thermoregulatory or exercise performance benefits of glycerol hyperhydration over pre-exercise hyperhydration with plain water. For example, exogenous glycerol diluted in 500 mL of water consumed 4 hours before exercise failed to promote fluid retention or ergogenic effects. Also, no cardiovascular or thermoregulatory advantages occurred when consuming glycerol with small volumes of water during exercise. Side effects of exogenous glycerol ingestion include nausea, dizziness, bloating, and lightheadedness.

SUMMARY

1. Ergogenic aids consist of substances or procedures that improve physical work capacity, physiologic function, or athletic performance.

2. Functional foods comprise foods and their bioactive components (e.g., olive oil, soy products, omega-3 fatty acids) that promote well-being, health, and optimal bodily function or reduce disease risk.

3. Increasing the body's alkaline reserve before anaerobic exercise by ingesting buffering solutions of sodium bicarbonate or sodium citrate improves performance. Buffer dosage and the cumulative anaerobic nature of the exercise interact to influence the ergogenic effect of bicarbonate or citrate loading.

4. Little scientific evidence exists to recommend exogenous phosphates as an ergogenic aid.

5. Cortisol decreases amino acid transport into cells, depressing anabolism and stimulating protein catabolism. Some believe that blunting cortisol's normal increase after exercise in healthy individuals augments muscular development with resistance training because muscle tissue synthesis progresses unimpeded in recovery.

6. An objective decision about the potential benefits and risks of glutamine, PS, and HMB to provide a "natural"

anabolic boost with resistance training for healthy individuals awaits further research.

7. Research fails to show any beneficial effect of chromium supplements on training-related changes in muscular strength, physique, fat-free body mass, or muscle mass.

8. In supplement form, creatine supplementation increases intramuscular creatine and phosphocreatine, enhances short-term anaerobic power output capacity, and facilitates recovery from repeated bouts of intense effort. Creatine loading occurs by ingesting 20 g of creatine monohydrate for 6 consecutive days. Thereafter, reducing intake to 2 g daily maintains elevated intramuscular levels.

9. Because of its role in energy metabolism, exogenous ribose ingestion has been touted as a means to quickly restore depleted ATP. No difference in any exercise performance and physiologic measure emerged between ribose and placebo exercise trials.

10. No compelling scientific evidence exists to conclude that ginseng supplementation offers positive benefits for physiologic function or performance during exercise.

11. Significant health risks accompany ephedrine use. Based on an analysis of existing data, the FDA

announced a ban on ephedra in 2004, which was upheld by the U.S. Supreme Court in 2007 after lower court challenges from lawsuits filed by the Utah-based manufacturer of ephedrine.

12. Many resistance-trained athletes supplement with amino acids, either singularly or in combination, to create a hormonal milieu to facilitate protein synthesis in skeletal muscle. Research generally shows no benefits of such general supplementation on levels of anabolic hormones or measures of body composition, muscle size, or exercise performance.

13. The proper timing of carbohydrate–protein–creatine supplementation immediately in recovery from resistance training produces a hormonal environment conducive to protein synthesis and muscle tissue growth (elevated plasma concentrations of insulin and GH).

14. CoQ$_{10}$ supplements in healthy individuals provide no ergogenic effect on aerobic capacity, endurance,

submaximal exercise lactate levels, or cardiovascular dynamics.

15. Because of their relatively rapid digestion, assimilation, and catabolism for energy, some believe that consuming MCTs enhances fat metabolism and conserves glycogen during endurance exercise. Ingesting about 86 g of MCTs enhances performance by an additional 2.5%.

16. Increasing plasma HCA availability via supplementation exerts no effect on skeletal muscle fat oxidation at rest or during exercise.

17. Pyruvate supplementation purportedly augments endurance performance and promotes fat loss. Body fat loss is attributed to its small effect on increasing metabolic rate.

18. Pre-exercise glycerol ingestion promotes hyperhydration. It remains controversial whether exogenous glycerol protects the individual from heat stress and heat injury during intense exercise.

THOUGHT QUESTIONS

1. Respond to the question: "If the government allows the chemicals in food supplements to be sold over the counter, how could they possibly be harmful to you?"

2. Discuss the importance of the psychological or "placebo" effect in evaluating claims for the effectiveness of particular nutrients, chemicals, or procedures as ergogenic aids.

Part 2   Pharmacologic Aids to Performance

Questions & Notes

Name 4 substances with high caffeine content.

1.

2.

3.

4.

Athletes at all levels of competition often use pharmacologic and chemical agents, believing that a specific drug positively influences their skill, strength, power, or endurance. When winning becomes all-important, cheating to win becomes pervasive. Despite scanty "hard" scientific evidence indicating a performance-enhancing effect of many of these chemicals, little can be done to prevent the use and abuse of drugs by athletes. This section discusses the most prominent of the pharmacologic chemical agents used by athletes to enhance performance.

CAFFEINE

In January 2004, the IOC removed **caffeine** from its list of restricted substances. Caffeine belongs to a group of compounds called *methylxanthines*, found naturally in coffee beans, tea leaves, chocolate, cocoa beans, and cola nuts and are added to carbonated beverages and nonprescription medicines (Table 4.3). Sixty-three plant species contain caffeine in their leaves, seeds, or fruit. In the United States, 75% of caffeine intake or 14 million kg comes from coffee, and 15% comes from tea. Depending on the preparation, 1 cup of brewed coffee contains between 60 to 150 mg of caffeine, instant coffee contains about

Table 4.3	Caffeine Content of Some Common Foods, Beverages, and Over-the-Counter and Prescription Medications

BEVERAGES AND FOOD		OVER-THE-COUNTER PRODUCTS	
SUBSTANCE	**CAFFEINE CONTENT, mg**	**SUBSTANCE**	**CAFFEINE CONTENT, mg**
Coffee[a]		**Soft Drinks**	
Coffee, Starbucks, grande, 16 oz	550	Jolt	100
Coffee, Starbucks, tall, 12 oz	375	Sugar Free Mr. Pibb	59
Coffee, Starbucks, short, 8 oz	250	Mellow Yellow, Mountain Dew	53–54
Coffee, Starbucks, Americano, tall, 12 oz	70	Tab	47
Coffee, Starbucks, Latte or Cappucinno, grande, 16 oz	70	Coca Cola, Diet Coke, 7-Up Gold	46
		Shasta-Cola, Cherry Cola, Diet Cola	44
Brewed, drip method	110–150	Dr. Pepper, Mr. Pibb	40–41
Brewed, percolator	64–124	Dr. Pepper, sugar free	40
Instant	40–108	Pepsi Cola	38
Expresso	100	Diet Pepsi, Pepsi Light, Diet RC, RC Cola, Diet Rite	36
Decaffeinated, brewed or instant; Sanka	2–5		
Tea, 5 oz cup[a]		**Stimulants**	
Brewed, 1 min	9–33	Vivarin tablet, NoDoz maximum strength caplet, Caffedrin	200
Brewed, 3 min	20–46	NoDoz tablet	100
Brewed, 5 min	20–50	Energets lozenges	75
Iced tea, 12 oz; instant tea	12–36		
Chocolate		**Weight Control Aids**	
Baker's semi-sweet, 1 oz; Baker's chocolate chips, and 5¼ cup	13	Dexatrim, Dietac	200
		Prolamine	140
Cocoa, 5 oz cup, made from mix	6–10	**Pain Drugs**[b]	
Milk chocolate candy, 1 oz	6	Cafergot	100
Sweet/dark chocolate, 1 oz	20	Migrol	50
Baking chocolate, 1 oz	35	Fiornal	40
Chocolate bar, 3.5 oz	12–15	Darvon compound	32
Jello chocolate fudge mousse	12		
Ovaltine	0		
Cold Remedies			
Dristan, Coryban-D, Triaminicin, Sinarest	30–31		
Excedrin	65		
Actifed, Contac, Comtrex, Sudafed	0		
Diuretics			
Aqua-ban	200		
Pre-Mens Forte	100		
Pain Remedies			
Vanquish	33		
Anacin, Midol	32		
Aspirin, any brand; Bufferin, Tylenol, Excedrin P.M.	0		

[a]Brewing tea or coffee for longer periods slightly increases the caffeine content.
[b]Prescription required.
Data from product labels and manufacturers.

100 mg, brewed tea contains between 20 and 50 mg, and caffeinated soft drinks contain about 50 mg. As a frame of reference, 2.5 cups of percolated coffee contains 250 to 400 mg, or generally between 3 and 6 mg per kg of body mass. Caffeine absorption by the small intestine occurs rapidly, reaching peak plasma concentrations between 30 and 120 minutes after ingestion to exert an influence on the nervous, cardiovascular, and muscular systems. Caffeine's metabolic half-life ranges between 3 to 8 hours,

which means that it clears from the body fairly rapidly, certainly after a night's sleep.

Caffeine's Ergogenic Effects

A strong base of evidence supports the use of caffeine to improve exercise performance. Ingesting the amount of caffeine (330 mg) in 2.5 cups of regularly percolated coffee 1 hour before exercising extends endurance in intense

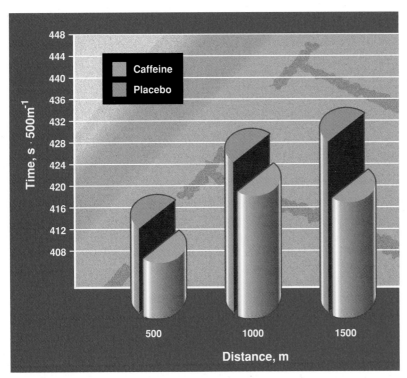

Figure 4.9 Split times for each 500 m of a 1500-m time trial for caffeine (*light purple*) and placebo (*dark purple*) trials. Caffeine produced significantly faster split times. (From MacIntosh, B.R., Wright, B.M.: Caffeine ingestion and performance of a 1,500-metre swim. *Can. J. Appl. Physiol.*, 20:168, 1995.)

 For Your Information

STOP CAFFEINE WHEN USING CREATINE

Caffeine blunts the ergogenic effect of creatine supplementation. To evaluate the effect of pre-exercise caffeine ingestion on intramuscular creatine stores and high-intensity exercise performance, subjects consumed a placebo, a daily creatine supplement ($0.5 \text{ g} \cdot \text{kg}^{-1}$ body mass), or the same daily creatine supplement plus caffeine ($5 \text{ mg} \cdot \text{kg}^{-1}$ body mass) for 6 days. Under each condition, they performed maximal intermittent knee extension exercise to fatigue on an isokinetic dynamometer. Creatine supplementation, with or without caffeine, increased intramuscular PCr by between 4% and 6%. Dynamic torque production also increased 10% to 23% with creatine only compared with the placebo. Taking caffeine, however, totally negated creatine's ergogenic effect. Thus, athletes who creatine load should refrain from caffeine-containing foods and beverages for several days before competition.

aerobic exercise. Subjects who consumed caffeine exercised for an average of 90.2 minutes compared with 75.5 minutes in subjects who exercised without caffeine. Even though heart rate and oxygen uptake were similar during the two trials, the caffeine made the work seem easier.

Caffeine also provides an ergogenic benefit during maximal swimming performances completed in less than 25 minutes. In a double-blind, cross-over study, seven male and four female distance swimmers (<25 min for 1500 m) consumed caffeine ($6 \text{ mg} \cdot \text{kg body mass}^{-1}$) 2.5 hours before swimming 1500 m. **Figure 4.9** illustrates that the split times improved with caffeine for each 500 m of the swim. Total swim time averaged 1.9% faster with caffeine than without it (20 min, 58.6 s vs. 21 min, 21.8 s). Lower plasma potassium concentration before exercise and higher blood glucose levels at the end of the trial accompanied enhanced performance with caffeine. This suggested that electrolyte balance and glucose availability might be key factors in caffeine's ergogenic effect.

Proposed Mechanism for Ergogenic Action

A precise explanation for the exercise-enhancing boost from caffeine remains elusive. In all likelihood, the ergogenic effect of caffeine (or other related methylxanthine compounds) in intense endurance exercise occurs from the facilitated use of fat as fuel, thus sparing the body's limited glycogen reserves. In quantities typically administered to humans, caffeine probably acts in one or more of the three following ways:

1. It acts directly by stimulating adipose tissues to release fatty acids.
2. Indirectly by stimulating epinephrine release from the adrenal medulla; epinephrine then facilitates fatty acid release from adipocytes into plasma. Increased plasma FFA levels, in turn, increase fat oxidation, thus conserving liver and muscle glycogen.
3. Produces analgesic effects on the central nervous system and enhances motoneuronal excitability, facilitating motor unit recruitment.

 For Your Information

ANOTHER USE FOR VIAGRA

Viagra (sildenafil citrate) represents the latest entry of drugs with purported ergogenic effects that athletes use to enhance exercise performance. The mechanism for ergogenic effects lies in its dilating effect on blood vessels to enhance oxygen delivery to muscles. Research on the climbers of Mt. Everest during acute hypoxia tends to support its effectiveness. No action has been taken regarding its use or the alternative tadalafil (phosphodiesterase-5 inhibitor; common name, Cialis) in athletic competition.

BOX 4.2   CLOSE UP

How to Recognize Warning Signs of Alcohol Abuse

Alcohol consumption has been a socially acceptable behavior for centuries. Alcohol is consumed at parties, religious ceremonies, dinners, and sport contests, and has been used as a mild sedative and as a pain killer for surgery. Some athletes possess a negative attitude about drinking, but they, as a group, are not immune to alcohol abuse.

Alcohol addiction develops slowly. Most people believe they can control their drinking habits and do not realize they have a problem until they become alcoholic; they develop a physical and emotional dependence on the drug, characterized by excessive use and constant preoccupation with drinking that leads to mental, emotional, physical, and social problems.

ALCOHOL ABUSE: ARE YOU DRINKING TOO MUCH?

The following checklist can help identify problem behaviors with alcohol. Two or more "Yes" answers on this questionnaire indicate a potential for jeopardizing health through excessive alcohol consumption.

Identifying Alcohol Abuse[a]		
YES	NO	QUESTION
☐	☐	When you are holding an empty glass at a party, do you always actively look for a refill instead of waiting to be offered one?
☐	☐	If given the chance, do you frequently pour out a more generous drink for yourself than seems to be the "going" amount for others?
☐	☐	Do you often have a drink or two when you are alone, either at home or in a bar?
☐	☐	Is your drinking ever the direct cause of a family quarrel, or do quarrels often seem to occur, if only by coincidence, after you have had a drink or two?
☐	☐	Do you feel that you must have a drink at a specific time every day (e.g., right after work, for your nerves)?
☐	☐	When worried or under unusual stress, do you almost automatically take a stiff drink to "settle your nerves?"
☐	☐	Are you untruthful about how much you have had to drink when questioned on the subject?
☐	☐	Does drinking ever cause you to take time off work or to miss scheduled meetings or appointments?
☐	☐	Do you feel physically deprived if you cannot have at least one drink every day?
☐	☐	Do you sometimes crave a drink in the morning?
☐	☐	Do you sometimes have "mornings after" when you cannot remember what happened the night before?

[a]Answer "yes" or "no" to each question. **Evaluation:** One "yes" answer should be viewed as a warning sign. Two "yes" answers suggests alcohol dependency. Three or more "yes" answers indicates a serious problem that requires immediate professional help.
From American Medical Association. *Family Medical Guide by the American Medical Association.* New York: Random House (1982).

Endurance Effects Often Inconsistent   Prior nutrition may partly account for variation in response to exercise after individuals consume caffeine. Although group improvements in endurance occur with caffeine, individuals who maintain high carbohydrate intake show a diminished effect on FFA mobilization. Individual differences in caffeine sensitivity, tolerance, and hormonal response from short- and long-term patterns of caffeine consumption also affect this drug's ergogenic qualities. Interestingly, the ergogenic effects of caffeine are less for caffeine in coffee than for an equivalent dose in capsule form. Apparently, components in coffee counteract caffeine's actions. Beneficial effects do not occur consistently in habitual caffeine users. This indicates that an athlete should consider "caffeine tolerance" rather than assume that caffeine provides a consistent benefit to all people. From a practical standpoint, athletes should omit caffeine-containing foods and beverages 4 to 6 days before competition to optimize caffeine's potential for ergogenic effects.

Effects on Muscle   Caffeine may act directly on muscles to enhance their capacity for exercise. A double-blind research design evaluated voluntary and electrically stimulated muscle actions under "caffeine-free" conditions and after oral administration of 500 mg of caffeine. Electrically stimulating the motor nerve enabled researchers to remove central nervous system control and quantify caffeine's direct effects on skeletal muscle. Caffeine produced no ergogenic effect on maximal muscle force during voluntary or electrically stimulated muscle actions. In contrast, for submaximal effort, caffeine increased force output for low-frequency electrical stimulation before and after muscle fatigue. This suggests that caffeine exerts a direct and specific ergogenic effect on skeletal muscle during repetitive low-frequency stimulation. Perhaps caffeine increases the sarcoplasmic reticulum's permeability to Ca^{++}, thus making this mineral readily available for contraction. Caffeine could also influence the myofibril's sensitivity to Ca^{++}.

ALCOHOL

Alcohol, more specifically ethyl alcohol or ethanol (a form of carbohydrate), is a depressant drug. Alcohol provides about 7 kCal of energy per gram (mL) of pure substance (100% or 200 proof). Adolescents and adults, both athletes and non-athletes, abuse alcohol more than any other drug in the United States. According to World Health Organization statistics, about 140 million people have alcohol-related disorders. A standard drink refers to one 12-oz bottle of beer or wine cooler, one 5-oz glass of wine, or 1.5 oz of 80-proof distilled spirits. Between 25% and 30% of men and 5% and 10% of

 For Your Information

CAFFEINE WARNING

Individuals who normally avoid caffeine may experience undesirable side effects when they consume it. Caffeine stimulates the central nervous system and can produce restlessness, headaches, insomnia and nervous irritability, muscle twitching, tremulousness, and psychomotor agitation and trigger premature left ventricular contractions. From the standpoint of temperature regulation, caffeine acts as a potent diuretic. Excessive consumption could cause an unnecessary pre-exercise fluid loss, negatively affecting thermal balance and exercise performance in a hot environment.

 For Your Information

MORE CAFFEINE IS NOT NECESSARILY BETTER

To study the effects of pre-exercise caffeine intake on endurance time trained, male cyclists received a placebo or a capsule containing 5, 9, or 13 mg of caffeine per kg of body mass 1 hour before cycling at 80% of maximal power output on a $\dot{V}O_{2max}$ test. All caffeine trials showed a 24% improvement in performance with *no additional benefit* from caffeine quantities above 5 mg·kg body mass^{-1}.

 For Your Information

ALCOHOL ABUSE

More young people in the United States use alcohol than tobacco or illicit drugs, which accounts for approximately 75,000 deaths yearly. Alcohol represents a major factor in about 41% of all deaths from motor vehicle accidents. Long-term alcohol abuse is associated with liver disease; cancer; cardiovascular disease; and neurologic damage, including psychiatric problems such as depression, anxiety, and antisocial personality disorder. All states prohibit people younger than age 21 years from purchasing alcohol, yet in 2007, 26% of high school students reported episodic heavy or binge drinking. Zero-tolerance laws make it illegal for youth younger than age 21 years to drive with any measurable amount of alcohol in their system (i.e., with a blood alcohol concentration ≥0.02 g/dL). In 2007, 11% of high school students reported driving a car or other vehicle during the past 30 days after drinking alcohol, and 29% of students reported riding in a car or other vehicle during the past 30 days driven by someone who had been drinking alcohol.

From U.S. Department of Health and Human Services. (2007). *The Surgeon General's Call to Action to Prevent and Reduce Underage Drinking.* Washington, DC: U.S. Department of Health and Human Services, Office of the Surgeon General. *http://ncadi.samhsa.gov.*

women abuse alcohol. About 16% of alcohol abusers report a family history of alcoholism in first-, second-, or third-degree relatives. Among college students in the United States, binge drinking (consumption of five or more drinks witin 2 h by men or four or more drinks by women) contributes to 1400 unintended student deaths yearly (including motor vehicle accidents), and approximately 600,000 students are assaulted by a drinking student. Of particular concern are the more than 70,000 students between the ages of 18 and 24 years who become victims of alcohol-related sexual assault or date rape each year.

Use Among Athletes

Statistics remain equivocal about alcohol use among athletes compared with the general population. In a study of athletes in Italy, 330 male high school non-athletes consumed more beer, wine, and hard liquor and had greater episodes of heavy drinking than 336 young athletes. Interestingly, the strongest predictor of a participant's alcohol consumption related to the drinking habits of his or her best friend and boyfriend or girlfriend. In other research, physically active men drank less alcohol than their sedentary counterparts. A self-reported questionnaire assessed alcohol intake of randomly selected students in a representative national sample of 4-year colleges in the United States. Compared with non-athletic students, athletes were at high risk for binge drinking, heavier alcohol use, and a greater number of drinking-related harms. Athletes were also more likely than non-athletes to surround themselves with others who binge drink and a social environment conducive to excessive alcohol consumption. These findings support the position that future alcohol prevention programs targeted to athletes should address the unique social and environmental influences that affect the current athletes' increased alcohol use.

Alcohol's Psychologic and Physiologic Effects

Some athletes use alcohol to enhance their performance because of its supposed "positive" psychologic and physiologic effects. In the psychologic realm, some have argued that alcohol before competition reduces tension and anxiety (**anxiolytic effect**), enhances self-confidence, and promotes aggressiveness. It also facilitates neurologic "disinhibition" through its initial, although transitory, stimulatory effect. Thus, athletes may believe that alcohol facilitates physical performance at or close to physiologic capacity, particularly for maximal strength and power activities. *Research does not substantiate any ergogenic effect of alcohol on muscular strength, short-term maximal anaerobic power, or longer term aerobic exercise performance.*

Although initially acting as a stimulant, alcohol ultimately depresses neurologic function (e.g., impaired memory, visual perception, speech, and motor coordination) in direct relationship to blood alcohol concentration. Damping of psychomotor function causes the anti-tremor effect of alcohol ingestion. Consequently, alcohol use has been particularly prevalent in sports that require extreme steadiness and accuracy such as rifle and pistol shooting and archery. Achieving an anti-tremor effect has also been the primary rationale among such athletes for using β-blockers (adrenergic receptor blocking agents such as propranolol), which blunt the arousal effect of sympathetic stimulation. Despite this specific potential for performance enhancement, the majority of research indicates that alcohol at best provides no ergogenic benefit; at worst, it can precipitate dangerous side effects that impair performance, termed an **ergolytic effect**. For example, alcohol's depression of nervous system function profoundly impairs almost all sports performances that require balance, hand–eye coordination, reaction time, and overall need for rapid information processing.

From a physiologic perspective, alcohol impairs cardiac function. Ingesting 1 g of alcohol per kg of body mass during 1 hour raises the blood alcohol level to just over $0.10 \, g \cdot dL^{-1}$ (1 dL = 100 mL). This level, often observed among social drinkers, acutely depresses myocardial contractility. In terms of metabolism, alcohol inhibits the liver's capacity to synthesize glucose from noncarbohydrate sources via gluconeogenesis. These effects could impair performance in intense aerobic activities that rely on cardiovascular capacity and energy from carbohydrate catabolism. Alcohol provides no benefit as an energy substrate and does not favorably alter the metabolic mixture in endurance exercise.

Alcohol Drinks for Fluid Replacement: Not a Good Idea
Alcohol exaggerates the dehydrating effect of exercise in a warm environment. It acts as a potent diuretic in two ways by:

1. Depressing antidiuretic hormone release from the posterior pituitary.
2. Diminishes the arginine-vasopressin response.

These effects impair thermoregulation during heat stress, placing the athlete at greater risk for heat distress.

Many athletes consume alcohol-containing beverages after exercising or sports competition; thus, one question concerns whether alcohol impairs rehydration in recovery. Alcohol's effect on rehydration has been studied after exercise-induced dehydration equal to approximately 2% of body mass. The subjects consumed a rehydration fluid volume equivalent to 150% of fluid lost and containing 0%, 1%, 2%, 3%, or 4% alcohol. Urine volume produced during the 6-hour study period was directly related to the beverages' alcohol concentration; greater alcohol consumed produced more urine. The increase in plasma volume in recovery compared with the dehydrated state averaged 8.1% when the rehydration fluid contained no alcohol but only 5.3% for the beverage with 4% alcohol content. *The bottom line—alcohol-containing beverages impede rehydration.*

Because of alcohol's action as a peripheral vasodilator, it should not be consumed during extreme cold exposure or to facilitate recovery from hypothermia. A good "stiff drink" does not warm you up. Current debate exists as to whether moderate alcohol intake exacerbates body cooling during mild cold exposure.

ANABOLIC STEROIDS

Anabolic steroids (available in oral, injectable, and transdermal forms) for therapeutic use became prominent in the early 1950s to treat patients deficient in natural androgens or with muscle-wasting diseases. Other legitimate steroid uses include treatment for osteoporosis and severe breast cancer and to counter the excessive decline in lean body mass and increase in body fat often observed among elderly men, people with HIV, and individuals undergoing kidney dialysis.

Anabolic steroids (popular trade names include Dianabol, Anadrol, Deca Durabolin, Parabolin, and Winstrol) became an integral part of the high-technology scene of competitive American sports, beginning with the 1955

U.S. weightlifting team's use of Dianabol (a modified, synthetic testosterone molecule, methandrostenolone). A new era of "drugging" competitive athletes was ushered in with the formulation of additional anabolic steroids.

Steroid Structure and Action

Anabolic steroids function similarly to testosterone. By binding with special receptor sites on muscle and other tissues, testosterone contributes to male secondary sex characteristics that include gender differences in muscle mass and strength that develop at puberty onset. The hormone's androgenic or masculinizing effects are minimized by synthetically manipulating the steroid's chemical structure to increase muscle growth from anabolic tissue building and nitrogen retention. Nevertheless, the masculinizing effect of synthetically derived steroids still occurs despite chemical alteration, particularly in women.

Athletes who take these drugs do so typically during the active years of their athletic careers. They combine multiple steroid preparations in oral and injectable form combined because they believe various androgens differ in their physiologic action. This practice, called **stacking**, progressively increases the drug dosage (**pyramiding**) during 6- to 12-week cycles. The drug quantity far exceeds the recommended medical dose. The athlete then alters the drug dosage or combines it with other prescription-only drugs before competition to minimize the chances of detection.

The difference between dosages used in research studies and the excess typically abused by athletes has contributed to a credibility gap between scientific findings (often, no effect of steroids) and what most in the athletic community believe to be true.

Estimates of Steroid Use

Estimates suggest that up to 4 million athletes (90% of male and 80% of female professional body builders) currently use androgens, often combined with stimulants, hormones, and diuretics. Even in the sport of professional baseball, interviews of strength trainers and current players estimate that up to 30% of the players use anabolic steroids in their quest to enhance their hitting and pitching performance. Male and female athletes usually combine anabolic steroid use with resistance training and augmented protein intake because they believe this combination

Questions & Notes

Is alcohol a stimulant or depressant?

Briefly discuss how alcohol acts as a dehydrating substance.

 ### For Your Information

ALCOHOL IN THE BODY

One alcoholic drink contains 1.0 oz (28.4 g or 28.4 mL) of 100-proof (50%) alcohol. This translates into 12 oz of regular beer (~4% alcohol by volume) or 5 oz of wine (11% to 14% alcohol by volume). The stomach absorbs between 15% and 25% of the alcohol ingested; the small intestine rapidly takes up the remainder for distribution throughout the body's water compartments (particularly the water-rich tissues of the central nervous system). The absence of food in the digestive tract facilitates alcohol absorption. The liver, the major organ for alcohol metabolism, removes alcohol at a rate of about 10 g per hour, equivalent to the alcohol content of one drink. Consuming two drinks in 1 hour produces a blood alcohol concentration of between 0.04 and 0.05 $g \cdot dL^{-1}$. Age, body mass, body fat content, and gender influence blood alcohol levels. The legal state limit for alcohol intoxication ranges between a blood alcohol concentration of 0.11 and 0.16 $g \cdot dL^{-1}$. A blood alcohol concentration of greater than 0.40 $g \cdot dL^{-1}$ (19 drinks or more in 2 hours) can lead to coma, respiratory depression, and eventual death.

 ### For Your Information

FDA ALERT FOR BODYBUILDERS

In October 2009, the FDA issued an alert to consumers to refrain from using body-building products sold as nutritional supplements because they may contain steroids or steroid-like substances that can cause stroke, pulmonary embolism, acute liver injury, and kidney failure. Particular emphasis was placed on products labeled with code words such as *anabolic* and *tren* or phrases such as *blocks estrogen* or *minimizes gyno*. The *gyno* and *estrogen* references indicate that the products aim to minimize feminizing effects such as breast swelling or shrinking testicles.

 ### For Your Information

IT'S AGAINST THE LAW

A federal law makes it illegal to prescribe, distribute, or possess anabolic steroids for any purpose other than treatment of disease or other medical conditions. First offenders face up to 5 years in prison and a fine up to $250,000.

improves sports performance that requires strength, speed, and power. The steroid abuser often has the image of a massively developed body builder; however, abuse also occurs frequently in competitive athletes participating in road cycling, tennis, track and field, and swimming.

Many competitive and recreational athletes obtain steroids on the black market, yet misinformed individuals take massive and prolonged dosages without medical monitoring. Particularly worrisome is steroid abuse among young boys and girls and its accompanying risks, including extreme masculinization and premature cessation of bone growth. Reports from the Centers for Disease Control and Prevention (CDC; *www.cdc.gov*) indicate that 4.4% to 5.7% of boys and 1.9% to 3.3% of girls grades 9 through 12 have used steroids. Both male and female teenagers cite improved athletic performance as the most common reason for taking steroids, although 25% acknowledged enhanced appearance as the main reason. Forty percent of those surveyed noted that obtaining steroids was relatively easy.

Effectiveness of Anabolic Steroids

Much of the confusion about the ergogenic effectiveness of anabolic steroids results from variations in experimental design, poor controls, differences in specific drugs and dosages (50 to >200 mg per day vs. the usual medical dosage of 5 to 20 mg), treatment duration, training intensity, measurement techniques, previous experience as subjects, individual variation in response, and nutritional supplementation. Also, the relatively small residual androgenic effect of the steroid can make the athlete more aggressive (so-called "roid rage"), competitive, and fatigue resistant. Such disinhibitory central nervous system effects allow the athlete to train harder for a longer time or believe that augmented training effects have actually occurred.

Abnormal alterations in mood, including psychiatric dysfunction, have been attributed to androgen use as well.

Research with animals suggests that anabolic steroid treatment, when combined with exercise and adequate protein intake, stimulates protein synthesis and increases muscle protein content. In contrast, other research shows no benefit from steroid treatment on the leg muscle weight of rats subjected to functional overload by surgically removing the synergistic muscle. The researchers concluded that anabolic steroid treatment did not complement functional overload to augment muscle development. Effects of steroids on humans remain difficult to interpret. Some studies show augmented body mass gains and reduced body fat with steroid use in men who train, but other studies show no effects on strength and power or body composition, even with sufficient energy and protein intake to support an anabolic effect. When steroid use produced body weight gains, the compositional nature of these gains (water, muscle, fat) remained unclear. The fact that steroid use remains widespread among top-level athletes including body builders and weight lifters suggests that it is a potent substance with considerable credibility.

Dosage Is an Important Factor

Variations in drug dosage contribute to the confusion and credibility gap between scientist and steroid user regarding the true effectiveness of anabolic steroids. Research studied 43 healthy men with some resistance training experience. Diet (energy and protein intake) and exercise (standard weight lifting, three times weekly) were controlled, with steroid dosage exceeding previous human studies (600 mg of testosterone enanthate injected weekly or placebo).

Figure 4.10 illustrates changes from baseline average values for FFM (assessed by hydrostatic weighing; refer to

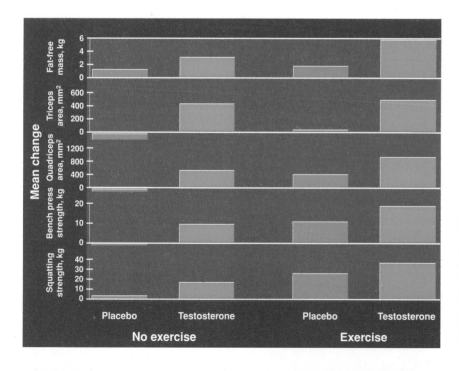

Figure 4.10 Changes from baseline in mean fat-free body mass, triceps, quadriceps cross-sectional areas, and muscle strength in bench-press and squatting exercises over 10 weeks of testosterone treatment. (Data from Bhasin, S., et al.: The effects of supraphysiological doses of testosterone on muscle size and strength in normal men. *N. Engl. J. Med.*, 335:1, 1996.)

Chapter 16), triceps and quadriceps cross-sectional muscle areas assessed by magnetic resonance imaging, and muscle strength repetition maximum (1-RM) after 10 weeks of testosterone treatment. The men who received the hormone and continued to train gained about 0.5 kg (1 lb) of lean tissue weekly, with no increase in body fat over the relatively brief treatment period. Even the group that received the drug but did not train increased their muscle mass and strength compared with the group receiving the placebo, although their increases were lower than the group that trained while taking testosterone.

Risks of Steroid Use

Table 4.4 lists some of the known harmful side effects from abuse of anabolic steroids. Prolonged high dosages of steroids (often at levels 10 to 200 times the therapeutic recommendation) can impair normal testosterone endocrine

Table 4.4	Steroid Use and Associated Detrimental Side Effects	
SYSTEM	**ADVERSE EFFECT**	**REVERSIBILITY**
Cardiovascular	Increased LDL cholesterol	Yes
	Decreased HDL cholesterol	Yes
	Hypertension	Yes
	Elevated triglycerides	Yes
	Arteriosclerotic heart disease	No
	High blood pressure	Possible
Reproductive– Male	Testicular atrophy	Possible
	Gynecomastia (breast enlargement)	Possible
	Impaired spermatogenesis	Yes
	Altered libido (impotence)	Yes
	Male pattern baldness	No
	Enlarged prostate gland	Possible
	Pain in urinating	Yes
Reproductive– Female	Menstrual dysfunction	Yes
	Altered libido	Yes
	Clitoral enlargement	No
	Deepening voice	No
	Male pattern baldness	No
	Breast reduction	No
Hepatic	Elevated liver enzymes	Yes
	Jaundice	Yes
	Hepatic tumors	No
	Peliosis	No
Endocrine	Altered glucose tolerance	Yes
	Decreased FSH, LH	Yes
	Acne	Yes
Musculoskeletal	Premature epiphyseal closure (stunted growth)	No
	Tendon degeneration, ruptures	No
	Swelling of feet or ankles	Yes
Central Nervous	Mood swings	Yes
	Violent behavior	Yes
	Depression	Yes
	Psychoses/delusions	Yes
Other	Hepatoma	Yes
	Bad breath	Yes
	Nausea and vomiting	Yes
	Sleep problems	Yes
	Impaired judgment	Yes
	Paranoid jealous	Yes
	Increased risk of blood poisoning and infections	No

*Q*uestions & Notes

Describe the magnitude of the differences between a typical medical and a typical athlete's dosage of steroids.

List 3 detrimental side effects of steroid abuse.

1.

2.

3.

List 2 adverse non-reversible side effects of steroid abuse.

1.

2.

For Your Information

COMPETITIVE ATHLETES BEWARE

Elite athletes who take androstenedione can fail a urine test for the banned anabolic steroid nandrolone. This occurs because the supplement often contains contaminates with trace amounts (as low as 10 mg) of 19-norandrosterone, the standard marker for nandrolone use. Many androstenedione preparations are grossly mislabeled. Analysis of nine different brands of 100-mg doses indicate wide fluctuations in overall content ranging from 0 to 103 mg of androstenedione, with one brand contaminated with testosterone.

function. A study of five male power athletes showed that 26 weeks of steroid administration reduced serum testosterone to less than half the level measured when the study began, with the effect lasting throughout a 12- to 16-week follow-up period. Infertility, reduced sperm concentrations (azoospermia), and decreased testicular volume pose additional problems for male steroid users.

Other accompanying hormonal alterations during steroid use in men include a sevenfold increase in estradiol concentration, the major female hormone. The higher estradiol level represents an average value for normal women and possibly explains the **gynecomastia** (excessive development of the male mammary glands, sometimes secreting milk) reported among men who take anabolic steroids. Furthermore, steroids have been shown to cause the following four responses:

1. Chronic stimulation of the prostate gland (increased size).
2. Injury and functional alterations in cardiovascular function and myocardial cell cultures.
3. Possible pathologic ventricular growth and dysfunction when combined with resistance training.
4. Increased blood platelet aggregation, which can compromise cardiovascular health and function and possibly increase the risk of stroke and acute myocardial infarction from blood clots.

Steroid Use and Life-Threatening Disease

Concern regarding the risk of chronic steroid use centers on evidence about possible links between androgen abuse and abnormal liver function. The liver almost exclusively metabolizes androgens, thus becoming susceptible to damage from long-term steroid use and toxic excess. One of the serious effects of androgens on the liver and sometimes splenic tissue occurs when it develops localized blood-filled lesions (cysts), a condition called **peliosis hepatis.** In extreme cases, the liver eventually fails or intraabdominal hemorrhage develops, and the patient dies. These outcomes emphasize the potentially serious side effects even when a physician prescribes the drug in the recommended dosage. Patients often take steroids for a longer duration than athletes, and some athletes take steroids on and off for years, with dosages exceeding typical therapeutic levels.

Steroid Use and Plasma Lipoproteins

Anabolic steroid use particularly the orally active 17-alkylated androgens in healthy men and women rapidly lowers high-density lipoprotein cholesterol (HDL-C), elevates both low-density lipoprotein cholesterol (LDL-C) and total cholesterol, and lowers the HDL-C:LDL-C ratio. Weight lifters who took anabolic steroids averaged an HDL-C of $26 \text{ mg} \cdot \text{dL}^{-1}$ compared with $50 \text{ mg} \cdot \text{dL}^{-1}$ for weight lifters not taking these drugs. Reduction of HDL-C to this level considerably increases risk of coronary artery disease.

Specific Risks for Females

Females have additional concerns about dangers from anabolic steroids. These include virilization (more apparent than in men), disruption of normal growth pattern by premature closure of the plates for bone growth, altered menstrual function, dramatic increase in sebaceous gland size, acne, hirsutism (excessive body and facial hair), generally irreversible deepening of the voice, decreased breast size, enlarged clitoris (clitoromegaly), and hair loss (alopecia areata). Serum levels of luteinziging hormone, follicle-stimulating hormone, progesterone, and estrogens also

---

BOX 4.3 CLOSE UP

American College of Sports Medicine (ACSM; *www.acsm.org*) Position Statement on Anabolic Steroids

Based on the world literature and a careful analysis of claims about anabolic-androgenic steroids, the ACSM issued the following statement:

1. Anabolic-androgenic steroids in the presence of an adequate diet and training can contribute to increases in body weight, often in the lean mass compartment.
2. The gains in muscular strength achieved through high-intensity exercise and proper diet can occur by the increased use of anabolic-androgenic steroids in some individuals.
3. Anabolic-androgenic steroids do not increase aerobic power or capacity for muscular exercise.

4. Anabolic-androgenic steroids have been associated with adverse effects on the liver, cardiovascular, reproductive system, and psychological status in therapeutic trials and in limited research on athletes. Until further research is completed, the potential hazards of the use of anabolic-androgenic steroids in athletes must include those found in therapeutic trials.
5. The use of anabolic-androgenic steroids by athletes is contrary to the rules and ethical principles of athletic competition as set forth by many of the sports governing bodies. The American College of Sports Medicine supports these ethical principles and deplores the use of anabolic-androgenic steroids by athletes.

decline. These may negatively affect follicle formation, ovulation, and menstrual function.

ANDROSTENEDIONE: A STEROID ALTERNATIVE

Many physically active individuals have taken the over-the-counter nutritional supplement **androstenedione** (also known as Andromax and Androstat 100), believing it produces endogenous testosterone to enable them to train harder, build muscle mass, and repair injury more rapidly. Initially marketed as a dietary supplement and anti-aging drug, androstenedione occurs naturally in meat and extracts of some plants and is touted on the internet as "a metabolite that is only one step away from the biosynthesis of testosterone." The NFL (*www.nfl.com*), National Collegiate Athletic Association (NCAA; *www.ncaa.com*), Men's Professional Tennis Association (*www.atpworldtour.com*), WADA, and IOC ban its use because these organizations believe it provides an unfair competitive advantage and may endanger health, similar to anabolic steroids. The IOC banned for life the 1996 Olympic shotput gold medalist because he used androstenedione, and it remains a banned substance by the IOC and U.S. Olympic Committee. In 2004, the FDA banned androstenedione because of its potent anabolic and androgenic effects and accompanying health risks.

$\mathcal{Q}$uestions & Notes

Briefly explain why steroid abuse relates to plasma lipoprotein levels.

BOX 4.4 CLOSE UP

2009–2010 NCAA List of Banned Substances:[a] Collegiate Athletes Beware

The NCAA bans the following classes of drugs: (Note: Any substance chemically related to these classes is also banned). The institution and the student-athlete shall be held accountable for all drugs within the banned drug class regardless of whether they have been specifically identified. There is no complete list of banned drug examples!

1. Stimulants
2. Anabolic agents
3. Alcohol and β-blockers (banned for rifle only)
4. Diuretics and other masking agents
5. Street drugs
6. Peptide hormones and analogues
7. Anti-estrogens
8. β$_2$ Agonists

Stimulants: Amphetamine (Adderall), caffeine (guarana), cocaine, ephedrine, fenfluramine (Fen), methamphetamine, methylphenidate (Ritalin), phentermine (Phen), Synephrine (bitter orange). **Exceptions:** Phenylephrine and pseudoephedrine are not banned.

Anabolic agents: Boldenone, clenbuterol, DHEA, nandrolone, stanozolol, testosterone, methasterone, androstenedione, norandrostenedione, methandienone, etiocholanolone, trenbolone

Alcohol and β-blockers (banned for rifle only): Alcohol, atenolol, metoprolol, nadolol, pindolol, propranolol, timolol

Diuretics and other masking agents: Bumetanide, chlorothiazide, furosemide, hydrochlorothiazide, probenecid, spironolactone (canrenone), triamterene, trichlormethiazide

Street drugs: Heroin, marijuana, tetrahydrocannabinol (THC)

Peptide hormones and analogues: Human growth hormone (hGH), human chorionic gonadotropin (hCG), erythropoietin (EPO)

Anti-estrogens: Anastrozole, clomiphene, tamoxifen, formestane

β$_2$ agonists: Bambuterol, formoterol, salbutamol, salmeterol

Available at www.ncaa.org

Action and Effectiveness

Androstenedione, an intermediate or precursor hormone between DHEA and testosterone, aids the liver to synthesize other biologically active steroid hormones. Normally produced by the adrenal glands and gonads, androstenedione converts to testosterone through enzymatic action in diverse tissues of the body. Some androstenedione also converts into estrogens.

Little scientific evidence supports claims about androstenedione's effectiveness or anabolic qualities. One study systematically evaluated whether short- and long-term oral androstenedione supplementation elevated blood testosterone concentrations and enhanced gains in muscle size and strength during resistance training. In one phase of the investigation, 10 young men received a single 100-mg dose of androstenedione or a placebo containing 250 mg of rice flour. With supplementation, serum androstenedione increased 175% during the first 60 minutes after ingestion and then increased further by about 350% above baseline values between minutes 90 and 270 minutes. No effect emerged for androstenedione supplementation on serum concentrations of either free or total testosterone.

In the experiment's second phase, 20 young, untrained men received either 300 mg of androstenedione daily or 250 mg of rice flour placebo daily during weeks 1, 2, 4, 5, 7, and 8 of an 8-week total body resistance training program. Serum androstenedione increased 100% in the androstenedione-supplemented group and remained elevated throughout training. Serum testosterone levels were higher in the androstenedione-supplemented group than the placebo group before and after supplementation, but serum free and total testosterone remained unaltered for both groups during the supplementation training period. Serum estradiol and estrone concentrations increased during the training period only for the group receiving the supplement, suggesting an increased aromatization of the ingested androstenedione to estrogens. Furthermore, resistance training increased muscle strength and lean body mass and reduced body fat for both groups, but *no synergistic effect* emerged for the group supplemented with androstenedione. The supplement did cause a 12% *reduction* in HDL-C after only 2 weeks, which remained lower for the 8 weeks of training and supplementation. Liver function enzymes remained within normal limits for both groups throughout the experimental period.

Taken together, these findings indicate *no effect* of androstenedione supplementation on (1) basal serum concentrations of testosterone or (2) training responsiveness in terms of muscle size and strength and body composition. A worrisome result relates to the potential negative effects of the reduction of HDL-C on overall heart disease risk and elevated serum estrogen levels on risk of gynecomastia and possibly pancreatic and other cancers. One must view these findings within the context of this specific study because test subjects took doses of androstenedione *far smaller* than those routinely taken by body builders and other athletes.

THG: THE HIDDEN STEROID

Tetrahydrogestrinone (THG), a relatively new drug listed by the FDA, represents an anabolic steroid specifically designed to escape detection by normal drug testing. This "designer drug" was made public in 2003 when the United States Anti-Doping Agency (USADA; *www.usantidoping.org*), which oversees drug testing for all sports federations under the U.S. Olympic umbrella, was contacted by an anonymous track and field coach claiming several top athletes used the drug. The same coach subsequently provided the USADA with a syringe containing THG that the USADA then used to develop a new test for its detection. They then reanalyzed 350 urine samples from participants at the June 2003 U.S. track and field championships and 100 samples from random out-of-competition tests. Six athletes tested positive.

The source of the THG was traced to the Bay Area Laboratory Cooperative (BALCO), a U.S. company that analyzed blood and urine from athletes and then prescribed a series of supplements to compensate for vitamin and mineral deficiencies. Among its clients were high-profile athletes in many professional and amateur sports. The ability to develop an undetectable steroid points to the disturbing ready market for such drugs among athletes who are prepared to try almost anything to achieve success.

CLENBUTEROL: ANABOLIC STEROID SUBSTITUTE

Extensive random testing of competitive athletes for anabolic steroid use has produced a number of steroid substitutes appearing on the illicit health food, mail order, and "black market" drug network. One such drug, the sympathomimetic amine **clenbuterol** (trade names Clenasma, Monores, Novegan, Prontovent, and Spiropent), is popular among athletes because of its purported tissue-building, fat-reducing benefits. Typically, when body builders discontinue steroid use before competition to avoid detection and possible disqualification, they substitute clenbuterol to maintain a steroid effect.

Clenbuterol, one of a group of chemical compounds classified as a β-adrenergic agonist (albuterol, clenbuterol, salbutamol, salmeterol, and terbutaline), is not approved for human use in the United States but is commonly prescribed abroad as an inhaled bronchodilator for treating obstructive pulmonary disorders. Clenbuterol facilitates responsiveness of adrenergic receptors to circulating epinephrine, norepinephrine, and other adrenergic amines. A review of available animal studies (no human studies exist) indicates that when sedentary, growing livestock receive clenbuterol in dosages in excess of those prescribed in

Europe for human use for bronchial asthma, clenbuterol increases skeletal and cardiac muscle protein deposition and slows fat gain by enhancing lipolysis. Clenbuterol has also been experimentally used in animals with some success to counter the muscle-wasting effects of aging, immobilization, malnutrition, and zero-gravity exposure. The enlarged muscle size from clenbuterol treatment came from decreases in protein breakdown and increases in protein synthesis. Reported short-term side effects in humans accidentally "overdosing" from eating animals that were treated with clenbuterol include muscle tremor, agitation, palpitations, muscle cramps, rapid heart rate, and headache. Despite such negative side effects, supervised use of clenbuterol may prove beneficial for humans with muscle wasting from disease, forced immobilization, and aging. Unfortunately, no data exist for its potential toxicity level in humans or its efficacy and safety in long-term use. Clearly, clenbuterol use cannot be justified or recommended as an ergogenic aid.

HUMAN GROWTH HORMONE: THE STEROID COMPETITOR

Human growth hormone (hGH), also known as somatotropic hormone, competes with anabolic steroids in the illicit market of alleged tissue-building, performance-enhancing drugs. This hormone, produced by the adenohypophysis of the pituitary gland, facilitates tissue-building processes and normal human growth. Specifically, hGH stimulates bone and cartilage growth, enhances fatty acid oxidation, and slows glucose and amino acid breakdown. Reduced hGH secretion (about 50% less at age 60 years than age 30 years) accounts for some of the decrease in FFM and increase in fat mass that accompany aging; reversal occurs with exogenous hGH supplements produced by genetically engineered bacteria.

Children with kidney failure or hGH-deficient children take this hormone to help stimulate long bone growth. hGH use appeals to strength and power athletes because at physiologic levels, it stimulates amino acid uptake and protein synthesis by muscle while enhancing fat breakdown and conserving glycogen reserves.

Research has produced equivocal results concerning the true benefits of hGH supplementation to counter the loss of muscle mass, thinning bones, increased body fat (particularly abdominal fat), and depressed energy levels. For example, 16 previously sedentary young men who participated in a 12-week resistance training program received daily recombinant hGH (40 g·kg^{-1}) or a placebo. FFM, total body water, and whole-body protein synthesis (attributed to increased nitrogen retention in lean tissue other than skeletal muscle) increased more in the hGH recipients, with no differences between groups in fractional rate of protein synthesis in skeletal muscle, torso and limb circumferences, or muscle function in dynamic and static strength measures.

One of the largest studies to date determined the effects of hGH on changes in the body composition and functional capacity of healthy men and women ranging in age from the mid-60s to the late 80s. Men who took hGH gained 7 pounds of lean body mass and decreased a similar amount of fat mass. Women gained about 3 pounds of lean body mass and lost 5 pounds of body fat compared with their counterparts who received a placebo. The subjects remained sedentary and did not change their diet over the 6-month study period. Unfortunately, serious side effects affected between 24% and 46% of the subjects. These included swollen feet and ankles, joint pain, carpal tunnel syndrome (swelling of tendon sheath over a nerve in the wrist), and the development of a diabetic or prediabetic condition. As in previous research, no effects occurred for hGH treatment on measures of muscular strength or endurance capacity despite increases in lean body mass.

 For Your Information

SUMMARY OF RESEARCH FINDINGS CONCERNING ANDROSTENEDIONE

- Elevates plasma testosterone concentrations
- No favorable effect on muscle mass
- No favorable effect on muscular performance
- No favorable alteration in body composition
- Elevates a variety of estrogen subfractions
- No favorable effects on muscle protein synthesis or tissue anabolism
- Impairs the blood lipid profile in apparently healthy men
- Increases the likelihood of testing positive for steroid use

 For Your Information

NASTY SIDE EFFECTS OF GH

Excessive GH production (or use) during skeletal growth produces **gigantism**, an endocrine and metabolic disorder characterized by abnormal size or overgrowth of the entire body or any of its parts. Excessive hormone production (or use) after growth cessation produces the irreversible disorder **acromegaly** that presents as enlarged hands, feet, and facial features.

Previously, healthy people could only obtain hGH on the black market, often in adulterated form. The use of human cadaver-derived hGH (discontinued by U.S. physicians in 1985) to treat children of short stature greatly increases the risk for contracting Creutzfeldt-Jakob disease, an infectious, incurable fatal brain-deteriorating disorder. A synthetic form of hGH (Protoropin and Humantrope) produced by genetic engineering currently treats hGH-deficient children. Undoubtedly, child athletes who take hGH believing they gain a competitive edge experience increased incidence of gigantism, and adults can develop acromegalic syndrome. Less visual side effects include insulin resistance leading to type 2 diabetes, water retention, and carpal tunnel compression.

DHEA: NEW "WONDER DRUG?"

Use of synthetic **dehydroepiandrosterone** (**DHEA**; marketed under the names Prastera, Fidelin, and Fluasterone) among athletes and the general population raises concerns because of issues related to safety and effectiveness. DHEA and its sulfated ester, DHEAS, are relatively weak steroid hormones synthesized from cholesterol in the adrenal cortex. The quantity of DHEA (commonly referred to as "mother hormone") produced by the body surpasses all other known steroids; its chemical structure closely resembles the sex hormones testosterone and estrogen, with a small amount of DHEA serving as a precursor for these hormones for men and women.

Because DHEA occurs naturally, the FDA has no control over its distribution or claims for its action and effectiveness. The lay press, mail order catalogs, and health food industry describe DHEA as a "superhormone" (even available as a chewing gum, each piece containing 25 mg) to increase testosterone production, preserve youth, protect against heart disease, cancer, diabetes, and osteoporosis, invigorate sex drive, facilitate lean tissue gain and body fat loss, enhance mood and memory, extend life, and boost immunity to a variety of infectious diseases (including AIDS). A Google search for "buy DHEA" returned almost 750,000 hits, and Yahoo! lists 2,720,027 (July, 2010) sites! The WADA and USOC include DHEA on their banned substance lists at zero-tolerance levels.

Figure 4.11 illustrates the generalized trend for plasma DHEA levels during a lifetime plus six common claims made by manufacturers for DHEA supplements. For boys and girls, DHEA levels are substantial at birth and then decline sharply. A steady increase in DHEA production occurs from age 6 to 10 years (an occurrence that some researchers believe contributes to the beginning of puberty and sexuality), followed by a rapid increase with peak production (higher in young men than young women) reached between ages 18 to 25 years.

In contrast to the glucocorticoid and mineralocorticoid adrenal steroids whose plasma levels remain relatively high with aging, a long, steady decline in DHEA

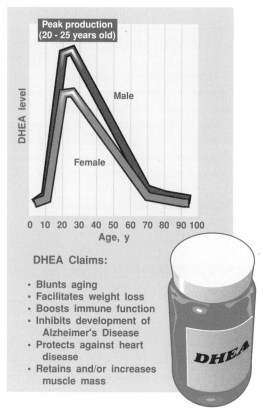

Figure 4.11 Generalized trend for plasma levels of DHEA (dehydroepiandrosterone) for men and women during a lifetime.

occurs after age 30 years. By age 75 years, plasma levels decrease to only about 20% of the value in young adulthood. This fact has fueled speculation that DHEA plasma levels might serve as a biochemical marker of biologic aging and disease susceptibility. Popular reasoning concludes that supplementing with DHEA diminishes the negative effects of aging by increasing plasma levels to more youthful concentrations. Many people supplement with this hormone "just in case" it proves beneficial without concern for safety.

Safety of DHEA

In 1994, the FDA reclassified DHEA from the category of unapproved new drug (prescription required for use) to a dietary supplement for sale over the counter without a prescription. Despite its quantitative significance as a hormone, researchers know little about DHEA's relationship to health and aging, cellular or molecular mechanisms of action, and possible receptor sites and the potential for negative side effects from exogenous dosage, particularly among young adults with normal DHEA levels. The appropriate DHEA dosage for humans has not been determined. Concern exists about possible harmful effects on blood lipids, glucose tolerance, and prostate gland health, particularly because medical problems associated with hormone supplementation often do not appear until years after their first use. *Despite its popularity among exercise enthusiasts, no data support an ergogenic effect of exogenous DHEA among young adult men and women.*

AMPHETAMINES

Amphetamines, or "pep pills," consist of pharmacologic compounds that exert a powerful stimulating effect on central nervous system function. Athletes most frequently use amphetamine (Benzedrine) and dextroamphetamine sulfate (Dexedrine). These compounds, referred to as **sympathomimetic**, mimic the actions of the sympathetic hormones epinephrine and norepinephrine to trigger increases in blood pressure, heart rate, cardiac output, breathing rate, metabolism, and blood glucose. Taking 5 to 20 mg of amphetamine usually produces an effect typically for 30 to 90 minutes. Amphetamines supposedly increase alertness, wakefulness, and augment work capacity by depressing sensations of muscle fatigue. The deaths of two famed cyclists in the 1960s during competitive road racing were attributed to amphetamine use for just such purposes. Soldiers in World War II commonly used amphetamines to increase their alertness and reduce fatigue; athletes frequently use amphetamines for the same purpose.

Dangers of Amphetamines

Dangers of amphetamine use include the following:

1. Continual use can lead to physiologic or emotional drug dependency. This often causes cyclical dependency on "uppers" (amphetamines) or "downers" (barbiturates). (Barbiturates blunt or tranquilize the "hyper" state brought on by amphetamines).
2. General side effects include headache, tremulousness, agitation, insomnia, nausea, dizziness, and confusion, all of which negatively impact sports performance.
3. Prolonged use eventually requires more of the drug to achieve the same effect because drug tolerance increases; this may aggravate and even precipitate cardiovascular and psychologic disorders. Medical risks include hypertension, stroke, sudden death, and glucose intolerance.
4. Amphetamines inhibit or suppress the body's normal mechanisms for perceiving and responding to pain, fatigue, and heat stress, severely jeopardizing health and safety.
5. Prolonged intake of high doses of amphetamines can produce weight loss, paranoia, psychosis, repetitive compulsive behavior, and nerve damage.

Amphetamines and Athletic Performance

Athletes take amphetamines to get "up" psychologically for competition. On the day or evening before a contest, competitors often feel nervous or irritable and have difficulty relaxing. Under these circumstances, a barbiturate induces sleep. The athlete then regains the "hyper" condition by taking an "upper." This undesirable cycle of depressant to stimulant becomes dangerous because the stimulant acts abnormally after barbiturate intake. Knowledgeable and prudent sports professionals urge banning amphetamines from athletic competition. Most athletic governing groups have rules regarding athletes who use amphetamines. Ironically, the majority of research indicates that amphetamines do not enhance physical performance. Perhaps their greatest influence includes the psychological realm, where naive athletes believe that taking any supplement contributes to superior performance. A placebo containing an inert substance often produces results identical to those of amphetamines.

Questions & Notes

Describe two negative side effects of using GH.

1.

2.

Briefly explain how DHEA supposedly acts as an ergogenic aid.

List 3 dangers of amphetamines.

1.

2.

3.

SUMMARY

1. Caffeine exerts an ergogenic effect in extending aerobic exercise duration by increasing fat utilization for energy, thus conserving glycogen reserves. These effects become less apparent in individuals who maintain a high-carbohydrate diet or habitually use caffeine.

2. Consuming ethyl alcohol produces an acute anxiolytic effect because it temporarily reduces tension and anxiety, enhances self-confidence, and promotes aggression. Other than the anti-tremor effect, alcohol conveys no ergogenic benefits and likely impairs overall athletic performance (ergolytic effect).

3. Anabolic steroids comprise a group of pharmacologic agents frequently used for ergogenic purposes. These drugs function similar to the hormone testosterone. Anabolic steroids may help to increase muscle size, strength, and power with resistance training in some individuals.

4. Side effects that accompany anabolic steroid use include infertility, reduced sperm concentrations, decreased testicular volume, gynecomastia, connective tissue damage that decreases the tensile strength and elastic compliance of tendons, chronic stimulation of the prostate gland, injury and functional alterations in cardiovascular function and myocardial cell cultures, possible pathologic ventricular growth and dysfunction, and increased blood platelet aggregation that can compromise cardiovascular system health and function and increase risk of stroke and acute myocardial infarction.

5. Research findings indicate no effect of androstenedione supplementation on basal serum concentrations of testosterone or training response in terms of muscle size and strength and body composition. Worrisome are the potentially negative effects of a lowered HDL-C on overall heart disease risk and the elevated serum estrogen level on risk of gynecomastia and possibly pancreatic and other cancers.

6. Tetrahydrogestrinone (THG) often escapes detection using normal drug testing. Its suspected use by competitive athletes caused the initiation of retesting urine samples from competitors in diverse sports.

7. The β_2-adrenergic agonist clenbuterol increases skeletal muscle mass and slows fat gain in animals to counter the effects of aging, immobilization, malnutrition, and tissue-wasting pathology. A negative finding showed hastened fatigue during short-term, intense muscle actions.

8. Debate exists about whether administration of GH to healthy people augments muscular hypertrophy when combined with resistance training. Significant health risks exist for those who abuse this chemical.

9. DHEA is a relatively weak steroid hormone synthesized from cholesterol by the adrenal cortex. DHEA levels steadily decrease throughout adulthood, prompting many individuals to supplement, hoping to counteract the effects of aging. Available research does not indicate an ergogenic effect of DHEA.

10. Little credible evidence exists that amphetamines ("pep pills") aid exercise performance or psychomotor skills any better than inert placebos. Side effects of amphetamines include drug dependency, headache, dizziness, confusion, and upset stomach.

THOUGHT QUESTIONS

1. Respond to the question: "If hormones, such as testosterone, GH, and DHEA, occur naturally in the body, what harm could exist in supplementing with these 'natural' compounds?"

2. Outline the main points you would make in a talk to a high school football team concerning whether they should consider using performance-enhancing chemicals and hormones.

3. A student swears that a chemical compound added to her diet profoundly improved her weight-lifting performance. Your review of the research literature indicates no ergogenic benefits for this compound. How would you reconcile this discrepancy?

4. What advice would you give to a collegiate football player who "sees no harm" in replacing fluid lost during the first half with a few beers at half time?

SELECTED REFERENCES

Abel, T., et al.: Influence of chronic supplementation of arginine aspartate in endurance athletes on performance and substrate metabolism: a randomized, double-blind, placebo-controlled study. *Int. J. Sports Med.*, 26:344, 2005.

Althuis, M.D., et al.: Glucose and insulin responses to dietary chromium supplements: a meta-analysis. *Am. J. Clin. Nutr.*, 76:148, 2002.

Alves, C., Lima, R.V.: Dietary supplement use by adolescents. *J. Pediatr.*, *(Rio J)*, 85:287, 2009.

American College of Sports Medicine: The use of anabolic–androgenic steroids in sports. *Sports Med. Bull.*, 19:13, 1984.

Bahrke, M., Morgan, W.P.: Evaluation of the ergogenic properties of ginseng. *Sports Med.*, 29:113, 2000.

Bahrke, M.S., Yesalis, C.E.: Abuse of anabolic androgenic steroids and related substances in sport and exercise. *Curr. Opin. Pharmacol.*, 4:614, 2004.

Battra, D.S., et al.: Caffeine ingestion does not impede the resynthesis of proglycogen and macroglycogen after prolonged exercise and carbohydrate supplementation in humans. *J. Appl. Physiol.*, 96:943, 2004.

Beedie, C., Foad, A.J.: The placebo effect in sports performance: a brief review. *Sports Med.*, 39:313, 2009.

Bell, D.G., et al.: Effect of caffeine and ephedrine ingestion on anaerobic performance. *Med. Sci. Sports Exerc.*, 33:1399, 2001.

Bell, D.G., McLellan, T.M.: Effect of repeated caffeine ingestion on repeated exhaustive exercise endurance. *Med. Sci. Sports Exerc.*, 35:1348, 2003.

Bemben, M.G., Lamont, H.S.: Creatine supplementation and exercise performance: recent findings. *Sports Med.*, 35:107, 2005.

Bent, S., et al.: The relative safety of ephedra compared with other herbal products. *Ann. Intern. Med.*, 138:468, 2003.

Berggren, A., et al.: Short-term administration of supraphysiological recombinant human growth hormone (GH) does not increase maximum endurance exercise capacity in healthy, active young men and women with normal GH-insulin-like growth factor I axes. *J. Clin. Endocrinol. Metab.*, 90:3268, 2005.

Bhasin, S., et al.: Older men are as responsive as young men to the anabolic effects of graded doses of testosterone on the skeletal muscle. *J. Clin. Endocrinol. Metab.*, 90:678, 2005.

Blackman, M.R., et al.: Growth hormone and sex steroid administration in healthy aged women and men: a randomized controlled trial. *JAMA*, 288:2282, 2002.

Blanchard, M.A., et al.: The influence of diet and exercise on muscle and plasma glutamine concentrations. *Med. Sci. Sports Exerc.*, 33:69, 2001.

Bohn, A.M., et al.: Ephedrine and other stimulants as ergogenic aids. *Curr. Sports Med. Rep.*, 2:220, 2003.

Bonnet, N., et al.: Doping dose of salbutamol and exercise: deleterious effect on cancellous and cortical bones in adult rats. *J. Appl. Physiol.*, 102:1502, 2007.

Branch, J.D.: Effect of creatine supplementation on body composition and performance: a meta-analysis. *Int. J. Sport Nutr. Exerc. Metab.*, 13:198, 2003.

Braun, H., et al.: Dietary supplement use among elite young German athletes. *Int. J. Sport Nutr. Exerc. Metab.*, 19:97, 2009.

Braun, H., et al.: Dietary supplement use among elite young German athletes. *Int. J. Sport Nutr. Exerc. Metab.*, 19:97, 2009.

Brown, G.A., et al.: Changes in serum testosterone and estradiol concentrations following acute androstenedione ingestion in young women. *Horm. Metab. Res.*, 36:62, 2004.

Brudnak, M.A.: Creatine: are the benefits worth the risk? *Toxicol. Lett.*, 150:123, 2004.

Burke, L.M., et al.: BJSM reviews: A–Z of nutritional supplements: dietary supplements, sports nutrition foods and ergogenic aids for health and performance. Part 7. *Br. J. Sports Med.*, 44:389, 2010.

Burke, L.M., et al.: BJSM reviews: A-Z of nutritional supplements: dietary supplements, sports nutrition foods and ergogenic aids for health and performance Part 4. *Br. J. Sports Med.*, 43:1088, 2009.

Burke, D.G., et al.: Effect of creatine and weight training on muscle creatine and performance in vegetarians. *Med. Sci. Sports Exerc.*, 35:1946, 2003.

Byars, A., et al.: The influence of a pre-exercise sports drink (PRX) on factors related to maximal aerobic performance. *J. Int. Soc. Sports Nutr.*, 7:12, 2010.

Cabral de Oliveira, A.C., et al.: Protection of Panax ginseng in injured muscles after eccentric exercise. *J. Ethnopharmacol.*, 28;97:211, 2005.

Candow, D.G., et al.: Effect of glutamine supplementation combined with resistance training in young adults. *Eur. J. Appl. Physiol.*, 86:142, 2001.

Castell, L.M., et al.: BJSM reviews: A-Z of nutritional supplements: dietary supplements, sports nutrition foods and ergogenic aids for health and performance Part 5. *Br. J. Sports Med.*, 44:77, 2010.

Castell, L.M., et al.: BJSM reviews: A-Z of nutritional supplements: dietary supplements, sports nutrition foods and ergogenic aids for health and performance. Part 8. *Br. J. Sports Med.* 44:468, 2010.

Castell, L.M., et al.: A-Z of nutritional supplements: dietary supplements, sports nutrition foods and ergogenic aids for health and performance. Part 9. *Br. J. Sports Med.*, 44:609, 2010.

Cheng, W., et al.: Beta-hydroxy-beta-methyl butyrate increases fatty acid oxidation by muscle cells. *FASEB J.* 11(3):A381, 1997.

Cheuvront, S.N., et al.: Branched-chain amino acid supplementation and human performance when hypohydrated in the heat. *J. Appl. Physiol.*, 97:1275, 2004.

Chilibeck, P.D., et al.: Effect of creatine ingestion after exercise on muscle thickness in males and females. *Med. Sci. Sports Exerc.*, 36:1781, 2004.

Collier, S.R., et al.: Oral arginine attenuates the growth hormone response to resistance exercise. *J. Appl. Physiol.* 101:848, 2006.

Davis, J.K., Green, J.M.: (2009). Caffeine and anaerobic performance: ergogenic value and mechanisms of action. *Sports Med.*, 39:813, 2009.

Dhar, R., et al.: Cardiovascular toxicities of performance-enhancing substances in sports. *Mayo Clin. Prod.*, 80:1307, 2005.

del Coso, J., et al.: Caffeine effects on short-term performance during prolonged exercise in the heat. *Med. Sci. Sports Exerc.*, 40:744, 2008.

Desbrow, B., et al.: Caffeine, cycling performance, and exogenous CHO oxidation: A dose-response study. *Med. Sci. Sports Exerc.*, 41:1744, 2009.

Doherty, M., et al.: Caffeine lowers perceptual response and increases power output during high-intensity cycling. *J. Sports Sci.*, 22:637, 2004.

Doherty, M., Smith, P.M.: Effects of caffeine ingestion on rating of perceived exertion during and after exercise: a meta-analysis. *Scand. J. Med. Sci. Sports*, 15:69, 2005.

Drakeley, A., et al.: Duration of azoospermia following anabolic steroids. *Fertil. Steril.*, 81:226, 2004.

Eckerson, J.M., et al.: Effect of two and five days of creatine loading on anaerobic working capacity in women. *J. Strength Cond. Res.*, 18:168, 2004.

Elliot, T.A., et al.: Milk ingestion stimulates net muscle protein synthesis following resistance exercise. *Med. Sci. Sports Exerc.*, 38:667, 2006.

El-Sayed, M.S., et al.: Interaction between alcohol and exercise: physiological and haematological implications. *Sports Med.*, 35:257, 2005.

Engels, H.J., et al.: Effects of ginseng on secretory IgA, performance, and recovery from interval exercise. *Med. Sci. Sports Exerc.*, 35:690, 2003.

Fomous, C.M., et al.: Symposium: conference on the science and policy of performance-enhancing products. *Med. Sci. Sports Exerc.*, 34:1685, 2002.

Fortunato, R.S., et al.: Chronic administration of anabolic androgenic steroid alters murine thyroid function. *Med. Sci. Sports Exerc.*, 38:256, 2006.

Gallagher, P.M., et al.: β-hydroxy-β-methylbutyrate ingestion, Part I: effects on strength and fat free mass. *Med. Sci. Sports Exerc.*, 32:2116, 2000.

Gallagher, P.M., et al.: β-hydroxy-β-methylbutyrate ingestion, Part II: effects on hematology, hepatic and renal function. *Med. Sci. Sports Exerc.*, 32:2116, 2000.

Ghofrani, H.A., et al.: Sidenafil increased exercise capacity during hypoxia at low altitudes and at Mt. Everest base camp: a randomized, double-blind, placebo-controlled crossover trial. *Ann. Intern. Med.*, 141:169, 2006.

Gibney, J., et al.: The growth hormone/insulin-like growth factor-I axis in exercise and sport. *Endocr. Rev.*, 28:603, 2007.

Gleeson, M.: Interrelationship between physical activity and branched-chain amino acids. *J. Nutr.*, 135(suppl):1591S, 2005.

Goldfield, G.S.: Body image, disordered eating and anabolic steroid use in female bodybuilders. *Eat. Disord.*, 17:200, 2009.

Gotshalk, L.A., et al.: Creatine supplementation improves muscular performance in older men. *Med. Sci. Sports Exerc.*, 34:537, 2002.

Hackney, A.C.: Effects of endurance exercise on the reproductive system of men: The "exercise-hypogonadal male condition." *J. Endocrinol. Invest.*, 31:932, 2008.

Harkey, M.R., et al.: Variability in commercial ginseng products: an analysis of 25 preparations. *Am. J. Clin. Nutr.*, 73:1101, 2001.

Hellsten, Y., et al.: Effect of ribose supplementation on resynthesis of adenine nucleotides after intense intermittent training in humans. *Am. J. Physiol. Regul. Integr. Comp. Physiol.*, 286:R182, 2004.

Herda, T.J., et al.: Effects of creatine monohydrate and polyethylene glycosylated creatine supplementation on muscular strength, endurance, and power output. *J. Strength Cond. Res.*, 23:818, 2009.

Hingson, R.W., et al.: Magnitude of alcohol-related mortality and morbidity among U.S. college students ages 18–24. *J. Stud. Alcohol*, 63:136, 2002.

Hingson, R.W., Howland, J.: Comprehensive community interventions to promote health: Implications for college-age drinking problems. *J. Stud. Alcohol Suppl.*, 14:226, 2002.

Hodges, A.N., et al.: Effects of pseudoephedrine on maximal cycling power and submaximal cycling efficiency. *Med. Sci. Sports Exerc.*, 35:1316, 2003.

Hoffman, J.R., et al.: Effect of low-dose, short-duration creatine supplementation on anaerobic exercise performance. *J. Strength Cond. Res.*, 19:260, 2005.

Hoffman, J.R., et al.: Nutritional supplementation and anabloic steroid use in adolescents. *Med. Sci. Sports Exerc.*, 40:15, 2008.

Hoffman, J.R., et al.: Position stand on androgen and human growth hormone use. *J. Strength Cond. Res.*, 23(5 suppl):S1, 2009.

Ivy, J.L.: Effect of pyruvate and dehydroxyacetone on metabolism and aerobic endurance capacity. *Med. Sci. Sports Exerc.*, 6:837, 1998.

Ivy, J.L., et al.: Improved cycling time-trial performance after ingestion of a caffeine energy drink. *Int. J. Sport Nutr. Exerc. Metab.*, 1:61, 2009.

Izquierdo, M., et al.: Effects of creatine supplementation on muscle power, endurance, and sprint performance. *Med. Sci. Sports Exerc.*, 34:332, 2002.

Jacobs, I., et al.: Effects of ephedrine, caffeine, and their combination on muscular endurance. *Med. Sci. Sports Exerc.*, 35:987, 2003.

Jowko, E., et al.: Creatine and beta-hydroxy-beta-methylbutyrate (HMB) additively increase lean body mass and muscle strength during a weight training program. *Nutrition*, 17:558, 2001.

Kam, P.C., Yarrow, M.: Anabolic steroid abuse: physiological and anaesthetic considerations. *Anaesthesia*, 60:685, 2005.

Kamber, M., et al.: Nutritional supplements as a source for positive doping cases? *Int. J. Sport Nutr. Exerc. Metab.*, 11:258, 2001.

Kearns, C. F., et al.: Chronic administration of therapeutic levels of clenbuterol acts as a repartitioning agent. *J. Appl. Physiol.*, 91:2064, 2001.

Kearns, C.F., McKeever, J.: Clenbuterol diminishes aerobic performance in horses. *Med. Sci. Sports Exerc.*, 34:1976, 2002.

Keisier, B.D., Armsey, T.D.: Caffeine as an ergogenic aid. *Curr. Sports Med. Rep.*, 5:215, 2006.

Kilduff, L.P., et al.: The effects of creatine supplementation on cardiovascular, metabolic, and thermoregulatory responses during exercise in the heat in endurance-trained humans. *Int. Jr. Sport Nutr. Exerc. Metab.*, 14:443, 2004.

Koh-Banerjee, P.K., et al.: Effects of calcium pyruvate supplementation during training on body composition, exercise capacity, and metabolic responses to exercise. *Nutrition.*, 21:312, 2005.

Kreider, R.B., et al.: ISSN exercise & sport nutrition review: research & recommendations. *J. Int. Soc. Sports Nutr.*, 7:7, 2010.

Kreider, R.B., et al.: Long-term creatine supplementation does not significantly affect clinical markers of health in athletes. *Mol. Cell. Biochem.*, 244:95, 2003.

Laure, P., et al.: Drugs, recreational drug use and attitudes towards doping of high school athletes. *Int. J. Sports Med.*, 25:133, 2004.

Liang, M.T., et al.: Panax notoginseng supplementation enhances physical performance during endurance exercise. *J. Strength Cond. Res.*, 19:108, 2005.

Liu, H., et al.: Systematic review: The effects of growth hormone on athletic performance. *Ann. Intern. Med.*, 148:747, 2008.

Lopez, R.M., Casa, D.J.: The influence of nutritional ergogenic aids on exercise heat tolerance and hydration status. *Curr. Sports Med. Rep.*, 8:192, 2009. Review.

Magkos, F., Kavouras, S.A.: Caffeine and ephedrine: physiological, metabolic and performance-enhancing effects. *Sports Med.*, 34:871, 2004.

Malvey, T., Armsey, T.: Tetrahydrogestrinone: the discovery of a designer steroid. *Curr. Sports Med. Rep.*, 4:227, 2005.

Mendes, R.R., et al.: Effects of creatine supplementation on the performance and body composition of competitive swimmers. *J. Nutr. Biochem.*, 15:473, 2004.

Miller, S.L., et al.: Independent and combined effects of amino acids and glucose after resistance exercise. *Med. Sci. Sports Exerc.*, 35:449, 2003.

Molinero, O., Márquez, S.: Use of nutritional supplements in sports: risks, knowledge, and behavioural-related factors. Review. *Nutr. Hosp.*, 24:128, 2009.

National Institute on Drug Abuse.: *Monitoring the Future. National Results on Adolescent Drug Use. Overview of Key Findings.* Washington, DC: National Institutes of Health, 2007. Available at *www.monitoringthefuture.org/pubs/monographs/overview2007.pdf.*

Noakes, T.D.: Tainted glory—doping and athletic performance. *N. Engl. J. Med.*, 351:847, 2004.

Paddon-Jones, D., et al.: Potential ergogenic effects of arginine and creatine supplementation. *J. Nutr.*, 134(suppl):2888S, 2004.

Parkinson, A.B, Evans, N.A.: Anabolic androgenic steroids: A survey of 500 users. *Med. Sci. Sports Exerc.*, 38:644, 2006.

Paul, G., et al.: Efficacy and safety of ephedra and ephedrine for weight loss and athletic performance: a meta-analysis. *JAMA*, 289:1537, 2003.

Percheron, G., et al.: Effect of 1-year oral administration of dehydroepiandrosterone to 60- to 80-year-old individuals on muscle function and cross-sectional area: a double-blind placebo-controlled trial. *Arch. Intern. Med.*, 163:720, 2003.

Porter, D.A., et al.: The effect of oral coenzyme Q10 on the exercise tolerance of middle-aged, untrained men. *Int. J. Sports Med.*, 16:421, 1995.

Rasmussen, B.B., Phillips, S.M.: Contractile and nutritional regulation of human muscle growth. *Exerc. Sport Sci. Rev.*, 31:127, 2003.

Raymer, G.H., et al.: Metabolic effects of induced alkalosis during progressive forearm exercise to fatigue. *J. Appl. Physiol.*, 96:2050, 2004.

Rennie, M.J., Tipton, K.D.: Protein and amino acid metabolism during and after resistance exercise and the effects of nutrition. *Ann. Rev. Nutr.*, 20:457, 2000.

Rodriguez, N.R., et al.: American College of Sports Medicine position stand. Nutrition and athletic performance. *Med. Sci. Sports Exerc.*, 41:709, 2009.

Rodriguez, N.R., et al.: Position of the American Dietetic Association, Dietitians of Canada, and the American College of Sports Medicine: Nutrition and athletic performance. American Dietetic Association; Dietetians of Canada; American College of Sports Medicine. *J. Am. Diet. Assoc.*, 109:509, 2009.

Rogers, N.L., Dinges, D.F.: Caffeine: implications for alertness in athletes. *Clin. Sports Med.*, 24:1, 2005.

Rogol, A.D.: Growth hormone and the adolescent athlete: What are the data for its safety and efficacy as an ergogenic agent? *Growth Horm., IGF Res.*, 19:294, 2009.

Rosell, M., et al.: The relation between alcohol intake and physical activity and the fatty acids 14:0, 15:0 and 17:0 in serum phospholipids and adipose tissue used as markers for dairy fat intake. *Br. J. Nutr.*, 93:115, 2005.

Rown, G.A., et al.: Testosterone prohormone supplements. *Med. Sci. Sports Exerc.*, 38:1451, 2006.

Roy, B.D., et al.: An acute oral dose of caffeine does not alter glucose kinetics during prolonged dynamic exercise in trained endurance athletes. *Eur. J. Appl. Physiol.*, 85:280, 2005.

Schilling, B.K., et al.: Creatine supplementation and health variables: a retrospective study. *Med. Sci. Sports Exerc.*, 33:183, 2001.

Sekera, M.H., et al.: Another designer steroid: discovery, synthesis, and detection of "madol" in urine. *Rapid Commun. Mass Spectrom.*, 19:781, 2005.

Selsby, J.T., et al.: Mg^{2+}-creatine chelate and a low-dose creatine supplementation regimen improve exercise performance. *J. Strength Cond. Res.*, 18:311, 2004.

Shekelle, P.G., et al.: Efficacy and safety of ephedra and ephedrine for weight loss and athletic performance: A meta-analysis. *JAMA*, 289:1537, 2003.

Schneiker, K.T., et al.: Effects of caffeine on prolonged intermittent-sprint ability in team-sport athletes. *Med. Sci. Sports Exerc.*, 38:578, 2006.

Shomrat, A., et al.: Effects of creatine feeding on maximal exercise performance in vegetarians. *Eur. J. Appl. Physiol.*, 82:321, 2000.

Slater, B., et al.: Beta-hydroxy-beta-methylbutyrate (HMB) supplementation does not affect changes in strength or body composition during resistance training in trained men. *Int. J. Sport Nutr. Exerc. Metab.*, 11:384, 2001.

Snow, R.J., Murphy, R.M.R.: Factors influencing creatine loading into human skeletal muscle. *Exerc. Sport Sci. Rev.*, 31:154, 2003.

Stacy, J. J., et al.: Ergogenic aids: Human growth hormone. *Curr. Sports Med. Rep.*, 3:229, 2004.

Stear, S.J., et al.: A-Z of nutritional supplements: dietary supplements, sports nutrition foods and ergogenic aids for health and performance. Part 10. *Br. J. Sports Med.*, 44:688, 2010.

Stear, S.J., et al.: BJSM reviews: A-Z of nutritional supplements: dietary supplements, sports nutrition foods and ergogenic aids for health and performance. Part 6. *Br. J. Sports Med.*, 44:297, 2010.

Stear, S.J., et al.: BJSM reviews: A-Z of nutritional supplements: dietary supplements, sports nutrition foods and Ergogenic aids for health and performance Part 3. *Br. J. Sports Med.*, 43:890, 2009.

Tagarakis, C.V., et al.: Anabolic steroids impair the exercise-induced growth of the cardiac capillary bed. *Int. J. Sports Med.*, 21:412, 2000.

Tian, H.H., et al.: Nutritional supplement use among university athletes in Singapore. Singapore *Med. J.*, 50:165, 2009.

Tipton, K.D., et al.: Acute response of net muscle protein balance reflects 24-h balance after exercise and amino acid ingestion. *Am. J. Physiol.*, 284:E76, 2003.

Tipton, K.D., et al.: Ingestion of casein and whey proteins result in muscle anabolism after resistance exercise. *Med. Sci. Sports Exerc.*, 36:2073, 2004.

Tokish, J.M., et al.: Ergogenic aids: a review of basic science, performance, side effects, and status in sports. *Am. J. Sports Med.*, 32:1543, 2004.

van Loon, L.J., et al.: Effects of creatine loading and prolonged creatine supplementation on body composition, fuel selection, sprint and endurance performance in humans. *Clin. Sci. (Lond)*, 104:153, 2003.

Vierck, J.L., et al.: The effects of ergogenic compounds on myogenic satellite cells. *Med. Sci. Sports Exerc.*, 35:769, 2003.

Villareal, D.T., Holloszy, J.O.: Effect of DHEA on abdominal fat and insulin action in elderly women and men: a randomized controlled trial. *JAMA*, 292:2243, 2004.

Vincent, J.B.: The potential value and toxicity of chromium picolinate as a nutritional supplement, weight loss agent and muscle development agent. *Sports Med.*, 33:213, 2003.

Vingren, J.L., et al.: Effect of resistance exercise on muscle steroidogenesis. *J. Appl. Physiol.*, 105:1754, 2008.

Vistisen, B., et al.: Minor amounts of plasma medium-chain fatty acids and no improved time trial performance after consuming lipids. *J. Appl. Physiol.*, 95:2434, 2003.

Volek, J.S.: Influence of nutrition on responses to resistance training. *Med. Sci. Sports Exerc.*, 36:689, 2004.

Vukovich, M.D., et al.: Body composition in 70-year-old adults responds to dietary beta-hydroxy-beta-methylbutyrate similarly to that of young adults. *J. Nutr.*, 131:2049, 2001.

Vuksan, V., et al.: American ginseng (*Panex quinquefolius* L.) attenuates postprandial glycemia in a time-dependent but not dose-dependent manner in healthy individuals. *Am. J. Clin. Nutr.*, 73:753, 2001.

Walker, J., Adams, B.: Cutaneous manifestations of anabolic-androgenic steroid use in athletes. *Int. J. Dermatol.*, 48:1044, 2009.

Walter, A.A., et al.: Acute effects of a thermogenic nutritional supplement on cycling time to exhaustion and muscular strength in college-aged men. *J. Int. Soc. Sports Nutr.*, 2009 13:6, 2009.

Willoughby, D.S., Rosene, J.: Effects of oral creatine and resistance training on myogenic regulatory factor expression. *Med. Sci. Sports Exerc.*, 35:923, 2003.

Wolfe, R.R.: Regulation of muscle protein by amino acids. *J. Nutr.*, 132(suppl):3219S, 2002.

Energy Transfer

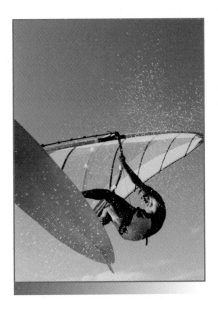

Biochemical reactions that do not consume oxygen generate considerable energy for short durations. This rapid energy generation becomes crucial in maintaining a high standard of performance in sprint activities and other bursts of all-out exercise. In contrast, longer duration (aerobic) exercise extracts energy more slowly from food catabolism through chemical reactions that require the continual use of oxygen. Planning effective training to enhance exercise performance requires the following:

1. Insight about how muscle tissue generates energy to sustain exercise.
2. The sources that provide that energy.
3. The energy requirements of diverse physical activities.

This section presents a broad overview of the fundamentals of human energy transfer during rest and exercise. We emphasize the means by which the body's cells extract chemical energy bound within food molecules and transfer it to a common compound that powers all forms of biologic work. The food nutrients and processes of energy transfer that play important roles in sustaining physiologic function during light, moderate, and strenuous exercise, is given special attention as are techniques to measure and evaluate the diverse human energy transfer capacities.

I often say that when you can measure what you are speaking about, and express it in numbers, you know something about it; but when you cannot measure it, when you cannot express it in numbers, your knowledge is of a meagre and unsatisfactory kind.

— Lord Kelvin
(William Thomson,
1st Baron) (1824–1907),
English physicist and
mathematician

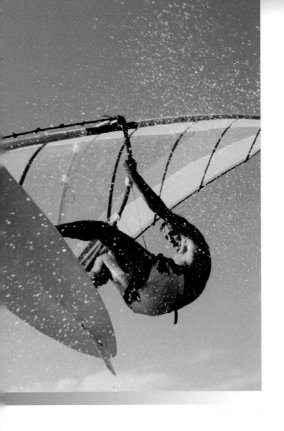

Chapter

5

Fundamentals of Human Energy Transfer

CHAPTER OBJECTIVES

- Describe the first law of thermodynamics related to energy balance and biologic work.

- Define the terms *potential energy* and *kinetic energy* and give examples of each.

- Give examples of exergonic and endergonic chemical processes within the body and indicate their importance.

- State the second law of thermodynamics and give a practical application.

- Identify and give examples of three forms of biologic work.

- Discuss the role of enzymes and coenzymes in bioenergetics.

- Identify the high-energy phosphates and discuss their contributions in powering biologic work.

- Outline the process of electron transport–oxidative phosphorylation.

- Explain oxygen's role in energy metabolism.

- Describe how anaerobic energy release occurs in cells.

- Describe lactate formation during progressively increasing exercise intensity.

- Outline the general pathways of the citric cycle during macronutrient catabolism.

- Contrast adenosine triphosphate yield from carbohydrate, fat, and protein catabolism.

- Explain the statement, "Fats burn in a carbohydrate flame."

The body's capacity to extract energy from food nutrients and transfer it to the contractile elements in skeletal muscle determines our capacity to move. Energy transfer occurs through thousands of complex chemical reactions that require the proper mixture of macro- and micronutrients continually fueled by oxygen. The term **aerobic** describes such oxygen-requiring energy reactions. In contrast, **anaerobic** chemical reactions generate energy rapidly from chemical reactions that do not require oxygen. *The anaerobic and aerobic breakdown of ingested food nutrients provides the energy source for synthesizing the chemical fuel that powers all forms of biologic work.*

This chapter presents an overview of the different forms of energy and the factors that affect energy generation. The chapter also discusses how the body obtains energy to power its diverse functions. A basic understanding of carbohydrate, fat, and protein breakdown (catabolism) and concurrent anaerobic and aerobic energy transfer forms the basis for much of the content of exercise physiology. Knowledge about human bioenergetics provides the practical basis for formulating sport-specific exercise training regimens, recommending activities for physical fitness and weight control, and advocating prudent dietary modifications for specific sport requirements.

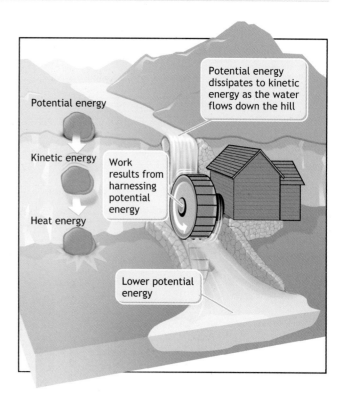

Figure 5.1 High-grade potential energy capable of performing work degrades to a useless form of kinetic energy. In the example of falling water, the waterwheel harnesses potential energy to perform useful work. For the falling boulder, all of the potential energy dissipates to kinetic energy (heat) as the boulder crashes to the surface.

Part 1	Energy—The Capacity for Work

Unlike the physical properties of matter, one cannot define energy in concrete terms of size, shape, or mass. Rather, the term *energy* suggests a dynamic state related to change; thus, the presence of energy emerges only when change occurs. Within this context, energy relates to the performance of work (as work increases, so does energy transfer) and the occurrence of change.

The **first law of thermodynamics**, one of the most important principles related to biologic work, states that energy cannot be created or destroyed; rather, it is transformed from one form to another without being depleted. In essence, this law describes the immutable principle of the **conservation of energy**. *In the body, chemical energy stored within the bonds of macronutrients does not immediately dissipate as heat during energy metabolism. Instead, a large portion remains as chemical energy, which the musculoskeletal system then changes into mechanical energy and then ultimately to heat energy.*

POTENTIAL AND KINETIC ENERGY

Potential energy and kinetic energy constitute the total energy of a system. **Figure 5.1** shows potential energy as energy of position, similar to a boulder tottering atop a cliff or water at the top of a mountain before it flows downstream. In the example of flowing water, the energy change is proportional to the water's vertical drop (i.e., the greater the vertical drop, the greater water's potential energy at the top). The waterwheel harnesses a portion of the energy from the falling water to produce useful work. In the case of the boulder, *all* potential energy transforms to kinetic energy and dissipates as useless heat as the boulder crashes to the ground.

Other examples of potential energy include bound energy within the internal structure of a battery, a stick of dynamite, or a macronutrient before release of its stored energy in metabolism. *Releasing potential energy transforms the basic ingredient into kinetic energy of motion.* In some cases, bound energy in one substance directly transfers to other substances to increase their potential energy. Energy transfers of this type provide the required energy for the body's chemical work of **biosynthesis**. In this process, specific building-block atoms of carbon, hydrogen, oxygen, and nitrogen become activated and join other atoms and molecules to synthesize important biologic compounds and tissues. Some newly created compounds provide structure as in bone or the lipid-containing plasma membrane that encloses each cell. The synthesized compounds ATP and phosphocreatine (PCr) serve the cell's energy requirements.

BOX 5.1 CLOSE UP

Adenosine Triphosphate—Nature's Powerful Ingredient

Animals and plants are as different as night and day, yet they share one important common biological trait—they each trap, store, and transfer energy through a complex series of chemical reactions that involve the compound adenosine triphosphate (ATP).

The history of the discovery of ATP reads like a mystery dating back to the 1860s in France and the work of Louis Pasteur (1822–1895), a leading scientist of the day. During one of his experiments with yeast, Pasteur proposed that this micro-organism's ability to degrade sugar to carbon dioxide and alcohol (ethanol) was strictly a living (Pasteur termed it "vitalistic") function of the yeast cell. He hypothesized that if the yeast cell died, the fermentation process would cease.

In 1897, the German chemist, Eduard Buchner (1860–1917) made a chance observation that proved Pasteur wrong. His discovery revolutionized the study of physiologic systems and represented the beginning of the modern science of **biochemistry**. Searching for therapeutic uses for protein, he concocted a thick paste of freshly grown yeast and sand in a large mortar and pressed out the yeast cell juice. The gummy liquid proved unstable and could not be preserved by techniques available at that time. One of the laboratory assistants suggested adding a large amount of sugar to the mixture—his wife used this technique to preserve fruit.

To everyone's surprise, what seemed like a silly solution worked; the nonliving juice from the yeast cells converted the sugar to carbon dioxide and alcohol directly contradicting Pasteur's prevailing theory. The epoch finding about noncellular fermentation earned Professor Buchner the 1907 Nobel Prize in Chemistry.

In 1905, British biochemist Arthur Harden (1865–1940) and Australian biochemist William Young (1878–1942) observed, as had their German predecessors, that the fermenting ability of yeast juice decreased gradually with

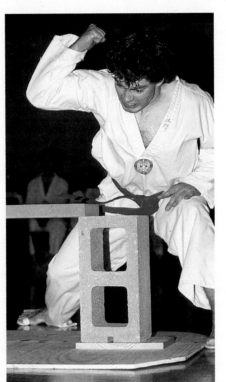

time and could be restored only by adding fresh boiled yeast juice or blood serum. What revitalized the mixture? After prolonged research, inorganic phosphate, present in both liquids, was identified as the activating agent.

Other British scientists working with eventual Nobel Laureate Sir Arthur Harden (1929 Nobel Prize in Chemistry) and William Young also played important roles in ATP's discovery. Crude yeast juice pressed through a gelatin film yielded a filtrate free of protein. The filtrate and protein were completely inert. Vigorous fermentation began when the filtrate and protein were recombined. They called this combination "zymase;" it consisted of the filtrate "cozymase" and the protein residue "apozymase." Many years passed before the two components were accurately analyzed and identified as containing "coenzyme" compounds. In addition, the apozymase consisted of many proteins, each a specific catalyst in sugar breakdown.

In 1929, young German scientist Karl Lohmann (1898–1978) working in Otto Meyerhoff's laboratory studied the "energy" source responsible for cellular reactions involving yeast and sugar. Working with yeast juice, Lohmann discovered that an unstable substance in the cozymase filtrate degraded the sugar. This energizing substance contained the nitrogen-containing compound adenine linked to the sugar ribose and three phosphate groups. We now call this compound ATP. The potential energy stored in the "high-energy bonds" link the phosphate groups in the ATP molecule. The splitting of these phosphate bonds releases the energy for *all* biologic work.

The function of ATP is truly amazing for the variety of processes it powers in all living cells. This ubiquitous compound, found in microorganisms, plants, and animals, ranges from nematodes to cockroaches to humans. Wherever ATP is found, it always has the same structure, regardless of the organism's complexity.

ENERGY-RELEASING AND ENERGY-CONSERVING PROCESSES

The term **exergonic** describes any physical or chemical process that releases (frees up) energy to its surroundings. Such reactions represent "downhill" processes; they produce a decline in free energy—"useful" energy for biologic work that encompasses all of the cell's energy-requiring, life-sustaining processes. In contrast, **endergonic** chemical processes store or absorb energy; these reactions represent "uphill" processes and proceed with an increase in free energy for biologic work. In some instances, exergonic processes link or couple with endergonic reactions to transfer some energy to the endergonic process.

Changes in free energy occur when the bonds in the reactant molecules form new product molecules but with different bonding. The equation that expresses these changes, under conditions of constant temperature, pressure, and volume, takes the following form:

$$\Delta G = \Delta H - T\Delta S$$

The symbol Δ designates change. The change in free energy represents a keystone of chemical reactions. In exergonic reactions, ΔG is negative ($-\Delta G$); the products contain *less* free energy than the reactants, with the energy differential released as heat. For example, when hydrogen unites with oxygen to form water, 68 kCal per mole (molecular weight of substance in g) of free energy are released in the following reaction:

$$H_2 + O \rightarrow H_2O - \Delta G \ 68 \ kCal \cdot mol^{-1}$$

In the reverse endergonic reaction, ΔG remains positive ($+\Delta G$) because the product contains *more* free energy than the

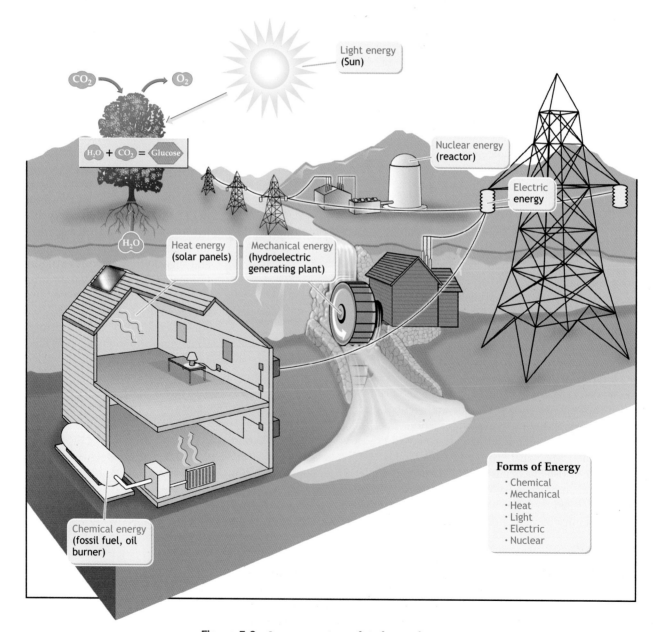

Figure 5.2 Interconversions of six forms of energy.

reactants. The infusion of 68 kCal of energy per mole of water causes the chemical bonds of the water molecule to split apart, freeing the original hydrogen and oxygen atoms. This "uphill" process of energy transfer provides the hydrogen and oxygen atoms with their original energy content to satisfy the principle of the first law of thermodynamics—energy conservation.

$$H_2 + O \leftarrow H_2O + \Delta G \; 68 \; kCal \cdot mol^{-1}$$

Energy transfer in cells follows the same principles in the waterfall–waterwheel example. Carbohydrate, lipid, and protein macronutrients possess considerable potential energy. The formation of product substances progressively reduces the nutrients' original potential energy with corresponding increases in kinetic energy. Enzyme-regulated transfer systems harness or conserve a portion of this chemical energy in new compounds for biologic work. In essence, living cells serve as transducers with the capacity to extract and use chemical energy stored within a compound's atomic structure. Conversely, and equally important, they also bond atoms and molecules together, raising them to a higher potential energy level.

The transfer of potential energy in any spontaneous process always proceeds in a direction that *decreases* the capacity to perform work. **Entropy** refers to the tendency of potential energy to convert to kinetic energy of motion with a lower capacity for work and reflects the **second law of thermodynamics.** A flashlight battery embodies this principle. The electrochemical energy stored within its cells slowly dissipates, even when the battery remains unused. The energy from sunlight also continually degrades to heat energy when light strikes and becomes absorbed by a surface. Food and other chemicals represent excellent stores of potential energy, yet this energy continually declines as the compounds decompose through normal oxidative processes. Energy, similar to water, always runs downhill to decrease the potential energy. *Ultimately, all of the potential energy in a system degrades to the unusable form of kinetic or heat energy.*

INTERCONVERSIONS OF ENERGY

During energy conversions, a loss of potential energy from one source often produces a temporary increase in the potential energy of another source. In this way, nature harnesses vast quantities of potential energy for useful purposes. Even under such favorable conditions, the net flow of energy in the biologic world still moves toward entropy, ultimately producing a loss of a system's total potential energy.

Figure 5.2 shows energy categorized into one of six forms:

1. Chemical
2. Mechanical
3. Heat
4. Light
5. Electric
6. Nuclear

Examples of Energy Conversions

Photosynthesis and **respiration** represent the most fundamental examples of energy conversion in living cells.

Photosynthesis   **Figure 5.3** depicts the dynamics of photosynthesis, an endergonic process powered by the sun's energy. The pigment chlorophyll located within the leaf's cells large organelles, the chloroplasts, absorbs radiant (solar) energy to synthesize glucose from carbon dioxide and water while oxygen flows to the environment. The plant also converts carbohydrates to

*Q*uestions & Notes

Describe the difference between kinetic and potential energy.

Kinetic energy:

Potential energy:

Complete the equation to indicate energy conservation:

$H_2 + O \leftrightarrow$

List the 6 forms of energy.

1.

2.

3.

4.

5.

6.

List 2 examples of energy conversion in living cells.

1.

2.

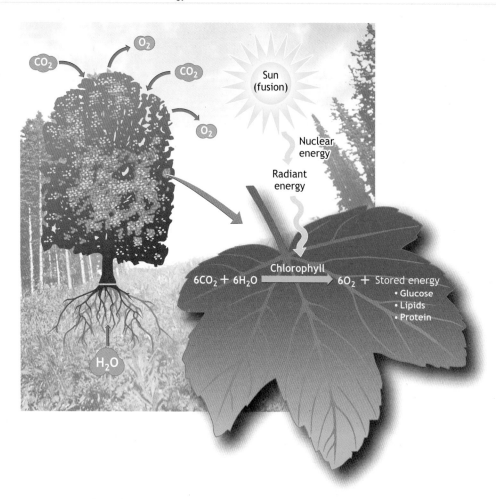

Figure 5.3 The endergonic process of photosynthesis in plants, algae, and some bacteria serves as the mechanism for synthesizing carbohydrates, lipids, and proteins. In this example, a glucose molecule forms from the union of carbon dioxide and water, with a positive free energy (useful energy) change ($+\Delta G$).

lipids and proteins for storage as a future reserve for energy and growth. Animals then ingest plant nutrients to serve their own energy needs. *In essence, solar energy coupled with photosynthesis powers the animal world with food and oxygen.*

Cellular Respiration **Figure 5.4** illustrates the reactions of respiration, the reverse of photosynthesis, as the plant's stored energy is recovered for biologic work. During these exergonic reactions, the cells extract the chemical energy stored in the carbohydrate, lipid, and protein molecules in the presence of oxygen. For glucose, this releases 689 kCal per mole (180 g) oxidized. *A portion of the energy released during cellular respiration becomes conserved in other chemical compounds in energy-requiring processes; the remaining energy flows to the environment as heat (loss).*

BIOLOGIC WORK IN HUMANS

Figure 5.4 also illustrates that biologic work takes one of three forms:

1. **Mechanical work** of muscle contraction.
2. **Chemical work** that synthesizes cellular molecules.
3. **Transport work** that concentrates various substances in the intracellular and extracellular fluids.

Mechanical Work

The most obvious example of energy transformation occurs from mechanical work generated by muscle action and subsequent movement. The molecular motors in a muscle fiber's protein filaments directly convert chemical energy into the mechanical energy of movement. The cell's nucleus represents another example of the body's mechanical work, where contractile elements literally tug at the chromosomes to produce cell division.

Chemical Work

All cells perform chemical work for maintenance and growth. Continuous synthesis of cellular components takes place as other components break down. The extreme muscle tissue synthesis that occurs in response to chronic overload in resistance training vividly illustrates chemical work.

Transport Work

Cellular materials normally flow from an area of higher concentration to one of lower concentration. This passive process of **diffusion** does not require energy. To maintain proper physiologic functioning, certain chemicals require

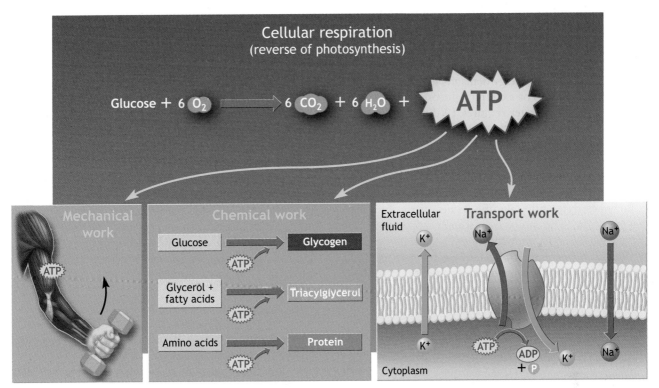

Figure 5.4 The exergonic process of cellular respiration. Exergonic reactions, such as the burning of gasoline or the oxidation of glucose, release potential energy. This results in a negative standard free energy change, that is, a reduction in total energy available for work, or $-\Delta G$. In this illustration, cellular respiration harvests the potential energy in food to form adenosine triphosphte (ATP). Subsequently, the energy in ATP powers all forms of biologic work.

transport "uphill," against their normal concentration gradients from an area of lower to higher concentration. **Active transport** describes this energy-requiring process. Secretion and reabsorption in the kidney tubules use active transport mechanisms, as does neural tissue in establishing the proper electrochemical gradients about its plasma membranes. These more "quiet" forms of biologic work require a continual expenditure of stored chemical energy.

FACTORS AFFECTING BIOENERGETICS

The limits of exercise intensity ultimately depend on the rate that cells extract, conserve, and transfer the chemical energy in the food nutrients to the contractile filaments of skeletal muscle. *The sustained pace of the marathon runner at close to 90% of maximum aerobic capacity or the speed achieved by the sprinter in all-out exercise directly reflects the body's capacity to transfer chemical energy into mechanical work.* Enzymes and coenzymes greatly affect the rate of energy release during chemical reactions.

Enzymes as Biological Catalysts

*An **enzyme**, a highly specific and large protein catalyst, accelerates the forward and reverse rates of chemical reactions within the body without being consumed or changed in the reaction.* Enzymes only govern reactions that would normally take place but at a much slower rate. Enzyme action takes place without altering the equilibrium constants and total energy released (free energy change) in the reaction.

Enzymes possess the unique property of not being readily altered by the reactions they affect. Consequently, enzyme turnover in the body remains relatively

Questions & Notes

Give the major difference between photosynthesis and respiration.

Describe the major function of enzymes.

Give one example of an enzyme and one example of a coenzyme.

Enzyme:

Coenzyme:

low, and the specific enzymes are continually reused. A typical mitochondrion may contain up to 10 billion enzyme molecules, each responsible for millions of cellular operations. During strenuous exercise, the rate of enzyme activity increases many fold as energy demands increase up to 100 times resting levels. For example, glucose breakdown to carbon dioxide and water requires 19 different chemical reactions, each catalyzed by its own specific enzyme. Enzymes activate precise locations on the surfaces of cell structures; they also operate within the structure itself. Many enzymes also function outside the cell—in the bloodstream, digestive mixture, or intestinal fluids.

Enzymes frequently take the names of the functions they perform. The suffix -*ase* usually appends to the enzyme whose prefix often indicates its mode of operation or the substance with which it interacts. For example, hydrol*ase* adds water during hydrolysis reactions, prote*ase* interacts with protein, oxid*ase* adds oxygen to a substance, and ribonucle*ase* splits ribonucleic acid (RNA).

Reaction Rates Enzymes do not all operate at the same rate—some operate slowly while others operate more rapidly. Consider the enzyme carbonic anhydrase, which catalyzes the hydration of carbon dioxide to form carbonic acid. Carbonic anhydrase's maximum **turnover number** of 800,000 represents the number of moles of substrate that react to form product per mole of enzyme per unit time. In contrast, the turnover number for tryptophan synthetase is only two to catalyzize the final step in tryptophan synthesis. Enzymes often work cooperatively. While one substance "turns on" at a particular site, its neighbor "turns off" until the process finishes. The operation can then reverse, with one enzyme becoming inactive and the other active. The pH and temperature of the cellular milieu dramatically affect enzyme activity. For some enzymes, peak activity requires relatively high acidity, but others function optimally on the alkaline side of neutrality. The pH opti-

mum for lipase in the stomach, for example, ranges from 4.0 to 5.0, but in the pancrease, the optimum lipase pH increases to 8.0.

Enzyme Mode of Action How an enzyme interacts with its specific substrate represents a unique characteristic of the enzyme's three-dimensional globular protein structure. Interaction works similiar to a key fitting a lock. The enzyme "turns on" when its **active site** (usually a groove, cleft, or cavity on the protein's surface) joins in a "perfect fit" with the substrate's active site. Upon forming an **enzyme–substrate complex**, the splitting of chemical bonds forms a new product with new bonds, freeing the enzyme to act on additional substrate. This lock-and-key mechanism serves a protective function so only the correct, specific enzyme activates a given substrate.

Coenzymes

Some enzymes remain totally dormant without activation by additional substances termed **coenzymes**. These complex nonprotein substances facilitate enzyme action by binding the substrate with its specific enzyme. Coenzymes then regenerate to assist in further similar reactions. The metallic ions iron and zinc play coenzyme roles as do the B vitamins or their derivatives. Whereas oxidation–reduction reactions use the B vitamins riboflavin and niacin, other vitamins serve as transfer agents for groups of compounds in other metabolic processes. A coenzyme requires less specificity in its action than an enzyme because the coenzyme affects a number of different reactions. Coenzymes either act as a "cobinder" or serve as a temporary carrier of intermediary products in the reaction. For example, the coenzyme **nicotinamide adenine dinucleotide (NAD^+)** forms NADH in transporting hydrogen atoms and electrons that split from food fragments during energy metabolism.

 S U M M A R Y

1. The first law of thermodynamics states that the body does not produce, consume, or use up energy; rather, it transforms it from one form into another as physiologic systems undergo continual change.

2. Potential energy and kinetic energy constitute the total energy of a system. Potential energy is the energy of position and form, and kinetic energy is the energy of motion. The release of potential energy transforms into kinetic energy of motion.

3. The term *exergonic* describes any physical or chemical process resulting in the release (freeing) of energy to its surroundings. Chemical processes that store or absorb energy are termed *endergonic*.

4. The second law of thermodynamics describes the tendency for potential energy to degrade to

kinetic energy with a lower capacity to perform work.

5. The total energy in an isolated system remains constant; a decrease in one form of energy matches an equivalent increase in another form.

6. Biologic work takes one of three forms: mechanical work (work of muscle contraction), chemical work (synthesizing cellular molecules), and transport work (concentrating various substances in the intracellular and extracellular fluids).

7. An enzyme, a highly specific and large protein catalyst, accelerates the forward and reverse rates of chemical reactions within the body without being consumed or changed in the reaction.

8. Enzymes do not all operate at the same rate; some operate slowly, and others operate more rapidly. Conditions of pH and temperature dramatically affect enzyme activity.

9. Coenzymes are nonprotein substances that facilitate enzyme action by binding the substrate with its specific enzyme.

THOUGHT QUESTIONS

1. From a metabolic perspective, why is the destruction of the rain forests throughout the world so bad for humans?

2. In terms of metabolism, why is body temperature maintained within a relatively narrow range?

Part 2   Phosphate-Bond Energy

The human body receives a continual chemical energy supply to perform its many functions. Energy derived from food oxidation does not release suddenly at some kindling temperature because the body, unlike a mechanical engine, cannot directly harness heat energy. Rather, complex, enzymatically controlled reactions within the cell's relatively cool, watery medium extract the chemical energy trapped within the bonds of carbohydrate, fat, and protein molecules. This extraction process reduces energy loss and enhances the efficiency of energy transformations. In this way, the body makes direct use of chemical energy for biologic work. **Adenosine triphosphate (ATP)**, the special carrier for free energy, provides the required energy for all cellular functions.

ADENOSINE TRIPHOSPHATE: ENERGY CURRENCY

The energy in food does not transfer directly to cells for biologic work. Rather, the "macronutrient energy" releases and funnels through the energy-rich compound ATP to power cellular needs. **Figure 5.5** shows how an ATP molecule forms from a molecule of adenine and ribose (called adenosine), linked to three phosphate molecules. The bonds linking the two outermost phosphates, termed **high-energy bonds**, represent considerable stored energy.

A tight linkage or coupling exists between the breakdown of the macronutrient energy molecules and ATP synthesis that "captures" a significant portion of the released energy. **Coupled reactions** occur in pairs; the breakdown of one compound provides energy for building another compound. To meet cellular energy needs, water binds ATP in the process of **hydrolysis**. This operation splits the outermost phosphate bond from the ATP molecule. The enzyme **adenosine triphosphatase** accelerates hydrolysis, forming a new compound **adenosine diphosphate (ADP)**. These reactions, in turn, couple to other reactions that incorporate the "freed" phosphate-bond chemical energy. The ATP molecules transfer the energy produced during catabolic reactions to power chemical reactions to

$\mathcal{Q}$uestions & Notes

In terms of energy use by the body, give the main difference between ATP and ADP.

Complete the equation:

$ATP + H_2O \rightarrow$

Give the amount of free energy liberated with the splitting of ATP to ADP.

Complete the following equations:

Glucose + Glucose →

Glycerol + Fatty acids →

Amino acids + Amino acids →

ⓘ For Your Information

HIGH-ENERGY PHOSPHATES

To appreciate the importance of the intramuscular high-energy phosphates in exercise, consider activities in which success requires short, intense bursts of energy. Football, tennis, track and field, golf, volleyball, field hockey, baseball, weight lifting, and wood chopping often require bursts of maximal effort for only up to 8 seconds.

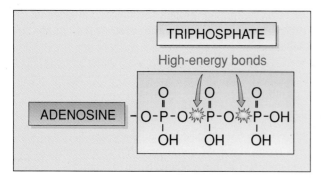

Figure 5.5 Adenosine triphosphate (ATP), the energy currency of the cell. The *starburst* represents the high-energy bonds.

synthesize new compounds. In essence, this energy receiver–energy donor cycle represents the cells' two major energy-transforming activities:

1. Form and conserve ATP from food's potential energy.
2. Use energy extracted from ATP to power all forms of biologic work.

Figure 5.6 illustrates examples of the anabolic and catabolic reactions that involve the coupled transfer of chemical energy. All of the energy released from catabolizing one compound does not dissipate as heat; rather, a portion remains conserved within the chemical structure of the newly formed compound. The highly "energized" ATP molecule represents the common energy transfer "vehicle" in most coupled biologic reactions.

Anabolism uses energy to synthesize new compounds. For example, many glucose molecules join together to form the larger more complex glycogen molecule; similarly, glycerol and fatty acids combine to make triacylglycerols, and amino acids bind together to form larger protein molecules. Each reaction starts with simple compounds and groups them as building blocks to form larger, more complex compounds.

Catabolic reactions release energy to form ADP. During this hydrolysis process, adenosine triphosphatase catalyzes the reaction when ATP joins with water. For each mole of

ATP degraded to ADP, the outermost phosphate bond splits and liberates approximately 7.3 kCal of **free energy**. This is the energy available for work.

$$\text{ATP} + \text{H}_2\text{O} \xrightarrow{\text{ATPase}} \text{ADP} + \text{P}_i - \Delta\text{G } 7.3 \text{ kCal} \cdot \text{mol}^{-1}$$

The symbol ΔG refers to the standard free energy change measured under laboratory conditions which seldom occur in the body (25°C; 1 atmosphere pressure; concentrations maintained at 1 molal at pH = 7.0). In the intracellular environment, the value may approach 10 kCal·mol^{-1}. The free energy liberated in ATP hydrolysis reflects the energy *difference* between the reactant and end products. This reaction generates considerable energy, so we refer to ATP as a **high-energy phosphate** compound.

The energy liberated during ATP breakdown directly transfers to other energy-requiring molecules. In muscle, this energy activates specific sites on the contractile elements that trigger muscle fibers to shorten. *Energy from ATP powers all forms of biologic work, so ATP may be thought of as constituting the cell's "energy currency."* **Figure 5.7** illustrates the general role of ATP as energy currency.

The splitting of ATP takes place immediately without oxygen. The cell's capability for ATP breakdown generates energy for rapid use. This anaerobic energy–producing process does not involve oxygen. Think of anaerobic energy release as a back-up power source relied on to deliver energy in *excess* of aerobic energy production. Examples of immediate anaerobic energy release include sprinting for a bus, lifting a fork, smashing a golf ball, spiking a volleyball, doing a pushup, or jumping up in the air. When you think of it, there literally are hundreds of examples you could list in your own daily routines. Lifting your hand to turn the page of this book occurs *without* the need for oxygen in the energy-requiring process. You can easily verify this by holding your breath when grasping the page—no external oxygen is required to execute the task. It takes less than 2 seconds to lift your hand to turn the page, and this act occurs anaerobically. In actuality, energy metabolism proceeds uninterrupted because intramuscular

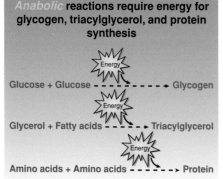

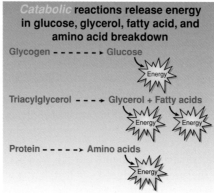

Figure 5.6 Anabolic and catabolic reactions.

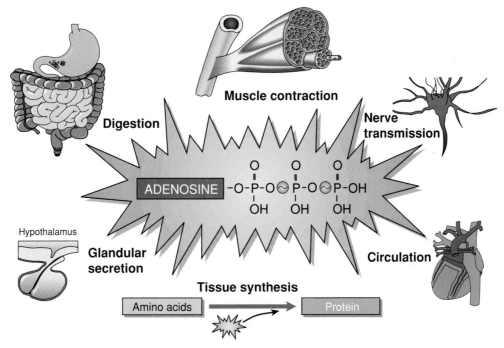

Figure 5.7 Adenosine triphosphate (ATP) represents the energy currency that powers all forms of biologic work.

anaerobic energy resources invariably provides the energy to perform these relatively short-duration activities.

Adenosine Triphosphate: A Limited Currency

A limited quantity of ATP serves as the energy currency for all cells. In fact, at any one time, the body stores only 80 to 100 g (3.5 oz) of ATP. This provides enough intramuscular stored energy for several seconds of explosive, all-out exercise. A limited quantity of "stored" ATP represents an additional advantage because of its molecule's heaviness. Biochemists estimate that a sedentary person each day uses an amount of ATP approximately equal to 75% of body mass. For an endurance athlete running a marathon race and generating 20 times the resting energy expenditure over 3 hours, the total equivalent ATP usage could amount to 80 kg.

Cells store only a small quantity of ATP so it must be resynthesized continually at its rate of use. This provides a biologically useful mechanism for regulating energy metabolism. By maintaining only a small amount of ATP, its relative concentration and corresponding concentration of ADP changes rapidly with any increase in a cell's energy demands. An ATP:ADP imbalance at the start of exercise immediately stimulates the breakdown of other stored energy-containing compounds to resynthesize ATP. As one might expect, increases in cellular energy transfer depend on exercise intensity. Energy transfer increases about fourfold in the transition from sitting in a chair to walking. Changing from a walk to an all-out sprint rapidly accelerates energy transfer rate within active muscle about 120 times within active muscle. Generating considerable energy output almost instantaneously demands ATP availability and a means for its rapid resynthesis.

PHOSPHOCREATINE: ENERGY RESERVOIR

The **hydrolysis** of a phosphate from another intracellular high-energy phosphate compound—**phosphocreatine (PCr)** (also known as creatine phosphate [CP]), provides some energy for ATP resynthesis. PCr, similar to ATP, releases

*Q*uestions & Notes

List the 6 forms of biologic work powered by ATP.

1.

2.

3.

4.

5.

6.

ⓘ For Your Information

TRAINING THE IMMEDIATE ENERGY SYSTEM

Exercise training increases the muscles' quantity of high-energy phosphates. The most effective training uses repeat 6- to 10-second intervals of maximal exercise in the specific activity requiring improved sprint-power capacity.

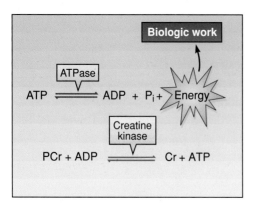

Figure 5.8 Adenosine triphosphate (ATP) and phosphocreatine (PCr) are anaerobic sources of phosphate-bond energy. The energy liberated from the hydrolysis (splitting) of PCr powers the union of ADP and P_i to reform ATP (the creatine kinase reaction).

a large amount of energy when the bond splits between the creatine and phosphate molecules. The hydrolysis of PCr begins at the onset of intense exercise, does not require oxygen, and reaches a maximum in about 8 to 12 seconds. Thus, PCr can be considered a "reservoir" of high-energy phosphate bonds. **Figure 5.8** illustrates the release and creation of phosphate-bond energy in ATP and PCr. The term **high-energy phosphates** or **phosphagens** describes these two stored intramuscular compounds.

In each reaction, the arrows point in both directions to indicate reversible reactions. In other words, creatine (Cr) and inorganic phosphate (from ATP) can join again to reform PCr. This also holds true for ATP where the union of ADP and P_i reforms ATP (top part of **Fig. 5.8**). ATP resynthesis occurs if sufficient energy exists to rejoin an ADP molecule with one P_i molecule. The hydrolysis of PCr "fuels" this energy.

Cells store PCr in considerably larger quantities than ATP. Mobilization of PCr for energy takes place almost instantaneously and does not require oxygen. Interestingly, the concentration of ADP in the cell stimulates the activity level of **creatine kinase**, the enzyme that facilitates PCr breakdown to Cr and ATP. This provides a crucial feedback mechanism known as the **creatine kinase reaction** that rapidly forms ATP from the high-energy phosphates.

The **adenylate kinase reaction** represents another single-enzyme–mediated reaction for ATP regeneration. The reaction uses two ADP molecules to produce one molecule of ATP and AMP as follows:

$$\text{2 ADP} \xrightleftharpoons[]{\text{Adenylate kinase}} \text{ATP + AMP}$$

The creatine kinase and adenylate kinase reactions not only augment how well the muscles rapidly increase energy output (i.e., increase ATP availability), they also produce the molecular byproducts (AMP, P_i, ADP) that activate the initial stages of glycogen and glucose breakdown in the cell fluids and the aerobic pathways of the mitochondrion.

INTRAMUSCULAR HIGH-ENERGY PHOSPHATES

The energy released from ATP and PCr breakdown within muscle can sustain all-out running, cycling, or swimming for 5 to 8 seconds. In the 100-m sprint, for example, the body cannot maintain maximum speed for longer than this duration. During the last few seconds, runners actually slow down, with the winner slowing the least. From an energy perspective, the winner most effectively supplies and uses the limited quantity of phosphate-bond energy.

In almost all sports, the energy transfer capacity of the ATP-PCr high-energy phosphates (termed the "**immediate energy system**") plays a crucial role in success or failure of some phase of performance. If all-out effort continues beyond about 8 seconds or if moderate exercise continues for much longer periods, ATP resynthesis requires an additional energy source other then PCr. Without this additional ATP resynthesis, the "fuel" supply diminishes, and high-intensity movement ceases. The foods we eat and store provide the energy to continually recharge cellular supplies of ATP and PCr.

Identifying Energy Sources is Important

Identifying the predominant source(s) of energy required for a particular sport or activities of daily living provides the basis for an effective exercise training program. Football and baseball, for example, require a high-energy output for only brief time periods. These performances rely almost exclusively on energy transfer from the intramuscular high-energy phosphates. Developing this immediate energy system becomes important when training to improve performance in movements of brief duration. Chapter 13 discusses specific training to optimize the power-output capacity of the different energy systems.

Phosphorylation: Chemical Bonds Transfer Energy In the body, biologic work occurs when compounds relatively low in potential energy "juice up" from the transfer of energy via high-energy phosphate bonds. ATP serves as the ideal energy-transfer agent. In one respect, the phosphate bonds of ATP "trap" a large portion of the original food molecules' potential energy. ATP then transfers this energy to other compounds to raise them to a higher activation level. **Phosphorylation** refers to energy transfer through phosphate bonds.

CELLULAR OXIDATION

The energy for phosphorylation comes from **oxidation** ("biologic burning") of the carbohydrate, lipid, and protein macronutrients in the body. A molecule becomes **reduced** when it accepts electrons from an electron donor. In turn, the molecule that gives up the electron becomes **oxidized**.

Oxidation reactions (donating electrons) and reduction reactions (accepting electrons) remain coupled because every oxidation coincides with a reduction. *In essence, cellular oxidation–reduction constitutes the mechanism for energy metabolism.* The stored carbohydrate, fat, and protein molecules continually provide hydrogen atoms for this process. The complex but highly efficient mitochondria (*micro.magnet.fsu.edu/cells*), the cell's "energy factories," contain carrier molecules that remove electrons from hydrogen (oxidation) and eventually pass them to oxygen (reduction). Synthesis of the high-energy phosphate ATP occurs during oxidation–reduction reactions.

Electron Transport

Figure 5.9 illustrates hydrogen oxidation and the accompanying electron transport to oxygen. During cellular oxidation, hydrogen atoms are not merely turned loose in cell fluid. Rather, highly specific **dehydrogenase enzymes** catalyze hydrogen's release from nutrient substrates. The coenzyme part of the dehydrogenase (usually the niacin-containing coenzyme, NAD^+) accepts pairs of electrons (energy) from hydrogen. While the substrate oxidizes and loses hydrogen (electrons), NAD^+ gains one hydrogen and two electrons and reduces to NADH; the other hydrogen appears as H^+ in cell fluid.

The riboflavin-containing coenzyme **flavin adenine dinucleotide (FAD)** is the other important electron acceptor that oxidizes food fragments. FAD also catalyzes dehydrogenations and accepts pairs of electrons. Unlike NAD^+, however, FAD becomes $FADH_2$ by accepting both hydrogens. This distinct difference between NAD^+ and FAD produces a different total number of ATP in the respiratory chain (see next section).

The NADH and $FADH_2$ formed in macronutrient breakdown represent energy-rich molecules because they carry electrons with a high-energy transfer potential. The cytochromes, a series of iron–protein electron carriers, then pass pairs of electrons carried by NADH and $FADH_2$ in "bucket brigade" fashion on the inner membranes of the mitochondria. The iron portion of each cytochrome exists in either its oxidized (ferric or Fe^{+++}) or reduced (ferrous or Fe^{++}) ionic state. By accepting an electron, the ferric portion of a specific cytochrome reduces to its ferrous form. In turn, ferrous iron donates electrons to the next cytochrome, and so on down the "bucket brigade." By shuttling between these two iron forms, the cytochromes transfer electrons to their ultimate destination, where they reduce oxygen to form water. The NAD^+ and FAD then recycle for subsequent reuse in energy metabolism.

Questions & Notes

Oxidation involves _____ of electrons.

Reduction involves _____ of electrons.

Name the cellular organelle where oxidation/reduction takes place.

Name the 2 specific coenzymes that catalyze hydrogen's release from nutrient substrates.

1.

2.

Fill-in:

For each pair of hydrogen atoms, _____ electrons flow down the respiratory chain and reduce _____ atoms of oxygen to form _____ .

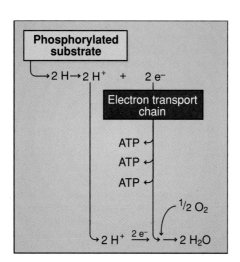

Figure 5.9 Oxidation (removal of electrons) of hydrogen and accompanying electron transport. In reduction, oxygen gains electrons and water forms.

Electron transport by specific carrier molecules constitutes the **respiratory chain**, the final common pathway where electrons extracted from hydrogen pass to oxygen. *For each pair of hydrogen atoms, two electrons flow down the chain and reduce one atom of oxygen to form water.* Of the five specific cytochromes, only the last one, cytochrome oxidase (cytochrome aa₃ with a strong affinity for oxygen), discharges its electron directly to oxygen. **Figure 5.10A** shows the respiratory chain route for hydrogen oxidation, electron transport, and energy transfer in the respiratory chain. The respiratory chain releases free energy in relatively small amounts. In several of the electron transfers, energy conservation occurs by forming high-energy phosphate bonds.

Oxidative Phosphorylation

Oxidative phosphorylation refers to how ATP forms during electron transfer from NADH and FADH₂ with the eventual involvement of molecular oxygen. This crucial cellular metabolic process represents cells' primary means for extracting and trapping chemical energy in the high-energy phosphates. *More than 90% of ATP synthesis takes place in the respiratory chain by oxidative reactions coupled with phosphorylation.*

Think of oxidative phosphorylation as a waterfall divided into several separate cascades by the waterwheels located at different heights. **Figure 5.10B** depicts the waterwheels harnessing the energy of the falling water; similarly, electrochemical energy generated via electron transport in the respiratory chain becomes harnessed and transferred (or coupled) to ADP. The energy in NADH transfers to ADP to reform ATP at three distinct coupling sites during electron transport (**Fig. 5.10A**). Oxidation of hydrogen and subsequent phosphorylation occurs as follows:

$$NADH + H^+ + 3ADP + 3P_i + \frac{1}{2}O_2 \rightarrow$$
$$NAD^+ + H_2O + 3ATP$$

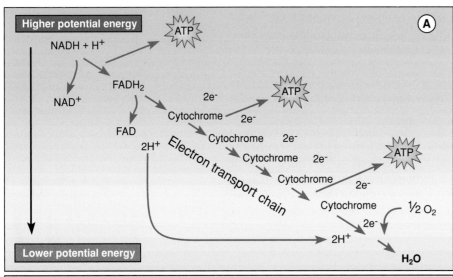

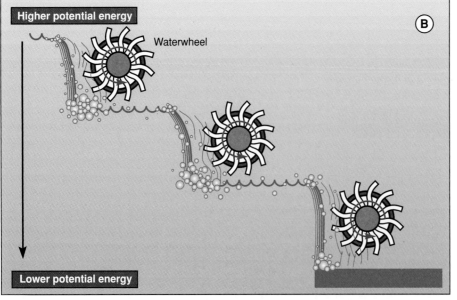

Figure 5.10 Examples of harnessing potential energy. **A.** In the body. The electron transport chain removes electrons from hydrogens and ultimately delivers them to oxygen. In this oxidation–reduction process, much of the chemical energy stored within the hydrogen atom does not dissipate to kinetic energy. Rather, it becomes conserved in forming adenosine triphosphate (ATP). **B.** In industry. The captured energy from falling water drives the waterwheel, which in turn performs mechanical work.

Thus, three ATP form for each NADH plus H^+ oxidized. However, if $FADH_2$ originally donates hydrogen, only two molecules of ATP form for each hydrogen pair oxidized. This occurs because $FADH_2$ enters the respiratory chain at a lower energy level at a point beyond the site of the first ATP synthesis.

Efficiency of Electron Transport and Oxidative Phosphorylation

Each mole of ATP formed from ADP conserves approximately 7 kCal of energy. Because 2.5 moles of ATP regenerate from the total of 52 kCal of energy released to oxidize 1 mole of NADH, about 18 kCal ($7 \; kCal \cdot mol^{-1} \times 2.5$) is conserved as chemical energy. This represents a relative efficiency of 34% for harnessing chemical energy via electron transport-oxidative phosphorylation ($18 \; kCal \div 52 \; kCal \times 100$). The remaining 66% of the energy dissipates as heat. If the intracellular energy change for ATP synthesis approaches $10 \; kCal \cdot mol^{-1}$, then efficiency of energy conservation approximates 50%. Considering that a steam engine transforms its fuel into useful energy at only about 30% efficiency, the value of 34% or above for the human body represents a relatively high-efficiency rate.

Role of Oxygen in Energy Metabolism

The continual resynthesis of ATP during coupled oxidative phosphorylation of the macronutrients has three prerequisites:

1. Availability of the reducing agents NADH or $FADH_2$.
2. Presence of a terminal oxidizing agent in the form of oxygen.
3. Sufficient quantity of enzymes and metabolic machinery in the tissues to make the energy transfer reactions "go" at the appropriate rate.

Satisfying these three conditions causes hydrogen and electrons to continually shuttle down the respiratory chain. The hydrogens combine with oxygen to form water, and the electrons pass on to form the high energy ATP molecule. During strenuous exercise, inadequacy in oxygen delivery (prerequisite 2, above) or its rate of utilization (prerequisite 3) creates a relative imbalance between hydrogen release and oxygen's final acceptance of them. If either of these conditions occurs, electrons flowing down the respiratory chain "back up," and hydrogens accumulate bound to NAD^+ and FAD. Without oxygen, the temporarily "free" hydrogens require another molecule to bind with. In a subsequent section, we explain how lactate forms when the compound pyruvate temporarily binds these excess hydrogens (electrons); lactate formation allows electron transport–oxidative phosphorylation to proceed relatively unimpeded at a particular exercise intensity.

Aerobic energy metabolism refers to the energy-generating catabolic reactions during which oxygen serves as the final electron acceptor in the respiratory chain and combines with hydrogen to form water. Some might argue that the term *aerobic metabolism* is misleading because oxygen does not participate directly in ATP synthesis. Oxygen's presence at the "end of the line," however, largely determines one's capability for ATP production via respiration.

Questions & Notes

How many kCal of energy conserve for each mole of ATP formed from ADP?

Does oxygen participate directly in ATP synthesis?

For Your Information

"OIL RIG"

To remember that oxidation involves the loss of electrons and reduction involves the gain of electrons, remember the phrase **OIL RIG**:

OIL: Oxidation **I**nvolves **L**oss
RIG: Reduction **I**nvolves **G**ain

For Your Information

A MODIFICATION IN ADENOSINE TRIPHOSPHATE ACCOUNTING

Biochemists have recently adjusted their accounting transpositions regarding conservation of energy in the resynthesis of an ATP molecule from carbohydrate in aerobic metabolism. Although it is true that energy provided by oxidation of NADH and $FADH_2$ resynthesizes ADP to ATP, additional energy (H^+) is also required to shuttle the NADH (and hence ATP exchanged for ADP and Pi) from the cell's cytoplasm across the mitochondrial membrane to deliver H^+ to electron transport. This added energy exchange of NADH shuttling across the mitochondrial membrane reduces the *net* ATP yield for glucose metabolism and changes the overall efficiency of ATP production. On average, only 2.5 ATP molecules form from oxidation of one NADH moloecule. This decimal value for ATP does not indicate formation of a one-half of an ATP molecule but rather indicates the average number of ATP produced per NADH oxidation with the energy for mitochondrial transport subtracted. When $FADH_2$ donates hydrogen, then on average only 1.5 molecules of ATP form for each hydrogen pair oxidized.

SUMMARY

1. Energy release occurs slowly in small amounts during complex, enzymatically controlled reactions to enable more efficient energy transfer and conservation.

2. About 40% of the potential energy in food nutrients transfers to the high-energy compound ATP.

3. Splitting of ATP's terminal phosphate bond liberates free energy to power all biologic work.

4. ATP represents the cell's energy currency, although its limited quantity amounts to only about 3.5 oz.

5. PCr interacts with ADP to form ATP; this nonaerobic, high-energy reservoir replenishes ATP rapidly. Collectively, ATP and PCr are referred to as "high-energy phosphates."

6. Phosphorylation represents energy transfer as energy-rich phosphate bonds. In this process, ADP and Cr continually recycle into ATP and PCr.

7. Cellular oxidation occurs on the inner lining of the mitochondrial membranes; it involves transferring electrons from NADH and $FADH_2$ to molecular oxygen. This releases and transfers chemical energy to combine ATP from ADP plus a phosphate ion.

8. During aerobic ATP resynthesis, oxygen (the final electron acceptor in the respiratory chain) combines with hydrogen to form water.

THOUGHT QUESTIONS

1. Based on the first law of thermodynamics, why is it imprecise to refer to energy "production" in the body?

2. Discuss the implications of the second law of thermodynamics for the measurement of energy expenditure.

Part 3	**Energy Release from Food**

The energy released from macronutrient breakdown serves one crucial purpose—to phosphorylate ADP to reform the energy-rich compound ATP (**Fig. 5.11**). Macronutrient catabolism favors generating phosphate-bond energy, yet the specific pathways of degradation differ depending on the nutrients metabolized.

Figure 5.12 outlines the following six macronutrient fuel sources that supply substrate for oxidation and subsequent ATP formation:

1. Triacylglycerol and glycogen molecules stored within muscle cells.
2. Blood glucose (derived from liver glycogen).
3. Free fatty acids (derived from triacylglycerols in liver and adipocytes).
4. Intramuscular- and liver-derived carbon skeletons of amino acids.
5. Anaerobic reactions in the cytosol in the initial phase of glucose or glycogen breakdown (small amount of ATP).
6. Phosphorylation of ADP by PCr under enzymatic control by creatine kinase and adenylate kinase.

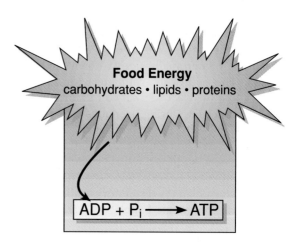

Figure 5.11 Potential energy in food powers adenosine triphosphate (ATP) resynthesis.

CARBOHYDRATE ENERGY RELEASE

Carbohydrates' primary function supplies energy for cellular work. Our discussion of nutrient energy metabolism begins with carbohydrates for five reasons:

1. Carbohydrate represents the *only* macronutrient whose potential energy generates ATP aerobically and anaerobically. This becomes important in vigorous exercise that requires rapid energy release above levels supplied by aerobic metabolic reactions.

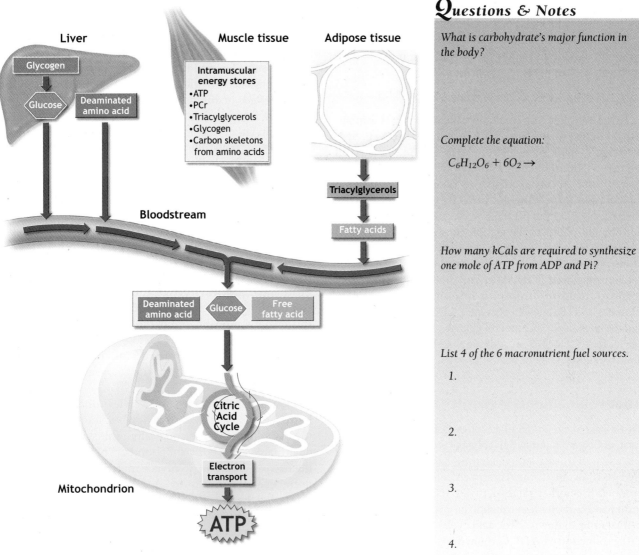

Figure 5.12 Macronutrient fuel sources that supply substrates to regenerate adenosine triphosphate (ATP). The liver provides a rich source of amino acids and glucose, and adipocytes generate large quantities of energy-rich fatty acid molecules. After their release, the bloodstream delivers these compounds to the muscle cell. Most of the cells' energy transfer takes place within the mitochondria. Mitochondrial proteins carry out their roles in oxidative phosphorylation on the inner membranous walls of this architechturally elegant complex. The intramuscular energy sources consist of the high-energy phosphates ATP and phosphocreatine and triacylglycerols, glycogen, and amino acids.

Questions & Notes

What is carbohydrate's major function in the body?

Complete the equation:

$$C_6H_{12}O_6 + 6O_2 \rightarrow$$

How many kCals are required to synthesize one mole of ATP from ADP and Pi?

List 4 of the 6 macronutrient fuel sources.

1.

2.

3.

4.

2. During light and moderate aerobic exercise, carbohydrate supplies about half of the body's energy requirements.
3. Processing fat through the metabolic mill for energy requires some carbohydrate catabolism.
4. Aerobic breakdown of carbohydrate for energy occurs at about *twice* the rate as energy generated from lipid breakdown. Thus, depleting glycogen reserves reduces exercise power output. In prolonged, high-intensity, aerobic exercise, such as marathon running, athletes often experience nutrient-related fatigue, a state associated with muscle and liver glycogen depletion.

ⓘ For Your Information

GLUCOSE IS NOT RETRIEVABLE FROM FATTY ACIDS

Cells can synthesize glucose from pyruvate and other 3-carbon compounds. However, glucose cannot form from the 2-carbon acetyl fragments of the β-oxidation of fatty acids. Consequently, fatty acids cannot readily provide energy for tissues (e.g., brain and nerve tissues) that use glucose almost exclusively for fuel. All dietary lipid occurs in triacylglycerol form. Triacylglycerol's glycerol component can yield glucose, but the glycerol molecule contains only 3 (6%) of the 57 carbon atoms in the molecule. Thus, fat from dietary sources or stored in adipocytes does not provide an adequate potential glucose source; about 95% of the fat molecule *cannot* be converted to glucose.

5. The central nervous system requires an uninterrupted stream of carbohydrates to function optimally.

The complete breakdown of one mole of glucose (180 g) to carbon dioxide and water yields a maximum of 686 kCal of chemical-free energy available for work.

$$C_6H_{12}O_6 + 6\,O_2 \rightarrow 6\,CO_2 + 6\,H_2O - \Delta G\; 686\; kCal \cdot mol^{-1}$$

In the body, glucose breakdown liberates the same quantity of energy, with a large portion conserved as ATP. Synthesizing 1 mole of ATP from ADP and phosphate ion requires 7.3 kCal of energy. Therefore, coupling all of the energy from glucose oxidation to phosphorylation could theoretically form 94 moles of ATP per mole of glucose (686 kCal ÷ 7.3 kCal per mole = 94 moles). In the muscles, however, the phosphate bonds only conserve 34% or 233 kCal of energy, with the remainder dissipated as heat. This loss of energy represents the body's metabolic *inefficiency* for converting stored potential energy into useful energy. In summary, glucose breakdown regenerates a net gain of 32 moles of ATP (net gain because 2 ATPs degrade to initiate glucose breakdown) per mole of glucose (233 kCal ÷ 7.3 kCal per mole = 32 ATP). An additional ATP forms if carbohydrate breakdown begins with glycogen.

Anaerobic versus Aerobic

Two forms of the initial phase of carbohydrate breakdown exist, collectively termed **glycolysis** (process of converting glucose to pyruvate and generating ATP). In one stage of glycolysis, lactate (formed from pyruvate) becomes the end product. In another stage, pyruvate remains the end substrate, and carbohydrate catabolism proceeds and couples to further breakdown (citric acid cycle) and electron transport production of ATP. Carbohydrate breakdown of this form (sometimes termed **aerobic** [with oxygen] **glycolysis**) is a relatively slow process resulting in substantial ATP formation. In contrast, glycolysis that results in lactate formation (referred to as **anaerobic** [without oxygen] **glycolysis**) represents *rapid* but limited ATP production. The net formation of either lactate or pyruvate depends more on the relative glycolytic and mitochondrial activities than on the presence of molecular oxygen. The relative demands for rapid or slow ATP production determines the form of glycolysis. The glycolytic process itself, from beginning substrate (glucose) to end substrate (lactate or pyruvate), does not involve oxygen. It has become common to call these two stages *rapid* (anaerobic) and *slow* (aerobic) glycolysis.

Anaerobic Energy From Glucose: Rapid Glycolysis

The first stage of rapid **glycolysis**, during which glucose is the substrate, is termed the *Embden-Meyerhoff pathway* (named for the two German scientist discoverers); the term **glycogenolysis** describes these reactions when they initiate from stored glycogen. These series of reactions, summarized in **Figure 5.13**, occur in the cell's cytoplasm, the watery medium outside of the mitochondrion. In a way, glycolytic reactions represent a more primitive form of energy transfer that is well developed in amphibians, reptiles, fish, and marine mammals. In humans, the cells' limited capacity for rapid glycolysis assumes a crucial role during physical activities that require maximal effort for up to 90 seconds in duration.

In the first reaction, ATP acts as a phosphate donor to phosphorylate glucose to **glucose 6-phosphate**. In most cells, this reaction "traps" the glucose molecule. In the presence of **glycogen synthase**, glucose links become **polymerized** with other glucose molecules to form glycogen. In energy metabolism, **glucose 6-phosphate** changes to **fructose 6-phosphate**. At this stage, no energy extraction occurs, yet energy incorporates into the original glucose molecule at the expense of one ATP molecule. In a sense, phosphorylation "primes the pump" for continued energy metabolism. The fructose 6-phosphate molecule gains an additional phosphate and changes to **fructose 1, 6-diphosphate** under control of **phosphofructokinase (PFK)**. The activity level of this enzyme probably limits the rate of glycolysis during maximum-effort exercise. Fructose 1, 6-diphosphate then splits into two phosphorylated molecules with 3-carbon chains; these further decompose to **pyruvate** in five successive reactions.

Figure 5.14 provides an overview of the glucose-to-pyruvate sequence in terms of carbon atoms. Essentially, the 6-carbon glucose compound splits into two interchangeable 3-carbon compounds. This ultimately produces two 3-carbon pyruvate molecules and generates useful energy as ATP.

Most of the energy generated in glycolysis does not resynthesize ATP but instead dissipates as heat. In reactions 7 and 10 in **Figure 5.13**, however, the energy released from the glucose intermediates stimulates the direct transfer of phosphate groups to ADPs, generating four molecules of ATP. Because two molecules of ATP were lost in the initial phosphorylation of the glucose molecule, glycolysis generates a *net gain* of 2 ATP molecules. Note that these specific energy transfers from substrate to ADP do not require molecular oxygen. Rather, energy directly transfers via phosphate bonds in the anaerobic reactions. Energy conservation during rapid glycolysis operates at an efficiency of about 30%.

Rapid glycolysis generates only about 5% of the total ATP during the glucose molecule's complete degradation. Examples of activities that rely heavily on ATP generated by rapid glycolysis include sprinting at the end of a mile run, swimming all-out from start to finish in a 50- and 100-m swim, routines on gymnastics apparatus, and sprint running up to 200 m.

Hydrogen Release During Rapid Glycolysis

During rapid glycolysis, two pairs of hydrogen atoms are stripped away from the substrate (glucose), and their electrons are passed to NAD^+ to form NADH (see **Fig. 5.13**). Normally, if the respiratory chain processed these electrons directly, 2.5 molecules of ATP would generate for each NADH molecule oxidized. The mitochondrion in

THE HENLEY COLLEGE LIBRARY

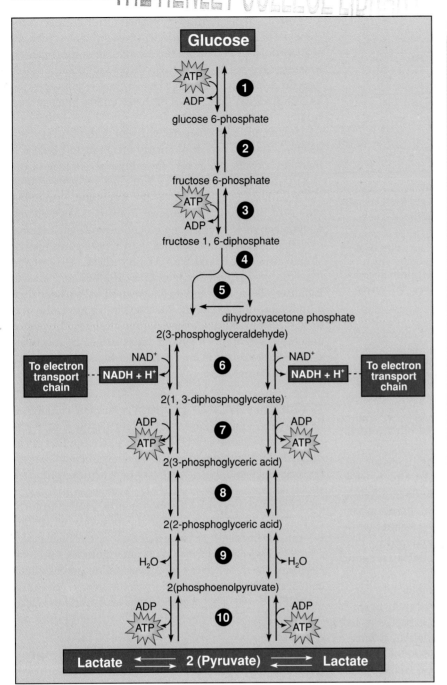

Figure 5.13 Glycolysis. Ten enzymatically controlled chemical reactions involve the anaerobic breakdown of glucose to two molecules of pyruvate. Lactate forms when NADH oxidation does not keep pace with its formation in glycolysis.

skeletal muscle remains impermeable to NADH formed in the cytoplasm during glycolysis. Consequently, the electrons from **extramitochondrial** NADH shuttle indirectly into the mitochondria. In skeletal muscle, this route ends with electrons passing to FAD to form $FADH_2$ at a point below the first ATP formation (see **Fig. 5.10A**). Thus, 1.5 rather than 2.5 ATP molecules form when the respiratory chain oxidizes cytoplasmic NADH. Because two molecules of NADH form in glycolysis, subsequent coupled electron transport–oxidative phosphorylation aerobically generates four ATP molecules.

Lactate Formation Sufficient oxygen bathes the cells during light to moderate levels of energy metabolism. The hydrogens (electrons) stripped from the substrate and carried by NADH oxidize within the mitochondria to form

Questions & Notes

Give the efficiency of energy conservation during glycolysis.

Give the percentage of energy stored within ATP molecules compared to the total energy released during glycolysis.

Give 2 examples of activities that rely heavily on ATP generated via glycolytic anaerobic reactions.

1.

2.

The total (net and gross) number of ATP molecules generated in glycolysis:

Net:

Gross:

In what tissue does the Cori cycle function?

ⓘ For Your Information

LINKS IN ENERGY TRANSFER

NAD^+ and FAD represent crucial oxidizing agents (electron acceptors) in energy metabolism. Oxidation reactions couple to reduction reactions, allowing electrons (hydrogens) picked up by NAD^+ and FAD to transfer to other compounds (reducing agents) during energy metabolism.

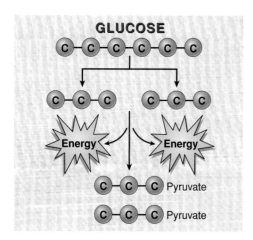

Figure 5.14 Glycolysis: the glucose-to-pyruvate pathway. A 6-carbon glucose splits into two 3-carbon compounds, which further degrade into two 3-carbon pyruvate molecules. Glucose splitting occurs under anaerobic conditions in the cells' watery medium.

water when they join with oxygen. In a biochemical sense, a "steady rate" exists because hydrogen oxidizes at about the same rate it becomes available. This condition of aerobic glycolysis forms pyruvate as the end product.

In strenuous exercise, when energy demands exceed either the oxygen supply or the utilization rate, the respiratory chain cannot process all of the hydrogen joined to NADH. Continued release of anaerobic energy in glycolysis depends on NAD^+ availability for oxidizing 3-phosphoglyceraldehyde (see reaction 6 in **Fig. 5.13**); otherwise, the rapid rate of glycolysis "grinds to a halt." During rapid or anaerobic glycolysis, NAD^+ "frees up" as pairs of "excess" non-oxidized hydrogens combine temporarily with pyruvate to form lactate, catalyzed by the enzyme lactate dehydrogenase in the reversible reaction shown in **Figure 5.15**.

During rest and moderate exercise, some lactate continually forms and readily oxidizes for energy in neighboring muscle fibers with high oxidative capacity or in more distant tissues such as the heart and ventilatory muscles. Lactate can also provide an indirect precursor of liver glycogen (see next section). Consequently, lactate does not accumulate because its removal rate equals its rate of production. One of the benefits of arduous, prolongled training for sports is that endurance athletes have an enhanced ability for lactate clearance or turnover during exercise.

A direct chemical pathway exists for liver glycogen synthesis from dietary carbohydrate. Liver glycogen synthesis also occurs indirectly from the conversion of the 3-carbon precursor lactate to glucose. Erythrocytes and adipocytes contain glycolytic enzymes, skeletal muscle possesses the largest quantity; thus, much of the lactate-to-glucose conversion likely occurs in muscle.

The temporary storage of hydrogen with pyruvate represents a unique aspect of energy metabolism because it provides a ready "collector" for temporary storage of the end product of rapid glycolysis. After lactate forms in muscle, it either (1) diffuses into the interstitial space and blood for buffering and removal from the site of energy metabolism or (2) provides a gluconeogenic substrate for glycogen synthesis. In this way, glycolysis continues to supply anaerobic energy for ATP resynthesis. This avenue for extra energy remains temporary if blood and muscle lactate levels increase and ATP formation fails to keep pace with its rate of use. Fatigue soon sets in, and exercise performance diminishes. Increased intracellular acidity under anaerobic conditions likely mediates fatigue by inactivating various enzymes in energy transfer impair the muscle's contractile properties.

A Valuable "Waste Product" Lactate should not be viewed as a metabolic waste product. To the contrary, it provides a valuable source of chemical energy that accumulates with intense exercise. When sufficient oxygen becomes available during recovery or when exercise pace slows or ceases (recovery), NAD^+ scavenges hydrogens attached to lactate, which subsequently oxidize to form ATP. The carbon skeletons of the pyruvate molecules reformed from lactate during exercise (one pyruvate molecule + 2 hydrogens forms one lactate molecule) become either oxidized for energy or synthesized to glucose (gluconeogenesis) in muscle itself or in the liver via the **Cori cycle** (**Fig. 5.16**). This cycle removes lactate and uses it to replenish glycogen reserves depleted from intense exercise.

Lactate Shuttle: Blood Lactate as an Energy Source Isotope tracer studies show that lactate produced in fast-twitch muscle fibers (and other tissues) circulates to other fast- or slow-twitch fibers for conversion to pyruvate. Pyruvate, in turn, converts to acetyl-CoA for entry into the citric acid cycle for aerobic energy metabolism. This process of **lactate shuttling** among cells enables

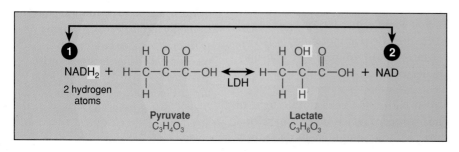

Figure 5.15 Lactate forms when excess hydrogens from NADH combine temporarily with pyruvate. This frees up NAD^+ to accept additional hydrogens generated in glycolysis. LDH = lactate dehydrogenase.

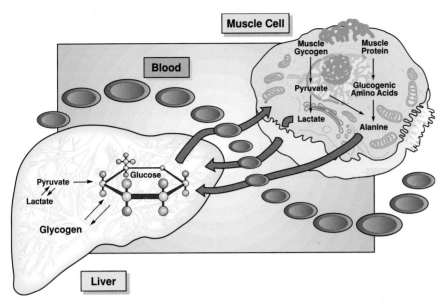

Figure 5.16 The Cori cycle in the liver synthesizes glucose from lactate released from active muscle. This gluconeogenic process maintains carbohydrate reserves.

glycogenolysis in one cell to supply other cells with fuel for oxidation. *This makes muscle not only a major site of lactate production but also a primary tissue for lactate removal via oxidation.*

Aerobic (Slow) Glycolysis: The Citric Acid Cycle

The anaerobic reactions of rapid glycolysis release only about 5% of the original potential energy within the original glucose molecule. This means that extracting the remaining energy must occur by another metabolic pathway. This occurs when pyruvate irreversibly converts to acetyl-CoA, a form of acetic acid. Acetyl-CoA enters the second stage of carbohydrate breakdown known as aerobic (slow) glycolysis (also termed the **citric acid cycle**, Krebs cycle, or tricarboxylic acid cycle).

Figure 5.17 shows the metabolic reactions of pyruvate to acetyl-CoA. Each 3-carbon pyruvate molecule loses a carbon when it joins with a CoA molecule to form acetyl-CoA and carbon dioxide. The reaction from pyruvate proceeds in one direction only.

Figure 5.18 illustrates that the citric acid cycle within the mitochondria degrades the acetyl-CoA substrate to carbon dioxide and hydrogen atoms. Hydrogen atoms oxidize during electron transport–oxidative phosphorylation that regenerates ATP.

Figure 5.19 shows pyruvate entering the citric acid cycle by joining with the vitamin B–derivative coenzyme A (A stands for acetic acid) to form the 2-carbon compound acetyl-CoA. This process releases two hydrogens and transfers their electrons to NAD^+, forming one molecule of carbon dioxide as follows:

$$\textbf{Pyruvate} + \textbf{NAD}^+ + \textbf{CoA} \rightarrow \textbf{Acetyl–CoA} + \textbf{CO}_2 + \textbf{NADH} + \textbf{H}^+$$

The acetyl portion of acetyl-CoA joins with oxaloacetate to form citrate (citric acid—the same 6-carbon compound found in citrus fruits) before proceeding through the citric acid cycle. The citric acid cycle continues to operate because it retains the original oxaloacetate molecule to join with a new acetyl fragment.

For each acetyl-CoA molecule that enters the citric acid cycle, the substrate releases two carbon dioxide molecules and four pairs of hydrogen atoms. One molecule of ATP also regenerates directly by substrate-level phosphorylation

Questions & Notes

Describe the major function of the citric acid cycle.

In what organale does the citric acid cycle occur?

 For Your Information

FREE RADICALS FORMED DURING AEROBIC METABOLISM

The passage of electrons along the electron transport chain sometimes forms free radicals, molecules with an unpaired electron in their outer orbital, making them highly reactive. These reactive free radicals bind quickly to other molecules that promote potential damage to the combining molecule. Free radical formation in muscle, for example, might contribute to muscle fatigue or soreness or a potential reduction in metabolic potential.

 For Your Information

CARBOHYDRATE DEPLETION REDUCES POWER OUTPUT

Carbohydrate depletion depresses exercise capacity (expressed as a percentage of maximum). This capacity progressively decreases after 2 hours to 50% of the initial exercise intensity. Reduced power directly results from the slow rate of aerobic energy release from fat oxidation, which now becomes the major energy pathway.

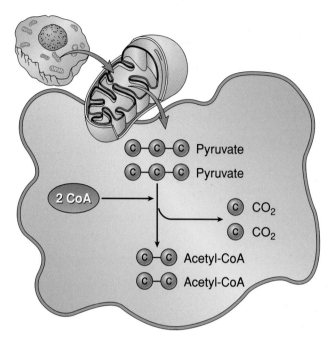

Figure 5.17 One-way reaction of pyruvate to acetyl-CoA. Two 3-carbon pyruvate molecules join with two coenzyme A molecules to form two 2-carbon acetyl-CoA molecules with 2 carbons lost as carbon dioxide.

from citric acid cycle reactions (see reaction 7 in **Fig. 5.19**). The bottom of **Figure 5.19** shows that four hydrogens release when acetyl-CoA forms from the two pyruvate molecules created in glycolysis, with an additional 16 hydrogens released in the citric acid cycle (acetyl-CoA hydrolysis). *Generating electrons for passage to the respiratory chain via NAD^+ and FAD represents the most important function of the citric acid cycle.*

Oxygen does not participate directly in citric acid cycle reactions. Instead, the aerobic process of electron transport–oxidative phosphorylation transfers a considerable portion of the chemical energy in pyruvate to ADP. With adequate oxygen, including enzymes and substrate, NAD^+ and FAD regeneration takes place, allowing citric acid cycle metabolism to proceed unimpeded.

Net Energy Transfer From Glucose Catabolism

Figure 5.20 summarizes the pathways for energy transfer during glucose breakdown in skeletal muscle. A net gain of two ATP molecules form from substrate-level phosphorylation in glycolysis; similarly, 2 ATP molecules come from

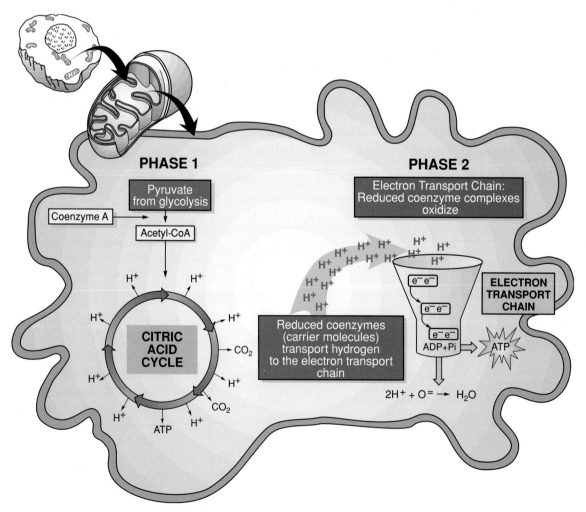

Figure 5.18 **Phase 1.** In the mitochondrion, citric acid cycle activity generates hydrogen atoms in acetyl-CoA breakdown. **Phase 2.** Significant adenosine triphosphate (ATP) regenerates when hydrogens oxidize via the aerobic process of electron transport–oxidative phosphorylation (electron transport chain).

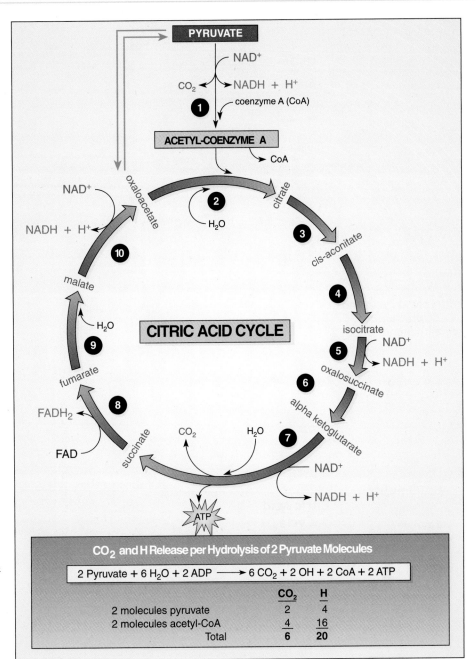

Figure 5.19 Release of H and CO_2 in the mitochondrion during breakdown of one pyruvate molecule. All values double when computing the net gain of H and CO_2 from pyruvate breakdown because glycolysis forms two molecules of pyruvate from one glucose molecule.

CO_2 and H Release per Hydrolysis of 2 Pyruvate Molecules

$$2\ Pyruvate + 6\ H_2O + 2\ ADP \longrightarrow 6\ CO_2 + 2\ OH + 2\ CoA + 2\ ATP$$

	CO_2	H
2 molecules pyruvate	2	4
2 molecules acetyl-CoA	4	16
Total	**6**	**20**

acetyl-CoA degradation in the citric acid cycle. The 24 released hydrogen atoms (and their subsequent oxidation) can be accounted for as follows:

1. Four extramitochondrial hydrogens (2 NADH) generated in rapid glycolysis yield 5 ATPs during oxidative phosphorylation.
2. Four hydrogens (2 NADH) released in the mitochondrion when pyruvate degrades to acetyl-CoA yield 5 ATPs.
3. The citric acid cycle via substrate-level phosphorylation produces two guanosine triphosphates (GTPs; a molecule similar to ATP).
4. Twelve of the 16 hydrogens (6 NADH) released in the citric acid cycle yield 15 ATPs (6 NADH × 2.5 ATPs per NADH = 15 ATPs).
5. Four hydrogens joined to FAD (2 FADH$_2$) in the citric acid cycle yield 3 ATPs.

The complete breakdown of glucose yields a total of 34 ATPs. Because 2 ATPs initially phosphorylate glucose, 32 ATP molecules equal the net ATP yield from glucose catabolism in skeletal muscle. Whereas four ATP molecules form directly from substrate-level phosphorylation (glycolysis and citric

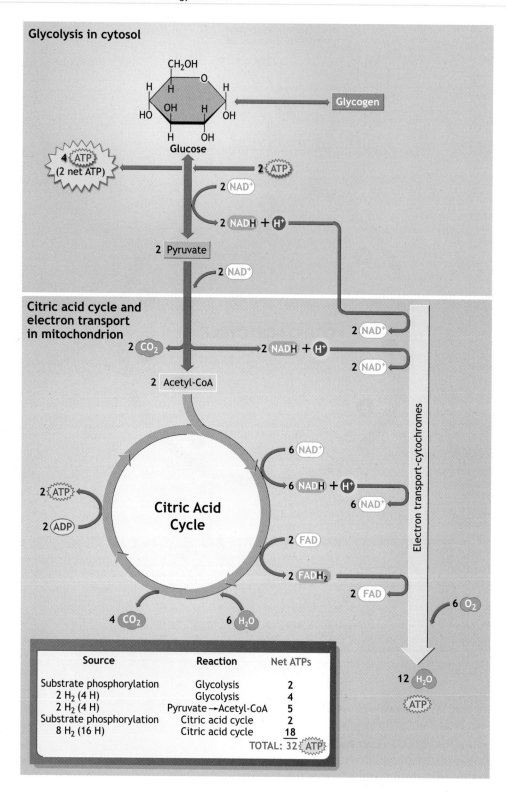

Glycolysis in cytosol

Citric acid cycle and electron transport in mitochondrion

Source	Reaction	Net ATPs
Substrate phosphorylation	Glycolysis	2
2 H₂ (4 H)	Glycolysis	4
2 H₂ (4 H)	Pyruvate →Acetyl-CoA	5
Substrate phosphorylation	Citric acid cycle	2
8 H₂ (16 H)	Citric acid cycle	18
	TOTAL:	32 ATP

Figure 5.20 A net yield of 32 ATPs from energy transfer during the complete oxidation of one glucose molecule in glycolysis, citric acid cycle, and electron transport.

acid cycle), 28 ATP molecules regenerate during oxidative phosphorylation.

Some textbooks quote a net yield of 36 to 38 ATP molecules from glucose catabolism. Depending on which shuttle system (the glycerol–phosphate or malate–aspartate) transports NADH with H$^+$ into the mitochondrion and the ATP yield per NADH oxidation used in the computations.

One must temper the *theoretical* values for ATP yield in energy metabolism in light of recent biochemical experiments that suggests an overestimate because only 30 to 32 ATP actually enter the cell's cytoplasm. The differentiation between theoretical versus actual ATP yield may result from the added energy cost to transport ATP out of the mitochondria.

ENERGY RELEASE FROM FAT

Stored fat represents the body's most plentiful source of potential energy. Relative to carbohydrate and protein, stored fat provides almost unlimited energy. The fuel reserves in an average young man represent between 60,000 and 100,000 kCal of energy from triacylglycerol in fat cells (adipocytes) and about 3000 kCal from intramuscular triacylglycerol stored in close proximity to muscle mitochondria. In contrast, the carbohydrate energy reserve only contributes about 2000 kCal to the total available energy pool.

Three specific energy sources for fat catabolism include:

1. Triacylglycerols stored directly within the muscle fiber in close proximity to the mitochondria (more in slow-twitch than in fast-twitch muscle fibers).
2. Circulating triacylglycerols in lipoprotein complexes that become hydrolyzed on the surface of a tissue's capillary endothelium.
3. Adipose tissue that provides circulating FFAs mobilized from triacylglycerols in adipose tissue.

Before energy release from fat, hydrolysis (**lipolysis**) in the cell's cytosol splits the triacylglycerol molecule into a glycerol molecule with three water-insoluble fatty acid molecules. **Hormone-sensitive lipase** (activated by cyclic AMP; see Chapter 12) catalyzes triacylglycerol breakdown as follows:

$$\text{Triacylglycerol} + 3\,H_2O \xrightarrow{\text{LIPASE}} \text{Glycerol} + 3\,\text{Fatty acids}$$

Adipocytes: Site of Fat Storage and Mobilization

All cells store some fat, but adipose tissue represents an active and major supplier of fatty acid molecules. Adipocytes synthesize and store triacylglycerol with these fat droplets occupying up to 95% of the cell's volume. When fatty acids diffuse from the adipocyte and enter the circulation, nearly all of them bind to plasma albumin for transport to the body's tissues as **free fatty acids** (**FFAs**). Fat utilization as an energy substrate varies in concert with blood flow in the active tissue. As blood flow increases with exercise, adipose tissue releases more FFA to active muscle for energy metabolism. The activity level of **lipoprotein lipase** (**LPL**), an enzyme synthesized within the cells and localized on the surface of its surrounding capillaries, facilitates the local cells' uptake of fatty acids for energy use or resynthesis (called re-esterification) of stored triacylglycerol in muscle and adipose tissue.

FFAs do not exist as truly "free" entities. At the muscle site, FFAs release from the albumin–FFA complex to move across the plasma membrane. Inside the muscle cell, FFAs either esterify to form intracellular triacylglycerol or bind with intramuscular proteins to enter the mitochondria for energy metabolism. Medium- and short-chain fatty acids do not depend on this carrier-mediated means of transport; most diffuse freely into the mitochondrion.

Breakdown of Glycerol and Fatty Acids

Figure 5.21 summarizes the pathways for the breakdown of the triacylglycerol molecule's glycerol and fatty acid components.

Glycerol The anaerobic reactions of glycolysis accept glycerol as 3-phosphoglyceraldehyde, which then degrades to pyruvate to form ATP by substrate-level phosphorylation. Hydrogen atoms pass to NAD^+, and the citric acid cycle oxidizes pyruvate. The complete breakdown of the single glycerol molecule in a triacylglycerol synthesizes 19 ATP molecules. Glycerol also provides carbon skeletons for glucose synthesis. *The gluconeogenic role of glycerol becomes prominent when*

Questions & Notes

Give the total ATP yield from the breakdown of one triacylglycerol (neutral fat) molecule.

Give the major function of β-oxidation.

Under what condition does gluconeogenesis predominate?

For Your Information

EXERCISE INTENSITY AND DURATION AFFECT FAT OXIDATION

Considerable fatty acid oxidation occurs during low-intensity exercise. For example, fat combustion almost totally powers exercise at 25% of aerobic capacity. Carbohydrate and fat contribute energy equally during more moderate-intensity exercise. Fat oxidation then gradually increases as exercise extends to 1 hour or more, and glycogen depletes. Toward the end of prolonged exercise (with glycogen reserves low), circulating FFAs supply nearly 80% of the total energy required.

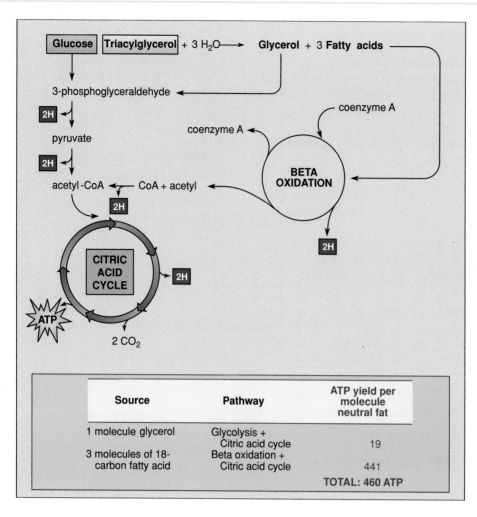

Source	Pathway	ATP yield per molecule neutral fat
1 molecule glycerol	Glycolysis + Citric acid cycle	19
3 molecules of 18-carbon fatty acid	Beta oxidation + Citric acid cycle	441
		TOTAL: 460 ATP

Figure 5.21 Breakdown of glycerol and fatty acid fragments of a triacylglycerol molecule. Glycerol enters the energy pathways of glycolysis. The fatty acid fragments enter the citric acid cycle via β-oxidation. The electron transport chain processes the released hydrogens from glycolysis, β-oxidation, and citric acid cycle metabolism to yield ATP.

glycogen reserves deplete from dietary restriction of carbohydrates, extended-duration exercise, or intense training.

Fatty Acids The fatty acid molecule transforms to acetyl-CoA in the mitochondrion during **β–oxidation** reactions (**Fig. 5.22**). This involves the successive release of 2-carbon acetyl fragments split from the fatty acid's long chain. ATP phosphorylates the reactions, water is added, hydrogens pass to NAD$^+$ and FAD, and acetyl-CoA forms when the acetyl fragment joins with coenzyme A. *This acetyl unit is the same as that generated from glucose breakdown.* β-oxidation continues until the entire fatty acid molecule degrades to acetyl-CoAs that directly enter the citric acid cycle. The respiratory chain oxidizes hydrogen released during fatty acid catabolism. Fatty acid breakdown relates directly with oxygen uptake. Oxygen must be present to join with hydrogen for β-oxidation to proceed; oxygen must also be present to join with hydrogen. Without oxygen (anaerobic conditions), hydrogen remains joined with NAD$^+$ and FAD and fat catabolism ceases.

Total Energy Transfer From Fat Catabolism

For each 18-carbon fatty acid molecule, 147 molecules of ADP phosphorylate to ATP during β-oxidation and citric acid cycle metabolism. Because each triacylglycerol molecule contains three fatty acid molecules, 441 ATP molecules (3 × 147 ATP) form from the triacylglycerol's fatty acid components. Also, 19 molecules of ATP form during glycerol breakdown to generate 460 molecules of ATP for each triacylglycerol molecule catabolized. This represents a considerable energy yield because only a net of 32 ATPs form when skeletal muscle catabolizes a glucose molecule.

Fats Burn in a Carbohydrate Flame

Interestingly, fatty acid breakdown depends in part on a continual background level of carbohydrate breakdown. Recall that acetyl-CoA enters the citric acid cycle by combining with oxaloacetate to form citrate (see **Fig. 5.19**). Depleting carbohydrate decreases pyruvate production during glycolysis. Diminished pyruvate further reduces citric acid cycle intermediates, slowing citric acid cycle activity. Fatty acid degradation in the citric acid cycle depends on sufficient oxaloacetate availability to combine with the acetyl-CoA formed during β-oxidation (see **Fig. 5.22**). When carbohydrate level decreases, the oxaloacetate level may become inadequate and reduce fat catabolism. In this sense, *fats burn in a carbohydrate flame.*

Metabolism Under Low-Carbohydrate Conditions   Oxaloacetate converts to pyruvate (see **Fig. 5.19**; note *two-way arrow*), which then can be synthesized to glucose. This occurs with inadequate carbohydrates perhaps from fasting, prolonged exercise, or diabetes due to their unavailability to combine with acetyl-CoA to form citrate. The liver converts the acetyl-CoA derived from the fatty acids into strong acid metabolites called *ketones* or ketone bodies. The three major ketone bodies include acetoacetic acid, β-hydroxybutyric acid, and acetone. Ketones are used as fuel primarily by muscles and to a more limited extent by nervous system tissues. Without ketone catabolism, they accumulate in the central circulation to produce the condition called **ketosis**. The high acidity of ketosis disrupts normal physiologic function, especially acid–base balance, which can ultimately be medically dangerous to health. Ketosis generally occurs more from an inadequate diet as in anorexia nervosa or diabetes than from prolonged exercise because muscle uses ketones as a fuel. During exercise, aerobically trained individuals use ketones more effectively than untrained individuals.

Slower Energy Release From Fat   A rate limit exists for how active muscle makes use of fatty acid. Aerobic training enhances this limit, but the

Questions & Notes

Briefly discuss what the phrase "fats burn in a carbohydrate flame" means.

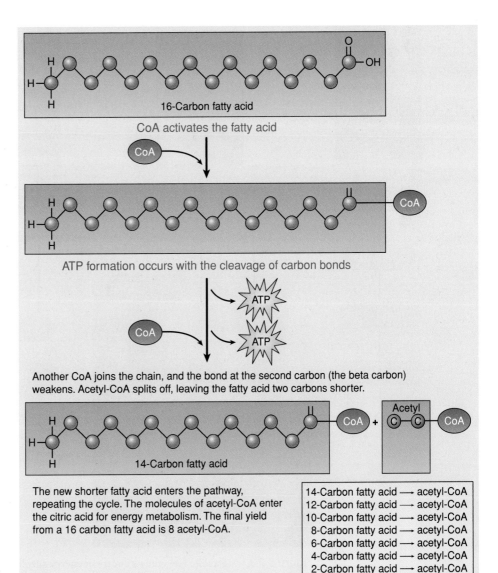

Figure 5.22   β-oxidation of a typical 16-carbon fatty acid. Fatty acids degrade to 2-carbon fragments that combine with CoA to form acetyl-CoA.

CoA activates the fatty acid

ATP formation occurs with the cleavage of carbon bonds

Another CoA joins the chain, and the bond at the second carbon (the beta carbon) weakens. Acetyl-CoA splits off, leaving the fatty acid two carbons shorter.

The new shorter fatty acid enters the pathway, repeating the cycle. The molecules of acetyl-CoA enter the citric acid for energy metabolism. The final yield from a 16 carbon fatty acid is 8 acetyl-CoA.

14-Carbon fatty acid ⟶ acetyl-CoA
12-Carbon fatty acid ⟶ acetyl-CoA
10-Carbon fatty acid ⟶ acetyl-CoA
8-Carbon fatty acid ⟶ acetyl-CoA
6-Carbon fatty acid ⟶ acetyl-CoA
4-Carbon fatty acid ⟶ acetyl-CoA
2-Carbon fatty acid ⟶ acetyl-CoA

rate of energy generated solely by fat breakdown still represents only about one-half of the value achieved with carbohydrate as the chief aerobic energy source. Thus, depleting muscle glycogen decreases the intensity that a muscle can sustain aerobic power output. Just as the hypoglycemic condition coincides with a "central" or neural fatigue, exercising with depleted muscle glycogen causes "peripheral" or local muscle fatigue.

Excess Macronutrients Regardless of Source Convert to Fat

Excess energy intake from any fuel source can be counterproductive. **Figure 5.23** shows how too much of any macronutrient converts to fatty acids, which then accumulate as body fat. Surplus dietary carbohydrate first fills the glycogen reserves. When these reserves fill, excess carbohydrate converts to triacylglycerols for storage in adipose tissue. Excess dietary fat calories move easily into the body's fat deposits. After they have been deaminated, the carbon residues of excess amino acids from protein readily convert to fat.

Hormones That Affect Fat Metabolism

Epinephrine, norepinephrine, glucagon, and growth hormone augment lipase activation and subsequent lipolysis and FFA mobilization from adipose tissue. Plasma concentrations of these lipogenic hormones increase during exercise to continually supply active muscles with energy-rich substrate. An intracellular mediator, **adenosine 3′,5′-cyclic monophosphate (cyclic AMP)**, activates hormone-sensitive lipase and thus regulates fat breakdown. Various lipid-mobilizing hormones that themselves do not enter the cell activate cyclic AMP. Circulating lactate, ketones, and particularly insulin inhibit cyclic AMP activation. Exercise training-induced increases in the activity level of skeletal muscle and adipose tissue lipases, including biochemical and vascular adaptations in the muscles themselves, enhance fat use for energy during moderate exercise. Paradoxically, excess body fat decreases the availability of fatty acids during exercise. Chapter 12 presents a more detailed evaluation of hormone regulation during exercise and training.

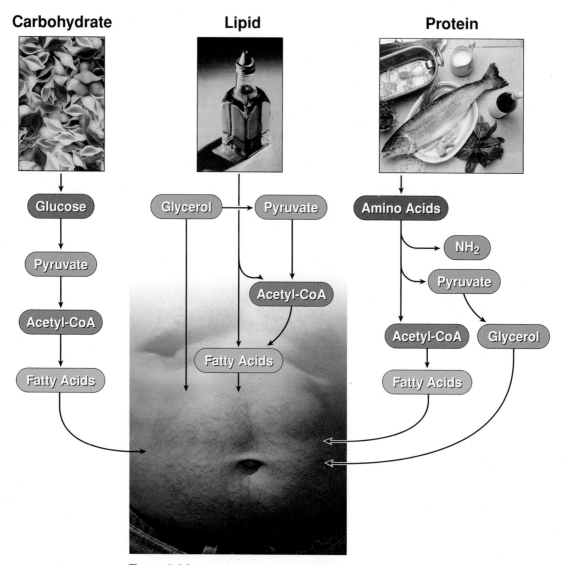

Figure 5.23 Metabolic fate of macronutrient energy surplus.

The availability of fatty acid molecules regulates fat breakdown or synthesis. After a meal, when energy metabolism remains relatively low, digestive processes increase FFA and triacylglycerol delivery to cells; this in turn stimulates triacylglycerol synthesis. In contrast, moderate exercise increases fatty acid use for energy, which reduces their cellular concentration. The decrease in intracellular FFAs stimulates triacylglycerol breakdown into glycerol and fatty acid components. Concurrently, hormonal release triggered by exercise stimulates adipose tissue lipolysis to further augment FFA delivery to active muscle.

ENERGY RELEASE FROM PROTEIN

Figure 5.24 illustrates how protein supplies intermediates at three different levels that have energy-producing capabilities. Protein acts as an energy substrate during long-duration, endurance-type activities. The amino acids (primarily the branched-chain amino acids leucine, isoleucine, valine, glutamine, and aspartic acid) first convert to a form that readily enters pathways for energy release. This conversion requires removing nitrogen from the amino acid molecule, a process known as deamination (refer to Chapter 2). The liver

Questions & Notes

Discuss the fate of excess energy intake.

Briefly describe the role of cyclic AMP in fat metabolism.

Briefly discuss the effects of exercise training on fat metabolism.

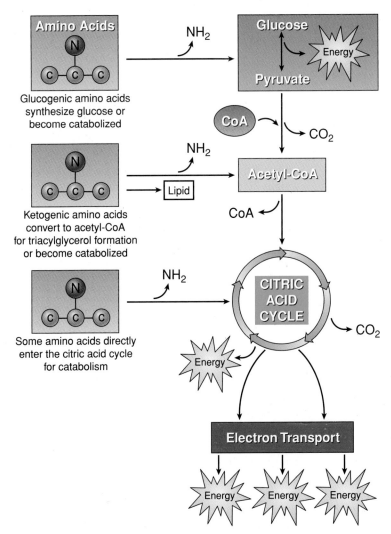

Figure 5.24 Protein-to-energy pathways.

BOX 5.2 CLOSE UP

How to Estimate Individual Protein Requirements

Total body protein remains constant when nitrogen intake from protein in food balances its excretion in the feces, urine, and sweat. An imbalance in the body's nitrogen content provides (1) an accurate estimate of either protein's depletion or accumulation and (2) a measure of the adequacy of dietary protein intake. Evaluating the nitrogen balance can estimate human protein requirements under various conditions, including intense exercise training.

The magnitude and direction of nitrogen balance in individuals engaged in exercise training depends on many factors, including training status; quality and quantity of protein consumed; total energy intake; the body's glycogen levels; and intensity, duration, and type of exercise performed.

MEASURING NITROGEN BALANCE

Nitrogen Intake. Estimate protein intake (in grams) by carefully measuring total food consumed over a 24-hour period. Determine nitrogen quantity (in grams) by assuming protein contains 16% nitrogen. Then:

$$\text{Total nitrogen intake (g)} = \text{Total protein intake (g)} \times 0.16$$

Nitrogen Output. Researchers determine nitrogen output by collecting all of the nitrogen excreted over the same period that assessed nitrogen intake. This involves collecting nitrogen loss from urine, lungs, sweat, and feces. A simplified method estimates nitrogen output by measuring urinary urea nitrogen (UUN; plus 4 g to account for other sources of nitrogen loss):

$$\text{Total nitrogen output} = \text{UUN} + 4\,\text{g}$$

Example
Male, age, 22 years; total body mass, 75 kg; total energy intake (food diary), 2100 kCal; protein intake (food diary), 63 g; UUN (collection and analysis of urine output), 8 g

$$\begin{aligned}
\text{Nitrogen balance} &= \text{nitrogen intake (g)} - \\
&\quad \text{nitrogen output (g)} \\
&= (63\,\text{g} \times 0.16) - (8\,\text{g} + 4\,\text{g}) \\
&= -1.92\,\text{g}
\end{aligned}$$

This example shows that a daily negative nitrogen balance of -1.92 g occurred because estimated protein catabolized in metabolism exceeded its replacement through dietary protein. To correct this deficiency and achieve nitrogen (protein) balance, the person would need to increase his daily protein intake.

Estimated Daily Protein Needs	
CONDITION	PROTEIN NEEDS g · kg BW
Normal, healthy	0.8–1.0
Fever, fracture, infection	1.5–2.0
Protein depleted	1.5–2.0
Extensive burns	1.5–3.0
Intensive training	0.8–1.5

ESTIMATING INDIVIDUAL PROTEIN REQUIREMENTS
The table above estimates average protein needs of adults under different conditions. For a healthy person who weighs 70 kg, the protein requirement equals 56 g.

$$0.8\,\text{g·kg}^{-1} \times 70\,\text{kg} = 56\,\text{g}$$

The same person with a chronic infection or in a protein-depleted state would require an upper-range estimate of 140 g of protein daily.

$$2.0\,\text{g·kg}^{-1} \times 70\,\text{kg} = 140\,\text{g}$$

serves as the main site of deamination. However, skeletal muscle also contains enzymes that remove nitrogen from an amino acid and pass it to other compounds during transamination (removal of nitrogen usually occurs when an amine group from a donor amino acid transfers to an acceptor acid from a new amino acid; refer to Chapter 1). In this way, the muscle directly uses for energy the carbon skeleton byproducts of donor amino acids. Enzyme levels for transamination favorably adapt to exercise training; this may further facilitate protein's use as an energy substrate. Only when an amino acid loses its nitrogen-containing amine group does the remaining compound (usually one of the citric acid cycle's reactive compounds) contribute to ATP formation. Some amino acids are **glucogenic**; when deaminated, they yield intermediate products for glucose synthesis via gluconeogenesis. In the liver, for example, pyruvate forms when alanine loses its amino group and gains a double-bond oxygen; this allows glucose synthesis from pyruvate. This gluconeogenic method is an important adjunct to the Cori cycle for providing glucose during prolonged exercise that depletes glycogen reserves. Similar to fat and carbohydrate, certain amino acids are **ketogenic**; they cannot synthesize to glucose, but instead when consumed in excess synthesize to fat.

Regulating Energy Metabolism

Electron transfer and subsequent energy release normally tightly couple to ADP phosphorylation. Without ADP availability for phosphorylation to ATP, electrons do not shuttle down the respiratory chain to oxygen. *Metabolites that either inhibit or activate enzymes at key control points in the oxidative pathways modulate regulatory control of glycolysis and the citric acid cycle.* Each pathway contains at least one enzyme considered *rate limiting* because the enzyme controls the overall speed of that pathway's reactions. *Cellular ADP concentration exerts the greatest effect on the rate-limiting enzymes that control macronutrient energy metabolism.* This mechanism for respiratory control makes sense because any increase in ADP signals a need to supply energy to restore depressed ATP levels. Conversely, high cellular ATP levels indicate a relatively low energy requirement. From a broader perspective, ADP concentrations function as a cellular *feedback mechanism* to maintain a relative constancy (homeostasis) in the level of energy currency required for biologic work. Other rate-limiting modulators include cellular levels of phosphate, cyclic AMP, AMP-activated protein kinase (AMPK), calcium, NAD^+, citrate, and pH. More specifically, ATP and NADH serve as enzyme inhibitors, and intracellular calcium, ADP, and NAD^+ function as activators. This form of chemical feedback allows rapid metabolic adjustment to the cells' energy needs. Within a resting cell, the ATP concentration considerably exceeds the concentration of ADP by about 500:1. A decrease in the ATP:ADP ratio and intramitochondrial $NADH:NAD^+$ ratio, as occurs when exercise begins, signals a need for increased metabolism of stored nutrients. In contrast, relatively low levels of energy demand maintain high ratios of ATP to ADP and NADH to NAD^+, which depress the rate of energy metabolism.

Independent Effects No single chemical regulator dominates mitochondrial ATP production. In vitro (artificial environment outside the living organism) and in vivo (in the living organism) experiments show that changes in each of these compounds independently alter the rate of oxidative phosphorylation. All compounds exert regulatory effects, each contributing differently depending on energy demands, cellular conditions, and the specific tissue involved.

THE METABOLIC MILL

The "metabolic mill" illustrated in **Figure 5.25** depicts the citric acid cycle as the essential "connector" between macronutrient energy and the chemical energy of ATP. The citric acid cycle plays a much more important role than simply degrading pyruvate produced during glucose catabolism. Fragments from other organic compounds formed from fat and protein breakdown provide energy during citric acid cycle metabolism. Deaminated residues of excess amino acids enter the citric acid cycle at various intermediate stages. In contrast, the glycerol fragment of triacylglycerol catabolism gains entrance via the glycolytic pathway. Fatty acids become oxidized via β-oxidation to acetyl-CoA, which then enters the citric acid cycle directly.

In addition to its role in energy metabolism, the citric acid cycle serves as a metabolic hub to provide intermediates to synthesize nutrients for tissue maintenance and growth. For example, excess carbohydrates provide glycerol and acetyl fragments to synthesize triacylglycerol. Acetyl-CoA also functions as the starting point for synthesizing cholesterol and many hormones. In contrast, fatty acids do not contribute to glucose synthesis because pyruvate's conversion to acetyl-CoA does not reverse (notice the *one-way arrow* in **Fig. 5.25**). Many of the carbon compounds generated in citric acid cycle reactions provide the organic starting points for synthesizing nonessential amino acids. Amino acids with carbon skeletons resembling citric acid cycle intermediates after deamination synthesize to glucose.

ℚuestions & Notes

Estimate the protein requirements for the following individuals:

1. Healthy 18 year old male:

2. Healthy 30 year old female athlete:

3. 60 year old male recovering from burns:

Briefly describe what is ment by the term "rate-limiting enzyme".

 For Your Information

EXCESS PROTEIN ACCUMULATES FAT

Athletes and others who believe that taking protein supplements builds muscle should beware. Extra protein consumed above the body's requirement (easily achieved with a well-balanced "normal" diet) ends up either catabolized for energy or converted to body fat! If an athlete wants to add fat, excessive protein intake achieves this end; this excess does *not* contribute to muscle tissue synthesis.

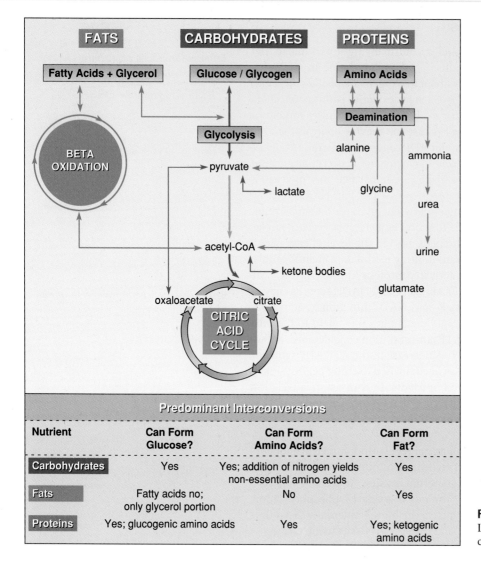

Figure 5.25 The "metabolic mill." Important interconversions between carbohydrates, fats, and proteins.

Predominant Interconversions

Nutrient	Can Form Glucose?	Can Form Amino Acids?	Can Form Fat?
Carbohydrates	Yes	Yes; addition of nitrogen yields non-essential amino acids	Yes
Fats	Fatty acids no; only glycerol portion	No	Yes
Proteins	Yes; glucogenic amino acids	Yes	Yes; ketogenic amino acids

SUMMARY

1. The complete breakdown of 1 mole of glucose liberates 689 kCal of energy. Of this total, ATP's bonds conserve about 233 kCal (34%), with the remainder dissipated as heat.

2. During glycolytic reactions in the cell's cytosol, a net of 2 ATP molecules form during anaerobic substrate-level phosphorylation.

3. In intense exercise, when hydrogen oxidation does not keep pace with its production, pyruvate temporarily binds hydrogen to form lactate.

4. In the mitochondrion, the second stage of carbohydrate breakdown converts pyruvate to acetyl-CoA. Acetyl-CoA then progresses through the citric acid cycle.

5. Hydrogen atoms released during glucose breakdown oxidize via the respiratory chain; the energy generated couples to ADP phosphorylation.

6. Oxidation of one glucose molecule in skeletal muscle yields a total of 32 ATP molecules (net gain).

7. Adipose tissue serves as an active and major supplier of fatty acid molecules.

8. The breakdown of a triacylglycerol molecule yields about 460 molecules of ATP. Fatty acid catabolism requires oxygen.

9. Protein can serve as an energy substrate. When deamination removes nitrogen from an amino acid molecule, the remaining carbon skeleton can enter metabolic pathways to produce ATP aerobically.

10. Numerous interconversions take place among the food nutrients. Fatty acids are an exception; they cannot be synthesized to glucose.

11. Fatty acids require a minimum level of carbohydrate breakdown for their continual catabolism for energy in the metabolic mill.

12. Cellular ADP concentration exerts the greatest effect on the rate-limiting enzymes that control energy metabolism.

THOUGHT QUESTIONS

1. How does aerobic and anaerobic energy metabolism affect optimal energy transfer capacity for a (1) 100-m sprinter, (2) 400-m hurdler, and (3) marathon runner?

2. How can elite marathoners run 26.2 miles at a pace of 5 minutes per mile, yet very few can run just 1 mile in 4 minutes?

3. In prolonged aerobic exercise such as marathon running, explain why exercise capacity diminishes when glycogen reserves deplete even though stored fat contains more than adequate energy reserves.

4. Is it important for weight lifters and sprinters to have a high capacity to consume oxygen? Explain.

5. From an exercise perspective, what are some advantages of having diverse sources of potential energy for synthesizing the cells' energy currency ATP?

SELECTED REFERENCES

Achten, J., Jeukendrup, A.E.: Optimizing fat oxidation through exercise and diet. *Nutrition*, 20(7–8):716, 2004.

Alberts, B., et al.: *Essential Cell Biology: An Introduction to the Molecular Biology of the Cell.* 2nd Ed. New York: Garland Publishers, 2003.

Åstrand, P.O., et al.: *Textbook of Work Physiology. Physiological Bases of Exercise.* 4th Ed. Champaign, IL: Human Kinetics, 2003.

Barnes, B.R., et al.: 5'-AMP-activated protein kinase regulates skeletal muscle glycogen content and ergogenics. *FASEB J.*, 19:773, 2005.

Berg, J.M., et al.: *Biochemistry.* 6th Ed. San Francisco: W.H. Freeman, 2006.

Binzoni, T.: Saturation of the lactate clearance mechanisms different from the "actate shuttle" determines the anaerobic threshold: prediction from the bioenergetic model. *J. Physiol. Anthropol. Appl. Human Sci.*, 24:175, 2005.

Brooks, G.A., et al.: *Exercise Physiology: Human Bioenergetics and Its Applications.* 4th Ed. New York: McGraw-Hill, 2004.

Brooks, G.A.: Cell-cell and intracellular lactate shuttles. *J. Physiol.*, 1;587:5591, 2009.

Brooks, G.A.: What does glycolysis make and why is it important. *J. Appl. Physiol.*, 108:1450, 2010.

Campbell, M.K., Farrell, S.O.: *Biochemistry.* 5th Ed. London: Thomson Brooks/Cole, 2007.

Campbell, P.N., et al.: *Biochemistry Illustrated.* 5th Ed. Philadelphia: Churchill Livingstone, 2005.

Carr, D.B., et al.: A reduced-fat diet and aerobic exercise in Japanese Americans with impaired glucose tolerance decreases intra-abdominal fat and improves insulin sensitivity but not beta-cell function. *Diabetes*, 54:340, 2005.

DiNuzzo, M., et al.: Changes in glucose uptake rather than lactate shuttle take center stage in subserving neuroenergetics: evidence from mathematical modeling. *J. Cereb. Blood Flow Metab.*, 30:586, 2010.

Enqvist, J.K., et al.: Energy turnover during 24 hours and 6 days of adventure racing. *Sports Sci.*, 28:947, 2010.

Fatouros, I.G., et al.: Oxidative stress responses in older men during endurance training and detraining. *Med. Sci. Sports Exerc.*, 36:2065, 2004.

Fox, S.I.: *Human Physiology.* 10th Ed. New York: McGraw-Hill, 2008.

Hashimoto, T., Brooks, G.A.: Mitochondrial lactate oxidation complex and an adaptive role for lactate production. *Med. Sci. Sports Exerc.*, 40:486, 2008.

Henderson, G.C., et al.: Pyruvate shuttling during rest and exercise before and after endurance training in men. *J. Appl. Physiol.*, 97:317, 2004.

Henderson G.C., et al.: Plasma triglyceride concentrations are rapidly reduced following individual bouts of endurance exercise in women. *Eur. J. Appl. Physiol.*, 109:721, 2010.

Horton, R.: *Principles of Biochemistry.* 4th Ed. Engelwood Cliffs, NJ: Prentice-Hall, 2005.

Jeukendrup, A.E., Wallis, G.A.: Measurement of substrate oxidation during exercise by means of gas exchange measurements. *Int. J. Sports Med.*, 26 Suppl 1:S28, 2005.

Jones D.E., et al.: Abnormalities in pH handling by peripheral muscle and potential regulation by the autonomic nervous system in chronic fatigue syndrome. *J. Intern. Med.*, 267:394, 2010.

Jorgensen, S.B., et al.: Role of AMPK in skeletal muscle metabolic regulation and adaptation in relation to exercise. *J. Physiol.*, 574 (Pt 1):17, 2006.

Kiens, B.: Skeletal muscle lipid metabolism in exercise and insulin resistance. *Physiol Rev.*, 86:205, 2006.

Lehninger, A.H., et al.: *Principles of Biochemistry.* 5th Ed. New York: WH Freeman, 2008.

Li, J., et al.: Interstitial ATP and norepinephrine concentrations in active muscle. *Circulation*, 111:2748, 2005.

Marieb, E.N.: *Human Anatomy and Physiology*. 8th Ed. Redwood City, CA: Pearson Education/Benjamin Cummings, 2009.

Peres, S.B., et al.: Endurance exercise training increases insulin responsiveness in isolated adipocytes through IRS/PI3-kinase/Akt pathway. *J. Appl. Physiol.*, 98:1037, 2005.

Petibois, C., Deleris, G.: FT-IR spectrometry analysis of plasma fatty acyl moieties selective mobilization during endurance exercise. *Biopolymers*, 77:345, 2005.

Revan, S., et al.: Short duration exhaustive running exercise does not modify lipid hydroperoxide, glutathione peroxidase and catalase. *J. Sports Med. Phys. Fitness.*, 50:235, 2010.

Ricquier, D.: Respiration uncoupling and metabolism in the control of energy expenditure. *Proc. Nutr. Soc.*, 64:47, 2005.

Roepstorff, C., et al.: Regulation of oxidative enzyme activity and eukaryotic elongation factor 2 in human skeletal muscle: influence of gender and exercise. *Acta. Physiol. Scand.*, 184:215, 2005.

Rose, A.J., Richter E.A.: Skeletal muscle glucose uptake during exercise: how is it regulated? *Physiology*, 20:260, 2005.

Widmaier, E.P.: *Vander's Human Physiology*. 11th ed. New York: McGraw-Hill, 2007.

Tarnopolsky, M.: Protein requirements for endurance athletes. *Nutrition*, 20:662, 2004.

Tauler, P., et al.: Pre-exercise antioxidant enzyme activities determine the antioxidant enzyme erythrocyte response to exercise. *J. Sports Sci.*, 23:5, 2005.

van Loon, L.J.: Use of intramuscular triacylglycerol as a substrate source during exercise in humans. *J. Appl. Physiol.*, 97:1170, 2004.

Veldhorst, M.A., et al.: Presence or absence of carbohydrates and the proportion of fat in a high-protein diet affect appetite suppression but not energy expenditure in normal-weight human subjects fed in energy balance. *Br. J. Nutr.*, 22:1, 2010.

Venables, M.C., et al.: Determinants of fat oxidation during exercise in healthy men and women: a cross-sectional study. *J. Appl. Physiol.*, 98:160, 2005.

Watson, J.D., Berry, A.: *DNA: The Secret of Life*. New York: Knopf, 2003.

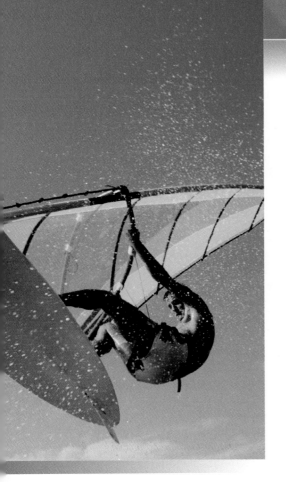

Chapter 6

Human Energy Transfer During Exercise

CHAPTER OBJECTIVES

- Identify the body's three energy systems and explain their relative contributions to exercise intensity and duration.

- Describe differences in blood lactate threshold between sedentary and aerobically trained individuals.

- Outline the time course for oxygen uptake during 10 minutes of moderate exercise.

- Draw a figure showing the relationship between oxygen uptake and exercise intensity during progressively increasing increments of exercise to maximum.

- Differentiate between the body's two types of muscle fibers.

- Explain differences in the pattern of recovery oxygen uptake from moderate and exhaustive exercise, and include factors that account for the excess post-exercise oxygen consumption or EPOC from each exercise mode.

- Outline optimal recovery procedures from steady-rate and non–steady-rate exercise.

Physical activity provides the greatest stimulus to energy metabolism. In sprint running and cycling, whole-body energy output in world-class competitors exceeds 40 to 50 times their resting energy expenditure. In contrast, during less intense but sustained marathon running, energy requirements still exceed resting level by 20 to 25 times. This chapter explains how the body's diverse energy systems interact to transfer energy during rest and different exercise intensities.

IMMEDIATE ENERGY: THE ADENOSINE TRIPHOSPHATE– PHOSPHOCREATINE SYSTEM

Performances of short duration and high intensity, such as the 100-m sprint, 25-m swim, smashing a tennis ball during the serve, or thrusting a heavy weight upward, require an immediate and rapid energy supply. The two high-energy phosphates adenosine triphosphate (ATP) and phosphocreatine (PCr) stored within muscles almost exclusively provide this energy. ATP and PCr are termed **phosphagens**.

Each kilogram (kg) of skeletal muscle stores approximately 5 millimoles (mmol) of ATP and 15 mmol of PCr. For a person with 30 kg of muscle mass, this amounts to between 570 and 690 mmol of phosphagens. If physical activity activates 20 kg of muscle, then stored phosphagen energy could power a brisk walk for 1 minute, a slow run for 20 to 30 seconds, or all-out sprint running and swimming for about 6 to 8 seconds. In the 100-m dash, for example, the body cannot maintain maximum speed for longer than this time, and the runner actually slows down toward the end of the race. *Thus, the quantity of intramuscular phosphagens substantially influences "all-out" energy for brief durations.* The enzyme creatine kinase, which triggers PCr hydrolysis to resynthesize ATP, regulates the rate of phosphagen breakdown.

SHORT-TERM ENERGY: THE LACTIC ACID SYSTEM

The intramuscular phosphagens must continually resynthesize rapidly for strenuous exercise to continue beyond a brief period. During intense exercise, intramuscular stored glycogen provides the energy source to phosphorylate ADP during anaerobic glycogenolysis, forming lactate (see Chapter 5, Figs. 5.13 and 5.15).

With inadequate oxygen supply and utilization, all of the hydrogens formed in rapid glycolysis fail to oxidize; in this case, pyruvate converts to lactate in the chemical reaction: Pyruvate + 2H → Lactate. This enables the continuation of rapid ATP formation by anaerobic substrate-level phosphorylation. Anaerobic energy for ATP resynthesis from glycolysis can be viewed as "reserve fuel" activated when the oxygen demand:oxygen utilization ratio exceeds 1.0, as

occurs during the last phase "sprint" of a 1-mile race. Rapid ATP production from rapid glycolysis remains crucial during a 440-m run or 100-m swim and in **multiple-sprint sports** such as ice hockey, field hockey, and soccer. These activities require rapid energy transfer that exceeds that supplied by stored phosphagens. If the intensity of "all-out" exercise decreases (thereby extending exercise duration), lactate buildup correspondingly decreases.

Blood Lactate Accumulation

Chapter 5 points out that some lactate continually forms even under resting conditions. However, lactate removal by heart muscle and nonactive skeletal muscle balances its production, yielding no "net" lactate buildup. Only when lactate removal fails to match production does blood lactate accumulate. *Aerobic activities produce cellular adaptations that increase rates of lactate removal so that only exercise at higher intensities produces lactate accumulation.* **Figure 6.1** illustrates the general relationship between oxygen uptake, expressed as a percentage of maximum, and blood lactate level during light, moderate, and strenuous exercise in endurance athletes and untrained individuals. During light and moderate exercise in both groups, aerobic metabolism adequately meets energy demands. Non-active tissues rapidly oxidize any lactate that forms, permitting blood lactate to remain fairly stable (i.e., no net blood lactate accumulates) even though oxygen uptake increases.

Blood lactate begins to increase exponentially at approximately 55% of a healthy, untrained person's maximal capacity for aerobic metabolism. The usual

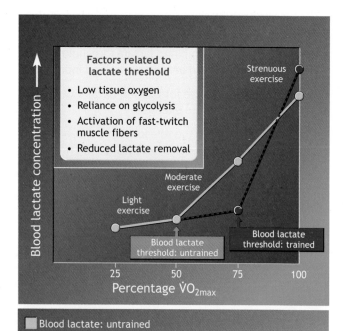

Figure 6.1 Blood lactate concentration for trained and untrained subjects at different levels of exercise expressed as a percentage of maximal oxygen consumption ($\dot{V}O_{2max}$).

explanation for increased blood lactate during intense exercise assumes a relative tissue hypoxia or lack of oxygen. Even though poor experimental evidence exists for direct exercise-induced hypoxia within muscle, indirect measures support the notion of reduced cellular oxygen content. During hypoxia, anaerobic rapid glycolysis partially meets any energy requirement, allowing hydrogen release to exceed its oxidation down the respiratory (electron transport) chain. Lactate forms as excess hydrogens produced during glycolysis attach to pyruvate (see Fig. 5.15). Lactate formation continues to increase at higher levels of exercise intensity when active muscle cannot meet the additional energy demands aerobically. *Blood lactate accumulates only when its disappearance (oxidation or substrate conversion) does not match its production rate.*

As **Figure 6.1** illustrates, trained individuals show a similar pattern of blood lactate accumulation as untrained individuals, except for the point at which blood lactate sharply increases. The point of abrupt increase in blood lactate, known as the **blood lactate threshold** also termed **onset of blood lactate accumulation or OBLA**, occurs at a higher percentage of an endurance athlete's $\dot{V}O_{2max}$. This favorable metabolic response could result from genetic endowment (e.g., muscle fiber type distribution) or specific local muscle adaptations with training that favor less lactate formation and its more rapid removal rate. For example, endurance training typically increases capillary density and mitochondria size and number. Training also increases the concentrations of various enzymes, and transfer agents involved in aerobic metabolism. Such alterations enhance the cells' capacity to generate ATP aerobically, particularly via fatty acid breakdown. These training adaptations also extend exercise intensity before the onset of blood lactate accumulation. For example, world-class endurance athletes sustain exercise intensities at 85% to 90% of their maximum capacity for aerobic metabolism before blood lactate accumulates.

The lactate formed in one part of an active muscle can be oxidized by other fibers in the same muscle or by less active neighboring muscle. Lactate uptake by less active muscle fibers depresses blood lactate levels during light to moderate exercise and conserves blood glucose and muscle glycogen in prolonged exercise. We discuss the concept of the blood lactate threshold and its relation to endurance performance in Chapter 13.

Lactate-Producing Capacity

Specific sprint-power anaerobic training produces high blood lactate levels during maximal exercise, which then decrease when training ceases. Sprint-power athletes often achieve 20% to 30% higher blood lactate levels than untrained counterparts during maximal short-duration exercise. One or more of the following three mechanisms explains this response:

1. Improved motivation that accompanies exercise training.
2. Increased intramuscular glycogen stores that accompany training probably allow a greater contribution of energy via anaerobic glycolysis.
3. Training-induced increase in glycolytic-related enzymes, particularly phosphofructokinase. The 20% increase in glycolytic enzymes falls well below the two- to threefold increase in aerobic enzymes with endurance training.

*Q*uestions & Notes

What 2 compounds comprise the high-energy phosphates?

1.

2.

List 3 examples of sporting events that rely almost exclusively on the immediate energy system.

1.

2.

3.

The point of abrupt increase in blood lactate concentration during exercise of increasing intensity is known as the_____ _____ _____.

Give the percentage of the maximal capacity for aerobic metabolism where blood lactate begins to increase in healthy, untrained persons.

Give the percentage of $\dot{V}O_{2max}$ where blood lactate begins to increase in world-class endurance athletes.

Give the percentage increase in blood lactate levels generated by anaerobic athletes compared to untrained individuals.

ⓘ For Your Information

LACTIC ACID AND pH

Hydrogen ions (H^+) dissociating from lactic acid, rather than undissociated lactate (La^-), present the primary problem to the body. At normal pH levels, lactic acid almost immediately completely dissociates to H^+ and La^- ($C_3H_5O_3^-$). There are few problems if the amount of free H^+ does not exceed the body's ability to buffer them and maintain the pH at a relatively stable level. The pH decreases when excessive lactic acid (H^+) exceeds the body's immediate buffering capacity. Discomfort occurs and performance decreases as the blood becomes more acidic.

Blood Lactate as an Energy Source

In Chapter 5 we pointed out how blood lactate serves as substrate for glucose retrieval (gluconeogenesis) and as a direct fuel source for active muscle. Isotope tracer studies of muscle and other tissues reveal that lactate produced in fast-twitch muscle fibers can circulate to other fast- or slow-twitch fibers for conversion to pyruvate. Pyruvate, in turn, converts to acetyl-CoA for entry to the citric acid cycle for aerobic energy metabolism. Such **lactate shuttling** between cells enables glycogenolysis in one cell to supply other cells with fuel for oxidation. *This makes muscle not only a major site of lactate production but also a primary tissue for lactate removal via oxidation.*

A muscle oxidizes much of the lactate produced by it without releasing lactate into the blood. The liver also accepts muscle-generated lactate from the bloodstream and synthesizes it to glucose through the Cori cycle's gluconeogenic reactions (see Chapter 5). Glucose derived from lactate takes one of two routes: (1) it returns in the blood to skeletal muscle for energy metabolism or (2) it synthesizes to glycogen for storage. These two uses of lactate make this anaerobic byproduct of intense exercise a valuable metabolic substrate and certainly not an unwanted product.

LONG-TERM ENERGY: THE AEROBIC SYSTEM

Glycolysis releases anaerobic energy rapidly, yet only a relatively small total ATP yield results from this pathway. In contrast, aerobic metabolic reactions provide for the greatest portion of energy transfer, particularly when exercise duration exceeds 2 to 3 minutes.

Oxygen Uptake During Exercise

The curve in **Figure 6.2** illustrates oxygen uptake during each minute of a 20-minute slow jog continued at a steady pace. The vertical y-axis indicates the uptake of oxygen by the body (referred to as oxygen uptake or oxygen consumption); the horizontal x-axis displays exercise time. The abbreviation $\dot{V}O_2$ indicates oxygen uptake, where the **V** denotes the volume consumed; the dot placed above the $\dot{V}$ expresses oxygen uptake as a per minute value. Oxygen uptake during any minute can be determined easily by locating time on the x-axis and its corresponding point for oxygen uptake on the Y-axis. For example, after running 4 minutes, oxygen uptake equals approximately $17 \text{ mL} \cdot \text{kg}^{-1} \cdot \text{min}^{-1}$.

Oxygen uptake increases rapidly during the first minutes of exercise and reaches a relative plateau between minutes 4 and 6. Oxygen uptake then remains relatively stable throughout the remainder of exercise. The flat portion, or plateau, of the oxygen uptake curve represents the **steady rate of aerobic metabolism**—a balance between energy required by the body and the rate of aerobic ATP production. Oxygen-consuming reactions supply the energy for steady-rate exercise; any lactate produced either oxidizes or reconverts to glucose in the liver, kidneys, and skeletal muscles. *No net accumulation of blood lactate occurs under these steady-rate metabolic conditions.*

Many Levels of Steady Rate For some individuals, lying in bed, working around the house, and playing an occasional round of golf represent the activity spectrum for steady-rate metabolism. In contrast, a champion marathon runner covers 26.2 miles in slightly more than 2 hours and can still maintain a steady rate of aerobic metabolism. This sub–5-minute-per-mile pace represents a magnificent physiologic–metabolic accomplishment. Maintenance of the required level of aerobic metabolism necessitates well-developed functional capacities to deliver adequate oxygen to active muscles and process oxygen within muscle cells for aerobic ATP production.

Oxygen Deficit Note that the upward curve of oxygen uptake shown in **Figure 6.2** does not increase

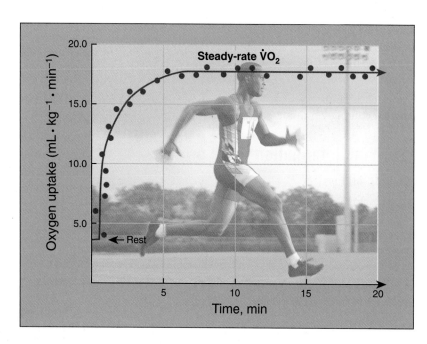

Figure 6.2 Time course of oxygen uptake during continuous jogging at a slow pace. The *dots* along the curve represent measured values of oxygen uptake determined by open-circuit spirometry.

instantaneously to a steady rate at the start of exercise. Instead, oxygen uptake remains considerably below the steady-rate level in the first minute of exercise even though the exercise energy requirement remains essentially unchanged throughout the activity period. The temporary "lag" in oxygen uptake occurs because ATP and PCr provide the muscles' immediate energy requirements without the need for oxygen. Even with experimentally increased oxygen availability and increased oxygen diffusion gradients at the tissue level, the initial increase in exercise oxygen consumption is *always* lower than the steady-rate oxygen consumption. Owing to the interaction of intrinsic inertia in cellular metabolic signals and enzyme activation and the relative sluggishness of oxygen delivery to the mitochondria, the hydrogens produced in energy metabolism do not immediately oxidize and combine with oxygen. Thus, a deficiency always exists in the oxygen uptake response to a new, higher steady-rate, regardless of activity mode or intensity.

The **oxygen deficit** *quantitatively represents the difference between the total oxygen consumed during exercise and an additional amount that would have been consumed if a steady-rate aerobic metabolism occurred immediately at the initiation of exercise.* Energy provided during the deficit phase of exercise represents, at least conceptually, a predominance of anaerobic energy transfer. Stated in metabolic terms, the oxygen deficit represents the quantity of energy produced from stored intramuscular phosphagens plus energy contributed from rapid glycolytic reactions. This yields phosphate-bond energy until oxygen uptake and energy demands reach steady rate.

Figure 6.3 depicts the relationship between the size of the oxygen deficit and the energy contribution from the ATP–PCr and lactic acid energy systems. Exercise that generates about a 3- to 4-L oxygen deficit substantially depletes

Questions & Notes

Explain oxygen deficit.

Briefly explain the benefits of lactate shuttling?

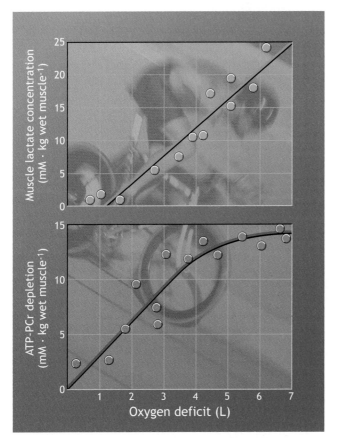

Figure 6.3 Muscle adenosine triphosphate (ATP) and phosphocreatine (PCr) depletion and muscle lactate concentration related to the oxygen deficit. (Adapted from Pernow, B., Karlsson, J.: Muscle ATP, CP and lactate in submaximal and maximal exercise. In: *Muscle Metabolism During Exercise.* Pernow, B., and Saltin, B. (eds.). New York: Plenum Press, 1971.)

For Your Information

LIMITED DURATION OF STEADY-RATE EXERCISE

Theoretically, exercise could continue indefinitely when performed at steady-rate aerobic metabolism. Factors other than motivation, however, limit the duration of steady-rate work. These include loss of important body fluids in sweat and depletion of essential nutrients, especially blood glucose and glycogen stored in the liver and active muscles.

BOX 6.1 CLOSE UP

Overtraining: Too Much of a Good Thing

With intense and prolonged training athletes can experience **overtraining**, **staleness**, or **burnout**. The overtrained condition reflects more than just a short-term inability to train as hard as usual or a slight dip in competition-level performance; rather, it involves a more chronic fatigue experienced during exercise workouts and subsequent recovery periods. Overtraining associates with sustained poor exercise performance, frequent infections (particularly of the upper respiratory tract), and a general malaise and loss of interest in high-level training. Injuries also are more frequent in the overtrained state. The specific symptoms of overtraining are highly individualized, with those outlined in the accompanying table most common. Little is known about the cause of this syndrome, although neuroendocrine alterations that affect the sympathetic nervous system, as well as alterations in immune function, are probably involved. These symptoms persist unless the athlete rests, with complete recovery requiring weeks or even months.

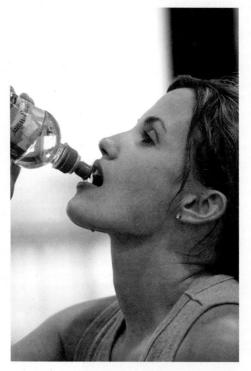

CARBOHYDRATES' POSSIBLE ROLE IN OVERTRAINING

A gradual depletion of the body's carbohydrate reserves with repeated strenuous training exacerbate the over-training syndrome. A pioneering study showed that after 3 successive days of running 16.1 km (10 miles), glycogen in the thigh muscle became nearly depleted. This occurred even though the runners' diets contained 40% to 60% of total calories as carbohydrates. In addition, glycogen use on the third day of the run averaged about 72% less than on day 1. The mechanism by which repeated occurrences of glycogen depletion may contribute to overtraining remains unclear.

TAPERING OFTEN HELPS

Overtraining symptoms may range from mild to severe. They more often occur in highly motivated individuals when a large increase in training occurs abruptly and when the overall training program does not include sufficient rest and recovery.

Overtraining symptoms often occur before season-ending competition. To achieve peak performance, athletes should reduce their training volume and increase their carbohydrate intake for at least several days before competition—a practice called **tapering**. The goal of tapering is to provide time for muscles to resynthesize glycogen to maximal levels and allow them to heal from training-induced damage.

OVERTRAINING SIGNS AND SYMPTOMS

Performance-Related Symptoms
1. Consistent performance decline
2. Persistent fatigue and sluggishness
3. Excessive recovery required after competitive events
4. Inconsistent performance

Physiologic-Related Symptoms
1. Decrease in maximum work capacity
2. Frequent headaches or stomach aches
3. Insomnia
4. Persistent low-grade stiffness and muscle or joint soreness

5. Frequent constipation or diarrhea
6. Unexplained loss of appetite and body mass
7. Amenorrhea
8. Elevated resting heart rate on waking

Psychologic-Related Symptoms
1. Depression
2. General apathy
3. Decreased self-esteem
4. Mood changes
5. Difficulty concentrating
6. Loss of competitive drive

the intramuscular high-energy phosphates. Consequently, this intensity of exercise continues only on a "pay-as-you-go" basis; ATP must be replenished continually through either glycolysis or the aerobic breakdown of carbohydrate, fat, and protein. Interestingly, lactate begins to increase in exercising muscle before the phosphagens attain their lowest levels. This means that glycolysis contributes anaerobic energy early in vigorous exercise before full utilization of the high-energy phosphates. *Energy for exercise does not merely result from a series of energy systems that "switch on" and "switch off" like a light switch. Rather, a muscle's energy supply represents a smooth transition between anaerobic and aerobic sources, with considerable overlap from one source of energy transfer to another.*

Oxygen Deficit in Trained and Untrained Individuals

Figure 6.4 shows the oxygen uptake response to submaximum cycle ergometer or treadmill exercise for a trained and an untrained person. Trained and untrained individuals show similar values for steady-rate oxygen uptake during light and moderate exercise. A trained person, however, achieves the steady-rate quicker; hence, this person has a smaller oxygen deficit for the same exercise duration compared with the untrained person. This indicates that the trained person consumes more total oxygen during exercise with a proportionately smaller anaerobic energy transfer component. A likely explanation relates to the trained person's more highly developed aerobic bioenergetic capacity. Greater aerobic power results from either improved central cardiovascular function or

For Your Information

OXYGEN UPTAKE AND BODY SIZE

To adjust for the effects of variations in body size on oxygen uptake (i.e., bigger people usually consume more oxygen), researchers frequently express oxygen uptake in terms of body mass (termed **relative oxygen uptake**) as milliliters of oxygen per kilogram of body mass per minute ($mL \cdot kg^{-1} \cdot min^{-1}$). At rest, this averages about 3.5 $mL \cdot kg^{-1} \cdot min^{-1}$ or of 1 metabolic equivalent (MET) or 245 $mL \cdot min^{-1}$ (**absolute oxygen uptake**) for a 70-kg person. Other means of relating oxygen uptake to aspects of body size and body composition include milliliters of oxygen per kilogram of fat-free body mass per minute ($mL \cdot kg\ FFM^{-1} \cdot min^{-1}$) and sometimes milliliters of oxygen per square centimeter of muscle cross-sectional area per minute ($mL \cdot cm\ MCSA^{-2} \cdot min^{-1}$).

Questions & Notes

List 2 symptoms of overtraining.

1.

2.

For the same level of work production (duration and intensity of effort), does a trained or an untrained person record a greater oxygen deficit? Explain.

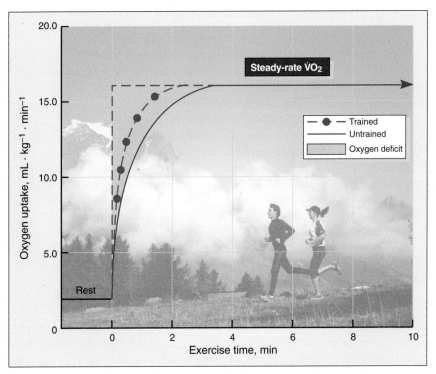

Figure 6.4 Oxygen uptake and oxygen deficit for trained and untrained individuals during submaximum cycle ergometer exercise. Both individuals reach the same steady-rate V̇O₂, but the trained person reaches it at a faster rate, reducing the oxygen deficit.

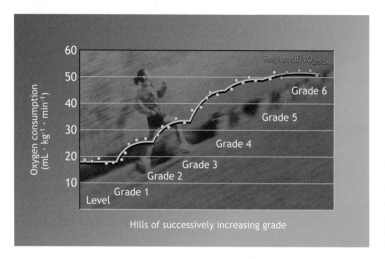

Figure 6.5 Attainment of maximal oxygen uptake ($\dot{V}O_{2max}$) while running up hills of increasing slope. This occurs in the region where a further increase in exercise intensity does not produce an additional or the expected increase in oxygen uptake. *Yellow and orange dots* represent measured values for oxygen uptake during the run up each hill.

training-induced local adaptations that increase a muscle's capacity to generate ATP aerobically. These adaptations for the trained person trigger an earlier onset of aerobic ATP production with less lactate formation.

MAXIMAL OXYGEN UPTAKE

Figure 6.5 depicts the curve for oxygen uptake during a series of constant-speed runs up six hills, each progressively steeper than the next. In the laboratory, these "hills" represent increasing treadmill elevations, raising the height of a step bench, providing greater resistance to pedaling a bicycle ergometer, or increasing the onward rush of water while a swimmer maintains speed in a swim flume. Each successive hill translates to an increase in exercise intensity requiring greater energy output and demand for aerobic metabolism. Increases in oxygen uptake relate linearly and in direct proportion to exercise intensity during the climb up the first several hills. The runner maintains speed up the last two hills, yet oxygen uptake does not increase by the same magnitude as in the prior hills. In fact, oxygen uptake does not increase during the run up the last hill. *The maximal oxygen uptake ($\dot{V}O_{2max}$) describes the highest oxygen uptake achieved despite increases in exercise intensity.* The $\dot{V}O_{2max}$ holds great physiologic significance because of its dependence on the functional capacity and integration of the many biologic systems required for oxygen supply, transport, delivery, and use.

The $\dot{V}O_{2max}$ indicates an individual's capacity to aerobically resynthese ATP. Exercise performed above $\dot{V}O_{2max}$ can only occur via energy transfer predominantly from anaerobic glycolysis with subsequent lactate formation. A large buildup of lactate, caused by the additional anaerobic muscular effort, disrupts the already high rate of energy transfer for the aerobic resynthesis of ATP. To borrow an analogy from business economics: supply (aerobic resynthesis of ATP) does not meet demand (aerobic energy required for muscular effort). An aerobic energy supply–demand imbalance impacts cellular processes so lactate accumulates with subsequent compromise of exercise performance.

Because of the importance of aerobic power in exercise physiology, subsequent chapters cover more detailed aspects of $\dot{V}O_{2max}$, including its measurement, physiologic significance, and role in endurance performance.

ENERGY TRANSFER IN FAST- AND SLOW-TWITCH MUSCLE FIBERS

Two distinct types of muscle fiber exist in humans. **Fast-twitch (FT)** or **type II muscle fibers** (with several subdivisions), possess rapid contraction speed and high capacity for glycolytic, anaerobic ATP production. Type II fibers become active during change-of-pace and stop-and-go activities such as basketball, soccer, and ice hockey. They also contribute increased force output when running or cycling up a hill while maintaining a constant speed or during all-out effort requiring rapid, powerful movements that depend almost exclusively on energy from anaerobic metabolism.

The second fiber-type, **slow-twitch (ST)** or **type I muscle fiber**, generates energy primarily through aerobic pathways. This fiber possesses relatively slow contraction speeds compared with type II fibers. Their capacity to generate ATP aerobically intimately relates to numerous large mitochondria and high levels of enzymes required for aerobic metabolism, particularly fatty acid catabolism. Slow-twitch muscle fibers primarily sustain continuous activities requiring a steady rate of aerobic energy transfer. Fatigue in endurance exercise associates with glycogen depletion in the muscles' type I and some type II muscle fibers. The predominance of slow-twitch muscle fibers contribute to high blood lactate thresholds among elite endurance athletes.

The preceding discussion suggests that a muscle's predominant fiber type contributes significantly to success in certain sports or physical activities. Chapter 14 explores this idea more fully, including other considerations concerning metabolic, contractile, and fatigue characteristics of each fiber type.

ENERGY SPECTRUM OF EXERCISE

Figure 6.6 depicts the relative contributions of anaerobic and aerobic energy sources for various durations of maximal exercise. The data represent estimates from laboratory experiments of all-out treadmill running and stationary bicycling. They also relate to other activities by juxaposing the appropriate time relationships. For example, a 100-m sprint run equates to any all-out 10-second activity, but an 800-m run lasts approximately 2 minutes. All-out exercise for 1 minute includes the 400-m sprint in track, the 100-m swim, and repeated full-court presses during a basketball game.

Intensity and Duration Determine the Blend

The body's energy transfer systems can be viewed along a continuum of exercise bioenergetics. Anaerobic sources supply most of the energy for fast movements and during increased resistance to movement at a given speed. Also, when movement begins at either fast or slow speed (from performing a front handspring to starting a marathon run), the intramuscular phosphagens provide immediate anaerobic energy for the required initial muscle actions.

At the short-duration extreme of maximum effort, the intramuscular phosphagens supply the major energy for the exercise. The ATP–PCr and lactic acid systems contribute about one-half of the energy required for "best-effort" exercise lasting 2 minutes; aerobic reactions contribute the remainder. Top performance in all-out, 2-minute exercise requires well-developed capacities for

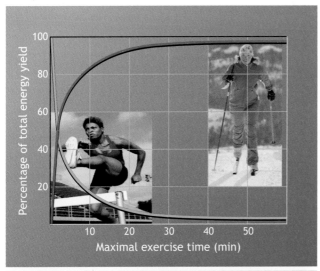

Duration of maximal exercise									
	Seconds				Minutes				
	10	30	60	2	4	10	30	60	120
Percentage anaerobic	90	80	70	50	35	15	5	2	1
Percentage aerobic	10	20	30	50	65	85	95	98	99

Figure 6.6 Relative contribution of aerobic and anaerobic energy metabolism during maximal physical effort of various durations; 2 minutes of maximal effort requires about 50% of the energy from both aerobic and anaerobic processes. At a world-class 4-minute mile pace, aerobic metabolism supplies approximately 65% of the energy, with the remainder generated from anaerobic processes. (Adapted from Åstrand, P.O., Rodahl, K.: *Textbook of Work Physiology.* New York: McGraw-Hill Book Company, 1977.)

Questions & Notes

Define maximal oxygen uptake ($\dot{V}O_{2max}$).

Give the amount of time that the ATP–PCr and lactic acid system can power maximal, all-out exercise.

List 2 factors that determine the energy system and metabolic mixture that predominate during exercise.

   1.

   2.

Compared to fat, carbohydrate generates about how much greater energy per unit of oxygen consumed?

Briefly explain the phenomenon known as "hitting the wall."

(i) For Your Information

IT'S DIFFICULT TO EXCEL IN ALL SPORTS

An understanding of the energy requirements of various physical activities partly explains why a world-record holder in the 1-mile run does not achieve similar success as a long-distance runner. Conversely, premier marathoners usually cannot run 1 mile in less than 4 minutes, yet they complete a 26-mile race averaging a 5-minute per mile pace.

aerobic *and* anaerobic metabolism. Five to 10 minutes of intense middle-distance running and swimming or stop-and-go sports such as basketball and soccer, demands greater aerobic energy transfer. Longer duration marathon running, distance swimming and cycling, recreational jogging, cross-country skiing, and hiking and backpacking require continual energy from aerobic resources without reliance on lactate's contribution.

Intensity and duration determine the energy system and metabolic mixture used during exercise. The aerobic system predominates in low-intensity exercise, with fat serving as the primary fuel source. The liver markedly increases its release of glucose to active muscle as exercise progresses from low to high intensity. Simultaneously, glycogen stored within muscle serves as the predominant carbohydrate energy source during the early stages of exercise and when exercise intensity increases. *The advantage of selective dependence on carbohydrate metabolism during near-maximum aerobic exercise lies in its two times more rapid energy transfer capacity compared with fat and protein fuels.* Compared with fat, carbohydrate also generates close to 6% greater energy per unit of oxygen consumed. As exercise continues with accompanying muscle glycogen depletion, progressively more fat (intramuscular triacylglycerols and circulating free fatty acids [FFAs]) serves as the substrate for ATP production. In maximal anaerobic effort, carbohydrate serves as the sole contributor to ATP production in mainstream glycolytic reactions.

A sound approach to exercise training first analyzes an activity for its specific energy components and then establishes a task-specific training regimen to ensure that optimal physiologic and metabolic adaptations occur. Improved capacity for energy transfer should translate to improved exercise performance.

Nutrient-Related Fatigue

Severe depletion of liver and muscle glycogen during intense aerobic exercise induces fatigue despite sufficient oxygen availability to muscle and an almost unlimited energy supply from stored fat. Endurance athletes commonly refer to this extreme sensation of fatigue as "bonking" or hitting the wall. The image of hitting the wall suggests an inability to continue exercising, which in reality does not occur, although pain exists in the active muscles and exercise intensity decreases markedly. Skeletal muscle does not contain the **phosphatase enzyme** present in the liver that helps release glucose from liver cells; this means that relatively inactive muscle retains all of its glycogen. Controversy exists as to why liver and muscle glycogen depletion during prolonged exercise reduces exercise capacity. Three factors are involved:

1. The central nervous system's use of blood glucose for energy.
2. Muscle glycogen's role as a "primer" in fat catabolism.
3. Significantly slower rate of energy release from fat compared with carbohydrate oxidation.

OXYGEN UPTAKE DURING RECOVERY: THE SO-CALLED "OXYGEN DEBT"

Bodily processes do not immediately return to resting levels after exercise. In light exercise (e.g., golf, archery, bowling), recovery to a resting condition takes place rapidly and often progresses unnoticed. Intense physical activity (e.g., running full speed for 800 m or trying to swim 200 m as fast as possible) requires considerable

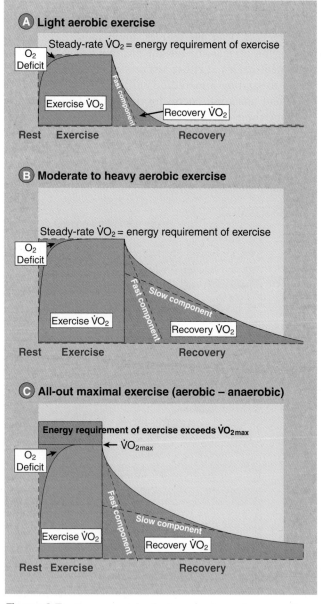

Figure 6.7 Oxygen uptake during exercise and recovery from light steady-rate exercise (**A**), moderate to intense steady-rate exercise (**B**), and exhaustive exercise with no steady rate of aerobic metabolism (**C**). The first phase (fast component) of recovery occurs rapidly; the second phase (slow component) progresses more slowly and may take considerable time to return to resting conditions. In exhaustive exercise, the oxygen requirement of exercise exceeds the measured exercise oxygen uptake.

time for the body to return to resting levels. The difference in recovery from light and strenuous exercise relates largely to the specific metabolic and physiologic processes in each exercise mode.

British Nobel physiologist A.V. Hill (1886–1977), referred to oxygen uptake during recovery as the **oxygen debt.** Contemporary researchers no longer uses this term. Instead, **recovery oxygen uptake** or **excess post-exercise oxygen consumption (EPOC)** now defines the excess oxygen uptake above the resting level in recovery. This specifically refers to the total oxygen consumed after exercise in excess of a pre-exercise baseline level.

Panel A in **Figure 6.7** illustrates that light exercise rapidly attains steady-rate with a small oxygen deficit. Rapid recovery ensues from such exercise with an accompanying small EPOC. In moderate to intense aerobic exercise (Panel B), it takes longer to achieve steady rate, so the oxygen deficit increases compared with light exercise. Oxygen uptake in recovery from relatively strenuous aerobic exercise returns more slowly to pre-exercise resting levels. Recovery oxygen uptake initially declines rapidly (similar to recovery from light exercise) followed by a gradual decline to baseline. In both Panels A and B, computation of the oxygen deficit and EPOC uses the steady-rate oxygen uptake to represent the exercise oxygen (energy) requirement. During exhausting exercise, illustrated in Panel C, a steady rate of aerobic metabolism cannot be attained. This produces a large accumulation of blood lactate; it takes oxygen uptake considerable time to return to the pre-exercise level. It is nearly impossible to determine the true oxygen deficit in such exercise without establishing a steady rate; in this instance the energy requirement exceeds the individual's maximal oxygen uptake.

No matter how intense the exercise (walking, bowling, golf, snowboarding, wrestling, cross-country skiing, or sprint running), an oxygen uptake in excess of the resting value always exists when exercise stops. The *shaded area* under the recovery curves in **Figure 6.7** indicates this quantity of oxygen; it equals the total oxygen consumed in recovery until attaining the baseline level minus the total oxygen normally consumed at rest for an equivalent duration. An assumption underlying discussions of the physiologic meaning of EPOC posits that resting oxygen uptake remains essentially unchanged during exercise and recovery. This assumption may be incorrect, particularly following strenuous exercise.

The recovery curves in **Figure 6.7** illustrate two fundamentals of EPOC:

1. **Fast component:** In low-intensity, primarily aerobic exercise with little increase in body temperature, about half of the total EPOC occurs within 30 seconds; complete recovery requires several minutes.
2. **Slow component:** A second slower phase occurs in recovery from more strenuous exercise (often accompanied by considerable increases in blood lactate and body temperature). The slower phase of recovery, depending on exercise intensity and duration, may require 24 hours or more before reestablishing the pre-exercise oxygen uptake.

*Q*uestions & Notes

Discuss possible reasons liver and/or muscle glycogen depletion reduces exercise capacity.

 For Your Information

EARLY RESEARCH ABOUT "OXYGEN DEBT": SPECIES DIFFERENCES

A.V. Hill and other researchers in the 1920s–1940s did not have a clear understanding of human bioenergetics. They frequently applied their knowledge of energy metabolism and lactate dynamics of amphibian and reptiles to observations on humans. In frogs, but not in humans for example, most of the lactate formed in active muscle reconverts to glycogen.

 For Your Information

SEVEN CAUSES OF EXCESS POSTEXERCISE OXYGEN CONSUMPTION WITH INTENSE EXERCISE

1. Resynthesis of ATP and PCr
2. Resynthesis of blood lactate to glycogen (Cori cycle)
3. Oxidation of blood lactate in energy metabolism
4. Restoration of oxygen to blood, tissue fluids, and myoglobin
5. Thermogenic effects of elevated core temperature
6. Thermogenic effects of hormones, particularly the catecholamines epinephrine and norepinephrine
7. Increased pulmonary and circulatory dynamics and other elevated levels of physiologic function

Metabolic Dynamics of Recovery Oxygen Uptake

Traditional View: A.V. Hill's 1922 Oxygen Debt Theory

A.V. Hill first coined the term "**oxygen debt**" in 1922, but Danish Nobel physiologist August Krogh (1874–1949; see Chapter 1) first reported the exponential decline in oxygen uptake immediately after exercise. Hill and others discussed the dynamics of metabolism in exercise and recovery in financial-accounting terms. Based on his work with frogs, Hill likened the body's carbohydrate stores to energy "credits," and thus, expending stored credits during exercise would incur a "debt." The larger the energy "deficit" (use of available stored energy credits) meant the larger the energy debt. The recovery oxygen uptake thus represented the added metabolic cost of repaying this debt, establishing the term "oxygen debt."

Hill hypothesized that lactate accumulation during the anaerobic component of exercise represented the use of stored glycogen energy credits. Therefore, the subsequent oxygen debt served two purposes: (1) reestablish the original carbohydrate stores (credits) by resynthesizing approximately 80% of the lactate back to glycogen in the liver (gluconeogenesis via the Cori cycle) and (2) catabolize the remaining lactate for energy through pyruvate–citric acid cycle pathways. ATP generated by this latter pathway presumably powered glycogen resynthesis from the accumulated lactate. The **lactic acid theory of oxygen debt** frequently describes this early explanation of recovery oxygen uptake dynamics.

Following Hill's work, researchers at Harvard's Fatigue Laboratory (1927–1946; see Chapter 1) in 1933 attempted to explain their observations that the initial fast component of the recovery oxygen uptake occurs before blood lactate decreases. In fact, they showed that an "oxygen debt" of almost 3 L could incur without appreciably elevated blood lactate levels. To resolve these discrepancies, they proposed two phases of oxygen debt. This model explained the energetics of oxygen uptake during recovery from exercise for the next 60 years.

1. Alactic or **alactacid oxygen debt** (without lactate buildup): The alactacid portion of the oxygen debt (depicted for steady-rate exercise in panels A and B of **Figure 6.7** or the rapid phase of recovery from strenuous exercise in panel C), restores the intramuscular high-energy phosphagens depleted toward the end of exercise. The aerobic breakdown of the stored macronutrients during recovery provides the energy for this restoration. A small portion of the alactacid recovery oxygen uptake reloads the muscles' myoglobin and hemoglobin in the blood returning from previously active tissues.

2. Lactic acid or **lactacid oxygen debt** (with lactate buildup): In keeping with A.V. Hill's explanation, the major portion of the lactacid oxygen debt represented reconversion of lactate to liver glycogen.

Testing Hill's Oxygen Debt Theory Acceptance of Hill's explanation for the lactacid phase of the oxygen debt requires evidence that in recovery, the major portion of lactate produced in exercise actually resynthesizes to glycogen. The evidence, however, indicates otherwise. When researchers infused radioactive-labeled lactate into rat muscle, more than 75% of it appeared as radioactive carbon dioxide, and only 25% synthesized to glycogen. In experiments with humans, no substantial replenishment of glycogen occurred 10 minutes after strenuous exercise even though blood lactate levels decreased significantly. Contrary to Hill's theory, the heart, liver, kidneys, and skeletal muscle use a major portion of blood lactate produced during exercise as an energy substrate during exercise and recovery.

Updated Explanation for EPOC

No doubt exists that the elevated aerobic metabolism in recovery helps restore the body's processes to pre-exercise conditions. Oxygen uptake after light and moderate exercise replenishes high-energy phosphates depleted in the preceding exercise, sustaining the cost of a somewhat elevated overall level of physiologic function. In recovery from strenuous exercise, some oxygen resynthesizes a portion of lactate to glycogen. *A considerable portion of recovery oxygen uptake supports physiologic functions that occur in recovery.* The considerably larger recovery oxygen uptake compared with oxygen deficit in exhaustive exercise results partly from an elevated body temperature. Core temperature frequently increases by about 3°C (5.4°F) during vigorous exercise and can remain elevated for several hours into recovery. This thermogenic "boost" directly stimulates metabolism and increases oxygen uptake *during* recovery.

In essence, all of the physiologic systems activated to meet the demands of muscular activity increase their need for oxygen during recovery. Two important factors characterize the recovery oxygen uptake:

1. Anaerobic metabolism of prior exercise.
2. Respiratory, circulatory, hormonal, ionic, and thermal disequilibriums caused by prior exercise.

Implications of EPOC for Exercise and Recovery

Understanding the dynamics of recovery oxygen uptake provides a basis for optimizing recovery from strenuous activity. Blood lactate does not accumulate considerably with either steady-rate aerobic exercise or brief 5- to 10-second bouts of all-out effort powered by the intramuscular high-energy phosphates. Recovery, reflecting the fast component proceeds rapidly, enabling exercise to begin again with only a brief pause. In contrast, anaerobic exercise powered mainly by rapid glycolysis causes lactate buildup and significant disruption in physiologic processes and the internal environment. This requires considerably more time for complete recovery (slow component). Incomplete recovery in basketball, hockey, soccer, tennis, and badminton hinders a performer when pushed to a high level of anaerobic metabolism. This may prevent full recovery even during brief rest periods and time-outs, between points, or even during half-time breaks.

Procedures for speeding recovery from exercise can classify as active or passive. **Active recovery** (often called "cooling down" or "tapering off") involves submaximum aerobic exercise performed immediately after exercise. Many believe that continued movement prevents muscle cramps and stiffness and facilitates the recovery process. In **passive recovery**, in contrast, a person usually lies down, assuming that inactivity during this time reduces the resting energy requirements and "frees" oxygen for metabolic recovery. Modifications of active and passive recovery have included cold showers, massages, specific body positions, ice application, and ingesting cold fluids. Research findings have been equivocal about these recovery procedures.

Optimal Recovery From Steady-Rate Exercise

Most people can easily perform exercise below 55% to 60% of $\dot{V}O_{2max}$ in steady rate with little or no blood lactate accumulation. The following occur during recovery from such exercise:

1. Resynthesis of high-energy phosphates.
2. Replenishment of oxygen in the blood.
3. Replenishment of bodily fluids.
4. Replenishment of muscle myoglobin.
5. Resupply of the small energy cost to sustain an elevated circulation and ventilation.

Passive procedures produce the most rapid recovery in such cases because exercise elevates total metabolism and delays recovery.

Optimal Recovery from Non–Steady-Rate Exercise

Exercise intensity that exceeds the maximum steady-rate level causes lactate formation to accumulate because its formation exceeds its rate of removal. As work intensity increases, the level of lactate increases sharply, and the exerciser soon feels "exhausted." The precise mechanisms of fatigue during intense anaerobic exercise are not fully understood, but the blood lactate level indicates the relative strenuousness of exercise, indirectly reflecting the adequacy of the recovery.

Active aerobic exercise in recovery accelerates lactate removal. The optimal level of exercise in recovery ranges between 30% and 45% of $\dot{V}O_{2max}$ for bicycle exercise and 55% and 60% of $\dot{V}O_{2max}$ when recovery involves treadmill running. The variation between these two forms of exercise probably results from the more localized nature of bicycling (i.e., more intense effort per unit muscle mass), which produces a lower lactate threshold compared with running.

Figure 6.8 illustrates blood lactate recovery patterns for trained men who performed 6 minutes of supermaximum bicycle exercise. Active recovery involved 40 minutes of continuous exercise at either 35% or 65% of $\dot{V}O_{2max}$. An exercise combination of 65% $\dot{V}O_{2max}$ performed for 7 minutes followed by 33 minutes at 35% $\dot{V}O_{2max}$ assessed whether a higher intensity exercise interval early in recovery expedited blood lactate removal. Moderate aerobic exercise in recovery clearly facilitated lactate removal compared with passive recovery. Combining higher intensity exercise followed by lower intensity exercise offered no greater benefit than a single exercise bout of moderate intensity. Recovery exercise above the lactate threshold might even prolong recovery by promoting lactate formation. In a practical sense, if left to their own choice,

Questions & Notes

List 3 factors that help explain increased $\dot{V}O_2$ during exercise recovery.

1.

2.

3.

Discuss advantages of active versus passive recovery.

For Your Information

THE SPECIFICITY OF SPEED

Haile Gebrselassie, the world record holder for the marathon (September 30, 2007), can run 1 mile in 4 minutes, 45 seconds and repeat the performance 26 times in a row yet cannot run 1 mile in less than 4 minutes.

For Your Information

KEEP MOVING IN RECOVERY FROM INTENSE EXERCISE

Active recovery most likely facilitates lactate removal because of increased perfusion of blood through the "lactate-using" liver and heart. Increased blood flow through the muscles in active recovery also enhances lactate removal because muscle tissue oxidizes this substrate during citric acid cycle metabolism.

BOX 6.2   CLOSE UP

How to Measure Work on a Treadmill, Cycle Ergometer, and Step Bench

An ergometer is an exercise apparatus that quantifies work, power output, or both. The most common ergometers include treadmills, cycle and arm-crank ergometers, stair steppers, and rowers.

WORK

Work (W) represents application of force (F) through a distance (D):

$$W = F \times D$$

For example, for a body mass of 70 kg and vertical jump score of 0.5 m, work accomplished equals 35 kilogram-meters (kg-m) (70 kg × 0.5 m). The most common units of measurement to express work include kg-m, foot-pounds (ft-lb), joules (J), Newton-meters (Nm), and kilocalories (kCal).

POWER

Power (P) represents work (W) performed per unit time (T):

$$P = F \times D \div T$$

In the above example, if the person were to accomplish work in the vertical jump of 35 kg-m in 500 msec (0.500 sec; 0.008 min), the power attained would equal 4375 kg-m·min^{-1}. The most common units of measurement for power are kg-m·min^{-1}, Watts (1 W = 6.12 kg-m·min^{-1}), and kCal·min^{-1}.

Calculation of Treadmill Work

The treadmill is a moving conveyor belt with variable angle of incline and speed. Work performed equals the product of the weight (mass) of the person (F) and the vertical distance (D) achieved walking or running up the incline. Vertical distance equals the sine of the treadmill angle (theta

or θ) multiplied by the distance traveled along the incline (treadmill speed × time).

$$W = \text{Body mass (F)} \times \text{Vertical distance (D)}$$

Example   For an angle θ of 8 degrees (measured with an inclinometer or determined by knowing the percent grade of the treadmill), the sine of angle θ equals 0.1392 (see table). The vertical distance represents treadmill speed multiplied by exercise duration multiplied by sine θ. For example, vertical distance on the incline while walking at 5000 m·h^{-1} for 1 hour equals 696 m (5000 × 0.1392). If a person with a body mass of 50 kg walked on a treadmill at an incline of 8 degrees (percent grade ~14%) for 60 minutes at 5000 m·h^{-1}, work accomplished computes as:

$$\begin{aligned} W &= F \times \text{Vertical distance (sine } \theta \times D) \\ &= 50 \text{ kg} \times (0.1392 \times 5000 \text{ m}) \\ &= 34{,}800 \text{ kg-m} \end{aligned}$$

The value for power equals 34,800 kg-m ÷ 60 minutes or 580 kg-m·min^{-1}.

Degree θ	Sine θ	Tangent θ	Percent Grade %
1	0.0175	0.0175	1.75
2	0.0349	0.0349	3.49
3	0.0523	0.0523	5.23
4	0.0698	0.0698	6.98
5	0.0872	0.0872	8.72
6	0.1045	0.1051	10.51
7	0.1219	0.1228	12.28
8	0.1392	0.1405	14.05
9	0.1564	0.1584	15.84
10	0.1736	0.1763	17.63
15	0.2588	0.2680	26.80
20	0.3420	0.3640	36.40

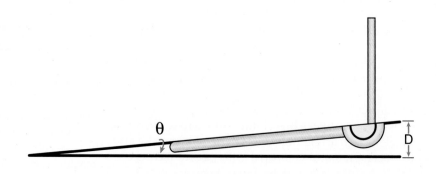

Calculation of Cycle Ergometer Work

The typical mechanically braked cycle ergometer contains a flywheel with a belt around it connected by a small spring at one end and an adjustable tension lever at the other end. A pendulum balance indicates the resistance against the flywheel as it turns. Increasing the tension on the belt increases flywheel friction, which increases pedaling resistance. The force (flywheel friction) represents braking load in kg or kilopounds (kp = force acting on 1-kg mass at the normal acceleration of gravity). The distance traveled equals number of pedal revolutions times flywheel circumference.

Example A person pedaling a bicycle ergometer with a 6-m flywheel circumference at 60 rpm for 1 minute covers a distance (D) of 360 m each minute (6 m × 60). If the frictional resistance on the flywheel equals 2.5 kg, total work computes as:

$$W = F \times D$$
$$= \text{Frictional resistance} \times \text{Distance traveled}$$
$$= 2.5 \text{ kg} \times 360 \text{ m}$$
$$= 900 \text{ kg-m}$$

Power generated by the effort equals 900 kg-m in 1 min or 900 kg-m·min^{-1} (900 kg-m ÷ 1 min).

Calculation of Bench Stepping Work

Only the vertical (positive) work can be calculated in bench stepping. Distance (D) computes as bench height times the number of times the person steps; force (F) equals the person's body mass (kg).

Example If a 70-kg person steps on a bench 0.375 m high at a rate of 30 steps per minute for 10 minutes, total work computes as:

$$W = F \times D$$
$$= \text{Body mass, kg} \times (\text{Vertical distance, m}$$
$$\times \text{Steps per min} \times 10 \text{ min})$$
$$= 70 \text{ kg} \times (0.375 \text{ m} \times 30 \times 10)$$
$$= 7875 \text{ kg-m}$$

Power generated during stepping equals 787 kg-m·min^{-1} (7875 kg-m ÷ 10 min).

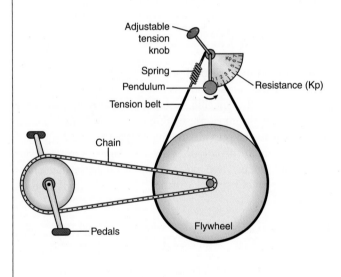

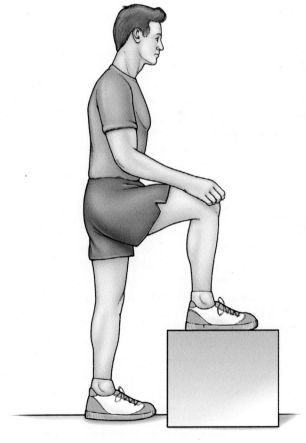

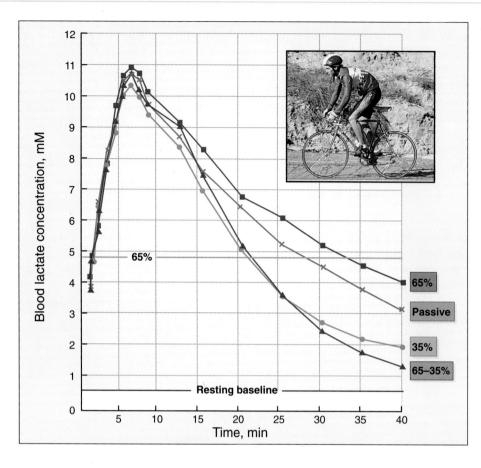

Figure 6.8 Blood lactate concentrations after maximal exercise during passive recovery and active exercise recoveries at 35% maximal oxygen consumption ($\dot{V}O_{2max}$), 65% $\dot{V}O_{2max}$, and a combination of 35% and 65% of $\dot{V}O_{2max}$. The *horizontal solid orange line* indicates the level of blood lactate produced by exercise at 65% of $\dot{V}O_{2max}$ without previous exercise. (Adapted from Dodd, S., et al.: Blood lactate disappearance at various intensities of recovery exercise. *J. Appl. Physiol.*, 57:1462, 1984.)

people voluntarily select their optimal intensity of recovery exercise for blood lactate removal.

Intermittent Exercise and Recovery: The Interval Training Approach

One can exercise at an intensity that normally proves exhausting within 3 to 5 minutes using preestablished spacing of exercise-to-rest intervals. This approach forms the basis of the **interval training** program. From a practical perspective, the exerciser applies various work-to-rest intervals using "supermaximum" effort to overload the specific systems of energy transfer. For example, in all-out exercise of up to 8 seconds, intramuscular phosphagens provide the major portion of energy, with little demand on glycolytic pathways. Rapid recovery ensues (fast component), and exercise can begin again after only a brief recovery. Chapter 13 further discusses interval training.

SUMMARY

1. The major energy pathway for ATP production differs depending on exercise intensity and duration. Intense exercise of short duration (100-m dash, weight lifting) derives energy primarily from the intramuscular phosphagens ATP and PCr (immediate energy system). Intense exercise of longer duration (1–2 min) requires energy mainly from the reactions of anaerobic glycolysis (short-term energy system). The long-term aerobic system predominates as exercise progresses beyond several minutes in duration.

2. The steady-rate oxygen uptake represents a balance between exercise energy requirements and aerobic ATP resynthesis.

3. The oxygen deficit represents the difference between the exercise oxygen requirement and the actual oxygen consumed.

4. The maximum oxygen uptake, or $\dot{V}O_{2max}$, represents quantitatively the maximum capacity for aerobic ATP resynthesis.

5. Humans possess different types of muscle fibers, each with unique metabolic and contractile properties. The two major fiber types include low glycolytic, high oxidative, slow-twitch fibers and low oxidative, high glycolytic, fast-twitch fibers.

6. Understanding the energy spectrum of exercise forms a sound basis for creating optimal training regimens.

7. Bodily processes do not immediately return to resting levels after exercise ceases. The difference in recovery from light and strenuous exercise relates largely to the specific metabolic and physiologic processes in each exercise.

8. Moderate exercise performed during recovery (active recovery) from strenuous physical activity facilitates recovery compared with passive procedures (inactive recovery). Active recovery performed below the point of blood lactate accumulation speeds lactate removal.

9. Proper spacing of exercise and rest intervals can optimize workouts geared toward training a specific energy transfer system.

THOUGHT QUESTIONS

1. If the maximal oxygen uptake represents such an important measure of a person's capacity to resynthesize ATP aerobically, why does the person with the highest $\dot{V}O_{2max}$ not always achieve the best marathon run performance?

2. How does an understanding of the energy spectrum of exercise help formulate optimal training to improve specific exercise performance?

3. Why is it so unusual to find athletes who excel at both short- and long-distance running?

SELECTED REFERENCES

Aisbett, B., Le Rossignol, P.: Estimating the total energy demand for supra-maximal exercise using the VO_2-power regression from an incremental exercise test. *J. Sci. Med. Sport*, 6:343, 2003.

Beneke, R.: Methodological aspects of maximal lactate steady state-implications for performance testing. *Eur. J. Appl. Physiol.*, 89:95, 2003.

Berg, K., et al.: Oxygen cost of sprint training. *J. Sports Med. Phys. Fitness*, 50:25, 2010.

Berger, N.J., et al.: Influence of continuous and interval training on oxygen uptake on-kinetics. *Med. Sci. Sports Exerc.*, 38:504, 2006.

Borsheim, E., Bahr, R.: Effect of exercise intensity, duration and mode on post-exercise oxygen consumption. *Sports Med.*, 33:1037, 2003.

Breen, L., et al.: No effect of carbohydrate-protein on cycling performance and indices of recovery. *Med. Sci. Sports Exerc.*, 42:1140, 2010.

Bourdin, M., et al.: Laboratory blood lactate profile is suited to on water training monitoring in highly trained rowers. *J. Sports Med. Phys. Fitness*, 44:337, 2004.

Carter, H., et al.: Effect of prior exercise above and below critical power on exercise to exhaustion. *Med. Sci. Sports Exerc.*, 37:775, 2005.

Chiappa, G.R., et al.: Blood lactate during recovery from intense exercise: Impact of inspiratory loading. *Med. Sci. Sports Exerc.*, 40:111, 2008.

Cleuziou, C., et al.: Dynamic responses of O_2 uptake at the onset and end of exercise in trained subjects. *Can. J. Appl. Physiol.*, 28:630, 2003.

Crommett, A.D., Kinzey, S.J.: Excess postexercise oxygen consumption following acute aerobic and resistance exercise in women who are lean or obese. *J. Strength Cond. Res.*, 18:410, 2004.

Da Silva, R.L., Brentano, M.A., et al.: Effects of different strength training methods on postexercise energetic expenditure. *J. Strength Cond. Res.*, 24:2255, 2010.

Dupont, G., et al.: Effect of short recovery intensities on the performance during two Wingate tests. *Med. Sci. Sports Exerc.*, 39:1170, 2007.

Ferguson, R.A., et al.: Effect of muscle temperature on rate of oxygen uptake during exercise in humans at different contraction frequencies. *J. Exp. Biol.*, 205:981, 2002.

Ferreira, L.F., et al.: Dynamics of skeletal muscle oxygenation during sequential bouts of moderate exercise. *Exp. Physiol.*, 90:393, 2005.

Gardner, A., et al.: A comparison of two methods for the calculation of accumulated oxygen deficit. *J. Sports Sci.*, 21:155, 2003.

Gordon, D., et al.: Influence of blood donation on oxygen uptake kinetics during moderate and heavy intensity cycle exercise. *Int. J. Sports Med.*, 31:298, 2010.

Hughson, R.L.: Oxygen uptake kinetics: historical perspective and future directions. *Appl. Physiol. Nutr. Metab.*, 34:840, 2009.

Ingham, S.A., et al.: Comparison of the oxygen uptake kinetics of club and Olympic champion rowers. *Med. Sci. Sports Exerc.*, 39:865, 2007.

Isaacs, K., et al.: Modeling energy expenditure and oxygen consumption in human exposure models: accounting for fatigue and EPOC. *Expo. Sci. Environ. Epidemiol.*, 18:289, 2008.

Kang, J., et al.: Evaluation of physiological responses during recovery following three resistance exercise programs. *J. Strength Cond. Res.*, 19:305, 2005.

Koppo, K., Bouckaert, J.: Prior arm exercise speeds the VO_2 kinetics during arm exercise above the heart level. *Med. Sci. Sports Exerc.*, 37:613, 2005.

LeCheminant, J.D., et al.: Effects of long-term aerobic exercise on EPOC. *Int. J. Sports Med.*, 29:53, 2008.

Lyons, S., et al.: Excess post-exercise oxygen consumption in untrained men following exercise of equal energy expenditure: comparisons of upper and lower body exercise. *Diabetes Obes. Metab.*, 9:889, 2007.

Markovitz, G.H., et al.: On issues of confidence in determining the time constant for oxygen uptake kinetics. *Br. J. Sports Med.*, 38:553, 2004.

McLaughlin, J.E., et al.: A test of the classic model for predicting endurance running performance. *Med. Sci. Sports Exerc.*, 42:991, 2010.

Nanas, S., et al.: Heart rate recovery and oxygen kinetics after exercise in obstructive sleep apnea syndrome. *Clin. Cardiol.*, 33:46, 2010.

Pringle, J.S., et al.: Effect of pedal rate on primary and slow-component oxygen uptake responses during heavy-cycle exercise. *J. Appl. Physiol.*, 94:1501, 2003.

Robergs, R., et al.: Influence of pre-exercise acidosis and alkalosis on the kinetics of acid-base recovery following intense exercise. *Int. J. Sport Nutr. Exerc. Metab.*, 15:59, 2005.

Sahlin, K., et al.: Prior heavy exercise eliminates $\dot{V}O_2$ slow component and reduces efficiency during submaximal exercise in humans. *J. Physiol.*, 564:765, 2005.

Scott, C.B., Kemp, R.B.: Direct and indirect calorimetry of lactate oxidation: implications for whole-body energy expenditure. *J. Sports Sci.*, 23:15, 2005.

Stupnicki, R., et al.: Fitting a single-phase model to the post-exercise changes in heart rate and oxygen uptake. *Physiol. Res.*, Aug 12., epub ahead of print. 2009.

Tahara, Y., et al.: Fat-free mass and excess post-exercise oxygen consumption in the 40 minutes after short-duration exhaustive exercise in young male Japanese athletes. *J. Physiol. Anthropol.*, 27:139, 2008.

Takken, T., et al.: Cardiopulmonary exercise testing in congenital heart disease: equipment and test protocols. *Neth. Heart J.*, 17:339, 2009.

Van Hall, G., et al.: Leg and arm lactate and substrate kinetics during exercise. *Am. J. Physiol. Endocrinol. Metab.*, 284:E193, 2003.

Whipp, B.J.: The slow component of O_2 uptake kinetics during heavy exercise. *Med. Sci. Sports Exerc.*, 26:1319, 1994.

Wilkerson, D.P., et al.: Effect of prior multiple-sprint exercise on pulmonary O_2 uptake kinetics following the onset of perimaximal exercise. *J. Appl. Physiol.*, 97:1227, 2004.

Winlove, M.A., et al.: Influence of training status and exercise modality on pulmonary O_2 uptake kinetics in pre-pubertal girls. *Eur. J. Appl. Physiol.*, 108:1169, 2010.

Wiltshire, E.V., et al.: Massage impairs post exercise muscle blood flow and "lactic acid" Removal. *Med. Sci. Sports Exerc.*, 42:1062, 2010.

Zhang, Z., et al.: Comparisons of muscle oxygenation changes between arm and leg muscles during incremental rowing exercise with near-infrared spectroscopy. *J. Biomed. Opt.*, 15:017007, 2010.

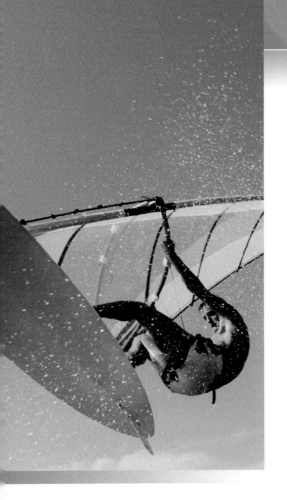

Chapter

7

Measuring and Evaluating Human Energy-Generating Capacities During Exercise

CHAPTER OBJECTIVES

- Compare and contrast the concepts of measurement, evaluation, and prediction.

- Explain specificity and generality applied to exercise performance and physiologic function.

- Describe procedures to administer two practical "field tests" to evaluate power output capacity of the intramuscular high-energy phosphates (immediate energy system).

- Describe a commonly used test to evaluate the power output capacity of glycolysis (short-term energy system).

- Explain the differences between direct and indirect calorimetry.

- Explain the differences between open- and closed-circuit spirometry.

- Describe different measurement systems used in open-circuit spirometry.

- Define the term *respiratory quotient* (RQ), including its use and importance.

- Explain factors that influence RQ and respiratory exchange ratio.

- Define *maximal oxygen uptake* ($\dot{V}O_{2max}$), including its physiological significance.

- Define *graded exercise stress test*.

- List criteria that indicate when a person reaches "true" $\dot{V}O_{2max}$ and $\dot{V}O_{2peak}$ during a graded exercise test.

- Outline three commonly used treadmill protocols to assess $\dot{V}O_{2max}$.

- Explain how each of the following affects $\dot{V}O_{2max}$: (1) mode of exercise, (2) heredity, (3) state of training, (4) gender, (5) body composition, and (6) age.

- Describe procedures to administer a submaximal walking "field test" to predict $\dot{V}O_{2max}$.

- Outline the procedure to administer a step test to predict $\dot{V}O_{2max}$.

- List three assumptions when predicting $\dot{V}O_{2max}$ from submaximal exercise heart rate.

All individuals possesses the capability for anaerobic and aerobic energy metabolism, although the *capacity* for each form of energy transfer varies considerably among individuals. These differences illustrate the concept of **individual differences** in metabolic capacity for exercise. A person's capacity for energy transfer (and for many other physiologic functions) does not exist as a general factor for all types of exercise; rather, it depends largely on exercise mode. A high maximal oxygen uptake ($\dot{V}O_{2max}$) in running, for example, does not necessarily ensure a similar $\dot{V}O_{2max}$ in swimming or rowing. The differences in $\dot{V}O_{2max}$ within an individual for different activities that activate different muscle groups emphasizes the **specificity of metabolic capacity**. In contrast, some individuals with high $\dot{V}O_{2max}$ in one form of exercise can also possess an above-average aerobic power in other diverse activities. This illustrates the **generality of metabolic capacity**. *For the most part, more specificity exists than generality in metabolic and physiologic functions.* In this chapter, we discuss different tests (and their evaluation) of the capacity of the various energy transfer systems discussed in Chapter 6 with reference to measurement, specificity, and individual differences.

OVERVIEW OF ENERGY TRANSFER CAPACITY DURING EXERCISE

Figure 7.1 illustrates the **specificity–generality concept** of energy capacities. The non-overlapped areas represent *specificity* of physiologic function, and the overlapped areas represent *generality* of function. For each of the energy systems, specificity exceeds generality; rarely do individuals excel in markedly different activities (e.g., sprinting and distance running). Although many world-class triathletes

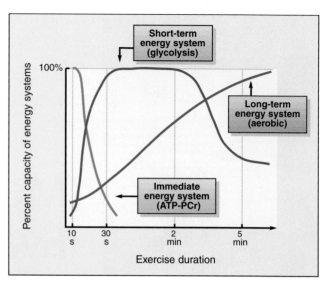

Figure 7.2 Three energy systems and their percentage contribution to total energy output during all-out exercise of different durations.

seem to possess "metabolically generalized" capacities for diverse aerobic activities, more than likely their performance results from hundreds of hours of highly specific training in *each* of the triathlon's three grueling events.

Based on the specificity principle, training for high aerobic power probably contributes little to one's capacity for anaerobic energy transfer and vice versa. *The effects of systematic exercise training remain highly specific for neurologic, physiologic, and metabolic responses.*

Figure 7.2 illustrates the involvement of anaerobic and aerobic energy transfer systems for different durations of all-out exercise. At the initiation of either high- or low-speed movements, the intramuscular phosphagens provide immediate and nonaerobic energy for muscle action. After the first few seconds of movement, the rapid-glycolytic energy system provides an increasingly greater proportion of the total energy requirements. Continuation of exercise, although at a lower intensity, places a progressively greater demand on aerobic metabolic pathways for ATP resynthesis.

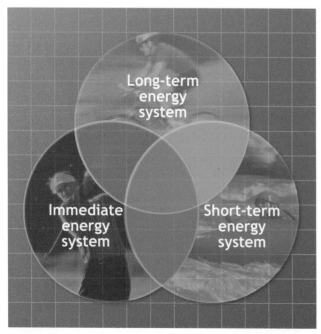

Figure 7.1 Specificity-generality concept of the three energy systems. The overlap of systems represents generality, and the remainder represents specificity.

Part 1	**Measuring and Evaluating the Immediate and Short-Term Anaerobic Energy Systems**

THE IMMEDIATE ENERGY SYSTEM

Two general approaches assess the anaerobic power and capacity responses of individuals:

1. Measure changes in ATP and PCr levels *metabolized* or lactate *produced* from anaerobic metabolism.
2. Quantify the amount of *external work performed* or *power generated* during short-duration, intense

activity (representing anaerobic energy transfer). This approach assumes that short-duration, intense activity could not be done without anaerobic energy; therefore, measuring such work or power indirectly measures (predicts) anaerobic energy utilization.

PERFORMANCE TESTS OF FAST AND SLOW ANAEROBIC POWER

Performance tests of anaerobic power and capacity have been developed as practical "field tests" to evaluate the **immediate energy system.** These maximal effort power tests that rely on maximal activation of the intramuscular ATP–PCr energy reserves evaluate the time rate of doing work (i.e., work accomplished per unit of time). The following formula computes power output (P):

$$P = (F \times D) \div T$$

where **F** equals force generated, **D** equals distance through which the force moves, and **T** equals exercise duration. **Watts** represent a common expression of power; 1 watt equals 0.73756 ft-lb·s^{-1} or 6.12 kg-m·min^{-1}.

Often tests of short term performance tests of maximal effort for 1 to 10 seconds reflect energy transfer of the immediate energy system, and maximal tests of longer duration (10–60 s) reflect utilization of the slow-glycolytic bioenergetic system.

Jumping Power Test

For years, physical fitness test batteries have included the jump-and-reach test (see Close Up Box 7.1: *Predicting Power of the Immediate Energy System Using a Vertical Jump Test,* on page 206) and standing broad jump to evaluate anaerobic power generated by the immediate energy system of ATP and PCr. The jump-and-reach test score equals the difference between a person's maximum standing reach and the maximum jump-and-touch height. For the broad jump, the score represents the horizontal distance covered in a leap from a semi-crouched position. Both tests purport to measure leg power, but they probably do not achieve the goal of evaluating a person's true ATP and PCr power output capacity.

Other Immediate Energy Power Tests

A 6- to 8-second performance involving all-out exercise measures a person's capacity for immediate power from the intramuscular high-energy phosphates (see **Fig. 7.2**). Examples of other similar tests include sprint running or cycling; shuttle runs; and more localized arm cranking or simulated stair climbing, rowing, or skiing. In the **Québec 10-second test** of leg cycling power, the subject performs two all-out, 10-second rides at a frictional resistance equal to 0.09 kg per kg of body mass with 10 minutes of rest between repeat bouts. Exercise begins by pedaling as fast as possible as the friction load is applied and continues all-out for 10 seconds. Performance represents the average of the two tests reported in peak joules (or kCal) per kg of body mass and total joules (or kCal) per kg of body mass.

The 40-yard sprint test is commonly used to test for "anaerobic performance of professional American football players." Unfortunately, this relates poorly to performance per se yet continues to be used. Several researchers have suggested replacing this test with a repeat, short-duration sprint test that includes changes in direction. Another alternative that would better represent an indvidual's true anaerobic power and capacity would include repeat testing to document anticipated performance decrements.

There are many concerns about short-duration tests. First, low interrelationships exist among different power output capacity test scores. Low interrelationships suggest a high degree of task specificity. This translates to mean that

Questions & Notes

Give an example of the generality of metabolic capacity.

Write the formula for calculating power.

Predict peak anaerobic power output in watts for a male weighing 80 kg who performs a vertical jump of 50 cm.

BOX 7.1 CLOSE UP

Predicting Power of the Immediate Energy System Using a Vertical Jump Test

Peak anaerobic power output underlies success in many sport activities. The vertical jump test has become a widely used test to assess "explosive" peak anaerobic power.

VERTICAL JUMP TEST

The vertical jump measures the highest distance jumped from a semi-crouched position. The specific protocol follows:

1. Establish standing reach height. The individual stands with the shoulder adjacent to a wall with the feet flat on the floor before reaching up as high as possible to touch the wall with the middle finger. Measure the distance (in centimeters) from the wall mark to the floor.
2. Bend the knees to roughly a 90 degree angle and place both arms back in a winged position.
3. Thrust forward and upward, touching as high as possible on the wall; no leg movement is permitted before jumping.
4. Perform three trials of the jump test and use the highest score to represent the individual's "best" vertical jump height.
5. Compute the vertical jump height as the difference between the standing reach height and the vertical jump height in centimeters.

ANAEROBIC POWER OUTPUT EQUATION

The following equation predicts **peak anaerobic power output from the immediate energy system** in watts (PAP_W) from vertical jump height in centimeters (VJ_{cm}) and body weight in kilograms (BW_{kg}). The equation applies to males and females:

$$PAP_W = (60.7 \times VJ_{cm}) + (45.3 \times BW_{kg}) - 2055$$

Example A 21-year-old man weighing 78 kg records a vertical jump height of 43 cm (standing reach height = 185 cm; vertical jump height = 228 cm); predict peak anaerobic power output in watts.

$$\begin{aligned} PAP_W &= (60.7 \times VJ_{cm}) + (45.3 \times BW_{kg}) - 2055 \\ &= (60.7 \times 43 \text{ cm}) + (45.3 \times 78 \text{ kg}) - 2055 \\ &= 4088.5 \text{ W} \end{aligned}$$

Applicability to Males and Females

For comparison purposes, average peak power output measured with this protocol averages 4620.2 W (SD = ±822.5 W) for males and 2993.7 W (SD = ±542.9 W) for females.

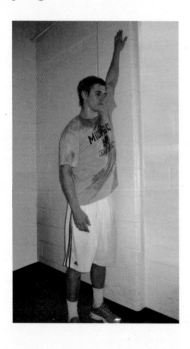 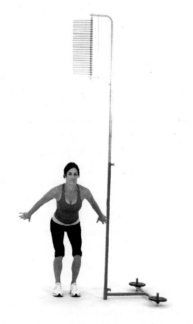 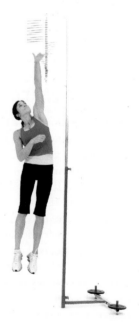

REFERENCES

Clark M.A., Lucett S.C., eds.: *NASM Essentials of Personal Fitness Training*. Baltimore: Lippincott Williams & Wilkins, 103, 2010.
Sayers, S., et al.: Cross-validation of three jump power equations. *Med. Sci. Sports Exerc.*, 31:572, 1999.

the best sprint runner may not necessarily be the best sprint swimmer, sprint cyclist, stair sprinter, repetitive volleyball leaper, or sprint arm cranker. Although the same metabolic reactions generate the energy to power each performance, energy transfer takes place within the specific muscles the exercise activates. Furthermore, each specific test requires different central nervous system (neurologic) skill components. The predominance of neuromuscular task specificity predicts that the outcome from any one test will likely differ from the results on another test.

Specific training can change an athlete's performance on anaerobic power tests. Such tests also serve as excellent self-testing and motivational tools and provide the actual movement-specific exercise for training the immediate energy system.

THE SHORT-TERM GLYCOLYTIC ENERGY SYSTEM

The anaerobic reactions of the **short-term energy system** do not imply that aerobic metabolism remains unimportant at this stage of exercise or that the oxygen-consuming reactions have failed to "switch on." To the contrary, the aerobic energy contribution begins very early in exercise. The energy requirement in brief, intense exercise significantly exceeds energy generated by hydrogen's oxidation in the respiratory chain. This means the anaerobic reactions of glycolysis predominate, presumably with large quantities of lactate accumulating within the active muscle and ultimately appearing in the blood.

No specific criteria exist to indicate when a person reaches a maximal anaerobic effort. In fact, one's level of self-motivation, including external factors in the test environment, likely influence test scores. *Researchers often use the blood lactate level to reveal the degree of activation of the short-term energy system.*

Physiologic Indicators of the Short-Term Glycolytic Energy System

Blood Lactate Levels
Considerable blood lactate accumulates from glycolytic energy pathway activation in maximal exercise. Establishing blood lactate levels reflect the capacity of the short-term energy system.

Figure 7.3 presents data obtained from 10 college men who performed 10 all-out bicycle ergometer rides of different durations on the Katch test (see Performance Tests of Glycolytic Power on pages 208 and 209) on different days. The subjects included men involved in physical conditioning programs and varsity athletics. Unaware of the duration of each test, the men were urged to turn as many revolutions as possible. The researchers measured the participants' venous blood lactate before and immediately after each test and throughout recovery. The plotted points represent the average peak blood lactate values at the end of exercise for each test. Blood lactate levels increased proportionally with duration (and total work output) of all-out exercise. The highest blood lactates occurred at the end of 3 minutes of cycling, averaging about 130 mg in each 100 mL of blood (~16 mmol).

Glycogen Depletion
Because the short-term energy system largely depends on glycogen stored within specific muscles activated by exercise, the pattern of glycogen depletion in these muscles provides an indication of the contribution of glycolysis to exercise.

Figure 7.4 shows that the rate of glycogen depletion in the quadriceps femoris muscle during bicycle exercise closely parallels exercise intensity. With steady-rate exercise at about 30% of $\dot{V}O_{2max}$, a substantial reserve of muscle glycogen remains even after cycling for 180 minutes because relatively light

$\mathcal{Q}$uestions & Notes

List 2 variables frequently used to indicate activation of the short-term energy system.

1.

2.

Complete the following:

1 kCal = _____ ft-lb

1 ft-lb = _____ kg-m

1 J = _____ Nm

1 watt = _____ m·min^{-1}

Give the duration of activity that requires substantial activation of the short-term energy system.

Give the duration and frictional resistance used in the popular Wingate test of anaerobic power and capacity.

For Your Information

INTERCHANGEABLE EXPRESSIONS FOR ENERGY AND WORK

1 foot-pound (ft-lb) = 0.13825 kilogram-meters (kg-m)

1 kg-m = 7.233 ft-lb = 9.8066 joules

1 kilocalorie (kCal) = 3.0874 ft-lb = 426.85 kg-m = 4.186 kilojoules (kJ)

1 joule (J) = 1 Newton-meter (Nm)

1 kilojoule (kJ) = 1000 J = 0.23889 kCal

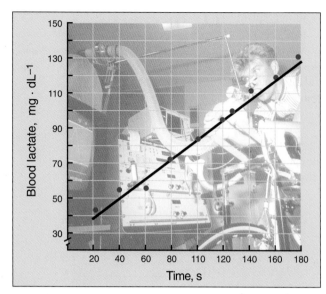

Figure 7.3 Pedaling a stationary bicycle ergometer at each subject's highest possible power output increases blood lactate in direct proportion to the duration of exercise for up to 3 minutes. Each value represents the average of 10 subjects. (Data from the Applied Physiology Laboratory, University of Michigan.)

exercise relies mainly on a low level of aerobic metabolism. This means large quantities of fatty acids provide energy with only moderate use of stored glycogen. The most rapid and pronounced glycogen depletion occurs at the two most intense workloads. This makes sense from a metabolic standpoint because glycogen provides the only stored nutrient for anaerobic ATP resynthesis. Thus, glycogen has high priority in the "metabolic mill" during such strenuous exercise.

Performance Tests of Glycolytic Power

Cycle Ergometer Tests   *Activities that require substantial activation of the short-term energy system demand maximal work for up to 3 minutes or longer in some individuals.* Testing anaerobic energy transfer capacity usually involves all-out runs and cycling exercise. Weight lifting (repetitive lifting of a certain percentage of maximum) and shuttle and agility runs also have been used. Age, gender, skill, motivation, and body size affect maximal physical performance. Thus, researchers have difficulty selecting a suitable criterion test to develop normative standards for glycolytic energy capacity. A test that maximally uses only leg muscles cannot adequately assess short-term anaerobic capacity for upper-body rowing or swimming. *Considered within the framework of exercise specificity, the performance test must be similar to the activity or sport for which energy capacity is evaluated. In most cases, the actual activity serves as the test.*

In the early 1970s, the **Katch test** performed on a Monarch bicycle ergometer used short-duration all-out leg cycling to generate the potential for fast and slow anaerobic energy. Subjects turned as many pedal revolutions as possible at a frictional resistance of 4.0 kg for men and 5.0 kg for women. The frictional resistance was established after the first pedal revolution and stabilized by the second or

third revolution. The peak power achieved during the test (always achieved during the first 10-second interval) represented **anaerobic power** or work per unit of time. This represented the immediate energy system potential, with total work accomplished reflecting **anaerobic capacity** or total work accomplished (representing the short-term energy system potential).

A subsequent modification, the **Wingate test**, involves 30 seconds of all-out exercise on either an arm-crank or leg-cycle ergometer. In this adaptation, the initial frictional resistance represents a function of the subject's body mass (0.075 kg of resistance per kg body mass) rather than a set value; the tester applies this resistance only after the subject overcomes the initial inertia and unloaded frictional resistance to pedaling (within ~3 s). Timing of the test then begins, with pedal revolutions counted continuously and usually reported every 5 seconds. **Peak power output** represents the highest mechanical power generated during any 3- to 5-second interval of the test; **average power output** equals the arithmetic average of total power generated during the 30-second test.

Anaerobic fatigue (the percentage of decline in power relative to the peak value) provides an index of anaerobic endurance; it represents the maximal capacity for ATP production via a combination of intramuscular phosphagen breakdown and glycolytic reactions. **Anaerobic capacity** represents the total work accomplished over the 30-second

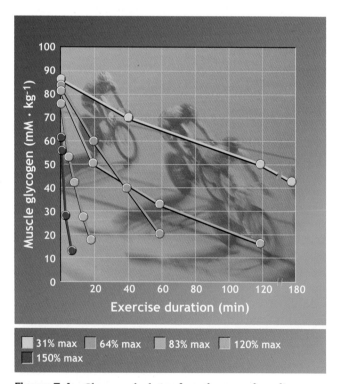

Figure 7.4 Glycogen depletion from the vastus lateralis portion of the quadriceps femoris muscle in bicycle exercise of different intensities and durations. Exercise at 31% of $\dot{V}O_{2max}$ (the lightest workload) caused some depletion of muscle glycogen, but the most rapid and largest depletion occurred with exercise that ranged from 83% to 150% of $\dot{V}O_{2max}$. (Adapted from Gollnick, P.D.: Selective glycogen depletion pattern in human muscle fibers after exercise of varying intensity and at varying pedaling rates. *J. Physiol.*, 241:45, 1974.)

exercise period (see Close Up Box 7.2: *Predicting Anaerobic Power and Capacity Using the Wingate Cycle Ergometer Test,* on page 210).

Interpretation of the Wingate test assumes that peak power output represents the energy-generating capacity of the intramuscular phosphagens and total power output reflects anaerobic (glycolytic) capacity. Elite volleyball and ice hockey players have recorded some of the highest cycle ergometer power scores. The Wingate and Katch tests elicit reproducible performance scores with acceptable validity. Modifications to the Wingate test include extending the duration to 60 seconds with use of variable resistance loadings.

Figure 7.5 presents estimates of the relative contribution of each metabolic pathway during three different duration all-out cycle ergometer tests. Part A presents the findings as a percentage of total work output, and part B shows the data in estimated kilojoules (kJ) and kCal of energy (1 kJ = 4.2 kCal). Note the progressive change in the percentage contribution of each of the energy systems to the total work output as the duration of effort increases.

Other Anaerobic Tests Running anaerobic power tests include all-out runs from 200 to 800 m and sport-specific run tests. For example, the evaluation of soccer players typically relies on repeat, 20-m all-out shuttle run-tests of varying distances and durations. Sport-specific, ultra-short tests exist for tennis, basketball, ice skating, and swimming. These tests attempt to mimic actual performance and can assess training success.

Questions & Notes

Define what is meant by anaerobic fatigue in the Wingate test.

Describe what happens to muscle fatigue during exhaustive bicycle riding for up to 180 min. (Hint: refer to Fig. 7.4).

State the differences between anaerobic power and anaerobic capacity.

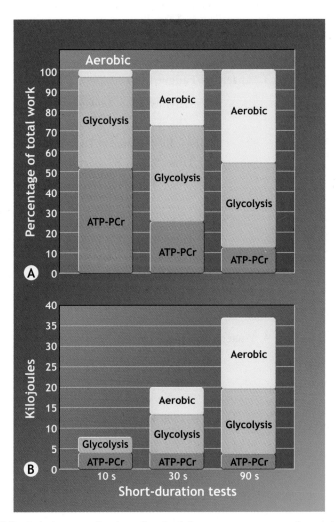

Figure 7.5 Relative contribution of each of the energy systems to the total work accomplished in three tests of short duration. **A.** Percent of total work output. **B.** Kilojoules of energy. Test results based on the Katch test protocol. (Data from the Applied Physiology Laboratory, University of Michigan.)

BOX 7.2 CLOSE UP

Predicting Anaerobic Power and Capacity Using the Wingate Cycle Ergometer Test

A mechanically braked bicycle ergometer serves as the testing device. After warming-up (3–5 min), the subject begins pedaling as fast as possible without resistance. Within 3 seconds, a fixed resistance is applied to the flywheel; the subject continues to pedal "all out" for 30 seconds. An electrical or mechanical counter continuously records flywheel revolutions in 5-second intervals.

RESISTANCE

Flywheel resistance equals 0.075 kg per kg body mass. For a 70-kg person, the flywheel resistance equals 5.25 kg (70 kg × 0.075). Higher resistances (1.0 to 1.3 kg × body mass) are often used to test power- and sprint-type athletes.

TEST SCORES

1. **Peak power output (PP):** The highest power output, observed during the first 5-second exercise interval, indicates the energy-generating capacity of the immediate energy system (intramuscular high-energy phosphates ATP and PCr). PP, expressed in watts (1 W = 6.12 kg-m·min^{-1}), computes as Force × Distance (Number of revolutions × Distance per revolution) ÷ Time in minutes (5 s = 0.0833 min).
2. **Relative peak power output (RPP):** Peak power output relative to body mass: PP ÷ Body mass (in kg).
3. **Anaerobic fatigue (AF):** Percentage decline in power output during the test; AF represents the total capacity to produce ATP via the immediate and short-term energy systems. AF computes as Highest 5-s PP − Lowest 5-s PP ÷ Highest 5-s PP × 100.
4. **Anaerobic capacity (AC):** Total work accomplished over 30 seconds; AC computes as the sum of each 5-second PP, or Force × Total distance in 30 seconds.

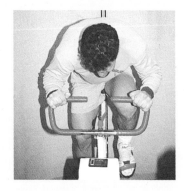

Example

A man weighing 73.3 kg (161.6 lb) performs the Wingate test on a Monark cycle ergometer (6.0 m traveled per pedal revolution) with an applied resistance of 5.5 kg (73.3 kg body mass × 0.075 = 5.497, rounded to 5.5 kg); pedal revolutions for each 5-second interval equal 12, 10, 8, 7, 6, and 5 (48 total revolutions in 30 s).

Calculations

1. Peak power output (PP)

$$PP = \text{Force} \times \text{Distance} \div \text{Time}$$
$$= 5.5 \times (12 \text{ rev} \times 6 \text{ m}) \div 0.0833$$
$$= 396 \div 0.0833$$
$$= 4753.9 \text{ kg-m·min}^{-1} \text{ or } 776.8 \text{ W}$$

2. Relative Peak Power Output (RPP)

$$RPP = PP \div \text{Body mass, kg}$$
$$= 776.8 \text{ W} \div 73.3 \text{ kg}$$
$$= 10.6 \text{ W·kg}^{-1}$$

3. Anaerobic Fatigue (AF)

$$AF = \text{Highest PP} - \text{Lowest PP} \div \text{Highest PP} \times 100$$

[Highest PP = Force × Distance ÷ Time: 5.5 kg × (12 rev × 6 m) ÷ 0.0833 min = 4753.9 kg-m·min^{-1} or 776.8 W]

[Lowest PP = Force × Distance ÷ Time: 5.5 kg × (5 rev × 6 m) ÷ 0.0833 min = 1980.8 kg-m·min^{-1} or 323.7 W]

$$= 776.8 \text{ W} - 323.7 \text{ W} \div 776.8 \text{ W} \times 100$$
$$= 58.3\%$$

4. Anaerobic Capacity (AC)

$$AC = \text{Force} \times \text{Total Distance (in 30 s)}$$
$$= 5.5 \times [(12 \text{ rev} + 10 \text{ rev} + 8 \text{ rev} + 7 \text{ rev} + 6 \text{ rev} + 5 \text{ rev}) \times 6 \text{ m}]$$
$$= 1584 \text{ kg-m·min}^{-1} \text{ or } 258.8 \text{ W}$$

Percentile Rankings for Average and Peak Power for Active Young Adults

| | AVERAGE POWER | | | | PEAK POWER | | | |
| | MALE | | FEMALE | | MALE | | FEMALE | |
% RANK	W	WKG	W	WKG	W	WKG	W	WKG
90	662	8.24	470	7.31	822	10.89	560	9.02
80	618	8.01	419	6.95	777	10.39	527	8.83
70	600	7.91	410	6.77	757	10.20	505	8.53
60	577	7.59	391	6.59	721	9.80	480	8.14
50	565	7.44	381	6.39	689	9.22	449	7.65
40	548	7.14	367	6.15	671	8.92	432	6.96
30	530	7.00	353	6.03	656	8.53	399	6.86
20	496	6.59	336	5.71	618	8.24	376	6.57
10	471	5.98	306	5.25	570	7.06	353	5.98

W = watts; WKG = watts per kg body mass.
From Maud, P.J., Schultz, B.B.: Norms for the Wingate anaerobic test with comparisons in another similar test. *Res. Q. Exerc. Sport.*, 60:144, 1989.

Anaerobic Power is Lower in Children   Children perform poorer on tests of short-term anaerobic power compared with adolescents and young adults. Perhaps children's lower muscle glycogen concentrations and rates of glycogen utilization partly account for this difference. Children have less lower leg muscle strength related to body mass compared with adults, which could also diminish their anaerobic exercise performance.

Gender Differences in Anaerobic Exercise Performance   *Differences in body composition, physique, muscular strength, or neuromuscular factors do not fully explain the considerable difference in anaerobic power capacity between women and men.* For example, supermaximal cycling exercise elicited a higher peak oxygen deficit (a measure of anaerobic capacity) in men than in women per unit of fat-free leg volume. This difference persisted even after considering gender differences in active muscle mass. Similar observations occur for gender differences in anaerobic exercise capacity in children and adolescents.

The above findings suggest the possibility of gender-related biologic differences in anaerobic exercise capacity. If this possibility proves correct, then physical testing that focuses on anaerobic exercise performance would further highlight performance differences between men and women to a greater degree than typically expected. Adjusting performance to body size or composition would not eliminate this effect. For physical testing in the occupational setting, justifiable concern exists that all-out anaerobic exercise testing exacerbates existing gender differences in performance scores; such testing adversely impacts females.

Factors Affecting Anaerobic Exercise Performance   Three factors influence individual differences in anaerobic exercise performance.

1. **Specific training:** Short-term supermaximal training produces higher levels of blood and muscle lactate and greater muscle glycogen depletion compared with untrained counterparts; better performances are usually associated with higher blood lactate levels, supporting the belief that training for brief, all-out exercise enhances the glycolytic system's capacity to generate energy.

2. **Buffering of acid metabolites:** Anaerobic training might enhance short-term energy transfer by increasing the body's buffering capacity (**alkaline reserve**) to enable greater lactate production; unfortunately,

Questions & Notes

Explain why children usually record poorer results than adults on tests of short-term anaerobic power.

List 3 factors that influence anaerobic performance.

1.

2.

3.

For Your Information

BENEFITS OF ENHANCED ALKALINE RESERVE

Pre-exercise altering of acid–base balance in the direction of alkalosis can temporarily but significantly enhance short-term, intense exercise performance. Run times improve by consuming a buffering solution of sodium bicarbonate before an anaerobic effort. This effect is accompanied by higher blood lactate and extracellular H^+ concentrations, which indicate increased anaerobic energy contribution.

no data confirm that trained individuals have a superior buffering capacity.

3. **Motivation:** Individuals with greater "pain tolerance," "toughness," or ability to "push"

beyond the discomforts of fatiguing exercise accomplish more anaerobic work and generate greater levels of blood lactate and glycogen depletion.

SUMMARY

1. The contribution of anaerobic and aerobic energy transfer depends largely on exercise intensity and duration. For sprint and strength-power activities, primary energy transfer involves the immediate and short-term anaerobic energy systems. The long-term aerobic energy system becomes progressively more important in activities that last longer than 2 minutes.

2. Appropriate physiologic measurements and performance tests provide estimates of each energy

system's capacity at a particular time or reveal changes consequent to specific training programs.

3. The 30-second, all-out Wingate test evaluates peak power and average power capacity from the glycolytic pathway. Interpretation of test results considers the exercise specificity principle.

4. Training status, motivation, and acid–base regulation contribute to differences among individuals in the capacities of the immediate and short-term energy systems.

THOUGHT QUESTIONS

1. Significant physiologic function and exercise performance specificity exist. How can one reconcile observations that certain individuals perform exceptionally well in multiple physical activity modes (i.e., they appear to be "natural" athletes)?

2. Give examples of how you would explain to an athlete the differences between the concepts of power and capacity.

3. How would you react to the coach who says, "You can't train for speed; it's a genetic gift"?

| **Part 2** | **Measuring and Evaluating the Aerobic Energy System** |

All of the metabolic processes within the body ultimately result in heat production. Thus, the rate of heat production from cells, tissues, or even the whole body operationally defines the rate of energy metabolism. The calorie represents the basic unit of heat measurement, and the term *calorimetry* defines the measurement of heat transfer. **Direct calorimetry** and **indirect calorimetry**, two different measurement

approaches illustrated in **Figure 7.6**, accurately quantify human energy transfer.

DIRECT CALORIMETRY

Direct calorimetry assesses human energy metabolism by measuring heat production similarly to the method for determining the energy value of foods in the bomb calorimeter (Fig. 3.1, Chapter 3). The early experiments of French chemist Antoine Lavoisier (1743–1794) and his contemporaries (*http://scienceworld.wolfram.com/biography/Lavoisier. html*) in the 1770s provided the impetus to directly measure energy expenditure during rest and physical activity.

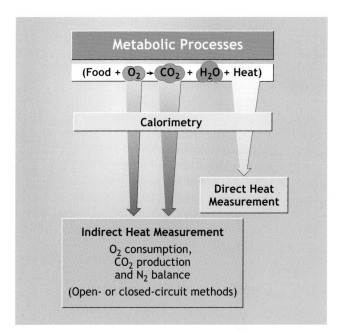

Figure 7.6 The measurment of the body's rate of heat production gives a direct assessment of metabolic rate. Heat production (metabolic rate) can also be estimated indirectly by measuring the exchange of gases (carbon dioxide and oxygen) during the breakdown of food macronutrients and the excretion of nitrogen.

*Q*uestions *&* Notes

Define calorimetry.

The calorie represents the basic unit for measuring _____.

The **human calorimeter** illustrated in **Figure 7.7** consists of an airtight chamber where a person lives and works for extended periods. A known volume of water at a specified temperature circulates through a series of coils at the top of the chamber. Circulating water absorbs the heat produced and radiated by the individual. Insulation protects the entire chamber, so any change in water temperature relates directly to the individual's energy metabolism. Chemicals continually remove moisture and absorb carbon dioxide from the person's exhaled air. Oxygen added to the air recirculates through the chamber.

Figure 7.7 A human calorimeter directly measures the body's rate of energy metabolism (heat production). In the Atwater-Rosa calorimeter, a thin sheet of copper lines the interior wall to which heat exchangers attach overhead and through which cold water passes. Water cooled to 2°C moves at a high flow rate, absorbing the heat radiated from the subject during exercise. As the subject rests, warmer water flows at a slower rate. In the original bicycle ergometer shown in the schematic, the rear wheel contacts the shaft of a generator that powers a light bulb. In later versions of ergometers, copper composed part of the rear wheel. The wheel rotated through the field of an electromagnet to produce an electric current for determining power output.

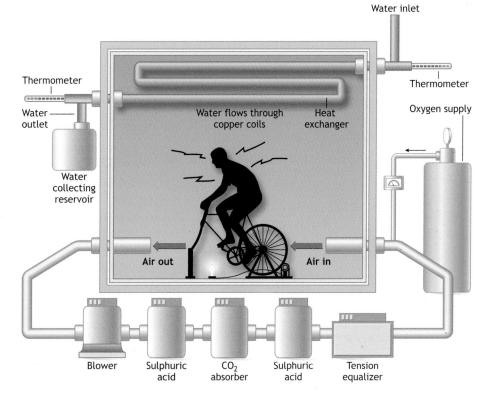

Professors W.O. Atwater (a chemist) and E.B. Rosa (a physicist) at Wesleyan University, Connecticut, in the 1890s built and perfected the first human calorimeter of major scientific importance. Their elegant human calorimetric experiments relating energy input to energy expenditure successfully verified the *law of the conservation of energy* and validated the relationship between direct and indirect calorimetry. The **Atwater-Rosa Calorimeter** consisted of a small chamber where the subject lived, ate, slept, and exercised on a bicycle ergometer. Experiments lasted from several hours to 13 days; during some experiments, subjects cycled continuously for up to 16 hours, expending more than 10,000 kCal. The calorimeter's operation required 16 people working in teams of eight for 12-hour shifts.

INDIRECT CALORIMETRY

All energy-releasing reactions in the body ultimately depend on the use of oxygen. By measuring a person's oxygen uptake, researchers obtain an *indirect* yet accurate estimate of energy expenditure. **Closed-circuit** and **open-circuit spirometry** represent the two methods of indirect calorimetry.

Closed-Circuit Spirometry

Figure 7.8 illustrates **closed-circuit spirometry**, which was developed in the late 1800s and currently used in

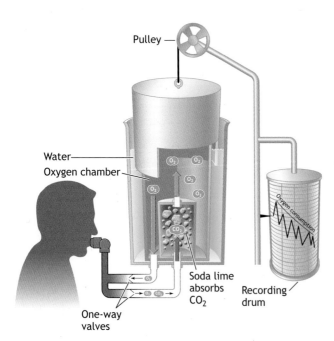

Figure 7.8 The closed-circuit method uses a spirometer prefilled with 100% oxygen. As the subject rebreathes from the spirometer, soda lime removes the expired air's carbon dioxide. The difference between the initial and final volumes of oxygen in the calibrated spirometer indicates oxygen consumption during the measurement interval.

hospitals and research laboratories to estimate resting energy expenditure. The subject breathes 100% oxygen from a prefilled container (spirometer). The spirometer in this application is a "closed system" because the person rebreathes only the gas in the spirometer with no outside air entering the system. A canister of soda lime (potassium hydroxide) placed in the breathing circuit absorbs the person's exhaled carbon dioxide. A drum attached to the spirometer revolves at a known speed and records the difference between the initial and final volumes of oxygen in the calibrated spirometer to indicate the oxygen uptake during the measurement interval. This system is unsuitable during exercise in which subject movement occurs with large volumes of air exchanged.

Open-Circuit Spirometry

Open-circuit spirometry represents the most widely used technique to measure oxygen uptake during exercise. A subject inhales ambient air that has a constant composition of 20.93% oxygen, 0.03% carbon dioxide, and 79.04% nitrogen. The nitrogen fraction also includes a small quantity of inert gases. Changes in oxygen and carbon dioxide percentages in expired air compared with inspired ambient air indirectly reflect the ongoing process of energy metabolism. The analysis of two factors—volume of air breathed during a specified time period and composition of exhaled air—measures oxygen uptake.

Three common open-circuit, indirect calorimetric procedures that measure oxygen uptake during physical activity are the bag technique, portable spirometry, and computerized instrumentation.

Bag Technique
Figure 7.9 depicts the **bag technique**. In this example, a subject rides a stationary bicycle ergometer wearing headgear containing a two-way, high-velocity, low-resistance breathing valve. Ambient air passes through one side of the valve and exits out the other side. The expired air then passes into either large canvas or plastic bags or rubber meteorologic balloons or directly through a gas meter to measure air volume. An aliquot of expired air is analyzed for its oxygen and carbon dioxide composition, with subsequent calculation of $\dot{V}O_2$ and calories.

Portable Spirometry
German scientists in the early 1940s perfected a lightweight, portable system to indirectly determine the energy expended during physical activity. The activities included war-related traveling over different terrain with full battle gear; operating transportation vehicles, including tanks and aircraft; and simulating tasks that soldiers would encounter during combat. Since then, many different portable systems have been designed, tested, and used in a variety of applications. For the most part, these portable systems use the latest advances in computer technology to produce acceptable results compared with more

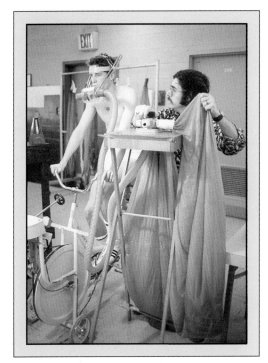

Figure 7.9 Oxygen uptake measurement by open-circuit spirometry (bag technique) during stationary cycle ergometer exercise.

Questions & Notes

Briefly describe the major difference between open- and closed-circuit spirometry procedures.

Give the percentage composition of oxygen, carbon dioxide, and nitrogen in ambient air.

fixed, dedicated desktop systems or the traditional bag system. **Figure 7.10** shows applications of a commerically available portable metabolic collections system. New systems on the horizon include a miniaturized system that can be worn on the wrist. In these applications, an onboard computer performs the metabolic calculations based on electronic signals it receives from micro-designed instruments that measure oxygen and carbon dioxide in expired air and repiratory flow dynamics and volumes. Data are stored on microchips for later analyses. More advanced systems include automated blood pressure, heart rate, and temperature monitors and preset instructions to regulate speed, duration, and workload of a treadmill, bicycle ergometer, stepper, rower, swim flume, resistance device, or other exercise apparatus.

ⓘ For Your Information

KILOCALORIE EQUIVALENT FOR 1 L OXYGEN

Assuming the combustion of a mixed diet, a rounded value of 5.0 kCal per liter of oxygen consumed designates the appropriate conversion factor for estimating energy expenditure from oxygen uptake under steady-rate conditions of aerobic metabolism.

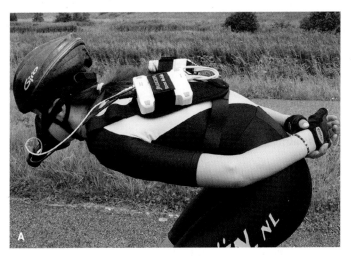

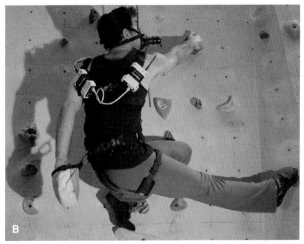

Figure 7.10 Portable micro-metabolic collection system using the latest in miniature computer technology. Built-in oxygen and carbon dioxide analyzer cells coupled with a highly sensitive micro-flow meter measure oxygen uptake by the open-circuit method during different activities such as (**A**) in-line skating and (**B**) wall climbing. (Photos courtesy of CareFusion Corporation, formerly VIASYS Healthcare [SensorMedics, Jaeger]).

BOX 7.3 CLOSE UP

How to Calibrate an Instrument

Most measuring instruments exhibit two types of errors, variable error and constant error.

Variable errors are unpredictable and produce inconsistent scores (i.e., scores fluctuate randomly in both positive and negative directions). Variable errors are caused by (1) instrument reading errors, (2) effects of uncontrolled environmental influences (temperature or barometric pressure), and (3) variable functioning inherent to the instrument's operation.

Constant errors include systematic errors that either add or subtract a consistent amount from the resulting score. Many scientific instruments exhibit a consistent drift of the zero so that it always reads consistently several units higher (or lower) than an established, criterion value.

CALCULATING ERRORS

Suppose you want to calibrate a new ventilation meter (NM) that can record expired air volumes (V_E) in $L \cdot min^{-1}$ during rest and up to maximum ventilation (e.g., from 12 to 120 $L \cdot min^{-1}$). Calculating constant and variable errors involves comparing volumes obtained using the NM versus volumes obtained using a criterion device (instrument known to yield correct values). In this example, a Tissot gasometer (TG) (see **Fig. 1**) serves as the criterion device for assessing gas volume.

To calibrate the NM, a subject breathes in ambient air through a two-way respiratory value, and the expired air passes into the NM and then into the TG, connected in series with low-resistance corrugated tubing.

Minute ventilation volumes are measured for 8 minutes under the following conditions: *rest* and *light*, *moderate*, and *intense* exercise. **Table 1** presents the $\dot{V}_E$ ($L \cdot min^{-1}$) for NM and TG and the difference between the two during the light exercise condition.

Constant Error

The mean absolute difference between the two methods (-5.13 $L \cdot min^{-1}$; last column, **Table 1**) represents the

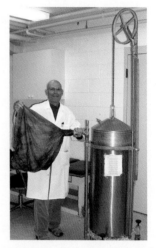

Figure 1 Tissot gasometer (water-filled and weight-balanced spirometer) capable of measuring up to 125 L of gas. The contents of a meteorologic balloon containing expired air are being transferred to the gasometer for precise measurement.

constant error (i.e., the NM, on average, consistently records 5.13 $L \cdot min^{-1}$ higher than the criterion TG). The constant error can be subtracted from each NM recording to more closely approximate TG values. The constant error is sometimes referred to as a **calibration factor**.

Variable Error

The standard deviation of the differences (± 1.38 $L \cdot min^{-1}$; last column, **Table 1**) represents the variable error of the NM. Expressed as a percentage of the mean criterion gas volume [$(1.38$ $L \cdot min^{-1} \div 32.99$ $L \cdot min^{-1}) \times 100$], the variable error represents $\pm 4.2\%$ of the actual gas volume. Because the variable error represents a random inconsistency in recording an accurate volume, it cannot be added or subtracted to more closely approximate the "true" TG volume; it will have to be determined whether this magnitude of variable error for the NM is small enough to warrant its use.

	Table 1 Ventilation Data for the New Meter (NM) and Criterion Tissot Gasometer (TG)		
MINUTE	TISSOT (TG) VOLUME, $L \cdot min^{-1}$	NEW METER (NM) VOLUME, $L \cdot min^{-1}$	TG − NM VOLUME, $L \cdot min^{-1}$
1	29.6	35.9	−6.2
2	33.8	38.5	−4.7
3	31.2	36.3	−5.1
4	31.2	34.7	−3.5
5	30.6	36.9	−6.3
6	40.5	43.0	−2.5
7	39.5	45.9	−6.4
8	27.5	33.8	−6.3
	$\bar{X} = 32.99$	$\bar{X} = 38.13$	$\bar{X}_{diff} = -5.13$
	SD = 4.37	SD = 3.95	$SD_{diff} = 1.38$

ERRORS AT DIFFERENT VOLUMES

The previous example illustrates constant and variable errors for a volume averaging about 30 L·min^{-1}. The same procedures are performed at different expiratory volumes to determine whether errors (constant and variable) change in relation to the size of the volume breathed into the meter. **Table 2** presents data for constant and variable errors for six ventilation volume ranges. (The data from **Table 1** are included in this table.)

In this example, note that the constant error remains stable throughout the different volume ranges. This is not the case with the variable error. A plot of the variable errors (L·min^{-1}) as a function of the mean criterion volume (L·min^{-1}) in **Figure 2** reveals that the new meter becomes progressively more inconsistent. It reaches ±12.3% (12.8 ÷ 104.1 × 100) of the criterion at the highest ventilation rate (see **Fig. 2**).

INTERPRETATION

Although constant errors can be corrected or accounted for, variable errors cannot. It becomes necessary to calculate the effects of a particular variable error before concluding if its magnitude reaches unacceptable levels. For example, a $\dot{V}_E$ variable error of ±2% to 4% by itself would

not be considered large, but when used for calculating oxygen consumption, it may represent an unacceptable level of error. This is the case at the highest ventilatory rates, where the calibration data show the new meter resulting in large and inconsistent errors. Therefore, this meter should not be used to determine ventilatory volume for computing oxygen uptake.

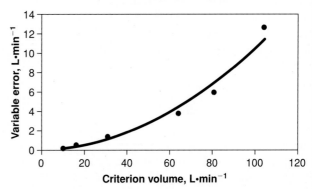

Figure 2 Plot of variables errors (L·min^{-1}) versus criterion volume. At the highest rate, % 100$^+$ L·min^{-1} the variable error of 12.8 L·min^{-1} amounts to 12.3% of the criterion volume (see Table 2).

Table 2 Constant and Variable Errors for Six Ventilation Ranges				
VENTILATION RANGE, L·min^{-1}	MEAN CRITERION VOLUME, L·min^{-1}	CONSTANT ERROR, L·min^{-1}	VARIABLE ERROR, L·min^{-1}	VARIABLE ERROR, % CRITERION
8–15	12.3	−5.0	0.113	0.92
15–25	18.4	−5.10	0.52	2.8
30–40	32.9	−5.13	1.38	4.2
50–75	65.2	−5.10	3.85	5.9
75–100	81.7	−5.0	6.05	7.4
+100	104.1	−5.2	12.80	12.3

Calibration Required

Regardless of the apparent sophistication of a particular automated system, the output data reflect the accuracy of the measuring device. Accuracy and validity of measurement devices require careful and frequent calibration using established reference standards. Metabolic measurements require frequent calibration of the meter that measures the air volume breathed and analyzers that measure oxygen and carbon dioxide. Most laboratories have criterion instruments for calibration purposes.

DIRECT VERSUS INDIRECT CALORIMETRY

Energy metabolism studied simultaneously using direct and indirect calorimetry provides convincing evidence for the validity of the indirect method. At the

List the 2 types of instrumental errors.

1.

2.

Which of the 2 errors can be corrected or accounted for?

turn of the century, the two calorimetric methods were compared by Atwater and Rosa for 40 days with three men who lived in calorimeters similar to the one shown in **Figure 7.7** on page 213. Their daily energy outputs averaged 2723 kCal when measured directly by heat production and 2717 kCal when computed indirectly using closed-circuit measures of oxygen uptake. Other experiments with animals and humans based on moderate exercise also demonstrated close agreement between direct and indirect methods; in most instances, the difference averaged less than ±1%. In the Atwater and Rosa calorimetry experiments, the ±0.2% method error represents a remarkable achievement, given that these experiments used handmade instruments.

DOUBLY LABELED WATER TECHNIQUE

The doubly labeled water technique provides an isotope-based method to safely estimate total and average daily energy expenditure of groups of children and adults in free-living conditions without the normal constraints imposed by laboratory procedures. Few studies routinely use this method because of the expense in using doubly labeled water and the need for sophisticated measurement equipment. Nevertheless, its measurement does serve as a criterion or standard to validate other methods that estimate total daily energy expenditure over prolonged periods.

The subject consumes a quantity of water with a known concentration of the heavy, non-radioactive forms of the stable isotopes of hydrogen (^{2}H or deuterium) and oxygen (^{18}O or oxygen-18)—hence the term **doubly labeled water**. The isotopes distribute throughout all bodily fluids. Labeled hydrogen leaves the body as water in sweat, urine, and pulmonary water vapor ($^{2}H_2O$), and labeled oxygen leaves as both water ($H_2{}^{18}O$) and carbon dioxide ($C^{18}O_2$) produced during macronutrient oxidation in energy metabolism. Differences between elimination rates of the two isotopes determined by an isotope ratio mass spectrometer relative to the body's normal background levels estimate total CO_2 production during the measurement period. Oxygen consumption is estimated on the basis of CO_2 production and an assumed (or measured) respiratory quotient (RQ) value of 0.85 (see next section).

Under normal circumstances, analysis of urine or saliva before consuming the doubly labeled water serves as the control baseline values for ^{18}O and ^{2}H. Ingested isotopes require about 5 hours to distribute throughout the body water. The researchers then measure the enriched urine or saliva sample initially and then every day (or week) thereafter for the study's duration, usually up to 3 weeks. The progressive decrease in the sample concentrations of the two isotopes permits computation of the CO_2 production rate and hence the $\dot{V}O_2$. The doubly labeled water technique provides an ideal way to assess total energy expenditure of individuals over prolonged periods, including bed rest and extreme activities such as climbing Mt. Everest, cycling the Tour de France, trekking across Antarctica,

military activities, extravehicular activities in space, and endurance running and swimming.

Caloric Transformation for Oxygen

Bomb calorimeter studies show that approximately 4.82 kCal release when a blend of carbohydrate, lipid, and protein burns in 1 L of oxygen. Even with large variations in the metabolic mixture, this **caloric value for oxygen** varies within ±2% to 4%.

An energy–oxygen equivalent of 5.0 kCal per liter provides a convenient yardstick to transpose any aerobic physical activity to a caloric (energy) frame of reference. Indirect calorimetry through oxygen uptake measurement provides the basis for quantifying the caloric cost of most physical activities.

RESPIRATORY QUOTIENT

Complete oxidation of a molecule's carbon and hydrogen atoms to carbon dioxide and water end products requires different amounts of oxygen because of inherent chemical differences in carbohydrate, lipid, and protein composition. Consequently, the substrate metabolized determines the quantity of carbon dioxide produced in relative to oxygen consumed. The **respiratory quotient (RQ)** refers to the following ratio of metabolic gas exchange:

$$\text{RQ} = \text{CO}_2 \text{ produced} \div \text{O}_2 \text{ consumed}$$

The RQ helps approximate the nutrient mixture catabolized for energy during rest and aerobic exercise. Also, the caloric equivalent for oxygen differs depending on the nutrients oxidized, so precisely determining the body's heat production (kCal) requires information about both oxygen uptake and RQ.

Respiratory Quotient for Carbohydrate

All of the oxygen consumed in carbohydrate combustion oxidizes carbon in the carbohydrate molecule to carbon dioxide. This occurs because the ratio of hydrogen to oxygen atoms in carbohydrates always exists in the same 2:1 ratio as in water. The complete oxidation of one glucose molecule requires six oxygen molecules and produces six molecules of carbon dioxide and water as follows:

$$C_6H_{12}O_6 + 6O_2 \rightarrow 6CO_2 + 6H_2O$$

Gas exchange during glucose oxidation produces an equal number of CO_2 molecules to O_2 molecules consumed; therefore, RQ for carbohydrate equals 1.00:

$$\text{RQ} = 6CO_2 \div 6O_2 = 1.00$$

Respiratory Quotient for Lipid

The chemical composition of lipids differs from carbohydrates because lipids contain considerably fewer oxygen atoms in proportion to hydrogen atoms and carbon.

Consequently, lipid catabolism for energy requires considerably more oxygen in relation to carbon dioxide production. Palmitic acid, a typical fatty acid, oxidizes to carbon dioxide and water to produce 16 carbon dioxide molecules for every 23 oxygen molecules consumed. The following equation summarizes this exchange to compute RQ:

$$C_{16}H_{32}O_2 + 23O_2 \rightarrow 16CO_2 + 16H_2O$$

$$RQ = 16CO_2 \div 23O_2 = 0.696$$

Generally, a value of 0.70 represents the RQ for lipid, ranging between 0.69 and 0.73 depending on the oxidized fatty acid's carbon chain length.

Respiratory Quotient for Protein

Proteins do not oxidize to carbon dioxide and water during energy metabolism. Rather, the liver first deaminates or removes nitrogen from the amino acid molecule; then the body excretes the nitrogen and sulfur fragments in the urine, sweat, and feces. The remaining "keto acid" fragment oxidizes to carbon dioxide and water to provide energy for biologic work. To achieve complete combustion, short-chain keto acids require more oxygen than carbon dioxide produced. For example, the protein albumin oxidizes as follows:

$$C_{72}H_{112}N_2O_{22}S + 77O_2 \rightarrow 63CO_2 + 38H_2O + SO_3 + 9CO(NH_2)_2$$

$$RQ = 63CO_2 \div 77O_2 = 0.818$$

The general value 0.82 characterizes the RQ for protein.

Respiratory Quotient for a Mixed Diet

During activities that range from complete bed rest to mild aerobic walking or slow jogging, the RQ seldom reflects the oxidation of pure carbohydrate or pure fat. Instead, metabolizing a mixture of nutrients occurs with an RQ intermediate between 0.70 and 1.00. *For most purposes, we assume an RQ of 0.82 from the metabolism of a mixture of 40% carbohydrate and 60% fat by applying the caloric equivalent of 4.825 kCal per liter of oxygen for the energy transformation.* Using 4.825 kCal, the maximum error possible in estimating energy metabolism from steady-rate oxygen uptake equals about ±4%.

Table 7.1 presents the energy expenditure per liter of oxygen uptake for different **non-protein RQ** values, including corresponding percentages and grams of carbohydrate and fat used for energy. *The non-protein RQ value assumes that the metabolic mixture comprises only carbohydrate and fat.* Interpret the table as follows:

Suppose oxygen uptake during 30 minutes of aerobic exercise averages 3.22 L·min^{-1} with CO_2 production of 2.78 L·min^{-1}. The RQ, computed as $\dot{V}CO_2 \div \dot{V}O_2$ (2.78 ÷ 3.22), equals 0.86. From Table 7.1, this RQ value (left column) corresponds to an energy equivalent of 4.875 kCal per liter of oxygen uptake, or an exercise energy output of 15.7 kCal·min^{-1} (3.22 L O_2·min^{-1} × 4.875 kCal). Based on a non-protein RQ, 54.1% of the calories come from the combustion of carbohydrate, and 45.9% come from fat. The total calories expended during the 30-minute exercise period equal 471 kCal (15.7 kCal·min^{-1} × 30).

RESPIRATORY EXCHANGE RATIO

Application of the RQ requires the assumption that the O_2 and CO_2 exchange measured at the lungs reflects cellular level gas exchange from

$\mathcal{Q}$*uestions & Notes*

Give the formula for computing RQ.

Give the "general" RQ values for the 3 macronutrients.

  Carbohydrate:

  Lipid:

  Protein:

Give the kCal per L O_2 uptake for a non-protein RQ = 0.86.

For Your Information

OXYGEN DRIFT

The $\dot{V}O_2$ increases under these exercise conditions: (1) while performing at an intensity level greater than about 70% $\dot{V}O_{2max}$; (2) at a lower percentage of $\dot{V}O_{2max}$ but for prolonged durations (>30 minutes); and (3) when performed in hot, humid environments for prolonged periods. These increases occur, although the energy requirement does not change. This *upward drift* in the $\dot{V}O_2$ results from increasing blood levels of catecholamines, lactate accumulation (if exercise is intense enough), shifting substrate utilization (to greater carbohydrate use), increased energy cost of ventilation, and increased body temperature.

For Your Information

RESPIRATORY QUOTIENT (RQ) VERSUS RESPIRATORY EXCHANGE RATIO (RER)

The respiratory exchange ratio or RER, (the ratio of the amount of CO_2 produced to the amount of O_2 consumed) represents occurrences on a total body level, while the RQ (ratio of CO_2 produced to O_2 consumed) represents the gas exchange from substrate metabolism on the cellular level.

Table 7.1 Thermal Equivalents of Oxygen for the Non-Protein Respiratory Quotient, Including Percentage kCal and Grams Derived From Carbohydrate and Fat

NON-PROTEIN RQ	KCAL PER LITER O_2 UPTAKE	PERCENTAGE KCAL DERIVED FROM		GRAMS PER LITER O_2 UPTAKE	
		CARBOHYDRATE	FAT	CARBOHYDRATE	FAT
0.707	4.686	0.0	100.0	0.000	.496
.71	4.690	1.1	98.9	.012	.491
.72	4.702	4.8	95.2	.051	.476
.73	4.714	8.4	91.6	.900	.460
.74	4.727	12.0	88.0	.130	.444
.75	4.739	15.6	84.4	.170	.428
.76	4.750	19.2	80.8	.211	.412
.77	4.764	22.8	77.2	.250	.396
.78	4.776	26.3	73.7	.290	.380
.79	4.788	29.9	70.1	.330	.363
.80	4.801	33.4	66.6	.371	.347
.81	4.813	36.9	63.1	.413	.330
.82	4.825	40.3	59.7	.454	.313
.83	4.838	43.8	56.2	.496	.297
.84	4.850	47.2	52.8	.537	.280
.85	4.862	50.7	49.3	.579	.263
.86	4.875	54.1	45.9	.621	.247
.87	4.887	57.5	42.5	.663	.230
.88	4.887	60.8	39.2	.705	.213
.89	4.911	64.2	35.8	.749	.195
.90	4.924	67.5	32.5	.791	.178
.91	4.936	70.8	29.2	.834	.160
.92	4.948	74.1	25.9	.877	.143
.93	4.961	77.4	22.6	.921	.125
.94	4.973	80.7	19.3	.964	.108
.95	4.985	84.0	16.0	1.008	.090
.96	4.998	87.2	12.8	1.052	.072
.97	5.010	90.4	9.6	1.097	.054
.98	5.022	93.6	6.4	1.142	.036
.99	5.035	96.8	3.2	1.186	.018
1.00	5.047	100.0	0	1.231	.000

From Zuntz, N.: Ueber die Bedeutung der verschiedenen Nährstoffe als Erzeuger der Muskelkraft. [*Arch. Gesamta Physiol.*, Bonn, Ger.: LXXXIII, 557–571, 1901], *Pflügers Arch. Physiol.*, 83:557, 1901.

nutrient metabolism. This assumption is reasonably valid for rest and during steady-rate mild to moderate aerobic exercise conditions without lactate accumulation. Various factors can alter the exchange of oxygen and carbon dioxide in the lungs so that the gas exchange ratio no longer reflects *only* the substrate mixture in cellular energy metabolism. For example, carbon dioxide elimination increases during hyperventilation because breathing increases to disproportionately high levels compared with the intrinsic metabolic demands. By overbreathing, the normal level of CO_2 in the blood decreases because the gas "blows off" in expired air. A corresponding increase in oxygen uptake does not accompany additional CO_2 elimination. Consequently, the exchange ratio often exceeds 1.00. *Respiratory physiologists refer to the ratio of carbon dioxide produced to oxygen consumed under such conditions as the* **respiratory exchange ratio, R or RER.** This ratio computes in exactly the same manner as RQ. An increase in the respiratory exchange ratio above 1.00 cannot be attributed to foodstuff oxidation.

Exhaustive exercise presents another situation in which R usually increases above 1.00. To maintain proper acid–base balance, sodium bicarbonate in the blood buffers or "neutralizes" the lactate generated during anaerobic metabolism in the following reaction:

$$HLa + NaHCO_3 \rightarrow NaLa + H_2CO_3 \rightarrow$$
$$H_2O + CO_2 \rightarrow Lungs$$

Lactate buffering produces the weaker carbonic acid. In the pulmonary capillaries, carbonic acid breaks down to its components carbon dioxide and water to allow carbon dioxide to readily exit through the lungs. The R increases above 1.00 because buffering adds "extra" CO_2 to expired air above the quantity normally released during cellular energy metabolism.

Relatively low R values occur after exhaustive exercise when carbon dioxide remains in body fluids to replenish bicarbonate that buffered the accumulating lactate. This action reduces expired carbon dioxide without affecting oxygen uptake; this decreases R to below 0.70.

MAXIMAL OXYGEN UPTAKE ($\dot{V}O_{2max}$)

The $\dot{V}O_{2max}$ (also called aerobic power) represents the greatest amount of oxygen a person can use to produce ATP aerobically on a per minute basis. This usually occurs during intense, endurance-type exercise. The data in **Figure 7.11** illustrate that persons who engage in sports that require sustained, intense exercise possess large aerobic energy transfer capacities.

Men and women who compete in distance running, swimming, bicycling, and cross-country skiing have nearly twice the aerobic capacity as sedentary individuals. This does not mean that only $\dot{V}O_{2max}$ determines endurance exercise capacity. Other factors at the muscle level, such as capillary density, enzymes, and muscle fiber type, strongly influence the capacity to sustain exercise at a high percentage of $\dot{V}O_{2max}$ (i.e., achieve a high blood lactate threshold). The $\dot{V}O_{2max}$ provides useful information about capacity of the long-term energy system. The attainment of $\dot{V}O_{2max}$ requires integration of the ventilatory, cardiovascular, and neuromuscular systems; this gives significant physiologic "meaning" to this metabolic measure. *In essence, $\dot{V}O_{2max}$ represents a fundamental measure in exercise physiology and serves as a standard to compare performance estimates of aerobic capacity and endurance fitness.*

Tests for $\dot{V}O_{2max}$ use exercise tasks that activate large muscle groups with sufficient intensity and duration to engage maximal aerobic energy transfer. Typical exercise includes treadmill walking or running, bench stepping, or

$\mathcal{Q}$uestions & Notes

Does an increase in the R above 1.00 directly reflect the mixture of macronutrients oxidized for energy?

Name the substance produced from lactate buffering.

What is the R value typically observed after exhaustive exercise?

BOX 7.4   CLOSE UP

Predicting $\dot{V}O_{2max}$ Using a Walking Test

A walking test devised in the 1980s for use on large groups predicts $\dot{V}O_{2max}$ (L·min^{-1}) from the following variables (see *Equation 1*): body weight (W) in pounds; age (A) in years; gender (G): 0 = female, 1 = male; time (T1) for the 1-mile track walk expressed as minutes and hundredths of a minute; and peak heart rate (HR$_{peak}$) in beats·min^{-1} at the end of the last quarter mile (measured as a 15-second pulse immediately after the walk × 4 to convert to b·min^{-1}). The test consisted of having individuals walk 1 mile as fast as possible without jogging or running.

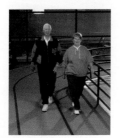

For most individuals, $\dot{V}O_{2max}$ ranged within ±0.335 L·min^{-1} (±4.4 mL·kg^{-1}·min^{-1}) of actual $\dot{V}O_{2max}$. This prediction method applies to a broad segment of the general population (ages 30 to 69 y).

EQUATIONS
Equation 1

Predicts $\dot{V}O_{2max}$ in L·min^{-1}:

$$\dot{V}O_{2max} = 6.9652 + (0.0091 \times W)$$
$$- (0.0257 \times A)$$
$$+ (0.5955 \times G) - (0.224 \times T1)$$
$$- (0.0115 \times HR_{peak})$$

Equation 2

Predicts $\dot{V}O_{2max}$ in mL·kg^{-1}·min^{-1}:

$$\dot{V}O_{2max} = 132.853 - (0.0769 \times W)$$
$$- (0.3877 \times A) + (6.315 \times G)$$
$$- (3.2649 \times T1)$$
$$- (0.1565 \times HR_{peak})$$

Example
Predict $\dot{V}O_{2max}$ (mL·kg^{-1}·min^{-1}) from the following data: gender, female; age, 30 years; body weight, 155.5 lb; T1, 13.56 min; HR$_{peak}$, 145 b·min^{-1}.

Substituting the above values in *equation 2*:

$$\dot{V}O_{2max} = 132.853 - (0.0769 \times 155.5)$$
$$- (0.3877 \times 30.0) + (6.315 \times 0)$$
$$- (3.2649 \times 13.56)$$
$$- (0.1565 \times 145)$$
$$= 132.853 - (11.96) - (11.63)$$
$$+ (0) - (44.27) - (22.69)$$
$$= 42.3 \text{ mL·kg}^{-1}\text{·min}^{-1}$$

REFERENCE

Kline, G., et al.: Estimation of $\dot{V}O_{2max}$ from a one-mile track walk, gender, age, and body weight. *Med. Sci. Sports Exerc.*, 19:253, 1987.

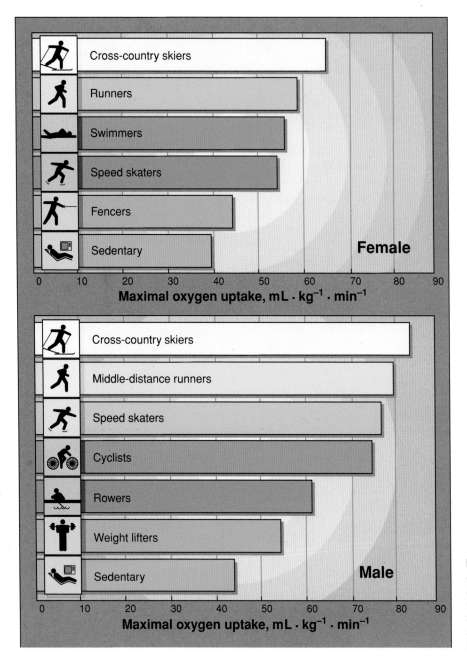

Figure 7.11 Maximal oxygen uptake of male and female Olympic-caliber athletes in different sport categories compared with healthy sedentary subjects. (Adapted from Saltin, B., and Åstrand, P.O.: Maximal oxygen uptake in athletes. *J. Appl. Physiol.*, 23:353, 1967.)

cycling; tethered and flume swimming and swim-bench ergometry; and simulated rowing, skiing, in-line skating, stair-climbing, ice skating, and arm-crank exercise. Considerable research effort has been directed toward (1) development and standardization of tests for $\dot{V}O_{2max}$ and (2) establishment of related age, gender, state of training, and body composition norms.

Criteria for $\dot{V}O_{2max}$

A leveling-off or peaking-over in oxygen uptake during increasing exercise intensity (**Fig. 7.12**) *signifies attainment of maximum capacity for aerobic metabolism (i.e., a "true" $\dot{V}O_{2max}$).* When this accepted criterion is not met or local

muscle fatigue in the arms or legs rather than central circulatory dynamics limits test performance, the term **peak oxygen uptake** ($\dot{V}O_{2peak}$) usually describes the highest oxygen uptake value during the test.

The data in **Figure 7.12** reflect oxygen uptake with progressive increases in treadmill exercise intensity; the test terminates when the subject decides to stop even when prodded to continue. For the average oxygen uptake values of 18 subjects plotted in this figure, the highest oxygen uptake occurred before subjects attained their maximum exercise level. The peaking-over criterion substantiates attainment of a true $\dot{V}O_{2max}$.

Peaking-over or slight decreases in oxygen uptake do not always occur as exercise intensity increases. The highest

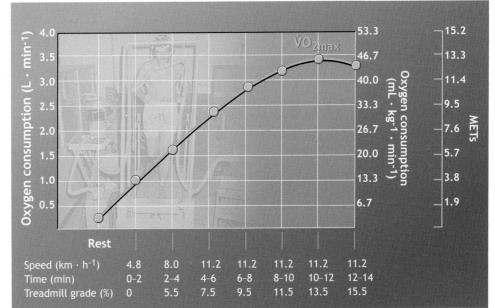

Figure 7.12 Peaking over in oxygen uptake with increasing intensity of treadmill exercise. Each point represents the average oxygen uptake of 18 sedentary men. The point at which oxygen uptake fails to increase the expected amount or even decreases slightly with increasing exercise intensity represents the maximal oxygen uptake ($\dot{V}O_{2max}$). (Data from the Applied Physiology Laboratory, University of Michigan.)

Speed (km · h⁻¹)	4.8	8.0	11.2	11.2	11.2	11.2	11.2
Time (min)	0–2	2–4	4–6	6–8	8–10	10–12	12–14
Treadmill grade (%)	0	5.5	7.5	9.5	11.5	13.5	15.5

oxygen uptake usually occurs during the last minute of exercise without the plateau criterion for $\dot{V}O_{2max}$. Additional criteria for establishing $\dot{V}O_{2max}$ (and $\dot{V}O_{2peak}$) are based on three metabolic and physiologic responses:

1. Failure for oxygen uptake versus exercise intensity to increase by some value usually expected from previous observations with the particular test ($\dot{V}O_{2max}$ criterion).
2. Blood lactate levels that attain at least 70 or 80 mg per 100 mL of blood or about 8 to 10 mmol to ensure the subject significantly exceeded the lactate threshold with near-maximal exercise effort ($\dot{V}O_{2peak}$ criterion).
3. Attainment of near age-predicted maximum heart rate, or a respiratory exchange ratio (R) in excess of 1.00 indicates that subject exercised at close to the maximum intensity ($\dot{V}O_{2peak}$ criterion).

Tests of Aerobic Power

Different standardized tests assess $\dot{V}O_{2max}$. Such tests remain independent of muscle strength, speed, body size, and skill, with the exception of specialized swimming, rowing, and ice skating tests.

The $\dot{V}O_{2max}$ test may require a continuous 3- to 5-minute "supermaximal" effort, but it usually consists of increments in exercise intensity, referred to as a **graded exercise test** or **GXT**, until the subject stops. Some researchers have imprecisely termed the end point "exhaustion," but the subject can terminate the test for a variety of reasons, with exhaustion only one possibility. A variety of psychologic or motivational factors can influence this decision instead of true physiologic exhaustion. It can take considerable urging and encouragement to convince subjects to attain their "real" $\dot{V}O_{2max}$. Children and adults encounter particular difficulty if they have little prior experience performing strenuous exercise with its associated central (cardiorespiratory) and peripheral (local muscular) discomforts. *Attaining a plateau in oxygen uptake during the $\dot{V}O_{2max}$ test requires high motivation and a large anaerobic component because of the maximal exercise requirement.*

Questions & Notes

State the major criterion for achieving $\dot{V}O_{2max}$ during graded exercise testing.

Name the 2 types of $\dot{V}O_{2max}$ tests.

1.

2.

Name 3 commonly used treadmill procedures to assess $\dot{V}O_{2max}$.

1.

2.

3.

BOX 7.5 CLOSE UP

Predicting $\dot{V}O_{2max}$ Using a Step Test

Recovery heart rate from a standardized stepping exercise can classify people on cardiovascular fitness and $\dot{V}O_{2max}$ with reasonable acceptable accuracy.

THE TEST

Individuals step to a four-step cadence ("up-up-down-down") on a bench $16\frac{1}{4}$ inches high (height of standard gymnasium bleachers). Women perform 22 complete step-ups per minute to a metronome set at 88 beats per minute; men use 24 step-ups per minute at a metronome setting of 96 beats per minute.

Stepping begins after a brief demonstration and practice period. After stepping, the person remains standing while another person measures the pulse rate (carotid or radial artery) for a 15-second period 5 to 20 seconds into recovery. Fifteen-second recovery heart rate converts to

beats per minute (15-s HR $\times$ 4), which converts to a percentile ranking for predicted $\dot{V}O_{2max}$ (see table).

Equations

The following equations predict $\dot{V}O_{2max}$ ($mL \cdot kg^{-1} \cdot min^{-1}$) from step-test heart rate recovery for men and women ages 18 to 24 years:

Men: $\dot{V}O_{2max} = 111.33 - (0.42 \times$ step-test pulse rate, $b \cdot min^{-1})$

Women: $\dot{V}O_{2max} = 65.81 - (0.1847 \times$ step-test pulse rate, $b \cdot min^{-1})$

The *Predicted $\dot{V}O_{2max}$* columns of the table present the $\dot{V}O_{2max}$ values for men and women from different recovery heart rate scores.

Percentile Ranking for Recovery Heart Rate and Predicted $\dot{V}O_{2max}$ ($mL \cdot kg^{-1} \cdot min^{-1}$) for Male and Female College Students

PERCENTILE	RECOVERY HR FEMALES	PREDICTED $\dot{V}O_{2max}$	RECOVERY HR MALES	PREDICTED $\dot{V}O_{2max}$
100	128	42.2	120	60.9
95	140	40.0	124	59.3
90	148	38.5	128	57.6
85	152	37.7	136	54.2
80	156	37.0	140	52.5
75	158	36.6	144	50.9
70	160	36.3	148	49.2
65	162	35.9	149	48.8
60	163	35.7	152	47.5
55	164	35.5	154	46.7
50	166	35.1	156	45.8
45	168	34.8	160	44.1
40	170	34.4	162	43.3
35	171	34.2	164	42.5
30	172	34.0	166	41.6
25	176	33.3	168	40.8
20	180	32.6	172	39.1
15	182	32.2	176	37.4
10	184	31.8	178	36.6
5	196	29.6	184	34.1

From McArdle, W.D., et al.: Percentile norms for a valid step test in college women. *Res. Q.*, 44:498, 1973; McArdle, W.D., et al.: Reliability and interrelationships between maximal oxygen uptake, physical work capacity, and step test scores in college women. *Med. Sci. Sports*, 4:182, 1972.

Comparisons Among $\dot{V}O_{2max}$ Tests

Two types of $\dot{V}O_{2max}$ tests are typically used:

1. **Continuous test:** No rest between exercise increments.
2. **Discontinuous test:** Several minutes of rest between exercise increments.

The data in Table 7.2 show a systematic comparison of $\dot{V}O_{2max}$ scores measured by six common continuous and discontinuous treadmill and bicycle procedures.

Only a small 8-mL difference occurred in $\dot{V}O_{2max}$ between continuous and discontinuous bicycle tests, with $\dot{V}O_{2max}$ averaging 6.4% to 11.2% below treadmill values.

Table 7.2	Average Maximal Oxygen Uptakes for 15 College Students During Continuous (Cont.) and Discontinuous (Discont.) Tests on the Bicycle and Treadmill					
VARIABLE	BIKE, DISCONT.	BIKE, CONT.	TREADMILL, DISCONT. WALK-RUN	TREADMILL, CONT. WALK	TREADMILL, DISCONT. RUN	TREADMILL, CONT. RUN
$\dot{V}O_{2max}$, mL·min^{-1}	3691 ± 453	3683 ± 448	4145 ± 401	3944 ± 395	4157 ± 445	4109 ± 424
$\dot{V}O_{2max}$, mL·kg^{-1}·min^{-1}	50.0 ± 6.9	49.9 ± 7.0	56.6 ± 7.3	56.6 ± 7.6	55.5 ± 7.6	55.5 ± 6.8

Values are means ± standard deviation.
$\dot{V}O_{2max}$ = maximal oxygen uptake.
Adapted from McArdle, W.D., et al.: Comparison of continuous and discontinuous treadmill and bicycle tests for max $\dot{V}O_2$. *Med. Sci. Sport*, 5:156, 1973.

The largest difference among any of the three treadmill tests equaled only 1.2%. The walking test, in contrast, elicited $\dot{V}O_{2max}$ scores about 7% above values achieved on the bicycle but 5% less than the average for the three run tests.

Subjects reported local discomfort in their thigh muscles during intense exercise on both bicycle tests. In walking, subjects reported discomfort in the lower back and calf muscles, particularly at higher treadmill elevations. The running tests produced little local discomfort, but subjects experienced general fatigue categorized as feeling "winded." A continuous treadmill run is the method of choice for ease of administration in healthy subjects. Total time to administer the test averaged slightly more than 12 minutes, whereas the discontinuous running test averaged about 65 minutes. $\dot{V}O_{2max}$ can also be achieved with a continuous exercise protocol during which exercise intensity increases progressively in 15-second intervals. With such an approach, the total test time for bicycle or treadmill exercise averages only about 5 minutes.

Commonly Used Treadmill Protocols

Figure 7.13 summarizes six commonly used treadmill protocols to assess $\dot{V}O_{2max}$ in healthy individuals and individuals with cardiovascular disease. Common features include manipulation of exercise duration and treadmill speed and grade. The Harbor treadmill test (example F), referred to as a **ramp test**, is unique because treadmill grade increases every minute up to 10 minutes by a constant amount that ranges from 1% to 4% depending on the subject's fitness. This quick procedure linearly increases oxygen uptake to the maximum level. Healthy individuals and monitored cardiac patients tolerate the protocol without problems.

Manipulating Test Protocol to Increase $\dot{V}O_{2max}$

On completion of a maximal oxygen uptake test, one assumes the tester has made every attempt to "push" the subject to near-limits of performance. This effort includes verbal encouragement from laboratory staff and peers or a monetary incentive. If the test meets the usual physiologic criteria, one assumes the test score represents the subject's "true" $\dot{V}O_{2max}$.

In one study, 44 sedentary and trained men and women performed a continuous treadmill $\dot{V}O_{2max}$ test to the point of so-called "exhaustion" in which they refused to continue exercising. They then recovered for 2 minutes before performing a second $\dot{V}O_{2max}$ test. During active recovery from test 1, the researchers lowered the treadmill grade at least 2.5% below the final grade of the previous test and reduced running speed from 11.0 km·h^{-1} to 9.0 km·h^{-1} for the trained subjects and from 9.0 km·h^{-1} to 6.0 km·h^{-1} for the sedentary subjects. After 2 minutes, treadmill speed increased to the test 1 speed for 30 seconds, at which time the percent grade increased to the final grade

Questions & Notes

Name 5 factors that affect $\dot{V}O_{2max}$.

1.

2.

3.

4.

5.

Briefly explain why different modes of exercise elicit different $\dot{V}O_{2max}$ values.

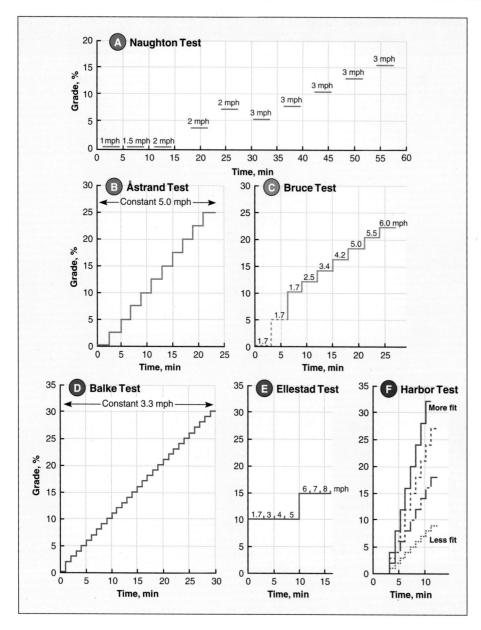

Figure 7.13 Six commonly used treadmill procedures. **A.** Naughton test. Three-minute exercise periods of increasing intensity alternate with 3 minutes of rest. The exercise periods vary in grade and speed. **B.** Åstrand test. Speed remains constant at 5 mph. After 3 minutes at 0% grade, grade increases 2.5% every 2 minutes. **C.** Bruce test. Grade, speed, or both change every 3 minutes. Healthy subjects do not perform grades 0% and 5%. **D.** Balke test. After 1 minute at 0% grade and 1 minute at 2% grade, grade increases 1% per minute (all at a speed of 3.3 mph). **E.** Ellestad test. The initial grade is 10%, the later grade 15%, and the speed increases every 2 or 3 minutes. **F.** Harbor test. After 3 minutes of walking at a comfortable speed, grade increases at a constant preselected amount each minute (1%, 2%, 3%, or 4%), so the subject reaches maximal oxygen uptake ($\dot{V}O_{2max}$) in approximately 10 minutes. (From Wasserman, K., et al.: *Principles of Exercise Testing and Interpretation*, 4th ed. Baltimore: Lippincott Williams & Wilkins, 2004.)

achieved in test 1. Treadmill grade increased every 2 minutes thereafter until the subjects again terminated the test. Subjects received strong verbal encouragement, particularly during the last minutes of exercise during both tests.

The $\dot{V}O_{2max}$ scores averaged a statistically significant 1.4% higher value on test 2. This small difference was almost double the difference typically measured between two final oxygen uptake readings on continuous or discontinuous tests. A "booster" test after a normally administered aerobic capacity test can increase the final oxygen uptake, illustrating the need to pay careful attention to $\dot{V}O_{2max}$ administrative techniques.

Factors Affecting $\dot{V}O_{2max}$

Many factors influence $\dot{V}O_{2max}$. The most important include exercise mode and the person's training state, heredity, gender, body composition, and age.

Exercise Mode *Variations in $\dot{V}O_{2max}$ during different modes of exercise reflect the quantity of activated muscle mass.* Experiments that measured $\dot{V}O_{2max}$ on the same subjects during treadmill exercise produced the highest values. Bench-stepping generates $\dot{V}O_{2max}$ scores nearly identical to treadmill values and significantly higher than bicycle ergometer values. With arm-crank exercise, a person's aerobic capacity reaches only about 70% of treadmill $\dot{V}O_{2max}$.

For skilled but untrained swimmers, $\dot{V}O_{2max}$ during swimming records about 20% below treadmill values. A definite test specificity exists in this form of exercise because trained collegiate swimmers achieved $\dot{V}O_{2max}$ values swimming only 11% below treadmill values; some elite competitive swimmers equal or even exceed their treadmill $\dot{V}O_{2max}$ scores during an aerobic capacity swimming test. Similarly, a distinct exercise and training specificity occurs among competitive racewalkers who achieve oxygen

BOX 7.6 CLOSE UP

Predicting $\dot{V}O_{2max}$ Using Age for Sedentary, Physically Active, and Endurance-Trained Individuals

$\dot{V}O_{2max}$ declines approximately 0.4 mL·kg^{-1}·min^{-1} each year for most individuals (4.0 mL·kg^{-1}·min^{-1} each decade). Sedentary individuals may have nearly twofold faster rates of decline in $\dot{V}O_{2max}$ aging. Heredity undoubtedly plays an important role, as does the well-documented decrement in muscle mass with age. Thus, for both active and sedentary persons, it is possible to predict $\dot{V}O_{2max}$ from age alone.

EQUATIONS

The accompanying table presents different equations to predict $\dot{V}O_{2max}$ using age as the predictor variable.

Example 1: Endurance-Trained Man, Age 55 y (Equation 3)

$$\text{Predicted } \dot{V}O_{2max} = 77.2 - 0.46 \, (\text{age, y})$$
$$= 77.2 - 0.46 \, (55)$$
$$= 51.7 \text{ mL·kg}^{-1}\text{·min}^{-1}$$

Example 2: Active Woman, Age 21 y (Equation 2)

$$\text{Predicted } \dot{V}O_{2max} = 61.4 - 0.39 \, (\text{age, y})$$
$$= 61.4 - 0.39 \, (21)$$
$$= 53.2 \text{ mL·kg}^{-1}\text{·min}^{-1}$$

Example 3: 23-Year-Old Woman of Unknown Fitness Status (Equation 4)

$$\text{Predicted } \dot{V}O_{2max} = 53.7 - 0.537 \, (\text{age, y})$$
$$= 53.7 - 0.537 \, (23)$$
$$= 41.4 \text{ mL·kg}^{-1}\text{·min}^{-1}$$

Equations to Predict $\dot{V}O_{2max}$ (mL·kg^{-1}·min^{-1}) from Age

GROUP	EQUATION	CORRELATION
1. Sedentary[a]	Predicted $\dot{V}O_{2max}$ = 54.2 − 0.40 (age, y)	r = 0.88
2. Moderately Active[b]	Predicted $\dot{V}O_{2max}$ = 61.4 − 0.39 (age, y)	r = 0.80
3. Endurance Trained[c]	Predicted $\dot{V}O_{2max}$ = 77.2 − 0.46 (age, y)	r = 0.89
4. Alternate equations (independent of relative fitness status)		
Males: Predicted $\dot{V}O_{2max}$ = 59.48 − 0.46 (age, y)		
Females: Predicted $\dot{V}O_{2max}$ = 53.7 − 0.537 (age, y)		

[a]No physical activity.
[b]Occasional physical activity, about 2 d·wk^{-1}.
[c]Physical activity = 3 d·wk^{-1} for at least 1 full year.

REFERENCES

1. Wilson, T.M., and Seals, D.R.: Meta-analysis of the age-associated decline in maximal aerobic capacity in men: Relation to habitual aerobic status. *Med. Sci. Sports Exerc.*, 31(suppl):S385, 1995.
2. Jackson, A.S., et al.: Changes in aerobic power of women age 20–64 y. *Med. Sci. Sports Exerc.*, 28:884, 1996.

uptakes during walking that equal $\dot{V}O_{2max}$ values during treadmill running. If competitive cyclists pedal at their fastest rate in competition, they also achieve $\dot{V}O_{2max}$ values equivalent to their treadmill scores.

The treadmill represents the laboratory apparatus of choice to determine $\dot{V}O_{2max}$ in healthy subjects. The treadmill easily quantifies and regulates exercise intensity. Compared with other exercise modes, subjects achieve one or more of the criteria on the treadmill to establish $\dot{V}O_{2max}$ or $\dot{V}O_{2peak}$ more easily. Bench stepping or bicycle exercise serve as suitable alternatives under non-laboratory "field" conditions.

Heredity A frequent question concerns the relative contribution of heredity to physiologic function and exercise performance. For example, to what extent does heredity determine the extremely high aerobic capacities of endurance athletes? Some researchers focus on the question of how genetic variability accounts for differences among individuals in physiologic and metabolic capacity.

Early studies were conducted on 15 pairs of identical twins (same heredity because they came from the same fertilized egg) and 15 pairs of fraternal twins (did not differ from ordinary siblings because they result from separate fertilization of two eggs) raised in the same city by parents with similar socioeconomic backgrounds. The researchers concluded that heredity alone accounted for up to 93% of the observed differences in $\dot{V}O_{2max}$. Subsequent investigations of larger groups of brothers, fraternal twins, and identical twins indicate a much smaller effect of inherited factors on aerobic capacity and endurance performance.

Current estimates of the genetic effect ascribe about 20% to 30% for $\dot{V}O_{2max}$, 50% for maximum heart rate, and 70% for physical working capacity. Future research will someday determine the exact upper limit of genetic determination, but present data show that inherited factors contribute *significantly* to physiologic functional capacity and exercise performance. A large genotype dependency also exists for the potential to improve aerobic and anaerobic power and adaptations of most muscle enzymes to training. In other words, members of the same twin pair show almost identical responses to exercise training.

Training State Maximal oxygen uptake must be evaluated relative to the person's state of training at the time of measurement. Aerobic capacity with training improves between 6% and 20%, although increases have been reported as high as 50% above pretraining levels. The largest $\dot{V}O_{2max}$ improvement occurs among the most sedentary individuals.

Gender $\dot{V}O_{2max}$ $(mL \cdot kg^{-1} \cdot min^{-1})$ for women typically averages 15% to 30% below values for men. Even among trained athletes, the disparity ranges between 10% and 20%. Such differences increase considerably when expressing $\dot{V}O_{2max}$ as an absolute value $(L \cdot min^{-1})$ rather than relative to body mass $(mL \cdot kg^{-1} \cdot min^{-1})$ or $mL \cdot FFM^{-1} \cdot min^{-1}$. Among world-class male and female cross-country skiers, a 43% lower $\dot{V}O_{2max}$ for women (6.54 vs. 3.75 $L \cdot min^{-1}$)

decreased to 15% (83.8 vs. 71.2 $mL \cdot kg^{-1} \cdot min^{-1}$) when using the athletes' body mass in the $\dot{V}O_{2max}$ ratio expression.

The apparent gender difference in $\dot{V}O_{2max}$ has been attributed to differences in body composition and the blood's hemoglobin concentration. Untrained young adult women possess about 25% body fat, the corresponding value for men averages 15%. Trained athletes have a lower body fat percentage, yet trained women still possess significantly more body fat than their male counterparts. Consequently, males generate more total aerobic energy simply because they possess a relatively large muscle mass and less fat than females.

Probably because of higher levels of testosterone, men also show a 10% to 14% greater concentration of hemoglobin than women. This difference in the blood's oxygen-carrying capacity enables males to circulate more oxygen during exercise to give them an edge in aerobic capacity.

Differences in normal physical activity level between an "average" male and "average" female also provide a possible explanation for the gender difference in $\dot{V}O_{2max}$. Perhaps less opportunity exists for women to become as physically active as men because of social structure and constraints. Even among prepubertal children, boys exhibit a higher physical activity level in daily life.

Despite these possible limitations, the aerobic capacity of physically active women exceeds that of sedentary men. For example, female cross-country skiers have $\dot{V}O_{2max}$ scores 40% higher than untrained men of the same age.

Body Composition *Differences in body mass explain roughly 70% of the differences in $\dot{V}O_{2max}$ $(L \cdot min^{-1})$ among individuals.* Thus, meaningful comparisons of $\dot{V}O_{2max}$ when expressed in $L \cdot min^{-1}$ become difficult among individuals who differ in body size or body composition. This has led to the common practice of expressing oxygen uptake in terms by body surface area, body mass (BM), fat-free body mass (FFM) or even limb volume (i.e., dividing the $\dot{V}O_{2max}$ scores by FFM or BM) in the hope that $\dot{V}O_{2max}$ will be expressed independent of the respective divisor.

Table 7.3 presents typical oxygen uptake values for an untrained man and woman who differ considerably in body mass. The percentage difference in $\dot{V}O_{2max}$ between these individuals, when expressed in $L \cdot min^{-1}$, amounts to 43%. The woman still exhibits about a 20% lower value when

Table 7.3	Different Ways of Expressing Oxygen Uptake		
VARIABLE	**FEMALE**	**MALE**	**% DIFFERENCE[a]**
$\dot{V}O_{2max}$, $L \cdot min^{-1}$	2.00	3.50	−43
$\dot{V}O_{2max}$, $mL \cdot min^{-1}$	40.0	50.0	−20
$\dot{V}O_{2max}$, $mL \cdot kg\ FFM^{-1} \cdot min^{-1}$	53.3	58.8	−9.0
Body mass, kg	50	70	−29
Percent body fat	25	15	+67
FFM, kg	37.5	59.5	−37

[a]Female minus male.
FFM, fat-free mass; $\dot{V}O_{2max}$ = maximal oxygen uptake.

expressing $\dot{V}O_{2max}$ related to body mass ($mL \cdot kg^{-1} \cdot min^{-1}$); when divided by FFM, the difference shrinks to 9%.

Similar findings occur for $\dot{V}O_{2peak}$ for men and women during arm-cranking exercise. Adjusting arm-crank $\dot{V}O_{2peak}$ for variations in arm and shoulder size equalize values between men and women. This suggests that gender differences in aerobic capacity largely reflect size of "acting" muscle mass. Such observations foster arguments that no gender difference exists in the capacity of active muscle mass to generate ATP aerobically. On the other hand, simply dividing $\dot{V}O_{2max}$ or $\dot{V}O_{2peak}$ by some measure of body composition does not automatically "adjust" for observable gender differences.

Age Changes in $\dot{V}O_{2max}$ relate to chronological age, yet limitations exist in drawing inferences from cross-sectional studies of different people at different ages. The available data provide insight into the possible effects of aging on physiologic function.

Absolute Values Maximal oxygen uptake ($L \cdot min^{-1}$) increases dramatically during the growth years. Longitudinal studies (measuring the same individual over a prolonged period) of children's $\dot{V}O_{2max}$ show that absolute values increase from about 1.0 $L \cdot min^{-1}$ at age 6 years to 3.2 $L \cdot min^{-1}$ at 16 years. $\dot{V}O_{2max}$ in girls peaks at about age 14 years and declines thereafter. At age 14 years, the differences in $\dot{V}O_{2max}$ ($L \cdot min^{-1}$) between boys and girls is approximately 25%, with the spread reaching 50% by age 16 years.

Relative Values When expressed relative to body mass, the $\dot{V}O_{2max}$ remains constant at about 53 $mL \cdot kg^{-1} \cdot min^{-1}$ between ages 6 and 16 years for boys. In contrast, relative $\dot{V}O_{2max}$ in girls gradually decreases from 52.0 $mL \cdot kg^{-1} \cdot min^{-1}$ at age 6 years to 40.5 $mL \cdot kg^{-1} \cdot min^{-1}$ at age 16 years. Greater accumulation of body fat in young women provides the most common explanation for this discrepancy.

A recent longitudinal study of a cohort of more than 3000 women and 16,000 men age 20 to 96 years from the Aerobics Center Longitudinal Study (*www.cooperinstitute.org/research/study/acls.cfm*) who completed serial health examinations including maximal treadmill testing during 1974 to 2006 illustrates the effects of age on aerobic capacity. *Beyond age 35 years, $\dot{V}O_{2max}$ declines at a non-linear rate that accelerates after age 45 years so that by age 60 years, it averages 11% below values for 35-year-old men and 15% below values for women* (**Fig. 7.14**). Although active adults retain a relatively high $\dot{V}O_{2max}$ at all ages, their aerobic power still declines with advancing years. However, research continues to show that one's habitual level of physical activity through middle age determines changes in $\dot{V}O_{2max}$ to a greater extent than chronological age per se.

$\dot{V}O_{2max}$ PREDICTIONS

Directly measuring $\dot{V}O_{2max}$ requires an extensive laboratory and equipment, including considerable motivation on the subject's part to perform "all out." In addition, maximal exercise can be hazardous to adults who have not received proper medical clearance or who are tested without appropriate safeguards or supervision (refer to Chapter 18).

In view of these requirements, alternative tests have been devised to predict $\dot{V}O_{2max}$ from submaximal performances (refer to Close Up Boxes 7.4–7.6 in this chapter). The most popular $\dot{V}O_{2max}$ predictions use walking and running performance. Easily administered, large groups can perform these tests without the need for a formal laboratory setting. Running tests assume that $\dot{V}O_{2max}$ largely determines the distance one runs in a specified time (>5 or 6 min). The first of the running tests required subjects to run-walk as far as possible in 15 minutes, and a 1968 revision of the test shortened the duration to 12 minutes or 1.5 miles.

*Q*uestions & Notes

Explain the rationale for expressing $\dot{V}O_2$ in $mL \cdot kg^{-1} \cdot min^{-1}$.

Briefly explain the effects of increasing age on $\dot{V}O_{2max}$.

Give the average $\dot{V}O_{2max}$ for the following individuals: (Hint see Figure 7.14)

1. 20 year old male:

2. 40 year old female:

3. 65 year old male:

4. 75 year old female:

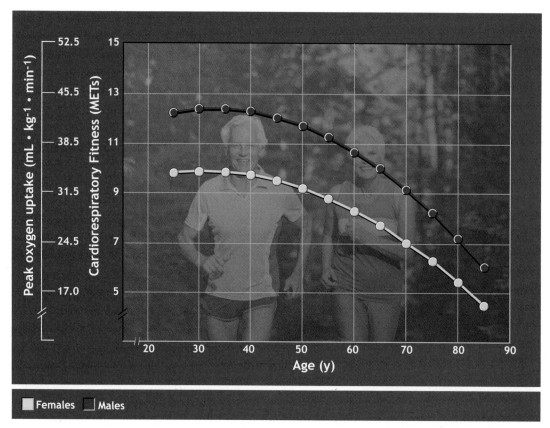

Figure 7.14   General trend for maximal oxygen uptake with age in a longitudinal study of a large cohort males and females. (Modified from Jackson, A., et al.: Role of lifestyle and aging on the longitudinal change in cardiorespiratory fitness. *Arch. Intern. Med.*, 169:1781, 2009.)

Findings from many research studies suggest that prediction of aerobic capacity should be approached with caution when using walking and running performance. Establishing a consistent level of motivation and effective pacing becomes critical for inexperienced subjects. Some individuals may run too fast early in the run and slow down or even stop as the test (and fatigue) progresses. Other individuals may begin too slowly and continue this way, so their final run score reflects inappropriate pacing or motivation, rather than physiologic and metabolic capacity.

Factors other than $\dot{V}O_{2max}$ determine walking-running performance. The following four factors contribute to the final $\dot{V}O_{2max}$ predicted score:

1. Body mass
2. Body fatness
3. Running economy
4. Percentage of aerobic capacity sustainable without blood lactate buildup

Heart Rate Predictions of V̇O2max

Common tests to predict $\dot{V}O_{2max}$ from exercise or postexercise heart rate use a standardized regimen of submaximal exercise on a bicycle ergometer, motorized

treadmill, or step test. Such tests make use of the essentially linear or straight-line relationship between heart rate and oxygen uptake for various intensities of light to moderately intense exercise. The slope of this relationship (rate of HR increase per unit of $\dot{V}O_2$ increase) reflects the individual's aerobic power ($\dot{V}O_{2max}$). It is estimated by drawing a best-fit straight line through several submaximum points that relate heart rate and oxygen uptake or exercise intensity, and then extending the line to an assumed maximum heart rate (HR_{max}) for the person's age.

Figure 7.15 for example, applies this **extrapolation procedure** for a trained and untrained subject. Four submaximal measures during bicycle exercise provided the data points to draw the heart rate–oxygen uptake (HR–$\dot{V}O_2$) line. Each person's HR–$\dot{V}O_2$ line tends to be linear, but the slope of the individual lines can differ considerably largely from variations in how much blood the heart pumps with each beat (stroke volume). A person with a relatively high aerobic power can accomplish more exercise and achieves a higher oxygen uptake before reaching their HR_{max} than a less "fit" person. The person with the lowest heart rate increase tends to have the highest exercise capacity and largest $\dot{V}O_{2max}$. The data in **Figure 7.15** predict $\dot{V}O_{2max}$ by extrapolating the HR–$\dot{V}O_2$ line to a heart

BOX 7.7 CLOSE UP

The Weir Method of Calculating Energy Expenditure

In 1949, J.B. Weir, a Scottish physician and physiologist from Glasgow University, presented a simple method to estimate caloric expenditure ($kCal \cdot min^{-1}$) from measures of pulmonary ventilation and expired oxygen percentage, accurate to within $\pm 1\%$ of the traditional RQ method.

BASIC EQUATION

Weir showed the following formula could calculate energy expenditure if total energy production from protein breakdown equaled 12.5% (a reasonable percentage for most people):

$$kCal \cdot min^{-1} = \dot{V}_{E(STPD)} \times (1.044 - 0.0499 \times \%O_{2E})$$

where $\dot{V}_{E(STPD)}$ represents expired minute ventilation ($L \cdot min^{-1}$) corrected to STPD conditions, and $\%O_{2E}$ represents expired oxygen percentage. The value in parentheses $(1.044 - 0.0499 \times \%O_{2E})$ represents the "Weir factor." The table displays Weir factors for different $\%O_{2E}$ values.

To use the table, locate the $\%O_{2E}$ and corresponding Weir factor. Compute energy expenditure in $kCal \cdot min^{-1}$ by multiplying the Weir factor by $\dot{V}_{E(STPD)}$.

Example

A person runs on a treadmill and $\dot{V}_{E(STPD)} = 50 \ L \cdot min^{-1}$ and $\%O_{2E} = 16.0\%$. Compute energy expenditure by the Weir method as follows:

$$
\begin{aligned}
kCal \cdot min^{-1} &= \dot{V}_{E(STPD)} \times (1.044 - [0.0499 \times \%O_{2E}]) \\
&= 50 \times (1.044 - [0.0499 \times 16.0]) \\
&= 50 \times 0.2456 \\
&= 12.3
\end{aligned}
$$

Weir also derived the following equation to calculate $kCal \cdot min^{-1}$ from RQ and $\dot{V}O_2$ in $L \cdot min^{-1}$:

$$kCal \cdot min^{-1} = ([1.1 \times RQ] + 3.9) \times \dot{V}O_2$$

Weir Factors			
WEIR	**$\%O_{2E}$ FACTOR**	**WEIR**	**$\%O_{2E}$ FACTOR**
14.50	0.3205	17.00	0.1957
14.60	0.3155	17.10	0.1907
14.70	0.3105	17.20	0.1857
14.80	0.3055	17.30	0.1807
14.90	0.3005	17.40	0.1757
15.00	0.2955	17.50	0.1707
15.10	0.2905	17.60	0.1658
15.20	0.2855	17.70	0.1608
15.30	0.2805	17.80	0.1558
15.40	0.2755	17.90	0.1508
15.50	0.2705	18.00	0.1468
15.60	0.2656	18.10	0.1408
15.70	0.2606	18.20	0.1368
15.80	0.2556	18.30	0.1308
15.90	0.2506	18.40	0.1268
16.00	0.2456	18.50	0.1208
16.10	0.2406	18.60	0.1168
16.20	0.2366	18.70	0.1109
16.30	0.2306	18.80	0.1068
16.40	0.2256	18.90	0.1009
16.50	0.2206	19.00	0.0969
16.60	0.2157	19.10	0.0909
16.70	0.2107	19.20	0.0868
16.80	0.2057	19.30	0.0809
16.90	0.2007	19.40	0.0769

If $\%O_{2E}$ (expired oxygen percentage) does not appear in the table, compute individual Weir factors as $1.044 - 0.0499 \times \%O_{2E}$.

From Weir, J.B.: New methods for calculating metabolic rates with special reference to protein metabolism. *J. Physiol.*, 109:1, 1949.

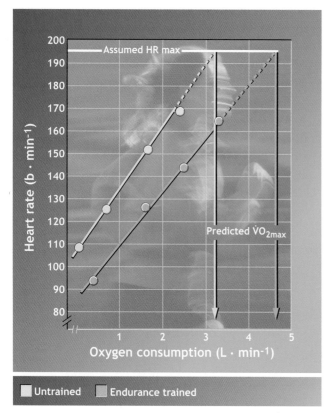

Untrained   Endurance trained

Figure 7.15 Prediction of maximal oxygen uptake ($\dot{V}O_{2max}$) by extrapolating the linear relationship between submaximal heart rate and oxygen uptake during graded exercise in an untrained and aerobically trained subject.

rate of 195 b·min^{-1} (the assumed maximum heart rate for these college-age subjects).

The following four assumptions limit the accuracy of predicting $\dot{V}O_{2max}$ from submaximal exercise heart rate:

1. **Linearity of the HR–$\dot{V}O_2$ (exercise intensity) relationship.** Various intensities of light to moderately intense exercise meet this assumption. For some subjects, the HR–$\dot{V}O_2$ line curves or asymptotes at the intense exercise levels in a direction that indicates a larger than expected increase in oxygen uptake per unit increase in heart rate. Oxygen uptake increases more than predicted through linear extrapolation of the HR–$\dot{V}O_2$ line, thus *under-estimating* the $\dot{V}O_{2max}$.

2. **Similar maximum heart rates for all subjects.** The standard deviation for the average maximum heart rate for individuals of the same age equals ±10 b·min^{-1}. The $\dot{V}O_{2max}$ of a 25-year-old person with a maximum heart rate of 185 b·min^{-1} would be *over-estimated* if the HR–$\dot{V}O_2$ line extrapolated to an assumed maximum heart rate for this age group of 195 b·min^{-1}. The opposite would occur if this subject's maximum heart rate equaled 210 b·min^{-1}. HR_{max} also decreases with age. Without considering the age effect, older subjects would consistently be *overestimated* by assuming a maximum heart rate of

195 b·min^{-1}, which represents the appropriate estimation for 25 year olds.

3. **Assumed constant exercise economy.** The predicted $\dot{V}O_{2max}$ can vary from variability in exercise economy when estimating submaximal oxygen uptake from an exercise level. A subject with low economy (submaximal $\dot{V}O_2$ higher than assumed) is *underestimated* for $\dot{V}O_{2max}$ because the heart rate increases from added oxygen cost of uneconomical exercise. The opposite occurs for a person with high exercise economy. The variation among individuals in oxygen uptake during walking, stepping, or cycling does not usually exceed ±6%. Seemingly small modifications in test procedures profoundly affect the metabolic cost of exercise. Allowing individuals to support themselves with treadmill handrails reduces exercise oxygen cost by up to 30%. Failure to maintain cadence on a bicycle ergometer or step test can dramatically alter the oxygen requirement.

4. **Day-to-day variation in exercise heart rate.** Even under highly standardized conditions, an individual's submaximal heart rate varies by about ±5 beats per minute with day-to-day testing at the same exercise intensity. This variation in exercise heart rate represents an additional error source.

Considering these four limitations, $\dot{V}O_{2max}$ predicted from submaximal heart rate generally falls within 10% to 20% of the person's actual $\dot{V}O_{2max}$. Clearly, this represents too large an error for research purposes. These tests are better suited for screening and classification of aerobic fitness.

A Word of Caution About Predictions

All predictions involve error. The error is referred to as the **standard error of estimate (SEE)** and computes from the original equation that generated the prediction. Errors of estimate are expressed in units of the predicted variable or a percentage. For example, say the $\dot{V}O_{2max}$ (mL·kg^{-1}·min^{-1}) prediction from a walking test equals 55 mL·kg^{-1}·min^{-1} and the SEE of the predicted score equals ±10 mL·kg^{-1}·min^{-1}. This means that in reality the actual $\dot{V}O_{2max}$ probably (68% likelihood) ranges within ±10 mL·kg^{-1}·min^{-1} of the predicted value, or between 45 and 65 mL·kg^{-1}·min^{-1}. This example represents a relatively large error (±18.2% of the actual value).

Obviously, a larger prediction error creates a less than useful predicted score because the true score falls within a broad range of possible values. One cannot judge the usefulness of the predicted score without knowing the magnitude of the error. Whenever predictions are made, one must interpret the predicted score in light of the magnitude of the prediction error. With a small error, prediction of $\dot{V}O_{2max}$ proves useful in appropriate situations in which direct measurement is not feasible.

SUMMARY

1. Direct and indirect calorimetry determine the body's rate of energy expenditure. Direct calorimetry measures the actual heat production in an insulated calorimeter. Indirect calorimetry infers energy expenditure from oxygen uptake and carbon dioxide production using closed- or open-circuit spirometry.

2. All energy-releasing reactions in the body ultimately depend on oxygen use. Measuring oxygen uptake during steady-rate exercise provides an indirect yet accurate estimate of energy expenditure.

3. Three common open-circuit, indirect calorimetric procedures to measure oxygen uptake during physical activity include portable spirometry, bag technique, and computerized instrumentation.

4. The complete oxidation of each nutrient requires a different quantity of oxygen uptake compared with carbon dioxide production. The ratio of carbon dioxide produced to oxygen consumed (the RQ) provides important information about the nutrient mixture catabolized for energy. The RQ averages 1.00 for carbohydrate, 0.70 for fat, and 0.82 for protein.

5. For each RQ value, a corresponding caloric value exists for 1 L of oxygen consumed. The RQ–kCal relationship determines energy expenditure during exercise with a high degree of accuracy.

6. During strenuous exercise, the RQ does not represent specific substrate use because of nonmetabolic production of carbon dioxide in lactate buffering.

7. The respiratory exchange ratio (R) reflects the pulmonary exchange of carbon dioxide and oxygen under various physiologic and metabolic conditions; R does not fully mirror the macronutrient mixture catabolized for energy.

8. $\dot{V}O_{2max}$ provides reliable and important information on the power of the long-term aerobic energy system, including the functional capacity of various physiologic support systems.

9. A leveling-off or peaking-over in oxygen uptake during increasing exercise intensity signifies attainment of maximum capacity for aerobic metabolism (i.e., a "true" $\dot{V}O_{2max}$). The term "peak oxygen uptake" ($\dot{V}O_{2peak}$) describes the highest oxygen uptake value when this accepted criterion is not met or local muscle fatigue in the arms or legs rather than central circulatory dynamics limits test performance.

10. Different standardized tests measure $\dot{V}O_{2max}$. Such tests remain independent of muscle strength, speed, body size, and skill, with the exception of specialized swimming, rowing, and ice skating tests.

11. The $\dot{V}O_{2max}$ test may require a continuous 3- to 5-minute "supermaximal" effort but usually consists of increments in exercise intensity referred to as a graded exercise test (GXT).

12. Two types of $\dot{V}O_{2max}$ tests are a continuous test without rest between exercise increments and a discontinuous test with several minutes of rest between exercise increments.

13. The most important factors that influence $\dot{V}O_{2max}$ include exercise mode, training state, heredity, gender, body composition, and age.

14. Differences in body mass explain roughly 70% of the differences among individuals in $\dot{V}O_{2max}$ ($L \cdot min^{-1}$).

15. Changes in $\dot{V}O_{2max}$ relate to chronological age.

16. Tests to predict $\dot{V}O_{2max}$ from submaximal physiologic and performance data can be useful for classification purposes. The validity of prediction equations relies on the following assumptions: linearity of the HR–$\dot{V}O_2$ line, similar maximal heart rate for individuals of the same age, a constant exercise economy, and a relatively small day-to-day variation in exercise heart rate.

17. Field methods to predict $\dot{V}O_{2max}$ provide useful information for screening purposes in the absence of the direct measurement of aerobic capacity with more elaborate testing.

THOUGHT QUESTION

1. Explain how oxygen uptake translates to heat production during exercise.

SELECTED REFERENCES

Aisbett, B., et al.: The influence of pacing during 6-minute supra-maximal cycle ergometer performance. *J. Sci. Med. Sport*, 6:187, 2003.

Amann, M., et al.: An evaluation of the predictive validity and reliability of ventilatory threshold. *Med. Sci. Sports Exerc.*, 36:1716, 2004.

Atwater, W.O., Rosa, E.B.: Description of a New Respiration Calorimeter and Experiments on the Conservation Of Energy in the Human Body. Bulletin No. 63, Washington, D.C., U.S. Department of Agriculture, Office of Experiment Stations, Government Printing Office, 1899.

Balmer, J., et al.: Mechanically braked Wingate powers: agreement between SRM, corrected and conventional methods of measurement. *J. Sports Sci.*, 22:661, 2004.

Bar-Or, O.: The Wingate anaerobic test: An update on methodology, reliability, and validity. *Sports Med.*, 4:381, 1987.

Bentley, D.J., McNaughton, L.R.: Comparison of W(peak), $\dot{V}O_2$(peak) and the ventilation threshold from two different incremental exercise tests: relationship to endurance performance. *J. Sci. Med. Sport*, 6:422, 2003.

Binzoni, T.: Saturation of the lactate clearance mechanisms different from the "lactate shuttle" determines the anaerobic threshold: prediction from the bioenergetic model. *J. Physiol. Anthropol. Appl. Human Sci.*, 24:175, 2005.

Blain, G., et al.: Assessment of ventilatory thresholds during graded and maximal exercise test using time varying analysis of respiratory sinus arrhythmia. *Br. J. Sports Med.*, 39:448, 2005.

Bosquet, L., et al.: Methods to determine aerobic endurance. *Sports Med.*, 32:675, 2002.

Bouchard, C., et al.: Familial resemblance for $\dot{V}O_{2max}$ in the sedentary state: The Heritage family study. *Med. Sci. Sports Exerc.*, 30:252, 1998.

Bouchard, C., et al.: Testing anaerobic power and capacity. In *Physiological Testing of the High Performance Athlete*. J. MacKougall, et al., eds. Champaign, IL: Human Kinetics Press; 175–222, 1991.

Brooks, G.A.: Intra- and extra-cellular lactate shuttles. *Med. Sci. Sports Exerc.*, 32:790, 2000.

Buresh, R., Berg, K.: Scaling oxygen uptake to body size and several practical applications. *J. Strength Cond. Res.*, 16:46, 2002.

Busso, T., et al.: A comparison of modelling procedures used to estimate the power-exhaustion time relationship. *Eur. J. Appl. Physiol.*, 108:257, 2010.

Cain, S.M.: Mechanisms which control $\dot{V}O_2$ near $\dot{V}O_{2max}$: An overview. *Med. Sci. Sports Exerc.*, 27:60, 1995.

Canavan, P.K., Vescovi, J.D.: Evaluation of power prediction equations: Peak vertical jumping power in women. *Med. Sci. Sports Exerc.*, 36:1589, 2004.

Castellani, J.W., et al.: Energy expenditure in men and women during 54h of exercise and caloric deprivation. *Med. Sci. Sports Exerc.*, 38:894, 2006.

Cooper, K.: Correlation between field and treadmill testing as a means for assessing maximal oxygen intake. *JAMA*, 203:201, 1968.

Cooper, S.M., et al.: A simple multistage field test for the prediction of anaerobic capacity in female games players. *Br. J. Sports Med.*, 38:784, 2004.

Coquart, J.B., et al.: Prediction of peak oxygen uptake from sub-maximal ratings of perceived exertion elicited during a graded exercise test in obese women. *Psychophysiology*, 46:1150, 2009.

Duncan, G.E., et al.: Applicability of $\dot{V}O_{2max}$ criteria: Discontinuous versus continuous protocols. *Med. Sci. Sports Exerc.*, 29:273, 1997.

Ekelund, U., et al.: Energy expenditure assessed by heart rate and doubly labeled water in young athletes. *Med. Sci. Sports Exerc.*, 34:1360, 2002.

Eston, R., et al.: Prediction of maximal oxygen uptake in sedentary males from a perceptually regulated, sub-maximal graded exercise test. *J. Sports Sci.*, 26:131, 2008.

Fleg, J.L., et al.: Accelerated longitudinal decline of aerobic capacity in healthy older adults. *Circulation*, 112:674, 2005.

Flouris, A.D., et al.: Prediction of $\dot{V}O_{2max}$ from a new field test based on portable indirect calorimetry. *J. Sci. Med. Sport*, 13:70, 2010.

Gladden, L.B.: Muscle as a consumer of lactate. *Med. Sci. Sports Exerc.*, 32:764, 2000.

Gladden, L.B.: The role of skeletal muscle in lactate exchange during exercise: introduction. *Med. Sci. Sports Exerc.*, 32:753, 2000.

Gore, J.C., et al.: CPX/D underestimates O_2 in athletes compared with an automated Douglas bag system. *Med. Sci. Sports Exerc.*, 35:1341, 2003.

Hagberg, J.M., et al.: Specific genetic markers of endurance performance and $\dot{V}O_{2max}$. *Exerc. Sport Sci. Rev.*, 29:15, 2001.

Haldane, J.S., Priestley, J.G.: *Respiration*. New York: Oxford University Press, 1935.

Hetzler, R.K., et al.: Development of a modified Margaria-Kalamen anaerobic power test for American football athletes. *Strength Cond. Res.*, 24:978, 2010.

Jackson, A., et al.: Role of lifestyle and aging on the longitudinal change in cardiorespiratory fitness. *Arch. Intern. Med.*, 169:1781, 2009.

Jéquier, E., Schutz, Y.: Long-term measurements of energy expenditure in humans using a respiration chamber. *Am. J. Clin. Nutr.*, 38:989, 1983.

Jo, E.: Influence of recovery duration after a potentiating stimulus on muscular power in recreationally trained individuals. *J. Strength Cond. Res.*, 24:343, 2010.

Jurca, R., et al.: Assessing cardiorespiratory fitness without performing exercise testing. *Am. J. Prev. Med.*, 29:185, 2005.

Katch, V.L., et al.: Optimal test characteristics for maximal anaerobic work on the bicycle ergometer. *Res. Q.*, 48:319, 1977.

Katch, V.: Kinetics of oxygen uptake and recovery for supramaximal work of short duration. *Eur. J. Appl. Physiol.*, 31:197, l973.

Katch, V.: Body weight, leg volume, leg weight and leg density as determiners of short duration work performance on the bicycle ergometer. *Med. Sci. Sports*, 6:267, 1974.

Katch, V., et al.: A steady-paced versus all-out cycling strategy for maximal work output of short duration. *Res. Q.*, 47:164, 1976.

Kohler, R.M., et al.: Peak power during repeated Wingate trials: Implications for testing. *J. Strength Cond. Res.*, 24:370, 2010.

Kounalakis, S.N., et al.: Oxygen saturation in the triceps brachii muscle during an arm Wingate test: the role of training and power output. *Res. Sports Med.*, 17:171, 2009.

Krustrup, P., et al.: The yo-yo intermittent recovery test: physiological response, reliability, and validity. *Med. Sci. Sports Exerc.*, 35:697, 2003.

Little, J.P., et al.: A practical model of low-volume high-intensity interval training induces mitochondrial biogenesis in human skeletal muscle: potential mechanisms. *J. Physiol.*, 588, 2010.

Margaria, R., et al.: Measurement of muscular power (anaerobic) in man. *J. Appl. Physiol.*, 21:1662, 1966.

McArdle, W.D., et al.: Specificity of run training on $\dot{V}O_{2max}$ and heart rate changes during running and swimming. *Med. Sci. Sports*, 10:16, 1978.

McLester, J.R., et al.: Effects of standing vs. seated posture on repeated Wingate performance. *J. Strength Cond. Res.*, 18:816, 2004.

McMurray, R.G., et al.: Predicted maximal aerobic power in youth is related to age, gender, and ethnicity. *Med. Sci. Sports Exerc.*, 34:145, 2002.

Molik, B., et al.: Relationship between functional classification levels and anaerobic performance of wheelchair basketball athletes. *Res. Q. Exerc. Sport*, 81:69, 2010.

Moore, A., Murphy, A.: Development of an anaerobic capacity test for field sport athletes. *J. Sci. Med. Sport*, 6:275, 2003.

Nikooie, R., et al.: Noninvasive determination of anaerobic threshold by monitoring the %SpO2 changes and respiratory gas exchange. *J. Strength Cond. Res.*, 23:2107, 2009.

Porszasz, J., et al.: A treadmill ramp protocol using simultaneous changes in speed and grade. *Med. Sci. Sports Exerc.*, 35:1596, 2003.

Potteiger, J.A., et al.: Relationship between body composition, leg strength, anaerobic power, and on-ice skating performance in division I men's hockey athletes. *J. Strength Cond. Res.*, 24:1755, 2010.

Ravussin, E., et al.: Determinants of 24-hour energy expenditure in man: Methods and results using a respiratory chamber. *J. Clin. Invest.*, 78:1568, 1986.

Rumpler, W., et al.: Repeatability of 24-hour energy expenditure measurements in humans by indirect calorimetry. *Am. J. Clin. Nutr.*, 51:147, 1990.

Seiler, S., et al.: The fall and rise of the gender difference in elite anaerobic performance 1952–2006. *Med. Sci. Sports Exerc.*, 39:534, 2007.

Sentija, D., et al.: The effects of strength training on some parameters of aerobic and anaerobic endurance. *Coll. Antropol.*, 33:111, 2009.

Snell, P.G., et al.: Maximal oxygen uptake as a parametric measure of cardiorespiratory capacity. *Med. Sci. Sports Exerc.*, 39:103, 2007.

Souissi, N., et al.: Diurnal variation in Wingate test performances: influence of active warm-up. *Chronobiol. Int.*, 27:640, 2010.

Speakman, J.R.: The history and theory of the doubly labeled water technique. *Am. J. Clin. Nutr.*, 68(Suppl):932S, 1998.

Spencer, M.R., Gastin, P.B.: Energy system contribution during 200-m to 1500-m running in highly trained athletes. *Med. Sci. Sports Exerc.*, 33:157, 2001.

Suminski, R.R., et al.: The effect of habitual smoking on measured and predicted $\dot{V}O_2(max)$. *J. Phys. Act. Health*, 6:667, 2009.

Tiainen, K., et al.: Heritability of maximal isometric muscle strength in older female twins. *J. Appl. Physiol.*, 96:173, 2004.

Uth, N., et al.: Estimation of $\dot{V}O_{2max}$ from the ratio between HR_{max} and HR_{rest}—the heart rate ratio method. *Eur. J. Appl. Physiol.*, 91:111, 2004.

Vandewalle, H., et al.: Standard anaerobic exercise test. *Sports Med.*, 4:268, 1987.

Wang, L., et al.: Time constant of heart rate recovery after low level exercise as a useful measure of cardiovascular fitness. *Conf. Proc. IEEE Eng. Med. Biol. Soc.*, 1:1799, 2006.

Wasserman, K., et al.: *Principles of Exercise Testing and Interpretation*, 3rd Ed. Baltimore: Lippincott Williams & Wilkins, 1999.

Weltman, A., et al.: The lactate threshold and endurance performance. *Adv. Sports Med. Fitness*, 2:91, 1989.

Weltman, A., et al.: Exercise recovery, lactate removal, and subsequent high intensity exercise performance. *Res. Q.*, 48:786, 1977.

Wiedemann, M.S., Bosquet, L.: Anaerobic Work Capacity derived from isokinetic and isoinertial cycling. *Int. J. Sports Med.*, 31:89, 2010.

Yoon, B.L., et al.: $\dot{V}O_{2max}$, protocol duration, and the $\dot{V}O_2$ plateau. *Med. Sci. Sports Exerc.*, 39:1186, 2007.

Zagatto, A.M., et al.: Validity of the running anaerobic sprint test for assessing anaerobic power and predicting short-distance performance. *J. Strength Cond. Res.*, 23:1820, 2009.

Zajac, A., et al.: The diagnostic value of the 10- and 30-second Wingate test for competitive athletes. *J. Strength Cond. Res.*, 13:16, 1999.

Zupan, M.F., et al.: Wingate anaerobic test peak power and anaerobic capacity classifications for men and women intercollegiate athletes. *J. Strength Cond. Res.*, 23:2598, 2009.

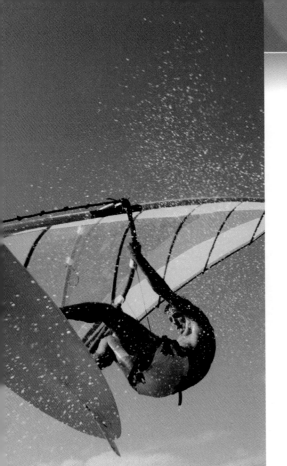

Chapter

8

Energy Expenditure During Rest and Physical Activity

CHAPTER OBJECTIVES

- Define *basal metabolic rate* and indicate factors that affect it.

- Explain the effect of body weight on the energy cost of different forms of physical activity.

- Identify factors that contribute to the total daily energy expenditure.

- Outline different classification systems for rating the intensity of physical activity.

- Describe two ways to predict resting daily energy expenditure.

- Explain the concepts of exercise efficiency and exercise economy.

- List three factors that affect the energy cost of walking and running.

- Identify factors that contribute to the lower exercise economy of swimming compared with running.

Part 1   Energy Expenditure During Rest

Three factors shown in **Figure 8.1** determine the **total daily energy expenditure** (TDEE):

1. Resting metabolic rate, which includes basal and sleeping conditions plus the added cost of arousal.
2. Thermogenic influence of consumed food.
3. Energy expended during physical activity and recovery.

BASAL (RESTING) METABOLIC RATE

For each individual, a minimum energy requirement sustains the body's functions in the waking state. Measuring oxygen uptake under the following three standardized conditions quantifies this requirement called the **basal metabolic rate** (BMR):

1. No food consumed for a minimum of 12 hours before measurement; the **postabsorptive state** describes this condition.
2. No undue muscular exertion for at least 12 hours before measurement.

3. Measured after the person has been lying quietly for 30 to 60 minutes in a dimly lit, temperature-controlled (thermoneutral) room.

Maintaining controlled conditions provides a way to study relationships among energy expenditure and body size, gender, and age. The BMR also establishes an energy baseline for implementing a prudent program of weight control by food restraint, exercise, or both. In most instances, basal values measured in the laboratory remain only marginally lower than values for **resting metabolic rate** measured under less strict conditions (e.g., 3 to 4 hours after a light meal without physical activity.) In these discussions, we use the terms *basal* and *resting metabolism* interchangeably.

INFLUENCE OF BODY SIZE ON RESTING METABOLISM

Body surface area frequently provides a common denominator for expressing basal metabolism. **Figure 8.2** shows BMR (expressed as kCal per body surface area (BSA) per hour, or $kCal \cdot m^{-2} \cdot h^{-1}$) averages 5% to 10% lower in females compared with males at all ages. A female's larger percentage body fat and smaller muscle mass in relation to body size helps explain her lower metabolic rate per unit surface area. From ages 20 to 40 years, average values for BMR equal $38 \, kCal \cdot m^{-2} \cdot h^{-1}$ for men and

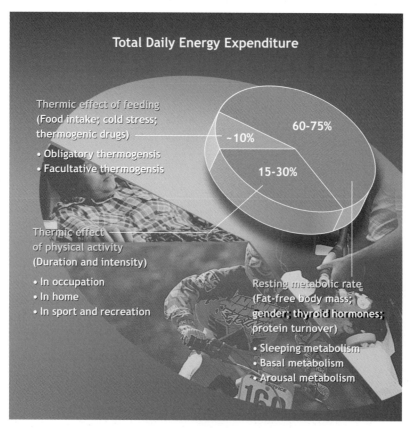

Figure 8.1 Components of daily energy expenditure.

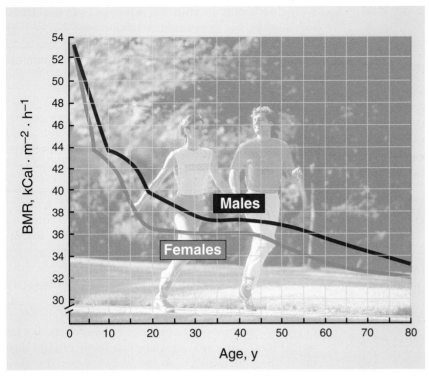

Figure 8.2 Basal metabolic rate as a function of age and gender. (Data from Altman, P.L., Dittmer, D.: *Metabolism*. Bethesda, MD: Federation of American Societies for Experimental Biology, 1968.)

Questions & Notes

Give 2 of the standardized conditions for measuring BMR.

1.

2.

Describe the general trend of the relationship between BMR and age.

What are the units of measurements for the BMR?

Write the formula for predicting body surface area.

List 3 factors that affect total daily energy expenditure.

1.

2.

3.

$36 \text{ kCal}\cdot\text{m}^{-2}\cdot\text{h}^{-1}$ for women. For a more precise BMR estimate, the actual average value for a specific age should be read directly from the curves. A person's resting metabolic rate in $\text{kCal}\cdot\text{min}^{-1}$ can be estimated and converted to a total daily resting requirement with the value for heat production (BMR) in **Figure 8.2** combined with the appropriate surface area value.

ESTIMATING RESTING DAILY ENERGY EXPENDITURE

The curves in **Figure 8.2** estimate a person's **resting daily energy expenditure** (**RDEE**). For example, between ages 20 and 40 years the BMR of men averages about 38 $\text{kCal}\cdot\text{m}^{-2}\cdot\text{h}^{-1}$; for women, the corresponding value equals 35 $\text{kCal}\cdot\text{m}^{-2}\cdot\text{h}^{-1}$. To estimate the total metabolic rate per hour, multiply the BMR value by the person's calculated BSA. This hourly total provides important information to estimate the daily energy baseline requirement for caloric intake.

Accurate measurement of the BSA poses a considerable challenge. Experiments in the early 1900s provided the data to determine BSA. The studies clothed eight men and two women in tight whole-body underwear and applied melted paraffin and paper strips to prevent modification of their body surface. After removing the treated cloth it was cut into flat pieces to allow precise measurements of BSA (length × width). The close relationship between height (stature) and body weight (mass) and BSA allowed the researcher to derive the following empirical formula to predict BSA:

$$\text{BSA, m}^2 = 0.20247 \times \text{Stature}^{0.725} \times \text{Body mass}^{0.425}$$

Stature is height in meters (multiply inches by 0.254 to convert to meters) and body mass is weight in kg (divide pounds by 2.205 to convert to kilograms).

For Your Information

CHILDREN EXHIBIT LOWER RUNNING ECONOMY THAN ADULTS

Children are less economical runners than adults; they require between 20% and 30% more oxygen per unit of body mass to run at a given speed. A larger ratio of surface area to body mass, greater stride frequency, shorter stride lengths, and anthropometric and biomechanical factors contribute to children's lower movement economy.

Example BSA computations for a man 70 inches tall (1.778 m) who weighs 165.3 lb (75 kg):

$$BSA = 0.20247 \times 1.778^{0.725} \times 75^{0.425}$$
$$= 0.20247 \times 1.51775 \times 6.2647$$
$$= 1.925 \ m^2$$

For a 20-year-old man the estimated BMR equals 36.5 $kCal \cdot m^{-2} \cdot h^{-1}$. If his surface area were 1.925 m^{-2} as in the calculation above, the hourly energy expenditure would equal 70.3 kCal (36.5 × 1.925 m^2). On a 24-hour basis, this amounts to an RDEE of 1686 kCal (70.3 × 24).

PREDICTING RESTING ENERGY EXPENDITURE

Body mass (BM), stature (S in centimeters), and age (A in years) can successfully predict RDEE with sufficient accuracy using the following equations.

Equations for women and men are:

Women: RDEE = 655 + (9.6 × BM) + (1.85 × S) − (4.7 × A)

Men: RDEE = 66.0 + (13.7 × BM) + (5.0 × S) − (6.8 × A)

Examples

Woman

BM = 62.7 kg; S = 172.5 cm; A = 22.4 y.

RDEE = 655 + (9.6 × 62.7)
+ (1.85 × 172.5) − (4.7 × 22.4)
= 655 + 601.92 + 319.13 − 105.28
= 1471 kCal

Man

BM = 80 kg; S = 189.0 cm; A = 30 y.

RDEE = 66.0 + (13.7 × 80) + (5.0 × 189.0)
− (6.8 × 30.0)
= 66.0 + 1096 + 945 − 204
= 1903 kCal

FACTORS AFFECTING TOTAL DAILY ENERGY EXPENDITURE

The three most important factors that affect total daily energy expenditure (TDEE) include physical activity, dietary-induced thermogenesis, and climate. Pregnancy also affects TDEE through its impact on the energy cost of many forms of physical activity.

Physical Activity

Physical activity profoundly affects human energy expenditure. World-class athletes nearly double their daily caloric outputs with 3 or 4 hours of physical training. Most people can sustain metabolic rates that average 10 times the resting value during "big muscle" exercises such as fast walking, running, cycling, and swimming. *Physical activity generally accounts for between 15% and 30% of TDEE.*

Dietary-Induced Thermogenesis

Consuming food increases energy metabolism from the energy-requiring processes of digesting, absorbing, and assimilating nutrients. **Dietary-induced thermogenesis (DIT;** also termed **thermic effect of food [TEF])** typically reaches maximum 1 hour after feeding, depending on food quantity and types of food consumed. The magnitude of DIT ranges between 10% and 35% of the ingested food energy. A meal of pure protein, for example, produces a thermic effect often equaling 25% of the meal's total energy content.

Advertisements routinely tout the high thermic effect of protein consumption to promote a high-protein diet for weight loss. Advocates maintain that fewer calories ultimately become available to the body compared with a lipid- or carbohydrate-rich meal of similar caloric value. This point has some validity, but other factors must be considered in formulating a prudent weight loss program. These include the potentially harmful strain on kidney and liver function induced by excessive protein and the cholesterol-stimulating effects of considerable saturated fatty acids contained in higher protein foods. Well-balanced nutrition requires a blend of macronutrients with appropriate quantities of vitamins and minerals. When combining exercise with food restriction for weight loss, carbohydrate not protein intake provides energy for exercise and conserves lean tissue invariably lost through dieting.

Individuals with poor control over their body weight often display a depressed thermic response to eating, an effect most likely related to genetic predisposition. This connection contributes to considerable body fat accumulation over many years. If a person's lifestyle includes regular moderate physical activity, then the thermogenic effect represents only a small percentage of TDEE. Also, exercising after eating further stimulates the normal thermic response to food consumption. This supports the wisdom of "going for a brisk walk" after a meal.

Climate

Environmental factors influence the resting metabolic rate. The resting metabolism of people living in tropical climates, for example, averages 5% to 20% higher than counterparts in more temperate regions. Exercise performed in hot weather also imposes a small 5% elevation in metabolic load that translates to correspondingly higher oxygen uptake compared with the same work performed in a thermoneutral environment. Three factors directly produce an increased thermogenic effect:

1. Elevated core temperature
2. Additional energy required for sweat-gland activity
3. Altered circulatory dynamics

Cold environments also increase energy metabolism depending on the body's fat content and thermal quality of clothing. During extreme cold stress, resting metabolism can triple because shivering generates heat to maintain a stable core temperature referred to as **shivering thermogenesis**. The effects of cold stress during exercise become most evident in cold water from extreme difficulty maintaining a stable core temperature in such a hostile environment.

Pregnancy

Maternal cardiovascular dynamics follow normal response patterns. Moderate exercise presents no greater physiologic stress to the mother than that imposed by the additional weight gain and possible encumbrance of fetal tissue. Pregnancy does not compromise the absolute value for aerobic capacity (L·min⁻¹). As pregnancy progresses, increases in maternal body weight add to the exercise effort during weight-bearing activities such as walking, jogging, and stair climbing and may reduce the economy of movement. Pregnancy, particularly in the later stages, increases pulmonary ventilation at a given submaximal exercise intensity. The hormone progesterone increases the sensitivity of the respiratory center to carbon dioxide and directly stimulates maternal hyperventilation.

Questions & Notes

List 3 factors responsible for producing an increased thermogenic effect.

1.

2.

3.

Explain how pregnancy effects metabolic and physiologic demands on the mother.

(i) For Your Information

REGULAR EXERCISE SLOWS DECREASES IN METABOLISM WITH AGE

Increases in body fat and decreases in fat-free mass (FFM) largely explain the 2% decline in BMR per decade through adulthood. Regular physical activity, blunts the decrease in BMR with aging. An accompanying 8% increase in resting metabolism occurs when 50- to 65-year-old men increase their FFM with intense resistance training. Endurance and resistance exercise training offsets the decrease in resting metabolism usually observed with aging.

SUMMARY

1. BMR reflects the minimum energy required for vital functions in the waking state. BMR relates inversely to age and gender, averaging 5% to 10% lower in women than men. FFM and the percentage of body fat largely account for the age and gender differences in BMR.

2. TDEE represents the sum of energy required in basal and resting metabolism, the thermic effect of food and energy generated in physical activity.

3. Body mass, stature, age, and FFM provide for accurate estimates of resting daily energy expenditure.

4. Physical activity, dietary-induced thermogenesis, environmental factors, and pregnancy significantly impact TDEE.

5. *Dietary-induced thermogenesis* refers to the increase in energy metabolism attributable to digestion, absorption, and assimilation of food nutrients.

6. Exposure to hot and cold environments slightly increases in TDEE.

THOUGHT QUESTIONS

1. Discuss the factors contributing to total daily energy expenditure. Explain which factor contributes the most.

2. Discuss the notion that for some individuals, a calorie ingested really is not a calorie in terms of its potential for energy storage.

3. What would be the ideal exercise prescription to optimize increases in total daily energy expenditure?

Part 2 Energy Expenditure During Physical Activity

An understanding of resting energy metabolism provides an important frame of reference to appreciate human potential to substantially increase daily energy output. According to numerous surveys, *physical inactivity* (e.g., watching television, lounging around the home, playing video games, and other sedentary activities) accounts for about one-third of a person's waking hours. This means that regular physical activity can considerably boost the TDEE of large numbers of men, women, and children. Actualizing this potential depends on the intensity, duration, and type of physical activity performed.

Researchers have measured energy expended during diverse activities such as brushing teeth, house cleaning, mowing the lawn, walking the dog, driving a car, playing ping-pong, bowling, dancing, swimming, rock climbing, and physical activity during space flight. Consider an activity such as rowing continuously at 30 strokes per minute for 30 minutes. How can we determine the number of calories "burned" during the 30 minutes? If the amount of oxygen consumed averages 2.0 L·min^{-1} during each minute of rowing, then in 30 minutes the rower would consume 60 L of oxygen. A reasonably accurate estimate of the energy expended in rowing can be made because 1 L of oxygen generates about 5 kCal of energy. In this example, the rower expends 300 kCal (60 L × 5 kCal) during the exercise. This value represents the **gross energy expenditure** for the exercise duration.

The 300 kCal of energy cannot all be attributed solely to rowing because this value also includes the resting requirement during the 30-minute row. The rower's BSA of 2.04 m^2, estimated from the formula BSA, m^2 = 0.20247 × Stature$^{0.725}$ × Body mass$^{0.425}$ (body mass = 81.8 kg; stature = 1.83 m), multiplied by the average BMR for gender (38 kCal·m^{-2}·h^{-1} × 2.04 m^2) gives the resting metabolism per hour, which is approximately 78 kCal per hour or

39 kCal "burned" over 30 minutes. Based on these computations, the **net energy expenditure** attributable solely to rowing equals gross energy expenditure (300 kCal) minus the requirement for rest (39 kCal), or approximately 261 kCal.

One estimates TDEE by determining the time spent in daily activities (using a diary) and determining the activities' corresponding energy requirements.

ENERGY COST OF RECREATIONAL AND SPORT ACTIVITIES

Table 8.1 illustrates the energy cost among diverse recreational and sport activities. Notice, for example, that volleyball requires about 3.6 kCal per minute (216 kCal per hour) for a person who weighs 71 kg (157 lb). The same person expends more than twice this energy, or 546 kCal per hour, swimming the front crawl. Viewed somewhat differently, 25 minutes spent swimming expends about the same number of calories as playing 1 hour of recreational volleyball. If the pace of the swim increases or the volleyball game becomes more intense, energy expenditure increases proportionately.

Effect of Body Mass   Body size plays an important contributing role in exercise energy requirements. **Figure 8.3** illustrates that heavier people expend more energy to perform the same activity than people who weigh less. This occurs because the energy expended during **weight-bearing exercise** increases directly with the body mass transported. *Such a strong relationship means that one can predict energy expenditure during walking or running from body mass with almost as much accuracy as measuring oxygen uptake under controlled laboratory conditions.* In non–weight-bearing or **weight-supported exercise** such as stationary cycling, little relationship exists between body mass and exercise energy cost.

From a practical standpoint, walking and other weight-bearing exercises require a substantial calorie burn for heavier people. Notice in Table 8.1 that playing tennis or volleyball requires considerably greater energy expenditure

Table 8.1	Gross Energy Cost for Selected Recreational and Sports Activities in Relation to Body Mass[a]											
ACTIVITY	kg 50 lb 110	53 117	56 123	59 130	62 137	65 143	68 150	71 157	74 163	77 170	80 176	83 183
Volleyball	2.5	2.7	2.8	3.0	3.1	3.3	3.4	3.6	3.7	3.9	4.0	4.2
Aerobic dancing	6.7	7.1	7.5	7.9	8.3	8.7	9.2	9.6	10.0	10.4	10.8	11.2
Cycling, leisure	5.0	5.3	5.6	5.9	6.2	6.5	6.8	7.1	7.4	7.7	8.0	8.3
Tennis	5.5	5.8	6.1	6.4	6.8	7.1	7.4	7.7	8.1	8.4	8.7	9.0
Swimming, slow crawl	6.4	6.8	7.2	7.6	7.9	8.3	8.7	9.1	9.5	9.9	10.2	10.6
Touch football	6.6	7.0	7.4	7.8	8.2	8.6	9.0	9.4	9.8	10.2	10.6	11.0
Running, 8-min/mile	10.8	11.3	11.9	12.5	13.11	3.6	14.2	14.8	15.4	16.0	16.5	17.1
Skiing, uphill racing	13.7	14.5	15.3	16.2	17.0	17.8	18.6	19.5	20.3	21.1	21.9	22.7

[a]Data from Katch F., et al.: *Calorie Expenditure Charts.* Ann Arbor, MI: Fitness Technologies Press, 1996.
Note: Energy expenditure computes as the number of minutes of participation multiplied by the kCal value in the appropriate body weight column. For example, the kCal cost of 1 hour of tennis for a person weighing 150 pounds equals 444 kCal (7.4 kCal × 60 min).

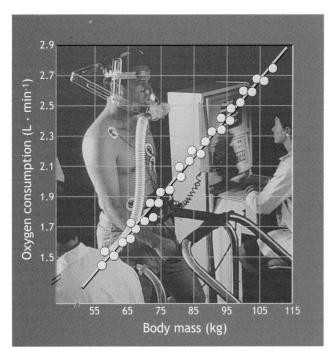

Figure 8.3 Relationship between body mass and oxygen uptake measured during submaximal, brisk treadmill walking. (From Applied Physiology Laboratory, Queens College, Flushing, NY. Photo courtesy of Dr. Jay Graves, University of Utah.)

for a person who weighs 83 kg than for someone who weighs 62 kg. Expressing caloric cost of weight-bearing exercise relative to body mass, as kilocalories per kilogram of body mass per minute ($kCal \cdot kg^{-1} \cdot min^{-1}$), greatly reduces the difference in energy expenditure among individuals of different body weights. Nonetheless, the absolute energy cost of the exercise ($kCal \cdot min^{-1}$) remains greater for the heavier person simply because of the extra body weight.

AVERAGE DAILY RATES OF ENERGY EXPENDITURE

A committee of the United States Food and Nutrition Board (*www.iom.edu/en*) proposed various norms to represent average rates of energy expenditure for men and women in the United States. These values apply to people with occupations considered between sedentary and active and who participate in some recreational activities such as weekend swimming, golf, hiking, and tennis. Table 8.2 shows that the average daily energy expenditure ranges between 2900 and 3000 kCal for men and 2200 kCal for women between the ages of 15 and 50 years. The lower part of the table reveals that the typical person spends about 75% of the day in sedentary activities. This predominance of physical *inactivity* has prompted some sociologists to refer to the modern-day American as *homosedentarius*.

CLASSIFICATION OF WORK BY ENERGY EXPENDITURE

All of us at one time or another have performed some type of physical work we would classify as exceedingly "difficult." This includes walking up a long flight of stairs, shoveling a snow-filled driveway, sprinting to catch a bus, loading and unloading furniture from a truck, digging trenches, skiing or snow-shoeing through a snowstorm, or running in soft beach sand. Two factors affect how researchers rate

Questions & Notes

If the $\dot{V}O_2$ averages 2.5 $L \cdot min^{-1}$ during skiing, how many kCal would be expended during 45 minutes?

Describe the difference between gross and net energy expenditure.

Compute the gross energy expenditure for a 62 kg person who plays touch football for 25 minutes. (refer to Table 8.1)

List 2 factors that determine the strenuousness of a particular exercise task.

1.

2.

Compute the $kCal \cdot min^{-1}$ for a 54-kg person who exercises at a 10-MET level.

Table 8.2	Average Rates of Energy Expenditure for Men and Women Living in the United States[a]					
	AGE (y)	BODY MASS		STATURE		ENERGY EXPENDITURE
		(kg)	(lb)	(cm)	(in)	(kCal)
Males	15–18	66	145	176	69	3000
	19–24	72	160	177	70	2900
	25–50	79	174	176	70	2900
	51+	77	170	173	68	2300
Females	15–18	55	120	163	64	2200
	19–24	58	128	164	65	2200
	25–50	63	138	163	64	2200
	50+	65	143	160	63	1900

ACTIVITY	AVERAGE TIME SPENT DURING THE DAY TIME (h)
Sleeping and lying down	8
Sitting	6
Standing	6
Walking	2
Recreational activity	2

[a]The information in this table was designed for the maintenance of practically all healthy people in the United States.
Data from Food and Nutrition Board, National Research Council: *Recommended Dietary Allowances*, revised. Washington, DC, National Academy of Sciences, 1989.

the difficulty of a particular task: *duration of activity* and *intensity of effort*. Both factors can vary considerably. Running a 26-mile marathon at various speeds illustrates this point. One runner maintains maximum pace and completes the race in a little more than 2 hours. Another runner of similar fitness selects a slower, more "leisurely" pace and completes the run in 3 hours. In these examples, the intensity of exercise differentiates the performance. In another situation, two people run at the same speed, but one runs twice as long as the other. Here, exercise duration differentiates performance.

METABOLIC EQUIVALENTS

Oxygen uptake and kilocalories commonly express differences in exercise intensity. As an alternative, a convenient way to express exercise intensity classifies physical effort as multiples of resting energy expenditure, with a unitless measure. To this end, scientists have developed the concept of **metabolic equivalents** (**METs**). One **MET** represents an adult's average seated resting oxygen consumption or energy expenditure—about 250 mL $O_2 \cdot min^{-1}$, 3.5 mL $O_2 \cdot kg^{-1} \cdot min^{-1}$, 1 $kCal \cdot kg^{-1} \cdot h^{-1}$, or 0.017 $kCal \cdot kg^{-1} \cdot min^{-1}$ (1 $kCal \cdot kg^{-1} \cdot h^{-1}$ ÷ 60 min $\cdot h^{-1}$ = 0.017). Using these data as a frame of reference, a 2-MET activity requires twice as much energy expended at rest, and so on.

The MET provides a convenient way to rate exercise intensity from a resting baseline (i.e., multiples of resting energy expenditure). Conversion from METs to $kCal \cdot min^{-1}$ requires knowledge of body mass and the

following conversion: 1.0 $kCal \cdot kg^{-1} \cdot h^{-1}$ = 1 MET. For example, if a person who weighs 70 kg bicycles at 10 mph, which is listed as a 10-MET activity, the corresponding kCal expenditure calculates as follows:

$$10.0 \text{ METs} = 10.0 \text{ kCal} \cdot kg^{-1} \cdot h^{-1} \times 70 \text{ kg} \div 60 \text{ min}$$
$$= 700 \text{ kCal} \div 60 \text{ min}$$
$$= 11.7 \text{ kCal} \cdot min^{-1}$$

Table 8.3 presents a five-level classification scheme of physical activity based on energy expenditure and corresponding MET levels for untrained men and women.

Heart Rate Estimates Energy Expenditure
For each person, heart rate (HR) and oxygen uptake relate linearly throughout a broad range of aerobic exercise intensities. By knowing this precise relationship, exercise HR provides an estimate of oxygen uptake (and thus energy expenditure) during physical activity. This approach has served as a substitute when oxygen uptake cannot be measured during the actual activity.

Figure 8.4 presents data for two members of a nationally ranked women's basketball team during a laboratory treadmill running test. The HR for each woman increased linearly with exercise intensity—a proportionate increase in HR accompanied each increase in oxygen uptake. However, a similar HR for each athlete did not correspond to the same level of oxygen uptake because the slope (rate of change) of the **HR–V̇O₂** line differed considerably between the women. For a given increase in oxygen uptake, the HR of subject B increased less

Table 8.3	Five-Level Classification of Physical Activity Based on Exercise Intensity

ENERGY EXPENDITURE[a]

MEN

LEVEL	$kCal \cdot min^{-1}$	$L \cdot min^{-1}$	$mL \cdot kg^{-1} \cdot min^{-1}$	METs
Light	2.0–4.9	0.40–0.99	6.1–15.2	1.6–3.9
Moderate	5.0–7.4	1.00–1.49	15.3–22.9	4.0–5.9
Heavy	7.5–9.9	1.50–1.99	23.0–30.6	6.0–7.9
Very heavy	10.0–12.4	2.00–2.49	30.7–38.3	8.0–9.9
Unduly heavy	12.5–	2.50–	38.4–	10.0–

WOMEN

LEVEL	$kCal \cdot min^{-1}$	$L \cdot min^{-1}$	$mL \cdot kg^{-1} \cdot min^{-1}$	METs
Light	1.5–3.4	0.30–0.69	5.4–12.5	1.2–2.7
Moderate	3.5–5.4	0.70–1.09	12.6–19.8	2.8–4.3
Heavy	5.5–7.4	1.10–1.49	19.9–27.1	4.4–5.9
Very heavy	7.5–9.4	1.50–1.89	27.2–34.4	6.0–7.5
Unduly heavy	9.5–	1.90–	34.5–	7.6–

[a]$L \cdot min^{-1}$ based on 5 kCal per liter of oxygen; $ml \cdot kg^{-1} \cdot min^{-1}$ based on 65-kg man and 55-kg woman; one MET equals average resting oxygen uptake of 3.5 $mL \cdot kg^{-1} \cdot min^{-1}$.

than for subject A. For player A, an exercise HR of 140 $b \cdot min^{-1}$ corresponds to an oxygen uptake of 1.08 $L \cdot min^{-1}$. The same HR for player B corresponds to an oxygen uptake of 1.60 $L \cdot min^{-1}$.

A major consideration when using HR to estimate oxygen uptake lies in the similarity between the laboratory assessment of the HR–$\dot{V}O_2$ line and the specific in vivo field activity applied to this relationship. It should be noted that factors other than oxygen uptake influence HR response to

Questions & Notes

List 3 factors that determine aerobic endurance performance.

1.

2.

3.

What is one assumption underlying predictions of $\dot{V}O_{2max}$ from HR?

Define the term MET.

Convert a 15 MET level exercise to $kCal \cdot min^{-1}$ for a 200 lb person.

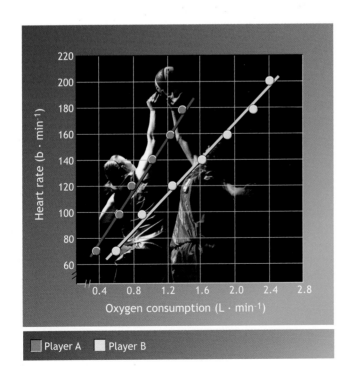

Figure 8.4 Linear relationship between heart rate and oxygen uptake during graded exercise on a treadmill in two collegiate basketball players of different aerobic fitness levels. (Data from Laboratory of Applied Physiology, Queens College, NY.)

exercise. These include environmental temperature, emotional state, previous food intake, body position, muscle groups exercised, continuous or discontinuous nature of the exercise, and whether the muscles act statically or more dynamically. During aerobic dance, for example, higher HRs occur while dancing at a specific oxygen uptake than at the same oxygen uptake while walking or running on a treadmill. Arm exercise, or when muscles act statically in a straining-type exercise, produces consistently higher HRs than dynamic leg exercise at any submaximum oxygen uptake. Consequently, applying HRs during upper-body or static exercise to a HR–$\dot{V}O_2$ line established during running or cycling *overpredicts* the criterion oxygen uptake.

SUMMARY

1. Energy expenditure can be expressed in gross or net terms. Gross or total values include the resting energy requirement during the activity phase, and the net energy expenditure reflects the energy cost of the activity that excludes resting metabolism over an equivalent time period.

2. Daily rates of energy expenditure classify different occupations and sports professions. Within any classification, variability exists from energy expended in recreational or on-the-job pursuits. Heavier individuals expend more energy in most physical activities than lighter counterparts simply because of the cost of moving the added body weight.

3. Average total daily energy expenditure ranges between 2900 and 3000 kCal for men and 2200 kCal for women age 15 to 50 years.

4. Different classification systems rate the strenuousness of physical activities. These include ratings based on energy cost expressed in $kCal \cdot min^{-1}$, oxygen requirement in $L \cdot min^{-1}$, or multiples of the resting metabolic rate (METs).

5. Exercise HR estimates energy expenditure during physical activity from a laboratory-determined individual's HR–$\dot{V}O_2$ line. Researchers then apply the HRs during recreational, sport, or occupational activity to the HR–$\dot{V}O_2$ line to estimate exercise oxygen uptake.

6. Diverse factors that influence HR act independent of the oxygen consumption so estimates of energy cost using HR response are limited to only select types of physical activities.

THOUGHT QUESTIONS

1. What circumstances would cause a particular exercise task to be rated "strenuous" in intensity by one person but only "moderate" by another?

2. Discuss the limitations of using exercise HR to estimate the energy cost of vigorous resistance training based on an HR–$\dot{V}O_2$ line determined from treadmill walking.

Part 3   Energy Expenditure During Walking, Running, and Swimming

Total daily energy expenditure depends largely on the type, intensity, and duration of physical activity. The following sections explore the energy expenditure for walking, running, and swimming. These activities play an important role in weight control, physical conditioning, and cardiac rehabilitation.

ECONOMY AND EFFICIENCY OF ENERGY EXPENDITURE

Three factors largely determine success in aerobic endurance performance:

1. Aerobic power ($\dot{V}O_{2max}$)
2. Ability to sustain effort at a large percentage of $\dot{V}O_{2max}$
3. Efficiency of energy use or movement economy

Exercise physiologists consider a high $\dot{V}O_{2max}$ as prerequisite for success in endurance activities. Among long-distance runners with nearly identical aerobic powers as often occurs at elite levels of competition, other factor(s) often explain success in competition. For example, a performance edge would clearly exist for an athlete able to run at a higher percentage of $\dot{V}O_{2max}$ than competitors. Similarly, the runner who maintains a given pace with relatively low energy expenditure or greater economy maintains a competitive advantage.

Efficiency of Energy Use

The energy expenditure related to external work represents only a portion of the total energy utilized when an individual exercises. The remainder appears as heat.

Mechanical efficiency (ME) indicates the percentage of the total chemical energy expended (denominator) that contributes to the external work output (numerator). Within this context:

$$ME (\%) = \frac{\text{Work Output}}{\text{Energy Expended}} \times 100$$

Force, acting through a vertical distance (F × D) and usually recorded as foot-pounds (ft-lb) or kilogram-meters (kg-m), yields the external work accomplished or work output. External work output is determined routinely during cycle ergometry or other exercises such as stair climbing or bench stepping that require lifting the body mass. In horizontal walking or running, work output cannot be computed because technically, external work does not occur. Reciprocal leg and arm movements negate each other, and the body achieves no net gain in vertical distance. If a person walks or runs up a grade, the work component can be estimated from body mass and vertical distance or lift achieved during the exercise period (see Close-Up Box in Chapter 6, page 198: *How to Measure Work on a Treadmill, Cycle Ergometer, and Step Bench*). Work output converts to kilocalories using these standard conversions:

1 kCal = 426.8 kg-m
1 kCal = 3087.4 ft–lb
1 kCal = 1.5593 10^{-3} hp·h^{-1}
1 watt = 0.01433 kCal·min^{-1}
1 watt = 6.12 kg-m·min^{-1}

Steady-rate oxygen uptake during exercise infers the energy input portion of the efficiency equation (denominator). To obtain common units, the oxygen uptake converts to energy units (1.0 L O_2 = 5.0 kCal; see Table 7.1 for precise calorific transformations based on the non-protein RQ).

Three terms express efficiency: **gross**, **net**, and **delta**. Each expression, calculated differently, exhibits a particular advantage. Each method assumes a submaximal steady-rate condition and requires that work output and energy expenditure be expressed in the same units—typically kilocalories. Applying the different calculation methods to the same exercise modality yields varying results for ME that range from 8% to 25% using gross calculations, 10% to 30% using net calculations, and 24% to 35% using delta calculations.

Gross Mechanical Efficiency

Gross ME, the most frequently calculated measure of efficiency, applies when one requires specific rates of work and speed or in nutritional studies that features energy expenditures over extended durations. Gross efficiency computations use the total oxygen uptake during the exercise.

For example, suppose a 15-minute ride on a stationary bicycle generated 13,300 kg-m of work or 31.2 kCal (13,300 kg-m ÷ 426.8 kCal per kg-m). The oxygen consumed to perform the work totaled 25 L with an RQ of 0.88. An RQ of 0.88 indicates that each liter of oxygen uptake generated an energy equivalent of 4.9 kCal (see Table 7.2). Thus, the exercise expended 122.5 kCal (25 L × 4.9 kCal). ME (%) computes as follows:

$$ME (\%) = \frac{\text{Work Output}}{\text{Energy Expended}} \times 100$$

$$= \frac{31.2 \text{ kCal}}{122.5 \text{ kCal}} \times 100$$

$$= 25.5\%$$

For Your Information

RUNNING ECONOMY IMPROVES WITH AGE

Running economy improves steadily from ages 10 to 18 years. This partly explains the relatively poor performance of young children in distance running and their progressive improvement throughout adolescence. Improved endurance occurs even though aerobic capacity relative to body mass (mL O_2·kg^{-1}·min^{-1}) remains relatively constant during this time.

Questions & Notes

Complete the following conversions:

1 kCal = _____ kg-m

1 kCal = _____ ft-lb

1 watt = _____ kCal·min^{-1}

1 watt = _____ kg-min·min^{-1}

Compute the mechanical efficiency for a 10-minute ride on a bicycle ergometer that generates 28 kCal of energy; oxygen uptake totaled 20 L with an RQ of 0.88.

Write the formula for gross mechanical efficiency.

Write the formula for delta efficiency.

List 3 factors that influence exercise efficiency.

1.

2.

3.

As with all machines, the human body's efficiency for producing mechanical work falls considerably below 100%. The energy required to overcome internal and external friction becomes the biggest factor affecting ME. Overcoming friction represents essentially wasted energy because it accomplishes no external work; consequently, work input *always* exceeds work output. The ME of human locomotion in walking, running, and cycling ranges between 20% and 30%.

Net Mechanical Efficiency

Net ME involves subtracting the resting energy expenditure from the total energy expended during exercise. This calculation indicates the efficiency of the work per se, unaffected by the energy expended to sustain the body at rest.

Net ME is calculated as follows:

$$\text{Net ME (\%)} = \frac{\text{Work Output}}{\text{Energy Expended Above Rest}} \times 100$$

Resting energy output is determined for the same time duration as the work output.

In the previous example for gross ME, if the resting oxygen uptake equaled 250 mL·min^{-1} (0.25 L·min^{-1}) and RQ equaled 0.91 (4.936 kCal·L O$_2^{-1}$; 0.250 L·min^{-1} × 4.936 = 1.234 kCal·min^{-1}), the net ME computes as:

Net ME (%)

$$= \frac{\text{Work Output}}{\text{Energy Expended Above Rest}} \times 100$$

$$= \frac{31.2 \text{ kCal}}{122.5 \text{ kCal} - (1.234 \text{ kCal} \cdot \text{min}^{-1} \times 15 \text{ min})} \times 100$$

$$= 30\%$$

Delta Efficiency

Delta efficiency calculates as the relative energy cost of performing an additional increment of work; that is, the ratio of the difference between work output at two levels of work output to the difference in energy expenditure determined for the two levels of work output.

Delta (Δ) Efficiency =

$$= \frac{\begin{array}{c}\text{Difference in Work Output}\\ \text{Between Two Exercise Levels}\end{array}}{\begin{array}{c}\text{Difference in Energy Expended}\\ \text{Between Two Exercise Levels}\end{array}} \times 100$$

For example, suppose an individual cycles at 100 watts for 5 minutes (100 W = 1.433 kCal·min^{-1}) at a steady-rate oxygen uptake of 1.70 L·min^{-1} with an RQ of 0.83 (4.838 kCal·L O$_2^{-1}$). This corresponds to an energy expenditure of 8.23 kCal·min^{-1}. The person then completes another 5 minutes at 200 watts (200 W = 2.866 kCal·min^{-1}) at a steady-rate oxygen uptake of 2.80 L·min^{-1} with an RQ of 0.90 (4.924 kCal·L O$_2^{-1}$). This results in an energy expenditure of 13.8 kCal·min^{-1}. Delta efficiency computes as:

Delta (Δ) Efficiency =

$$= \frac{\begin{array}{c}\text{Difference in Work Output}\\ \text{Between Two Exercise Levels}\end{array}}{\begin{array}{c}\text{Difference in Energy Expended}\\ \text{Between Two Exercise Levels}\end{array}} \times 100$$

$$= \frac{2.866 \text{ kCal·min}^{-1} - 1.433 \text{ kCal·min}^{-1}}{13.79 \text{ kCal·min}^{-1} - 8.23 \text{ kCal·min}^{-1}} \times 100$$

$$= \frac{1.433 \text{ kCal·min}^{-1}}{5.56 \text{ kCal·min}^{-1}} \times 100$$

$$= 25.8\%$$

Delta efficiency remains the calculation of choice when assessing efficiency of treadmill exercise because it is impossible to determine work output accurately during horizontal movement.

Factors Influencing Exercise Efficiency

Seven factors influence exercise efficiency:

1. **Work rate:** Efficiency generally decreases as work rate increases because the relationship between energy expenditure and work rate is curvilinear rather than linear. Thus, as work rate increases, total energy expenditure increases disproportionately to work output, resulting in a lowered ME.

2. **Movement speed:** Every individual has an optimum speed of movement for any given work rate. Generally, the optimum movement speed increases as power output increases (i.e., higher power outputs require greater movement speed to create optimum efficiency). Any deviation from the optimal movement speed decreases efficiency. Low efficiencies at slow speeds most likely result from inertia (increased energy expended to overcome internal starting and stopping). A decline in efficiency at high speeds might result from increases in muscular friction, with resulting increases in internal work and energy expenditure.

3. **Extrinsic factors:** Improvements in equipment design have increased efficiency in many physical activities. For example, changes in shoe design (lighter, softer) permit running at a given speed with a lower energy expenditure, thus increasing efficiency of movement; changes in clothing (lighter more absorbent fabrics and more hydrodynamic full-body swim suits) have produced a similar effect.

4. **Muscle fiber composition:** Activation of slow-twitch muscle fibers produces greater efficiency than the same work accomplished by fast-twitch fibers (slow-twitch fibers require less ATP per unit work than fast-twitch fibers). Thus, individuals with a higher percentage of slow-twitch muscle fibers display increased ME.

5. **Fitness level:** More fit individuals perform a given task at a higher efficiency because of decreased energy expenditure for non–exercise-related functions such as temperature regulation, increased circulation, and waste product removal.

6. **Body composition:** Fatter individuals perform a given exercise task (particularly weight-bearing exercises such as walking and running) at a lower efficiency. This results from an increased energy cost of transporting extra body fat.

7. **Technique:** Improved technique produces fewer extraneous body movements, resulting in a lower energy expenditure and hence higher efficiency. The golf swing is a prime example. Millions of men and women expend considerable "energy" trying to hit the ball where they want it to go—most of the time with less than perfect execution. In contrast, a golf pro expends seemingly little "energy" in coordinating the legs, hips, shoulders, and arms to strike the ball 250 to 300 yards on a perfect trajectory.

ECONOMY OF MOVEMENT

The concept of exercise economy also can be viewed as the relationship between energy input and energy output. For **economy of human movement**, the quantity of energy to perform a particular task relative to performance quality represents an important concern. In a sense, many of us assess economy by visually comparing the ease of movement among highly trained athletes. It does not require a trained eye to discriminate the ease of effort in comparisons of elite swimmers, skiers, dancers, gymnasts, and divers with less proficient counterparts who seem to expend considerable "wasted energy" to perform the same tasks. Anyone who has learned a new sport recalls the difficulties encountered performing basic movements that with practice, became automatic and seemingly "effortless."

Exercise Oxygen Uptake Reflects Economy

A common method to assess differences between individuals in economy of movement evaluates the steady-rate oxygen uptake during a specific exercise at a set power output or speed. This approach only applies to steady-rate exercise in which oxygen uptake closely mirrors energy expenditure. *At a given submaximum speed of running, cycling, or swimming, an individual with greater movement economy consumes less oxygen.* Economy takes on importance during longer duration exercise during which the athlete's aerobic capacity and the oxygen requirements of the task largely determine success. *All else being equal, a training adjustment that improves economy of effort directly translates to improved exercise performance.* **Figure 8.5** relates running economy to endurance performance in elite athletes of comparable aerobic fitness. Clearly, athletes with greater running economies (lower oxygen uptake at the same running pace) achieve better performance.

No single biomechanical factor accounts for individual differences in running economy. Significant variation in economy at a particular running speed occurs even among trained runners. In general, improved running economy results from years of arduous run training. Short-term training that emphasizes only the "proper techniques" of running (e.g., arm movements and body alignment) probably does not improve running economy. Distance runners who lack an economical stride-length pattern benefit from a short-term program of audiovisual feedback that focuses on optimizing their stride length.

$\mathcal{Q}$**uestions & Notes**

List the 4 factors that influence movement efficiency.

1.

2.

3.

4.

Define economy of movement.

 For Your Information

ELITE RUNNERS RUN MORE ECONOMICALLY

At a particular speed, elite endurance runners run at a lower oxygen uptake than less trained or less successful counterparts of similar age. This holds for 8- to 11-year-old cross-country runners and adult marathoners. Elite distance athletes, as a group, run with 5% to 10% greater economy than well-trained middle-distance runners.

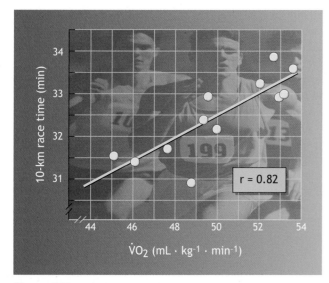

Figure 8.5 Relationship between submaximum maximal oxygen consumption ($\dot{V}O_2$) at 16.1 km·h^{-1} and 10-km race time in elite male runners of comparable aerobic capacity.

WALKING ECONOMY

For most individuals, the most common form of exercise, walking, represents the major type of physical activity that falls outside the realm of sedentary living. **Figure 8.6** displays the curvilinear relationship between energy expendi-ture versus walking at slow and fast speeds. A linear rela-tionship exists between walking speeds of 3.0 and 5.0 km·h^{-1} (1.9–3.1 mph) and oxygen uptake; at faster speeds, walking becomes less economical, so the relation-ship curves upward to indicate a disproportionate increase in energy cost related to walking speed. In general, the **crossover velocity** (note intersection of two straight lines) appears to be about 6.5 km·h^{-1} (4.0 mph) at which run-ning becomes more economical than walking.

Competition Walking

The energy expenditure of Olympic-caliber walkers has been studied at various speeds while walking and running on a treadmill. Their competitive walking speeds average a remarkable 13.0 km·h^{-1} (11.5–14.8 km·h^{-1} or 7.1–9.2 mph) over distances ranging from 1.6 to 50 km. (The current world record [as of January 2010] 20-km speed walk is 1:16:43 for men [set June 2008] and 1:24:50 for women [set March 2001]. This equals a speed of 15.64 km·h^{-1} [9.718 mph] for men, and 14.15 km·h^{-1} [8.79 mph] for men.) The cross-over velocity during which running becomes more economical than walking for these competitive race walkers occurs at about 8.0 km·h^{-1} (4.97 mph). The oxygen uptake of race walkers during treadmill walking at competition speeds averages only slightly lower than the highest oxygen uptake measured

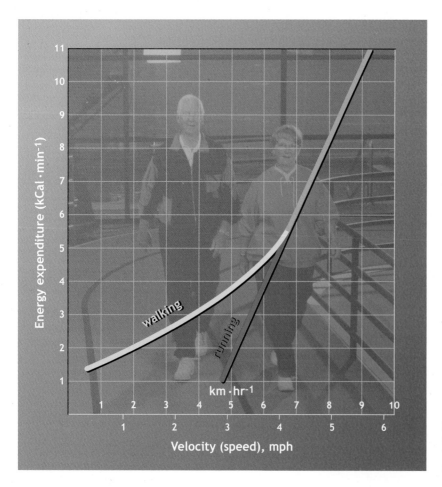

Figure 8.6 Energy expenditures while walking on a level surface at different speeds. The *line* represents a compilation of values reported in the literature.

Table 8.4	Prediction of Energy Expenditure (kCal·min⁻¹) from Speed of Level Walking and Body Mass							

		BODY MASS						
SPEED		kg	36	45	54	64	73	82	91
mph	km·h⁻¹	lb	80	100	120	140	160	180	200
2.0	3.22		1.9	2.2	2.6	2.9	3.2	3.5	3.8
2.5	4.02		2.3	2.7	3.1	3.5	3.8	4.2	4.5
3.0	4.83		2.7	3.1	3.6	4.0	4.4	4.8	5.3
3.5	5.63		3.1	3.6	4.2	4.6	5.0	5.4	6.1
4.0	6.44		3.5	4.1	4.7	5.2	5.8	6.4	7.0

How to use the chart: A 54-kg (120-lb) person who walks at 3.0 mph (4.83 km·h⁻¹) expends 3.6 kCal·min⁻¹. This person would expend 216 kCal during a 60-min walk (3.6 × 60).

for these athletes during treadmill running. Also, a linear relationship exists between oxygen uptake and walking at speeds above 8 km·h⁻¹, but the slope of the line was *twice* as steep compared with running at the same speeds. The athletes could walk at velocities up to 16 km·h⁻¹ (9.94 mph) and attain oxygen uptakes as high as those while running; the economy of walking faster than 8 km·h⁻¹ averaged half of running at similar speeds.

Effects of Body Mass

Body mass can predict energy expenditure with reasonable accuracy at horizontal walking speeds ranging from 3.2 to 6.4 km·h⁻¹ (~2.0–4.0 mph) for people of diverse body size and composition. The predicted values for energy expenditure during walking listed in **Table 8.4** fall within ±15% of the actual energy expenditure for men and women of different body weights up to 91 kg (200 lb). On a daily basis, the estimated energy expended while walking would only be in error by about 50 to 100 kCal, assuming the person walks 2 hours daily. Extrapolations can be made for heavier individuals but with some loss in accuracy.

Effects of Terrain and Walking Surface

Table 8.5 summarizes the influence of terrain and surface on the energy cost of walking. Similar economies exist for level walking on a grass track or paved surface. Not surprisingly, the energy cost almost doubles walking in sand compared with walking on a hard surface; in soft snow, the metabolic cost increases threefold compared with treadmill walking. A brisk walk along a beach or in freshly fallen snow provides excellent exercise for programs designed to "burn up" calories or improve physiologic fitness.

Table 8.5	Effect of Different Terrain on the Energy Expenditure of Walking Between 5.2 and 5.6 km·h⁻¹

TERRAIN[a]	CORRECTION FACTOR[b]
Paved road (similar to a grass track)	0.0
Plowed field	1.5
Hard snow	1.6
Sand dune	1.8

[a]First entry from Passmore, R., Dumin, J.V.G.A.: Human energy expenditure. *Physiol. Rev.*, 35:801, 1955. Last three entries from Givoni, B., Goldman, R.F.: Predicting metabolic energy cost. *J. Appl. Physiol.*, 30:429, 1971.
[b]The correction factor represents a multiple of the energy expenditure for walking on a paved road or grass track. For example, the energy cost of walking in a plowed field averages 1.5 times the cost of walking on the paved road.

Questions & Notes

Energy cost almost _____ walking in sand compared with walking in soft snow.

Which muscle fiber acts with greater mechanical efficiency?

It requires _____ energy to carry added weight in the hands or on the torso than to carry a similar weight on the feet or ankles.

What is the impact force on the legs during running?

What is the increase in energy expenditure walking in hard snow compared with walking on a hard, paved road?

List the 3 ways to increase running speed.

1.

2.

3.

BOX 8.1 CLOSE UP

Predicting Energy Expenditure During Treadmill Walking and Running

An almost linear relationship exists between oxygen consumption (energy expenditure) and walking speeds between 3.0 and 5.0 $km \cdot h^{-1}$ (1.9 and 3.1 mph) and running at speeds faster than 8.0 $km \cdot h^{-1}$ (5–10 mph; see **Fig. 8.6**). Adding the resting oxygen consumption to the oxygen requirements of the horizontal and vertical components of the walk or run makes it possible to estimate total (gross) exercise oxygen consumption ($\dot{V}O_2$) and energy expenditure.

BASIC EQUATION

$\dot{V}O_2$ ($mL \cdot kg^{-1} \cdot min^{-1}$) = Resting component (1 MET [3.5 mL $O_2 \cdot kg^{-1} \cdot min^{-1}$]) + Horizontal component (speed, [$m \cdot min^{-1}$] $\times$ Oxygen consumption of horizontal movement) + Vertical component (percentage grade $\times$ speed [$m \cdot min^{-1}$] $\times$ oxygen consumption of vertical movement)

To convert mph to $m \cdot min^{-1}$, multiply by 26.82; to convert $m \cdot min^{-1}$ to mph, multiply by 0.03728.

Walking

Oxygen consumption of the horizontal component of movement equals 0.1 $mL \cdot kg^{-1} \cdot min^{-1}$ and 1.8 $mL \cdot kg^{-1} \cdot min^{-1}$ for the vertical component.

Running

Oxygen consumption of the horizontal component of movement equals 0.2 $mL \cdot kg^{-1} \cdot min^{-1}$ and 0.9 $mL \cdot kg^{-1} \cdot min^{-1}$ for the vertical component.

PREDICTING ENERGY EXPENDITURE OF TREADMILL WALKING

A 55-kg person walks on a treadmill at 2.8 mph (2.8 $\times$ 26.82 = 75 $m \cdot min^{-1}$) up a 4% grade. Calculate (1) $\dot{V}O_2$ ($mL \cdot kg^{-1} \cdot min^{-1}$), (2) METs, and (3) energy expenditure ($kCal \cdot min^{-1}$). *Note: express % grade as a decimal value (i.e., 4% grade = 0.04).*

Solution

1. $\dot{V}O_2$ ($mL \cdot kg^{-1} \cdot min^{-1}$) = Resting component + Horizontal component + Vertical component

$\dot{V}O_2$ = Resting $\dot{V}O_2$ ($mL \cdot kg^{-1} \cdot min^{-1}$)
+ [speed ($m \cdot min^{-1}$)
$\times$ 0.1 $mL \cdot kg^{-1} \cdot min^{-1}$]
+ [% grade $\times$ speed ($m \cdot min^{-1}$)
$\times$ 1.8 $mL \cdot kg^{-1} \cdot min^{-1}$]
= 3.5 + (75 $\times$ 0.1)
+ (0.04 $\times$ 75 $\times$ 1.8)
= 3.5 + 7.5 + 5.4
= 16.4 $mL \cdot kg^{-1} \cdot min^{-1}$

2. METs = $\dot{V}O_2$ ($mL \cdot kg^{-1} \cdot min^{-1}$)
$\div$ 3.5 $mL \cdot kg^{-1} \cdot min^{-1}$
= 16.4 $\div$ 3.5
= 4.7

3. $kCal \cdot min^{-1}$ = $\dot{V}O_2$ ($mL \cdot kg^{-1} \cdot min^{-1}$)
$\times$ Body mass (kg)
$\times$ 5.05 $kCal \cdot LO_2^{-1}$
= 16.4 $mL \cdot kg^{-1} \cdot min^{-1}$
$\times$ 55 kg $\times$ 5.05 $kCal \cdot L^{-1}$
= 0.902 $L \cdot min^{-1}$
$\times$ 5.05 $kCal \cdot L^{-1}$
= 4.6

PREDICTING ENERGY EXPENDITURE OF TREADMILL RUNNING

Problem

A 55-kg person runs on a treadmill at 5.4 mph (5.4 $\times$ 126.82 = 145 $m \cdot min^{-1}$) up a 6% grade. Calculate (1) $\dot{V}O_2$ in $mL \cdot kg^{-1} \cdot min^{-1}$, (2) METs, and (3) energy expenditure ($kCal \cdot min^{-1}$).

Solution

1. $\dot{V}O_2$ ($mL \cdot kg^{-1} \cdot min^{-1}$) = Resting component + Horizontal component + Vertical component

$\dot{V}O_2$ = Resting $\dot{V}O_2$ ($mL \cdot kg^{-1} \cdot min^{-1}$)
+ [speed ($m \cdot min^{-1}$)
$\times$ 0.2 $mL \cdot kg^{-1} \cdot min^{-1}$]
+ [% grade $\times$ speed ($m \cdot min^{-1}$)
$\times$ 0.9 $mL \cdot kg^{-1} \cdot min^{-1}$]
= 3.5 + (145 $\times$ 0.2) + (0.06 $\times$ 145 $\times$ 0.9)
= 3.5 + 29.0 + 7.83
= 40.33 $mL \cdot kg^{-1} \cdot min^{-1}$

2. METs = $\dot{V}O_2$ ($mL \cdot kg^{-1} \cdot min^{-1}$)
$\div$ 3.5 $mL \cdot kg^{-1} \cdot min^{-1}$
= 40.33 $\div$ 3.5
= 11.5

3. $kCal \cdot min^{-1}$ = $\dot{V}O_2$ ($mL \cdot kg^{-1} \cdot min^{-1}$)
$\times$ Body mass (kg)
$\times$ 5.05 $kCal \cdot LO_2^{-1}$
= 40.33 $mL \cdot kg^{-1} \cdot min^{-1}$ $\times$ 55 kg
$\times$ 5.05 $kCal \cdot L^{-1}$
= 2.22 $L \cdot min^{-1}$
$\times$ 5.05 $kCal \cdot L^{-1}$
= 11.2

Footwear Effects

It requires considerably more energy to carry added weight on the feet or ankles than to carry similar weight attached to the torso. For a weight equal to 1.4% of body mass placed on the ankles, for example, the energy cost of walking increases an average of 8% or nearly six times more than with the same weight carried on the torso. In a practical sense, the energy cost of locomotion during walking and running increases when wearing boots compared with running shoes. Simply adding an additional 100 g to each shoe increases oxygen uptake by 1% during moderate running. The implication of these findings seems clear for the design of running shoes, hiking and climbing boots, and work boots traditionally required in mining, forestry, fire fighting, and the military; small changes in shoe weight produce large changes in economy of locomotion (energy expenditure). The cushioning properties of shoes also affect movement economy. A softer-soled running shoe reduced the oxygen cost of running at moderate speed by about 2.4% compared with a similar shoe with a firmer cushioning system, even though the softer-soled shoes weighed an additional 31 g or only 1.1 oz. The preceding observations about terrain, footwear, and economy of locomotion indicate that, at the extreme, one could dramatically elevate energy cost by walking in soft sand at rapid speed wearing heavy work boots and ankle weights. Another more prudent approach would involve unweighted race walking or running on a firm surface.

Use of Handheld and Ankle Weights

The impact force on the legs during running equals about three times body mass, the amount of leg shock with walking reaches only about 30% of this value.

Ankle weights increase the energy cost of walking to values usually observed for running. This benefits people who want to use only walking as a relatively low-impact training modality yet require intensities of effort higher than at normal walking speeds. Handheld weights also increase the energy cost of walking, particularly when arm movements accentuate a pumping action. Despite this apparent benefit, this procedure may disproportionately elevate systolic blood pressure perhaps because of increased intramuscular tension while gripping the weight. For individuals with hypertension or coronary heart disease, an unnecessarily "induced" elevated blood pressure contraindicates the use of handheld weights. For these individuals, increasing running speed (or distance) offers a more desirable alternative to increase energy expenditure than handheld or ankle weights.

ENERGY EXPENDITURE DURING RUNNING

Terrain, weather, training goals, and the performer's fitness level influence the speed of running. Two ways quantify running energy expenditure:

1. During performance of the actual activity
2. On a treadmill in the laboratory, with precise control over running speed and grade

Jogging and *running* represent qualitative terms related to speed of locomotion. This difference relates largely to the relative aerobic energy demands required in raising and lowering the body's center of gravity and accelerating and decelerating the limbs during the run. At identical running speeds, a trained distance runner moves at a lower percentage of aerobic capacity than an untrained runner, even though the oxygen uptake during the run may be similar for both. The demarcation between jogging and running depends on the participant's fitness; a jog for one person represents a run for another.

Questions & Notes

Write the basic equation to predict energy expenditure during treadmill walking or running up an incline.

What is the increase in energy expenditure by adding ankle weights during walking?

List 4 factors that influence running speed.

  1.

  2.

  3.

  4.

For the average person, at what speed is it more economical to run than walk?

For Your Information

A CONSIDERABLE ENERGY OUTPUT

During a marathon, elite athletes generate a steady-rate energy expenditure of about 25 kCal per minute for the duration of the run. Among elite rowers, a 5- to 7-minute competition generates about 36 kCal per minute!

*Independent of fitness, it becomes more economical from an energy standpoint to discontinue walking and begin to jog or run at speeds greater than about 6.5 km·h^{-1} (~4.0 mph) (**Fig. 8.6**).*

Running Economy

The data in **Figure 8.6** also illustrate an important principle in relation to running speed (e.g., >5 mph or 8 km·h^{-1}) and energy expenditure. Oxygen uptake relates linearly to running speed; thus, the same total caloric cost results when running a given distance at a steady-rate oxygen uptake at a fast or slow pace. In simple terms, if one runs a mile at a 10-mph pace (16.1 km·h^{-1}), it requires about twice as much energy per minute as a 5-mph pace (8 km·h^{-1}). The runner finishes the mile in 6 minutes, but running at the slower speed requires twice the time, or 12 minutes. Consequently, the *net* energy cost for the mile remains about the same regardless of the pace (±10%).

For horizontal running, the net energy cost (i.e., excluding the resting requirement) per kilogram of body mass per kilometer traveled averages approximately 1 kCal or 1 kCal· kg^{-1}· km^{-1}. For an individual who weighs 78 kg, the net energy requirement for running 1 km equals about 78 kCal, regardless of running speed. Expressed as oxygen uptake, this amounts to 15.6 L of oxygen consumed per kilometer (1 L O$_2$ = 5 kCal; 5.0 × 15.6).

Energy Cost of Running

Table 8.6 presents values for net energy expended during running for 1 hour at various speeds. The table expresses running speed as kilometers per hour, miles per hour, and number of minutes required to complete 1 mile at a given running speed. The boldface values represent net calories expended to run 1 mile for a person of a given body mass; this energy requirement remains independent of running speed. For example, for a person who weighs 62 kg, running a 26.2-mile marathon requires about 2600 net kCal whether the run takes just over 2 hours or 4 hours.

The energy cost per mile increases proportionally with the runner's body mass (refer to column 3). This observation certainly supports the role of weight-bearing exercise as a caloric stress for overweight individuals who wish to increase energy expenditure for weight loss. For example, a 102-kg person who jogs 5 miles daily at any comfortable pace expends about 163 kCal for each mile completed, or a total of 815 kCal for the 5-mile run. Increasing or decreasing the speed (within the broad range of steady-rate paces) simply alters the length of the exercise period required to burn a given number of calories.

Table 8.6	**Net Energy Expenditure per Hour for Horizontal Running in Relation to Velocity and Body Mass**[a,b]									
	km·h^{-1}	8	9	10	11	12	13	14	15	16
	mph	4.97	5.60	6.20	6.84	7.46	8.08	8.70	9.32	9.94
BODY MASS	min per mile	12:00	10:43	9:41	8:46	8:02	7:26	6:54	6:26	6:02
kg lb	kCal per mile									
50 110	**80**	400	450	500	550	600	650	700	750	800
54 119	**86**	432	486	540	594	648	702	756	810	864
58 128	**93**	464	522	580	638	696	754	812	870	928
62 137	**99**	496	558	620	682	744	806	868	930	992
66 146	**106**	528	594	660	726	792	858	924	990	1056
70 154	**112**	560	630	700	770	840	910	980	1050	1120
74 163	**118**	592	666	740	814	888	962	1036	1110	1184
78 172	**125**	624	702	780	858	936	1014	1092	1170	1248
82 181	**131**	656	738	820	902	984	1066	1148	1230	1312
86 190	**138**	688	774	860	946	1032	1118	1204	1290	1376
90 199	**144**	720	810	900	990	1080	1170	1260	1350	1440
94 207	**150**	752	846	940	1034	1128	1222	1316	1410	1504
98 216	**157**	784	882	980	1078	1176	1274	1372	1470	1568
102 225	**163**	816	918	1020	1122	1224	1326	1428	1530	1632
106 234	**170**	848	954	1060	1166	1272	1378	1484	1590	1696

[a]Interpret the table as follows: For a 50-kg person, the *net* energy expenditure for running for 1 hour at 8 km·h^{-1} (4.97 mph) equals 400 kCal; this speed represents a 12-minute per mile pace. Thus, 5 miles would be run in 1 hour and 400 kCal would be expended. If the pace increased to 12 km·h^{-1} (7.46 mph), 600 kCal would be expended during the 1-hour run.
[b]Running speeds expressed as kilometers per hour (km·h^{-1}), miles per hour (mph), and minutes required to complete each mile (min per mile). The values in **boldface type** equal *net* calories (resting energy expenditure subtracted) expended to run 1 mile for a given body mass, independent of running speed.

Stride Length and Stride Frequency Effects on Running Speed

Running speed can increase in three ways:

1. Increase the number of steps each minute (stride frequency)
2. Increase the distance between steps (stride length)
3. Increase stride length and stride frequency

Although the third option may seem the obvious way to increase running speed, several experiments provide objective data concerning this question.

In 1944, researchers studied the stride pattern for the Danish champion in the 5- and 10-km running events. At a running speed of 9.3 km·h^{-1} (5.8 mph), this athlete's stride frequency equaled 160 per minute with a corresponding stride length of 97 cm (38.2 in). When running speed increased 91% to 17.8 km·h^{-1} (11.1 mph), stride frequency increased only 10% to 176 per minute, whereas an 83% increase to 168 cm occurred in stride length. These data illustrate that running speed increases predominantly by lengthening the stride length. Only at faster speeds does stride frequency become important.

Optimum Stride Length An optimum combination of stride length and frequency exists for running at a particular speed. The optimum combination depends largely on the person's "style" of running and cannot be determined from objective body measurements. Running speed chosen by the person incorporates the most economical stride length. Lengthening the stride above the optimum increases oxygen uptake more than a shorter-than-optimum stride length. Urging a runner who shows signs of fatigue to "lengthen stride" to maintain speed proves counterproductive for exercise economy.

Well-trained runners run at a stride length "selected" through years of training. This produces the most economical running performance, in keeping with the concept that the body naturally attempts to achieve a level of "**minimum effort**." No "best" style exists to characterize elite runners. Instead, individual differences in body size, inertia of limb segments, and anatomic development interact to vary one's stride to the one most economical.

Effects of Air Resistance

Anyone who has run into a strong headwind knows it requires more energy to maintain a given pace compared with running in calm weather or with the wind at one's back. Three factors influence how air resistance affects energy cost of running:

1. Air density
2. Runner's projected surface area
3. Square of headwind velocity

Depending on running speed, overcoming air resistance accounts for 3% to 9% of the total energy requirement of running in calm weather. Running into a headwind creates an additional energy expense. In one study, for example, running at 15.9 km·h^{-1} (9.9 mph) in calm conditions produced an oxygen uptake of 2.92 L·min^{-1}. This increased by 5.5% to 3.09 L·min^{-1} against a 16-km·h^{-1} (9.9 mph) headwind and to 4.1 L·min^{-1} while running against the strongest wind (41 mph); running into the strongest wind represents a 40% additional expenditure of energy to maintain running velocity.

Questions & Notes

What major factor determines optimum stride length and frequency.

List 2 factors that determine how air resistance affects the energy cost of running.

1.

2.

What is the net energy cost per kg body weight per km travelled?

List 2 factors that contribute to the lower economy of effort in swimming compared to running?

1.

2.

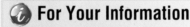

ⓘ For Your Information

EXERCISE ECONOMY AND MUSCLE FIBER TYPE

Muscle fiber type affects the economy of cycling effort. During submaximal cycling, the exercise economies of trained cyclists vary up to 15%. Differences in muscle fiber types in the active muscles account for an important component of this variation. Cyclists exhibiting the most economical cycling pattern possess the greater percentage of slow-twitch (type I) muscle fibers in their legs. This suggests that the type I fiber acts with greater ME than the faster acting type II fiber.

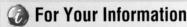

ⓘ For Your Information

CALORIES ADD UP WITH REGULAR EXERCISE

For distance runners who train up to 100 miles a week, or slightly less than the distance of four marathons, at close to competitive speeds, the weekly caloric expenditure from exercise averages about 10,000 kCal. For the serious marathon runner who trains year round, the total energy expended in training for 4 years before an Olympic competition exceeds 2 million calories—the caloric equivalent of 555 pounds of body fat. This more than likely contributes to the low levels of body fat (3% to 5% of body mass for men; 12% to 17% for women) typical for these athletes.

Some may argue that the negative effects of running into a headwind counterbalance on one's return with the tailwind. This does not occur because the energy cost of cutting through a headwind exceeds the reduction in exercise oxygen uptake with an equivalent wind velocity from the rear. Wind tunnel tests show that running performance increases by wearing form-fitting clothing; even shaving body hair improves aerodynamics and reduces wind resistance effects by up to 6%. In competitive cycling, manufacturers continually modify clothing and helmets to reduce the effects of air resistance on energy cost. This includes frame redesign to optimize the rider's body position on the bicycle.

At altitude, wind velocity affects energy expenditure less than at sea level because of reduced air density at higher elevations. Speed skaters experience a lower oxygen requirement while skating at a particular speed at altitude compared with sea level. Overcoming air resistance at altitude only becomes important at the faster skating speeds. An altitude effect also applies to competitive cycling, where the impeding effect of air resistance increases at the high speeds achieved by these athletes.

Drafting   Athletes use "**drafting**" by following directly behind a competitor to counter the negative effects of air resistance and headwind on energy cost. For example, running 1 m behind another runner at a speed of 21.6 km·h^{-1} (13.4 mph) decreases the total energy expenditure by about 7%. Drafting at this speed could save about 1 second for each 400 m covered during a race. The beneficial aerodynamic effect of drafting on the economy of effort also exists for cross-country skiing, speed skating, and cycling. About 90% of the power generated when cycling at 40 km·h^{-1}

(24.9 mph) on a calm day goes to overcome air resistance. At this speed, energy expenditure decreases between 26% and 38% when a competitor follows closely behind another cyclist.

Treadmill versus Track Running

Researchers use the treadmill almost exclusively to evaluate the physiology of running. A question concerns the association between treadmill running and running performance on a track or road race. For example, does it require the same energy to run a given speed or distance on a treadmill and a track in calm weather? To answer this question, researchers studied distance runners on both a treadmill and track at three submaximum speeds of 10.8, 12.6, and 15.6 km·h^{-1} (6.7, 7.8, and 9.7 mph). They also measured the athletes during a graded exercise test to determine possible differences between treadmill and track running on submaximal and maximal oxygen uptake.

From a practical standpoint, no meaningful differences occurred in aerobic requirements of submaximal running (up to 17.2 km·h^{-1}) on the treadmill or track or between the $\dot{V}O_{2max}$ measured in both exercise forms under similar environmental conditions. At the faster running speeds of endurance competition, air resistance could negatively impact outdoor running performance and oxygen cost may exceed that of "stationary" treadmill running at the same speed.

Marathon Running

Figure 8.7 shows the world and olympic *best times* for men and women. The world marathon record for men is 2 h,

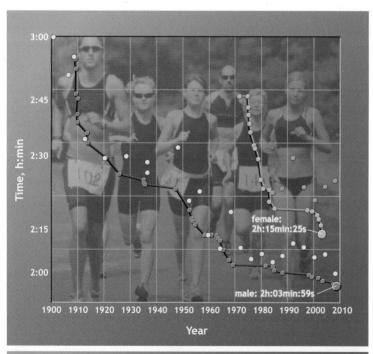

Figure 8.7   Male and female world record and Olympic record marathon run times. The male record, set in 2008 at the Berlin, Germany, marathon is 2 h, 3 min, 59 s, and the female record set at the London, England, marathon in 2003 is 2 h, 15 min, 25 s.

3 min, 59 s (set on September 28, 2008, at the Berlin, Germany, marathon.) The record holder, Haile Gebrselassie, became the first man to break the 2:04 barrier at an average pace of 4:44 per mile. The women's world record of 2 h, 15 min, 25 s set on April 19, 2003, at the London, England, Marathon by Paula Radcliffe from Great Britain who posted 5 min, 10 s; 5 min, 08 s; and 4 min, 57 s splits for the first 3 miles. Radcliffe also set world-record marks for 20 miles (1:43:44) and 30 km (1:36:36) during this run. The amazingly fast paces for both athletes not only require a steady-rate aerobic metabolism that greatly exceeds the aerobic capacity of the average male college student, it also represents about 85% of the marathoners' $\dot{V}O_{2max}$, maintained for over 2 hours. Aerobic capacity of these athletes ranges between 70 and 84 mL·kg^{-1}·min^{-1}. The energy expenditure required to run the marathon averages about 2400 kCal, excluding any elevated energy expenditure during recovery, which can persist for up to 24 to 48 hours.

ENERGY EXPENDITURE DURING SWIMMING

Swimming differs in several important respects from walking and running. For one thing, swimmers must expend energy to maintain buoyancy while generating horizontal movement at the same time using the arms and legs, either in combination or separately. Other differences include the energy requirements for overcoming drag forces that impede the movement of an object through a water medium. The amount of drag depends on the characteristics of the medium and the object's size, shape, and velocity. *These factors all contribute to a considerably lower economy swimming compared with running. More specifically, it requires about four times more energy to swim a given distance than to run the same distance.* Energy expenditure has been computed from oxygen uptake measured by open-circuit spirometry during swimming (**Fig. 8.8**). In measurement in the pool, the researcher walks alongside the swimmer while carrying the portable gas collection equipment.

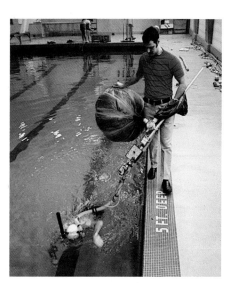

Figure 8.8 Open-circuit spirometry (bag technique) to measure oxygen consumption during front-crawl swimming.

 For Your Information

MARATHON DISTANCE

The current marathon distance (26 mi, 385 yd) was set for the 1908 London Olympics so that the course could start at Windsor Castle and end in front of the Royal Box. Not until 1921 was this distance adopted as the "official" marathon distance by the International Association of Athletics Federations (IAAF, *www.iaaf.org*).

 For Your Information

MARATHON RECORDS ARE DIFFICULT TO REPEAT

Only five men and eight women have been able to follow one marathon world record with another. James Peters set four marathon records between 1952 and 1954, and Abebe Bikila, Derek Clayton, Khalid Khannouchi, and most recently Haile Gebrselassie each set two world records back-to-back. On the women's side, Greta Weitz set four consecutive world records from 1978 to 1983 (the last stood only for 1 day!), and Chantal Langlace, Jacqueline Hansen, Christa Vahlensieck, Joyce Smith, Tegla Loroupe, and most recently Paula Radcliffe each broke the marathon record twice. Perhaps the most famous of all of the world records were the races of Abebe Bikila, the barefoot Ethiopian, who set world records 4 years apart while winning Olympic Marathons in 1960 (barefoot) and 1964 (wearing shoes).

Questions & Notes

List 3 components of swimming drag.

1.

2.

3.

About how much can wet suits reduce swimming drag?

Elite swimmers swim a given distance with a _____ $\dot{V}O_{2max}$.

True or False:

Women have higher buoyancy than men.

Energy Cost and Drag

Three components comprise the total drag force that impedes a swimmer's forward movement:

1. **Wave drag** caused by waves that build up in front of and form hollows behind the swimmer moving through the water. This component of drag only becomes a significant factor at fast speeds.
2. **Skin friction drag** produced as the water slides over the skin's surface. Removal of body hair reduces drag to slightly decrease the energy cost and physiologic demands during swimming.
3. **Viscous pressure drag** contributes substantially to counter the propulsive efforts of the swimmer at slow velocities. It results from the separation of the thin sheet of water (boundary layer) adjacent to the swimmer. The pressure differential created in front of and behind the swimmer represents viscous pressure drag. Highly skilled swimmers who "streamline" their stroke reduce this component of total drag. Streamlining with improved stroke mechanics reduces the separation region by moving the separation point closer to the water's trailing edge. This also occurs when an oar slices through the water with the blade parallel rather than perpendicular to water movement.

Differences in total drag force between swimmers can make the difference between winning and losing, particularly in longer distance competitions. Wet suits worn during the swim portion of a triathlon can reduce body drag by 14%. Improved swimming economy largely explains the faster swim times of athletes who wear wet suits. Proponents of the neck-to-body suits worn by pool swimmers maintain that the technology-driven approach to competitive swimming maximizes swimming economy and allows swimmers to achieve 3% faster times than those with standard swimsuits. As in running, cross-country skiing, and cycling, drafting in ocean swimming (following closely behind the wake of a lead swimmer) reduces energy expenditure. This enables an endurance swimmer to conserve energy and possibly improve performance toward the end of competition.

Energy Cost, Swimming Velocity, and Skill

Elite swimmers swim a particular stroke at a given velocity at a lower oxygen uptake than either less elite or recreational swimmers. Elite swimmers swim a given speed with a lower oxygen uptake than untrained yet skilled swimmers. For different swimming strokes in terms of energy expenditure, swimming the breaststroke "costs" the most at any speed followed by the backstroke. The front crawl represents the least "expensive" (calorie-wise) among the three strokes.

Effects of Buoyancy: Men versus Women

Women of all ages possess, on average, more total body fat than men. Because fat floats and muscle and bone sink, the average woman gains a hydrodynamic lift and floats more easily than the average man. This difference in buoyancy can help to explain women's greater swimming economy compared with men. For example, women swim a given distance at a lower energy cost than men; expressed another way, women achieve a higher swimming velocity than men for the same level of energy expenditure.

Whereas the distribution of body fat toward the periphery in women causes their legs to float higher in the water, making them more horizontal or "streamlined," men's leaner legs tend to swing down in the water. Lowering the legs to a deeper position increases body drag and thus reduces swimming economy. The potential hydrodynamic benefits enjoyed by women become noteworthy in longer distances during which swimming economy and body insulation assume added importance. For example, the women's record for swimming the 21-mile English Channel from England to France is 7 h, 40 min. The men's record equals 7 h, 17 min, a difference of only 5.2%. In several instances, as displayed in **Table 8.7**, women actually swim faster than men. In fact, American Gertrude Ederle (*http://en.wikipedia.org/wiki/Gertrude_Ederle*), the first woman to swim the English Channel (14 h, 31 min) on August 6, 1926, was faster by more than 2 hours than British Capt. Matthew Webb (*http://en.wikipedia.org/wiki/Matthew_Webb*), the first man without a life vest to complete the swim (21 h, 45 min on August 25, 1875).

Table 8.7	Comparisons of English Channel World Record Swimming Times Between Men and Women

ENGLISH CHANNEL RECORDS (H:MIN): MALE VS. FEMALE

RECORD	MALE	FEMALE	% DIFFERENCE (MALE:FEMALE)
First attempt–one way	21:45 (1875)	14:39 (1926)	34.9
Fastest–one way	07:17 (1994)	7:40 (1978)	−5.26
Youngest–one way	11:54 (11 y, 11 mo; 1988)	15:28 (12 y, 11 mo; 1983)	−29.9
Oldest–one way	18:37 (67 y; 1987)	12:32 (57 y; 1999)	32.69
Fastest–2 way	16:10 (1987)	17:14 (1991)	−6.6
Fastest–3 way	28:21 (1987)	34:40 (1990)	−22.2

Note that for two records (first attempt, oldest) females bettered the male record by more than 30%.

SUMMARY

1. Mechanical efficiency represents the percentage of total chemical energy expended that contributes to external work, with the remainder representing lost heat.

2. Exercise economy refers to the relationship between energy input and energy output commonly evaluated by oxygen uptake while exercising at a set power output or speed.

3. Walking speed relates linearly to oxygen uptake between speeds of 1.9 and 3.1 mph; walking becomes less economical at speeds faster than 4.0 mph.

4. Walking surface impacts energy expenditure; walking on sand requires about twice the energy expenditure as walking on hard surfaces. The energy cost of such weight-bearing exercise becomes proportionally larger for heavier people.

5. Handheld and ankle weights increase the energy cost of walking to values usually observed for running.

6. It is more energetically economical to jog-run than to walk at speeds that exceed 8 km·h^{-1} (5 mph).

7. The total energy cost for running a given distance remains independent of running speed. For horizontal running, the net energy expenditure averages about 1 kCal·kg^{-1}·km^{-1}.

8. Shortening the running stride and increasing the stride frequency to maintain a constant running speed requires less energy than lengthening the stride and reducing the stride frequency.

9. Overcoming air resistance accounts for 3% to 9% of the total energy cost of running in calm weather.

10. Running directly behind a competitor, a favorable aerodynamic technique called "drafting," counters the negative effect of air resistance and headwind on the energy cost of running.

11. It requires the same amount of energy to run a given distance or speed on a treadmill as on a track under identical environmental conditions.

12. Children run at a given speed with less economy than adults because they require between 20% and 30% more oxygen per unit of body mass.

13. It takes about four times more energy to swim than to run the same distance because a swimmer expends considerable energy to maintain buoyancy and overcome the various drag forces that impede movement.

14. Elite swimmers expend fewer calories to swim a given stroke at any velocity.

15. Significant gender differences exist for body drag, economy, and net oxygen uptake during swimming. Women swim a given distance at approximately 30% lower energy cost than men.

THOUGHT QUESTIONS

1. A 60-kg (132-lb) elite marathoner who trains year round expends about 4000 kCal daily over a 4-year training period before Olympic competition. Assuming the athlete's body mass remains unchanged and 70% of daily caloric intake comes from carbohydrate and 1.4 g per kg body mass comes from protein, compute the runner's total 4-year calorie intake and total grams consumed from carbohydrate and protein.

2. Respond to this question, "Why do children who run in 10-km races never seem to perform as well as adults?"

3. Explain why it is untrue that it takes more total calories to run a given distance faster. In what way does correcting this misunderstanding contribute to a recommendation for the use of exercise for weight loss?

4. An elite 120-lb runner claims that she consistently consumes 12,000 kCal daily simply to maintain her body weight owing to the strenuousness of her training. Using examples of exercise energy expenditures, discuss whether this intake level could reflect a plausible regular energy intake requirement.

SELECTED REFERENCES

ACSM's Guidelines for Exercise Testing and Prescription. 8th Ed. Baltimore: Lippincott Williams & Wilkins, 2009.

ACSM's Resource Manual for Guidelines for Exercise Testing and Prescription. 6th Ed. Baltimore: Lippincott Williams & Wilkins, 2009.

ACSM's Guidelines for Exercise Testing and Prescription. 8th Ed. Baltimore: Lippincott Williams & Wilkins, 2010.

ACSM's Resource Manual for Guidelines for Exercise Testing and Prescription. 6th Ed. Baltimore: Lippincott Williams & Wilkins, 2010.

ACSM's Resources for Clinical Exercise Physiology. 6th Ed. Baltimore: Lippincott Williams & Wilkins, 2010.

Alexander, R.M.: Physiology: enhanced: walking made simple. *Science*, 308:58, 2005.

Alfonzo-Gonzalez, G., et al.: Estimation of daily energy needs with the FAO/WHO/UNU 1985 procedures in adults: comparison to whole-body indirect calorimetry measurements. *Eur. J. Clin. Nutr.*, 58:1125, 2004.

Barbosa, T.M., et al.: Energy cost and intracyclic variation of the velocity of the centre of mass in butterfly stroke. *Eur. J. Appl. Physiol.*, 93:519, 2005.

Barbosa, T.M., et al.: Energetics and biomechanics as determining factors of swimming performance: updating the state of the art. *J. Sci. Med. Sport.*, 13:262, 2010.

Bertram, J.E.: Constrained optimization in human walking: cost minimization and gait plasticity. *J. Exp. Biol.*, 208:979, 2005.

Blanc, S., et al.: Energy requirements in the eighth decade of life. *Am. J. Clin. Nutr.*, 79:303, 2004.

Browning, R.C., et al.: Pound for pound: Working out how obesity influences the energetics of walking. *J. Appl. Physiol.*, 106:1755, 2009.

Browning, R.C., et al.: The effects of adding mass to the legs on the energetics and biomechanics of walking. *Med. Sci. Sports Exerc.*, 39:515, 2007.

Butte, N.F., et al.: Energy requirements of women of reproductive age. *Am. J. Clin. Nutr.*, 77:630, 2003.

Byrne, N.M., et al.: Metabolic equivalent: One size does not fit all. *J. Appl. Physiol.*, 99:1112, 2005.

Chasan-Taber, L., et al.: Development and validation of a pregnancy physical activity questionnaire. *Med. Sci. Sports Exerc.*, 36:1750, 2004.

Chatard, J.C., Wilson, B.: Effect of fastskin suits on performance, drag, and energy cost of swimming. *Med. Sci. Sports Exerc.*, 40:1149, 2008.

Chatard, J-C., et al.: Drafting distance in swimming. *Med. Sci. Sports Exerc.*, 35:1176, 2003.

Coyle, E.F.: Improved muscular efficiency displayed as Tour de France champion matures. *J. Appl. Physiol.*, 98:2191, 2005.

Crouter, S.E., et al.: Accuracy of polar S410 heart rate monitor to estimate energy cost of exercise. *Med. Sci. Sports Exerc.*, 36:1433, 2004.

da Rocha, E.E., et al.: Can measured resting energy expenditure be estimated by formulae in daily clinical nutrition practice? *Curr. Opin. Clin. Nutr. Metab. Care*, 8:319, 2005.

Das, S.K., et al.: Energy expenditure is very high in extremely obese women. *J. Nutr.*, 134:1412, 2004.

DeLany, J.P., et al.: Energy expenditure in African American and white boys and girls in a 2-y follow-up of the Baton Rouge Children's Study. *Am. J. Clin. Nutr.*, 79:268, 2004.

Delextrat, A., et al.: Drafting during swimming improves efficiency during subsequent cycling. *Med. Sci. Sports Exerc.*, 35:1612, 2003.

Dennis, S.C., Noakes, T.D.: Advantages of a smaller body mass in humans when distance-running in warm, humid conditions. *Eur. J. Appl. Physiol.*, 79:280, 1999.

Doke, J., et al.: Mechanics and energetics of swinging the human leg. *J. Exp. Biol.*, 208:439, 2005.

Donahoo, W.T., et al.: Variability in energy expenditure and its components. *Curr. Opin. Clin. Nutr. Metab. Care*, 7:599, 2004.

Duffield, R., et al.: Energy system contribution to 100-m and 200-m track running events. *J. Sci. Med. Sport*, 7:302, 2004.

Edwards, A.G., Byrnes, W.C.: Aerodynamic characteristics as determinants of the drafting effect in cycling. *Med. Sci. Sports Exerc.*, 39:170, 2007.

Farshchi, H.R., et al.: Decreased thermic effect of food after an irregular compared with a regular meal pattern in healthy lean women. *Int. J. Obes. Relat. Metab. Disord.*, 28:653, 2004.

Flodmark, C.E.: Calculation of resting energy expenditure in obese children. *Acta. Paediatr.*, 93:727, 2004.

Garet, M., et al.: Estimating relative physical workload using heart rate monitoring: a validation by whole-body indirect calorimetry. *Eur. J. Appl. Physiol.*, 94:46, 2005.

Gottschall, J.S., Kram, R.: Ground reaction forces during downhill and uphill running. *J. Biomech.*, 38:445, 2005.

Hall, C., et al.: Energy expenditure of walking and running: comparison with prediction equations. *Med. Sci. Sports Exerc.*, 36:2128, 2004.

Hausswirth, C., et al.: Effects of cycling alone or in a sheltered position on subsequent running performance during a triathlon. *Med. Sci. Sports Exerc.*, 31:599, 1999.

Helseth, J., et al.: How do low horizontal forces produce disproportionately high torques in human locomotion? *J. Biomech.*, 41:1747, 2008.

Hiilloskorpi, H.K., et al.: Use of heart rate to predict energy expenditure from low to high activity levels. *Int. J. Sports Med.*, 24:332, 2003.

Hoyt, R.W., et al.: Total energy expenditure estimated using foot-ground contact pedometry. *Diabetes Technol. Ther.*, 6:71, 2004.

Keytel, L.R., et al.: Prediction of energy expenditure from heart rate monitoring during submaximal exercise. *J. Sports Sci.*, 23:289, 2005.

Kien, C.L., Ugrasbul, F.: Prediction of daily energy expenditure during a feeding trial using measurements of resting energy expenditure, fat-free mass, or Harris-Benedict equations. *Am. J. Clin. Nutr.*, 80:876, 2004.

Kram, R.: Muscular force or work: what determines the metabolic energy cost of running? *Exer. Sport Sci. Rev.*, 28:138, 2000.

Kyrölälinen, H., et al.: Interrelationships between muscle structure, muscle strength, and running economy. *Med. Sci. Sports Exerc.*, 35:45, 2003.

Larsson, L., Lindqvist, P.G.: Low-impact exercise during pregnancy study of safety. *Acta. Obstet. Gynecol. Scand.*, 84:34, 2005.

Lätt, E., et al.: Longitudinal development of physical and performance parameters during biological maturation of young male swimmers. *Percept. Mot. Skills.*, 108:297, 2009.

Lätt, E., et al.: Physical development and swimming performance during biological maturation in young female swimmers. *Coll. Antropol.*, 33:117, 2009.

Lin, P.H., et al.: Estimation of energy requirements in a controlled feeding trial. *Am. J. Clin. Nutr.*, 77:639, 2003.

Malison, E.R., et al.: Running performance in middle-school runners. *J. Sports Med. Phys. Fitness*, 44:383, 2004.

Manini, T.M.: Energy expenditure and aging. *Ageing Res. Rev.*, 9:1, 2010.

McArdle, W.D., et al.: Aerobic capacity, heart rate and estimated energy cost during women's competitive basketball. *Res. Q.*, 42:178, 1971.

McArdle, W.D., Foglia, G.F.: Energy cost and cardiorespiratory stress of isometric and weight training exercise. *J. Sports Med. Phys. Fitness.*, 9:23, 1969.

Mollendorf, J.C., et al.: Effect of swim suit design on passive drag. *Med. Sci. Sports Exerc.*, 36:1029, 2004.

Morgan, D.W., et al.: Longitudinal stratification of gait economy in young boys and girls: the locomotion energy and growth study. *Eur. J. Appl. Physiol.*, 91:30, 2004.

Morgan, D.W., et al.: Prediction of the aerobic demand of walking in children. *Med. Sci. Sports Exerc.*, 34:2097, 2002.

Pendergast, D., et al.: Energy balance of human locomotion in water. *Eur. J. Appl. Physiol.*, 90:377, 2003.

Pendergast, D., et al.: The influence of drag on human locomotion in water. *Undersea Hyperb. Med.*, 32:45, 2005.

Pendergast, D.R., et al.: Evaluation of fins used in underwater swimming. *Undersea Hyperb. Med.*, 30:57, 2003.

Pontzer, H.: A new model predicting locomotor cost from limb length via force production. *J. Exp. Biol.*, 208:1513, 2005.

Puthoff, M.L., et al.: The effect of weighted vest walking on metabolic responses and ground reaction forces. *Med. Sci. Sports Exerc.*, 38:746, 2006.

Ramirez-Marrero, F.A., et al.: Comparison of methods to estimate physical activity and energy expenditure in African American children. *Int. J. Sports Med.*, 26:363, 2005.

Ratel, S., Poujade, B.: Comparative analysis of the energy cost during front crawl swimming in children and adults. *Eur. J. Appl. Physiol.*, 105:543, 2009.

Ray, A.D., et al.: Respiratory muscle training reduces the work of breathing at depth. *Eur. J. Appl. Physiol.*, 108:811, 2010.

Reis, V.M., et al.: Examining the accumulated oxygen deficit method in front crawl swimming. *Int. J. Sports Med.*, 31:421, 2010.

Rosenberger, F., et al.: Running 8000 m fast or slow: Are there differences in energy cost and fat metabolism? *Med. Sci. Sports Exerc.*, 37:1789, 2005.

Rotstein, A., et al.: Preferred transition speed between walking and running: Effects of training status. *Med. Sci. Sports Exerc.*, 37:1864, 2006.

Roy, J-P.R., Stefanyshyn, D.J.: Shoe midsole longitudinal bending stiffness and running economy, joint energy, and EMG. *Med. Sci. Sports Exerc.*, 38:562, 2006.

Royer, T.D., Martin, P.E.: Manipulations of leg mass and moment of inertia: effects on energy cost of walking. *Med. Sci. Sports Exerc.*, 37:649, 2005.

Saunders, P.U., et al.: Reliability and variability of running economy in elite distance runners. *Med. Sci. Sports Exerc.*, 36:1972, 2004.

Sazonov, E.S., Schuckers, S.: The energetics of obesity: a review: monitoring energy intake and energy expenditure in humans. *IEEE Eng. Med. Biol. Mag.*, 29:31, 2010. Review.

Scott, C.B., Devore, R.: Diet-induced thermogenesis: variations among three isocaloric meal-replacement shakes. *Nutrition*, 21:874, 2005.

Slawinski, J.S., Billat, V.L.: Difference in mechanical and energy cost between highly, well, and nontrained runners. *Med. Sci. Sports Exerc.*, 36:1440, 2004.

Speakman, J.R.: Body size, energy metabolism and lifespan. *J. Exp. Biol.*, 208:1717, 2005.

Srinivasan, M.: Optimal speeds for walking and running, and walking on a moving walkway. *Chaos.*, 19:026112, 2009.

Støren, ø., et al.: Maximal strength training improves running economy in distance runners. *Med. Sci. Sports Exerc.*, 40:1087, 2008.

Tharion, W.J., et al.: Energy requirements of military personnel. *Appetite*, 44:47, 2005.

Unnithan, V., et al.: Aerobic cost in elite female adolescent swimmers. *Int. J. Sports Med.*, 30:194, 2009.

Vasconcellos, M.T., Anjos, L.A.: A simplified method for assessing physical activity level values for a country or study population. *Eur. J. Clin. Nutr.*, 57:1025, 2003.

Vercruyssen, F., et al.: Cadence selection affects metabolic responses during cycling and subsequent running time to fatigue. *Br. J. Sports Med.*, 39:267, 2005.

Weissgerber, T.L., et al.: The role of regular physical activity in preeclampsia prevention. *Med. Sci. Sports Exerc.*, 36:2024, 2004.

Weyand, P.G., Bundle, M.W.: Energetics of high-speed running: integrating classical theory and contemporary observations. *Am. J. Physiol. Regul. Integr. Comp. Physiol.*, 288:R956, 2005.

Zamparo, P., et al.: The interplay between propelling efficiency, hydrodynamic position and energy cost of front crawl in 8 to 19-year-old swimmers. *Eur. J. Appl. Physiol.*, 104:689, 2008.

The Physiologic Support Systems

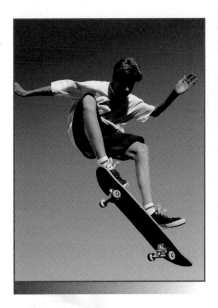

Most sport, recreational, and occupational activities require a moderately intense yet sustained energy release. The aerobic breakdown of carbohydrates, fats, and proteins generates this energy from adenosine diphosphate (ADP) phosphorylation to adenosine triphosphate (ATP). Without a steady rate between oxidative phosphorylation and the energy requirements of physical activity, an anaerobic–aerobic energy imbalance develops, lactate accumulates, tissue acidity increases, and fatigue quickly ensues. Two factors limit an individual's ability to sustain a high level of exercise intensity without undue fatigue:

1. The capacity for oxygen delivery to active muscle cells
2. The capacity of active muscle cells to generate ATP aerobically

Understanding the roles of the ventilatory, circulatory, muscular, and endocrine systems during exercise explains the broad range of individual differences in exercise capacity. Knowing the energy requirements of exercise and the corresponding physiologic adjustments necessary to meet these requirements helps formulate an effective physical fitness program to properly evaluate physiologic and fitness status before and during such a program.

All the problems of the world could be settled easily if men were only willing to think. The trouble is that men very often resort to all sorts of devices in order not to think, because thinking is such hard work.

— Thomas J. Watson
President of IBM (1924–1952)

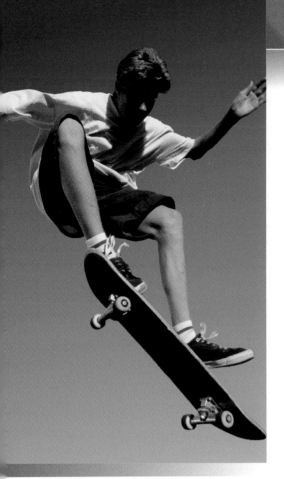

The Pulmonary System and Exercise

CHAPTER OBJECTIVES

- Diagram the ventilatory system and show the glottis, larynx, trachea, bronchi, bronchioles, and alveoli.

- Describe the dynamics of inspiration and expiration during rest and exercise.

- Describe the Valsalva maneuver and its physiologic consequences.

- Define *minute ventilation*, *alveolar minute ventilation*, *ventilation–perfusion ratio*, and *anatomic and physiologic dead spaces*.

- Explain the Bohr effect and its benefit during physical activity.

- List and quantify three means for carbon dioxide transport in blood.

- Identify major factors that regulate pulmonary ventilation during rest and exercise.

- Describe how hyperventilation extends breath-holding time but can have dangerous consequences in sport diving.

- Graph relationships among pulmonary ventilation, blood lactate concentrations, and oxygen uptake during incremental exercise. Indicate the demarcation points for the lactate threshold and onset of blood lactate accumulation.

- Explain what triggers exercise-induced asthma and identify factors that affect its severity.

Part 1

Pulmonary Structure and Function

If oxygen supply depended only on diffusion through skin, it would be impossible to support the basal energy requirement, let alone the 4- to 6-L oxygen uptake each minute to sustain a world-class 5 minute per mile marathon pace. The remarkably effective **ventilatory system** meets the body's needs to maintain efficient gas exchange. This system, depicted in **Figure 9.1**, regulates the gaseous state of our "external" environment for aerating fluids of the "internal" environment during rest and exercise. The major functions of the ventilatory system include:

1. Supply oxygen required in metabolism
2. Eliminate carbon dioxide produced in metabolism
3. Regulate hydrogen ion concentration $[H^+]$ to maintain acid–base balance

ANATOMY OF VENTILATION

The term **pulmonary ventilation** describes how ambient atmospheric air moves into and exchanges with air in the lungs. A distance of about 0.3 m (1 ft) separates ambient air just outside the nose and mouth from the blood flowing through the lungs. Air entering the nose and mouth flows into the conductive portion of the ventilatory system, where it adjusts to body temperature and is filtered and almost completely humidified as it passes through the trachea. The trachea, a short 1-inch-diameter tube that extends from the larynx, divides into two tubes of smaller diameter called **bronchi**. The bronchi serve as primary conduits within the right and left lungs. They further subdivide into numerous **bronchioles** that conduct inspired air through a narrow route until eventually mixing with air in the **alveoli**, the terminal branches of the respiratory tract.

Lungs

The lungs provide the surface between blood and the external environment. Lung volume varies between 4 and 6 L (amount of air in a basketball) and provides an exceptionally large moist surface. The lungs of an average-sized person weigh about 1 kg, yet if spread out, they would cover a surface of 60 to 80 m², about 35 times the external surface of the person, and almost half the size of a tennis court or an entire badminton court. This represents a considerable interface for aeration of blood because during any 1 second of maximal exercise, no more than 1 pint of blood

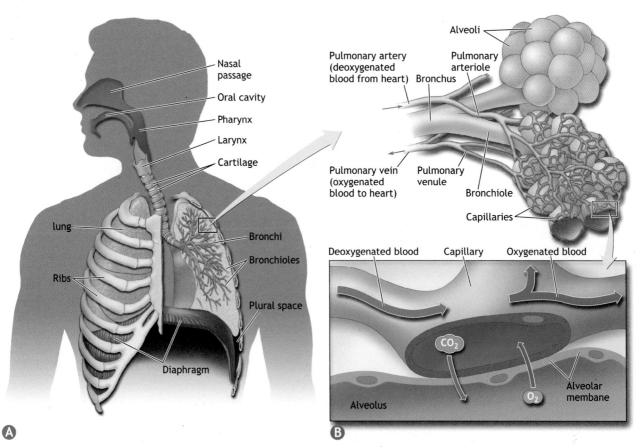

Figure 9.1 **A.** Major pulmonary structures within the thoracic cavity. **B.** Respiratory passages, alveoli, and gas exchange function in an alveolus.

flows in the lung tissue's weblike, intricate, and interlaced network of blood vessels.

Alveoli

Lung tissue contains more than 600 million alveoli. These elastic, thin-walled, membranous sacs provide the vital surface for gas exchange between the lungs and blood. Alveolar tissue has the largest blood supply of any organ in the body. Millions of thin-walled capillaries and alveoli lie side by side, with air moving on one side and blood on the other. The capillaries form a dense, meshlike cover that almost encircles the entire outside of each alveolus (**Fig. 9.2A**). This web becomes so dense that blood flows as a sheet over each alveolus. When blood reaches the pulmonary capillaries, only a single cell barrier, the **respiratory membrane**, separates blood from air in the alveolus (**Fig. 9.2B**). This thin tissue–blood barrier permits rapid diffusion between alveolar and blood gases.

During rest, approximately 250 mL of oxygen *leave* the alveoli each minute and enter the blood, and about 200 mL of carbon dioxide diffuse *into* the alveoli. When trained endurance athletes perform intense exercise, about 20 times the resting oxygen uptake transfers across the respiratory membrane into the blood each minute. The primary function of pulmonary ventilation during rest and exercise is to maintain relatively constant and favorable concentrations of oxygen and carbon dioxide in the alveolar chambers. This ensures effective alveolar gaseous exchange before the blood exits the lungs for transit throughout the body.

Mechanics of Ventilation

Figure 9.3 illustrates the physical principle underlying breathing dynamics. The example shows two balloons connected to a jar whose glass bottom has been replaced by a thin rubber membrane. When the membrane lowers, the jar's volume increases, and air pressure within the jar becomes less than air pressure outside the jar. Consequently, air rushes into the balloons, and they inflate. Conversely, if the elastic membrane recoils, the pressure within the jar temporarily increases, and air rushes out. Air exchange occurs within the

Questions & Notes

Define pulmonary ventilation.

List 2 functions of the ventilatory system.

1.

2.

How many liters of oxygen leave the alveoli and enter the blood each minute during rest?

How many liters of carbon dioxide leave the blood and enter the alveoli each minute at rest.

List 2 factors that determine lung filling.

1.

2.

BOX 9.1   CLOSE UP

Common Symbols Used by Pulmonary Physiologists

PULMONARY VENTILATION	EXTERNAL RESPIRATION	INTERNAL RESPIRATION
$\dot{V}_E$ = Minute ventilation	$\dot{V}_A$ = Alveolar minute ventilation	a–$\bar{v}$O$_{2diff}$ = Quantity of oxygen carried in the arteries minus the amount carried in the veins
V_d = Dead space	$P_{A}O_2$ = Partial pressure of oxygen in the alveoli	
V_T = Tidal volume	PaO_2 = Partial pressure of oxygen in arterial blood	PaO_2 = Partial pressure of oxygen in arterial blood
F = Breathing frequency	(A–a)PO$_{2diff}$ = Oxygen or PO$_2$ pressure gradient between the alveoli and arteries	$PacO_2$ = Partial pressure of carbon dioxide in arterial blood
V_d/V_T = Ratio of dead space to tidal volume	SaO$_{2\%}$ = Percent saturation of arterial blood with oxygen	$PvcO_2$ = Partial pressure of carbon dioxide in venous blood
	$P_{A}CO_2$ = Partial pressure of carbon dioxide in the alveoli	SvO$_{2\%}$ = Percent saturation of venous blood with oxygen
		PvO_2 = Partial pressure of oxygen in venous blood

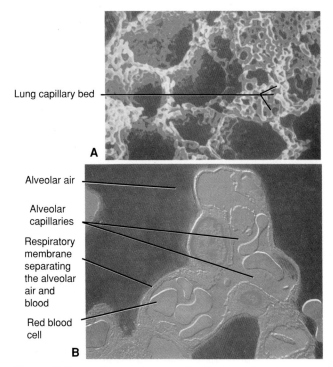

Lung capillary bed

A

Alveolar air

Alveolar capillaries

Respiratory membrane separating the alveolar air and blood

Red blood cell

B

Figure 9.2 **A.** Electron micrograph of lung capillaries (×1300). Note the extremely dense capillary bed; the dark areas represent the alveolar chambers. **B.** Electron micrograph of a pulmonary capillary (×6000). Note the extremely thin respiratory membrane layer separating alveolar air from red blood cells.

balloons as the distance and rate of descent and ascent of the rubber membrane increases.

The lungs are not merely suspended in the chest cavity as depicted with the balloons and jar. Rather, the difference in pressure within the lungs and the lung–chest wall interface causes the lungs to adhere to the chest wall interior and literally follow its every movement. Any change in thoracic cavity volume thus produces a corresponding change in lung volume. Skeletal muscle action during inspiration and expiration alters thoracic dimensions to change lung volume.

Inspiration

The **diaphragm**, a large, dome-shaped sheet of muscle, serves the same purpose as the jar's rubber membrane in **Figure 9.3**. The diaphragm muscle makes an airtight separation between the abdominal and thoracic cavities. During **inspiration**, the diaphragm contracts, flattens out, and moves downward up to 10 cm toward the abdominal cavity. This enlarges and elongates the chest cavity. The air in the lungs then expands, reducing its pressure (referred to as **intrapulmonic pressure**) to about 5 mm Hg below atmospheric pressure. *The pressure differential between the lungs and ambient air literally sucks air in through the nose and mouth and inflates the lungs.* The degree of lung filling depends on two factors:

1. The magnitude of inspiratory movements
2. The pressure gradient between the air inside and the air outside the lung

Inspiration concludes when thoracic cavity expansion ceases and intrapulmonic pressure increases to equal atmospheric pressure.

During exercise, the scaleni and external intercostal muscles between the ribs contract. This causes the ribs to rotate and lift up and away from the body—an action similar to the movement of the handle lifted up and away from the side of the bucket at the right in **Figure 9.3**. Air moves into the lungs when chest cavity volume increases from three factors: (1) descent of the diaphragm, (2) upward lift of the ribs, and (3) outward thrust of the sternum.

Expiration

Expiration, a predominantly passive process, occurs as air moves out of the lungs from the recoil of stretched lung tissue and relaxation of the inspiratory muscles. This causes the sternum and ribs to swing down while the diaphragm moves toward the thoracic cavity. These movements decrease chest cavity volume and compress alveolar gas; this forces it out through the respiratory tract to the atmosphere. During ventilation in moderate to intense exercise, the internal intercostal muscles and abdominal muscles act powerfully on the ribs and abdominal cavity to produce a rapid and greater depth of exhalation. Greater involvement of the pulmonary musculature during progressively intense exercise causes larger pressure differentials and concomitant increases in air movement.

LUNG VOLUMES AND CAPACITIES

Figure 9.4 presents a lung volume tracing with average values for men and women. To obtain these measurements, the subject rebreathes through a water-sealed, volume-displacement spirometer similar to the one described in Chapter 7 for measuring oxygen consumption with the closed-circuit method. As with many anatomic and physiologic measures, lung volumes vary with age, gender, and body size and composition, but particularly with stature. Common practice evaluates lung volumes by comparing them with established standards that consider these factors.

Two types of measurements, static and dynamic, provide information about lung volume dimensions and capacities. **Static lung volume** tests evaluate the *dimensional component* for air movement within the pulmonary tract and impose no time limitation on the subject. In contrast, **dynamic lung volume** measures evaluate the *power component* of pulmonary performance during different phases of the ventilatory excursion.

Static Lung Volumes

During static lung function measurement, the spirometer bell falls and rises with each inhalation and exhalation to provide a record of the ventilatory volume and breathing

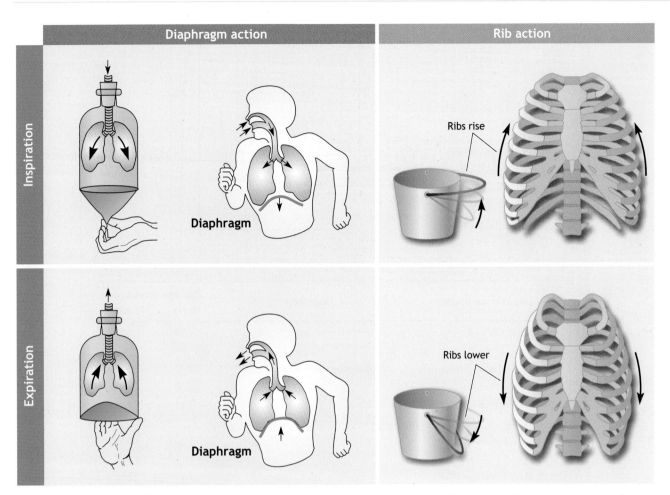

Figure 9.3 Mechanics of breathing. During inspiration, the chest cavity increases in size because the ribs rise and the muscular diaphragm lowers. During exhalation, the ribs swing down, and the diaphragm returns to a relaxed position. This reduces the thoracic cavity volume, and air rushes out. The movement of the jar's rubber bottom causes air to enter and leave the two balloons, simulating the diaphragm's action. The movement of the bucket handle simulates rib action.

rate. **Tidal volume (TV)** describes air moved during either the inspiratory or expiratory phase of each breathing cycle. For healthy men and women, TV under resting conditions ranges between 0.4 and 1.0 L of air per breath.

After recording several representative TVs, the subject breathes in normally and then inspires maximally. An additional volume of 2.5 to 3.5 L above TV air represents the reserve for inhalation, termed the **inspiratory reserve volume (IRV)**. The normal breathing pattern begins once again following the IRV. After a normal exhalation, the subject continues to exhale and forces as much air as possible from the lungs. This additional volume, the **expiratory reserve volume (ERV)**, ranges between 1.0 and 1.5 L for an average-size man (10%–20% lower for a woman). During exercise, TV increases considerably because of encroachment on IRV and ERV but particularly IRV.

Forced vital capacity (FVC) represents total air volume moved in one breath from full inspiration to maximum expiration or vice versa. FVC varies with body size and body position during measurement; values usually average 4 to 5 L in healthy young men and 3 to 4 L in healthy young women. FVCs of 6 to 7 L are common for tall individuals, and values above 8 L have been reported for some large-size professional athletes. These large lung volumes probably reflect genetic endowment because exercise training does not change appreciably static lung volumes.

Residual Lung Volume After a maximal exhalation, a volume of air remains in the lungs that cannot be exhaled. This volume, called the **residual**

 For Your Information

BODY POSITION FACILITATES BREATHING

Athletes frequently bend forward from the waist to facilitate breathing after intense exercise. This body position serves two purposes:

1. Facilitates blood flow to the heart
2. Minimizes antagonistic effects of gravity on respiratory movements

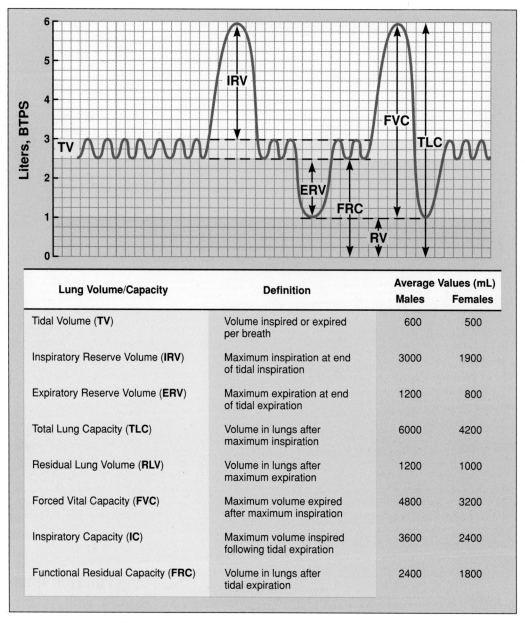

Figure 9.4 Static measures of lung volume and capacity.

Lung Volume/Capacity	Definition	Average Values (mL)	
		Males	**Females**
Tidal Volume (**TV**)	Volume inspired or expired per breath	600	500
Inspiratory Reserve Volume (**IRV**)	Maximum inspiration at end of tidal inspiration	3000	1900
Expiratory Reserve Volume (**ERV**)	Maximum expiration at end of tidal expiration	1200	800
Total Lung Capacity (**TLC**)	Volume in lungs after maximum inspiration	6000	4200
Residual Lung Volume (**RLV**)	Volume in lungs after maximum expiration	1200	1000
Forced Vital Capacity (**FVC**)	Maximum volume expired after maximum inspiration	4800	3200
Inspiratory Capacity (**IC**)	Maximum volume inspired following tidal expiration	3600	2400
Functional Residual Capacity (**FRC**)	Volume in lungs after tidal expiration	2400	1800

lung volume (RLV), averages between 1.0 and 1.2 L for young adult women and 1.2 and 1.6 L for men.

Aging changes lung volumes because of decreases in lung tissue elasticity and a decline in pulmonary muscle power. These two factors do not entirely result from aging per se but more from the effects of a sedentary lifestyle. *Sedentary living, rather than true aging, most likely accounts for the largest changes in lung volumes and pulmonary function.*

Dynamic Lung Volumes

Dynamic measures of pulmonary ventilation depend on two factors:

1. The maximum lung volume expired (FVC)
2. The speed of moving a volume of air

Airflow speed depends on the pulmonary airways' resistance to the smooth flow of air and resistance ("stiffness") offered by the chest and lung tissue to changes in shape during breathing termed **lung compliance.**

Ratio of Forced Expiratory Volume to Forced Vital Capacity

Normal values for vital capacity occur in severe lung disease if no time limit exists to expel air. For this reason, a dynamic lung function measure, such as the **percentage of FVC expelled in 1 second (FEV$_{1.0}$)**, serves a more useful diagnostic purpose than static measures. The *forced expiratory volume-to-FVC ratio (FEV$_{1.0}$ / FVC) reflects expiratory power and overall resistance to air movement in the lungs.* Normally, the FEV$_{1.0}$ / FVC averages about 85%. With severe obstructive pulmonary disease (e.g., emphysema, bronchial asthma), the FEV$_{1.0}$ / FVC often decreases below 40% of vital capacity. *The clinical demarcation for airway obstruction represents the point where a person can expel less than 70% of the FVC in 1 second.*

Maximum Voluntary Ventilation Another dynamic assessment of ventilatory capacity requires rapid, deep breathing for 15 seconds. Extrapolation of this 15-second volume to the volume breathed for 1 minute represents the **maximum voluntary ventilation (MVV)**. For healthy young men, the MVV ranges between 140 and 180 L·min^{-1}. The average for women is 80 to 120 L·min^{-1}. Male members of the United States Nordic Ski Team averaged 192 L·min^{-1}, with an individual high MVV of 239 L·min^{-1}. Patients with obstructive lung disease achieve only about 40% of the MVV predicted normal for their age and stature. Specific pulmonary therapy benefits these patients because training the muscles used in breathing increases the strength and endurance of the respiratory muscles and enhances MVV.

PULMONARY VENTILATION

Minute Ventilation

During quiet breathing at rest, an adult's breathing rate averages 12 breaths per minute, and the TV averages about 0.5 L of air per breath. Under these conditions, the volume of air breathed each minute, termed **minute ventilation**, equals 6 L.

$$\text{Minute ventilation } (\dot{V}_E) = \text{Breathing rate} \times \text{TV}$$
$$6.0 \text{ L·min}^{-1} = 12 \times 0.5 \text{ L}$$

An increase in the depth or rate of breathing or both increases minute ventilation. During maximal exercise, the breathing rate of healthy young adults increases to 35 to 45 breaths per minute, while elite athletes often achieve 60 to 70 breaths per minute. In addition, TV commonly increases to 2.0 L and greater during intense exercise. This causes exercise minute ventilation in adults to reach 100 L or about 17 times the resting value. In well-trained male endurance athletes, ventilation can increase to 160 L·min^{-1} during maximal exercise, with several studies of elite endurance athletes reporting ventilation volumes exceeding 200 L·min^{-1}. *Even with these large minute ventilations, the TV rarely exceeds 55% to 65% of vital capacity.*

Alveolar Ventilation

Alveolar ventilation refers to the portion of minute ventilation that mixes with the air in the alveolar chambers. A portion of each breath inspired does not enter the alveoli and does not engage in gaseous exchange with blood. The air that fills the nose, mouth, trachea, and other non-diffusible conducting portions of the respiratory tract constitutes the **anatomic dead space**. In healthy people, this volume equals 150 to 200 mL, or about 30% of the resting TV. Almost equivalent composition exists between dead-space air and ambient air except for dead-space air's full saturation with water vapor.

Because of dead-space volume, approximately 350 mL of the 500 mL of ambient air inspired in each TV at rest mixes with existing alveolar air. This does not mean

Questions & Notes

List an average tidal volume for men and women.

Men:

Women:

List the average vital capacity for men and women.

Men:

Women:

List an average residual lung volume for men and women.

Men:

Women:

List the average FEV$_{1.0}$ / FVC for healthy adults.

Compute $\dot{V}_E$ for an individual with a tidal volume of 0.6 L and a breathing rate of 15 breaths per minute.

 For Your Information

VENTILATORY MUSCLES RESPOND TO TRAINING

Specific exercise training of the ventilatory muscles improves their strength and endurance and increases both inspiratory muscle function and MVV. Ventilatory training in patients with chronic pulmonary disease enhances exercise capacity and reduces physiologic strain. Patients with chronic obstructive lung disease receive benefits from ventilatory muscle training and regular large muscle low-intensity aerobic exercise. This occurs from progressive desensitization to the feeling of breathlessness and greater self-control of respiratory symptoms.

BOX 9.2 CLOSE UP

Predicting Pulmonary Function Variables from Stature and Age

Pulmonary function variables do not directly relate to measures of physical fitness in healthy individuals, but their measurement often forms part of a standard medical, health, or fitness examination, particularly for individuals at risk for limited pulmonary function (e.g., chronic cigarette smokers, people with asthma). Measurement of diverse components of pulmonary dimension and lung function with a water-filled spirometer or electronic spirometer (see Fig. 7.8) provide the framework to discuss pulmonary dynamics during rest and exercise. Proper evaluation of measured values for pulmonary function requires comparison with norms from the clinical literature. Stature and age are two variables that predict the lung function value expected to be average (normal) for a particular individual.

EXAMPLES

Predictions use cm for stature (ST) and years for age (A).

Data
Woman: Age, 22 y; stature, 165.1 cm (65 in)
   Man: Age, 22 y; stature, 182.9 cm (72 in)

Woman
1. FVC

$$FVC, L = (0.0414 \times ST) - (0.0232 \times A) - 2.20$$
$$= 6.835 - 0.5104 - 2.20$$
$$= 4.12\,L$$

2. $FEV_{1.0}$

$$FEV_{1.0}, L = (0.0268 \times ST) - (0.0251 \times A) - 0.38$$
$$= 4.425 - 0.5522 - 0.38$$
$$= 3.49\,L$$

3. $FEV_{1.0} / FVC$

$$FEV_{1.0} / FVC, \% = (-0.2145 \times ST) - (0.1523 \times A) + 124.5$$
$$= -35.41 - 3.35 + 124.5$$
$$= 85.7\%$$

4. Maximum voluntary ventilation (MVV)

$$MMV, L \cdot min^{-1} = 40 \times FEV_{1.0}$$
$$= 40 \times 3.49 \text{ (from eq. 2)}$$
$$= 139.6\,L \cdot min^{-1}$$

Man
1. FVC

$$FVC, L = (0.0774 \times ST) - (0.0212 \times A) - 7.75$$
$$= 14.156 - 0.4664 - 7.75$$
$$= 5.49\,L$$

2. $FEV_{1.0}$

$$FEV_{1.0}, L = (0.0566 \times ST) - (0.0233 \times A) - 0.491$$
$$= 10.35 - 0.5126 - 4.91$$
$$= 4.93\,L$$

3. $FEV_{1.0} / FVC$

$$FEV_{1.0} / FVC, \% = (-0.1314 \times ST) - (0.1490 \times A) + 110.2$$
$$= -24.03 - 3.35 + 110.2$$
$$= 82.8\%$$

4. MVV

$$MMV, L \cdot min^{-1} = 40 \times FEV_{1.0}$$
$$= 40 \times 4.93 \text{ (from eq. 2)}$$
$$= 197.2\,L \cdot min^{-1}$$

REFERENCES

1. Miller, A. *Pulmonary Function Tests in Clinical and Occupational Disease.* Philadelphia: Grune & Stratton. 1986.
2. Wasserman, K., et al. *Principles of Exercise Testing.* Baltimore: Lippincott Williams & Wilkins. 1999.

that only 350 mL of air enters and leaves the alveoli with each breath. To the contrary, if the TV equals 500 mL, then 500 mL of air enters the alveoli but only 350 mL represents fresh air (about one-seventh of the total air in the alveoli). This relatively small, seemingly inefficient alveolar ventilation prevents drastic changes in alveolar air composition. This ensures a consistency in arterial blood gases throughout the breathing cycle.

Table 9.1 shows that minute ventilation does not always reflect the actual alveolar ventilation. In the first example of shallow breathing, the TV decreases to 150 mL, yet a 6-L minute ventilation occurs when the breathing rate increases to 40 breaths per minute. The same 6-L minute volume can be achieved by decreasing the breathing rate to 12 breaths per minute and increasing the TV to 500 mL. Doubling the TV and reducing ventilatory rate by half, as in the example of deep breathing, again produces a 6-L minute ventilation. Each ventilatory adjustment drastically affects alveolar ventilation. In the example of shallow breathing, dead-space air represents the entire air volume moved

Table 9.1	Relationships Among Tidal Volume, Breathing Rate, and Minute and Alveolar Minute Ventilation					
CONDITION	TIDAL VOLUME (mL)	× BREATHING RATE (breaths·min^{-1})	= MINUTE VENTILATION (mL·min^{-1})	− DEAD SPACE VENTILATION (mL·min^{-1})	= ALVEOLAR VENTILATION (mL·min^{-1})	
Shallow breathing	150	40	6000	(150 mL × 40)	0	
Normal breathing	5000	12	6000	(150 mL × 12)	4200	
Deep breathing	1000	6	6000	(150 mL × 6)	5100	

(no alveolar ventilation has taken place). The other examples involve deeper breathing; thus, a larger portion of each breath mixes with existing alveolar air. *Alveolar ventilation, not dead-space ventilation, determines gaseous concentrations at the alveolar–capillary membrane.*

Physiologic Dead Space

Some alveoli may not function adequately in gas exchange because of under-perfusion of blood or inadequate ventilation relative to alveolar surface area. The term **physiologic dead space** describes the portion of the alveolar volume with poor tissue regional perfusion or inadequate ventilation. **Figure 9.5** illustrates that only a negligible physiologic dead space exists in healthy lungs.

Physiologic dead space can increase to 50% of resting TV. This occurs because of two factors:

1. Inadequate perfusion during hemorrhage or blockage of the pulmonary circulation from an embolism or blood clot
2. Inadequate alveolar ventilation in chronic pulmonary disease

Adequate gas exchange and aeration of blood are **impossible** *when the lung's total dead space exceeds 60% of lung volume.*

Depth Versus Rate

Adjustments in breathing rate and depth maintain alveolar ventilation as exercise intensity increases. In moderate exercise, trained endurance athletes maintain adequate alveolar ventilation by increasing the TV and only minimally by increasing the breathing rate. With deeper breathing, alveolar ventilation

*Q*uestions & Notes

TV rarely exceeds _____% to _____% of vital capacity.

Give the normal range for the anatomic dead space (volume) for healthy adults.

Why do novice exercisers sometimes experience dyspnea during exercise?

i For Your Information

THE GAS LAWS

The four laws governing gas behavior include:

- **Boyle's law:** If temperature remains constant, the pressure of a gas varies inversely with its volume.
- **Gay–Lussac's law:** If gas volume remains constant, its pressure increases in direct proportion to its absolute temperature.
- **Law of partial pressures:** In a mixture of gases, each gas exerts a partial pressure proportional to its concentration.
- **Henry's law:** If temperature remains constant, the quantity of a gas dissolved in a liquid varies in direct proportion to its partial pressure.

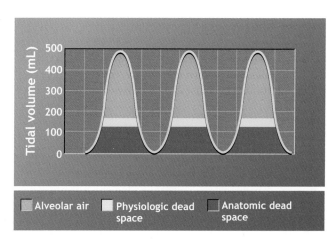

Figure 9.5 Distribution of tidal volume in the lungs of a healthy subject at rest. Tidal volume includes about 350 mL of ambient air that mixes with alveolar air, 150 mL of air in the larger air passages (anatomic dead space), and a small portion of air distributed to either poorly ventilated or poorly perfused alveoli (physiologic dead space).

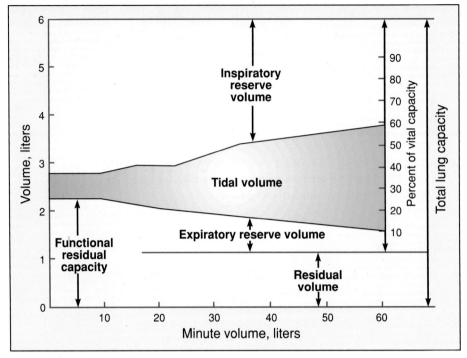

Figure 9.6 Tidal volume and subdivisions of pulmonary air during rest and exercise.

usually increases from 70% of minute ventilation at rest to more than 85% of the total ventilation in exercise. *This increase occurs because a greater percentage of incoming TV enters the alveoli with deeper breathing.*

Figure 9.6 shows increasing TV during in exercise results largely from encroachment on IRV, with an accompanying but smaller decrease in end-expiratory level. As exercise intensity increases, TV plateaus at about 60% of vital capacity; further increases in minute ventilation result from increases in breathing rate. These ventilatory adjustments occur unconsciously; each individual develops a "style" of breathing by blending the breathing rate and TV so alveolar ventilation matches alveolar perfusion. *Conscious attempts to modify breathing during running and other general physical activities do not benefit exercise performance. In most instances, conscious manipulation of breathing detracts from the exquisitely regulated ventilatory adjustments to exercise.* During rest and exercise each individual should breathe in the manner that seems "most natural." Most individuals who perform rhythmical walking, running, cycling, and rowing naturally synchronize breathing frequency with limb movements. This breathing pattern, termed **entrainment**, reduces the energy cost of the activity.

DISRUPTIONS IN NORMAL BREATHING PATTERNS

Breathing patterns during exercise generally progress in an effective and highly economical manner, yet some pulmonary responses negatively impact exercise performance.

Dyspnea

Dyspnea refers to shortness of breath or subjective distress in breathing. The sense of inability to breathe during exercise, particularly in novice exercisers, usually accompanies elevated arterial carbon dioxide and $[H^+]$. Both chemicals excite the inspiratory center to increase breathing rate and depth. Failure to adequately regulate arterial carbon dioxide and $[H^+]$ most likely relates to low aerobic fitness levels and a poorly conditioned ventilatory musculature. The strong neural drive to breathe during exercise causes poorly conditioned respiratory muscles to fatigue, disrupting normal plasma levels of carbon dioxide and $[H^+]$. This accelerates the pattern of shallow, ineffective breathing, and the individual senses an inability to breathe sufficient air.

Hyperventilation

Hyperventilation refers to an increase in pulmonary ventilation that exceeds the oxygen needs of metabolism. This "overbreathing" quickly lowers normal alveolar carbon dioxide concentration, which causes excess carbon dioxide to leave body fluids via the expired air. An accompanying decrease in $[H^+]$ increases plasma pH. Several seconds of hyperventilation generally produces lightheadedness; prolonged hyperventilation can lead to unconsciousness from excessive carbon dioxide unloading from the blood (see page 288).

BOX 9.3　CLOSE UP

The Valsalva Maneuver Impedes Blood Flow Return to the Heart

With quiet breathing, intrapulmonic pressure within the airways and alveoli decreases by only about 3 to 5 mm Hg below atmospheric pressure during the inspiratory cycle; exhalation produces a similar pressure increase (**A**). Closing the glottis after a full inspiration and then activating the expiratory muscles causes the compressive forces of exhalation to increase considerably (**B**). Maximal exhalation force against a closed glottis can increase pressure within the thoracic cavity (**intrathoracic pressure**) by more than 150 mm Hg above atmospheric pressure, with somewhat higher pressures within the abdominal cavity. A **Valsalva maneuver** describes this forced exhalation against a closed glottis. This ventilatory maneuver occurs commonly in weight lifting and other activities requiring a rapid, maximum application of force for short duration. The fixation of the abdominal and thoracic cavities with a Valsalva optimizes the force-generating capacity of the chest musculature.

PHYSIOLOGIC CONSEQUENCES

With the onset of a Valsalva maneuver (in straining-type exercises; see figure), blood pressure *briefly increases* abruptly as elevated intrathoracic pressure forces blood from the heart into the arterial system (**C**). Simultaneously, the inferior vena cava compresses because pressure within the thoracic and abdominal cavities exceeds the relatively low pressures within the venous system. This significantly reduces blood flow into the heart (venous return). Reduced venous return and subsequent *large decrease* in arterial blood pressure diminish the brain's blood supply, producing dizziness, "spots before the eyes," and even fainting. Normal blood flow reestablishes (with perhaps even an "overshoot") when the glottis opens and intrathoracic pressure decreases.

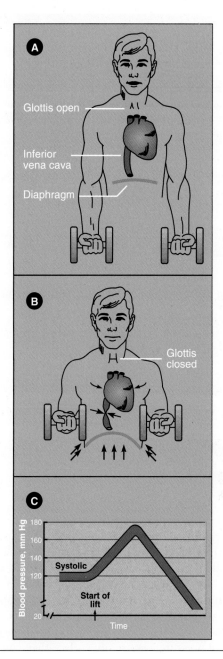

SUMMARY

1. The healthy lung provides a large interface between the body's internal fluid environment and the gaseous external environment. No more than 1 pint of blood flows in the pulmonary capillaries during any 1 second.

2. Pulmonary ventilation adjustments maintain favorable concentrations of alveolar oxygen and carbon dioxide to ensure adequate aeration of lung blood flow.

3. Pulmonary airflow depends on small pressure differences between ambient air and air within the lungs. The action of muscles that alter the dimensions of the thoracic cavity produces these pressure differences.

4. Lung volumes vary with age, gender, body size, and stature; they should be evaluated only relative to norms based on these variables.

5. TV increases during exercise by encroachment on inspiratory and expiratory reserve volumes.

6. When a person breathes to vital capacity, air remains in the lungs at maximal exhalation. This RLV allows for an uninterrupted gas exchange during the breathing cycle.

7. $FEV_{1.0}$ and MVV provide a dynamic assessment of the ability to sustain high airflow levels. They serve as excellent screening tests to detect lung disease.

8. Minute ventilation equals breathing rate times TV. It averages about 6 L at rest. In maximum exercise, increases in the breathing rate and TV produce minute ventilations as high as 200 L in large, endurance-trained individuals.

9. Alveolar ventilation represents the portion of minute ventilation entering the alveoli for gaseous exchange with the blood.

10. Healthy people exhibit their own unique breathing styles during rest and exercise. Conscious attempts to modify the breathing pattern during aerobic exercise confer no physiologic or performance benefits.

11. Disruptions in normal breathing patterns during exercise include dyspnea (shortness of breath), hyperventilation (overbreathing), and the Valsalva maneuver (forcefully trying to exhale against a closed glottis).

THOUGHT QUESTIONS

1. Advise a track athlete trying to change her breathing pattern in the hope of becoming a more economical runner.

2. How might regular resistance and aerobic exercise training blunt the typical decline in lung function with advancing age?

3. After straining to "squeeze out" a maximum lift in the standing press, the person states: "I feel slightly dizzy and see spots before my eyes." Provide a plausible physiologic explanation. What can be done to prevent this from happening?

Part 2	Gas Exchange

Oxygen supply depends on oxygen concentration in ambient air and its pressure. Ambient air composition remains constant: 20.93% oxygen, 79.04% nitrogen (including small quantities of inert gases that behave physiologically like nitrogen), 0.03% carbon dioxide, and usually small quantities of water vapor. The gas molecules move quickly and exert a pressure against any surface they contact. At sea level, the pressure of air's gas molecules raises a column of mercury to an average height of 760 mm (29.9 in). This barometric reading varies somewhat with changing weather conditions and decreases predictably at increased altitude.

RESPIRED GASES: CONCENTRATIONS AND PARTIAL PRESSURES

Gas concentration should not be confused with gas pressure:

- **Gas concentration** reflects the amount of gas in a given volume, which is determined by the product of the gas' partial pressure and solubility.
- **Gas pressure** represents the force exerted by the gas molecules against the surfaces they encounter.

A mixture's total pressure equals the sum of the partial pressures of the individual gases, which computes as follows:

$$\text{Partial pressure} = \text{Percentage concentration} \times \text{Total pressure of gas mixture}$$

Ambient Air

Table 9.2 presents the percentages, partial pressures, and volumes of the specific gases in 1 L of dry, ambient air at sea level. The partial pressure (the letter P before the gas symbol denotes partial pressure) of oxygen equals 20.93% of the total 760 mm Hg pressure exerted by the air mixture, or 159 mm Hg (0.2093×760 mm Hg); the random movement of the minute quantity of carbon dioxide exerts a pressure of only 0.2 mm Hg (0.0003×760 mm Hg), and nitrogen molecules exert a pressure that raises the

Table 9.2	Percentages, Partial Pressures, and Volumes of Gases in 1 L of Dry Ambient Air at Sea Level		
GAS	PERCENTAGE	PARTIAL PRESSURE (at 760 mm Hg)	VOLUME OF GAS (mL·L^{-1})
Oxygen	20.93	159 mm Hg	209.3
Carbon dioxide	0.03	0.2 mm Hg	0.4
Nitrogen	79.04[a]	600 mm Hg	790.3

[a]Includes 0.93% argon and other trace rare gases.

mercury in a manometer about 600 mm Hg (0.7904 × 760 mm Hg). For sea level ambient air:

$$P_{O_2} = 159 \text{ mm Hg}; \quad P_{CO_2} = 0.2 \text{ mm Hg}; \quad \text{and} \quad P_{N_2} = 600 \text{ mm Hg}$$

Tracheal Air

Air entering the nose and mouth passes down the respiratory tract; it completely saturates with water vapor, which slightly dilutes the inspired air mixture. At body temperature, the pressure of water molecules in humidified air equals 47 mm Hg; this leaves 713 mm Hg (760 mm Hg − 47 mm Hg) as the total pressure exerted by the inspired dry air molecules at sea level. This decreases the effective P_{O_2} in tracheal air by about 10 mm Hg from its dry ambient value of 159 mm Hg to 149 mm Hg (0.2093 × [760 mm Hg − 47 mm Hg]). Humidification has little effect on inspired P_{CO_2} because of carbon dioxide's near negligible concentration in inspired air.

Alveolar Air

Alveolar air composition differs considerably from the incoming breath of ambient air because carbon dioxide continually enters the alveoli from the blood and oxygen leaves the lungs for transport throughout the body. Table 9.3 shows that moist alveolar air contains approximately 14.5% oxygen, 5.5% carbon dioxide, and 80.0% nitrogen.

After subtracting water vapor pressure in moist alveolar gas, the average alveolar P_{O_2} equals 103 mm Hg (0.145 × [760 mm Hg − 47 mm Hg]), and P_{CO_2} equals 39 mm Hg (0.055 × [760 mm Hg − 47 mm Hg]). These values represent the average pressures exerted by oxygen and carbon dioxide molecules against the alveolar side of the respiratory membrane. They do not exist as physiologic constants but vary slightly with the phase of the ventilatory cycle and adequacy of ventilation in different lung segments.

Table 9.3	Percentages, Partial Pressures, and Volumes of Gases in 1 L of Moist Alveolar Air at Sea Level (37°C)		
GAS	PERCENTAGE	PARTIAL PRESSURE (at 760 − 47 mm Hg)	VOLUME OF GAS (mL·L^{-1})
Oxygen	14.5	103 mm Hg	145
Carbon dioxide	5.5	39 mm Hg	55
Nitrogen	80.00	571 mm Hg	800
Water vapor		47 mm Hg	

Questions & Notes

List the ambient air percentages for oxygen, carbon dioxide, and nitrogen are:

O_2:

CO_2:

N_2:

Give the formula for computing partial pressure.

What determines gas concentration?

List the P_{O_2} in ambient air at sea level.

List alveolar's air concentration for oxygen and carbon dioxide at rest:

O_2:

CO_2:

MOVEMENT OF GAS IN AIR AND FLUIDS

Knowledge of how gases act in air and fluids allows us to understand the mechanism for gas movement between the external environment and the body's tissues. In accord with **Henry's law**, the amount of a specific gas dissolved in a fluid depends on two factors:

1. Pressure differential between the gas above the fluid and gas dissolved in the fluid
2. Solubility of the gas in the fluid

Pressure Differential

Figure 9.7 shows three examples of gas movement between air and fluid. Oxygen molecules continually strike the water surface in each of the three chambers. Pure water in container A contains no oxygen, so a large number of oxygen molecules dissolve in water. Some oxygen molecules also leave the water because the dissolved molecules move continuously in random motion. In chamber B, the pressure gradient between air and water still favors oxygen's net movement (diffusion) into the fluid from the gaseous state, but the quantity of additional oxygen dissolving in the fluid remains less than in chamber A. Eventually, the pressures for gas movement attain equilibrium, and the number of molecules entering and leaving the fluid equalize (chamber C). Conversely, if pressure of dissolved oxygen molecules exceeds the air's oxygen pressure, oxygen leaves the fluid until it attains a new pressure equilib-

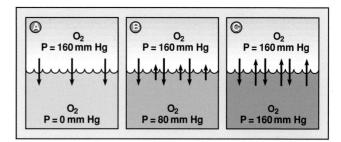

Figure 9.7 Solution of oxygen in water when oxygen first comes in contact with pure water (**A**); dissolved oxygen halfway to equilibrium with gaseous oxygen (**B**); and equilibrium established between the oxygen in air and oxygen dissolved in water (**C**).

rium. These examples illustrate that the net diffusion of a gas occurs only when a *difference* exists in gas pressure. Specific gas' partial pressure gradient represents the driving force for its diffusion. Similarly, concentration gradients provide the driving force for diffusion of nongaseous molecules (e.g., glucose, sodium, and calcium).

Solubility

Gas solubility, or its dissolving power, reflects the quantity of a gas dissolved in fluid at a particular pressure. A gas with greater solubility has a higher concentration at a specific pressure. For two different gases at identical pressure differentials, the solubility of each gas determines the number of molecules moving into or out of a fluid. *For each unit of pressure favoring diffusion, approximately*

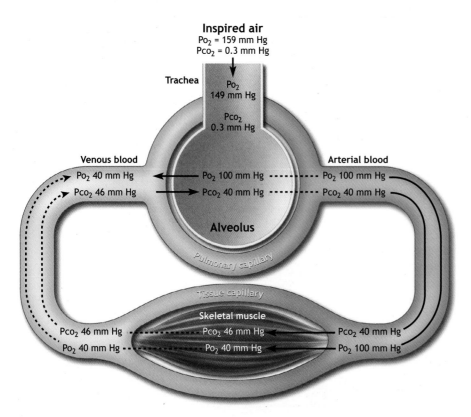

Figure 9.8 Pressure gradients for gas transfer within the body at rest. The P_{O_2} and P_{CO_2} of ambient, tracheal, and alveolar air and these gas pressures in venous and arterial blood and muscle tissue. Gas movement at the alveolar–capillary and tissue–capillary membranes always progresses from an area of higher partial pressure to lower partial pressure.

BOX 9.4 CLOSE UP

Exercise-Induced Asthma

Asthma, a **chronic obstructive pulmonary disease (COPD)**, affects more than 300 million individuals around the world and is the most common chronic disease in children (*http://www.who.int/mediacentre/factsheets/fs307/en/index.html*). Asthma is a public health problem not just for high-income countries; it occurs in all countries regardless of the level of development, although most asthma-related deaths occur in low- and lower middle income countries. Asthma is underdiagnosed and undertreated and often restricts individuals' activities for a lifetime.

A high fitness level does not confer immunity from this ailment. Hyperirritability of the pulmonary airways, usually manifested by coughing, wheezing, and shortness of breath, characterizes an asthmatic condition.

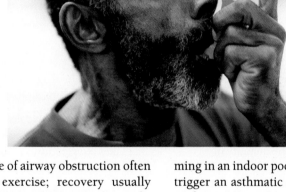

With exercise, catecholamines released from the sympathetic nervous system produce a relaxation effect on smooth muscle that lines the pulmonary airways. Everyone experiences initial bronchodilation with exercise. For people with asthma, however, bronchospasm and excessive mucus secretion occur after normal bronchodilation. An acute episode of airway obstruction often appears 10 minutes after exercise; recovery usually occurs spontaneously within 30 to 90 minutes. One technique for diagnosing EIA uses progressive increments of exercise on a treadmill or bicycle ergometer. During a 10- to 20-minute recovery after each exercise bout, a spirometer evaluates $FEV_{1.0}$ / FVC. A 15% reduction in pre-exercise values confirms the diagnosis of EIA.

SENSITIVITY TO THERMAL GRADIENTS

An attractive theory to explain EIA relates to the rate and magnitude of alterations in pulmonary heat exchange as ventilation increases in exercise. As the incoming breath of air moves down the pulmonary pathways, heat and water transfer from the respiratory tract as air warms and humidifies. This form of "air conditioning" cools and dries the respiratory mucosa; an abrupt airway rewarming occurs during recovery. The thermal gradient from cooling and subsequent rewarming and loss of water from mucosal tissue stimulates the release of proinflammatory chemical mediators that cause bronchospasm.

ENVIRONMENT MAKES A DIFFERENCE

Exercising in a humid environment, regardless of ambient air temperature, diminishes the EIA response. This is perplexing because conventional belief maintains that a dry climate best suits people with asthma. In fact, inhaling ambient air fully saturated with water vapor in exercising patients often abolishes the bronchospastic response. This also explains why people with asthma tolerate walking or jogging on a warm, humid day or swimming in an indoor pool, but outdoor winter sports usually trigger an asthmatic attack. People with asthma should perform 15 to 30 minutes of continuous warm-up because it initiates a "refractory period" that minimizes the severity of a bronchoconstrictive response during subsequent, more intense exercise.

Currently, medications offer considerable relief from bronchoconstriction for individuals who want to exercise on a regular basis without affecting their performance. Exercise training cannot "cure" the asthmatic condition, but it can increase airway reserve and reduce the work of breathing during all modes of physical activity.

---

25 times more carbon dioxide than oxygen moves into or from a fluid.

GAS EXCHANGE IN THE BODY

The exchange of gases between lungs and blood and their movement at the tissue level takes place passively by diffusion. **Figure 9.8** illustrates the pressure gradients favoring gas transfer in the body.

 For Your Information

EVEN FIT ATHLETES CAN HAVE ASTHMA

Champions are not immune from asthma. One of the most famous examples is 1984 Olympic marathon champion Joan Benoit Samuelson, who experienced breathing problems during several races in 1991 that led to the discovery of her asthmatic condition. Despite breathing difficulties during the 1991 New York Marathon she finished with a time of 2 h:33 min:40 s!

Gas Exchange in the Lungs

The first step in oxygen transport involves the transfer of oxygen from the alveoli into the blood. Three factors account for the dilution of oxygen in inspired air as it passes into the alveolar chambers:

1. Water vapor saturates relatively dry inspired air.
2. Oxygen continually leaves alveolar air.
3. Carbon dioxide continually enters alveolar air.

Considering these three factors, alveolar PO_2 averages about 100 mm Hg, a value considerably below the 159 mm Hg in dry ambient air. Despite this reduced PO_2, the pressure of oxygen molecules in alveolar air still averages about 60 mm Hg higher than the PO_2 in venous blood that enters pulmonary capillaries. This allows oxygen to diffuse through the alveolar membrane into the blood. Carbon dioxide exists under slightly greater pressure in returning venous blood than in the alveoli, causing carbon dioxide to diffuse from the blood to the lungs. Although only a small pressure gradient of 6 mm Hg exists for carbon dioxide diffusion compared with oxygen, adequate carbon dioxide transfer occurs rapidly because of carbon dioxide's high solubility. Nitrogen, an inert gas in metabolism, remains unchanged in alveolar–capillary gas.

Gas Exchange in Tissues

In tissues where energy metabolism consumes oxygen at a rate equal to carbon dioxide production, gas pressures differ from arterial blood (see **Fig. 9.8**). At rest, the average PO_2 within the muscle rarely drops below 40 mm Hg; intracellular PCO_2 averages about 46 mm Hg. In contrast, whereas vigorous exercise reduces the pressure of oxygen molecules in active muscle tissue to 3 mm Hg, carbon dioxide pressure approaches 90 mm Hg. *The large pressure differential between gases in plasma and tissues establishes the diffusion gradient—oxygen leaves capillary blood and flows toward metabolizing cells, and carbon dioxide flows from the cell into the blood.* Blood then enters the veins and returns to the heart for delivery to the lungs. Diffusion rapidly begins when venous blood enters the lung's dense capillary network.

S U M M A R Y

1. The partial pressure of a specific gas in a gas mixture varies proportionally to its concentration in the mixture and the total pressure exerted by the mixture.

2. Pressure and solubility determine the quantity of gas that dissolves in a fluid. Because of carbon dioxide's 25 times greater solubility than oxygen in plasma, more carbon dioxide molecules move down relatively small pressure gradients in body fluids.

3. Gas molecules diffuse in the lungs and tissues down their concentration gradients from higher concentration (higher pressure) to lower concentration (lower pressure).

4. Alveolar ventilation adjusts during intense exercise so the composition of alveolar gas remains similar to resting conditions. Alveolar and arterial oxygen pressures equal about 100 mm Hg, and carbon dioxide pressure remains at 40 mm Hg.

5. Compared with alveolar gas, venous blood contains oxygen at lower pressure than carbon dioxide; this makes oxygen diffuse into the blood and carbon dioxide diffuse into the lungs.

6. Diffusion gradients in the tissues favor oxygen movement from the capillaries to the tissues and carbon dioxide movement from the cells to the blood. Exercise expands these gradients, making oxygen and carbon dioxide diffuse rapidly.

7. EIA represents a relatively common obstructive lung disorder associated with the rate and magnitude of airway cooling (and drying) and subsequent rewarming. Breathing humidified air during exercise often eliminates EIA.

T H O U G H T   Q U E S T I O N S

1. Discuss the driving forces for the exchange of respiratory gases in the lungs and active muscles.

2. One technique during "natural" childbirth requires rapid breathing to effectively "work with" the normal ebb and flow of uterine contractions. How can a person accelerate the breathing rate at rest without disrupting normal alveolar ventilation?

Part 3	Oxygen and Carbon Dioxide Transport

OXYGEN TRANSPORT IN THE BLOOD

The blood transports oxygen in two ways:

1. **In physical solution**—dissolved in the fluid portion of the blood
2. **Combined with hemoglobin (Hb)**—in loose combination with the iron–protein Hb molecule in the red blood cell

Oxygen Transport in Physical Solution

Oxygen does not dissolve readily in fluids. At an alveolar P_{O_2} of 100 mm Hg, only about 0.3 mL of gaseous oxygen dissolves in the plasma of each 100 mL of blood (3 mL·L^{-1}). Because the average adult's total blood volume equals about 5 L, 15 mL of oxygen dissolves for transport in the fluid portion of the blood (3 mL·L^{-1} × 5 = 15 mL). This amount of oxygen sustains life for about 4 seconds. Viewed somewhat differently, the body would need to circulate 80 L of blood each minute just to supply the resting oxygen requirements if oxygen were transported only in physical solution.

Despite its limited quantity, oxygen transported in physical solution serves a vital physiologic function. Dissolved oxygen establishes the P_{O_2} of the blood and tissue fluids to help regulate breathing and determines the magnitude that Hb loads with oxygen in the lungs and unloads it in the tissues.

Oxygen Combined with Hemoglobin

The blood of many animal species contains a metallic compound to augment its oxygen-carrying capacity. In humans, the iron-containing protein pigment Hb constitutes the main component of the body's 25 trillion red blood cells. *Hb increases the blood's oxygen-carrying capacity 65 to 70 times above that normally dissolved in plasma.* For each liter of blood, Hb temporarily "captures" about 197 mL of oxygen. Each of the four iron atoms in a Hb molecule loosely binds one molecule of oxygen to form oxyhemoglobin in the reversible **oxygenation reaction:**

$$Hb + 4O_2 \rightarrow Hb_4O_8$$

This reaction requires no enzymes; it progresses without a change in the valance of Fe^{++}, as occurs during the more permanent process of oxidation. *The partial pressure of oxygen in solution solely determines the oxygenation of Hb to oxyhemoglobin.*

Oxygen-Carrying Capacity of Hemoglobin
In men, each 100 mL of blood contains approximately 15 to 16 g of Hb. The value averages 5% to 10% less for women, or about 14 g per 100 mL of blood. The gender difference in Hb concentration contributes to the lower aerobic capacity of women even after adjusting statistically for gender-related differences in body mass and body fat.

Each gram of Hb can combine loosely with 1.34 mL of oxygen. Thus, the oxygen-carrying capacity of the blood from its Hb concentration computes as follows:

Oxygen-carrying capacity = Hb (g·100 mL blood^{-1}) × Oxygen capacity of Hb

If the blood's Hb concentration equals 15 g, then approximately 20 mL of oxygen (15 g per 100 mL × 1.34 mL = 20.1) combine with the Hb in each 100 mL of blood if Hb achieved full oxygen saturation (i.e., if all Hb existed as Hb_4O_8).

Questions & Notes

List 2 ways oxygen transports in blood.

1.

2.

At an alveolar P_{O_2} of 100 mm Hg, the amount of oxygen dissolved in each 100 mL of blood plasma equals _____.

List the amount of hemoglobin in each 100 mL of blood for normal men and women.

Men:

Women:

Complete the following for hemoglobin:

O_2 carrying capacity =

Percentage saturation =

Name the vertical and horizontal axes for the oxyhemoglobin dissociation curve.

The alveolar-capillary oxygen partial pressure equals _____ mm Hg.

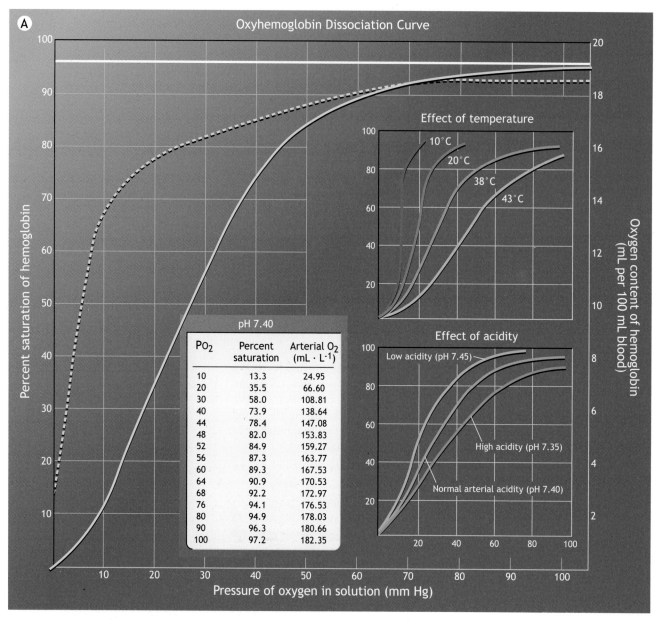

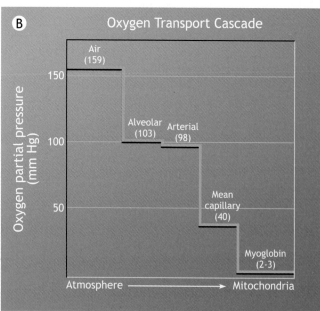

Figure 9.9 Oxyhemoglobin dissociation curve. The *two yellow lines* indicate the percentage saturation of Hb (*solid line*) and myoglobin (*dashed line*) in relation to oxygen pressure. The *right ordinate* shows the quantity of oxygen carried in each deciliter of blood under normal conditions. The *two inset curves* within the figure illustrate the effects of temperature and acidity in altering Hb's affinity for oxygen (Bohr effect). The *light-blue inset box* presents oxyhemoglobin saturation and arterial blood's oxygen-carrying capacity for different P_{O_2} values with Hb concentration of $14 \, g \cdot dL^{-1}$ blood at a pH of 7.40. The *white horizontal line* at the top of the graph indicates percentage saturation of Hb at the average sea-level alveolar P_{O_2} of 100 mm Hg. **B.** Partial pressures as oxygen moves from ambient air at sea level to the mitochondria of maximally active muscle tissue (oxygen transport cascade).

Po$_2$ and Hemoglobin Saturation   The discussion of the blood's oxygen-carrying capacity assumes that Hb achieves full saturation with oxygen when exposed to alveolar gas. **Figure 9.9A** shows the relationship between percentage saturation of Hb (*left vertical axis*) at various Po$_2$s under normal resting physiologic conditions (arterial pH 7.4, 37°C) and the effects of changes in pH and temperature (inset curves) on Hb's affinity for oxygen. The percentage saturation of Hb computes as follows:

$$\text{Percentage saturation} = (\text{Total O}_2 \text{ combined with Hb} \div \text{Oxygen-carrying capacity of Hb}) \times 100$$

This curve, termed the **oxyhemoglobin dissociation curve**, also quantifies the amount of oxygen carried in each 100 mL of blood in relation to plasma Po$_2$ (*right vertical axis*, **Fig. 9.9A**). For example, at a Po$_2$ of 90 mm Hg (95% Hb saturation), the normal complement of Hb in 100 mL of blood carries about 19 mL of oxygen; at a Po$_2$ of 40 mm Hg (75% Hb saturation), the oxygen quantity decreases to about 15 mL, and the oxygen quantity is only slightly more than 2 mL at a Po$_2$ of 10 mm Hg. These values indicate that at relatively low oxygen partial pressures at the capillary–tissue membrane, oxygen readily dissociates (unloads) from Hb for use by the cell. **Figure 9.9B** also shows the partial pressure gradients as oxygen moves from ambient air at sea level into the mitochondria. The "**oxygen transport cascade**" describes the downward steps in oxygen partial pressures from ambient air at sea level to the mitochondria of maximally active muscle, with the progressively lowering of Po$_2$ facilitating the unloading of oxygen.

Po$_2$ in the Lungs

At the alveolar–capillary Po$_2$ of 100 mm Hg, Hb remains 98% saturated with oxygen; under these conditions, the Hb in each 100 mL of blood contains about 19.7 mL of oxygen. An additional increase in alveolar Po$_2$ contributes little to how much oxygen combines with Hb. Each 100 mL of plasma in arterial blood contains about 0.3 mL of oxygen in physical solution. For healthy individuals who breathe ambient air at sea level, 100 mL of arterial blood carries 20.0 mL of oxygen (19.7 mL bound to Hb and 0.3 mL dissolved in plasma).

Careful examination of **Figure 9.9A** shows that the Hb saturation changes little until the oxygen pressure decreases to about 60 mm Hg. This relatively flat upper portion of the oxyhemoglobin dissociation curve provides a margin of safety to ensure near full loading of Hb despite relatively large decreases in alveolar Po$_2$. Alveolar Po$_2$ reduction to 75 mm Hg as occurs in certain lung diseases or when one travels to moderate altitude only decreases arterial Hb saturation by about 6%. In contrast, when Po$_2$ drops below 60 mm Hg, a sharp decrease occurs in how much oxygen combines with Hb.

Tissue Po$_2$

The Po$_2$ in the cell fluids at rest averages 40 mm Hg. Thus, dissolved oxygen in arterial plasma (Po$_2$ = 100 mm Hg) readily diffuses across the capillary membrane through tissue fluids into cells. This reduces plasma Po$_2$ below that in the red blood cells causing Hb to release its oxygen in the reaction HbO$_2 \rightarrow$ Hb + O$_2$. The oxygen then moves from the blood cells through the capillary membrane into the tissues.

At the tissue–capillary Po$_2$ of 40 mm Hg at rest, Hb holds 75% of its total capacity for oxygen (see *solid line* in **Fig. 9.9A**). Thus, each 100 mL of blood leaving the resting tissues carries 15 mL of oxygen; nearly 5 mL has been released to cells for energy metabolism. The **arteriovenous–oxygen difference** (a–v O$_2$ difference) describes this difference in oxygen content between arterial and venous blood (expressed in mL per 100 mL blood).

Questions & Notes

At what Po$_2$ does percentage saturation of hemoglobin begin to dramatically decrease?

Give the average Po$_2$ in most cell fluids under resting conditions.

Give the units of measurement for a-v O$_2$ difference.

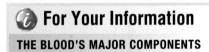

ℹ **For Your Information**

THE BLOOD'S MAJOR COMPONENTS

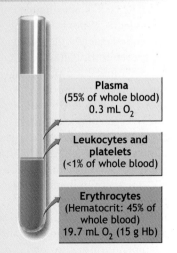

Plasma
(55% of whole blood)
0.3 mL O$_2$

Leukocytes and platelets
(<1% of whole blood)

Erythrocytes
(Hematocrit: 45% of whole blood)
19.7 mL O$_2$ (15 g Hb)

Major components of centrifuged whole blood, including the quantity of oxygen carried in each 100 mL (dL) of blood (Hb, hemoglobin) in healthy, untrained individuals.

The a–v O_2 difference in tissues at rest averages 5 mL · 100 mL^{-1}. The large quantity of oxygen still remaining with Hb provides an "automatic" reserve for cells to immediately obtain oxygen if oxygen demands suddenly increase. As the cells' need for oxygen increases with exercise above rest, tissue P_{O_2} rapidly decreases. This forces Hb to release greater quantities of oxygen to meet metabolic requirements. In vigorous exercise, tissue P_{O_2} decreases to 15 mm Hg, and Hb retains about 5 mL of oxygen. This expands the tissue a–v O_2 difference to 15 mL of oxygen per 100 mL of blood. When active muscles' P_{O_2} decreases to about 3 mm Hg during exhaustive exercise, Hb releases all of its remaining oxygen to active tissues. Even without any increase in local blood flow, the amount of oxygen released to active muscle increases three times above that supplied at rest simply by a more complete unloading of Hb.

Bohr Effect   The inset curves in **Figure 9.9** show that increases in acidity ([H$^+$] and CO_2) and temperature cause the oxyhemoglobin dissociation curve to shift downward and to the right (enhanced unloading), particularly in the P_{O_2} range of 20 to 50 mm Hg. This phenomenon, known as the **Bohr effect** (named after its discoverer, Danish physician and physiologist Christian Bohr [1855–1911]), results from alterations in Hb's molecular structure.

The existence of the Bohr effect becomes particularly important in vigorous exercise because increased metabolic heat and acidity in active tissues augments oxygen release. For example, at a P_{O_2} of 20 mm Hg and normal body temperature (37°C), percentage saturation of Hb with oxygen equals 35%. At the same P_{O_2}, but with body temperature increased to 43°C (a temperature often recorded at the end of a marathon run), Hb's percentage saturation decreases to about 23%. This means that more oxygen unloads from Hb for use in cellular metabolism. Similar effects take place with increased acidity during intense exercise. The lack of a negligible Bohr effect in pulmonary capillary blood at normal alveolar P_{O_2} means that Hb becomes fully loaded with oxygen as blood passes through the lungs, even during maximal exercise.

The compound **2,3-diphosphoglycerate (2,3-DPG)**, the anaerobic metabolite produced in red blood cells during glycolysis, also affects Hb's affinity for oxygen. 2,3-DPG facilitates oxygen dissociation by combining with subunits of Hb to reduce its affinity for oxygen. Individuals with cardiopulmonary disease and high-altitude inhabitants have increased levels of this metabolic intermediate. Elevated 2,3-DPG for these individuals represents a compensatory adjustment that facilitates oxygen release to the cells. In general, adaptations in 2,3-DPG occur relatively slowly compared with the immediate Bohr effect from increased tissue temperature, acidity, and carbon dioxide.

Myoglobin and Muscle Oxygen Storage

Skeletal and cardiac muscle contain the iron–protein compound **myoglobin**. Myoglobin, similar to Hb, combines reversibly with oxygen; however, each myoglobin molecule contains only 1 iron atom in contrast to Hb, which contains 4 atoms. Myoglobin adds additional oxygen to the muscle in the following reaction:

$$MbO_2 \rightarrow MbO_2$$

Myoglobin facilitates oxygen transfer to the mitochondria, notably at the start of exercise and during intense exercise when cellular P_{O_2} decreases considerably. **Figure 9.9A** reveals that the dissociation curve for myoglobin (*dashed yellow line*) forms a rectangular hyperbola, not the S-shaped curve for Hb. This makes myoglobin bind and retain oxygen at low pressures much more readily than Hb. During rest and moderate exercise when cellular P_{O_2} remains relatively high, myoglobin remains highly saturated with oxygen. At a P_{O_2} of 40 mm Hg, for example, myoglobin retains 85% of its oxygen. MbO_2 releases its greatest quantity of oxygen when tissue P_{O_2} decreases to less than 10 mm Hg. Unlike Hb, myoglobin does not exhibit a Bohr effect.

CARBON DIOXIDE TRANSPORT IN BLOOD

Once carbon dioxide forms in cells, diffusion and transport to the lungs in venous blood provides its only means for "escape." **Figure 9.10** illustrates that blood transports carbon dioxide to the lungs in three ways:

1. Physical solution in plasma (7%–10%)
2. Loose combination with Hb (20%)
3. Combined with water as bicarbonate (70%)

Carbon Dioxide in Solution

Plasma transports 7% to 10% of carbon dioxide produced in energy metabolism as free carbon dioxide in physical solution (**Fig. 9.10A**). The random movement of this relatively small quantity of dissolved carbon dioxide molecules establishes the P_{CO_2} of the blood.

Carbon Dioxide as Carbamino Compounds

About 20% of carbon dioxide reacts directly with the amino acid molecules of blood proteins to form carbamino compounds (**Fig. 9.10B**). The globin portion of Hb carries a significant amount of carbon dioxide in the blood as follows:

$$\underset{\text{Hemoglobin}}{CO_2 + HbNH} \rightarrow \underset{\text{Carbaminohemoglobin}}{HbNHCOOH}$$

Formation of carbamino compounds reverses in the lungs as plasma P_{CO_2} decreases. This moves carbon dioxide into solution for diffusion into the alveoli. Concurrently, Hb's oxygenation reduces its capacity to bind carbon dioxide. The interaction between oxygen loading and carbon dioxide release, termed the **Haldane effect**, facilitates carbon dioxide removal from the lungs.

A CO₂ dissolved in plasma

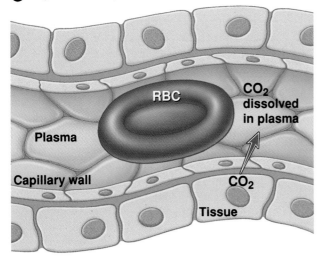

B CO₂ chemically bound to hemoglobin

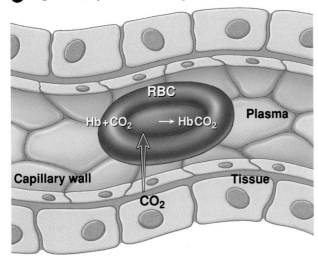

C CO₂ combined with water as bicarbonate

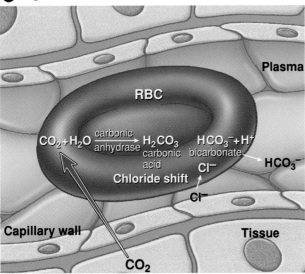

Figure 9.10 Carbon dioxide transport in blood. **A.** Physically dissolved in blood plasma. **B.** Chemically bound to hemoglobin (Hb). **C.** Combined with water as bicarbonate.

Questions & Notes

Briefly describe the Bohr effect.

What is the % saturation of Hb at a Po₂ of 20 mm Hg at normal body temperature?

What is the function of 2,3-DPG?

ⓘ **For Your Information**

EXERCISE TRAINING AND MYOGLOBIN

As might be expected, slow-twitch muscle fibers with high capacity to generate ATP aerobically contain relatively large quantities of myoglobin. Among animals, a muscle's myoglobin content relates to their level of physical activity. The leg muscles of hunting dogs, for example, contain more myoglobin than the muscles of sedentary house pets; similar findings exist for grazing cattle compared with penned animals.

Carbon Dioxide as Bicarbonate

The major portion (70%) of carbon dioxide in solution combines with water to form carbonic acid (**Fig. 9.10C**).

$$CO_2 + H_2O \leftrightarrow H_2CO_3^-$$

Because of the slow rate of this reaction, little carbon dioxide transports in this form without **carbonic anhydrase**, a zinc-containing enzyme within red blood cells. This catalyst accelerates interaction of carbon dioxide and water about 5000 times.

In the Tissues

When carbonic acid forms in the tissues, most of it ionizes to hydrogen ions (H^+) and bicarbonate ions (HCO_3^-) as follows:

$$CO_2 + H_2O \xrightarrow{\text{Carbonic anhydrase}} H_2CO_3 \rightarrow H^+ + HCO_3^-$$

The protein portion of the Hb molecule then buffers H^+ to maintain blood pH within narrow limits. Because of bicarbonate's high solubility, it diffuses from red blood cells into plasma in exchange for a chloride ion (Cl^-), which then moves into the blood cell to maintain ionic equilibrium. The term **chloride shift** describes this exchange of Cl^- for HCO^-; it accounts for the higher Cl^- content of erythrocytes in venous blood compared with arterial blood.

In the Lungs

As tissue P_{CO_2} increases, carbonic acid forms rapidly. Conversely, in the lungs, carbon dioxide diffuses from plasma into the alveoli; this lowers plasma P_{CO_2} and disturbs the equilibrium between carbonic acid and the formation of bicarbonate ions. The H^+ and HCO_3^- recombine to form carbonic acid. In turn, carbon dioxide and water reform, allowing carbon dioxide to exit through the lungs as follows:

$$H^+ + HCO_3^- \rightarrow H_2CO_3 \xrightarrow{\text{Carbonic anhydrase}} CO_2 + H_2O$$

Plasma bicarbonate concentration decreases in the pulmonary capillaries, permitting the Cl^- to move from the red blood cell back into plasma.

SUMMARY

1. Hb, the iron–protein pigment in red blood cells, increases the oxygen-carrying capacity of whole blood about 65 times compared with the amount dissolved in physical solution in plasma.

2. The small quantity of oxygen dissolved in plasma exerts molecular movement and establishes the blood's P_{O_2}. Plasma P_{O_2} determines the loading of Hb at the lungs (oxygenation) and its unloading at the tissues (deoxygenation).

3. The blood's oxygen transport capacity changes only slightly with normal variations in Hb content.

4. Gender differences in Hb concentration contribute to the lower aerobic capacity of women even after adjusting for gender-related differences in body mass and body fat.

5. The S-shaped nature of the oxyhemoglobin dissociation curve dictates that Hb-oxygen saturation changes little until P_{O_2} decreases below 60 mm Hg. Oxygen releases rapidly from capillary blood and flows into the cells to meet metabolic demands.

6. About 25% of the blood's total oxygen releases to the tissues at rest; the remaining 75% returns "unused" to the heart in the venous blood.

7. Increases in acidity, temperature, and carbon dioxide concentration alter Hb's molecular structure, reducing its effectiveness to hold oxygen (Bohr effect). Because exercise accentuates these factors, oxygen release to tissues becomes further facilitated.

8. Myoglobin stores "extra" oxygen in skeletal and cardiac muscle. Myoglobin releases its oxygen only at a low P_{O_2}, thus facilitating oxygen transfer to the mitochondria during strenuous exercise.

9. About 7% of carbon dioxide dissolves as free carbon dioxide in plasma to establish the blood's P_{CO_2}.

10. About 20% of the body's carbon dioxide combines with blood proteins (including Hb) to form carbamino compounds.

11. Approximately 70% of carbon dioxide combines with water to form bicarbonate. This reaction reverses in the lungs to allow carbon dioxide to leave the blood and diffuse into the alveoli.

THOUGHT QUESTIONS

1. Discuss whether it would be advantageous for runners to breathe 100% oxygen immediately before running a marathon to "load-up" on oxygen.

2. Why do minute amounts of impurities such as CO_2 and CO in a breathing mixture exert profound physiologic effects?

| Part 4 | Regulation of Pulmonary Ventilation |

VENTILATORY CONTROL DURING REST

The body regulates the rate and depth of breathing exquisitely in response to metabolic needs. During all exercise intensities in healthy individuals, arterial pressures for oxygen, carbon dioxide, and pH remain essentially at resting values. Neural information from higher centers in the brain, from the lungs, and from mechanical and chemical sensors throughout the body regulates pulmonary ventilation. The gaseous and chemical state of the blood that bathes the brain (medulla) and the aortic and carotid chemoreceptors also affect alveolar ventilation. **Figure 9.11** presents the primary factors in ventilatory control.

Neural Factors

*The normal respiratory cycle comes from inherent, automatic activity of inspiratory neurons whose cell bodies reside in the **medial medulla** of the brain.* The lungs inflate because neurons activate the diaphragm and intercostal muscles. The inspiratory neurons cease firing from their own self-limitation and from inhibitory influence from the medulla's expiratory neurons. Inflation of lung tissue stimulates stretch receptors in the bronchioles that inhibit inspiration and stimulate expiration.

Exhalation begins by the passive recoil of the stretched lung tissue and raised ribs when the inspiratory muscles relax. Activation of expiratory neurons and associated muscles that further facilitate expiration synchronizes with this passive phase. As expiration proceeds, the inspiratory center is released again from inhibition and progressively becomes more active.

Humoral Factors

The chemical state of the blood largely regulates pulmonary ventilation at rest. Variations in arterial P_{O_2}, P_{CO_2}, acidity, and temperature activate sensitive

Name 2 neurogenic factors that regulate pulmonary ventilation.

1.

2.

Complete the following:

$Hb + CO_2 \rightarrow$

$CO_2 + H_2O \rightarrow$

$H^+ + HCO_3^- \rightarrow$

Name 2 humoral factors that regulate pulmonary ventilation.

1.

2.

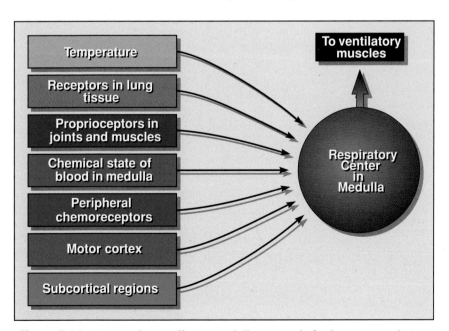

Figure 9.11 Primary factors affecting medullary control of pulmonary ventilation.

neural units in the medulla and arterial system to adjust ventilation to maintain arterial blood chemistry within narrow limits.

Plasma Po₂ and Chemoreceptors

Plasma Po₂ and Chemoreceptors   Inhaling a gas mixture of 80% oxygen increases alveolar Po_2 and reduces minute ventilation by about 20%. Conversely, reducing the inspired oxygen concentration increases minute ventilation, particularly if alveolar Po_2 decreases below 60 mm Hg. Recall that at 60 mm Hg, Hb's oxygen saturation dramatically decreases. The point at which decreasing arterial Po_2 stimulates ventilation has been termed the **hypoxic threshold**; it usually occurs at an arterial Po_2 between 60 and 70 mm Hg.

Sensitivity to reduced arterial oxygen pressure (arterial hypoxia) results from stimulation of small structures located outside the central nervous system called **chemoreceptors**. **Figure 9.12** shows these specialized neurons located in the arch of the aorta (**aortic bodies**) and at the branching of the carotid arteries in the neck (**carotid bodies**). The carotid bodies, which are about 5 mm in diameter, maintain a strategic position to monitor arterial blood status just before it perfuses brain tissues. Nerves from carotid and aortic bodies activate the brain's respiratory neurons.

Peripheral chemoreceptors provide an "early warning system" to alert against reduced oxygen pressure. These structures also stimulate ventilation in response to increased carbon dioxide, temperature, and acidity; a decrease in blood pressure; and perhaps a decline in circulating potassium.

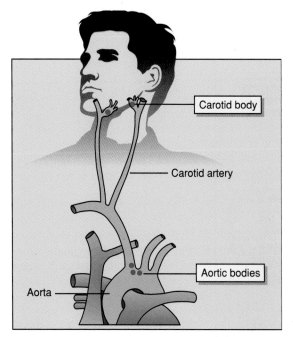

Figure 9.12   Aortic and carotid cell bodies (sensitive to a reduced plasma Po_2) located in the aortic arch and bifurcation of carotid arteries. These peripheral receptors defend against arterial hypoxia.

Plasma Pco₂ and H⁺ Concentration

Plasma Pco₂ and H⁺ Concentration   *Carbon dioxide pressure in arterial plasma provides the most important respiratory stimulus at rest.* Small increases in the Pco_2 of inspired air stimulate the medulla and peripheral chemoreceptors to initiate large increases in minute ventilation. For example, resting ventilation almost doubles when inspired Pco_2 increases to just 1.7 mm Hg (0.22% CO_2 in inspired air).

Molecular carbon dioxide does not entirely account for its effect on ventilatory control. Recall that carbonic acid formed from the union of carbon dioxide and water rapidly dissociates to bicarbonate ions and hydrogen ions. The increase in $[H^+]$, which varies directly with the blood's CO_2 content in the cerebrospinal fluid bathing the respiratory areas, stimulates inspiratory activity. The resulting increase in ventilation eliminates carbon dioxide, which lowers arterial $[H^+]$.

Hyperventilation and Breath-Holding

If a person breath-holds after a normal exhalation it takes about 40 seconds before breathing commences. This urge to breathe results mainly from the stimulating effects of increased arterial Pco_2 and $[H^+]$, not from a decreased arterial Po_2. *The "break point" for breath-holding generally corresponds to an increase in arterial Pco_2 to about 50 mm Hg.*

If this same person consciously increased alveolar ventilation above the normal level before breath-holding, the composition of alveolar air becomes more similar to ambient air. Alveolar Pco_2 with hyperventilation may decrease to 15 mm Hg, creating a considerable diffusion gradient for carbon dioxide run-off from venous blood that enters the pulmonary capillaries. Consequently, a larger than normal amount of carbon dioxide leaves the blood, decreasing arterial Pco_2 below normal levels. Reduced arterial Pco_2 extends the breath-hold until the arterial Pco_2, $[H^+]$, or both increase to a level that stimulates ventilation.

Swimmers and sport divers hyperventilate and breath-hold to improve their physical performance. In sprint swimming, it is biomechanically undesirable to roll the body and turn the head during the stroke's breathing phase. These swimmers hyperventilate on the starting blocks to prolong their breath-hold time during the swim. Snorkel divers hyperventilate to extend breath-hold time, but often with tragic results. As the length and depth of the dive increase, the oxygen content of the blood can decrease to critically low values before arterial Pco_2 increases to stimulate breathing and signal the need to ascend to the surface. Reduced arterial Po_2 can cause a loss of consciousness before the diver reaches the surface.

VENTILATORY CONTROL DURING EXERCISE

Chemical Factors

Chemical stimuli cannot fully explain the increased ventilation (**hyperpnea**) during physical activity. For example,

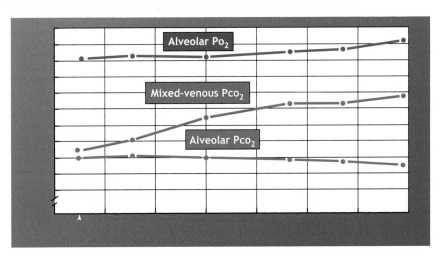

Figure 9.13 Values for P_{CO_2} in mixed-venous blood entering the lungs, and alveolar P_{O_2} and P_{CO_2} related to oxygen uptake during graded exercise. Despite increased metabolism with exercise, alveolar P_{O_2} and P_{CO_2} remain near resting levels. Increases in mixed-venous P_{CO_2} result from increased carbon dioxide production in metabolism. (Data from the Laboratory of Applied Physiology, Queens College.)

manipulating arterial P_{O_2}, P_{CO_2}, and acidity does not increase minute ventilation nearly as much as vigorous exercise.

Arterial P_{O_2} in exercise does not decrease to the point that it stimulates ventilation by chemoreceptor activation. In fact, large breathing volumes in vigorous exercise actually increase alveolar (and arterial) P_{O_2} above the average resting value of 100 mm Hg. **Figure 9.13** illustrates the dynamics of venous and alveolar P_{CO_2} and alveolar P_{O_2} related to oxygen uptake in men during a graded exercise test. During light and moderate exercise ($\dot{V}O_2$ = <2000 mL·min^{-1}), pulmonary ventilation closely couples to oxygen uptake and carbon dioxide production in a manner that maintains alveolar P_{O_2} at about 100 mm Hg and P_{CO_2} at 40 mm Hg. Increases in acidity and subsequent increases in CO_2 and $[H^+]$ during strenuous exercise provide an additional ventilatory stimulus that reduces alveolar P_{CO_2} to below 40 mm Hg and sometimes to as low as 25 mm Hg. This eliminates carbon dioxide and decreases arterial P_{CO_2}. Concurrently, augmented ventilation slightly increases alveolar P_{O_2} to facilitate oxygen loading.

Nonchemical Factors

Ventilation increases so rapidly when exercise begins that it occurs almost within the first ventilatory cycle. A plateau lasting about 20 seconds follows this abrupt increase in ventilation; thereafter, minute ventilation gradually increases and approaches a steady level in relation to the demands for metabolic gas exchange. When exercise stops, ventilation decreases rapidly to a point about 40% of the final exercise value and then slowly returns to resting levels. The rapidity of the ventilatory response at the onset and cessation of exercise shows that input other than from changes in arterial P_{CO_2} and $[H^+]$ mediate these components of exercise and recovery hyperpnea.

Neurogenic Factors

Cortical and peripheral factors regulate pulmonary ventilation in exercise.

- **Cortical influence:** Neural outflow from regions of the motor cortex during exercise and cortical activation in anticipation of exercise stimulate respiratory neurons in the medulla. Cortical outflow acting in concert with the demands of exercise abruptly increases ventilation when exercise begins.

$\mathcal{Q}$uestions & Notes

What P_{O_2} corresponds to the break point for breath-holding?

Why do some swimmers hyperventilate on the starting blocks?

Arterial P_{O_2} in exercise _____ to stimulate ventilation by chemoreceptor activation.

List the 2 factors that regulate pulmonary ventilation during exercise.

1.

2.

Briefly explain what happens during breadth holding.

 For Your Information

LESS BREATHING DURING SWIMMING

Lower ventilatory equivalents from restrictive breathing occur at all levels of energy expenditure during prone swimming. Depressed ventilation may hinder gas exchange during maximal swimming and contribute to the lower $\dot{V}O_{2max}$ with swimming compared with running.

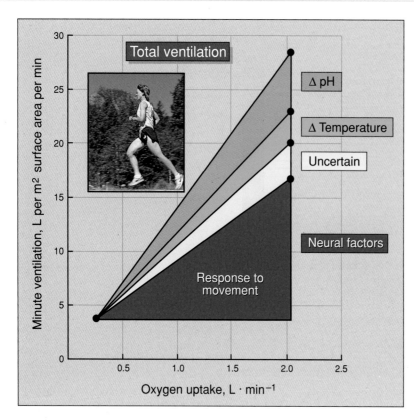

Figure 9.14 Generalized illustration of the composite of factors that influence pulmonary ventilation in exercise. The different colors estimate the contribution of changes in acidity (pH), temperature, and the effects of neurogenic stimuli from cerebral regions or joints and muscles. The *yellow-shaded wedge* represents ventilatory change not quantitatively accounted for by the other three factors. (From Lambertson, C.J.: Interactions of physical, chemical, and nervous factors in respiratory control. In: *Medical Physiology*. Mountcastle, V.B. (ed.), St. Louis: C.V. Mosby Co., 1974.)

- **Peripheral influence:** Sensory input from joints, tendons, and muscles adjusts ventilation during exercise. The specific peripheral receptors remain unknown, but experiments involving passive limb movements, electrical muscle stimulation, and voluntary exercise with the muscle's blood flow occluded support the existence of **mechanoreceptors** in peripheral tissues that produce reflex hyperpnea.

Influence of Temperature   An increase in body temperature directly excites neurons of the respiratory center and likely helps regulate ventilation in prolonged exercise. The rapidity of ventilatory changes at the onset and end of exercise, however, cannot be explained by the relatively *slow* changes in core temperature.

Integrated Regulation   *No single factor controls breathing during exercise; rather, it depends on the combined* *and perhaps simultaneous effects of several chemical and neural stimuli* (**Fig. 9.14**). The current model suggests the following scenario for ventilatory control during exercise:

1. Neurogenic stimuli from the cerebral cortex (**central command**) and active limbs cause the initial, abrupt increase in breathing when exercise begins (**phase I ventilation**).
2. After a short (about 20 s) plateau, minute ventilation gradually increases to a steady level that adequately meets the demands for metabolic gas exchange (**phase II ventilation**). Central command input plus factors intrinsic to medullary control system neurons and peripheral stimuli from chemoreceptors and mechanoreceptors contribute to the control of this phase of ventilation.
3. The final phase of control (**phase III ventilation**) involves "fine tuning" of ventilation through peripheral sensory feedback mechanism (e.g., temperature, CO_2, and $[H^+]$).

SUMMARY

1. Inherent activity of neurons in the medulla controls the normal respiratory cycle. Neural circuits that relay information from higher brain centers, the lungs themselves, and other sensors throughout the body modulate medullary activity.

2. Arterial P_{CO_2} and acidity $[H^+]$ act directly on the respiratory center or modify its activity reflexly through chemoreceptors to control alveolar ventilation at rest.

3. Peripheral chemoreceptor activation stimulates breathing when arterial P_{O_2} decreases during high-altitude ascent or in severe pulmonary disease.

4. Hyperventilation lowers arterial P_{CO_2} and $[H^+]$ to prolong breath-hold time until carbon dioxide and acidity increase to levels that stimulate breathing.

5. Extended breath-hold by hyperventilation should not be practiced during underwater swimming because it could produce deadly consequences.

6. Nonchemical regulatory factors augment ventilatory adjustments to exercise. These include cortical activation in anticipation of exercise and outflow from the motor cortex when exercise begins; peripheral sensory input from mechanoreceptors in joints and muscles; and elevation in body temperature.

7. Neural and chemical factors that operate either singularly or in combination effectively regulate exercise alveolar ventilation. Each factor adjusts a particular phase of the ventilatory response to exercise.

THOUGHT QUESTION

Outline the mechanism by which hyperventilation extends breath-hold duration. Why is hyperventilation ill-advised in breath-hold diving?

| Part 5 | Pulmonary Ventilation During Exercise |

PULMONARY VENTILATION AND ENERGY DEMANDS

Physical activity increases oxygen uptake and carbon dioxide production more than any other physiologic stress. Large amounts of oxygen diffuse from the alveoli into the blood returning to the lungs during exercise. Conversely, considerable carbon dioxide moves from the blood into the alveoli. Concurrently, increases in pulmonary ventilation maintain stable alveolar gas concentrations, so oxygen and carbon dioxide exchange proceeds unimpeded. **Figure 9.15** illustrates the relationship between minute ventilation and oxygen uptake through the range of steady-rate and non–steady-rate exercise levels up to $\dot{V}O_{2max}$.

Ventilation in Steady-Rate Exercise

During light and moderate exercise ($\dot{V}O_2 < 2.5$ L·min^{-1} in this example), pulmonary ventilation increases linearly with oxygen uptake; ventilation mainly increases by increases in TV.

The **ventilatory equivalent for oxygen** ($\dot{V}_E / \dot{V}O_2$) represents the ratio of minute ventilation to oxygen uptake. This index indicates breathing economy because it reflects the quantity of air breathed per amount of oxygen consumed. Healthy young adults usually maintain $\dot{V}_E / \dot{V}O_2$ at about 25 (i.e., 25 L air breathed per L oxygen consumed) during submaximal exercise up to about 55% of $\dot{V}O_{2max}$. Higher ventilatory equivalents occur in children, averaging about 32 in 6-year-old children. Despite individual differences in the ventilatory equivalent for oxygen of healthy children and adults during steady-rate exercise, complete aeration of blood takes place because of two factors:

1. Alveolar P_{O_2} and P_{CO_2} remain at near-resting values
2. Transit time for blood flowing through the pulmonary capillaries proceeds slowly enough to permit complete gas exchange

Questions & Notes

Briefly discuss the difference between phase I and phase II ventilation.

Define and briefly explain the importance of the $\dot{V}E/\dot{V}O_2$.

1.

2.

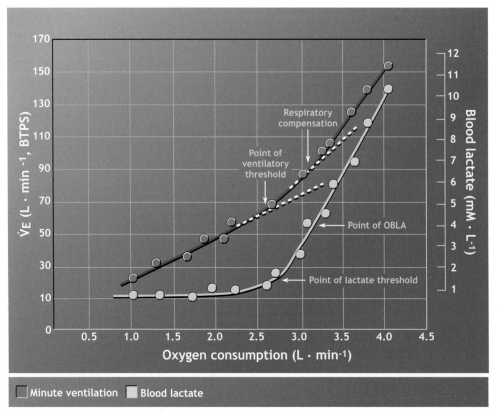

Figure 9.15 Pulmonary ventilation, blood lactate concentration, and oxygen consumption during graded exercise to maximum. The *lower dashed white line* extrapolates the linear relationship between $\dot{V}_E$ and $\dot{V}O_2$ during submaximal exercise. The lactate threshold (not necessarily the threshold for anaerobic metabolism) represents the highest exercise intensity (oxygen consumption) not associated with elevated blood lactate concentration. It occurs at the point at which the relationship between $\dot{V}_E$ and $\dot{V}O_2$ deviates from linearity, indicated as the point of ventilatory threshold. The onset of blood lactate accumulation (OBLA) represents the point of lactate increase just above a 4.0-mM baseline. Respiratory compensation represents a further disproportionate increase in ventilation (indicated by deviation from *the upper dashed white line*) to counter the decrease in plasma pH in intense exercise.

During steady-rate exercise, the **ventilatory equivalent for carbon dioxide** ($\dot{V}_E$ / $\dot{V}CO_2$) also remains relatively constant because pulmonary ventilation eliminates the carbon dioxide produced during cellular respiration.

Ventilation in Non–Steady-Rate Exercise

Ventilatory Threshold Note in **Figure 9.15** that as exercise oxygen uptake increases, minute ventilation eventually increases disproportionately to the increase in oxygen uptake. This increases the ventilatory equivalent above the steady-rate exercise value; it may reach as high as 35 or 40 in maximal exercise. The point at which pulmonary ventilation increases disproportionately with oxygen uptake during graded exercise has been termed **ventilatory threshold** (V_T). At this exercise intensity, pulmonary ventilation no longer links tightly to oxygen demand at the cellular level. Rather, the "excess" ventilation relates directly to carbon dioxide's increased output from the buffering of lactate that begins to accumulate from anaerobic metabolism.

Recall that sodium bicarbonate in the blood buffers the lactate generated during anaerobic metabolism in the following reaction:

$$\text{Lactate} + \text{NaHCO}_3 \rightarrow \text{Na lactate} + \text{H}_2\text{CO}_3 \rightarrow \text{H}_2\text{O} + \text{CO}_2$$

Excess, non-metabolic carbon dioxide liberated in this buffering reaction stimulates pulmonary ventilation that disproportionately increases $\dot{V}_E$ / $\dot{V}O_2$. The respiratory exchange ratio ($\dot{V}CO_2$ / $\dot{V}O_2$) exceeds 1.00 when additional carbon dioxide is exhaled because of acid buffering.

The term **anaerobic threshold** originally defined the abrupt increase in ventilatory equivalent caused by nonmetabolic carbon dioxide production from lactate buffering. Some researchers believed this point signaled the body's shift to anaerobic metabolism (lactate formation). The researchers proposed the anaerobic threshold as a noninvasive ventilatory measure of the onset of anaerobiosis. Subsequent research showed that the ratios of $\dot{V}_E$ / $\dot{V}O_2$ or $\dot{V}CO_2$ / $\dot{V}O_2$ did not necessarily link in a *causal* manner with lactate production (or accumulation) in exercise. Even if the association between ventilatory dynamics and cellular metabolic events remains noncausal, useful information can be obtained about exercise performance by applying these indirect procedures. **Figure 9.16** outlines possible underlying factors that relate to anaerobic threshold detected from pulmonary gas exchange dynamics during graded exercise.

Onset of Blood Lactate Accumulation Steady-rate exercise indicates that oxygen supply and utilization

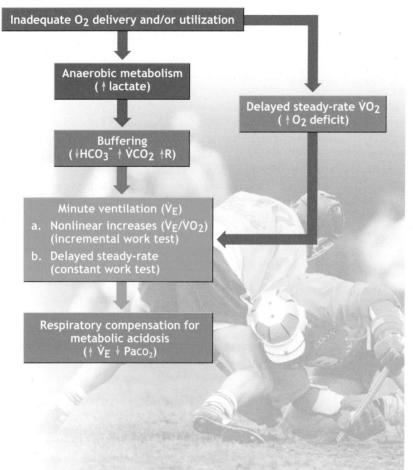

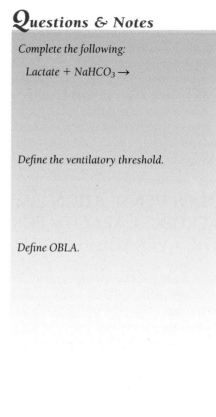

Complete the following:

Lactate + $NaHCO_3 \rightarrow$

Define the ventilatory threshold.

Define OBLA.

Figure 9.16 Factors that relate to pulmonary gas exchange dynamics for detecting the lactate threshold.

satisfy the energy requirements of muscular effort. When this occurs, lactate production does *not* exceed its removal, and blood lactate does not accumulate. **Figure 9.15** showed that exercise intensity or oxygen uptake where blood lactate begins to increase above a baseline level of about 4 mM·L^{-1} indicates the point of **onset of blood lactate accumulation (OBLA)**. OBLA normally occurs between 55% and 65% of $\dot{V}O_{2max}$ in healthy, untrained subjects and often equals more than 80% $\dot{V}O_{2max}$ in highly trained endurance athletes.

Causes of OBLA   The exact cause of the OBLA remains controversial. Many believe it represents the point of muscle hypoxia (inadequate oxygen) and therefore anaerobiosis. Muscle lactate accumulation does not necessarily coincide with hypoxia because lactate forms even in the presence of adequate muscle oxygenation. The OBLA does imply an imbalance between the rate of blood lactate appearance and disappearance. The imbalance may not result from muscle hypoxia; rather, it may result from decreased lactate clearance in total or increased lactate production only in specific muscle fibers. Practitioners should cautiously interpret the specific metabolic significance of the OBLA and its possible relationship to tissue hypoxia.

OBLA and Endurance Performance   The point of OBLA often increases with aerobic training without an accompanying increase in $\dot{V}O_{2max}$. This suggests that separate factors influence OBLA and $\dot{V}O_{2max}$. Traditionally, exercise physiologists have applied $\dot{V}O_{2max}$ as the main yardstick to gauge capacity

ⓘ For Your Information

AN ADDED STIMULUS TO BREATHING

Lactate produced during intense exercise places an added demand on pulmonary ventilation, causing "over-breathing." This results from the buffering of lactate to the weaker carbonic acid. In the lungs, carbonic acid splits into its water and carbon dioxide components; this "non-metabolic" carbon dioxide provides an added stimulus to pulmonary ventilation.

for endurance exercise. This measure generally relates to long-duration exercise performance but does not fully explain all aspects of success. Experienced distance athletes generally compete at an exercise intensity slightly above the point of OBLA. Exercise intensity at the OBLA has emerged as a consistent and powerful predictor of aerobic exercise performance. *Changes in endurance performance with training often relate more closely to training-induced changes in the exercise level for OBLA than to changes in $\dot{V}O_{2max}$.*

DOES VENTILATION LIMIT AEROBIC CAPACITY FOR THE AVERAGE PERSON?

With inadequate breathing capacity, the line relating pulmonary ventilation and oxygen uptake in **Figure 9.15** would not curve upward (increase in ventilatory equivalent) during heavy exercise; instead, it would level off or slope downward to the right to reflect a decrease in ventilatory equivalent. Such a response would indicate a *failure* for ventilation to keep pace with increasing oxygen demands; in this case, a person truly would "run out of wind." Actually, healthy individuals tend to overbreathe in relation to oxygen uptake with increasing exercise intensity. **Figure 9.13** demonstrates that the ventilatory adjustment to strenuous exercise decreases alveolar P_{CO_2} concomitant with small increases in alveolar P_{O_2}. Arterial P_{O_2} and Hb oxygen saturation remain at near-resting values during intense exercise for most individuals. This means that pulmonary function does not represent the "weak link" in the oxygen transport system of healthy individuals with average to moderately high aerobic capacities.

Work of Breathing

Two major factors determine the energy requirements of breathing:

1. Compliance of the lungs and thorax
2. Resistance of the airways to the smooth flow of air

Lung and thorax **compliance** refers to how "easily" these tissues stretch. The radius of the bronchi primarily establishes resistance to airflow. More specifically, airflow resistance varies inversely with a vessel's radius raised to the fourth power in accordance with Poiseuille's law. Reducing airway radius by half causes airway resistance to increase 16 times. Normally, bronchi and bronchiole dimensions do not impede smooth air flow, so breathing requires relatively little energy. In some lung diseases, airways constrict or lung tissues themselves lose compliance; this imposes considerable resistance to airflow. Trying to breathe through a drinking straw gives some indication of breathing difficulties with severe obstructive lung disease.

A healthy person rarely senses the breathing effort, even during moderate exercise. In contrast, respiratory disease often makes the work of breathing during exercise an exhausting physical task. For patients with **chronic obstructive pulmonary disease** (COPD; e.g., asthma, emphysema), breathing effort at rest can reach three times that of healthy individuals. In severe pulmonary disease, breathing's energy requirement may easily reach 40% of the total exercise oxygen uptake. This obviously encroaches on the oxygen available to the active, nonrespiratory muscles and seriously limits the exercise capacity of these patients.

Figure 9.17 shows the relationship in healthy subjects between pulmonary ventilation and oxygen uptake during rest and submaximal exercise and its division into respiratory and nonrespiratory components. At rest and in light exercise, the relatively small oxygen requirement of breathing averages between 1.9 and 3.1 mL of oxygen per liter of air breathed, or about 4% of the total energy expenditure. As the rate and depth of breathing increase during exercise, the energy cost of breathing increases to about 4 mL of oxygen per liter of ventilation. It can increase to 9 mL of oxygen in maximal exercise when pulmonary ventilation exceeds 100 L·min^{-1}. *At these exercise intensities, the oxygen cost of breathing represents between 10% and 20% of the total oxygen uptake.*

Exercise and Cigarette Smoking

Since the initial 1964 release of the *Surgeon General's Report on Smoking and Health*, numerous review articles have concluded that a **causal** link exists between smoking and lung cancer; chronic bronchitis and emphysema;

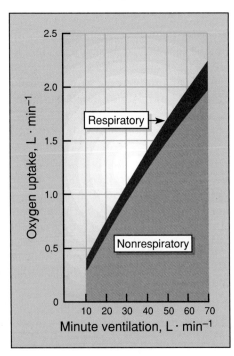

Figure 9.17 Relationship between oxygen uptake and pulonary ventilation and the respiratory and nonrespiratory oxygen cost components during submaximal exercise in healthy individuals.

cardiovascular disease; and cancers of the lip, larynx, esophagus, and urinary bladder. Unfortunately, little research relates cigarette smoking habits to exercise performance. Most endurance participants avoid cigarettes for fear of hindering performance from what they consider "loss of wind." Chronic cigarette smokers exhibit decreases in dynamic lung function, which in severe cases, manifests as obstructive lung disorders. Such pathologic processes usually take years to develop. Teenage and young adult smokers rarely exhibit chronic lung function deterioration of a magnitude to significantly impair their exercise performance. Unfortunately, young, fit smokers often believe they are immune from smoking's crippling effects.

Other more acute effects of cigarette smoking adversely affect exercise capacity. For example, airway resistance at rest can increase threefold in chronic smokers and nonsmokers after 15 puffs on a cigarette during a 5-minute period. Added resistance to breathing lasts an average of 35 minutes, with only minor negative effects in light exercise during which the oxygen cost of breathing remains small. In vigorous exercise, however, the residual effect of smoking on airway resistance proves detrimental because the additional cost of breathing becomes physiologically significant. In one study of habitual cigarette smokers who exercised at 80% of $\dot{V}O_{2max}$, the energy requirement of breathing averaged 14% of the exercise oxygen uptake after smoking but averaged only 9% in the "nonsmoking" trials. Also, exercise heart rates averaged 5% to 7% lower after 1 day of smoking abstinence; all subjects reported that they felt better exercising in the nonsmoking condition. Almost complete reversibility of the increased oxygen cost of breathing with smoking can occur in chronic smokers with only 1 day of abstinence. *Thus, athletes who cannot conquer the smoking habit should at least stop 24 hours before competition.*

BUFFERING

Whereas **acids** dissociate in solution and release H^+, **bases** accept H^+ to form hydroxide ions (OH^-). The term **buffering** designates reactions that minimize changes in H^+ concentration; **buffers** refer to chemical and physiologic mechanisms that prevent this change.

The symbol **pH** designates a quantitative measure of acidity or alkalinity (basicity) of a liquid solution. Specifically, pH refers to the concentration of protons or H^+. Acid solutions have more H^+ than OH^- at a pH below 7.0 and vice versa for basic solutions whose pH exceeds 7.0. Chemically pure (distilled) water, considered neutral, has equal H^+ and OH^- and thus a pH of 7.0.

The pH of bodily fluids ranges from a low of 1.0 for the digestive acid hydrochloric acid to a slightly basic pH between 7.35 and 7.45 for arterial and venous blood and most other bodily fluids. The acid–base characteristics of bodily fluids fluctuate within narrow limits because metabolism remains highly sensitive to H^+ concentrations in the reacting medium. Three mechanisms regulate the pH of the internal environment:

1. Chemical buffers
2. Pulmonary ventilation
3. Renal function

Chemical Buffers

The chemical buffering system consists of a weak acid and salt of that acid. Bicarbonate buffer, for example, consists of the weak acid **carbonic acid** and its salt, **sodium bicarbonate.** Carbonic acid forms when bicarbonate binds H^+. When H^+ concentration remains elevated, the reaction produces the weak acid because excess H^+ ions bind in accord with the general reaction:

$$H^+ + Buffer \rightarrow H\text{-}Buffer$$

Questions & Notes

Discuss the importance of OBLA to endurance performance success.

For Your Information

STITCH IN THE SIDE

During intense exercise, individuals frequently experience a severe, sharp pain in the lower, lateral aspects of the chest wall. This pain, called a "stitch in the side," has no universally accepted explanation nor has it been possible to duplicate its occurrence in the laboratory. It usually occurs during adjustment to new metabolic demands and occurs most frequently in untrained individuals, it seems reasonable to speculate insufficient blood flow (ischemia) to either the diaphragm or intercostal muscles as the cause.

For Your Information

CIGARETTE SMOKE CONSTRICTS AIRWAYS

The increase in peripheral airway resistance and subsequent increased oxygen cost of breathing with cigarette smoking results mainly from a vagal reflex possibly triggered from sensory stimulation by minute particles in smoke and partially from nicotine's stimulation of parasympathetic nerves.

In contrast, when H^+ concentration decreases the buffering reaction moves in the opposite direction and releases H^+ as follows:

$$H^+ + Buffer \leftarrow H\text{-}Buffer$$

During hyperventilation, plasma carbonic acid declines because carbon dioxide leaves the blood and exits through the lungs.

Most of the carbon dioxide generated in energy metabolism reacts with water to form the relatively weak carbonic acid that dissociates into H^+ and HCO_3^-. Likewise, the stronger lactic acid reacts with sodium bicarbonate to form sodium lactate and carbonic acid; in turn, carbonic acid dissociates and increases H^+ concentration of the extracellular fluids. Other organic acids such as fatty acids dissociate and liberate H^+, as do sulfuric and phosphoric acids generated during protein catabolism. Bicarbonate, phosphate, and protein chemical buffers provide the rapid first line of defense to maintain consistency in the acid–base character of the internal environment.

Bicarbonate Buffer

The bicarbonate buffer system consists of carbonic acid and sodium bicarbonate in solution. During buffering, hydrochloric acid (a strong acid) converts to the much weaker carbonic acid by combining with sodium bicarbonate in the following reaction:

$$HCl + NaHCO_3 \rightarrow NaCl + H_2CO_3 \leftrightarrow H^+ + HCO_3^-$$

The buffering of hydrochloric acid produces only a slight reduction in pH. Sodium bicarbonate in plasma exerts a strong buffering action on lactic acid to form sodium lactate and carbonic acid. Any additional increase in H^+ concentration from carbonic acid dissociation causes the dissociation reaction to move in the opposite direction to release carbon dioxide into solution.

Result of Acidosis

$$H_2O + CO_2 \leftarrow H_2CO_3 \leftarrow H^+ + HCO_3^-$$

An increase in plasma carbon dioxide or H^+ concentration immediately stimulates ventilation to eliminate "excess" carbon dioxide.

Conversely, a decrease in plasma H^+ concentration inhibits the ventilatory drive and retains carbon dioxide that then combines with water to increase acidity (carbonic acid) and normalize pH.

Result of Alkalosis

$$H_2O + CO_2 \rightarrow H_2CO_3 \rightarrow H^+ + HCO_3^-$$

Phosphate Buffer

The phosphate buffering system consists of phosphoric acid and sodium phosphate. These chemicals act similarly to the bicarbonate buffers. Phosphate buffer exerts an important effect on acid–base balance in the kidney tubules and intracellular fluids where phosphate concentration remains high.

Protein Buffer

Venous blood buffers the H^+ released from the dissociation of relatively weak carbonic acid produced from $H_2O + CO_2$. *By far, Hb provides the most important H^+ acceptor for this buffering function.* Hb is almost six times more potent in regulating acidity than the other plasma proteins. Hb's release of oxygen to the cells makes Hb a weaker acid, thereby increasing its affinity to bind H^+. The H^+ generated when carbonic acid forms in the erythrocyte combines readily with deoxygenated Hb (Hb^-) in the reaction:

$$H^+ + Hb^- \text{ (Protein)} \rightarrow HHb$$

Intracellular tissue proteins also regulate plasma pH. Some amino acids possess free acidic radicals. When dissociated, they form OH^-, which readily reacts with H^+ to form water.

Physiologic Buffers

The pulmonary and renal systems present the second line of defense in acid–base regulation. Their buffering function occurs only when a change in pH has already occurred.

Ventilatory Buffer

When the quantity of free H^+ in extracellular fluid and plasma increases, it directly stimulates the respiratory center to immediately increase alveolar ventilation. This rapid adjustment reduces alveolar P_{CO_2} and causes carbon dioxide to be "blown off" from the blood. Reduced plasma carbon dioxide levels accelerate the recombination of H^+ and HCO_3^-, lowering free H^+ concentration in plasma. For example, doubling alveolar ventilation by hyperventilation at rest increases blood alkalinity and pH by 0.23 units from 7.40 to 7.63. Conversely, reducing normal alveolar ventilation (hypoventilation) by half increases blood acidity by approximately 0.23 pH units. The potential magnitude of ventilatory buffering equals twice the combined effect of all the body's chemical buffers.

Renal Buffer

Chemical buffers only temporarily affect excess acid buildup. Excretion of H^+ by the kidneys, although relatively slow, provides an important longer term defense that maintains the body's buffer reserve known as **alkaline reserve**. To this end, the kidneys stand as final guardians to preserve normal function. The renal tubules regulate acidity through complex chemical reactions that secrete ammonia and H^+ into the urine and then reabsorb alkali, chloride, and bicarbonate.

Effects of Intense Exercise

Increased H^+ concentration from carbon dioxide production and lactate formation during strenuous exercise makes pH regulation progressively more difficult. Acid–base regulation becomes exceedingly difficult during repeated, brief bouts of all-out exercise that elevate blood lactate values to 30 mM (270 mg of lactate per dL of blood) or higher.

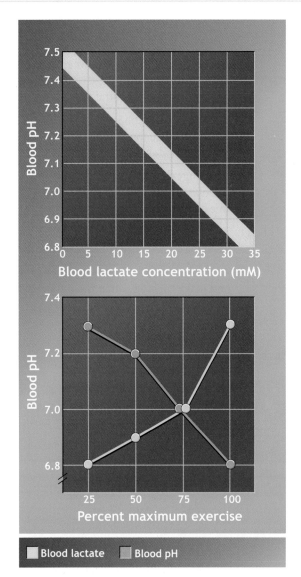

Figure 9.18 *Top.* General relationship between blood pH and blood lactate concentration during rest and increasing intensities of short-duration exercise up to maximum. *Bottom.* Blood pH and blood lactate concentration related to exercise intensity expressed as a percentage of the maximum. Decreases in blood pH accompany increases in blood lactate concentration.

Questions & Notes

Complete the following:

$H^+ + Buffer \leftarrow$

$H^+ + Hb^- \; (protein) \rightarrow$

Identify the 2 substances of the bicarbonate buffer system.

1.

2.

Describe the immediate effects of an increase in plasma CO_2 or H^+ concentration.

Identify the 2 substances of the phosphate buffering system.

1.

2.

Figure 9.18 illustrates the inverse linear relationship between blood lactate concentration and blood pH. Blood lactate concentration varied between a pH of 7.43 at rest and 6.80 during exhaustive exercise. This response indicates that humans *temporarily* tolerate pronounced disturbances in acid–base balance during maximal exercise, at least to an overall blood pH as low as 6.80. A plasma pH below 7.00 does not occur without consequences; this level of acidosis produces nausea, headache, and dizziness in addition to discomfort and pain that ranges from mild to severe within active muscles.

SUMMARY

1. Pulmonary ventilation increases linearly with oxygen uptake during light and moderate exercise. The ventilatory equivalent at these exercise intensities averages 20 to 25 L of air breathed per liter of oxygen consumed.

2. In non–steady-rate exercise, pulmonary ventilation increases disproportionately with increases in oxygen uptake, and the ventilatory equivalent may reach 35 or 40.

3. The eventual sharp upswing in pulmonary ventilation related to oxygen uptake during incremental exercise indicates the point of OBLA.

4. OBLA effectively predicts endurance performance and can be measured without significant metabolic acidosis or cardiovascular strain.

5. Breathing normally requires a relatively small oxygen cost even during exercise. In respiratory disease, the work of breathing becomes excessive, and exercise alveolar ventilation often becomes inadequate.

6. Pulmonary ventilation does not limit optimal alveolar gas exchange in healthy individuals who perform maximal exercise.

7. Airway resistance increases significantly after cigarette smoking. The added oxygen cost of breathing can impair high-intensity, aerobic exercise performance.

Reversibility of these effects occurs with 1 day of cigarette smoking abstinence.

8. Buffers consist of a weak acid and the salt of that acid. Their action during acidosis converts a strong acid to a weaker acid and a neutral salt.

9. The bicarbonate, phosphate, and protein chemical buffers provide the rapid first line of defense to maintain acid–base regulation.

10. The lungs contribute to pH regulation. Changes in alveolar ventilation rapidly alter free H^+ concentration in extracellular fluids.

11. The renal tubules act as the body's final defense by secreting H^+ into the urine and reabsorbing bicarbonate.

12. Anaerobic exercise increases the demand for buffering and makes pH regulation progressively more difficult.

THOUGHT QUESTIONS

1. How would the relationship change between $\dot{V}_E/\dot{V}O_2$ under the following conditions: (1) an aging person who remains sedentary versus an aging person who performs regular aerobic exercises; (2) during the transition from adolescence to young adulthood; and (3) a person training for American football?

2. Present two arguments to justify that pulmonary ventilation does not limit aerobic exercise performance for most healthy people.

3. In what ways are the terms *lactate threshold* and *OBLA* biochemically more precise than the term *anaerobic threshold*?

SELECTED REFERENCES

Abu-Hasan, M., et al.: Exercise-induced dyspnea in children and adolescents: if not asthma then what? *Ann. Allergy Asthma Immunol.*, 94:366, 2005.

Ainslie, P.N., Duffin, J.: Integration of cerebrovascular CO_2 reactivity and chemoreflex control of breathing: mechanisms of regulation, measurement, and interpretation. *Am. J. Physiol. Regul. Integr. Comp. Physiol.*, 265: R1473, 2009.

Amann, M., et al.: An evaluation of the predictive validity and reliability of ventilatory threshold. *Med. Sci. Sports Exerc.*, 36:1716, 2004.

BABB, T.G., et. al., short- and long-term modulation of Exercise Ventilatory Response. *Med. Sci. Sports Exerc.*, 42:1691, 2010.

Bassett, D.R. Jr., Howley, E.T.: Limiting factors for maximum oxygen uptake and determinants of endurance performance. *Med. Sci. Sports Exerc.*, 32:270, 2000.

Bernaards, C.M., et al.: A longitudinal study in smoking in relationship top fitness and heart rate response. *Med. Sci. Sports Exerc.*, 35:793, 2003.

Boulet, L.P., et al.: Lower airway inflammatory responses to high-intensity training in athletes. *Clin. Invest. Med.*, 28:15, 2005.

Buchheit, M., et al.: Improving acceleration and repeated sprint ability in well-trained adolescent handball players: speed

versus sprint interval training. *Int. J. Sports Physiol. Perform.*, 5:152, 2010.

Cannon, D.T., et al.: On the determination of ventilatory threshold and respiratory compensation point via respiratory frequency. *Int. J. Sports Med.*, 30:157, 2009.

Chmura, J., Naza, K.: Parallel changes in the onset of blood lactate accumulation (OBLA) and threshold of psychomotor performance deterioration during incremental exercise after training in athletes. *Int. J. Psychophysiol.*, 75:287, 2010.

Chung, Y., et al.: Control of respiration and bioenergetics during muscle contraction. *Am. J. Physiol. Cell. Physiol.*, 288:C730, 2005.

Dantas De Luca, R., et al.: The lactate minimum test protocol provides valid measures of cycle ergometer $\dot{V}O_{2peak}$. *J. Sports Med. Phys. Fitness*, 4:279, 2003.

Dekerle, J., et al.: Maximal lactate steady state, respiratory compensation threshold and critical power. *Eur. J. Appl. Physiol.*, 89:281, 2003.

Del Coso, J., et al.: Respiratory compensation and blood pH regulation during variable intensity exercise in trained and untrained subjects. *Eur. J. Appl. Physiol.*, 107:83, 2009.

Dempsey, J.A.: Crossing the apnoeic threshold: causes and consequences. *Exp. Physiol.*, 90:13, 2005.

Dempsey, J.A.: Challenges for future research in exercise physiology as applied to the respiratory system. *Exerc. Sport Sci. Rev.*, 34:92, 2006.

Dempsey, J.A., et al.: Respiratory system determinants of peripheral fatigue and endurance performance. *Med. Sci. Sports Exerc.*, 40:457, 2008.

DePalo, V.A., et al.: Respiratory muscle strength training with nonrespiratory maneuvers. *J. Appl. Physiol.*, 96:731, 2004.

Faude, O., et al.: Lactate threshold concepts: how valid are they? *Sports Med.*, 39:469, 2009.

Fontana, P., et al.: Time to exhaustion at maximal lactate steady state is similar for cycling and running in moderately trained subjects. *Eur. J. Appl. Physiol.*, 107:187, 2009.

Gross, M.A., et al.: Seasonal variation of $\dot{V}O_2$ max and the $\dot{V}O_2$-work rate relationship in elite Alpine skiers. *Med. Sci. Sports Exerc.*, 41:2084. 2009.

Harms, C.A., Rosenkranz, S: Sex differences in pulmonary function during exercise. *Med. Sci. Sports Exerc.*, 40:664, 2008.

Hashizume, K., et al.: Effects of abstinence from cigarette smoking on the cardiorespiratory capacity. *Med. Sci. Sports Exerc.*, 32:386, 2000.

Haykowsky, J., et al.: Resistance exercise, the Valsalva maneuver, and cerebrovascular transmural pressure. *Med. Sci. Sports Exerc.*, 35:65, 2003.

Haverkamp, H.C., Dempsey, J.A.: On the normal variability of gas exchange efficiency during exercise: does sex matter? *J. Physiol.*, 557:345, 2004.

Hinton, P.S., et al.: Iron supplementation improves endurance after training in iron-depleted women. *J. Appl. Physiol.*, 88:1103, 2000.

Hopkins, S.R., Harms, C.A.: Gender and pulmonary gas exchange during exercise. *Exerc. Sport Sci. Rev.*, 32:50, 2004.

Kowalchuk, J.M., et al.: The effect of resistive breathing on leg muscle oxygenation using near-infrared spectroscopy during exercise in men. *Exp. Physiol.*, 87:601, 2002.

Laplaud, D., Menier, R.: Reproducibility of the instant of equality of pulmonary gas exchange and its physiological significance. *J. Sports Med. Phys. Fitness*, 43:437, 2003.

Lomax, M.: Inspiratory muscle training, altitude, and arterial oxygen desaturation: a preliminary investigation. *Aviat. Space Environ. Med.*, 81:498, 2010.

Lucas, S.R., Platts-Mills, T.A.: Physical activity and exercise in asthma: relevance to etiology and treatment. *J. Allergy Clin. Immunol.*, 115:928, 2005.

Mahler, D.A., et al.: Responsiveness of continuous ratings of dyspnea during exercise in patients with COPD. *Med. Sci. Sports Exerc.*, 37:529, 2005.

Miller, J.D., et al.: Skeletal muscle pump versus respiratory muscle pump: modulation of venous return from the locomotor limb in humans. *J. Physiol.*, 563:925, 2005.

Morris, D.M., Shafer, R.S.: Comparison of power outputs during time trialing and power outputs eliciting metabolic variables in cycle ergometry. *Int. J. Sport Nutr. Exerc. Metab.*, 20:115, 2010.

Nybo, L., Rasmussen, O.: Inadequate cerebral oxygen delivery and central fatigue during strenuous exercise. *Exer. Sport Sci. Rev.*, 35:110, 2007.

Ozcelik, O., Kelestimur, H.: Effects of acute hypoxia on the determination of anaerobic threshold using the heart rate-work rate relationships during incremental exercise tests. *Physiol. Res.*, 53:45, 2004.

Prabhakar, N.R., Peng, Y-J.: Peripheral chemoreceptors in health and disease. *J. Appl. Physiol.*, 96:359, 2004.

Puente-Maestu, L., et al.: Effects of training on the tolerance to high-intensity exercise in patients with severe COPD. *Respiration*, 70:367, 2003.

Randolph, C.: The challenge of asthma in adolescent athletes: exercise induced bronchoconstriction (EIB) with and without known asthma. *Adolesc. Med. State Art Rev.*, 21:44, viii. 2010. Review.

Richardson, R.S., et al.: Skeletal muscle intracellular PO_2 assessed by myoglobin desaturation: response to graded exercise. *J. Appl. Physiol.*, 91:2679, 2001.

Ricquier, D.: Respiration uncoupling and metabolism in the control of energy expenditure. *Proc. Nutr. Soc.*, 64:47, 2005.

Scherer, T.A., et al.: Respiratory muscle endurance training in chronic obstructive pulmonary disease. Impact on exercise capacity, dyspnea, and quality of life. *Am. J. Respir. Crit. Care Med.*, 162:1709, 2000.

Schumann, A.Y., et al.: Aging effects on cardiac and respiratory dynamics in healthy subjects across sleep stages. *Sleep*, 33:943, 2010.

Smith, C.A., et al.: Ventilatory responsiveness to CO_2 above & below eupnea: relative importance of peripheral chemoreception. *Adv. Exp. Med. Biol.*, 551:65, 2004.

Steiner, J.L., et al.: Effect of carbohydrate supplementation on the RPE-blood lactate relationship. *Med. Sci. Sports Exerc.*, 41:1326, 2009.

Strickland, M.K., Lovering, A.T.: Exercise-induced intrapulmonary arteriovenous shunting and pulmonary gas exchange. *Exerc. Sport Sci. Rev.*, 34:99, 2006.

Svedahl, K., MacIntosh, B.R.: Anaerobic threshold: the concept and methods of measurement. *Can. J. Appl. Physiol.*, 28:299, 2003.

Torchio, R., et al.: Mechanical effects of obesity on airway responsiveness in otherwise healthy humans. *J. Appl. Physiol.*, 107:408, 2009.

van der Vlist, J., Janssen, T.W.: The potential anti-inflammatory effect of exercise in chronic obstructive pulmonary disease. *Respiration*, 79:160, 2010.

Van Schuylenbergh, R., et al.: Correlations between lactate and ventilatory thresholds and the maximal lactate steady state in elite cyclists. *Int. J. Sports Med.*, 25:403, 2004.

Wagner, P.D.: Why doesn't exercise grow the lungs when other factors do? *Exerc. Sport Sci. Rev.*, 33:3, 2005.

Wasserman, K., et al.: *Principles of Exercise Testing and Interpretation*. 3rd Ed. Baltimore: Lippincott Williams & Wilkins, 1999.

West, J.B.: Vulnerability of pulmonary capillaries during exercise. *Exer. Sport Sci. Rev.*, 32:24, 2004.

Zuo, Y.Y., Possmayer, F.: How does pulmonary surfactant reduce surface tension to very low values? *J. Appl. Physiol.*, 102:1733, 2007.

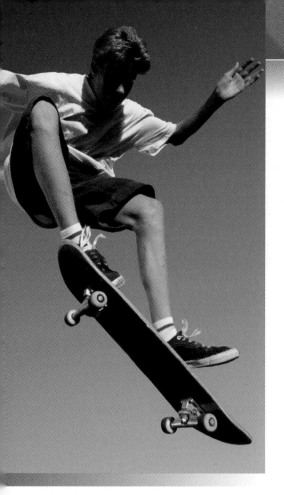

Chapter

10

The Cardiovascular System and Exercise

CHAPTER OBJECTIVES

- List important functions of the cardiovascular system.

- Describe how to use the auscultatory method to measure blood pressure and give average values for systolic and diastolic blood pressure during rest and moderate aerobic exercise.

- Describe the blood pressure response during resistance exercise, upper-body exercise, and exercise in the inverted position.

- State the potential benefits of aerobic exercise for treating moderate hypertension.

- Identify intrinsic and extrinsic factors that regulate heart rate during rest and exercise.

- Identify neural and local metabolic factors that regulate blood flow during rest and exercise.

- Compare average values of cardiac output during rest and maximal exercise for an endurance-trained athlete and a sedentary person.

- Explain three physiologic mechanisms that affect the heart's stroke volume.

- Describe the relationship between maximal cardiac output and maximal oxygen uptake among individuals with varied aerobic fitness levels.

- List the Mayo Clinic's seven benefits of regular physical activity.

The Greek physician Galen theorized that blood flowed like ocean tides, surging and abating into arteries, away from the heart and back again. In Galen's view, fluid carried with it "humors," good and evil that determined well-being. If a person became ill, the standard practice required "blood-letting"—to drain off the diseased humors and restore health. This theory prevailed until the seventeenth century when physician William Harvey (see Chapter 1) proposed a different theroy of blood flow. Experimenting with frogs, cats, and dogs, Harvey demonstrated the existence of heart valves that provided for a one-way flow of blood through the body, a finding incompatible with Galen's "ebb-and-flow" view. In a set of ingenious experiments, Harvey measured the volume of the heart's chambers and counted the number of times the heart contracted in 1 hour. He concluded that if the heart emptied only one-half of its volume with each beat, the body's total blood volume would be pumped in minutes. This finding led Harvey to hypothesize that blood moved (*circulated*) within a closed system in a circular, unidirectional pattern throughout the body. Harvey, of course, was correct; the heart pumps the entire 5-L blood volume in 1 minute. Harvey's experiments changed medical science forever, yet it would take nearly 200 more years for his theories to play important roles in physiology and medicine.

From Harvey's early experiments to sophisticated research at the dawn of the twenty-first century, we know that the highly efficient ventilatory system described in Chapter 9 complements a rapid blood ransport and delivery system composed of blood, the heart, and more than 60,000 miles of blood vessels that integrate the body as a unit. The circulatory system serves five important functions during physical activity:

1. Delivers oxygen to active tissues
2. Aerates blood returned to the lungs
3. Transports heat, a byproduct of cellular metabolism, from the body's core to the skin
4. Delivers fuel nutrients to active tissues
5. Transports hormones, the body's chemical messengers

Part 1   The Cardiovascular System

COMPONENTS OF THE CARDIOVASCULAR SYSTEM

The cardiovascular system consists of an interconnected, continuous vascular circuit containing a pump (heart), a high-pressure distribution system (arteries), exchange vessels (capillaries), and a low-pressure collection and return system (veins). **Figure 10.1** presents a schematic view of the cardiovascular system.

Heart

The heart provides the force to propel blood throughout the vascular circuit. This four-chambered organ, a fist-sized pump, beats at rest an average of 70 b·min^{-1}, 100,800 times a day, and 36.8 million times a year. Even for a healthy person of average fitness, maximum output of blood from this remarkable organ exceeds fluid output from a household faucet turned wide open.

The heart muscle (**myocardium**) consists of striated muscle similar to skeletal muscle. Unlike skeletal muscle, individual fibers interconnect in latticework fashion. As a result, stimulation (depolarization) of one myocardial cell spreads an action potential throughout the myocardium, causing the heart to function as a unit. **Figure 10.2** details the heart as a pump. Functionally, the heart consists of two separate pumps.

The hollow chambers of the *right heart pump* perform two crucial functions:

1. Receive deoxygenated blood returning from all parts of the body
2. Pump blood to the lungs for aeration via the **pulmonary circulation**

The chambers of *left heart pump* also perform two crucial functions:

1. Receive oxygenated blood from the lungs
2. Pump blood into the thick-walled, muscular aorta for distribution throughout the body via the **systemic circulation**

A thick, solid muscular wall (septum) separates the left and right sides of the heart. The **atrioventricular (AV) valves** situated within the heart direct the one-way flow of blood from the right atrium to the right ventricle (**tricuspid valve**) and from the left atrium to the left ventricle (**mitral valve** or **bicuspid valve**). The **semilunar valves** located in the arterial wall just outside the heart prevent blood from flowing back (regurgitation) into the heart between ventricular contractions.

The relatively thin-walled, saclike atrial chambers receive and store blood returning from the lungs and body during ventricular contraction. About 70% of the blood returning to the atria flows directly into the ventricles before the atria contract. Simultaneous contraction of both atria forces the remaining blood into the respective ventricles directly below. Almost immediately after atrial contraction, the ventricles contract and force blood into the arterial systems. To learn more, visit this excellent website that deals with important aspects of heart function: *www.pbs.org/wgbh/nova/eheart/human.html*.

Arteries

The arteries are the high-pressure tubing that conducts oxygen-rich blood to the tissues. **Figure 10.3** shows the arteries composed of layers of connective tissue and smooth muscle. Because of their thickness, no gaseous exchange takes place between arterial blood and surrounding tissues.

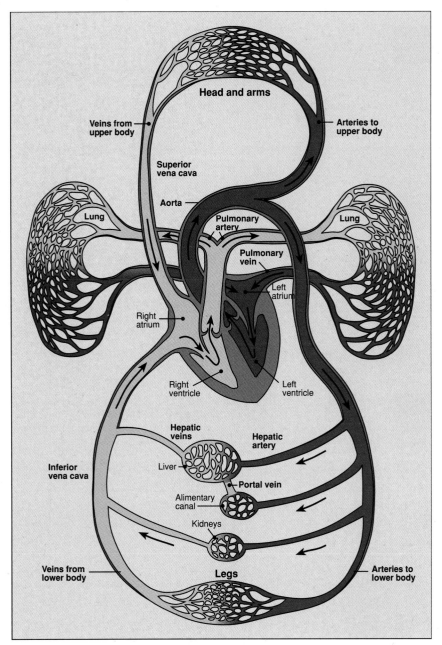

Figure 10.1 Schematic view of the cardiovascular system consisting of the heart and the pulmonary and systemic vascular circuits. The *darker red shading* shows oxygen-rich arterial blood; deoxygenated venous blood appears somewhat paler. In the pulmonary circuit, the situation reverses, and oxygenated blood returns to the heart via the right and left pulmonary veins.

Blood pumped from the left ventricle into the highly muscular yet elastic aorta circulates throughout the body via a network of arteries and **arterioles** (smaller arterial branches). *The arteriole walls contain circular layers of smooth muscle that either constrict or relax to regulate peripheral blood flow.* The redistribution function of arterioles becomes important during exercise because blood diverts to active muscles from areas that can temporarily compromise their blood supply.

Capillaries

The arterioles continue to branch and form smaller and less muscular vessels called *metarterioles*. These tiny vessels merge into **capillaries** (see bottom of **Fig. 10.3**), a network of microscopic blood vessels so thin they provide only

$\mathcal{Q}$*uestions & Notes*

List the 4 major components of the cardio-vascular system.

1.

2.

3.

4.

The myocardium consists of what type of muscle?

List 2 functions of the left and right sides of the heart.

Left heart

1.

2.

Right heart

1.

2.

Describe the main function of arteries and arterioles.

The capillaries contain approximately _____ percent of the total blood volume.

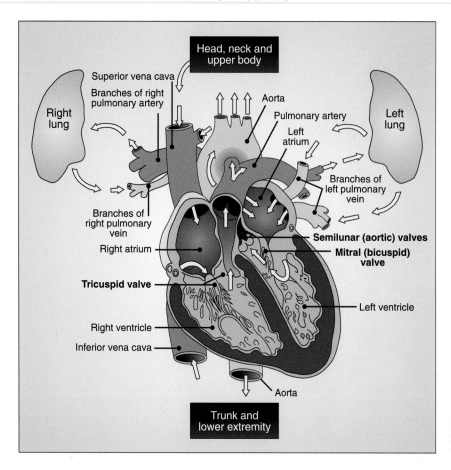

Figure 10.2 The heart's valves provide for the one-way flow of blood indicated by the *yellow arrows*.

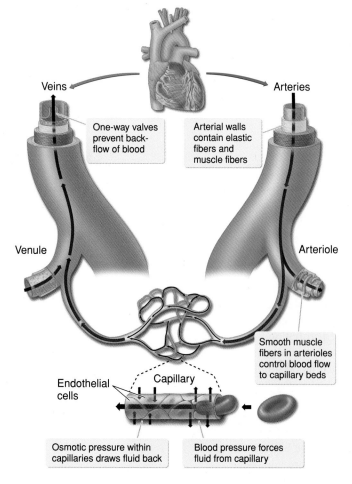

Figure 10.3 The structure of the walls of the various blood vessels. A single layer of endothelial cells lines each vessel. Fibrous tissue, wrapped in several layers of smooth muscle, surrounds the arterial walls. A single layer of muscle cells sheaths the arterioles; capillaries consist of only one layer of endothelial cells. In the venule, fibrous tissue encases the endothelial cells; veins also possess a layer of smooth muscle. A vessel's resistance to flow depends on its diameter. Decreasing vessel diameter by one-half increases resistance 16-fold.

enough room for blood cells to squeeze through in single file. Capillaries contain about 5% of the body's total blood volume at any time. Gases, nutrients, and waste products rapidly transfer across the thin, porous capillary walls. A ring of smooth muscle called the **precapillary sphincter** encircles the capillary at its origin to control the vessel's internal diameter. This sphincter provides a local means for regulating capillary blood flow within a specific tissue to meet metabolic requirements that change rapidly and dramatically in exercise.

Capillary branching increases the total cross-sectional area of the microcirculation 800 times more than the 1-inch diameter aorta. Blood flow velocity relates inversely to the vasculature's total cross section, making velocity progressively decrease as blood moves toward and into the capillaries.

Veins

The vascular system maintains continuity of blood flow as capillaries feed deoxygenated blood at almost a trickle into the small veins or **venules** (**Fig. 10.3**). Blood flow then increases slightly because the venous system's cross-sectional area becomes less than for capillaries. The lower body's smaller veins eventually empty into the largest vein, the **inferior vena cava**, which travels through the abdominal and thoracic cavities toward the heart. Venous blood draining the head, neck, and shoulder regions empties into the **superior vena cava** and moves downward to join the inferior vena cava at heart level. The mixture of blood from the upper and lower body then enters the **right atrium** and descends into the **right ventricle** for delivery through the pulmonary artery to the lungs. Gas exchange takes place in the lungs' alveolar–capillary network, where the pulmonary veins return oxygenated blood to the left heart pump, and the journey through the body resumes.

Venous Return A unique characteristic of veins solves a potential problem related to the low pressure of venous blood. **Figure 10.4** shows that thin,

*Q***uestions** *&* **Notes**

What structures are present in veins but not arteries? What purpose do these structures serve?

Briefly discuss the role of veins as blood reservoirs.

Where do varicose veins usually appear? Why?

Discuss the major differences between arteries and veins.

What determines blood vessel's resistance to flow?

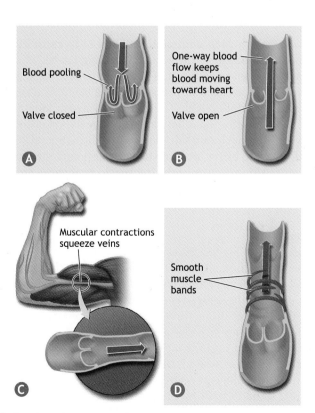

Figure 10.4 The valves in veins (**A**) prevent the back flow of blood but do not hinder the normal one-way flow of blood (**B**). Blood moves through veins by the action of nearby active muscle (muscle pump) (**C**) or contraction of smooth muscle bands within the veins (**D**).

membranous, flaplike valves spaced at short intervals within the vein permit one-way blood flow back to the heart. Because of low venous blood pressure, veins compress from muscular contractions or minor pressure changes within the chest cavity during breathing. Alternate venous compression and relaxation, combined with the one-way action of valves, provides a "milking" effect similar to the action of the heart. Whereas venous compression imparts considerable energy for blood flow, "diastole" or relaxation allows these vessels to refill as blood moves toward the heart. Without valves, blood would stagnate or pool (as it sometimes does) in extremity veins, and people would faint every time they stood up because of reduced blood flow to the brain.

A Significant Blood Reservoir The veins do not merely function as passive conduits. At rest, the venous system normally contains about 65% of total blood volume; hence, veins serve as capacitance vessels or blood reservoirs. A slight increase in tension (tone) by the veins' smooth muscle layer alters the diameter of the venous tree. A generalized increase in **venous tone** rapidly redistributes blood from peripheral veins toward the central blood volume returning to the heart. *In this manner, the venous system plays an important role as an active blood reservoir to either retard or enhance blood flow to the systemic circulation.*

Varicose Veins Sometimes valves within a vein become defective and do not maintain one-way blood flow. This condition of **varicose veins** usually occurs in superficial veins of the lower extremities from the force of gravity that retards blood flow in an upright posture. As blood accumulates, these veins distend excessively and become painful, often impairing circulation from surrounding areas. In severe cases, the venous wall inflames and degenerates, a condition called **phlebitis**, which often requires surgical removal of the damaged vessel.

Individuals with varicose veins should avoid excessive straining exercises such as heavy resistance training. During sustained, nonrhythmic muscle actions, the muscle and ventilatory "pumps" do not contribute to venous return. Increased abdominal pressure with straining also impedes blood flow return. These factors cause blood to pool (i.e., temporarily stagnate) in the veins of the lower body, which could aggravate existing varicose veins. Whether regular aerobic exercise prevents the occurrence of varicose veins remains unknown. Rhythmic physical activity could minimize complications because dynamic muscle actions continually propel peripheral blood toward the heart.

Venous Pooling The fact that people faint when forced to maintain an upright posture without movement (e.g., standing at attention for a prolonged period) demonstrates the importance of muscle contraction's ability to augment venous return. Also, changing from a lying to a standing position affects the dynamics of venous return and triggers physiologic responses. If a person suddenly rises and remains erect without movement, an uninterrupted column of blood exists from heart level to the toes, creating a hydrostatic force of 80 to 100 mm Hg. Swelling (edema) occurs from pooling of blood in the lower extremities and creates "back pressure" that forces fluid from the capillary bed into surrounding tissues. Concurrently, impaired venous return decreases blood pressure; at the same time, heart rate (HR) accelerates and venous tone increases to counter the hypotensive condition. Maintaining an upright position without movement leads to dizziness and eventual fainting from insufficient cerebral blood supply. Resuming a horizontal or head-down position restores circulation and consciousness.

Active Cool-Down The potential for venous pooling justifies continued slow jogging or walking immediately following strenuous exercise. "Cooling down" with rhythmic exercise facilitates blood flow through the vascular circuit including the heart during recovery. An "active recovery" of light to moderate exercise also speeds lactate removal from the blood (see Chapter 6). Pressurized suits worn by test pilots and special support stockings also retard hydrostatic shifts of blood to veins of the lower extremities in the upright position. A similar supportive effect occurs in upright exercise in a swimming pool because the water's external support facilitates venous return.

BLOOD PRESSURE

With each contraction of the left ventricle, a surge of blood enters the aorta, distending the vessel and creating pressure within it. The stretch and subsequent recoil of the aortic wall propagates as a wave through the entire arterial system. The pressure wave readily appears as a pulse in the following areas: the superficial radial artery on the thumb side of the wrist, the temporal artery (on the side of the head at the temple), and the carotid artery along the side of the trachea. In healthy persons, the pulse rate equals the HR.

At Rest

The highest pressure generated by left ventricular contraction (**systole**) to move blood through a healthy, resilient arterial system at rest usually reaches 120 mm Hg. As the heart relaxes (**diastole**) and the aortic valves close, the natural elastic recoil of the aorta and other arteries provides a continuous head of pressure to move blood into the periphery until the next surge from ventricular systole. During the cardiac cycle's diastole, arterial blood pressure decreases to 70 to 80 mm Hg. Arteries "hardened" by mineral and fatty deposits within their walls or arteries with excessive peripheral resistance to blood flow from kidney malfunction induce systolic pressures as high as 300 mm Hg and diastolic pressures above 120 mm Hg.

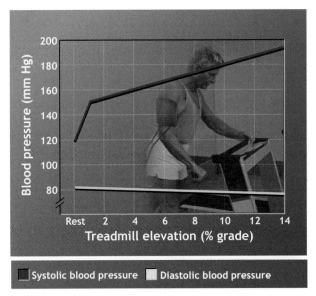

Figure 10.5 Generalized response for systolic and diastolic blood pressures during continuous, graded treadmill exercise up to maximum.

Questions & Notes

Give a normal blood pressure at rest.

  Systolic:

  Diastolic:

Systolic blood pressure estimates what physiologic factor?

Describe the relationship between systolic blood pressure and cardiac output during exercise of increasing intensity.

What does diastolic blood pressure estimate?

High blood pressure (**hypertension**) imposes a chronic strain on normal cardiovascular function. If left untreated, severe hypertension leads to heart failure as the heart muscle weakens, unable to maintain its normal pumping ability. Degenerating, brittle vessels can obstruct blood flow or can burst, cutting off vital blood flow to brain tissue to precipitate a stroke.

During Exercise

Rhythmic Exercise   During rhythmic brisk walking, hiking, jogging, swimming, and bicycling, dilatation of the active muscles' blood vessels increases the vascular area for blood flow. The alternate, rhythmic contraction and relaxation of skeletal muscles forces blood through the vessels and returns it to the heart. Increased blood flow during moderate exercise increases systolic pressure in the first few minutes; it then levels off, usually between 140 and 160 mm Hg. Diastolic pressure remains relatively unchanged.

Figure 10.5 reveals the general pattern for systolic and diastolic blood pressures during continuous, graded treadmill exercise. After an initial rapid increase from the resting level, systolic blood pressure increases linearly with exercise intensity, and diastolic pressure remains stable or decreases slightly at the higher exercise levels. Healthy, sedentary, and endurance-trained subjects

ⓘ For Your Information

DETERMINANTS OF BLOOD PRESSURE AND TOTAL PERIPHERAL RESISTANCE

Arterial blood pressure relates to arterial blood flow per minute (cardiac output) and peripheral vascular resistance to blood flow in the following relationships:

Blood pressure = Cardiac output × Total peripheral resistance

Rearranging terms:

Total peripheral resistance = Blood pressure ÷ Cardiac output

ⓘ For Your Information

RACIAL DIFFERENCES IN BLOOD PRESSURE

The prevalence of hypertension in black and white men and women differs significantly. The total prevalence is only slightly higher in blacks than whites (28.1% vs. 23.2%), yet in young adults, hypertension occurs much more frequently in blacks, particularly black women. In the 35 to 44 age range, hypertension occurs in one-third as many white women (8.5%) as black women (22.9%). The fact that African Americans have a much greater incidence than blacks in Africa compounds the issue of race and hypertension and perhaps emphasizes non-genetic, lifestyle contributory factors to hypertension. Ongoing research focuses on diet, stress, cigarette smoking, and other lifestyle and environmental factors that trigger this chronic blood pressure response in genetically susceptible blacks (*http://www.ash-us.org/*). The American College of Sports Medicine's "Position Stand on Physical Activity, Physical Fitness, and Hypertension" can be accessed at *www.acsm-msse.org*.

BOX 10.1 CLOSE UP

How to Measure Blood Pressure

Blood pressure represents the force or pressure exerted by blood against the arterial walls during a cardiac cycle. Systolic blood pressure, the higher of the two pressure measurements, occurs during ventricular contraction (systole) as the heart propels 70 to 100 mL of blood into the aorta. After systole, the ventricles relax (diastole), the arteries recoil, and arterial pressure continually declines as blood flows into the periphery and the heart refills with blood. The lowest pressure reached during ventricular relaxation represents the diastolic blood pressure. Normal systolic blood pressure in an adult varies between 110 and 130 mm Hg, and diastolic pressure varies between 60 and 85 mm Hg. Elevated systolic or diastolic blood pressure (termed stage 1 hypertension) is defined as a resting systolic blood pressure of 139 mm Hg or greater and diastolic pressure 90 mm Hg and above. The accompanying table (next page) lists the latest adult guidelines for classification and management of hypertension.

Pulse pressure reflects the difference between systolic and diastolic pressures.

MEASUREMENT PROCEDURES

Blood pressure is measured indirectly by **auscultation** (listening to sounds termed *Korotkoff sounds*, described in 1902 by Russian physician N.S. Korotkoff [1874–1920]), which uses a stethoscope and sphygmomanometer consisting of a blood pressure cuff and an aneroid or mercury column pressure gauge.

1. Have the subject sit in a quiet room with the upper arm exposed.
2. Have the subject bend the arm to bring the elbow to heart level.
3. Locate the brachial artery at the inner side of the upper arm, approximately 1 inch above the bend in the elbow.
4. Take the free end of the cuff and gently slide it through the metal loop (or wrap over exposed Velcro) and flap it back over so the cuff wraps around the upper arm at heart level. Align the arrows on the cuff with the brachial artery. Secure the Velcro parts of the cuff. The sphygmomanometer cuff should fit snugly, but not tight, to obtain accurate readings. Use appropriate-sized cuffs for children and obese individuals.
5. Place the stethoscope bell below the antecubital space over the brachial artery.
6. The cuff should now have the connecting tube from the sphygmomanometer bulb and gauge exiting the cuff towards the arm.
7. Before inflating the cuff, make sure the air release valve remains closed by turning the knob clockwise.

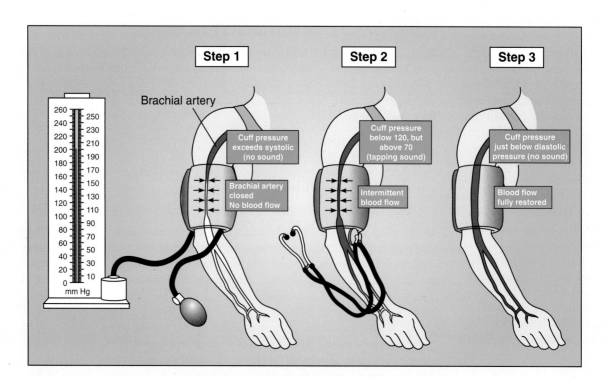

8. Inflate the cuff with quick, even pumps to about 180 mm Hg.
9. Gradually release cuff pressure about 3 mm·s⁻¹ by slowly opening the air release knob (counterclockwise turn), noting the first sound that results from turbulence from the rush of blood as the formerly closed artery briefly opens during the highest pressure in the cardiac cycle. *This represents the systolic blood pressure.*

10. Continue to reduce the pressure, noting when the sound becomes muffled (*fourth phase diastolic pressure*) and when the sound disappears (*fifth phase diastolic pressure*). Clinicians usually record the fifth phase as the diastolic blood pressure.
11. If the measured pressure exceeds 140/90 mm Hg, allow a 10-minute rest and repeat the procedure.

Blood Pressure Classification and Management for Adults

BP CLASSIFICATION	SBPa mm Hg	DBPa mm Hg	WITHOUT LIFESTYLE MODIFICATION	WITHOUT COMPELLING INDICATION	WITH COMPELLING INDICATIONb
Normal	<120	and <80	Encourage		
Prehypertension	120–139	or 80–89	Yes	No drugs indicated	Drug(s) for compelling indications
Stage 1 Hypertension	140–159	or 90–99	Yes	Thiazide-type diuretics for most. May consider ACEI, ARB, BB, CCB, or combination	Drug(s) for compelling indications.b Other antihypertensive drugs (diuretics, ACEI, ARB, BB, CCB) as needed.
Stage 2 Hypertension	≥160	or ≥100	Yes	Two-drug combination for mostc (usually thiazide-type diuretic and ACEI or ARB or BB or CCB)	

DBP = diastolic blood pressure; SBP = systolic blood pressure
aTreatment determined by highest BP category.
bCompelling indications include individuals with heart failure, postmyocardial infarction, high coronary disease risk and diabetes.
cInitial combined therapy should be used cautiously for those at risk for orthostatic hypotension; treat patients with chronic kidney disease or diabetes to BP goal of <130/80 mmHg.
ACEI = angiotensin converting enzyme inhibitor; ARB = angiotensin receptor blocker; BB = beta blocker; CCB = calcium channel blocker.
From: Seventh report of the joint committee on prevention, detection, evaluation, and treatment of high blood pressure (JNCV): US Department of Health and Human Services. National Institutes of Health, National Heart, Lung, and Blood Institute. National High Blood Pressure Education Program. NIH Publication No. 03-5233, May, 2003.

demonstrate similar blood pressure responses. But during maximum exercise by healthy, fit men and women, systolic blood pressure may increase to 200 mm Hg or higher despite reduced total peripheral resistance. This level of arterial blood pressure most likely reflects the heart's large cardiac output during maximal exercise by individuals with high aerobic capacity.

Resistance Exercise
Figure 10.6 contrasts the blood pressure responses during rhythmic aerobic exercise and intense resistance exercises that engage small and large amounts of muscle mass. Straining-type exercise (e.g., heavy resistance exercise, shoveling wet snow) increases blood pressure dramatically because sustained muscular force compresses peripheral arterioles, considerably increasing the resistance to blood flow. The heart's additional workload from acute elevations in blood pressure increases the risk for individuals with existing hypertension or coronary heart disease. In such cases, rhythmic forms of moderate physical activity provide less risk and greater health benefits. On a more positive note, those who regularly engage in resistance training show less dramatic blood pressure increases than untrained counterparts, particularly when each exerts the same absolute muscle force.

Questions & Notes

The _____ method measures changes in sound to estimate blood pressure.

Give the three blood pressure classifications and the cut-off values for each:

Class   SBP Cut-off   DBP Cut-off
1.

2.

3.

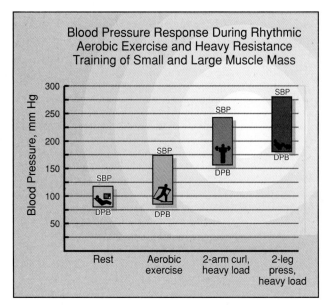

Figure 10.6 Blood pressure response during rhythmic aerobic exercise and heavy resistance training of a small (arms) and large (legs) muscle mass. The *top of each bar* represents systolic blood pressure; the *bottom* represents diastolic blood pressure.

Upper-Body Exercise Exercise at a given percentage of $\dot{V}O_{2max}$ increases systolic and diastolic blood pressures substantially more in rhythmic (upper arm) compared with rhythmic leg (lower body) exercise. The smaller arm muscle mass and vasculature offer greater resistance to blood flow than the larger and more vascularized lower-body regions. This means that blood flow to the arms during exercise requires a much larger systolic head of pressure and accompanying increase in myocardial workload and vascular strain. For individuals with cardiovascular dysfunction, more prudent exercise involves larger muscle groups, as in walking, running, bicycling, and stair climbing, rather than unregulated exercises of a limited muscle mass, as in shoveling, overhead hammering, or even arm-crank ergometry.

In Recovery

After a bout of sustained light- to moderate-intensity exercise, systolic blood pressure temporarily decreases below pre-exercise levels for up to 12 hours in normal and hypertensive subjects. Pooling of blood in the visceral organs and lower limbs

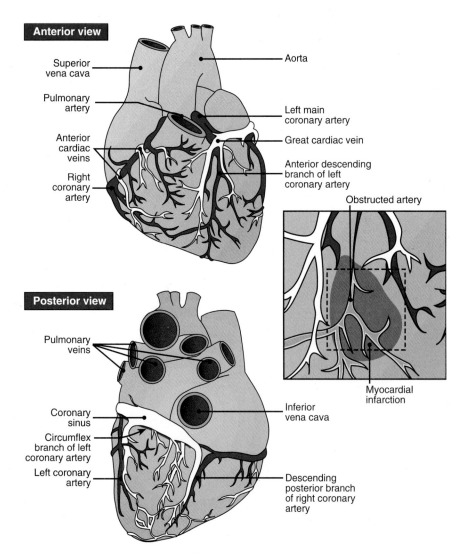

Figure 10.7 Anterior and posterior views of the coronary circulation, with arteries *shaded dark red* and veins *unshaded*. The *inset figure* illustrates a myocardial infarction resulting from the blockage (occlusion) of a coronary vessel.

during recovery reduces central blood volume, which contributes to lower blood pressure. This **hypotensive recovery response** further supports exercise as an important nonpharmacologic hypertension therapy. A potentially effective approach spreads several bouts of moderate physical activity throughout the day.

THE HEART'S BLOOD SUPPLY

Nearly 2000 gallons of blood flow from the heart each day, but none of its oxygen or nutrients pass directly to the myocardium from the heart's chambers. The myocardium maintains its own elaborate circulatory system. **Figure 10.7** illustrates these vessels as a visible, crownlike network, the **coronary circulation**, that arises from the top portion of the heart.

The openings for the left and right coronary arteries emerge from the aorta just above the semilunar valves where oxygenated blood leaves the left ventricle. The arteries then curl around the heart's surface; the **right coronary artery** supplies predominantly the right atrium and ventricle, and the greatest blood volume flows in the **left coronary artery** to the left atrium and ventricle and a small portion of the right ventricle. These vessels divide to eventually form a dense capillary network within the myocardium. Blood leaves the tissues of the left ventricle through the coronary sinus; blood from the right ventricle exits through the anterior cardiac veins and empties directly into the right atrium.

Myocardial Oxygen Utilization

Oxygen utilization by the heart muscle remains high in relation to its blood flow. At rest, the myocardium extracts 70% to 80% of the oxygen from the blood flowing in the coronary vessels. In contrast, most other tissues use only about 25% of the blood's available oxygen at rest. Because near-maximal oxygen extraction occurs in the myocardium at rest, increases in coronary blood flow provide the primary means to meet myocardial oxygen demands in exercise. In vigorous exercise, coronary blood flow increases four to six times above the resting level because of elevated myocardial metabolism and increased aortic pressure.

Profuse myocardial vascularization supplies each muscle fiber with at least one capillary. Adequate oxygenation becomes so crucial that impairment in coronary blood flow triggers chest discomfort and pain, a condition termed **angina pectoris**. The pain increases during exercise when myocardial oxygen demand rises considerably and supply remains limited. A blood clot (**thrombus**) lodged in one of the coronary vessels can severely impair normal heart function. This form of "heart attack," termed **myocardial infarction**, often injures the myocardium; severe damage to this muscle can result in death.

Rate-Pressure Product: An Estimate of Myocardial Work   Three important mechanical factors determine myocardial oxygen uptake:

1. Tension development within the myocardium
2. Myocardial contractility
3. Heart rate

𝒬uestions & Notes

Give one possible explanation for the post-exercise hypotensive response.

At rest, how much oxygen is extracted from the coronary blood flow?

List 2 factors that increase coronary blood flow during vigorous exercise.

1.

2.

Write the equation for the rate-pressure product (RPP).

ⓘ For Your Information

LIFESTYLE CHOICES THAT LOWER BLOOD PRESSURE

Advice	Details	Decrease in Systolic Blood Pressure (mm Hg)
Lose excess weight	For every 20 lb you lose	5–20
Follow the DASH diet	Eat a lower fat diet rich in vegetables, fruits, and low-fat dairy foods	8–14
Exercise daily	Get 30 minutes a day of aerobic activity (e.g., brisk walking)	4–9
Limit sodium	Eat no more than 2400 mg a day (1500 mg is better)	2–8
Limit alcohol	Have no more than 2 drinks a day for men or 1 drink a day for women (1 drink = 12 oz beer, 5 oz wine, or 1.5 oz 80-proof liquor)	2–4

DASH, Dietary Approaches to Stop Hypertension. *www.dashdiet.org.*

When each of these factors increases during exercise, myocardial blood flow adjusts to balance oxygen supply with demand. The product of systolic blood pressure (SBP; measured at the brachial artery) and HR provides a convenient estimate of myocardial workload (oxygen uptake). This index of *relative* cardiac work, called the **double product** or **rate-pressure product (RPP)**, closely reflects directly measured myocardial oxygen uptake and coronary blood flow in healthy subjects over a range of exercise intensities. RPP computes as:

$$RPP = SBP \times HR$$

Exercise studies of people with coronary heart disease have linked the RPP to the onset of angina or electrocardiographic (ECG) abnormalities. RPP has also assessed various clinical, surgical, and exercise interventions for their effects on cardiac performance. The reductions in exercise heart rate and systolic blood pressure at a specific level of submaximal effort with endurance training improve cardiac patients' exercise capacity (before angina onset) because of the reduced myocardial oxygen requirement. In addition, aerobic training increases the RPP of patients before they experience the onset of heart disease symptoms. In nine patients who were followed over 7 years of exercise training, RPP increased 11.5% before ischemic abnormalities appeared. These important findings provide indirect evidence for a training-induced improvement in myocardial oxygenation, perhaps from greater coronary vascularization, reduced obstruction, or a combination of both factors. Typical values for RPP range from 6000 at rest (HR, 50 b·min^{-1}; SBP, 120 mm Hg) to 40,000 during intense exercise (HR, 200 b·min^{-1}; SBP, 200 mm Hg).

Changes in heart rate and blood pressure contribute equally to a change in RPP.

The Heart's Energy Supply

The myocardium relies almost exclusively on energy released from aerobic reactions; not surprisingly then, myocardial tissue has a threefold higher oxidative capacity than skeletal muscle. Its muscle fibers contain the greatest mitochondrial concentration of all tissues, with exceptional capacity for long-chain fatty acid catabolism as a primary means for adenosine triphosphate (ATP) resynthesis.

Glucose, fatty acids, and lactate formed from glycolysis in skeletal muscle all provide the energy for myocardial functioning. At rest, these three substrates contribute to ATP resynthesis, with the most energy from free fatty acid breakdown (60%–70%). After a meal, glucose becomes the heart's preferred energy substrate. In essence, the heart uses for energy whatever substrate it "sees" on a physiologic level. During intense exercise when lactate efflux from active skeletal muscle into the blood increases dramatically, the heart derives its major energy by oxidizing circulating lactate. In more moderate exercise, equal amounts of fat and carbohydrate provide the energy fuel. In prolonged submaximal exercise, myocardial metabolism of free fatty acids increases to almost 80% of the total energy requirement. Similar patterns of myocardial metabolism exist for trained and untrained individuals. An endurance-trained person, however, demonstrates considerably greater myocardial reliance on fat catabolism in submaximal exercise. This difference, similar to the effect for skeletal muscle, illustrates the "carbohydrate-sparing effect" of aerobic training.

SUMMARY

1. The heart functions as two separate pumps: one pump receives blood from the body and pumps it to the lungs for aeration (pulmonary circulation); the other pump accepts oxygenated blood from the lungs and pumps it throughout the body (systemic circulation).

2. Pressure changes during the cardiac cycle act on the heart's valves to provide one-way blood flow through the vascular circuit.

3. The dense capillary network provides a large, effective surface for exchange between blood and tissues. These microscopic vessels adjust blood flow in response to the tissue's metabolic activity.

4. Vein compression and relaxation through muscle actions impart considerable energy for venous return. "Muscle-pump" action justifies use of active recovery from vigorous exercise.

5. Nerves and hormones constrict or stiffen the smooth muscle layer in venous walls. Alterations in venous tone profoundly affect redistribution of total blood volume.

6. Systolic blood pressure represents the highest pressure generated during the cardiac cycle; diastolic blood pressure describes the lowest pressure before the next ventricular contraction.

7. Hypertension imposes a chronic stress on cardiovascular function. Regular aerobic training modestly reduces systolic and diastolic blood pressures during rest and submaximal exercise.

8. During graded exercise, systolic blood pressure increases in proportion to oxygen uptake and cardiac output, but diastolic pressure remains essentially unchanged. The same relative exercise intensity (%$\dot{V}O_{2max}$) produces a larger blood pressure response with upper-body compared with lower-body exercise.

9. During recovery from light and moderate exercise, blood pressure decreases below pre-exercise levels, called a hypotensive response, and remains lower for up to 12 hours.

10. Peak systolic and diastolic blood pressures mirror the hypertensive state during resistance exercises. Inordinately high blood pressure and RPP in such exercise poses a risk to individuals with hypertension and coronary heart disease.

11. Regular resistance exercise training blunts the hypertensive response to straining-type exercise.

12. At rest, the myocardium extracts about 80% of the oxygen from coronary blood flow. Consequently, increased myocardial oxygen demands in exercise depend on proportionate increases in coronary blood flow.

13. Impaired coronary blood flow causes chest discomfort and pain (angina pectoris); blockage of a coronary artery (myocardial infarction) can irreversibly damage the myocardium.

14. The product of heart rate and systolic blood pressure (RPP) estimates relative myocardial workload. Clinicians use this index to study exercise-training effects on cardiac performance in patients with heart disease.

15. Glucose, fatty acids, and lactate represent the heart's main substrates for energy metabolism. The percentage utilization varies with nutritional status and exercise intensity and duration.

 THOUGHT QUESTION

1. What advantage does a "closed" circulatory system provide to a physically active individual?

Part 2	Cardiovascular Regulation and Integration

At rest in a comfortable environment, the skin receives 250 mL (5%) of the 5 L of blood pumped from the heart each minute. In contrast, 20% of the total cardiac output flows to the body's surface for heat dissipation with exercise in a hot, humid environment. The rapid redistribution or "shunting" of blood to meet metabolic and physiologic requirements with appropriate maintenance of blood pressure requires a closed circulatory system with both central and local control of pump output and vascular dimensions.

HEART RATE REGULATION

Cardiac muscle possesses intrinsic rhythmicity. Without external stimuli, the adult heart would beat steadily between 50 and 80 times each minute. Within the body, nerves that directly supply the myocardium and chemicals within the blood rapidly alter heart rate. Extrinsic control of cardiac function causes the heart to speed up in "anticipation" even before exercise begins. To a large extent, extrinsic regulation can adjust heart rate to as slow as 40 b·min^{-1} at rest in endurance athletes and as fast as 215 to 220 b·min^{-1} during maximum exercise.

Intrinsic Regulation

A mass of specialized muscle tissue, the **sinoatrial (SA) node**, lies within the posterior wall of the right atrium. The SA node spontaneously depolarizes and

Questions & Notes

Name the heart's "pacemaker."

Trace the route of the electrical impulse from the SA node into the ventricles. (Hint: see Figure 10.8)

For Your Information

THE AMAZING HEART

Here's a straightforward calculation with an amazing answer about the heart. "How many cars with 20-gallon capacity gas tanks would 60 years of resting cardiac output fill up?" (Hint: Use an average resting cardiac output of 5 L·min^{-1}.)

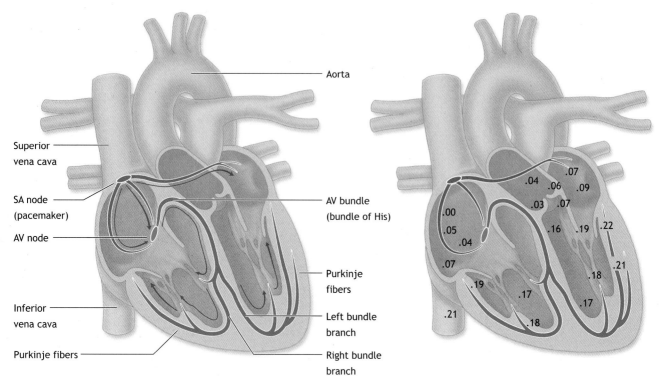

Figure 10.8 *Left.* The *red arrows* denote the normal route for excitation and conduction of the cardiac impulse. The impulse originates at the sinoatrial (SA) node, travels to the atrioventricular (AV) node, and then spreads throughout the ventricular mass. *Right.* Time sequence in seconds for electrical impulse transmission from the SA node throughout the myocardium.

repolarizes to provide an "innate" stimulus to the heart. For this reason, the term "**pacemaker**" describes the SA node. **Figure 10.8** (*left*) shows the normal route for impulse transmission within the myocardium.

The Heart's Electrical Impulse

Figure 10.8 (*right*) illustrates the time sequence of the propagation of the electrical impulse from the SA node throughout the myocardium. Rhythms originating at the SA node spread across the atria to another small knot of tissue, the **AV node**. This node delays the impulse about 0.10 seconds to provide sufficient time for the atria to contract and force blood into the ventricles. The AV node gives rise to the **AV bundle (bundle of His)**, which speeds the impulse rapidly through the ventricles over specialized conducting fibers called the **Purkinje system.** Purkinje fibers form distinct branches that penetrate the right and left ventricles. Each ventricular cell becomes stimulated within 0.06 seconds from passage of the impulse into the ventricles; this causes simultaneous contraction of both ventricles. Cardiac impulse transmission progresses as follows:

SA node → Atria → AV node →
AV bundle (Purkinje fibers) → Ventricles

Electrocardiography

The electrical activity generated by the myocardium creates an electrical field throughout the body. Salty body fluid conducts electricity well so electrodes placed on the skin's surface detect the sequence of electrical events during each cardiac cycle. The **ECG** provides a graphic record of voltage changes during the heart's electrical activity. **Figure 10.9** illustrates a normal ECG with important sequences of major myocardial electrical activity.

The ECG provides a means to monitor heart rate during exercise. Radiotelemetry allows ECG transmission while a person freely performs diverse physical activities, including football, weight lifting, basketball, ice hockey, dancing, and even swimming. The ECG can uncover abnormalities in heart function related to cardiac rhythm, electrical conduction, myocardial oxygen supply, and actual tissue damage (see Close Up Box 10.2, *How to Place Electrodes for Bipolar and 12-Lead ECG Recordings*, page 316).

Extrinsic Regulation

Neural impulses override the inherent myocardial rhythmicity. The signals originate in the cardiovascular center in the medulla and travel through the sympathetic and parasympathetic components of the autonomic nervous system.

Sympathetic Influence   Stimulation of sympathetic cardioaccelerator nerves releases the **catecholamines** epinephrine and norepinephrine. These neural hormones increase myocardial contractility and accelerate SA node depolarization to increase heart rate, a response termed **tachycardia.** Epinephrine, released from the medullary

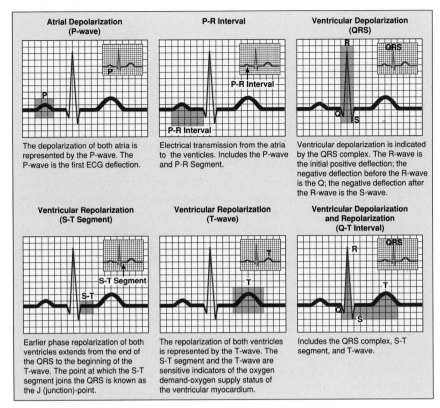

Figure 10.9 Different phases of the normal electrocardiogram from atrial depolarization (*upper left*) to repolarization of the ventricles (*lower three figures*).

portion of the adrenal glands in response to general sympathetic activation, also produces a similar though slower acting effect on cardiac function.

Parasympathetic Influence   Acetylcholine, the parasympathetic nervous system hormone, retards the sinus discharge rate to slow the heart. This response, termed **bradycardia**, comes from the **vagus nerve** whose cell bodies originate in the cardioinhibitory portion of the medulla. Vagal stimulation does not affect myocardial contractility. **Table 10.1** summarizes the effects of the autonomic nervous system on cardiovascular function.

Vascular smooth muscles also contract and relax in response to chemical substances released by endothelium tissue (cells comprising the inner lining of the blood vessels). Relaxing factors include the most potent factor, nitric oxide (NO). NO, released from endothelial cells in large arteries that supply muscle, appears particularly important in supplying the muscles with adequate blood during exercise. The endothelium releases NO in response to pulsatile blood flow and blood vessel wall stress, both of which increase during exercise. Other relaxing factors include protacyclin and endothelium-derived

Table 10.1	The Autonomic Nervous System and Cardiovascular Function	
SYMPATHETIC INFLUENCE		**PARASYMPATHETIC INFLUENCE**
Increase heart rate		Decrease heart rate
Increase myocardial contraction force		Decrease myocardial contraction force
Dilate coronary blood vessels		Constrict coronary blood vessels
Constrict pulmonary blood vessels		Dilate pulmonary blood vessels
Constrict blood vessels in abdomen, muscle, skin, and kidneys		Dilate blood vessels in abdomen, muscle, skin, and kidneys

Questions & Notes

Draw and label a typical ECG tracing.

What autonomic neural fibers stimulate atria and ventricles?

List 2 uses for the ECG.

1.

2.

List 2 effects of sympathetic and 2 effects of parasympathetic stimulation on cardiovascular function.

Sympathetic:

1.

2.

Parasympathetic:

1.

2.

ⓘ For Your Information

HEART'S REST PERIOD

The heart's relatively long depolarization period requires about 0.30 seconds before the myocardium can receive another impulse and contract again. This "rest" or refractory period provides sufficient time for ventricular filling between beats.

BOX 10.2 CLOSE UP

How to Place Electrodes for Bipolar and 12-Lead ECG Recordings

The ECG represents a composite record of the heart's electrical events during a cardiac cycle. These events provide a means to monitor heart rate during different physical activities and exercise stress testing. The ECG can detect contraindications to exercise, including previous myocardial infarction, ischemic S-T segment changes, conduction defects, and left ventricular enlargement (hypertrophy). A valid ECG tracing requires proper electrode placement. The term **ECG lead** indicates the specific placement of *a pair* of electrodes on the body that transmits the electrical signal to a recorder. The record of electrical differences across diverse ECG leads creates the composite electrical "picture" of myocardial activity.

SKIN PREPARATION

Proper skin preparation reduces extraneous electrical "noise" (interference and skeletal muscle artifact). The skin should be abraded with fine sandpaper or commercially available pads and alcohol to remove surface epidermis and oil; the skin should appear red, slightly irritated, dry, and clean.

BIPOLAR (THREE-ELECTRODE) CONFIGURATION

The *left figure* shows the typical electrode placement for a bipolar configuration. This positioning provides less sensitivity for diagnostic testing but proves useful for routine ECG monitoring in functional exercise testing and radiotelemetry of the ECG during physical activity. The ground (green or black) electrode attaches over the sternum, the positive (red) electrode attaches on the left side of the chest in the V_5 position (level of the 5th intercostal space adjacent to the midaxillary line), and the positive (white) electrode attaches on the right side of the chest just below the nipple at the level of the fifth intercostal space. Placement of the positive electrode can be altered to optimize the recording (e.g., third and fourth intercostal spaces, anterior portion of the right shoulder, or near the clavicle). Correct electrode placement can be remembered as follows: *white to right, green to ground, red to left*.

MODIFIED 12-LEAD (10-ELECTRODE, TORSO-MOUNTED) CONFIGURATION FOR EXERCISE STRESS TESTING

The standard 12-lead ECG consists of three limb leads, three augmented unipolar leads, and six chest leads. For improved exercise ECG recordings, electrodes mounted on the torso at the abdominal level replace the conventional ankle (leg) and wrist electrodes. This "torso-mounted limb lead system" (*right figure*) reduces electrical artifact introduced by limb movement during exercise.

Electrode Positioning in the Modified 10-Electrode Torso-Mounted System

1. RL (right leg): Just above right iliac crest on the midaxillary line
2. LL (left leg): Just above the left iliac crest on the midaxillary line
3. RA (right arm): Just below right clavicle medial to deltoid muscle
4. LA (left arm): Just below left clavicle medial to deltoid muscle
5. V_1: On the right sternal border in the fourth intercostal space
6. V_2: On the left sternal border in the fourth intercostal space
7. V_3: At the midpoint of a straight line between V_2 and V_4
8. V_4: On the midclavicular line in the fifth intercostal space
9. V_5: On the anterior axillary line and horizontal to V_4
10. V_6: On the midaxillary line and horizontal to V_4 and V_5

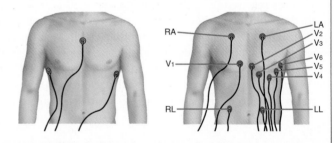

REFERENCE

Phibbs, B., Buckels, L.: Comparative yields of ECG leads in multistage stress testing. *Am. Heart. J.*, 90:275, 1985.

hyperpolarizing factor. Contracting factors include endothelin and vasoconstrictor protaglandins.

Endurance training creates an imbalance between sympathetic accelerator and parasympathetic depressor activity to favor greater vagal parasympathetic dominance. The effect occurs primarily from increased parasympathetic activity, with some decrease in sympathetic discharge. Training may also decrease the SA node's intrinsic firing rate. These adaptations account for the bradycardia frequently observed among highly conditioned endurance athletes and sedentary individuals who undertake aerobic training.

Cortical Influence

Impulses originating in the brain's higher somato-motor **central command system** pass via small afferent nerves to directly modulate the activity of the cardiovascular center in the ventrolateral medulla. This provides the coordinated and rapid response of the heart and blood vessels to optimize tissue perfusion and maintain central blood pressure in relation to motor cortex involvement. *Central command provides the greatest control over heart rate.* It exerts its effect not only during exercise but also at rest and in the immediate pre-exercise period. Thus, variation in emotional state can considerably affect cardiovascular responses, often obscuring "true" resting values for heart rate and blood pressure. Cortical input also causes the heart rate to increase rapidly in anticipation of exercise. The combined effects of an increase in sympathetic discharge and reduction of vagal tone produce the **anticipatory heart rate**, which becomes particularly apparent before all-out physical effort.

The heart "turns on" for exercise from four sources:

1. Increased sympathetic activity
2. Decreased parasympathetic activity combined with
3. Input from the brain's central command
4. Feedback information from activation of receptors in joints and muscles as exercise begins

Even for non-sprint events, the heart rate reaches 180 b·min^{-1} within 30 seconds of 1- and 2-mile runs. Further heart rate increases progress gradually, with plateaus attained several times during the runs.

Figure 10.10 depicts major factors controlling heart rate and myocardial contractility. The medulla receives continual input about blood pressure from baroreceptors within the carotid arteries and aorta. The medulla also acts as an integrating and coordinating center, receiving stimuli from the cortex and peripheral tissues and routing an appropriate response to the heart and blood vessels.

Peripheral Input   The cardiovascular center in the medulla receives sensory input from mechanical receptors (**mechanoreceptors**) and chemical receptors called **chemoreceptors** in blood vessels, joints, and muscles. Stimuli from these peripheral receptors monitor the state of active muscle; they modify either vagal or sympathetic outflow to create an appropriate cardiovascular response. Reflex neural input from active muscle, termed the **exercise pressor reflex**, in conjunction with output originating in the brain's higher motor areas, assesses the nature and intensity of exercise and the quantity of muscle recruited. Input from mechanoreceptors provides important feedback for the central nervous system's regulation of blood flow and blood pressure during dynamic exercise. Receptors in the aortic arch and carotid sinus respond to changes in arterial blood pressure. As blood pressure increases, the stretch of arterial vessels activates these **baroreceptors**, which reflexly slows heart rate and dilates peripheral vasculature. This lowers blood pressure toward normal levels. Exercise overrides this particular feedback mechanism because both heart rate and blood pressure increase. Baroreceptors likely prevent abnormally high blood pressure levels in exercise.

Questions & Notes

Name the cardiovascular control center that regulates the output of blood from the heart.

Briefly describe the anticipatory heart rate response.

Briefly describe the role of the medulla in controlling the heart.

Briefly identify and describe the role of the chemoreceptors.

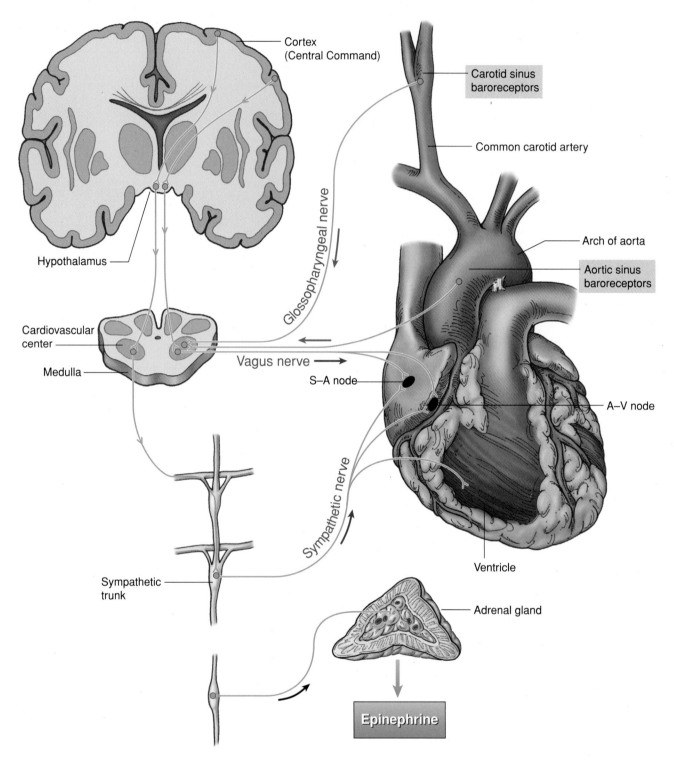

Figure 10.10 Pathways in reflex control of heart rate. The cardiovascular center in the medulla receives input from (1) baroreceptors in the carotid sinus and aortic arch and (2) cortical stimulation (central command). Efferent pathways from the medulla activate the heart by the vagus (parasympathetic) and sympathetic nerves.

Carotid Artery Palpation For healthy adults and cardiac patients, **carotid artery palpation** has little effect on heart rate during rest, exercise, and recovery. Under these conditions, strong external pressure against the carotid artery slows heart rate, probably from direct stimulation of carotid artery baroreceptors.

Accurate heart rate measurement provides the basis for establishing "target heart rates" during exercise training (see Chapter 13). If heart rate measurement consistently underestimated actual values, the person would exercise at higher levels than prescribed, which is certainly an undesirable effect when prescribing exercise for cardiac patients. An excellent substitute method involves determining the pulse rate at the radial or temporal arteries (see Close Up Box 10.3, *Assessing Heart Rate by Palpation and Auscultation Methods,* pages 320–322) because palpation at these sites does not change the heart rate.

Arrhythmias

The exquisite regulation of heart rate by intrinsic and extrinsic mechanisms generally progresses unnoticed and without adverse consequence. ECG and heart rate irregularities do occur and can herald myocardial disease. The term **arrhythmia** describes heart rhythm irregularities.

Heart Rhythm Irregularities
Interruption of regular heart rate pattern often occurs as extra beats (**extrasystoles**). Parts of the atria can become prematurely electrically active and depolarize spontaneously before SA node excitation, a condition called **premature atrial contraction (PAC)**. Premature excitation of ventricles (**premature ventricular contraction [PVC]**) also occurs during the interval between two regular beats. Occasional extrasystoles appear during rest and usually progress unnoticed. Psychological stress, anxiety, and caffeine consumption can trigger extrasystoles, probably from the effects of catecholamines on the rate of change of the SA node's membrane potential. Removal of such stimuli usually reestablishes normal heart rhythm. If this fails, medication blocking norepinephrine's action on the beta-receptors of atrial cells (**beta-blockers**) effectively treats this condition. Atrial arrhythmias do not compromise the heart's pumping ability (recall that atrial contraction contributes little to ventricular filling). A potentially dangerous situation arises when PACs link successively to create **atrial fibrillation.**

Ventricular fibrillation is the most serious cardiac arrhythmia. With this condition, foci of stimulation continually affect different parts of the ventricle rather than the normal single stimulus from the AV node. *Portions of the ventricle contract in an uncoordinated manner with repetitive PVCs, thus hindering the ventricle's ability to pump blood. Cardiac output and blood pressure decrease and the person rapidly loses consciousness.*

Resuscitation takes two forms: (1) reestablish normal heart pumping action to restore blood pressure and blood flow and (2) halt fibrillation and reestablish normal electrical rhythm. **Cardiopulmonary resuscitation (CPR)** mechanically simulates the heart's pumping action and often reverses fibrillation. If this fails, a defibrillator applies a strong burst of electric current across the entire myocardium. This depolarizes the heart so that a normal rhythm can initiate from the SA node upon repolarization. All exercise specialists need to be CPR certified (and recertified each year). The American Red Cross maintains CPR testing and certification programs for all interested persons *(www.redcross.org/; depts.washington.edu/learncpr/).*

BLOOD DISTRIBUTION

Exercise Effects

Increased energy expenditure requires rapid readjustments in blood flow that affect the entire cardiovascular system. For example, nerves and local metabolic conditions act on the smooth muscle bands of arteriole walls, causing them to alter their internal diameter almost instantaneously. Concurrently, neural stimulation of venous capacitance vessels causes them to "stiffen," moving blood from peripheral veins into the central circulation.

During exercise, the vascular portion of active muscles increases through dilatation of local arterioles; at the same time, other vessels constrict to "shut

---

Questions & Notes

List 3 common heart rate palpation sites.

1.

2.

3.

Define ventricular fibrillation.

Name 2 different heart rate rhythm irregularities.

1.

2.

Name and describe the most serious cardiac arrhythmia condition.

ⓘ For Your Information

ECG OR EKG?

ECG sometimes appears abbreviated as EKG. The "K" comes from the German spelling of the word for *electrocardiograph*. In 1895, Dutch physiologist Wilhelm Einthoven (1860–1927), 1924 Noble Prize winner in Physiology or Medicine for his pioneering work in myocardial electrophysiology, made the first tracings of the heart's electrical activity. He used his invention of a 500-lb string galvanometer consisting of a thin quartz wire in a magnetic field to record the heart's electrical activity.

BOX 10.3 CLOSE UP

Assessing Heart Rate by Palpation and Ascultation Methods

The rate of the cardiac cycle (i.e., heart rate) provides a fundamental tool to set exercise intensity and assess changes from exercise training. Four methods can measure heart rate: (1) by ear (auscultation), (2) by touch (palpation), (3) with a heart rate monitor, or (4) an ECG recorder. The auscultation and palpation methods are practical and useful.

HEART RATE BY THE ASCULTATION METHOD

The auscultation method uses a stethoscope to amplify and direct sound waves, thus bringing the ear of the listener closer to the sound source (heart).

Using the Stethoscope

1. With the ear tips of the stethoscope pointing forward, insert them directly down each ear canal.
2. Gently tap the diaphragm of the stethoscope to be sure you can hear the sound adequately.
3. Position the stethoscope just below the left breast at the pectoralis major muscle over the third intercostal space to the left of the sternum.
4. Hold the diaphragm of the stethoscope firmly against the skin, not over clothing.

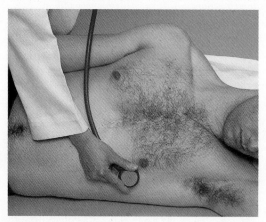

(Reprinted with permission from Bickely, L.S. (2003). *Bate's Guide to Physical Examination and History Taking*, 8th ed. Philadelphia: Lippincott Williams & Wilkins.)

HEART RATE BY PALPATION

The pulse wave generated by the pumping of blood through the arteries is most often measured over the radial or carotid arteries with a finger or hand. Use the tip of the middle and index fingers; do not use the thumb because it has a pulse of its own. Press lightly to avoid obstructing blood flow. An **apical beat** (vibration pulse) generated by the left ventricle hitting the chest wall near the left fifth rib becomes prominent immediately following exercise in lean individuals. Position the entire hand over the left side of the chest at heart level to palpate an apical beat.

Location for the Palpation Method

The four common palpation sites include:

1. Temporal artery: At the temple around the hairline of the head- (see Figure A, next page).
2. Carotid artery: Just lateral to the larynx (do not apply excessive pressure at this site because it may trigger a reflex that slows the heart rate)- (see Figure B, next page).
3. Radial artery: Anterolateral aspect of the wrist directly in line with the base of the thumb- (see Figure C, next page).
4. Brachial artery: Anteromedial aspect of the arm below the belly of the biceps brachii, 2 to 3 cm (1 in) above the antecubital fossa.

COUNTING HEART RATE

Record the HR as a rate per minute (e.g., 150 b·min^{-1}). Two common methods for counting heart rate include the timed heart rate method and the 30-beat heart rate method.

Timed Heart Rate Method

This method counts the number of pulses in a specific amount of time. Usually, pulse counts are taken for 6, 10, or 15 seconds. If palpating the pulse for 6 seconds, multiply by 10 to express as a per-minute rate; for a 10-second palpation, multiply by 6; and if palpating for 15 seconds, multiply the pulse count by 4. **Table 1** presents the heart rate conversion for each of the above 6-, 10-, or 15-second multiplications. Obviously, the 6-second count produces the least accurate pulse count.

Table 1 Heart Rate (in beats per minute; bpm) Conversion. Find the Number of Pulse Counts for 6, 10, or 15 Seconds; Read Across for the bpm

6-S COUNT	PER MIN RATE	10-S COUNT	PER MIN RATE	15-S COUNT	PER MIN RATE
4	40	7	42	10	40
5	50	8	48	11	44
6	60	9	54	12	48
7	70	10	60	13	52
8	80	11	66	14	56
9	90	12	72	15	60
10	100	13	78	16	64
11	110	14	84	17	68
12	120	15	90	18	72
13	130	16	96	19	76
14	140	17	102	20	80
15	150	18	108	21	84
16	160	19	114	22	88
17	170	20	120	23	92
18	180	21	126	24	96
19	190	22	132	25	100
20	200	23	138	26	104
21	210	24	144	27	108
22	220	25	150	28	112
		26	156	29	116
		27	162	30	120
		28	168	31	124
		29	174	32	128
		30	180	33	132
		31	186	34	136
		32	192	35	140
		33	198	36	144
		34	204	37	148
		35	210	38	152
		36	216	39	156
		37	222	40	160
				41	164
				42	168
				43	172
				44	176
				45	180
				46	184
				47	188
				48	192
				49	196
				50	200
				51	204
				52	208
				53	212
				54	216
				55	220

Three typical locations for palpating pulse: (**A**) temporal; (**B**) carotid; and (**C**) radial arteries.

(*continued*)

BOX 10.3 CLOSE UP

Assessing Heart Rate by Palpation and Ascultation Methods *(Continued)*

Thirty-Beat Heart Rate Method

This method counts the time in seconds (s) for 30 pulse beats to occur. Count the first beat as "zero" and simultaneously begin to record the time to count 30-pulse beats. The computational formula for computing heart rate in beats per min (bpm) follows:

$$HR \text{ (bpm)} = 30 \text{ b} \div \text{Time (s)} \times 60 \text{ s} \div 1 \text{ min}$$

For example, if 30 beats (b) occur in 20 s:

$$\begin{aligned} HR \text{ (bpm)} &= 30 \text{ b} \div \text{time (s)} \times 60 \text{ s} \div 1 \text{ min} \\ &= 30 \text{ b} \div 20 \text{ s} \times 60 \text{ s} \div 1 \text{ min} \\ &= 1.5 \times 60 \\ &= 90 \text{ bpm} \end{aligned}$$

Table 2 presents a conversion chart for the above method, with heart rate rounded to the nearest whole number. Find the time for recording 30 beats and the corresponding heart rate (bpm).

Table 2 Conversion Chart for 30-Beat Heart Rate Method					
TIME FOR 30 BEATS, S	HR, BPM	TIME FOR 30 BEATS, S	HR, BPM	TIME FOR 30 BEATS, S	HR, BPM
8	225	21	86	34	53
9	200	22	82	35	51
10	180	23	78	36	50
11	164	24	75	37	49
12	150	25	72	38	47
13	138	26	69	39	46
14	129	27	67	40	45
15	120	28	64	41	44
16	113	29	62	42	43
17	106	30	60	43	42
18	100	31	58	44	41
19	95	32	56	45	40
20	90	33	55		

REFERENCE

The Online Journal of Cardiology. Available at *http://sprojects.mmi.mcgill.ca/heart/egcyhome.html.*

down" blood flow to tissues that can temporarily compromise blood supply. Kidney function vividly illustrates regulatory capacity for adjusting regional blood flow. Renal circulation at rest normally averages 1100 mL·min^{-1} or about 20% of the total cardiac output. In maximal exercise, renal blood flow decreases to 250 mL·min^{-1}, which represents only 1% of a 25-L exercise cardiac output.

Blood Flow Regulation

Pressure differentials and resistances determine fluid movement through a vessel. Resistance varies directly with the length of the vessel and inversely with its diameter; greater driving force increases flow, and increased resistance impedes it. The following equation expresses the interaction between pressure, resistance, and fluid flow:

$$\textbf{Flow} = \textbf{Pressure} \div \textbf{Resistance}$$

Three factors determine resistance to blood flow:

1. Viscosity or blood thickness
2. Length of conducting tube
3. Radius of blood vessel

The following equation, referred to as **Poiseuille's law**, expresses the general relationship among pressure differential (gradient), resistance, and flow in a cylindrical vessel:

$$\textbf{Flow} = \textbf{Pressure gradient} \times \textbf{Vessel radius}^4 \div \\ \textbf{Vessel length} \times \textbf{Fluid viscosity}$$

Blood viscosity and transport vessel length remain relatively constant in the body. Consequently, blood vessel radius represents the most important factor affecting blood flow. *Resistance to flow changes with vessel radius raised to the fourth power.* Reducing a vessel's radius by half decreases flow by a factor of 16; conversely, doubling the radius increases volume 16-fold. This means that a relatively small degree of vasoconstriction or vasodilation dramatically impacts regional blood flow.

Local Factors

One of every 30 to 40 capillaries actually remains open in muscle tissue at rest. Thus, opening of large numbers of "dormant" capillaries with exercise serves three important functions:

1. Increases muscle blood flow
2. Only a small increase in velocity accompanies an increase in blood-flow volume
3. Increases effective surface for gas and nutrient exchange between blood and individual muscle fibers

A decrease in tissue oxygen supply stimulates local vasodilation in skeletal and cardiac muscle. Local increases in temperature, carbon dioxide, acidity, adenosine, NO, and magnesium and potassium ions also enhance regional blood flow. These **autoregulatory mechanisms** for blood flow make sense physiologically because they reflect elevated tissue metabolism and increased oxygen need. Rapid, local vasodilation provides the most effective, immediate step for increasing a tissue's oxygen supply.

Neural Factors

Central vascular control via sympathetic and, to a minor degree, parasympathetic portions of the autonomic nervous system override vasoregulation afforded by local factors. For example, muscles contain small sensory nerve fibers highly sensitive to chemical substances released in active muscle during exercise. Stimulation of these fibers provides input to the central nervous system to bring about appropriate cardiovascular responses. With central regulation, blood flow in one area cannot dominate when a concurrent oxygen need exists in other, more "needy" tissues.

Sympathetic nerve fibers end in the muscular layers of small arteries, arterioles, and precapillary sphincters. Norepinephrine acts as a general vasoconstrictor released at certain sympathetic nerve endings (**adrenergic fibers**). Other sympathetic neurons in skeletal and heart muscle release acetylcholine; these **cholinergic fibers** dilate the blood vessel. Continual sympathetic constrictor neuron activity maintains a relative state of vasoconstriction termed **vasomotor tone**. Dilatation of blood vessels regulated by adrenergic neurons results more from reduced vasomotor tone than increased sympathetic or parasympathetic dilator fiber activity. Powerful local vasodilation induced by metabolic byproducts also maintains blood flow in active tissue.

Hormonal Factors

Sympathetic nerves terminate in the medullary portion of the adrenal glands. With sympathetic activation, this glandular tissue releases large quantities of epinephrine and a small amount of norepinephrine into the blood. These hormones cause a general constrictor response *except* in blood vessels of the heart and skeletal muscles. Adrenal hormones provide relatively minor control of regional blood flow during exercise compared with the more rapid and powerful local sympathetic neural drive.

INTEGRATED RESPONSE IN EXERCISE

Table 10.2 summarizes the integrated chemical, neural, and hormonal adjustments immediately before and during exercise.

Questions & Notes

Complete the following equations:

Flow = pressure gradient ÷

_____

Flow = pressure gradient × _____ ÷ _____

_____ × _____

_____

What is another name for the sympathetic constrictor fibers?

Name the substances cholinergic nerve fibers release.

Name the substance(s) that provide an autoregulatory mechanism for blood flow within muscle.

Table 10.2	Summary of Integrated Chemical, Neural, and Hormonal Adjustments Before and During Exercise	
CONDITION	**ACTIVATOR**	**RESPONSE**
Pre-exercise "anticipatory" response	Activation of motor cortex and higher areas of brain causes increase in sympathetic outflow and reciprocal inhibition of parasympathetic activity	Acceleration of heart rate; increased myocardial contractility; vasodilation in skeletal and heart muscle (cholinergic fibers); vasoconstriction in other areas, especially skin, gut, spleen, liver, and kidneys (adrenergic fibers); increase in arterial blood pressure
Exercise	Continued sympathetic cholinergic outflow; alterations in local metabolic conditions due to hypoxia ($\downarrow$pH, $\uparrow P_{CO_2}$, $\uparrow$ADP, $\uparrow Mg^{++}$, $\uparrow Ca^{++}$, $\uparrow$NO, $\uparrow$temperature)	Further dilation of muscle vasculature
	Continued sympathetic adrenergic outflow in conjunction with epinephrine and norepinephrine from the adrenal medulla	Concomitant constriction of vasculature in inactive tissues to maintain, adequate perfusion pressure throughout the arterial system
		Venous vessels stiffen to reduce their capacity
		Venoconstriction facilitates venous return and maintains the central blood volume

At the start of exercise or even slightly before exercise begins, nerve centers above the medullary region initiate cardiovascular activity. The adjustments increase the rate and pumping strength of the heart and alter regional blood flow in direct proportion to exercise intensity. As exercise continues and becomes more intense, sympathetic cholinergic outflow plus local metabolic factors acting on chemosensitive nerves and directly on blood vessels dilate resistance vessels in the active musculature. Reduced peripheral resistance permits muscle tissue to accommodate greater blood flow. Constrictor adjustments in less active tissues maintain adequate perfusion pressure despite dilatation of the muscle's vasculature. Vasoconstriction in non-active areas (e.g., kidneys and gastrointestinal tract) also promotes blood redistribution to meet specific tissues' metabolic requirements during exercise.

Factors that affect venous return play an equally important role as those regulating arterial flow. Muscle and ventilatory pump action and stiffening of veins through neural stimulation propel blood into the central circulation and toward the right ventricle. This balances cardiac output and venous return.

SUMMARY

1. The cardiovascular system rapidly regulates heart rate and distributes blood while maintaining blood pressure in response to the metabolic and physiologic demands of increased physical activity.

2. The cardiac impulse originates at the SA node. It then travels across the atria to the AV node; after a brief delay, it spreads rapidly across the large ventricular mass. With a normal conduction pattern, the atria and ventricles contract effectively to provide the impetus for blood flow.

3. The ECG displays a record of the sequence of myocardial electrical events during a cardiac cycle.

4. The majority of heart rhythm irregularities (arrhythmias) involve extra beats (extrasystoles). Atrial arrhythmias generally do not compromise the heart's pumping ability. Ventricular fibrillation, the most serious arrhythmia, results from repetitive, spontaneous discharge of portions of the ventricular mass.

5. The sympathetic catecholamines epinephrine and norepinephrine accelerate heart rate and increase myocardial contractility. Acetylcholine, a parasympathetic neurotransmitter, slows heart rate via the vagus nerve.

6. Increases in temperature, carbon dioxide, acidity, adenosine, NO, and magnesium and potassium ions provide potent stimuli to autoregulate blood flow in active tissues. Of these, NO occupies a role of considerable importance as a "relaxer" of arteriole smooth muscle.

7. The heart "turns on" in transition from rest to exercise from increased sympathetic and decreased parasympathetic activity.

8. Neural and hormonal extrinsic factors modify the heart's inherent rhythmicity. The heart can accelerate rapidly in anticipation of exercise and increase to more than 200 b·min^{-1} in maximum exercise.

9. Carotid artery palpation accurately measures heart rate during and immediately after exercise. In certain medical conditions, pressure against the carotid artery reflexly slows the heart, which underestimates the actual exercise heart rate.

10. Cortical stimulation immediately before and during the initial stages of physical activity accounts for a substantial part of the heart rate adjustment to exercise.

11. Regulation of blood flow occurs when nerves, hormones, and local metabolic factors alter the internal diameter of smooth muscle bands in blood vessels.

12. Vasoconstriction occurs when adrenergic sympathetic fibers release norepinephrine; cholinergic sympathetic neurons secrete acetylcholine that triggers vasodilation.

 T H O U G H T   Q U E S T I O N S

1. Give a physiologic rationale for biofeedback and relaxation techniques to treat hypertension and stress-related disorders.

2. If heart transplantation surgically removes all nerves to the myocardium, explain why heart rate increases for these patients during exercise.

3. The Romans executed criminals by tying their arms and legs to a cross mounted in the vertical position. Discuss the physiologic responses that would cause death under these circumstances.

| **Part 3** | **Cardiovascular Dynamics During Exercise** |

CARDIAC OUTPUT

Cardiac output provides the most important indicator of the circulatory system's functional capacity to meet the demands for physical activity. As with any pump, the rate of pumping (**heart rate**) and quantity of blood ejected with each stroke (**stroke volume**) determine the heart's output of blood:

$$\text{Cardiac output} = \text{Heart rate} \times \text{Stroke volume}$$

The relationship between cardiac output, oxygen uptake, and difference between the oxygen content of arterial and mixed-venous blood (a–$\bar{v}$O$_2$ difference) embodies the principle discovered by German physiologist Adolph Fick (1829–1901) in 1870.

$$\text{Cardiac output, mL} \cdot \text{min}^{-1} = [\dot{V}O_2, \text{mL} \cdot \text{min}^{-1} \div$$
$$\text{a–}\bar{v}O_2 \text{ diff, mL} \cdot \text{dL blood}^{-1}] \times 100$$

RESTING CARDIAC OUTPUT: UNTRAINED VERSUS TRAINED

Each minute, the left ventricle ejects the entire 5-L blood volume of an average-sized man. This value pertains to most individuals, but stroke volume and heart rate vary considerably depending on cardiovascular fitness status. A heart rate of about 70 b·min^{-1} sustains the average adult's 5-L (5000 mL) resting cardiac output. Substituting this heart rate value in the cardiac output equation (Cardiac output = Stroke volume × Heart rate; Stroke volume = Cardiac output ÷ Heart rate) yields a calculated stroke volume of 71 mL·b^{-1}.

Questions & Notes

Cardiac output = _____ ×

_____ .

Blood flow from the heart increases in direct proportion to exercise

_____ .

Give typical cardiac output values for untrained versus trained during rest and maximal exercise.

	Trained	Untrained
Rest	_____	_____
Maximal Exercise	_____	_____

Draw and label the relationship between stroke volume and percent $\dot{V}O_{2max}$.

The resting heart rate for an endurance athlete averages close to 50 b·min⁻¹. The athlete's resting cardiac output also averages 5 L·min⁻¹ as blood circulates with a proportionately larger stroke volume of 100 mL per beat (5000 mL ÷ 50 b). Stroke volumes for women usually average 25% below values for men with equivalent training. The smaller body size of the typical woman chiefly accounts for this "gender difference."

The table in the box below summarizes average values for cardiac output, heart rate, and stroke volume for endurance-trained and untrained men at rest:

	Cardiac Output (mL·min⁻¹)	Heart Rate (b·min⁻¹)	Stroke Volume (mL·b⁻¹)
Untrained	5000	70	71
Trained	5000	50	100

The underlying mechanisms for the heart rate and stroke volume differences between trained and untrained individuals remain unclear. Does the bradycardia that accompanies increased aerobic fitness "cause" a larger stroke volume, or vice versa, because the myocardium becomes strengthened and internal ventricular dimensions increase with training? The following two factors probably interact as aerobic fitness improves:

1. Increased vagal tone slows the heart, allowing more time for ventricular filling
2. Enlarged ventricular volume and a more powerful myocardium eject a larger volume of blood with each systole

EXERCISE CARDIAC OUTPUT: UNTRAINED VERSUS TRAINED

Blood flow from the heart increases in direct proportion to exercise intensity for both trained and untrained individuals. From rest to steady-rate exercise, cardiac output increases rapidly, followed by a more gradual increase until it plateaus as blood flow matches exercise metabolic requirements.

In sedentary, college-age men, cardiac output in maximal aerobic exercise increases about four times the resting level to an average maximum of 22 L of blood per minute. Maximum heart rate for these young adults averages 195 b·min⁻¹. Consequently, stroke volume averages 113 mL of blood per beat during exercise (22,000 mL ÷ 195 b). In contrast, world-class endurance athletes generate maximum cardiac outputs of 35 L·min⁻¹, with a similar or slightly lower maximum heart rate than untrained counterparts. The difference between maximum cardiac output of both individuals relates *solely* to differences in

stroke volume. The table in the box below summarizes average values for cardiac output, heart rate, and stroke volume of endurance-trained and untrained men during maximal exercise:

	Cardiac Output (mL·min⁻¹)	Heart Rate (b·min⁻¹)	Stroke Volume (mL·b⁻¹)
Untrained	22,000	195	113
Trained	35,000	195	179

EXERCISE STROKE VOLUME

Figure 10.11 relates stroke volume and percentage $\dot{V}O_{2max}$ (to better equate exercise intensity among subjects) for eight healthy college-age men during graded exercise on a cycle ergometer. Stroke volume increases progressively with exercise to about 50% $\dot{V}O_{2max}$ and then gradually levels off until termination of exercise. For several subjects, stroke volume decreased slightly at near-maximal exercise intensities.

Stroke Volume and $\dot{V}O_{2max}$

Stroke volume clearly differentiates people with high and low $\dot{V}O_{2max}$. For example, three groups of subjects were studied: (1) patients with mitral stenosis, a valvular disease that causes inadequate emptying of the left ventricle; (2) healthy but sedentary men; and (3) athletes. Differences in $\dot{V}O_{2max}$ among the groups closely paralleled differences in maximal stroke volume. Aerobic capacity and maximum stroke volume of mitral stenosis patients averaged half the values of sedentary subjects. This close linkage also emerges in comparisons among healthy subjects; a 60% larger stroke volume in athletes compared with sedentary men paralleled the 62% larger $\dot{V}O_{2max}$. All groups showed fairly similar maximum heart rates; thus, stroke

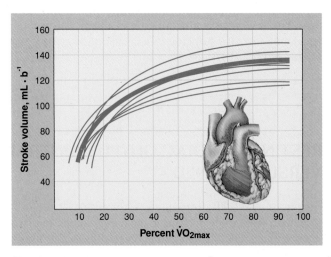

Figure 10.11 Stroke volume (mL·b⁻¹) related to increasing exercise intensity (percent maximal oxygen consumption [$\dot{V}O_{2max}$]) for eight healthy male subjects. (Data from the Applied Physiology Laboratory, University of Michigan.)

volume differences accounted for the variations in maximum cardiac output and $\dot{V}O_{2max}$ among groups.

Stroke Volume Increases During Rest and Exercise

Three physiologic mechanisms increase the heart's stroke volume during exercise.

1. The first, intrinsic to the myocardium, involves enhanced cardiac filling in diastole followed by a more forceful systolic contraction.
2. Neurohormonal influence governs the second mechanism, which involves normal ventricular filling with a subsequent forceful ejection and emptying during systole.
3. The third mechanism comes from training adaptations that expand blood volume and reduce resistance to blood flow in peripheral tissues.

Greater Systolic Emptying Versus Enhanced Diastolic Filling

Greater ventricular filling in diastole during the cardiac cycle occurs through any factor that increases venous return (**preload**) or slows heart rate. An increase in end-diastolic volume stretches myocardial fibers, causing a powerful ejection stroke as the heart contracts. This expels the normal stroke volume plus the additional blood that entered the ventricles and stretched the myocardium.

German physiologist Otto Frank (1865–1944) and British colleague Ernest H. Starling's (1866–1927) experiments with animals in the early 1900s first described relationships between muscle force and resting fiber length. Improved contractility of a stretched muscle (within a limited range) probably relates to a more optimum arrangement of intracellular myofilaments as the muscle stretches. **Frank-Starling's law of the heart** describes this phenomenon applied to the myocardium.

For many years, physiologists taught the Frank-Starling mechanism as the main cause of increases in stroke volume during exercise. They believed that enhanced venous return in exercise caused greater cardiac filling, which stretched the ventricles in diastole to produce a more forceful ejection. In all likelihood, this pattern describes stroke volume response in transition from rest to exercise or when a person moves from the upright to recumbent position. Enhanced diastolic filling probably also occurs in activities such as swimming, in which the body's horizontal position optimizes venous return and myocardial preload.

Body position affects circulatory dynamics. Cardiac output and stroke volume reach the highest and most stable levels in a horizontal position. *Near-maximal stroke volume occurs at rest in a horizontal position and increases only slightly during exercise.* In contrast, gravity's effect in the upright position counters venous return and lowers stroke volume. This postural effect becomes prominent when comparing circulatory dynamics at rest in the upright and supine positions. As upright exercise intensity increases, stroke volume also increases to approach the maximum value in the supine position.

In most forms of upright exercise, the heart does not fill to an extent that increases cardiac volume to values observed in the recumbent position. The increase in stroke volume during exercise likely results from the *combined effects* of enhanced diastolic filling *and* more complete systolic emptying. In both the recumbent and upright positions, the heart's stroke volume increases in exercise despite resistance to flow from increased systolic pressure, called **afterload**.

At rest in the upright position, 40% to 50% of the total end-diastolic blood volume remains in the left ventricle after systole; this **functional residual volume of the heart** amounts to 50 to 70 mL of blood. The sympathetic hormones epinephrine and norepinephrine increase myocardial stroke power and systolic emptying during exercise; this reduces the heart's residual blood volume from enhanced systolic ejection.

More than likely, endurance training also increases compliance of the left ventricle (reduced cardiac stiffness) to facilitate its ability to accept blood in the

$\mathcal{Q}$*uestions & Notes*

Name the 3 physiologic mechanisms that increase the heart's stroke volume during exercise.

1.

2.

3.

Briefly describe Frank-Starling's law of the heart.

Describe the body position that produces near-maximal for stroke volume at rest.

The functional residual volume of the heart at rest in the upright position averages _____ mL.

Briefly describe the relationship between stroke volume and exercise

What is another name for increased venous return?

diastolic phase of the cardiac cycle. Whether endurance training enhances the myocardium's *innate* contractile state remains unclear. This adaptation would contribute to a larger stroke volume.

Cardiovascular Drift: Reduced Stroke Volume and Increased Heart Rate During Prolonged Exercise

Submaximal exercise for more than 15 minutes, particularly in the heat, produces progressive water loss through sweating and a fluid shift from plasma to tissues. A rise in core temperature also causes redistribution of blood to the periphery for body cooling. At the same time, the progressive decrease in plasma volume decreases central venous cardiac filling pressure that reduces stroke volume. A reduced stroke volume initiates a compensatory heart rate increase to maintain a nearly constant cardiac output as exercise progresses. The term **cardiovascular drift** describes this gradual time-dependent downward "drift" in several cardiovascular responses, most notably stroke volume with concomitant heart rate increase, during prolonged steady-rate exercise. Under these circumstances, a person usually must exercise at a lower intensity than if cardiovascular drift did not occur.

One explanation for cardiovascular drift suggests that a stroke volume decline during prolonged exercise in a thermoneutral environment relates to an increased exercise heart rate and not increased cutaneous blood flow, as hypothesized by some researchers. More than likely, the progressive increase in exercise heart rate with cardiovascular drift decreases end-diastolic volume, subsequently reducing the heart's stroke volume.

EXERCISE HEART RATE

Graded Exercise

Figure 10.12 depicts the relationship between heart rate and oxygen uptake during increasing intensity exercise (graded exercise) to maximum for endurance trained individuals and sedentary counterparts. Heart rate for the untrained person accelerates relatively rapidly with increasing exercise demands; a much smaller heart rate increase occurs for the trained person. The trained person achieves a higher level of exercise oxygen uptake at a particular submaximal heart rate than a sedentary person. Maximum heart rate and the heart rate–oxygen uptake relationship remain fairly consistent for a particular individual from day to day, although the slope of the relationship decreases considerably from the stroke volume increases with aerobic training.

Submaximum Exercise

Heart rate increases rapidly and levels off within several minutes during submaximum steady-rate exercise. A subsequent increase in exercise intensity increases heart rate to a new plateau as the body attempts to match the cardio-

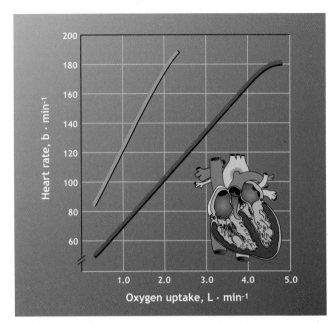

Figure 10.12 Generalized response for heart rate in relation to oxygen uptake during exercise for endurance-trained individuals (*red line*) and sedentary counterparts (*green line*).

vascular response to the metabolic demands. Each increment in exercise intensity requires progressively more time to achieve heart rate stabilization.

CARDIAC OUTPUT DISTRIBUTION

Blood flow to specific tissues increases in proportion to their metabolic activities.

At Rest

Figure 10.13A shows the approximate distribution of a 5-L cardiac output at rest. More than one-fourth of the cardiac output flows to the liver; one-fifth flows to kidneys and muscles; and the remainder diverts to the heart, skin, brain, and other tissues.

During Exercise

Figure 10.13B illustrates the distribution of cardiac output to various tissues during intense aerobic exercise. *Regional blood flow varies considerably depending on environmental conditions, level of fatigue, and exercise mode, yet active muscles receive a disproportionately large portion of the cardiac output in exercise.* Each 100 g of muscle receives 4 to 7 mL of blood per minute during rest. Muscle blood flow increases steadily during exercise to reach a maximum of between 50 to 75 mL per 100 g of active muscle tissue.

Blood Flow Redistribution The increase in muscle blood flow with exercise comes largely from increased cardiac output. Neural and hormonal vascular regulation,

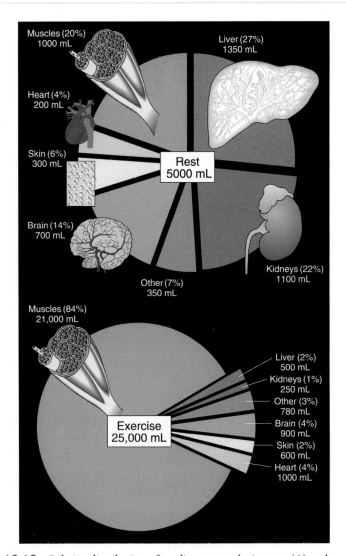

Figure 10.13 Relative distribution of cardiac output during rest (**A**) and strenuous endurance exercise (**B**). The *numbers in parentheses* indicate the percent of total cardiac output. Despite its large mass, muscle tissue receives about the same amount of blood as the much smaller kidneys at rest. In strenuous exercise, however, nearly 85% of the total cardiac output diverts to active muscles.

*Q*uestions & Notes

Describe the difference in blood flow distribution between rest and exercise.

What is cardiovascular drift?

Describe the general relationship between HR and $\dot{V}O_2$, up to maximum levels.

including local metabolic conditions within muscles moves blood through active muscles from areas that temporarily tolerate a reduction in normal blood flow. Shunting of blood away from specific tissues occurs primarily in intense exercise. Blood flow to the skin increases during light and moderate exercise, so metabolic heat generated in muscle can dissipate at the skin's surface. During intense, short-duration exercise, however, cutaneous blood flow decreases even when exercising in a hot environment.

In some tissues, blood flow during exercise decreases four-fifths of the flow at rest. The kidneys and splanchnic tissues use only 10% to 25% of the oxygen available in their blood supply at rest. Consequently, these tissues tolerate a considerably reduced blood flow before oxygen demand exceeds supply and compromises organ function. With reduced blood flow, increased oxygen extraction from available blood maintains the tissue's oxygen needs. The visceral organs tolerate substantially reduced blood flow for more than 1 hour during intense exercise. This "frees" as much as 600 mL of oxygen each minute for use by active musculature.

Blood Flow to the Heart and Brain The myocardium and brain cannot compromise their blood supplies. At rest, the myocardium normally uses

75% of the oxygen in the blood flowing through the coronary circulation. With such a limited "margin of safety," increased coronary blood flow primarily meets the heart's oxygen demands. Cerebral blood flow increases up to 30% with exercise compared with rest; the largest portion of any "extra" blood probably moves to areas related to motor functions.

CARDIAC OUTPUT AND OXYGEN TRANSPORT

At Rest

Each 100 mL (deciliter [dL]) of arterial blood normally carries about 20 mL of oxygen or 200 mL of oxygen per liter of blood at sea level conditions (see Chapter 9). Trained and untrained adults circulate 5 L of blood each minute at rest, so potentially 1000 mL of oxygen becomes available during 1 minute (5 L blood × 200 mL O_2). Resting oxygen uptake averages only about 250 mL·min^{-1}; this means 750 mL of oxygen returns "unused" to the heart. This does not represent an unnecessary waste of cardiac output. To the contrary, extra oxygen in the blood above the resting needs maintains oxygen in reserve—a margin of safety for immediate use if the need arises.

During Exercise

A person with a maximum heart rate of 200 b·min^{-1} and a stroke volume of 80 mL per beat generates a maximum cardiac output of 16 L (200 b·min^{-1} × 0.080 L). Even during maximum exercise, hemoglobin remains fully saturated with oxygen, so each liter of arterial blood carries about 200 mL of oxygen. Consequently, 3200 mL of oxygen circulate each minute via a 16-L cardiac output (16 L × 200 mL O_2). If the body extracted all of the oxygen delivered in a 16-L cardiac output, $\dot{V}O_{2max}$ would equal 3200 mL. This represents the theoretical upper limit for this person because the oxygen needs of tissues such as the brain do not increase greatly with exercise, yet they require an uninterrupted blood supply.

An increase in maximum cardiac output directly improves a person's capacity to circulate oxygen and profoundly impacts the maximal oxygen consumption. If the heart's stroke volume increased from 80 to 200 mL while the maximum heart rate remained unchanged at 200 b·min^{-1}, the maximum cardiac output would dramatically increase to 40 L·min^{-1}. This means that the amount of oxygen circulated in maximum exercise each minute increases approximately 2.5 times from 3200 to 8000 mL (40 L × 200 mL O_2).

Maximum Cardiac Output and $\dot{V}O_{2max}$

Figure 10.14 displays the relationship between maximum cardiac output and $\dot{V}O_{2max}$ and includes values representative of sedentary individuals and elite endurance athletes. An unmistakable relationship emerges. Whereas a low aerobic capacity links closely to a low maximum cardiac

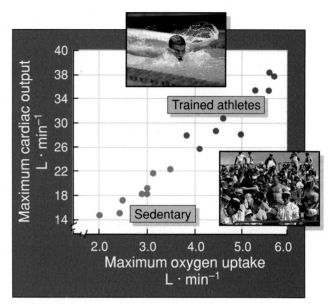

Figure 10.14 Relationship between maximal cardiac output and maximal oxygen uptake in trained and untrained individuals. Maximal cardiac output relates to maximal oxygen consumption ($\dot{V}O_{2max}$) in a ratio of about 6:1. (Swimmer photo courtesy of Jim Richardson, University of Michigan.)

output, a 30- to 40-L cardiac output always accompanies the ability to generate a 5- or 6-L $\dot{V}O_{2max}$.

Cardiac Output Differences Among Men, Women, and Children

Cardiac output and oxygen consumption remain linearly related during graded exercise for boys and girls and men and women. Teenage and adult females generally exercise at any level of submaximal oxygen consumption with a 5% to 10% larger cardiac output than males. Any apparent gender difference in submaximal cardiac output most likely results from the 10% lower hemoglobin concentration in women than in men. A proportionate increase in submaximal cardiac output compensates for this small gender-related decrease in the blood's oxygen-carrying capacity.

Higher heart rates in children than in adults during submaximal treadmill and cycle ergometer exercise do not fully compensate for their smaller stroke volume. This produces a smaller cardiac output for children at a given submaximal exercise oxygen consumption. Consequently, the a–$\bar{v}O_2$ difference expands to satisfy the oxygen requirements. The biologic significance of this difference in central circulatory function between children and adults remains unclear.

EXTRACTION OF OXYGEN: THE a–$\bar{v}O_2$ DIFFERENCE

If blood flow were the only means for increasing a tissue's oxygen supply, cardiac output would need to increase from 5 L·min^{-1} at rest to 100 L in maximum exercise to achieve a 20-fold increase in oxygen uptake, an oxygen uptake increase common among endurance athletes. Fortunately, intense exercise does not require such a large cardiac output because hemoglobin releases its considerable "extra" oxygen from blood perfusing active tissues.

Two mechanisms for oxygen supply increase a person's oxygen uptake capacity:

1. Increased tissue blood flow
2. Use of the relatively large quantity of oxygen that remains unused by tissues at rest (i.e., expand the a–$\bar{v}O_2$ difference)

The following rearrangement of the Fick equation summarizes the important relationship between maximum cardiac output, maximum a–$\bar{v}O_2$ difference, and $\dot{V}O_{2max}$:

$$\dot{V}O_{2max} = \textbf{Maximum cardiac output} \times \textbf{Maximum a–}\bar{v}O_2 \textbf{ difference}$$

The a–$\bar{v}O_2$ Difference During Rest and Exercise

Figure 10.15 shows a representative pattern for changes in a–$\bar{v}O_2$ difference from rest to maximum exercise for physically active men. A similar pattern emerges for women except that the arterial oxygen content averages 5% to 10% lower because of lower hemoglobin concentrations. The figure includes values for the oxygen content of arterial blood and mixed-venous blood during different exercise intensities. Arterial blood oxygen content varies little from its value of 20 mL·dL^{-1} at rest throughout the full exercise intensity range. In contrast, mixed-venous oxygen content varies between 12 and 15 mL·dL^{-1} at rest to a low of 2 to 4 mL·dL^{-1} during maximum exercise. The difference between arterial and mixed-venous blood oxygen content (a–$\bar{v}O_2$ difference) at any time represents oxygen extraction from blood as it circulates through the body's tissues. At rest, for example, a–$\bar{v}O_2$ difference equals 5 mL of oxygen, or only

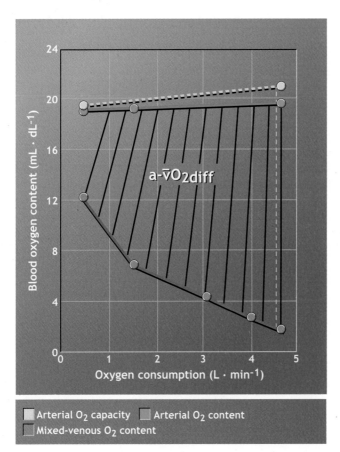

Figure 10.15 Changes in a–$\bar{v}O_2$ difference from rest of maximal exercise in physically active men.

Questions & Notes

Describe the relationship between $\dot{V}O_{2max}$ and maximum cardiac output.

Give one reason why females have a larger cardiac output compared to males at the same absolute sub-maximum $\dot{V}O_2$.

List 2 mechanisms for how oxygen supply leads to an increase in oxygen uptake capacity.

1.

2.

How much O_2 is carried in each dL of blood?

Describe the relationship between maximum cardiac output, maximum a–$\bar{v}O_2$ difference and $\dot{V}O_{2\,max}$.

25% of the blood's oxygen content (5 mL ÷ 20 mL × 100); 75% of the oxygen returns "unused" to the heart bound to hemoglobin.

The progressive expansion of the a–$\bar{v}O_2$ difference to at least three times the resting value occurs from a reduced venous oxygen content, which, in maximal exercise, approaches 20 mL in the active muscle (all oxygen extracted). The oxygen content of a true mixed-venous sample from the pulmonary artery rarely falls below 2 to 4 mL·dL^{-1} because blood returning from active tissues mixes with oxygen-rich venous blood from metabolically less active regions.

Figure 10.15 also indicates that the capacity of each dL of arterial blood to carry oxygen actually increases during exercise. This results from an increased concentration of red blood cells (hemoconcentration) from the progressive movement of fluid from the plasma to the interstitial space because of two factors:

1. Increases in capillary hydrostatic pressure as blood pressure increases
2. Metabolic byproducts of exercise metabolism create an osmotic pressure that draws fluid from the plasma into tissue spaces

FACTORS AFFECTING THE EXERCISE a–$\bar{v}O_2$ DIFFERENCE

Central and peripheral factors interact to increase oxygen extraction in active tissue during exercise. Diverting a large portion of the cardiac output to active muscles influences the magnitude of the a–$\bar{v}O_2$ difference in maximal exercise. As mentioned previously, some tissues temporarily compromise blood supply during exercise by redistributing blood to make more oxygen available for muscle metabolism. Exercise training facilitates redirection of the central circulation to active muscle.

Increases in skeletal muscle microcirculation with endurance training also increase tissue oxygen extraction. Muscle biopsy specimens from the quadriceps femoris show a relatively large ratio of capillaries to muscle fibers in individuals who exhibit large a–$\bar{v}O_2$ differences in intense exercise. An increase in the capillary-to-fiber ratio reflects a positive training adaptation that enlarges the interface for nutrient and gas exchange during exercise. Individual muscle cells' ability to generate energy aerobically represents another important factor governing oxygen extraction capacity.

CARDIOVASCULAR ADJUSTMENTS TO UPPER-BODY EXERCISE

The highest oxygen uptake during upper-body exercise generally averages between 70% to 80% of the $\dot{V}O_{2max}$ in bicycle and treadmill exercise. Similarly, maximal heart rate and pulmonary ventilation remain lower in exercise with the arms. The relatively smaller muscle mass of the upper body largely accounts for these physiologic differences. The lower maximal heart rate in exercise that activates a smaller muscle mass most likely results from the following:

1. Reduced output stimulation from the motor cortex central command to the cardiovascular center in the medulla (less feedforward stimulation)
2. Reduced feedback stimulation to the medulla from the smaller active musculature

In submaximal exercise, the metabolic and cardiovascular response pattern between upper- and lower-body exercise reverses. **Figure 10.16** shows that any level of submaximal power output produces a higher oxygen uptake with arm compared with leg exercise. This difference remains small during light exercise but becomes progressively larger as intensity of effort increases. Lower economy of effort in arm-crank exercise probably results

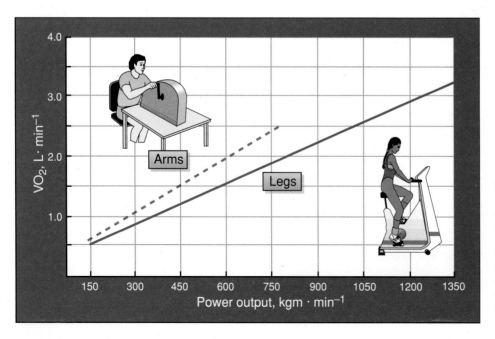

Figure 10.16 Arm (upper-body) exercise requires a greater oxygen uptake compared with leg (lower-body) exercise at any power output throughout the comparison range. The largest differences occur during intense exercise. Average data for men and women. (From Laboratory of Applied Physiology, Queens College, NY.)

from static muscle actions that do not produce external work but consume extra oxygen. In addition, the extra musculature activated to stabilize the torso during most forms of arm exercise adds to the oxygen requirement. Upper-body exercise also produces greater physiologic strain (heart rate, blood pressure, pulmonary ventilation, and perception of physical effort) for any level of oxygen uptake (or percentage of maximal oxygen uptake) than lower-body leg exercise.

Understanding differences in physiologic response between upper- and lower-body exercise enables the clinician to formulate prudent exercise programs using both exercise modes. A standard exercise load (e.g., power output or oxygen consumption) produces greater physiologic strain with the arms, so exercise prescriptions based on running and bicycling *cannot* be applied to upper-body exercise. Also, $\dot{V}O_{2max}$ for arm exercises does not strongly correlate with leg exercise $\dot{V}O_{2max}$; thus, one cannot predict accurately one's aerobic capacity for arm exercise from a test using the legs and vice versa. *This further substantiates the concept of aerobic fitness specificity.*

 For Your Information

IMPORTANT LOCAL ADAPTATIONS

Increasing the size and number of mitochondria and augmenting aerobic enzyme activity with regular exercise improves a muscle's metabolic capacity in exercise. Local vascular and metabolic improvements within muscle ultimately enhance its capacity to produce ATP aerobically. These local training adaptations translate to an increased oxygen extraction capacity of the active muscles.

SUMMARY

1. Cardiac output reflects the functional capacity of the circulatory system. Heart rate and stroke volume determine the heart's output capacity in the following relationship: Cardiac output = Heart rate × Stroke volume.

2. Cardiac output increases in proportion to exercise intensity from about 5 L·min^{-1} at rest to an exercise maximum of 20 to 25 L·min^{-1} in untrained college-age men and to 35 to 40 L·min^{-1} in elite male endurance athletes.

3. Differences in maximum cardiac output primarily relate to individual differences in the heart's maximum stroke volume.

4. During upright exercise, stroke volume increases during the transition from rest to moderate exercise, reaching maximum at about 50% $\dot{V}O_{2max}$. Thereafter, increases in heart rate increase cardiac output.

5. Stroke volume increases in upright exercise generally result from interactions between greater ventricular filling during diastole and more complete emptying during systole. Sympathetic hormones that augment myocardial force generated during systole increase stroke volume.

6. Training adaptations that expand blood volume and reduce resistance to blood flow in peripheral tissues also contribute to an enhanced stroke volume.

7. Heart rate and oxygen uptake relate linearly throughout the major portion of the exercise range in trained and untrained individuals. Endurance training shifts the heart rate–oxygen uptake line to the right because of an improved stroke volume.

8. Local metabolism generally determines blood flow in specific tissues; it causes substantial diversion of cardiac output to active muscles during exercise. Kidneys and splanchnic regions temporarily compromise their blood supplies to reroute blood to active muscles.

9. Maximum cardiac output and maximum a–$\bar{v}O_2$ difference determine $\dot{V}O_{2max}$ in the following relationship: $\dot{V}O_{2max}$ = Maximum cardiac output × Maximum a–$\bar{v}O_2$ difference.

10. Large cardiac outputs clearly differentiate endurance athletes from untrained counterparts. Training also expands the maximum a–$\bar{v}O_2$ difference.

11. Upper-body arm cranking exercise generates about a 25% lower $\dot{V}O_{2max}$ than exercise with the lower body (running or cycling).

12. For any level of submaximal power output or oxygen uptake, exercise with the arms produces greater physiologic strain than lower-body exercise.

THOUGHT QUESTIONS

1. Moderate increases in hemoglobin concentration increase $\dot{V}O_{2max}$ during maximal exercise at sea level. This effect supports the contention that what component of the maximal oxygen consumption equation, oxygen delivery or oxygen utilization becomes the limiting factor in $\dot{V}O_{2max}$? Discuss.

2. How would factors that influence the a–$\bar{v}O_2$ difference in maximal exercise explain the specificity of $\dot{V}O_{2max}$ improvement with different modes of aerobic training?

SELECTED REFERENCES

ACSM position stand: Exercise and hypertension. *Med. Sci. Sports Exerc.*, 36:533, 2004.

Beckett, N., et al.: Treatment of hypertension in patients 80 years of age or older. *N. Engl. J. Med.*, 358:1887, 2008.

Bolad, I., Delafontaine, P.: Endothelial dysfunction: its role in hypertensive coronary disease. *Curr. Opin. Cardiol.*, 20:270, 2005.

Buckwalter, J.B., et al.: Role of nitric oxide in exercise sympatholysis. *J. Appl. Physiol.*, 97:417, 2004.

Carter, J.B., et al.: The effect of age and gender on heart rate variability after endurance training. *Med. Sci. Sports Exerc.*, 35:1333, 2003.

Chobanian, A.V., et al.: The Seventh Report of the Joint National Committee on Prevention, Detection, Evaluation, and Treatment of High Blood Pressure: the JNC 7 report. *JAMA*, 289:2560, 2003.

Clifford, P.S., Hellsten, Y.: Vasodilatory mechanisms in contracting skeletal muscle: *J. Appl. Physiol.*, 97:393, 2004.

Coyle, E.F., González-Alonso, J.: Cardiovascular drift during prolonged exercise: new perspectives. *Exer. Sport Sci. Rev.*, 28:88, 2001.

DeVan, A.E., et al.: Acute effects of resistance exercise on arterial compliance. *J. Appl. Physiol.*, 98:2287, 2005.

Dibrezzo, R., et al.: Exercise intervention designed to improve strength and dynamic balance among community-dwelling older adults. *J. Aging Phys. Act.*, 13:198, 2005.

Dujic, Z., et al.: Postexercise hypotension in moderately trained athletes after maximal exercise. *Med. Sci. Sports Exerc.*, 38:318, 2006.

Farias, M. 3rd, et al.: Plasma ATP during exercise: possible role in regulation of coronary blood flow. *Am. J. Physiol. Heart Circ. Physiol.*, 288:H1586, 2005.

Fu, Q., et al.: Cardiac origins of the postural orthostatic tachycardia syndrome. *J. Am. Coll. Cardiol.*, 22;55:2858, 2010.

Ganio, M.S., et al.: Fluid ingestion attenuates the decline in $\dot{V}O_{2peak}$ associated with cardiovascular drift. *Med. Sci. Sports Exerc.*, 38:901, 2006.

Goodman, J.M., et al.: Left ventricular adaptations following short-term endurance training. *J. Appl. Physiol.*, 2005;98:454.

González-Alonso, J.: Point:Counterpoint: Stroke volume does/does not decline during exercise at maximal effort in healthy individuals. *J. Appl. Physiol.*, 104:275, 2008.

Halliwill, J.R., et al.: Peripheral and baroreflex interactions in cardiovascular regulation in humans. *J. Physiol.*, 1:552(Pt 1), 2003.

Harvey, P.J., et al.: Hemodynamic after-effects of acute dynamic exercise in sedentary normotensive postmenopausal women. *J. Hypertens.*, 23:285, 2005.

Heinonen, I., et al.: Role of adenosine in regulating the heterogeneity of skeletal muscle blood flow during exercise in humans. *J. Appl. Physiol.*, 103:2042, 2007.

Houzi, P., et al.: Sensing vascular distension in skeletal muscle by slow conducting afferent fibers: neurophysiological basis and implication for respiratory control. *J. Appl. Physiol.*, 96:407, 2004.

Izquierdo, M., et al.: Effects of combined resistance and cardiovascular training on strength, power, muscle cross-sectional area, and endurance markers in middle-aged men. *Eur. J. Appl. Physiol.*, 94:70, 2005.

Jakovljevic, D.G., et al.: Comparison of cardiac power output and exercise performance in patients with left ventricular assist devices, explanted (recovered) patients, and those with moderate to severe heart failure. *Am. J. Cardiol.*, 105:1780, 2010.

Ketelhut, G., et al.: Regular exercise as an effective approach in antihypertensive therapy. *Med. Sci. Sports Exerc.*, 36:4, 2004.

Keramidas, M.E., et al.: Enhancement of the finger cold-induced vasodilation response with exercise training. *Eur. J. Appl. Physiol.*, 109:133, 2010.

Lafrenz, A.J., et al.: Effect of ambient temperature on cardiovascular drift and maximal oxygen uptake. *Med. Sci. Sports Exerc.*, 40:1065, 2008.

Lawes, C.M., et al.: Blood pressure and stroke: an overview of published reviews. *Stroke*, 35:1024, 2004.

Lee, S.M., et al.: Aerobic exercise deconditioning and countermeasures during bed rest. *Aviat. Space Environ. Med.*, 81:52, 2010.

Lockwood, J.M., et al.: Postexercise hypotension is not explained by a prostaglandin-dependent peripheral vasodilation. *J. Appl. Physiol.*, 98:447, 2005.

Lott, M.E., Sinoway, L.I.: What has microdialysis shown us about the metabolic milieu within exercising skeletal muscle? *Exerc. Sport Sci. Rev.*, 32:69, 2004.

Lucas, J.W., et al.: Summary health statistics for U.S. adults: National Health Interview Survey, 2001. *Vital Health Stat.*, 10. 218:1, 2004.

MacDonnell, S.M., et al.: Improved myocardial beta-adrenergic responsiveness and signaling with exercise training in hypertension. *Circulation*, 111:3420, 2005.

Marwood, S., et al.: Faster pulmonary oxygen uptake kinetics in trained versus untrained male adolescents. *Med. Sci. Sports Exerc.*, 42:127, 2010.

Mattsson, C.M., et al.: Reversed drift in heart rate but increased oxygen uptake at fixed work rate during 24 h ultra-endurance exercise. *Scand. J. Med. Sci. Sports*, 20:298, 2010.

Mortensen, S.P., et al.: Limitations to systemic and locomotor limb muscle oxygen delivery and uptake during maximal exercise in humans. *J. Physiol.*, 566:273, 2005.

Nottin, S., et al.: Central and peripheral cardiovascular adaptations during maximal cycle exercise in boys and men. *Med. Sci. Sports Exerc.*, 34:456, 2002.

Padilla, J., et al.: Accumulation of physical activity reduces blood pressure in pre- and hypertension. *Med. Sci. Sports Exerc.*, 37:1264, 2005.

Pavlik, G., et al.: Echocardiographic data in Hungarian top-level water polo players. *Med. Sci. Sports Exerc.*, 37:323, 2005.

Patterson, J.A., et al.: Case report on PWC of a competitive cyclist before and after heart transplant. *Med. Sci. Sports Exerc.*, 39:1447, 2007.

Pricher, M.P., et al.: Regional hemdodynamics during postexercise hypotension. I. Splanchnic and renal circulations. *J. Appl. Physiol.*, 97:2065, 2004.

Rakobowchuk, M., et al.: Effect of whole body resistance training on arterial compliance in young men. *Exp. Physiol.*, 90:645, 2005.

Rankinen, T., et al.: Cardiorespiratory fitness, BMI, and risk of hypertension: The HYPGENE Study. *Med. Sci. Sports Exerc.*, 39:1687, 2007.

Rowell, L.B., et al.: Integration of cardiovascular control systems in dynamic exercises. In: *Handbook of Physiology.* Rowell, L.B., and Shepard, J. (eds.). New York: Oxford University Press, 1996.

Rowland, T., et al.: Cardiac responses to exercise in normal children: a synthesis. *Med. Sci. Sports Exerc.*, 32:253, 2000.

Sagiv, M., et al.: Left ventricular function at peak all-out anaerobic exercise in older men. *Gerontology*, 51:122, 2005.

Scharf, M., et al.: Cardiac magnetic resonance assessment of left and right ventricular morphologic and functional adaptations in professional soccer players. *Am. Heart J.*, 159:911, 2010.

Swain, D.P., Franklin, B.A.: Comparison of cardioprotective benefits of vigorous versus moderate intensity aerobic exercise. *Am. J. Cardiol.*, 97:141, 2006.

Thomas, G.D., Segal, S.S.: Neural control of muscle blood flow during exercise. *J. Appl. Physiol.*, 97:731, 2004.

Tordi, N., et al.: Intermittent versus constant aerobic exercise: effects on arterial stiffness. *Eur. J. Appl. Physiol.,* 108:801, 2010.

Tune, J.D., et al.: Matching coronary blood flow to myocardial oxygen consumption. *J. Appl. Physiol.*, 97:404, 2004.

Vieira, G.M., et al.: Intraocular pressure during weight lifting. *Arch. Ophthalmol.,* 124:1251, 2006.

Walther, C., et al.: The effect of exercise training on endothelial function in cardiovascular disease in humans. *Exerc. Sport Sci. Rev.*, 32:129, 2004.

Warburton, D.E., Haykowsky, M.J.: Impaired pulmonary oxygen uptake kinetics and reduced peak aerobic power during small muscle mass exercise in heart transplant recipients. *J. Appl. Physiol.*, 103:1722, 2007.

Williams, P.T.: Reduced diabetic, hypertensive, and cholesterol medication use with walking. *Med. Sci. Sports Exerc.*, 40:433, 2008.

Williams, P.T., Franklin, B.: Vigorous exercise and diabetic, hypertensive, and hypercholesterolemia medication use. *Med. Sci. Sports Exerc.*, 39:1933, 2007.

Wingo, J.E., et al.: Cardiovascular drift is related to reduced maximal oxygen uptake during heat stress. *Med. Sci. Sports Exerc.*, 37:248, 2005.

Young, D.R., et al.: Physical activity, cardiorespiratory fitness, and their relationship to cardiovascular risk factors in African Americans and non-African Americans with above-optimal blood pressure. *J. Comm. Health*, 30:107, 2005.

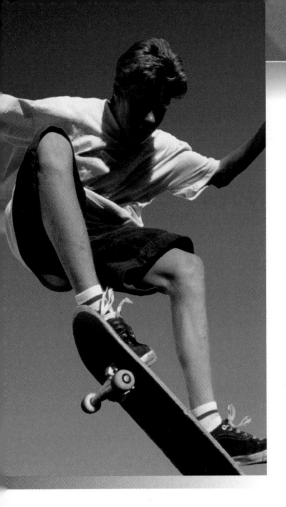

II

The Neuromuscular System and Exercise

CHAPTER OBJECTIVES

- Identify the major structural components of the central nervous system that control human movement.

- Diagram the anterior motoneuron and discuss its role in human movement.

- Draw and label the basic components of a reflex arc.

- Define *motor unit, neuromuscular junction, autonomic nervous system, excitatory postsynaptic potential,* and *inhibitory postsynaptic potential*.

- Explain factors associated with neuromuscular fatigue.

- Describe the function of muscle spindles and Golgi tendon organs.

- Draw and label a skeletal muscle fiber's ultrastructural components.

- Describe the sequence of chemical and mechanical events during skeletal muscle contraction and relaxation.

- Contrast slow- and fast-twitch muscle fiber characteristics including subdivisions.

- Outline muscle fiber-type distribution patterns among diverse groups of elite athletes.

- Explain how exercise training modifies muscle fibers and fiber types.

<table>
<tr><td>

Part 1

Neural Control of Human Movement

</td></tr>
</table>

Similarities exist between the most advanced supercomputer and the brain's highly sophisticated and intricate multiple-layer system of neurons and their interconnections to the muscular system. Not surprisingly, the integrative and organizational complexity of the human nervous system far exceeds the capacity of many clusters of supercomputers. Interactive neural control mechanisms selectively process bits of sensory input in response to ever-changing internal and external stimuli. Human movements that require little force, and sophisticated movements that require large force, depend on the coordinated reception and integration of sensory neural input to transmit and coordinate signals to the effector organs—the muscles.

This chapter describes the neural control of human movement that includes:

1. Structural organization of the neuromotor system, with emphasis on the central and peripheral nervous systems
2. Neuromuscular transmission
3. Sensory input for muscular activity
4. Motor unit type, function, and activation

NEUROMOTOR SYSTEM ORGANIZATION

The human nervous system consists of two major components: (1) the **central nervous system (CNS)**, which includes the brain and spinal cord, and (2) the **peripheral nervous system (PNS)** composed of cranial and spinal nerves. **Figure 11.1** presents an overview of these two components of the human nervous system.

Central Nervous System—The Brain

Figure 11.2A illustrates a lateral view of the brain's six main divisions:

1. Medulla oblongata
2. Pons
3. Midbrain
4. Cerebellum
5. Diencephalon
6. Telencephalon

Each of the 12 cranial nerves originates in one of these anatomic areas. **Figure 11.2B** shows a superior view of the brain. The longitudinal fissure runs down the midline and separates the brain's right and left sides, which are called *hemispheres*. Below the fissure, a large tract of nerve fibers (corpus callosum, not shown) connects the two hemi-

spheres. The outer portion of the brain, the **cerebral cortex** or **gray matter** (gray because nerve fibers lack a white myelin coating), consists of a series of folded convolutions. The bottom panel in **Fig. 11.2C** depicts the four lobes of the cerebral cortex (**occipital, parietal, temporal,** and **frontal**) and the sensory and motor areas and cerebellum.

The bony skull and a composite of four tough membranes called *meninges,* which contain a jelly-like cushioning substance, surround the brain to protect it from external trauma as occurs in sports-related traumatic brain injuries (*www.headinjury.com/sports.htm*).

Central Nervous System—The Spinal Cord

Figure 11.3A illustrates the spinal cord (about 45 cm long and 1 cm in diameter) encased by 33 vertebrae (seven cervical, 12 thoracic, five lumbar, five sacral, and four coccygeal). The 12 pairs of peripheral nerves, grouped into cervical, thoracic, lumbar, and sacral sections according to their location along the spine, exit the spinal cord through a small hole or foramen at the juncture between each pair of vertebrae (**Fig. 11.3C**).

This unique anatomical design allows extreme vertebral movement without affecting spinal nerve function. **Intervertebral discs** separate adjacent vertebrae and under normal circumstances provide a cushioning surface. Unfortunately, a disc can bulge into the space occupied by that segment's spinal nerve, compressing it and causing pain in an area the nerve innervates (e.g., lower back, buttocks, or full length of the leg). This unfortunate cascade of events can cause loss of motor control. If the condition persists with significant muscle weakness (e.g., inability to raise and lower the body vertically off the ball of one foot), surgical repair or removal of the offending disc often relieves the pressure and pain, but this is not a foolproof solution.

When viewed in cross-section (**Fig. 11.3B**), the spinal cord shows its H-shaped core of gray matter. The limbs of this core, the ventral (anterior) and dorsal (posterior) horns, contain principally three types of nerves:

1. Interneurons
2. Sensory neurons
3. Motoneurons (motor neurons)

Motor or **efferent neurons** conduct impulses outward from the brain or spinal cord. They exit the cord through the ventral root to supply extrafusal and intrafusal skeletal muscle fibers. **Sensory** or **afferent neurons** enter the spinal cord via the dorsal root. An area of white matter that contains ascending and descending nerve tracts within the cord surrounds the gray core. The ascending nerve tracts within the spinal cord transmit sensory information from peripheral sensory receptors to the brain. Tracts of nerve tissue descend from the brain and terminate at neurons in the spinal cord. One key tract of neurons, the **pyramidal tract**, transmits impulses downward through the spinal cord. By direct routes and interconnecting spinal cord neurons, these nerves eventually excite motoneurons that control skeletal muscles. **Extrapyramidal tract** nerves originate in the brain stem and connect at all levels of the

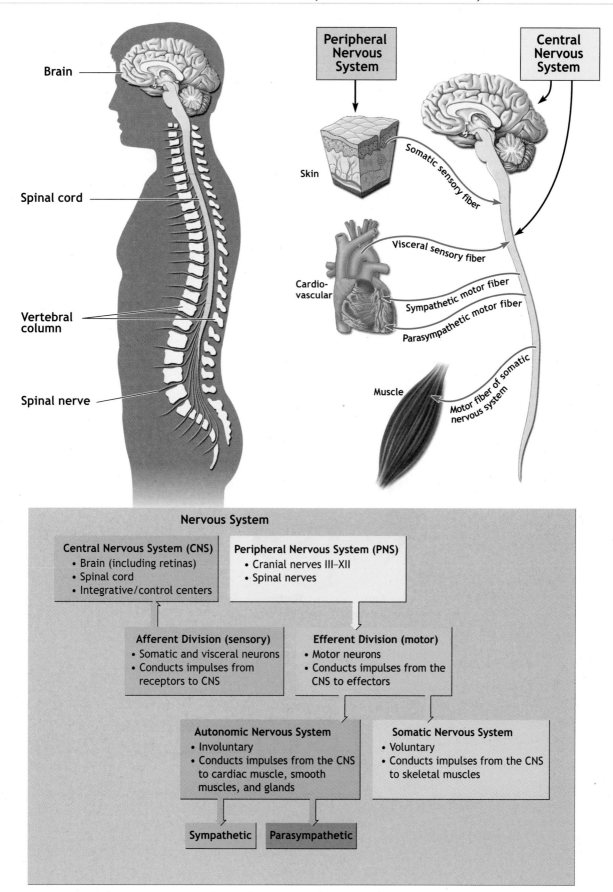

Figure 11.1 The two divisions of the human nervous system. The central nervous system (CNS) contains the brain (including the retinas), spinal cord, and integrating and control centers; the cranial nerves and spinal nerves make up the peripheral nervous system (PNS). The PNS further subdivides into the afferent (sensory) and efferent (motor) divisions. The efferent division consists of the somatic nervous system and autonomic nervous system (sympathetic and parasympathetic divisions).

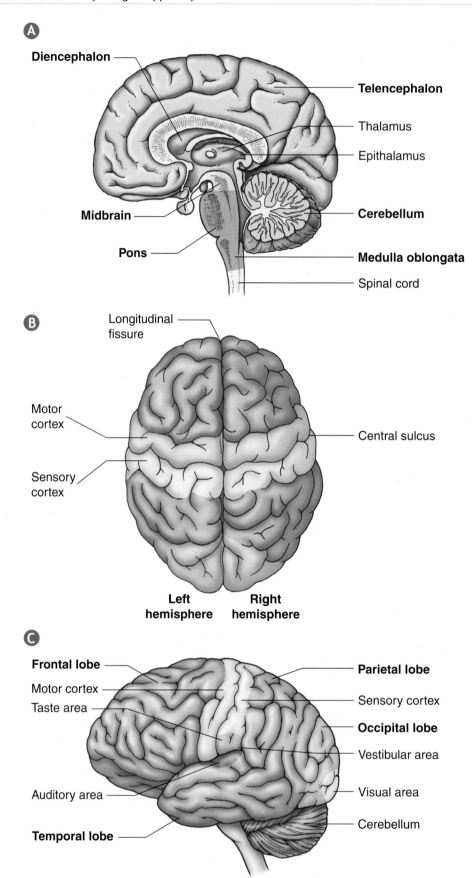

Figure 11.2 (A) Principal six divisions of the brain, lateral view. (B) Superior view of the brain. (C) Four lobes of the cerebral cortex.

spinal cord. These neurons control posture and provide a continual background level of neuromuscular tone in contrast to discrete movements stimulated by the pyramidal tract nerves.

Brain Neurotransmitters   Nerves communicate by releasing at their terminal ends chemical messengers called **neurotransmitters** that diffuse across the **synapse** or junction between one nerve end and the cell body of another nerve. The neurotransmitter combines with a targeted receptor molecule on the postsynaptic membrane to facilitate depolarization or, in some instances, hyperpolarization. Many of the neurons of the CNS particularly in the brain release or respond to these neurotransmitters. Three important brain neurotransmitter categories include:

1. **Monoamines:** Modified amino acids include epinephrine, norepinephrine, serotonin, histamine, and dopamine.
2. **Neuropeptides:** Short chains of amino acids include arginine, vasopressin, and angiotensin II (also act as hormones [see Chapter 12]). Enkephalins and endorphins (sometimes called opioid neurotransmitters) represent other neuropeptides that produce a general sense of well-being. Release of endogenous opioid neurotransmitters with exercise contributes to the exercise "high."
3. **Nitric oxide (NO):** Neurons in the CNS and other cell types contain NO receptors that serve as signalling molecules in the cardiovascular system.

Peripheral Nervous System

The PNS consists of 31 pairs of spinal nerves (eight cervical, 12 thoracic, five lumbar, five sacral, and one coccygeal) and 12 pairs of cranial nerves. Numbers identify these nerves (e.g., C1 is the first nerve from cervical region). Careful experiments have tracked the exact location of the spinal nerves and mapped the muscles they innervate. Injury to a specific spinal cord area produces predictable neurologic consequences. For example, quadriplegia almost always results from damage to the upper thoracic vertebra and corresponding descending nerve tract. The PNS includes afferent nerves that relay sensory information from muscles, joints, skin, and bones *toward* the brain and efferent nerves that transmit information *away* from the brain to glands and muscles. The somatic and autonomic nervous systems consist of efferent neurons.

Somatic Nervous System   The **somatic nervous system** innervates skeletal muscle (voluntary muscle). Somatic efferent nerve firing excites muscle activation, and autonomic nerve firing discussed in the next section can excite or inhibit activation.

Autonomic Nervous System   Efferent nerves of the autonomic nervous system activate the viscera and other tissues on a subconscious level. Autonomic nerves innervate smooth muscle (involuntary muscle) in the intestines, sweat and salivary glands, myocardium, and some endocrine glands. The heart and intestines display automatic excitability, but one can also exert conscious control over these tissues under some circumstances. For example, individuals who practice yoga or meditation can modify their heart rate and regional blood flow on command. In hypnosis (from the Greek word "sleep") a state of heightened awareness and focused concentration can manipulate pain perception, access repressed material, and "reprogram" some behaviors. Some champion weight lifters apply self-hypnosis before attempting heavy lifts to focus all their muscular efforts on the lift without the possible distraction of discomfort in attempting the lift (just prior to the lift as the muscles tense and prepare for an all-out effort). This self-induced "trance" blocks out superfluous neural input that might interfere with a maximal effort.

Questions & Notes

List the 2 major components of the human nervous system.

1.

2.

List the 2 parts of the autonomic nervous system.

1.

2.

List the 2 parts of the somatic nervous system.

1.

2.

The number of cranial nerves = _____

List the 4 brain lobes.

1.

2.

3.

4.

State the primary function of intervertebral discs.

List 3 types of neurons in the human nervous system.

1.

2.

3.

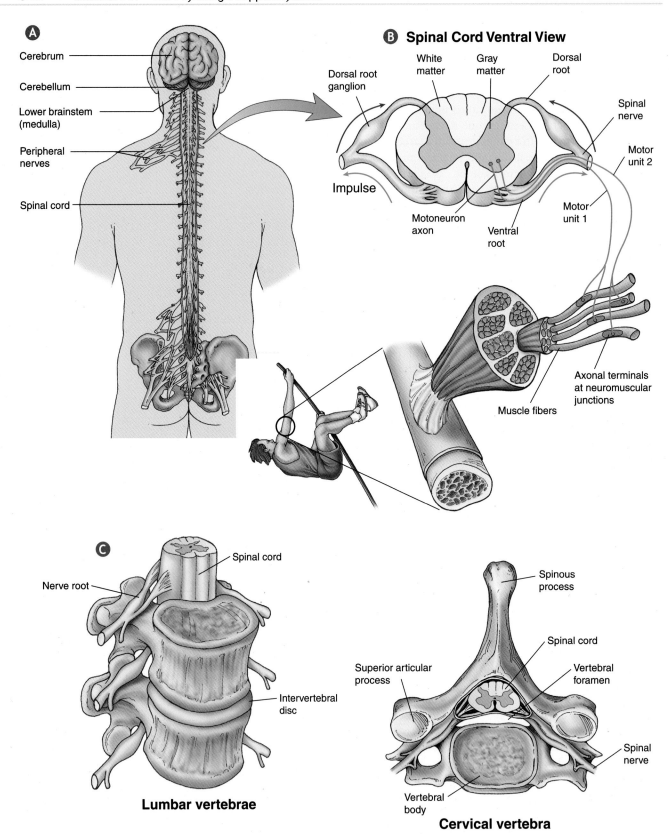

A

- Cerebrum
- Cerebellum
- Lower brainstem (medulla)
- Peripheral nerves
- Spinal cord

B **Spinal Cord Ventral View**

- Dorsal root ganglion
- White matter
- Gray matter
- Dorsal root
- Spinal nerve
- Motor unit 2
- Motor unit 1
- Impulse
- Motoneuron axon
- Ventral root
- Axonal terminals at neuromuscular junctions
- Muscle fibers

C

- Nerve root
- Spinal cord
- Intervertebral disc

Lumbar vertebrae

- Spinous process
- Superior articular process
- Spinal cord
- Vertebral foramen
- Spinal nerve
- Vertebral body

Cervical vertebra

Figure 11.3 (**A**) Human spinal cord showing the peripheral nerves. (**B**) Ventral view of a spinal cord section to illustrate dorsal and ventral root neural pathways and nerve impulse direction. (**C**) Junction of two lumbar vertebral bodies and a cross-section through one cervical vertebra.

Conscious modulation of aspects of the autonomic nervous system offers alternative treatment in medicine, such as control of hypertension and stress-related disorders through biofeedback techniques and applies to certain sports. Competitors in archery and other target-shooting events consciously modify their cardiovascular and respiratory patterns so normal breathing and pulse rate temporarily "stop" during the crucial steadying phase of performance.

The autonomic nervous system functions as a unit to maintain constancy in the internal environment. **Figure 11.4** illustrates the **sympathetic** and **parasympathetic** divisions of the autonomic nervous system. Sympathetic nerve fibers mediate excitation and parasympathetic activation inhibits excitation except for vagal parasympathetic excitation of gastrointestinal motility and tone and pancreatic insulin secretion. In contrast to the somatic nervous system, some cell bodies or ganglia of sympathetic and parasympathetic neurons exist outside the CNS.

Sympathetic Nervous System Sympathetic nerve fibers supply the heart, smooth muscle, sweat glands, and viscera. These neurons exit the spinal cord and enter a series of ganglia near the cord's **sympathetic chain**. The nerves terminate relatively far from the target organ in **adrenergic fiber** endings that release norepinephrine. Excitation of the sympathetic nervous system occurs during fight-or-flight situations that require whole-body arousal for emergencies. Autonomic sympathetic stimulation accelerates breathing and heart rate almost instantaneously; the pupils dilate, and blood flows from the skin to deeper tissues in anticipation of a perceived bodily challenge.

Parasympathetic Nervous System Parasympathetic nerve fibers exit the brain stem and sacral segments of the spinal cord to supply the thorax, abdomen, and pelvic regions. Parasympathetic nerve endings release acetylcholine (**ACh; cholinergic fibers**). The postganglionic parasympathetic nerve fibers located close to the organs they innervate produce effects *opposite* of sympathetic fibers. For example, parasympathetic neural stimulation via the vagus nerve slows heart rate while sympathetic stimulation accelerates heart rate.

Most organs receive simultaneous sympathetic and parasympathetic stimulation. Both systems maintain a constant degree of activation called *neural tone*. Depending on physiologic need, one system becomes more active while the other becomes inhibited. Dual innervation of this type permits a finer level of control at the end organs. This can be likened to hot and cold faucets being open at the same time; minor adjustments in both faucets rapidly and precisely change the temperature compared with alternately turning each of the faucets on or off.

Autonomic Reflex Arc

Figure 11.5 illustrates a typical neural arrangement for a monosynaptic **reflex arc** in the spinal cord. Sensory input (e.g., a knee tap with a percussion reflex hammer and subsequent excitation of muscle spindles within the quadriceps muscle) initiates transmission of afferent impulses to the spinal cord via the sensory (dorsal) root. This in turn stimulates the anterior motoneuron to the quadricep femoris to contract and extend the lower leg, counteracting the initial stretch. The "knee-jerk" reaction only takes a few milliseconds because the triggered impulse has to make a return trip via the spinal cord without going to the brain. A delay or absence of the stretch reflex can indicate possible neurologic or neuromuscular dysfunction to spinal nerves and their innervations or injuries to the knee and leg. In a polysynaptic reflex arc the nerves synapse in the cord through interneurons that distribute information to various cord levels. The impulse then passes over the motor root pathway through anterior motoneurons to the effector organ.

Questions & Notes

Name the 2 divisions of the autonomic nervous system.

1.

2.

Describe the function of sympathetic nerve fibers.

Describe the function of parasympathetic nerve fibers.

Indicate areas of the body innervated by the sympathetic and parasympathetic nervous system.

Sympathetic:

Parasympathetic:

 For Your Information

INNERVATION RATIO

The finger contains 120 motor units that control 41,000 muscle fibers. In contrast, the medial gastrocnemius muscle (calf) has 580 motor units that innervate 1,030,000 fibers. The ratio of muscle fibers per motor unit averages 340 for finger muscles and 1800 for the gastrocnemius muscle.

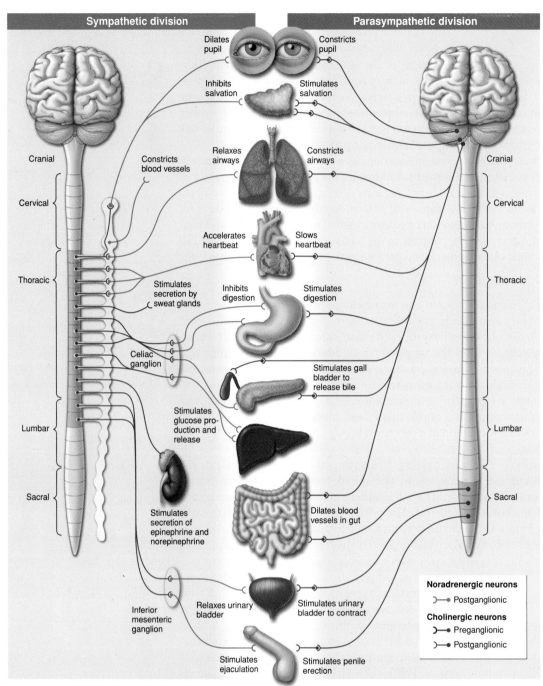

Figure 11.4 The sympathetic and parasympathetic divisions of the autonomic nervous system: comparisons of effects of activation of each. The preganglionic inputs of both divisions use acetylcholine (Ach; colored red) as a neurotransmitter. The postganglionic parasympathetic innervation of the visceral organs also uses Ach, but postganglionic sympathetic innervation uses norepinephrine (NE; colored blue), with the exception of innervation of the sweat glands, which use Ach. The adrenal medulla receives preganglionic sympathetic innervation and secretes epinephrine into the bloodstream when activated. In general, sympathetic stimulation produces catabolic effects that prepare the body to "fight" or "flee," and parasympathetic stimulation produces anabolic responses that promote normal function and conserve energy. (Modified from Bear, M.F., et al.: *Neuroscience: Exploring the Brain*, 3rd ed. Baltimore: Lippincott Williams & Wilkins, 2006.)

Within the figure:

Sympathetic division | **Parasympathetic division**

- Dilates pupil / Constricts pupil
- Inhibits salvation / Stimulates salvation
- Constricts blood vessels
- Relaxes airways / Constricts airways
- Accelerates heartbeat / Slows heartbeat
- Stimulates secretion by sweat glands
- Inhibits digestion / Stimulates digestion
- Celiac ganglion
- Stimulates gall bladder to release bile
- Stimulates glucose production and release
- Stimulates secretion of epinephrine and norepinephrine
- Dilates blood vessels in gut
- Inferior mesenteric ganglion
- Relaxes urinary bladder / Stimulates urinary bladder to contract
- Stimulates ejaculation / Stimulates penile erection

Labels: Cranial, Cervical, Thoracic, Lumbar, Sacral

Noradrenergic neurons
>—• Postganglionic

Cholinergic neurons
>—• Preganglionic
>—• Postganglionic

Comparison of effects of sympathetic and parasympathetic activation on end organs		
End organ	**Sympathetic effects**	**Parasympathetic effects**
Skeletal muscle	Increase blood flow	Decrease blood flow
Ventilation	Increase	Decrease
Sweat glands	Increase perspiration	No effect
Heart	Increase force and contraction rate	Decrease force and contraction rate
GI tract motility	Decrease	Increase
Eyes	Dilate pupils	Constrict pupils
Secretion of digestive juices	Decrease	Increase
Blood pressure	Increase mean pressure	Decrease mean pressure
Airways	Increase diameter	Decrease diameter

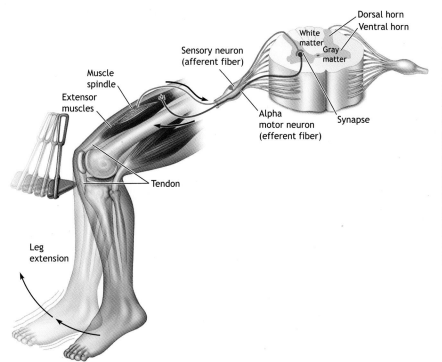

Figure 11.5 text labels: Dorsal horn; Ventral horn; White matter; Gray matter; Sensory neuron (afferent fiber); Muscle spindle; Extensor muscles; Alpha motor neuron (efferent fiber); Synapse; Tendon; Leg extension

Questions & Notes

Draw and label a typical autonomic reflex arc in the spinal cord.

Briefly describe the main differences between a simple and complex spinal reflex.

Figure 11.5 Schematic of the patella tendon stretch reflex (also called the patellar reflex). Firm percussion or tapping of the patellar tendon with the reflex hammer shown at the left draws the patella momentarily down, stimulating the muscle spindles' afferents and Golgi tendon organs (GTOs) by altering the stretch and length of the muscle that provokes a preprogrammed reflex contraction. The "knee-jerk" reaction only takes a few milliseconds because the triggered impulse only has to make a return trip to the spinal cord without going to the brain. A delay or absence of the stretch reflex can indicate possible neurologic or neuromuscular dysfunction to spinal nerves and their innervations or injuries to the knee and leg. The diagram only shows one side of the spinal nerve complex.

Another example of a simple reflex arc occurs when a person accidentally touches a hot object. Stimulation of pain receptors in the fingers fires sensory information over afferent fibers to the spinal cord to activate efferent motor fibers to remove the hand from the hot object. Concurrently, the signal transmits via interneurons up the cord to the sensory area in the brain that actually "feels" the pain. The various operational levels for sensory input, processing, and motor output, including the reflex action just described, explain how the hand withdraws from the hot object *before* the person perceives pain. Reflex actions in the spinal cord and other subconscious areas of the CNS control many muscle functions. These reflex actions even operate for people who have had their spinal cords severed above the level required for the reflex.

Complex Reflexes

Complex spinal reflexes that involve multiple synapses and muscle groups also exist. Consider the situation of stepping on a tack with the left foot. Almost simultaneously as the tack pierces the skin, the right leg straightens to remove weight from the injured foot, which lifts off the ground. **Figure 11.6** illustrates the neural and motor pathways activated in this complex action, termed the **crossed-extensor reflex**, in the following five-step sequence:

Step 1. The tack stimulates pain receptors in the skin. The receptors transmit the message to the spinal cord via the sensory nerve.

Step 2. Sensory neurons branch to each side of the cord to activate interneurons in the gray matter.

Step 3. Interneurons synapse with motoneurons, innervating both flexor and extensor muscles in each leg.

 For Your Information

TYPES OF MOTONEURONS

The large diameters of anterior motoneurons, termed type A α fibers, range between 8 and 20 μm (1 μm = one-millionth [0.000001] of a meter). Diameters of other smaller type A fibers (γ efferent motoneurons) do not exceed 10 μm. Their conduction velocities equal about half of α fibers. γ Efferent fibers connect with proprioreceptors (special stretch sensors) in skeletal muscle to detect minute changes in muscle fiber length.

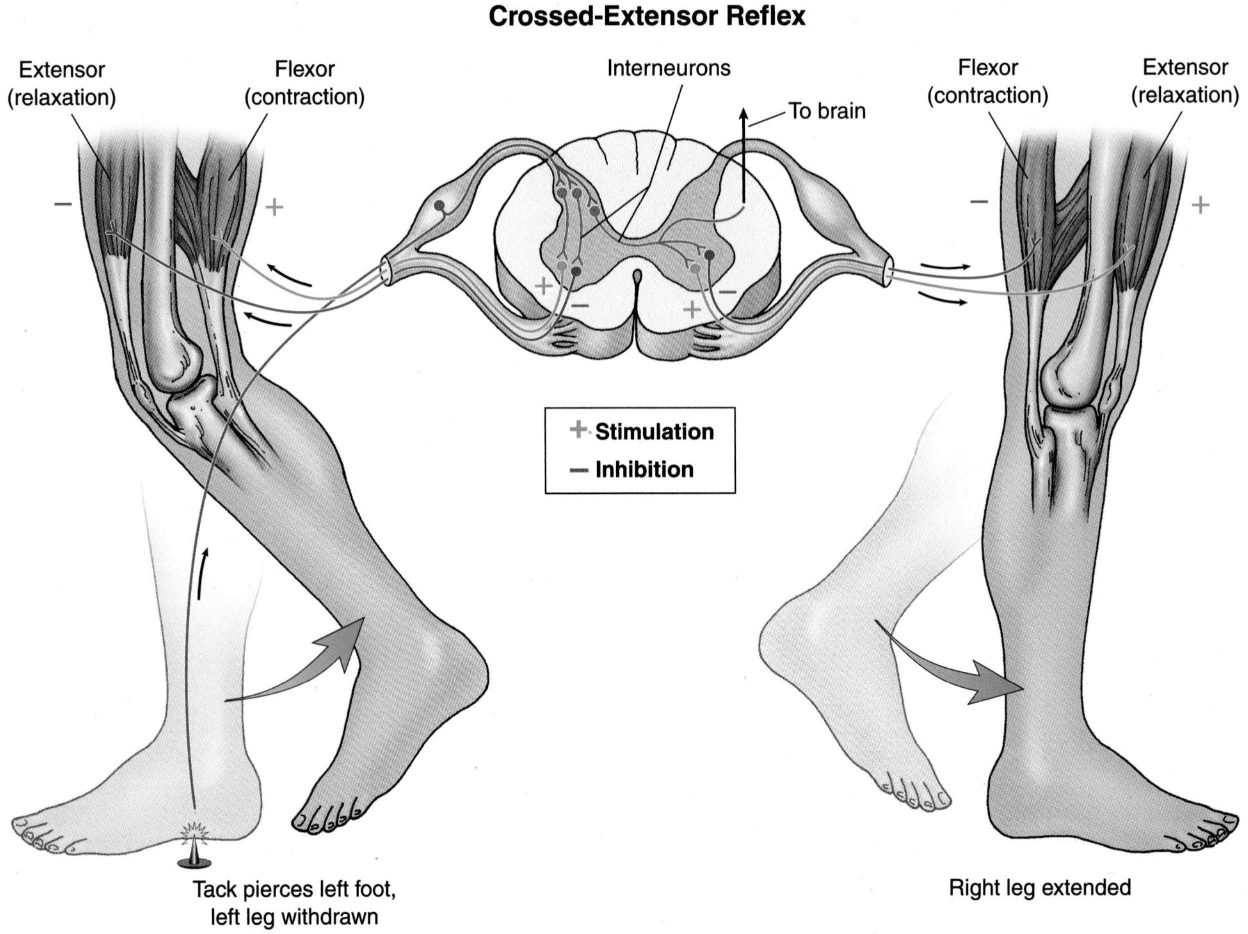

Crossed-Extensor Reflex

Figure 11.6 Crossed-extensor reflex in both legs represents a more complex reflex with multiple synapses and muscle groups.

Step 4. Inhibition and stimulation of appropriate leg flexor and extensor muscles cause concurrent rapid extension of the uninjured limb and flexion to remove the injured limb.

Step 5. Interneuron connections simultaneously activate neural pathways to transmit information to appropriate sensory areas of the brain where the pain is "felt."

Learned Reflexes The knee-jerk and crossed-extensor reflexes occur automatically and require no learning. Practice facilitates other more complex reflex patterns such as most sports performances and occupational tasks. Consider a trained office worker who types 90 words a minute. At an average of five letters per word, this requires six to eight keystrokes per second. For this person, the sight of a word to type initiates a series of rapid hand and finger movements that require little conscious effort. A beginning typist, in contrast, proceeds slowly since thought must be directed to the position of each key along the keyboard and proper execution and sequencing of wrist and finger movements. As neuromuscular pathways become "ingrained" through proper or meaningful practice the typing movements progressively become reflex actions as the beginner approaches expert status. People who routinely send text messages have mastered the proper sequencing of finger and hand movements so the desired outcome occurs essentially automatically. Perfecting a sports skill, no matter how simple it may appear like swinging a baseball bat to contact a "fast" pitch or kicking a soccer ball with just the right speed into the right or left side of the net, requires hundreds or even thousands of practice hours to *engrain* the movement until it becomes automatic and flawless in execution. Unfortunately, improper practice also can automate a task to engrain less than optimal neuromuscular actions. Most individuals who practice the golf swing, for example, do so by reinforcing poor habits. It starts with the grip and the first 6 inches of the takeaway in the backswing. Setting up with an improper grip, followed by a rapid cocking of the wrists at the start of the backswing, fuels a recipe for disaster. This means that continual "poor" practice reinforces nonoptimal mechanics and poor shots. Instead of hitting one ball after another, hours on end, the aspiring golfer must practice correct swing mechanics under the watchful eye of a trained professional, ideally with video feedback. The adage "practice makes perfect" should be amended to "perfect practice leads to more perfect performance."

Nerve Supply to Muscle The terminal branches of one neuron innervate at least one of the body's approximately

250 million muscle fibers. About 420,000 motor nerves exist yet a single nerve usually supplies numerous individual muscle fibers. In general, the branches of a nerve within a muscle pass to specific localized groups of motor units. In multiple group muscles, for example, the quadriceps with four separate muscles act in concert to perform the main muscle action with no single muscle responsible for the full movement. *The ratio of muscle fibers to nerves generally relates to a muscle's particular movement function.* Delicate, precise eye muscle movements require one neuron to control fewer than 10 muscle fibers (ratio of 10:1). The ratio in the larynx is an even lower 1:1. For less complex movements of the large leg muscles, a motoneuron may innervate as many as 3000 muscle fibers (ratio of 3000:1).

A basic rule states that **less complex movements** like forearm supination and elbow flexion have a higher ratio of muscle fibers to motor nerves. **Complex eye and hand movements** that require more specialized movements have a much lower ratio. The next sections review how information processed in the CNS activates specific muscles to cause an appropriate, specialized motor response.

THE MOTOR UNIT

A *motor unit* describes skeletal muscle fibers and their corresponding innervating anterior motoneuron. The motor unit thus represents the funtional unit of movement. A whole muscle contains many motor units, each containing a single motoneuron and its composite muscle fibers.

The muscle fibers belonging to a particular motor unit are scattered over subregions of the muscle; fibers from one motor unit are interspersed among fibers of other motor units. The consequence of this disperson results in forces being spread over a large muscle area to minimize mechanical stress.

Motor Unit Anatomy

Anterior Motoneuron **Figure 11.7** illustrates that an **anterior (alpha) motoneuron** with its three main parts: cell body, axon, and dendrites. The cell's unique architectural design permits the transmission of electrochemical impulses from the spinal cord to muscle. The **cell body,** located within the spinal cord's gray matter, houses the *control center,* the structures involved in replicating and transmitting the genetic code. The **axon** extends from the cord and delivers an impulse to the muscle fibers it innervates. Short neural branches called **dendrites** receive impulses through numerous spinal cord connections and conduct them toward the cell body.

Nerve cells conduct impulses *in one direction only,* akin to a one-way street, down the axon away from the stimulation point. As the axon approaches the muscle, it branches with each terminal branch to innervate a single muscle fiber. A whole muscle contains numerous motor units, each with a single motoneuron and its complement of muscle fibers.

The **myelin sheath** encircles the axon of nerve fibers that are either long in length or large in diameter. A large part of this sheath acts as an electrical insulator that envelops the axon akin to the plastic coating around a copper electrical wire. The lipid-protein membrane myelin consists of approxomately 75% lipids (cholesterol and phospholipid) and 25% proteins. Myelin's main function increases the speed of neural impulses along the myelinated fiber. This occurs because myelin increases electrical resistance across the cell membrane by a factor of 5000 and decreases capacitance by 10-fold this number. Fiber myelination thus keeps the electrical current from leaving the bare axon while at the same time allowing a high signal transmission speed. The fat-containing molecules inhibit the propagation of electricity to make the signals jump from one section of myelin to the next. In the PNS, specialized **Schwann cells** encase the bare axon and then spiral around it. Myelin forms a large part of this sheath to insulate the axon. A thinner membrane, the **neurilemma,** covers the myelin

Questions & Notes

The ratio of muscle fibers to neurons relates to a muscle's particular

_____ _____.

Describe the anatomy of a motor unit.

Describe an anterior motoneuron.

Describe the main function of the axon's myelin sheath.

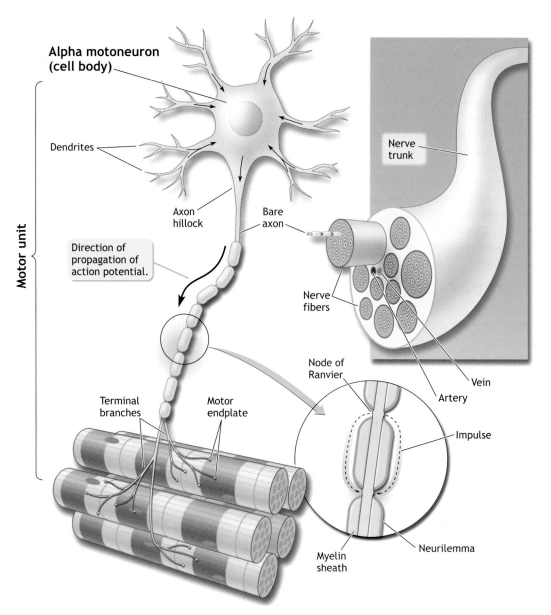

Figure 11.7 The anterior α-motoneuron consists of a cell body, axons, and dendrites. The round *inset* at the bottom right illustrates a node of Ranvier that permits impulses to jump from one node to the next as the electrical current travels toward the terminal branches at the motor end-plate.

sheath. **Nodes of Ranvier** interrupt the Schwann cells and myelin every 1 or 2 mm along the axon's length. The myelin sheath insulates the axon to ion flow allowing the nodes of Ranvier axon to depolarize along their axon segments. The alternating sequence of myelin sheath and node of Ranvier (termed *saltatory conduction*) allows impulses to "jump" from node to node (similar to signals progressing from one telephone pole to the next) as electrical current travels toward the terminal branches at the motor end-plate. Nerve conduction in this manner accounts for the higher transmission velocity in myelinated compared with unmyelinated fibers. Degenertion of the myelin sheath produces peripheral neuropathy and disease. In multiple sclerosis, an autoimmune disease that affects approximately 200 people each week in the United States, destruction of the myelin sheath surrounding nerve fibers adversely affects neural pathways to the brain, spinal cord, and optic nerves. This interferes with vision, sensation, and body movements.

Neuromuscular Junction (Motor End-Plate)

Figure 11.8 highlights the microanatomy of the **neuromuscular junction** or **motor end-plate** that provides interface between the end of a myelinated motoneuron and a muscle fiber. It functions to transmit nerve impulses to muscle fibers. Each muscle fiber usually has one neuromuscular junction. The inset table in **Figure 11.8** lists representative values for ionic concentrations across the motoneuron membrane.

The terminal portion of the axon forms several smaller axon branches whose endings, called **presynaptic terminals**, lie close to but not in contact with the muscle fiber's plasma membrane or **sarcolemma**. The **synaptic gutter**, the region of the postsynaptic membrane, contains infoldings that increase its surface area. Between the synaptic gutter

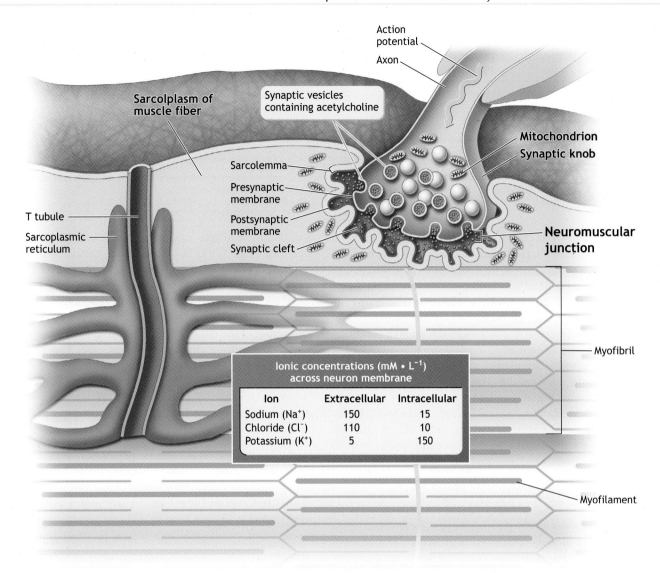

Figure 11.8 Microanatomy of the neuromuscular junction, including details of the presynaptic and postsynaptic contact area between the motoneuron and the muscle fiber it innervates. The *inset table* shows representative values for ionic concentrations across the motoneuron membrane.

and the presynaptic terminal of the axon lies the **synaptic cleft**, the region where neural impulse transmission occurs.

Excitation *Excitation normally occurs only at the neuromuscular junction.* The neurotransmitter ACh provides the chemical stimulus to change an electrical neural impulse into a chemical stimulus at the motor end-plate. Acetylcholine, released from small, saclike vesicles within the terminal axon, increases the postsynaptic membrane's permeability to sodium and potassium ions. This spreads the impulse over the entire muscle fiber as a distinct wave of depolarization. As depolarization progresses, the muscle fiber's contractile machinery primes for its major function—to contract or shorten.

The enzyme **cholinesterase**, purified and crystallized from electric eels in 1968 and concentrated at the borders of the synaptic cleft, degrades acetylcholine within 5 millisecond (ms) of its release from the synaptic vesicles. This action immediately repolarizes the postsynaptic membrane. The axon resynthesizes acetylcholine from acetic acid and choline, byproducts of cholinesterase action, so the entire process can repeat with the arrival of successive nerve impulses.

*Q*uestions & Notes

Describe the primary function of the neuromuscular junction.

Describe the role of acetylcholine in neuromuscular excitation.

Table 11.1	Characteristics and Correspondence Between Motor Units and Muscle Fiber Types				
MOTOR UNIT DESIGNATION	**FORCE PRODUCTION**	**CONTRACTION SPEED**	**FATIGUE RESISTANCE**[a]	**SAG**[b]	**MOTOR UNIT MUSCLE FIBER TYPE**
Fast fatigable (FF)	High	Fast	Low	Yes	Fast glycolytic (FG)
Fast fatigue-resistance (FR)	Moderate	Fast	Moderate	Yes	Fast oxidative-glycolytic (FOG)
Slow (S)	Low	Slow	High	No	Slow oxidative (SO)

[a]How much the muscle tension declined with repetitive stimulation.
[b]Under repetitive stimuli, some motor units respond smoothly with a systematic increase in tension, but others first increase tension and then decrease or "sag" slightly in response to the same tetanic stimulus. These sag characteristics can classify the different motor units. Only the slow (S) motor units do not exhibit sag, which probably relates more to their lower force-generating capabilities than their fatigue characteristics.
Modified from Lieber, R.L.: *Skeletal Muscle Structure, Function, and Plasticity*, 3rd ed. Baltimore: Lippincott Williams & Wilkins, 2010.

Facilitation A motoneuron generates an action potential when its microvoltage decreases sufficiently to reach its threshold for excitation. With a subthreshold action potential, the neuron does not discharge, but its resting membrane potential still lowers, temporarily increasing its "tendency" to fire. A neuron fires when many subthreshold excitatory impulses arrive in rapid succession, a condition termed **temporal summation**. **Spatial summation** describes the simultaneous stimulation of different presynaptic terminals on the same neuron. The "summing" of each excitatory effect often initiates an action potential.

Removing inhibitory neural influences becomes important under certain exercise conditions. In all-out strength and power activities like maximal bench press or vertical leap, disinhibition and maximal activation of all motoneurons required for a movement enhances performance. *Effective disinhibition fully activates muscle groups during maximal lifting, an effect that accounts for the rapid, highly specific strength increases observed during the first few days and weeks of resistance training.* Enhanced neuromuscular activation accounts for considerable improvements in muscular strength *without* concurrent increases in muscle size. CNS excitation (also called "neuronal facilitation") explains why intense concentration, or "psyching," can substantially "supercharge" maximal strength and power efforts.

Inhibition Some presynaptic terminals generate inhibitory impulses by releasing chemicals that increase postsynaptic membrane permeability to potassium and chloride ions. The efflux of positively charged potassium ions or influx of negatively charged chloride ions increases the membrane's resting electrical potential to create an **inhibitory postsynaptic potential (IPSP)** that makes the neuron more difficult to fire. No action potential occurs when a motoneuron encounters excitatory and inhibitory influences or encounters a large IPSP. For example, one can usually override or inhibit the reflex to pull the hand away when removing a splinter.

The neurotransmitter γ-aminobutyric acid (GABA) and glycine exert inhibitory effects. Neural inhibition serves protective functions and reduces the input of unwanted stimuli to produce smooth, purposeful responses.

Motor Unit Physiology

Identifying Muscle Fibers with Motor Units

A whole muscle contains many possible motor units containing a single motoneuron; thus, it is difficult to identify which fibers belong to which motor unit without ambiguity. The classic motor unit physiology experiments performed in the late 1960s and early 1970s were on isolated cat hindlimb motor units using intracellular motoneuron stimulation to measure different electrophysiologic properties of the motoneuron and mechanical properties of the motor units within the whole muscle. This research, still used today, describes motor unit differences based on the physiologic properties of the respective muscle fibers innervated. Table 11.1 and **Figure 11.9** describe and illustrate the three physiologic and mechanical properties of motor units and the muscle fibers they innervate:

1. Twitch (speed of contraction) characteristics
2. Tension-generating (force) characteristics
3. Neuromuscular fatigability

Twitch Characteristics Early motor unit studies revealed that in response to a single electrical impulse, some units developed high-twitch tensions but others develped "relatively" low-twitch tensions whereas others generated intermediate tension. The differences between motor units were judged on a relative rather than absolute basis, sometimes making comparisons between studies difficult. Motor units with low-twitch tensions also tended to have "slower" contraction times but those with higher tensions tended to have "faster" contraction times.

Tension-Generating Characteristics Different motor units and the muscles they innervate can develop different amounts of tension based on many factors. For example, fast motor units and their corresponding fast muscle fibers are able to generate more tension than a slow motor unit and its corresponding slow muscle fiber. Alternatively, perhaps fast and slow fibers generate the same tension, but fast motor units simply innervate a greater number of fibers then slow motor units. Or fast and slow units have the same number of fibers of equal intrinsic strength, but fast fibers are larger and therefore generate more tension. Each of these possibilities is supported by research, but current thinking indicates that fast and slow muscle fibers within a motor unit have about the same specific tension capacity but that fiber size and innervation ratio differ between motor unit types. Differences in tension generation are governed by three factors: the all-or-none principle, graduation of force principle, and level of motor unit recruitment patterns.

All-or-None Principle If a stimulus triggers an action potential in the motoneuron, all of the accompanying muscle fibers contract synchronously. A single motor unit cannot generate strong and weak contractions; either the impulse elicits a contraction or it does not. Once the neuron fires and the impulse reaches the neuromuscular junction, the muscle cells always contract to the fullest extent in accord with the **all-or-none principle** first described by Henry Pickering Bowditch in 1871, American physiologist at Harvard's Medical School and Department of Anatomy, Physiology, and Physical Training (see Chapter 1).

Gradation of Force Principle The force of muscle action varies from slight to maximal in one of two mechanisms:

1. Increasing the *number* of motor units recruited
2. Increasing the *frequency* of motor unit discharge

Activation of all motor units in a muscle generates considerable force compared with activating only a few units. Total tension also increases if repetitive stimuli

Questions & Notes

Describe 2 situations when temporal summation could enhance exercise performance.

1.

2.

Describe what happens when a motor neuron encounters both excitatory and inhibitory influences but the IPSP is larger.

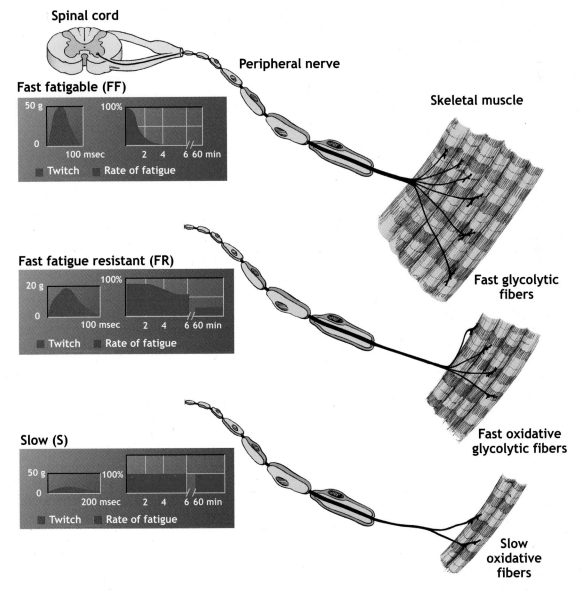

Figure 11.9 Schematic reprsentation of the anatomic, physiologic, and histochemical properties of the three motor unit types. Fast fatigable (FF) motor units (*top*) have large axons that innervate many large muscle fibers. The units generate large tensions but fatigue rapidly (see the tension and fatigue graphs to the left). Fast-fatigue resistant (FR) units (*middle*) have modertely sized axons that innervate many muscle fibers. The units generate moderte tensions and do not fatigue much. Slow units (S) (*bottom*) composed of small axons innervate few small fibers. These units generate low forces but maintain force for a prolonged time period.

reach a muscle before it relaxes. Blending recruitment of motor units and their firing rate permits a wide variety of graded muscle actions. These range from the delicate touch of an eye surgeon reparing a retinal blood vessel to the maximal effort in throwing a baseball from deep left field to throw out a runner rounding third base and heading to home plate. The golf swing provides a good example of force gradation. Tension in the fingers, hands, arms, and legs continually adjusts during the backswing, swing initiation and acceleration, club-ball contact, and follow-through. Similarly, the seemingly simple task of writing with a pen involves innumerable highly complex and coordinated neuromuscular forces and actions. Think about picking up a grape and bringing it to your mouth. Without exquisite neuromuscular control, the fingers would literally crush the grape when grasped, and your hand and arm, without exhibiting precise control and coordination over their movements, might thrust what remains of the grape forcibly into your nose or eye, totally missing your mouth not to mention the pain of the jab!

Motor Unit Recruitment Low-force muscle actions activate only a few motor units, whereas higher force actions progressively enlist more units. **Motor unit recruitment** describes the process of adding motor units to increase muscle force. Motoneurons with progressively larger axons become recruited as muscle force increases. This response, termed the **size principle**, provides an anatomic basis for the orderly recruitment of specific motor units to produce a smooth action.

All of a muscle's motor units do not fire at the same time. If they did, it would be virtually impossible to control muscle force output. *From the standpoint of neuromotor control, selective recruitment and firing pattern of the fast- and slow-twitch motor units that control movement (and perhaps other stabilizing regions) provide the mechanism to produce the desired coordinated response.*

In accordance with the size principle, slow-twitch motor units with low activation thresholds become selectively recruited during light to moderate effort. Activation of more powerful, higher threshold, fast-twitch units progresses as force requirements increase. Sustained, submaximal jogging, cycling, cross-country skiing on a level grade, and lifting a light weight at slow speed involve selective recruitment of slow-twitch motor units. Rapid, powerful movements such as sprint running, cycling, and swimming progressively activate fast-twitch, fatigue-resistant motor units up through the fast-twitch fatigable units at peak force.

The differential control of the motor unit firing pattern distinguishes specific athletic groups and skilled from unskilled performers. Weight lifters, for example, generally demonstrate a synchronous pattern of motor-unit firing (i.e., many motor units recruited simultaneously during a lift). Endurance athletes generally exhibit an asynchronous firing pattern (i.e., some motor units fire while others recover). The synchronous firing of fast-twitch motor units allows the weight lifter to generate high force quickly for the desired lift. In contrast, for endurance athletes, the asynchronous firing of predominantly slow-

twitch, fatigue-resistant motor units serves as a built-in recuperative period so performance continues with minimal fatigue. This becomes possible because motor units share the burden of "cooperation" during multiple movements and changing exercise intensities.

Neuromuscular Fatigability Fatigability represents the decline in muscle tension or force capacity with repeated stimulation during a given time period. Resistance to fatigue (maintenance of muscle tension with repeated stimulation) represents another important quality to distinguish differences in motor units.

These four factors can decrease a muscle's force-generating capacity:

1. Exercise-induced alterations in levels of CNS neurotransmitters serotonin, 5-hydroxytryptamine (5-HT), dopamine, and ACh, including the neuromodulators ammonia and cytokines secreted by immune cells. The latter alter one's psychic or perceptual state to disrupt ability to exercise.
2. Reduced glycogen content in active muscle fibers during prolonged exercise. Such "nutrient-related fatigue" occurs despite availability of sufficient oxygen and fatty acid substrate for adenosine triphosphate (ATP) regeneration through aerobic metabolic pathways. Depletion of phosphocreatine (PCr) and decline in the total adenine nucleotide pool (ATP + Adenosine diphosphate [ADP] + Adenosine monophosphate [AMP]) accompanies the fatigue state during prolonged submaximal exercise.
3. A lack of oxygen and increased levels of blood and muscle lactate relate to muscle fatigue in short-term, maximal exercise. The dramatic increase in [H^+] in the active muscle disrupts the intracellular environment and the process of energy transfer.
4. Fatigue at the neuromuscular junction does not allow the action potential to traverse from the motoneuron to the muscle fiber.

If muscle function declines during prolonged submaximal exercise, additional motor unit recruitment occurs to maintain the crucial force output necessary to provide a relatively constant level of performance. During all-out exercise that presumably activates the available number of motor units, fatigue occurs when accompanied by an objectively measured decline in neural activity to those motor units. Similar to the dimming of a light bulb, reduced neural activity probably indicates that failure in neural or myoneural transmission produces fatigue in activities that involve maximal effort muscle actions.

PROPRIOCEPTORS IN MUSCLES, JOINTS, AND TENDONS

Muscles, joints, and tendons contain specialized sensory receptors sensitive to stretch, tension, and pressure. These **proprioceptor** end organs almost instantaneously relay critical information about muscular dynamics, limb position, and kinesthesia and proprioception to conscious and subconscious portions of the central nervous system. Proprioception allows continual monitoring of the progress of any movement or sequence of movements and serves as the basis for modifying subsequent motor actions. Individuals with chronic low back pain, or individuals who have undergone successful low back surgery, often temporarily lose full proprioception in the ankles, predisposing them to possible balance issues (e.g., an inability to easily balance with the eyes open or closed on one leg without swaying for more than 3 to 5 s).

Muscle Spindles

Muscle spindles provide mechanosensory information about changes in muscle fiber length and tension. They primarily respond to muscle stretch through reflex action by initiating a stronger muscle action to counteract the stretch.

Structural Organization   **Figure 11.10 A–C** illustrates the general location of the fusiform-shaped muscle spindle attached in parallel to regular muscle fibers (called **extrafusal fibers**) and Golgi tendon end organs. Any elongation of the muscle stretches the spindle. The number of spindles per gram of muscle varies depending on the muscle group. More spindles exist in muscles that routinely perform complex movements. The spindle contains two types of specialized fibers with contractile capabilities called **intrafusal fibers**.

Questions & Notes

Briefly describe the advantage of selective motor recruitment.

Describe the major factor(s) that distinguishes a skilled from an unskilled individual.

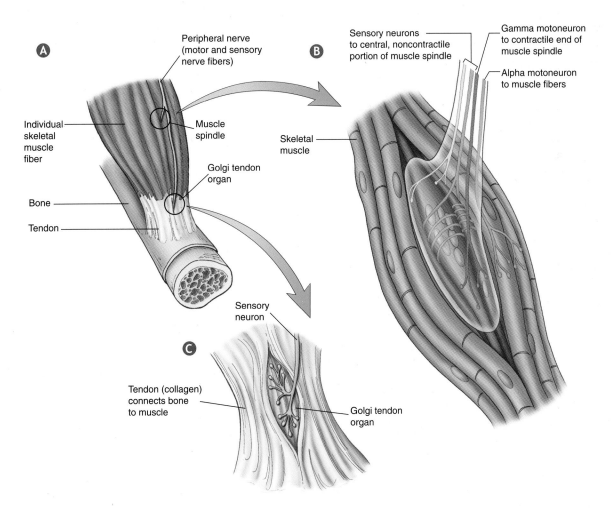

Figure 11.10   (A) General location of muscle spindles and Golgi tendon end organs. (B) Muscle spindle surrounded by skeletal muscle fibers. Two types of sensory neurons innervate the spindle's central portion: (1) fast-adapting neurons with spiral endings and (2) slow-adapting neurons with branched endings. γ motoneurons innervate the contractile ends of muscle spindle cells, and α-motoneurons activate skeletal muscle cells. (C) Slow-adapting sensory neurons innervate Golgi tendon organs (see also Fig. 11.12).

BOX 11.1 CLOSE UP

Proprioceptive Neuromuscular Facilitation Stretching

Static stretching techniques include **passive** (relaxation of all voluntary and reflex muscular resistance followed by passive assistance from another person or device during voluntary movement), **active assistive** (involves assistance from another person as the segment moves through its normal range of motion [ROM]), **active** (a muscle or joint actively moves through its ROM), and **proprioceptive neuromuscular facilitation** (PNF; an inverse stretch reflex induces relaxation in a muscle prior to its being stretched, allowing for increased stretch).

PROPRIOCEPTIVE NEUROMUSCULAR FACILITATION STRETCHING

PNF stretching increases ROM by augmenting prior muscle relaxation through spinal reflex mechanisms using these techniques:

1. **Contract–relax stretch** (hold–relax stretch). This stretching technique involves a prior isometric action of the muscle group to be stretched followed by a slow, static stretch (relaxation phase).
2. **Contract–relax–contract stretch** (hold–relax–contract stretch), also referred to as the **contract–relax with agonist contraction (CRAC)** technique. This approach involves an isometric action of the muscle group to be stretched; the relax stretching phase is accompanied by a submaximal action of the opposing (agonist) muscle group.

Both PNF techniques use **reciprocal inhibition**, the isometric action of the antagonists muscle group being stretched to induce a reflex facilitation and contraction of the agonist. This suppresses the contractile activity in the antagonist muscle during the slow, static stretch phase. Inhibition allows for an increased stretch of the antagonist muscle and connective tissue harness. The technique induces additional inhibitory input to the antagonist through reciprocal inhibition, allowing for greater stretch of the antagonist.

PERFORMING PNF STRETCHES

1. Stretch the target muscle group by moving the joint to the end of its ROM (**Fig. 1A**).
2. Isometrically contract the prestretched muscle group against an immovable resistance (e.g., partner) for 5 to 6 seconds.
3. Relax the contracted muscle group as the partner stretches the muscle group to a new, increased ROM (**Fig. 1B**). With CRAC, the opposing muscle group (agonist) contracts submaximally for 5 to 6 seconds to facilitate relaxation and produce further stretching of the muscle group.

PNF Example: To stretch the hamstring and lower back muscles, the individual lies on the floor with the arms extended to the side (**Fig. 1A**). The person contracts the lower back muscle isometrically as the partner offers resistance to horizontal extension (**Fig. 1A**). After the isometric action, the partner stretches the hamstrings to a new increased ROM (**Fig. 1B**).

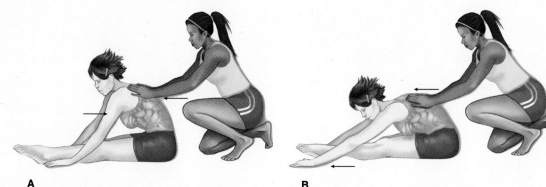

A   B

Figure 1   Proprioceptive neuromuscular facilitation (PNF) stretching technique: isometric phase (**A**); stretching phase (**B**).

GUIDELINES FOR PROPER STRETCHING USING PNF

1. Determine the appropriate posture or position to ensure proper position and alignment.
2. Emphasize proper breathing. Inhale through the nose and exhale during the stretch through pursed lips with the eyes closed to increase concentration and awareness of the stretch.
3. Hold end-points progressively for 30 to 90 seconds followed by another deep breath.
4. Exhale and feel the muscle being stretched and relaxed to achieve further ROM.
5. Do *not* bounce or spring during stretching.
6. Do *not* force a stretch during breath-holding.
7. Increasing stretching range during exhalation encourages full-body relaxation.
8. Slowly reposition from the stretch posture and allow the muscles to recover to their natural resting length.

REFERENCES

Fasen, J.M., et al.: A randomized controlled trial of hamstring stretching: comparison of four techniques. *J. Strength Cond. Res.,* 23:660, 2009.

Kreun, M.K., et al.: The efficacy of two modified proprioceptive neuromuscular facilitation stretching techniques in subjects with reduced hamstring muscle length. *Physiother. Theory Pract.,* 26:240, 2010.

Ryan, E.E., et al.: The effects of the contract-relax-antagonist-contract form of proprioceptive neuromuscular facilitation stretching on postural stability. *J. Strength Cond. Res.,* 24:1888, 2010.

Streepey, J.W., et al.: Effects of quadriceps and hamstrings proprioceptive neuromuscular facilitation stretching on knee movement sensation. *J. Strength Cond. Res.,* 24:1037, 2010.

SELECTED INTERNET SITES

1. *www.thestretchinghandbook.com/archives/pnf-stretching.php* (PNF stretching explained)
2. *www.youtube.com/watch?v=791XXiYzNbE* (PNF stretching for hamstrings)
3. *www.canadaspace.com/crwb.php?q=PNF+Stretching* (resources for PNF stretching)

Two afferent (sensory) and one efferent (motor) nerve fibers innervate the spindles. The motor spindles consist of thin γ (gamma) efferent fibers that innervate the contractile, striated ends of intrafusal fibers. These fibers, activated by higher brain centers, maintain the spindle at peak operation at all muscle lengths.

Stretch Reflex Muscle spindles lodged in parallel with the main fibers in the belly of a muscle detect, respond to, and modulate changes in the length of the extrafusal muscle fibers. This provides an important regulatory control function for total body movement and maintenance of posture. Postural muscles continuously receive neural input to sustain their readiness to respond to conscious (voluntary) movements. These muscles require continual subconscious activity to adjust to the pull of gravity in upright posture. Without this monitoring and feedback mechanism, the body would literally collapse into a heap from the absence of tension in the neck muscles, spinal muscles, hip flexors, abdominal muscles, and large leg musculature. The patella tendon **stretch reflex** in **Figure 11.5** serves as a fundamental controlling mechanism in human movement. The stretch reflex consists of three main components:

1. Muscle spindle that responds to stretch
2. Afferent nerve fiber that carries the sensory impulse from the spindle to the spinal cord
3. Efferent spinal cord motoneuron that activates the stretched muscle fibers

This simplest autonomic monosynaptic reflex arc involves only one synapse. Spindles lie parallel to the extrafusal fibers and stretch when these fibers elongate as the relfex hammer strikes the patellar tendon. The spindle's sensory receptors fire when its intrafusal fibers stretch, directing impulses through the dorsal root into the spinal cord to directly activate the anterior motoneurons.

Questions & Notes

What is the major function of a muscle spindle?

List the 3 main components of the stretch reflex.

1.

2.

3.

The gray matter contains neuron cell bodies; the white matter carries longitudinal columns of nerve fibers. Stimulation of a single α-motoneuron affects up to 3000 muscle fibers. The reflex also activates interneurons within the spinal cord to facilitate the appropriate motor response. For example, excitatory impulses activate synergistic muscles that support the desired movement, and inhibitory impulses flow to motor units that normally counter the movement. In this way, the stretch reflex acts as a self-regulating, compensating mechanism. This salient feature allows the muscle to adjust automatically to differences in load and length without requiring immediate information processing through higher CNS centers. Humans are indeed fortunate to have this CNS system of checks and balances. Without it, the human body could not perform relatively "simple" muscular movements like touching the tip of your index finger to the tip of your thumb let alone the highly complex, coordinated movement patterns such as smashing a volleyball over a net or trying to hit a stationary golf ball 155 yards straight at the pin.

Golgi Tendon Organs

Golgi tendon organs (GTOs), named to honor Italian physician Camillo Golgi (1843–1926) who first identified these proprioceptors in 1898, connect in series to as many as 25 extrafusal fibers in contrast to muscle spindles that lie parallel to extrafusal muscle fibers. These tiny sensory receptors also are located in ligaments of joints to primarily detect differences in muscle tension rather than length. **Figure 11.11** shows details of the GTOs that respond as a feedback monitor to discharge impulses when muscle shortens or stretches.

When activated by excessive muscle tension or stretch, Golgi receptors immediately transmit signals to cause reflex inhibition of the muscles they supply. This occurs because of an overriding influence of inhibitory spinal interneurons on the motoneurons supplying muscle. With extreme tension or stretch, the Golgi "sensor" discharge increases to further depress motoneuron activity and reduce tension in

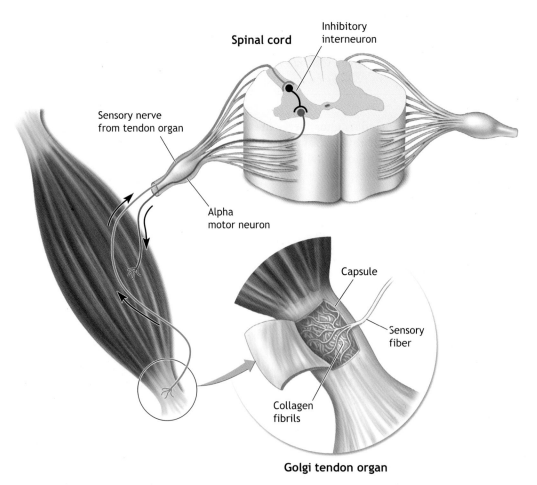

Figure 11.11 The Golgi tendon organ (GTO). Excessive tension or stretch on a muscle activates the tendon's Golgi receptors, which brings about a reflex inhibition of the muscles they supply. In this way, the GTO functions as a protective sensory mechanism to detect and subsequently inhibit undue strain within the muscle-tendon structure.

the muscle fibers. Ultimately, the GTOs protect muscle and its connective tissue harness from injury by sudden, excessive load or stretch.

Pacinian Corpuscles

Pacinian corpuscles are small, ellipsoidal bodies located close to the GTOs and embedded in a single, unmyelinated nerve fiber. They are located in the subcutaneous tissue on the nerves of the soles of the feet and palms of the hands, in the mucous membranes, in male and female genital organs, and in close proximity with the nerves of joints. The ends of the corpuscles are covered by a sensitive receptor membrane whose sodium channels open with any membrane deformation or vibration. Several concentric capsules of connective tissue with a viscous gel between them surround each corpuscle, which attaches to and encloses the termination of a single nerve fiber.

These sensitive sensory receptors respond to quick movement and deep pressure. Deformation or compression of the onionlike capsule by any mechanical stimulus transmits pressure to the sensory nerve ending within its core to change the electric potential of the sensory nerve ending. If this generator potential achieves sufficient magnitude, a sensory signal propagates down the myelinated axon that leaves the corpuscle and enters the spinal cord. Think of Pacinian corpuscles as fast-adapting mechanical sensors. They discharge a few impulses at the onset of a steady stimulus and then remain electrically silent or discharge another volley of impulses when the stimulus ceases. Pacinian corpuscles detect *changes* in movement or pressure rather than the magnitude of movement or the quantity of pressure applied.

$\mathcal{Q}$uestions & Notes

What is the main function of pacinian corpuscles?

Describe the major function of Golgi tendon organs.

For Your Information

CAMILLO GOLGI

In 1878, Camillo Golgi (1843–1926), an Italian neurohistochemist, discovered the minute tendon organs that now bear his name using a silver nitrate stain described in his masterful text, *On the Fine Anatomy of the Nervous System*. Golgi received the Nobel Prize in Physiology or Medicine in 1906 with Santiago Ramón y Cajal (1852–1934) for their insightful contributions about the structures of the nervous system. One of Golgi's greatest contributions was his creative method of staining individual nerve and cell structures using a weak solution of silver nitrate. This invaluable method traced the tiny processes and intricate structures of cells (*nobelprize.org/nobel_prizes/medicine/laureates/ 1906/golgi-bio.html*).

SUMMARY

1. CNS neural control mechanisms finely regulate human movement. In response to internal and external stimuli, bits of sensory input are automatically and rapidly routed, organized, and retransmitted to the muscles.

2. The cerebellum serves as the major comparing, evaluating, and integrating center to fine tune muscular activity.

3. The spinal cord and other subconscious areas of the CNS control numerous muscular functions.

4. The reflex arc processes and initiates automatic (subconscious) muscular movements and responses.

5. The number of muscle fibers in a motor unit depends on the muscle's movement function. Intricate movement patterns require a relatively small fiber-to-neuron ratio, but for gross movements, a single neuron may innervate several thousand muscle fibers.

6. The anterior motoneuron (cell body, axon, and dendrites) transmits the electrochemical neural impulse from the spinal cord to the muscle. Dendrites receive impulses and conduct them toward the cell body; the axon transmits the impulse in one direction only—down the axon to the muscle.

7. The neuromuscular junction provides the interface between the motoneuron and its muscle fibers. ACh release at this junction activates the muscle.

8. Excitatory and inhibitory impulses continually bombard synaptic junctions between neurons. These alter a neuron's threshold for excitation by increasing or decreasing its tendency to fire.

9. In all-out, high-power output exercise, a large degree of disinhibition benefits performance because it allows for maximal activation of a muscle's motor units.

10. Gradation of muscle force results from an interaction of factors that regulate the number and type of motor units recruited and their frequency of discharge.

11. In accordance with the size principle, light exercise predominantly recruits slow-twitch motor units followed by activation of fast-twitch units when force output requirements increase.

12. Sensory receptors in muscles, tendons, and joints relay information about muscular dynamics and limb movement to specific portions of the CNS.

13. Golgi tendon organ receptors respond to quick movement and deep pressure.

14. Pacinian corpuscles detect changes in movement or pressure.

THOUGHT QUESTIONS

1. Discuss why fatigue may not relate to"only" muscular factors.

2. Discuss factors to explain why some individuals are "faster learners" of certain tasks.

3. How might drugs that mimic neurotransmitters affect physiologic response and performance in maximal exercise?

Part 2 — **Muscular System:** Organization and Activation

Skeletal muscles transform the chemical energy within ATP molecules into the mechanical energy of motion. Part 2 presents the architectural organization of skeletal muscle and focuses on its gross and microscopic structure. The discussion includes the sequence of chemical and mechanical events in muscular contraction and relaxation and the differences in muscle fiber characteristics among elite performers in different sports.

COMPARISON OF SKELETAL, CARDIAC, AND SMOOTH MUSCLE

Humans possess three types of muscle—cardiac, smooth, and skeletal, which each have functional and anatomical differences. Cardiac muscle occurs only in the heart. It shares several common features with skeletal muscle; both appear striated (striped) under microscopic examination and contract (shorten) in a similar manner. Smooth muscle lacks a striated appearance but shares cardiac muscle's characteristic of nonconscious regulation. Table 11.2 contrasts the structural and functional characteristics of the three types of muscle.

GROSS STRUCTURE OF SKELETAL MUSCLE

Each of the more than 430 voluntary muscles in the body contains various wrappings of fibrous connective tissue.

Figure 11.12 shows a skeletal muscle cross-section that consists of thousands of cylindrical cells called fibers. These long, slender multinucleated fibers lie parallel to one another whose number largely becomes fixed by the second trimester of fetal development, with the force of contraction occurring mainly along the fiber's long axis.

A fine layer of connective tissue, the **endomysium**, wraps each fiber and separates it from neighboring fibers. Another layer of connective tissue, the **perimysium**, surrounds a bundle of up to 150 fibers to form a **fasciculus**. The **epimysium** surrounds the entire muscle with a fascia of fibrous connective tissue. This protective sheath tapers at its distal end as it blends into and joins the intramuscular tissue sheaths to form the dense, strong connective tissue of **tendons**. Tendons connect each end of the muscle to the **periosteum**, the outermost covering of the skeleton. The force of muscle action transmits directly from the muscle's connective tissue harness to the tendons at their bony points of attachment.

The **sarcolemma**, a thin, elastic membrane that encloses the fiber's cellular contents, lays beneath the endomysium and surrounds each muscle fiber. **Sarcoplasm** (the fiber's aqueous protoplasm) contains enzymes, fat and glycogen particles, nuclei that contain the genes, mitochondria, and other specialized organelles. The sarcoplasm includes an extensive interconnecting network of tubular channels and vesicles called the **sarcoplasmic reticulum**. This highly specialized system enhances the cell's structural integrity. It allows the wave of depolarization to spread rapidly from the fiber's outer surface to its inner environment through the T-tubule system to initiate muscle action. The sarcoplasmic reticulum that surrounds each myofibril contains biologic "pumps" that take up Ca^{++} from the fiber's sarcoplasm. This produces a calcium concentration gradient between the sarcoplasmic reticulum (higher Ca^{++}) and the sarcoplasm surrounding the filaments (lower Ca^{++}).

Table 11.2	Characteristics of the Three Types of Human Muscle		
	TYPE OF MUSCLE		
CHARACTERISTICS	**SKELETAL**	**CARDIAC**	**SMOOTH**
Location	Attached to bones	Heart only	Part of blood vessel structure: surrounds many internal hollow organs
Function	Movement	Pumps blood	Constricts blood vessels; moves contents of internal organs
Anatomical description	Large cylindrical, multinucleated cells arranged in parallel	Quadrangular cells	Small, spindle-shaped cells with long axis oriented in the same direction
Striated	Yes	Yes	No
Initiation of action potential	By neuron only	Spontaneous (pacemaker cells)	Spontaneous
Duration of electrical activity	Short (1–2 ms)	Long (~200 ms)	Very long, slow (~300 ms)
Energy source	Anaerobic, Aerobic	Aerobic	Aerobic
Energy efficiency	Low	Moderate	High
Fatigue resistance	Low to high	Low	Very low
Rate of shortening	Fast	Moderate	Very slow
Duration of action	As brief as 100 ms; prolonged tetanus	Short (~300 ms); summation and tetanus not possible	Very long; may be sustained indefinitely

Chemical Composition

Skeletal muscle contains about 75% water and 20% protein, with the remaining 5% comprising inorganic salts and high-energy phosphates, urea, lactate, calcium, magnesium, and phosphorus; enzymes and pigments; sodium, potassium, and chloride ions; and amino acids, fats, and carbohydrates.

Blood Supply

Intense dynamic muscle actions often require an oxygen uptake of 4000 mL·min^{-1} and higher, and the oxygen consumed by active muscle increases at least 70 times above its resting level to about 3400 mL·min^{-1}. To accommodate the increased oxygen requirement, the local vascular bed redirects blood flow through active tissues similar to a traffic officer rerouting congested traffic. In continuous, rhythmic running, swimming, and cycling, muscle blood flow fluctuates; it decreases during the shortening action and increases during muscle relaxation. Alternating contraction and relaxation provides a "milking action" to propel blood through the muscles back to the heart. Concurrently, the rapid dilation of previously dormant capillaries complements the pulsatile blood flow. Between 200 and 500 capillaries deliver blood to each square millimeter of active muscle cross-section, with up to four capillaries directly contacting each fiber. In endurance athletes, five to seven capillaries surround each fiber; this adaptation ensures greater local blood flow and adequate tissue oxygenation when needed.

Straining-type activities, such as trying to lift a heavy weight, present a somewhat different picture. When a muscle contracts at about 60% of its force-generating capacity, elevated intramuscular pressure begins to restrict the muscle's blood supply. The muscle's compressive force with a maximal isometric action literally retards blood flow. This changes the energy dynamics so the breakdown of stored intramuscular phosphagens and anaerobic glycolytic reactions now provide the energy stream to sustain the muscular effort.

Muscle Capillarization   Capillary microcirculation expedites removal of heat and metabolic byproducts from active tissues. A rich network of these tiny

Questions & Notes

Discuss why the sarcoplasmic reticulum important.

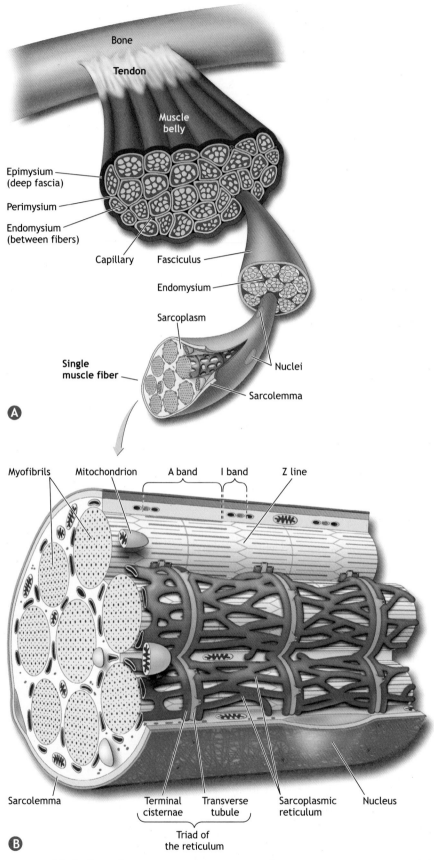

Figure 11.12 Cross-section of skeletal muscle structures and arrangement of connective tissue wrappings. (**A**) Endomysium covers individual fibers. Perimysium surrounds groups of fibers called fasciculi, and epimysium wraps the entire muscle in a sheath of connective tissue. The sarcolemma, a thin, elastic membrane, covers the surface of each muscle fiber. (**B**) A cross-section of the sarcoplasmic reticulum and T-tubule system that surrounds the myofibrils. Note the close contact of the mitochondria and network of intracellular membranes and tubules.

exchange vessels provides a large surface area to exchange not only metabolically generated heat but fluids, electrolytes, gases, and macromolecules as well. In contracting muscles, microvessels immediately after stimulation exhibit increased flow of blood and perfused capillary surface area transport. In regards to exercise training, electron microscopy reveals that the total number of capillaries per muscle (and capillaries per mm^2 of muscle tissue) averages about 40% higher in endurance-trained athletes than untrained counterparts. A positive association also exists between $\dot{V}O_{2max}$ (maximal oxygen consumption) and the average number of muscle capillaries. Enhanced vascularization on the capillary level proves particularly beneficial during exercise that requires a high level of steady-rate aerobic metabolism.

ULTRASTRUCTURE OF SKELETAL MUSCLE

Electron microscopy, laser diffraction, and histochemical staining techniques have revealed the ultrastructure of skeletal muscle (*http://muscle.ucsd.edu/musintro/jump.shtml*). **Figure 11.13A** to **11.13F** show the gross and subcellular microscopic organization of skeletal muscle.

Each muscle fiber contains smaller functional units that lie parallel to the fiber's long axis. The **myofibrils**, approximately 1 μ in diameter, contain even smaller subunits called **myofilaments** that also run parallel to the myofibril's long axis. The myofilaments consist mainly of the proteins **actin** and **myosin** that constitute about 84% of the myofibrillar complex.

The Sarcomere

At low magnification under a light microscope, the alternating light and dark bands along the length of the skeletal muscle fiber appear **striated**. **Figure 11.14** illustrates the structural details of the myofibril's cross-striation pattern. In the resting state, the length of each sarcomere averages 2.5 μm. Thus, a myofibril that is 15 mm long contains about 6000 sarcomeres joined end to end. The length of the sarcomere largely determines a muscle's functional properties.

The **I band** shows up as the lighter area and darker zone the **A band**. The **Z line** bisects the I band and adheres to the sarcolemma to stabilize the entire structure. *The sarcomere, the repeating unit between two Z lines, comprises the functional unit of the muscle cell.* The actin and myosin filaments within a sarcomere provide the mechanical mechanism for muscle action (i.e., contraction and relaxation).

The position of the sarcomere's thin actin and thicker myosin proteins overlaps the two filaments. The center of the A band contains the **H zone**, a region of lower optical density because of the absence of actin filaments in this region. The **M line** bisects the central portion of the H zone and delineates the sarcomere's center. The M line contains the protein structures that support the arrangement of myosin filaments.

Actin–Myosin Orientation

Thousands of myosin filaments lie along the line of actin filaments in a muscle fiber. **Figure 11.15** illustrates the ultrastructure of actin–myosin orientation within a sarcomere at resting length. Six thin actin filaments, each about 50 angstroms (Å; 1 Å = 100 millionths of a centimeter) in diameter and 1 μ long, surround a thicker myosin filament (150 Å in diameter and 1.5 μ long). This forms an impressive muscular substructure. For example, a myofibril that is 1 μ in diameter contains about 450 thick filaments in the center of the sarcomere and 900 thin filaments at each end. Consequently, a single muscle fiber 100 μ in diameter and 1 cm long contains about 8000 myofibrils, each with 4500 sarcomeres. In a single muscle fiber, this translates to a total of 16 billion thick and 64 billion thin filaments in a single muscle fiber.

Questions & Notes

Which cellular component gives the muscle fiber its striated appearance?

Name the functional unit of the muscle fiber.

Name the sarcomere's 2 contractile proteins.

1.

2.

Describe the structural link between thin and thick myofilaments.

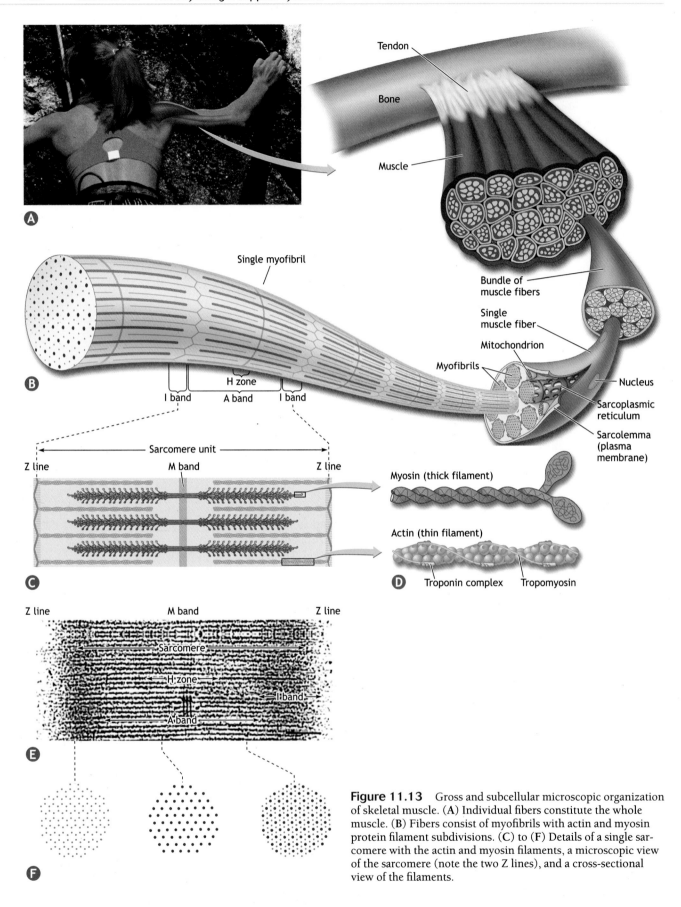

Figure 11.13 Gross and subcellular microscopic organization of skeletal muscle. (**A**) Individual fibers constitute the whole muscle. (**B**) Fibers consist of myofibrils with actin and myosin protein filament subdivisions. (**C**) to (**F**) Details of a single sarcomere with the actin and myosin filaments, a microscopic view of the sarcomere (note the two Z lines), and a cross-sectional view of the filaments.

Figure 11.16 details the spatial orientation of various proteins that form the contractile filaments. Projections or **crossbridges** spiral around the myosin filament in the region where the actin and myosin filaments overlap. Crossbridges repeat at intervals of 450 Å along the filament. Their globular, "lollipop-like" heads extend perpendicularly to latch onto the thinner, double-twisted actin strands to create structural and functional links between myofilaments. The unique feature of myosin's two heads concerns their opposite orientation at the ends of the thick filament. ATP hydrolysis activates the two heads, placing them in an optimal orientation to bind actin's active sites. This pulls the thin filaments and Z lines of the sarcomere toward the middle.

Tropomyosin and **troponin**, the two most important core constituents of the actin helix structure, regulate the make-and-break contacts between myofilaments during muscle action. Tropomyosin distributes along the length of the actin filament in a groove formed by the double helix. It inhibits actin and myosin interaction (coupling) to prevent their permanent bonding. Troponin, which is embedded at fairly regular intervals along the actin strands, exhibits a high affinity for calcium ions (Ca^{++}). Troponin which play a crucial role in

*Q**uestions & Notes*

What activates crossbridge activity?

List the 2 components of the Actin helix

  1.

  2.

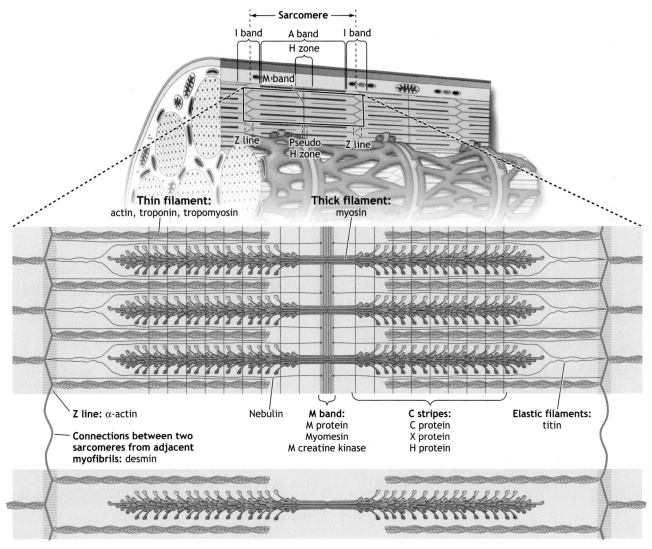

Figure 11.14 (*Top*) Structural position of the filaments in a sarcomere. The Z line bounds a sarcomere at both ends. (*Bottom*) Detailed view of a sarcomere, including the additional proteins nebulin (major regulator of force production with three subunits that lie in the groove of each actin filament that block myosin's binding site in the absence of ionic calcium) and titin (closely associated with the myosin molecule, it appears to anchor the myosin network to the actin network).

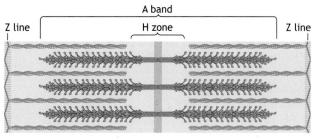

A Resting sarcomere

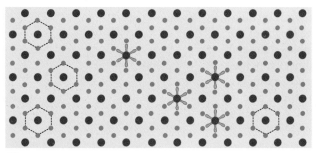

B Cross-section of myofibrils

Figure 11.15 (**A**) Ultrastructure of actin–myosin orientation within a resting sarcomere. (**B**) Representation of electron micrograph through a cross-section of myofibrils in a single muscle fiber. Note the hexagonal orientation of the smaller actin and larger myosin filaments, including crossbridges that extend from a thick to thin filament.

muscle function and fatigue. The action of Ca^{++} and troponin triggers myofibrils to interact and slide past each other. During muscle fiber stimulation, troponin molecules undergo a conformational change that "tugs" on tropomyosin protein strands. Tropomyosin then moves

Figure 11.16 Details of the thick and thin protein filaments, including tropomyosin, troponin complex, and M bridge. The globular heads of myosin contain myosin ATPase; these "active" heads free the energy from adenosine triphosphate (ATP) to power muscle actions.

deeper into the groove between the two actin strands, "uncovering" actin's active sites so muscle action proceeds.

The M line consists of transverse and longitudinally oriented proteins that maintain proper orientation of the thick filament within a sarcomere. The perpendicular oriented M-bridges connect with six adjacent thick myosin filaments in a hexagonal pattern.

Intracellular Tubule Systems

Figure 11.17 illustrates a three-dimensional representation of the intricate tubule system within a muscle fiber. The sarcoplasmic reticulum's complex network of interconnecting tubular channels runs parallel to the myofibrils. The lateral end of each tubule terminates in a saclike vesicle that stores Ca^{++}. Another network of tubules, the transverse-tubule system or **T-tubule system**, runs perpendicular to the myofibril. The T tubules lie between the lateral-most portion of two sarcoplasmic channels; the vesicles of these structures abut the T tubule. The repeating pattern of two vesicles and T tubules in the region of each Z line forms a **triad**. Each sarcomere contains two triads; this pattern repeats regularly throughout the myofibril's length.

The T tubules pass through the fiber and open externally from the inside of the muscle cell. *The triad and T-tubule system function as a microtransportation or plumbing network for spreading the action potential or wave of depolarization from the fiber's outer membrane inward to the deeper cell regions.* The triad sacs release Ca^{++} during depolarization; this diffuses a relatively short distance to activate the actin filaments. Contraction begins when the myosin filaments' crossbridges interact with the active sites on actin filaments. When electrical excitation ceases, cytoplasmic free Ca^{++} concentration decreases and the muscle relaxes.

CHEMICAL AND MECHANICAL EVENTS DURING MUSCLE ACTION AND RELAXATION

Sliding-Filament Theory

Two British biologists with the same last name, Hugh Huxley (1924–) and Sir Andrew Fielding Huxley (1917–), unrelated and working independently in the early 1950s, received the 1963 Nobel Prize in physiology or medicine for work on ionic mechanisms involved in excitation and inhibition in the peripheral and central portions of the nerve cell membrane. Their work led to a proposed sliding-filament model of muscle action.

*This theory proposes that muscle fibers shorten or lengthen because thick and thin myofilaments glide past each other without the filaments themselves changing length. The myosin crossbridges, which cyclically attach, rotate, and detach from the actin filaments with energy from ATP hydrolysis, provide the **molecular motor** to drive fiber shortening (http://muscle. ucsd.edu/musintro/Bridge.shtml).* Muscle action changes

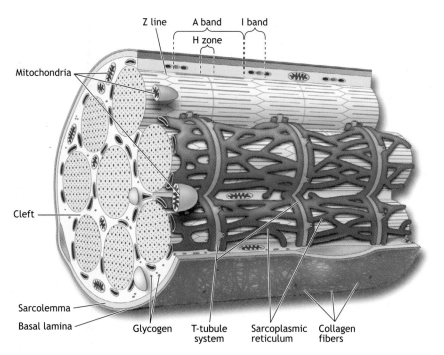

Z line   A band   I band
H zone

Mitochondria

Cleft

Sarcolemma
Basal lamina

Glycogen   T-tubule   Sarcoplasmic   Collagen
system   reticulum   fibers

Figure 11.17 Three-dimensional representation of the sarcoplasmic reticulum and interlocking mesh T-tubule system within a muscle fiber.

*Q*uestions & Notes

Describe the major function of the intracellular tubule system.

In which muscle band region does major structural rearrangement take place during muscle action?

List the structure that provides the mechanical power stroke for actin and myosin filaments to slide past each other.

Briefly summerize the major points of the sliding filament theory of muscle action.

the relative size of the sarcomere's various zones and bands. **Figure 11.18** shows the structural rearrangment of actin and myosin filaments as the thin actin myofilaments slide past the myosin myofilaments and move into the region of the A band during muscle action and move out in relaxation.

The major structural rearrangement during muscle action occurs in the I band region. The I band decreases markedly in size as the Z bands become pulled toward each sarcomere's center. No change occurs in A band width, although the H zone can disappear when the actin filaments contact at the center of the sarcomere. An isometric muscle action generates force, but the fiber's length remains relatively unchanged. In this situation, the relative spacing of I and A bands remains constant to allow the same molecular groups to repeatedly interact with each other. The A band widens when a muscle generates force while lengthening in an eccentric action.

Mechanical Action of Crossbridges
Myosin plays a dual enzymatic and structural role in muscle action. *The globular head of the myosin crossbridge provides the mechanical power stroke for actin and myosin filaments to glide past each other.* **Figure 11.19** shows the oscillating to-and-fro action of the crossbridges, which move similar to the action of oars knifing through water. But unlike oars, the crossbridges do not move synchronously. If they did, the muscle action would produce a series of uneven actions instead of finely graded, smoothly modulated movements and force outputs. During muscle activation, each crossbridge undergoes repeated but independent cycles of attachment

(i) For Your Information

MUSCULAR CONTRACTION OR MUSCULAR ACTION?

During the previous 50 years or so, the term **muscular contraction** commonly referred to processes involving generation of muscular tension associated with muscle shortening. In striated muscle, three types of actions can occur during muscle tension: (1) the muscle can shorten (concentric action), (2) it can remain the same length (static action), or (3) it can lengthen (eccentric action). Thus, the term **muscular action** seems preferable to refer to tension development in skeletal muscle. In this text, we use the terms "contraction" and "action" interchangably to refer to the same event.

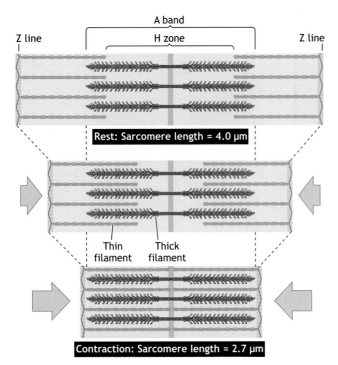

Figure 11.18 Structural rearrangement of actin and myosin filaments at rest (sarcomere length, 4.0 μm) and during muscle shortening (contracted sarcomere length, 2.7 μm).

crossbridge movement. One of the reacting sites on the globular head of the myosin crossbridge binds to a reactive site on actin. The other myosin active site acts as the enzyme myofibrillar adenosine triphosphatase (**myosin–ATPase**) that splits ATP to release its energy for force production. ATP splits "slowly" if myosin and actin remain apart; when joined, the ATP hydrolysis rate increases tremendously. Energy released from ATP changes the shape of the

and detachment to actin. A single crossbridge moves only a short distance, so crossbridges must attach, produce movement, and detach thousands of times to shorten the sarcomere. The process resembles the movement of a person climbing a rope. The arms and legs represent the crossbridges. Climbing progresses by first reaching with the arms; then grabbing, pulling, and breaking contact while the legs extend; and then repeating this procedure throughout the climb as the person traverses from one point to the next point and so on. Only about 50% of the crossbridges contact the actin filaments at any instant to form the contractile protein complex **actomyosin**; the remaining crossbridges maintain some other position during their vibrating cycle.

Link Among Actin, Myosin, and Adenosine Triphosphate

The interaction and movement of the protein filaments during a muscle action require the myosin crossbridges to continually oscillate by combining, detaching, and recombining to new sites along the actin strands (or the same sites in a static action). When an ATP molecule joins the actomyosin complex, it detaches the myosin crossbridges from the actin filament. This chemical reaction allows the myosin crossbridge to resume its original state so it can again bind to a new active actin site. The dissociation of actomyosin occurs in the following reaction:

Actomyosin + ATP → Actin + Myosin–ATP + Force

ATP serves an important function in muscle action. *Splitting the terminal phosphate from ATP provides energy for*

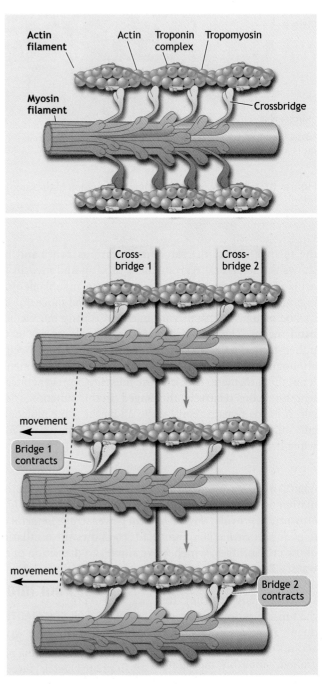

Figure 11.19 (*Top*) Relative positioning of actin and myosin filaments during the oscillating to-and-fro action of the crossbridges. (*Bottom*) The action of each crossbridge contributes a small displacement of movement. For clarity, we show only one actin strand.

globular head of the myosin crossbridge so it interacts and oscillates with the appropriate actin molecule.

Excitation–Contraction Coupling

Excitation–contraction coupling provides the physiologic mechanism so an electrical discharge at the muscle initiates chemical events responsible for activation.

An inactive muscle's Ca^{++} concentration remains relatively low. When stimulated to contract, arrival of the action potential at the transverse tubules releases Ca^{++} from lateral sacs of the sarcoplasmic reticulum, dramatically increasing intracellular Ca^{++} levels. The rapid binding of Ca^{++} to troponin in actin filaments releases troponin's inhibition of actin–myosin interaction. In a sense, muscle "turns on" for action.

Myosin–ATPase splits ATP when the active sites of actin and myosin join together. Energy transfer from ATP breakdown moves the myosin crossbridges, allowing the muscle to generate tension as follows:

$$\text{Actin} + \text{Myosin ATPase} \rightarrow \text{Actomyosin ATPase}$$

The crossbridges uncouple from actin when ATP binds to the myosin bridge. Coupling and uncoupling continue as long as Ca^{++} concentration remains at a level sufficient to inhibit the troponin–tropomyosin system. Discontinuing the nerve stimulus to the muscle moves Ca^{++} back into the lateral sacs of the sarcoplasmic reticulum. This restores the inhibitory effect of troponin–tropomyosin; the presence of ATP maintains actin and myosin separation as follows:

$$\text{Actomyosin-ATPase} \rightarrow \text{Actomyosin} + \text{ADP} + \text{Pi} + \text{Energy}$$

Figure 11.20 illustrates the interaction among actin and myosin filaments, Ca^{++}, and ATP in relaxed and contracted skeletal muscle fibers. In essence, the magnitude and duration of contraction relates directly to the presence of

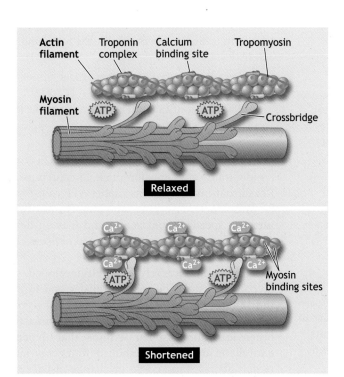

Figure 11.20 Interaction among actin-myosin filaments, Ca^{++}, and ATP in relaxed and contracted muscle. In the relaxed state, troponin and tropomyosin interact with actin, preventing the myosin crossbridge from coupling to actin. During muscle action, the crossbridge couples with actin from Ca^{++} binding with troponin–tropomyosin.

Questions & Notes

Write the formula for the dissociation of actomyosin.

Name the substance that provides energy for crossbridge movement.

Complete the equation:

Actomyosin-ATPase →

List 2 purposes of "deactivation" during a muscle fiber's relaxation period.

1.

2.

List the 2 muscle fiber types.

1.

2.

ⓘ For Your Information

LIKE A COCKED SPRING

Before the muscle action the elongated, flexible myosin head literally bends around the ATP molecule and becomes cocked, almost like a spring. Myosin then interacts with the adjacent action filament, producing a sliding motion that initiates muscle shortening.

calcium. Contraction ceases and relaxation begins when calcium moves back into the sarcoplasmic reticulum, allowing the troponin–tropomyosin complex to inhibit myosin and actin interaction.

Relaxation

When muscle stimulation ceases, active transport mechanisms pump Ca^{++} into the sarcoplasmic reticulum, concentrating Ca^{++} in the lateral vesicles. Calcium retrieval from the myofilament proteins "turns off" the active sites on the actin filament. Deactivation serves two purposes:

1. Prevents any mechanical link between the myosin crossbridges and actin filaments
2. Inhibits myosin ATPase activity to curtail ATP splitting

Muscle relaxation occurs when the actin and myosin filaments return to their original states.

Sequence of Events in Muscle Excitation–Contraction

Figure 11.21 provides a schematic view of the nine important steps in muscle action and relaxation. The numbers correspond to the sequence of nine steps outlined in the figure.

Step 1: Generation of an action potential in the motor neuron causes the small, saclike vesicles within the terminal axon to release ACh. ACh diffuses across the synaptic cleft and attaches to specialized ACh receptors on the sarcolemma. Almost perfect symmetry exists between the "imprint" of the presynaptic vesicles that contain ACh and the "imprint" of the postsynaptic receptors that capture ACh.

Step 2: The muscle action potential depolarizes the transverse tubules at the sarcomere's A–I junction.

Step 3: Depolarization of the T-tubule system causes Ca^{++} release from the lateral sacs (terminal cisternae) of the sarcoplasmic reticulum.

Step 4: Ca^{++} binds to troponin–tropomyosin in the actin filaments. This releases the inhibition that prevented actin from combining with myosin.

Step 5: During muscle action, actin combines with myosin–ATP. Actin also activates the enzyme myosin ATPase, which then splits ATP. The reaction's energy produces myosin crossbridge movement and creates tension.

Step 6: ATP binds to the myosin crossbridge; this breaks the actin–myosin bond and allows the crossbridge to dissociate from actin. The thick and thin filaments then slide past each other, and the muscle shortens.

Step 7: Crossbridge activation continues when Ca^{++} concentration remains high enough from membrane depolarization to inhibit the troponin–tropomyosin system.

Step 8: When muscle stimulation ceases, intracellular Ca^{++} concentration rapidly decreases as Ca^{++} moves back into the lateral sacs of the sarcoplasmic reticulum through active transport that requires ATP hydrolysis.

Step 9: Ca^{++} removal restores the inhibitory action of troponin–tropomyosin. In the presence of ATP, actin and myosin remain in the dissociated, relaxed state.

MUSCLE FIBER TYPES

Through the years, different researchers have used different schemes to classify skeletal muscle fiber types (see Close-up Box 11.2: *Histochemical Staining Assays,* page 370). To date, the so-called metabolic classification emerges as the most useful to make the connection between fiber type and function. Moreover, different researchers have used different nomenclature to describe different fibers.

In general, two distinct fiber types have emerged for classification, termed fast twitch and slow twitch. The proportions of each type of muscle fiber vary from muscle to muscle and person to person. Table 11.3 lists characteristics of these fiber types and their different subdivisions, and **Figure 11.22** shows serial cross-sections obtained by muscle biopsy of human vastus lateralis muscle with identification of type I and type IIa, IIx, and IIc fiber subdivisions.

Fast-Twitch Muscle Fibers

Fast-twitch muscle fibers exhibit the following four characteristics:

1. Rapidly transmit action potentials
2. High activity level of myosin ATPase
3. Rapid rate of calcium release and uptake by the sarcoplasmic reticulum
4. Generate rapid crossbridge turnover

These four qualities relate to how well a fast-twitch fiber rapidly transfers energy for quick, forceful muscle actions. Recall that myosin–ATPase splits ATP to provide energy for muscle action (force generation). The fast-twitch fiber's intrinsic speed of contraction and tension development averages two to three times the speed of fibers classified as slow twitch.

Fast-twitch fibers rely on a well-developed, short-term glycolytic system for energy transfer and force production. Labeled as FG fibers, they signify fast glycogenolytic capabilities. Short-term, high-power output activities and other forceful muscular actions that depend almost entirely on anaerobic metabolism for energy activate fast-twitch fibers. Stop-and-go or change-of-pace sports like basketball, soccer, rugby, lacrosse, and field hockey also require rapid energy from anaerobic pathways in fast-twitch fibers.

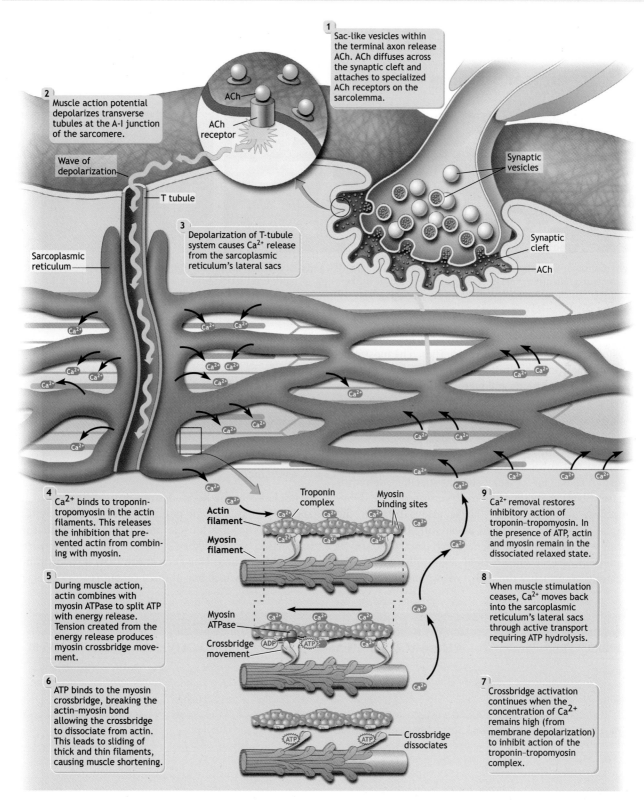

1 Sac-like vesicles within the terminal axon release ACh. ACh diffuses across the synaptic cleft and attaches to specialized ACh receptors on the sarcolemma.

2 Muscle action potential depolarizes transverse tubules at the A-I junction of the sarcomere.

Wave of depolarization

T tubule

ACh

ACh receptor

Synaptic vesicles

Synaptic cleft

ACh

Sarcoplasmic reticulum

3 Depolarization of T-tubule system causes Ca²⁺ release from the sarcoplasmic reticulum's lateral sacs

Ca²⁺

Troponin complex

Myosin binding sites

Actin filament

Myosin filament

Myosin ATPase

Crossbridge movement

ADP ATP

Crossbridge dissociates

ATP ATP

4 Ca²⁺ binds to troponin-tropomyosin in the actin filaments. This releases the inhibition that prevented actin from combining with myosin.

5 During muscle action, actin combines with myosin ATPase to split ATP with energy release. Tension created from the energy release produces myosin crossbridge movement.

6 ATP binds to the myosin crossbridge, breaking the actin-myosin bond allowing the crossbridge to dissociate from actin. This leads to sliding of thick and thin filaments, causing muscle shortening.

9 Ca²⁺ removal restores inhibitory action of troponin-tropomyosin. In the presence of ATP, actin and myosin remain in the dissociated relaxed state.

8 When muscle stimulation ceases, Ca²⁺ moves back into the sarcoplasmic reticulum's lateral sacs through active transport requiring ATP hydrolysis.

7 Crossbridge activation continues when the concentration of Ca²⁺ remains high (from membrane depolarization) to inhibit action of the troponin-tropomyosin complex.

Figure 11.21 Schematic view of the nine main events in muscle contraction and relaxation. Numbers correspond to the sequence of nine steps outlined on p. 368. The neurotransmitter acetylcholine (ACh), released from saclike vesicles within the terminal axon, initiates transmission at the myoneural junction where the electrochemical signal "jumps" across the 0.05-μm cleft between neuron and muscle fiber. The electrical impulse traveling at a velocity of 1 m·s⁻¹ or faster, spreads through the fiber's architecturally elegant tubule system to the myofibril's inner contractile "machinery."

BOX 11.2 CLOSE UP

Histochemical Staining Assays to Assess Muscle Fiber Types

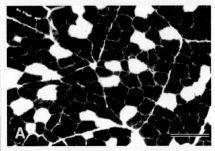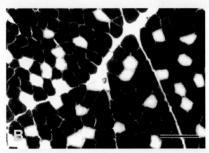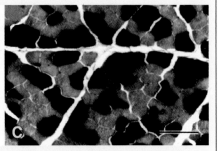

Light micrographs of the vastus lateralis (**A**), vastus medialis (**B**), and rectus femoris muscles (**C**). All micrographs were taken at the same magnification. Fast fibers appear dark, and slow fibers appear light. Calibration bars = 100 μm. (From Lieber R.L. *Skeletal Muscle Structure, Function, and Plasticity: The Physiological Basis of Rehabilitation*, 3rd ed. Baltimore: Lippincott Williams & Wilkins, 2010.)

Many schemes classify skeletal muscle histochemical, physiologic, and morphologic properties. The most relevant schemes rely on physiologic, biochemical, and histochemical experiments and methodologies combined to develop a iterative and unified understanding of human skeletal muscle types.

The term "histochemical" (histo = tissue) implies that the chemical reaction occurs in the tissue itself rather than in a test tube. The three main assays include the myosin ATPase (mATPase) assay, the succinate dehydrogenase (SDH) assay, and the α-glycerophosphate dehydrogenase (α-GPD) assay. These assays rely on the premise that enzymes located in carefully biopsied, thin frozen sections of muscle fibers (6 to 8 μm; [1000 μm = 1 mm thick]) react when treated chemically to allow the researcher to visualize the extent of enzyme activity. The

biochemical assay methods rely on the following basic requirements:

1. Introduction of a biological fuel to serve as one of many enzymes for analyses
2. Addition of an energy source to activate the enzyme so it joins with the substrate
3. Formation of a reaction product to link to another product to form a precipitate for final microscopic assessment

Histochemical methods identify muscle fibers into fast and slow, oxidative or nonoxidative, and glycolytic or nonglycolytic. If a muscle fiber is stained for all three properties, any of eight (2^3) fiber types could theoretically be obtained. However, more than 95% of human muscle classify into one of three categories.

Human Fiber Type by Histochemical Assay

FIBER TYPE	ATPase ACTIVITY (FAST OR SLOW)	SDH ACTIVITY	α-GPD ACTIVITY
Fast-glycolytic (FG)	High	Low	High
Fast-glycolytic-oxidative (FOG)	High	High	High
Slow-oxidative (SO)	Low	High	Low

GPD, glycerophosphate dehydrogenase; SDH, succinate dehydrogenase.

Fast-Twitch Type II Subdivisions   Type II fibers distribute in three primary subtypes, types IIa, IIx, and IIb. Recent studies show that human skeletal muscle contains types I, IIa, and IIx fibers, previously referred to as type IIb and a new type IIb subtype. Types IIa, IIx, and IIb fibers appear in skeletal muscle of rodents and cats.

The type **IIa fiber** exhibits fast shortening speed and a moderately well-developed capacity for energy transfer from both aerobic (high level of aerobic enzyme suc-

cinic dehydrogenase [SDH]) and anaerobic (high level of anaerobic enzyme phosphofructokinase, [PFK]) sources. These fibers represent the **fast–oxidative–glycolytic (FOG) fibers**. The **type IIx fiber** possesses the greatest anaerobic potential and most rapid shortening velocity; it represents the "true" **fast–glycolytic (FG) fiber**. A **type IIc fiber**, normally rare and undifferentiated, may contribute to reinnervation and motor unit transformation.

Slow-Twitch Muscle Fibers

Slow-twitch muscle fibers generate energy for ATP resynthesis predominantly by aerobic energy transfer. They possess a low activity level of myosin ATPase, a slow speed of contraction, and a glycolytic capacity less well developed than fast-twitch counterparts (Table 11.3). Slow-twitch fibers contain relatively large and numerous mitochondria and iron-containing cytochromes of the electron transport chain (which contribute to their red appearance). A high concentration of mitochondrial enzymes supports the enhanced aerobic metabolic machinery. Consequently, slow-twitch fibers resist fatigue and power prolonged aerobic exercise. These fibers are labeled **slow-oxidative (SO) fibers**, which describes their slow contraction speed and predominant reliance on oxidative metabolism.

Studies of muscle glycogen depletion patterns indicate that slow-twitch muscle fibers exclusively power prolonged, moderate intensity exercise. Even after exercising for 12 hours, the limited but still available glycogen exists in the unused fast-twitch fibers. Differences in the oxidative capacity of the two fiber types also determine blood flow capacity through muscle tissues during exercise; slow-twitch fibers receive considerably more blood than fast-twitch counterparts. Exercise at near-maximum aerobic and anaerobic levels like middle-distance running, swimming, or multiple-sprint sports like field hockey, lacrosse, basketball, ice hockey, and soccer, activate both muscle fiber types.

Muscle Fiber Type Differences Among Athletic Groups

Several interesting observations emerge concerning muscle fiber type variation among individuals and sport categories and the possible influence of specific exercise training on fiber composition and metabolic capacity. On average, sedentary children and adults possess about 50% slow-twitch fibers. The percentage of fast-twitch fibers probably distributes equally between subdivisions, yet fiber-type distribution varies considerably among individuals. Generally, one's muscle fiber-type

Questions & Notes

List 3 characteristics of FT muscle fibers.

1.

2.

3.

List 2 subdivisions of FT muscle fibers.

1.

2.

(i) For Your Information

MULTIMEDIA MUSCLE ACTION VIDEOS

The following 10 multimedia video animations present many aspects of muscle action processes. These videos, produced by students for students, are complementary to our presentation of muscle action dynamics.

1. *www.youtube.com/watch?v=iMD7wNhWdc8&feature=related*
2. *www.youtube.com/watch?v=zC0cd45W0oI&feature=related*
3. *www.youtube.com/watch?v=FdV4_PBSVy0&feature=related*
4. *www.youtube.com/watch?v=ren_IQPObJc&feature=related*
5. *www.youtube.com/watch?v=IZjZAutXzbw&feature=related*
6. *www.youtube.com/watch?v=EdHzKYDxrKc&feature=related*
7. *www.youtube.com/watch?v=WRxsOMenNQM&feature=related*
8. *www.youtube.com/watch?v=InIba7bCTjM&feature=related*
9. *www.youtube.com/watch?v=DFDbq4KPVBE&feature=related*
10. *www.youtube.com/watch?v=BCUVDE_Bng8&feature=related*

Table 11.3 — Classification of Human Skeletal Muscle Fiber Types

FIBER TYPE	TYPE I FIBERS	TYPE IIa FIBERS	TYPE IIx FIBERS	TYPE IIb FIBERS
Contraction time	Slow	Moderately fast	Fast	Very fast
Size of motor neuron	Small	Medium	Large	Very large
Resistance to fatigue	High	Fairly high	Intermediate	Low
Activity used for	Aerobic	Long-term anaerobic	Short-term anaerobic	Short-term anaerobic
Maximum duration of use	Hours	<30 minutes	<5 minutes	<1 minute
Force production	Low	Medium	High	Very high
Mitochondrial density	High	High	Medium	Low
Capillary density	High	Intermediate	Low	Low
Oxidative capacity	High	High	Intermediate	Low
Glycolytic capacity	Low	High	High	High
Major storage fuel	Triacylglycerol	Creatine phosphate, glycogen	Creatine phosphate, glycogen	Creatine phosphate, glycogen
Myosin-heavy chains, human genes	MYH7[a]	MYH2	MYH1	MYH4

[a]MYH7 is also known as myosin or myosin heavy chain 4.

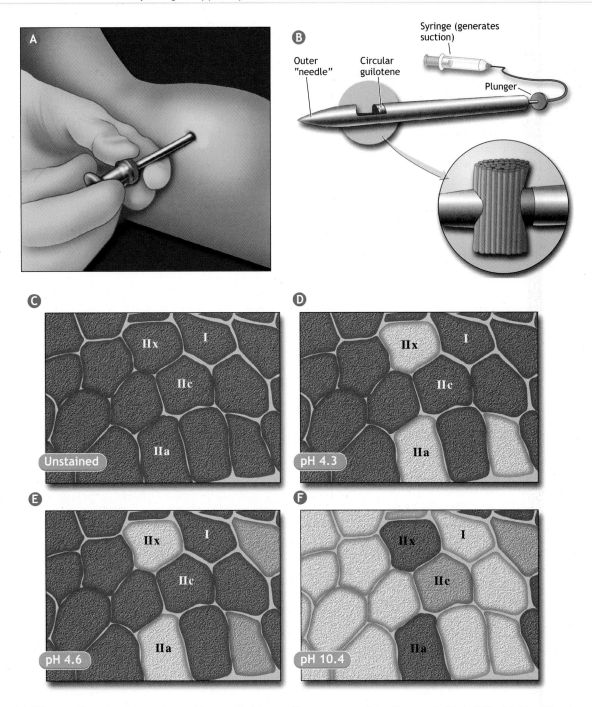

Figure 11.22 Serial cross-sections obtained by muscle biopsy of human vastus lateralis muscle (**A** and **B**) with identification of type I and type IIA, X, and C fiber subdivisions. (**C**) Thick unstained section (40–50 μm) where all fibers appear similar. Three other panels indicate same fibers stained for myosin–ATPase activity at a preincubation pH of 4.3 (highly acidic) (**D**), 4.6 (intermediate acidity) (**E**), and 10.6 (alkaline) (**F**).

distribution remains consistent for the body's major muscle groups.

Elite athletes possess distinct patterns of fiber distribution. Successful endurance athletes, for example, possess a predominance of slow-twitch fibers in the muscles routinely activated in their sport; the fast-twitch muscle fiber predominates for sprint athletes. **Figure 11.23** illustrates sport-specific tendencies for muscle fiber type among top Nordic competitors from different sports. Distance runners and cross-country skiers with the highest aerobic and endurance

capacities possess the greatest percentages of slow-twitch fibers, often as high as 90%. In contrast, weight lifters, ice-hockey players, and sprinters typically have more fast-twitch fibers and a relatively lower $\dot{V}O_{2max}$. As might be expected, male and female middle-distance specialists show approximately equal percentages of the two muscle fiber types. Equal fiber-type distribution also exists for throwers, jumpers, and high jumpers (i.e., power athletes).

Relatively clear-cut distinctions between performance and muscle fiber composition emerge only for elite athletes

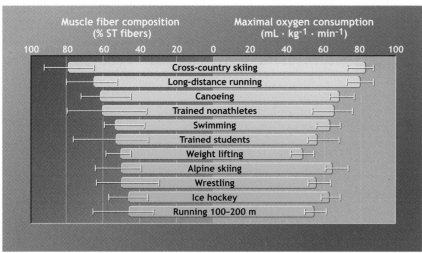

Figure 11.23   Muscle fiber composition (percent slow-twitch fibers, *left side*) and maximal oxygen uptake (*right side*) in athletes representing different sports. The outer *lightly shaded bars* denote the range. (Fom Bergh, U., et al.: Maximal oxygen uptake and muscle fiber types in trained and untrained humans. *Med. Sci. Sports*, 10:151, 1978.)

 For Your Information

RIGOR MORTIS

Muscles become stiff and rigid about 3 hours after death, a condition termed *rigor mortis* (Latin *mors*, **mortis** meaning "of death"). This occurs because ATP no longer functions in the membrane of the sarcoplasmic reticulum to pump calcium ions into the terminal cisternae. When Ca^{++} diffuses from a higher concentration in the terminal cisternae and extracellular fluid to an area of lower concentration in the sarcomere, it binds with troponin to allow crossbridging between the actin and myosin proteins. In essence, without ATP, the myosin crossbridges and actin remain attached so the muscle cannot return to a relaxed state.

who have achieved prominence in a specific sport category. Regardless of performance status, muscle fiber composition does not exclusively determine success. Within groups of trained or untrained individuals, knowledge of predominant fiber type provides limited value in predicting performance outcome. Achievement depends on a blending of many physiologic, biochemical, neurologic, and biomechanical support systems and not simply on a single factor such as muscle fiber type.

 For Your Information

MUSCLE FIBER TRAINING SPECIFICITY

Why do some highly trained athletes who switch to a sport requiring different muscle groups feel essentially untrained for the new activity? The answer is fairly straightforward—only the specific fibers activated in training adapt metabolically and physiologically to the specific exercise regimen. Thus, swimmers or canoeists do not necessarily transfer their upper-body "fitness" to a running sport unless they specifically train the muscles required for that sport.

 SUMMARY

1. Various wrappings of connective tissue that encase skeletal muscle eventually blend into and join the tendinous attachment to bone. With this harness, muscles act on the bony levers to transform ATP's chemical energy into mechanical energy and motion.

2. Skeletal muscle contains approximately 75% water and 20% protein, with the remaining 5% containing inorganic salts, enzymes, minerals, pigments, fats, proteins, and carbohydrates.

3. Vigorous aerobic exercise increases the active muscle's oxygen uptake nearly 70 times above its resting level. Aerobic training augments a muscle's oxygen supply by increasing capillary density up to 40%.

4. The sarcomere contains the contractile proteins actin and myosin, the muscle fiber's functional unit. An average-sized muscle fiber contains about 4500 sarcomeres and a total of 16 billion thick (myosin) and 64 billion thin (actin) filaments. The actin and myosin filaments within the sarcomere provide the mechanical mechanism for muscle action.

5. Crossbridge projections link thin and thick contractile filaments. The globular head of the myosin crossbridge provides the mechanical power stroke for actin and myosin filaments to slide past each other.

6. Tropomyosin and troponin, two core myofibrillar proteins, regulate the make-and-break contacts between filaments during muscle action. Tropomyosin inhibits actin and myosin interaction; troponin with

calcium triggers the myofibrils to interact and glide past each other.

7. The triad and T-tubule microtransportation system network spreads the action potential from the fiber's outer membrane inward to deeper cell regions.

8. Muscle action occurs when calcium activates actin, attaching the myosin crossbridges to active sites on the actin filaments. Relaxation occurs when calcium concentration decreases.

9. The sliding-filament theory proposes that a muscle fiber shortens or lengthens because its protein filaments slide past each other without changing length. Excitation–contraction coupling initiates an electrical discharge that triggers the chemical events for contraction.

10. Two types of muscle fibers are classified according to contractile and metabolic characteristics: (1) fast-twitch fibers (type II), which predominantly generate energy anaerobically for quick, powerful contractions; and (2) slow-twitch fibers (type I), which contract at relatively slow speeds and generate energy for ATP resynthesis largely by aerobic metabolism.

11. Muscle fiber-type distribution differs among individuals. A person's genetic code largely determines his or her predominant fiber type.

12. Specific exercise training improves the metabolic capacity of each fiber type.

THOUGHT QUESTIONS

1. Show how knowledge about neuromuscular exercise physiology can enhance an athlete's (1) muscular strength and power and (2) sports skill performance.

2. In terms of neuromuscular physiology, discuss the validity of the adage "practice makes perfect."

3. Discuss the meaning of *molecular motor* to describe how the myofilament crossbridges contribute to muscle fiber action.

SELECTED REFERENCES

Armstrong, R.B.: Muscle fiber recruitment patterns and their metabolic correlates. In: *Exercise, Nutrition, and Energy Metabolism.* Horton, E.S., Terjung, R.L. (eds.). New York: Macmillan, 1988.

Asmussen, E.: Muscle fatigue. *Med. Sci. Sports Exerc.,* 25:412, 1993.

Asp, S., et al.: Muscle glycogen accumulation after a marathon: Roles of fiber type and pro- and macroglycogen. *J. Appl. Physiol.,* 86:474, 1999.

Baldwin, J., et al.: Muscle IMP accumulation during fatiguing submaximal exercise in endurance trained and untrained men. *Am. J. Physiol.,* 277:R295, 1999.

Barash, I.A., et al.: Rapid muscle-specific gene expression changes after a single bout of eccentric contractions in the mouse. *Am. J. Physiol. Cell. Physiol.,* 286:C355, 2004.

Baron, B., et al.: The eccentric muscle loading influences the pacing strategies during repeated downhill sprint intervals. *Eur. J. Appl. Physiol.,* 105:749, 2009.

Basmajian, J.V., Deluca, C.J.: *Muscles Alive. Their Functions Revealed by Electromyography,* 5th Ed. Baltimore: Williams & Wilkins, 1985.

Billeter, R., Hoppler, H.: Muscular basis of strength. In: *Strength and Power in Sport.* Komi, P. (ed.). London: Blackwell Scientific Publications, 1992.

Boe, S.G., et al.: Decomposition-based quantitative electromyography: effect of force on motor unit potentials and motor unit number estimates. *Muscle Nerve,* 31:365, 2005.

Booth, F.W., et al.: Viewpoint: Gold standards for scientists who are conducting animal-based exercise studies. *J. Appl. Physiol.* 108:219, 2010.

Caiozzo, V.J., et al.: MHC polymorphism in rodent plantaris muscle: effects of mechanical overload and hypothyroidism. *Am. J. Physiol. Cell Physiol.,* 278:C709, 2000.

Caiozzo, V.J., et al.: Single-fiber myosin heavy chain polymorphism: how many patterns and what proportions? *Am. J. Physiol. Regul. Integr. Comp. Physiol.,* 285:R570, 2003.

Carins, S.P., et al.: Role of extracellular $[Ca^{2+}]$ in fatigue of isolated mammalian skeletal muscle. *J. Appl. Physiol.,* 84:1395, 1998.

Crew, J.R., et al.: Muscle fiber type specific induction of slow myosin heavy chain 2 gene expression by electrical stimulation. *Exp. Cell Res.,* 316:1039, 2010.

Davis, J.M., Bailey, S.P.: Possible mechanisms of central nervous system fatigue during exercise. *Med. Sci. Sports Exerc.,* 29:45, 1997.

Dawson, B., et al.: Changes in performance, muscle metabolites, enzymes and fiber types after short sprint training. *Eur. J. Appl. Physiol.,* 78:163, 1998.

Delbono, O., et al.: Loss of skeletal muscle strength by ablation of the sarcoplasmic reticulum protein JP45. *Proc. Natl. Acad. Sci. U.S.A.* 104:20108, 2007.

Demirel, H.A., et al.: Exercise induced alterations in skeletal muscle myosin heavy chain phenotype: Dose-response relationship. *J. Appl. Physiol.*, 86:1002, 1999.

Ennion, S., et al.: Characterization of human skeletal muscle fibers according to the myosin heavy chain they express. *J. Muscle Res. Cell Motil.*, 16:35, 1995.

Farina, D., et al.: Spike-triggered average torque and muscle fiber conduction velocity of low-threshold motor units following submaximal endurance contractions. *J. Appl. Physiol.*, 98:1495, 2005.

Fisher, S., et al.: Structural mechanism of the recovery stroke in the myosin molecular motor. *Proc. Natl. Acad. Sci.*, 102:6873, 2005.

Fong, A.J., et al.: Recovery of control of posture and locomotion after a spinal cord injury: solutions staring us in the face [review]. *Prog. Brain Res.*, 175:393, 2009.

Fowles, J.R., Green, H.J.: Coexistence of potentiation and low-frequency fatigue during voluntary exercise in human skeletal muscle. *Can. J. Physiol. Pharmacol.*, 81:1092, 2003.

Gordon, T., et al.: The resilience of the size principle in the organization of motor unit properties in normal and reinnervated adult skeletal muscles. *Can. J. Physiol. Pharmacol.*, 82:645, 2004.

Green, H.J., et al.: Malleability of human skeletal muscle Na+-K+-ATPase pump with short-term training. *J. Appl. Physiol.*, 97:143, 2004.

Green, H., et al.: Regulation of fiber size, oxidative potential, and capillarization in human muscle by resistance exercise. *Am. J. Physiol.*, 276:R591, 1999.

Green, H.J., et al.: Reversal of muscle fatigue during 16-h of heavy intermittent cycle exercise. *J. Appl. Physiol.*, 97:2166, 2004.

Gregory, C.M., Bickel, C.S.: Recruitment patterns in human skeletal muscle during electrical stimulation. *Phys. Ther.*, 85:358, 2005.

Hawke, T.J.: Muscle stem cells and exercise training. *Exerc. Sport Sci. Rev.*, 33:63, 2005.

Heckmann, C.J., et al.: Persistent inward currents in motoneuron dendrites: Implications for motor output. *Muscle Nerve*, 31:135, 2005.

Hintz, C.S., et al.: Comparison of muscle fiber typing by quantitative enzyme assays and by myosin ATPase staining. *J. Histochem. Cytochem.*, 32:655, 1984.

Hochachka, P.W.: *Muscles as Molecular and Metabolic Machines.* Boca Raton, FL: CRC Press, 1994.

Holloszy, J.O., Coyle, E.F.: Adaptations of skeletal muscle to endurance training and their metabolic consequences. *J. Appl. Physiol.*, 56:831, 1984.

Huxley, H.E.: The fine structure of striated muscle and its functional significance. *Harvey Lectures*, 60:85, 1966.

Huxley, H.E., Kress, M.: Crossbridge behaviour during muscle contraction. *J. Muscle Res. Cell Motil.*, 6:153, 1985.

Keenan, K.G., et al.: Influence of amplitude cancellation on the simulated surface electromyogram. *J. Appl. Physiol.*, 98:120, 2005.

Keller P, et al.: Using systems biology to define the essential biological networks responsible for adaptation to endurance exercise training. *Biochem. Soc. Trans.*, 35:1306, 2007.

Kernell, D.: Principles of force gradation in skeletal muscles. *Neural Plast.*, 10:69, 2003.

Kraus, W.E., et al.: Skeletal muscle adaptation to chronic low-frequency motor nerve stimulation. *Exerc. Sport Sci. Rev.*, 22:313, 1994.

Lambert, E.V., et al.: Complex systems model of fatigue: integrative homeostatic control of peripheral physiological systems during exercise in humans. *Br. J. Sports Med.*, 39:52, 2005.

Lewis, S.F., Fulco, C.S.: A new approach to studying muscle fatigue and factors affecting performance during dynamic exercise in humans. *Exerc. Sport Sci. Rev.*, 26:91, 1998.

Lieber, R.L.: *Skeletal Muscle Structure, Function, and Plasticity: The Physiological Basis of Rehabilitation*, 3rd ed. Baltimore: Williams & Wilkins, 2010.

Lieber, R.L., et al.: Biomechanical properties of the brachioradialis muscle: Implications for surgical tendon transfer. *J. Hand Surg. [Am].*, 30:273, 2005.

Lin, J., et al.: Transcriptional co-activator PGC-1 alpha drives the formation of slow-twitch muscle fibers. *Nature*, 418:797, 2002.

Lucas, C.A., et al.: Monospecific antibodies against the three mammalian fast limb myosin heavy chains. *Biochem. Biophys. Res. Comm.*, 272:303, 2000.

Lutz, G.J., Lieber, R.L.: Skeletal muscle myosin II structure and function. *Exerc. Sport Sci. Rev.*, 27:63, 1999.

Mottram, C.J., et al.: Motor-unit activity differs with load type during a fatiguing contraction. *J. Neurophysiol.*, 93:1381, 2005.

Nielsen, O.B., Clausen, T. The Na/K-pump protects muscle excitability and contractility during exercise. *Exerc. Sport Sci. Rev.*, 28:159, 2000.

Noakes, T.D., et al.: From catastrophe to complexity: a novel model of integrative central neural regulation of effort and fatigue during exercise in humans: summary and conclusions. *Br. J. Sports Med.*, 39:120, 2005.

Otten, E.: Concepts and models of functional architecture in skeletal muscle. In: *Exercise and Sport Sciences Reviews*, vol. 16. Pandolf, K.B. (ed.). New York: Macmillan, 1988.

Patel, T.J., Lieber, R.L.: Force transmission in skeletal muscle: From actomyosin to external tendons. *Exer. Sport Sci. Rev.*, 25:321, 1997.

Roy, R.R., et al.: Modulation of myonuclear number in functionally overloaded and exercised rat plantaris fibers. *J. Appl. Physiol.*, 87:634, 1999.

Russell AP, et al.: Endurance training in humans leads to fiber type-specific increases in levels of peroxisome proliferator-activated receptor-gamma coactivator-1 and peroxisome proliferator-activated receptor-alpha in skeletal muscle. *Diabetes*, 52: 2874–2881, 2003.

Schunk, K., et al.: Contributions of dynamic phosphorus-31 magnetic resonance spectroscopy to the analysis of muscle fiber distribution. *Invest. Radiol.*, 34:348, 1999.

Sieck, G.C. Neural control of movement. *J. Appl. Physiol.*, 96:1247, 2004.

Smerdu, V., et al.: Type IIx myosin heavy chain transcripts are expressed in type IIb fibers of human skeletal muscle. *Am. J. Physiol. Cell Physiol.* 267:C1723, 1994.

Smith, M.F., The role of physiology in the development of golf performance. *Sports Med.,* 40:635, 2010.

Sweeney, L.J., et al.: An introductory biology lab that uses enzyme histochemistry to teach students about skeletal muscle fiber types. *Adv. Physiol. Educ.,* 28:23, 2004.

Ward, S.R., et al.: Are current measurements of lower extremity muscle architecture accurate? *Clin. Orthop. Relat. Res.,* 467:1074, 2009.

Weston, A.R., et al.: African runners exhibit greater fatigue resistance, lower lactate accumulation, and higher oxidative enzyme activity. *J. Appl. Physiol.,* 86:915, 1999.

Wickham, J.B., Brown, J.M.: Muscles within muscles: The neuromotor control of intra-muscular segments. *Eur. J. Appl. Physiol.,* 78:219, 1998.

Zawadowska, B., et al.: Characteristics of myosin profile in human vastus lateralis muscle in relation to training background. *Folia. Histochem. Cytobiol.,* 42:181, 2004.

Zhou, P., Rymer, W.Z.: An evaluation of the utility and limitations of counting motor unit action potentials in the surface electromyogram. *J. Neural. Eng.,* 1:238, 2004.

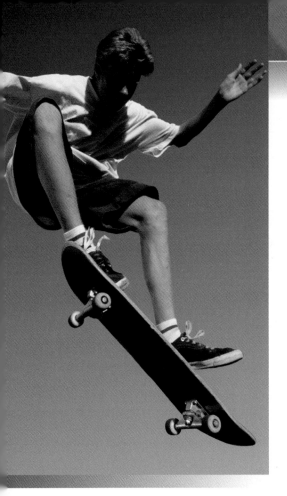

Chapter

12

Hormones,
Exercise,
and Training

CHAPTER OBJECTIVES

- Draw the location of the major endocrine glands within an outline of the human body.

- Describe how hormones alter cellular reaction rates of specific target cells.

- Describe how hormonal, humoral, and neural factors stimulate endocrine glands.

- List the hormones secreted by the anterior and posterior pituitary glands and explain how acute and chronic physical activity affects their release.

- List the thyroid gland hormones, their functions, and how acute and chronic physical activity affects their release.

- List the hormones of the adrenal medulla and adrenal cortex, their functions, and how acute and chronic physical activity affects their release.

- List the hormones of the pancreas' α and β cells, their functions, and how acute and chronic physical activity affects their release.

- Define type 1 and type 2 diabetes mellitus and give three differences between these two diabetes subdivisions.

- List five risk factors for type 2 diabetes.

- Outline the benefits of regular physical activity for a type 2 diabetic.

- Explain the general effects of exercise training on endocrine function.

- Characterize the functions of opioid peptides, their response to physical activity, and possible role in the "exercise high."

The endocrine system (the term endocrine *means* **hormone secreting***) consists of a host organ (gland), minute quantities of chemical messengers (hormones), and a target or receptor organ.* This system integrates and regulates body functions to stabilize the internal environment. **Hormones** produced by endocrine glands affect all aspects of human function; they regulate growth, metabolism, and reproduction, with heightened acute and chronic response to physical and psychological stress. Hormones maintain internal homeostasis by modulating electrolyte and acid–base balance and adjusting energy metabolism to power biologic work.

The endocrine system works in tandem with the nervous system to provide hormonal secretions throughout the body. The hormones produced within endocrine glands serve as "chemical messengers" in the bloodstream, and the nervous system serves as the "electrical" system. The nervous system works almost instantaneously with short-lived results, but endocrine system hormones act slower and often with longer lasting effects.

This chapter reviews aspects of the endocrine system, including its functions during rest and physical activity and response to acute and chronic exercise.

ENDOCRINE SYSTEM OVERVIEW

Figure 12.1 shows the location of the major endocrine organs: the pituitary, thyroid, parathyroid, adrenal, pineal,

and thymus glands. Several organs contain discrete areas of endocrine tissue that also produce hormones. These include the pancreas, gonads (ovaries and testes), and hypothalamus, also a major organ of the nervous system.

Table 12.1 lists the different endocrine glands and nonglandular endocrine cells and their major hormonal secretions, target tissue(s), and main bodily effects.

ENDOCRINE SYSTEM ORGANIZATION

Three components characterize the endocrine system:

1. Host gland
2. Hormones
3. Target (receptor) cells or organs

Glands classify as either endocrine, exocrine, or both. **Endocrine glands** secrete hormones; they lack ducts (*ductless*) but discharge their substances directly into the extracellular space around the gland. **Figure 12.2** shows that hormones diffuse into the blood for transport to target tissue throughout the body. Similar to neuromuscular responses, hormone secretion adjusts rapidly to changing

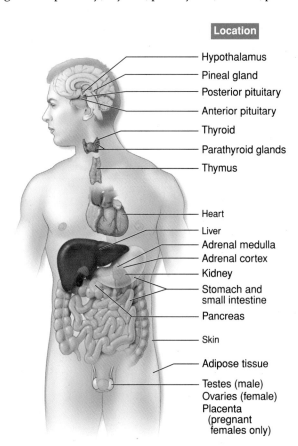

Figure 12.1 Location of the hormone-producing endocrine glands.

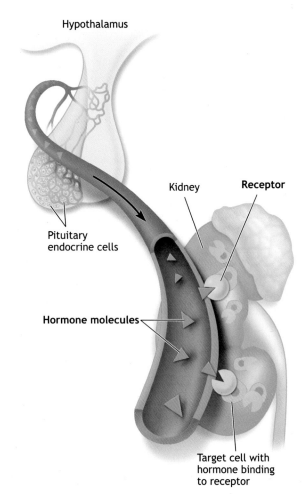

Figure 12.2 Hormones secreted from endocrine glands travel in the bloodstream to exert influence on body tissues.

Table 12.1 **Endocrine Organs and Their Secretions**

LOCATION	GLAND OR CELL	CHEMICAL TYPE	HORMONE	TARGET	MAIN EFFECT
Adipose tissue	Cells	Peptide	Leptin; adiponectin (resistin)	Hypothalamus, other tissues	Food intake, metabolism, reproduction
Adrenal cortex	Gland	Steroid	Mineralocorticoids (aldosterone)	Kidney	Stimulates Na^+ reabsorption and K^+ secretion
			Glucocorticoids (Cortisol; corticosterone)	Many tissues	Promotes protein and fat catabolism; raises blood glucose levels; adapts body to stress
			Androgens (androstenedione; dehydroepiandrosterone [DHEA]; estrone)	Many tissues	Promotes sex drive
Adrenal medulla	Gland	Amine	Epinephrine, norepinephrine	Many tissues	Facilitates sympathetic activity; increases cardiac output; regulates blood vessels; increases glycogen catabolism and fatty acid release
Gastrointestinal tract (stomach and small intestine)	Cells	Peptide	Gastrin; cholecystokinin (CCK); secretin; glucose-dependent insulinotropic peptide (GIP)	GI tract and pancreas	Assists digestion and absorption of nutrients; regulates gastrointestinal motility
Heart	Cells	Peptide	Atrial natriuretic peptide (ANP)	Kidney tubules	Inhibits sodium reabsorption
Hypothalamus	Clusters of neurons	Peptide	Trophic hormones (releasing and release-inhibiting hormones: corticotrophin-releasing hormone [CHR]; thyrotrophin-releasing hormone [TRH]; growth hormone-releasing hormone [GHRH]; gonadrotrophin-releasing hormone [GnRH])	Anterior pituitary	Releases or inhibits anterior pituitary hormones
Kidney	Cells	Peptide Steroid	Erythropoietin (EPO) 1,25 Dihydroxy-vitamin D_3 (calciferol)	Bone marrow Intestine	Red blood cell production Increase calcium absorption
Liver	Cells	Peptide	Angiotensinogen	Adrenal cortex, blood vessels, brain	Aldosterone secretion; increase blood pressure
			Insulin-like growth factors (IGF-1)	Many tissues	Growth
Muscle	Cells	Peptide	Insulin-like growth factors (IGF-1, IGF-II); myogenic regulatory factors (MRFs)	Many tissues	Growth

(continued)

Table 12.1	Endocrine Organs and Their Secretions (*Continued*)				
LOCATION	**GLAND OR CELL**	**CHEMICAL TYPE**	**HORMONE**	**TARGET**	**MAIN EFFECT**
Pancreas	Gland	Peptide	Insulin	Many tissues	Lowers blood glucose levels; promotes protein, lipid, and glycogen synthesis
			Glucagon	Many tissues	Raises blood glucose levels; promotes glycogenolysis and gluconeogenesis
			Somatostatin (SS)	Many tissues	Inhibits secretion of pancreatic hormones; regulates digestion and absorption of nutrients by GI system
Parathyroid	Gland	Peptide	Parathyroid hormone (PTH)	Bone, kidney	Promotes Ca^{++} release from bone, Ca^{++} absorption by intestine and Ca^{++} reabsorption by kidney; raises blood Ca^{++} levels; stimulates vitamin D_3 synthesis
Pineal gland	Gland	Amine	Melatonin	Unknown	Controls circadian rhythms
Pituitary-anterior	Gland	Peptides	Growth hormone (GH)	Many tissues	Growth; stimulates bone and soft tissue growth; regulates protein, lipid, and CHO metabolism
			Adrenocorticotropic hormone (ACTH)	Adrenal cortex	Stimulates glucocorticoid secretion
			Thyroid-stimulating hormone (TSH)	Thyroid gland	Stimulates secretion of thyroid hormones
			Prolactin	Breast	Milk secretion
			Follicle-stimulating hormone (FSH)	Gonads	Females: stimulates growth and development of ovarian follicles and estrogen secretion; Males: sperm production by testis
			Luteinizing hormone (LH)	Gonads	Females: stimulates ovulation, secretion of estrogen and progesterone; Males: testosterone secretion by testis
Pituitary-posterior	Extension of hypo-thalamic neurons	Peptide	Oxytocin (OT)	Breast and uterus	Females: stimulates uterine contractions and milk ejection by mammary glands; Males: unknown function
			Antidiuretic hormone (ADH or vasopressin)	Kidney	Decreases urine output by kidneys; promotes blood vessel (arterioles) constriction
Placenta (pregnant female)	Gland	Steroid	Estrogens and progesterone	Many tissues	Fetal and maternal development
		Peptide	Chorionic somatomammotropin (CS)		Metabolism
			Chorionic gonadotropin (CG)		Hormone secretion

Table 12.1	Endocrine Organs and Their Secretions (*Continued*)				
LOCATION	GLAND OR CELL	CHEMICAL TYPE	HORMONE	TARGET	MAIN EFFECT
Skin	Cells	Steroid	Vitamin D$_3$	Intermediate form of hormone	Precursor of 1,25 dihydroxy-vitamin D$_3$
Ovaries (female)	Glands	Steroid	Estrogens (estradiol)	Many tissues	Egg production; secondary sex characteristics
			Progestins (progesterone)	Uterus	Promotes endometrial growth to prepare uterus for pregnancy
Testes (male)	Glands	Peptide Steroid	Ovarian inhibin Androgen	Anterior pituitary Many tissues	Inhibits FSH secretion Sperm production; secondary sex characteristics
		Peptide	Inhibin	Anterior pituitary	Inhibit FSH secretion
Thymus	Gland	Peptide	Thymosin, thymopoietin	Lymphocytes	Stimulates proliferation and function of T lymphocytes
Thyroid	Gland	Iodinated amines	Triiodothyronine (T$_3$); thyroxine (T$_4$)	Many tissues	Increases metabolic rate; normal physical development
		Peptide	Calcitonin (CT)	Bone	Promotes calcium deposition in bone; lowers blood calcium levels

bodily functions. For this reason, many hormone secretions occur in a pulsatile manner rather than at a constant rate.

Exocrine glands include sweat glands and upper digestive tract glands; in contrast, contain secretory ducts that lead directly to the specific compartment or surface that requires the hormone. The nervous system controls most exocrine glands.

What Makes a Chemical a Hormone?

The term *hormone* was coined from the Greek word meaning "impetus." An accepted operational definition describes a hormone as *a chemical, usually a peptide or a steroid secreted by a cell or group of cells into the blood for transport to a distant target, where it exerts its effect at low concentrations.* Recent findings suggest that this may be too broad a definition because many different non-hormone substances also function as chemical messengers.

Must Hormones Be Transported to Distant Targets?   Physiologists have questioned whether a chemical must be transported to distant targets to classify as a hormone. For example, the different hypothalamic-regulating hormones, the trophic chemical messengers that include releasing and release-inhibiting chemicals, and the different "growth factors" seem to lack widespread distribution in the circulation, yet they meet the other qualifications for hormone classification.

Hormones Exert Effects at Low Concentrations   With the discovery of new signal molecules and receptors, the boundary between hormone and non-hormone molecules becomes blurred, particularly at physiologically effective concentrations. Although some hormones act at concentrations in the nanomolar (10^{-9} M) to picomolar (10^{-12} M) range, other chemicals transported

Questions & Notes

List 3 components that comprise the endocrine system.

1.

2.

3.

ⓘ **For Your Information**

SMALL BUT CRITICAL

Endocrine glands are small compared with other body organs; combined, they weigh only about 0.5 kg. Endocrine hormone secretions occur in minute amounts, measured in micrograms (μg; 10^{-6} g), nanograms (ng; 10^{-9} g), and picograms (pg; 10^{-12} g).

in the blood exist in higher concentrations before an effect occurs. For example, cytokines, a group of regulatory peptides that control cell development, differentiation, and the immune response, act on target cells at a much higher concentration than a typical hormone. Erythropoietin, the molecule that controls red blood cell synthesis, classifies as a hormone but functionally behaves as a cytokine.

Hormones Bind to Receptors   All hormones bind to target cell receptors and initiate biochemical responses. This characteristic varies from one hormone to another and from one tissue to another. Some hormones act on multiple tissues in different ways or have no effect at different times. Insulin, for example, exhibits varied effects depending on the target tissue; in muscle and adipose cells, insulin alters glucose and protein transport and enzymes for glucose metabolism. In the liver, insulin modulates enzyme activity without directly affecting glucose and protein transport, and in brain tissues, glucose metabolism does not require insulin.

Hormone Classification

Hormones typically classify according to several different systems: their sources, their receptor type, or their chemical structure (the most common classification scheme). Three different chemical structures or hormones exist: (1) *peptide hormones* composed of linked amino acids, (2) *steroid hormones* derived from cholesterol and amine hormones, and (3) *amine hormones* derived from a single type of amino acid.

Table 12.2 compares the storage, synthesis, release mechanism, transport medium, receptor location and receptor-ligand binding, and target organ response of the peptide, steroid, and amine hormones.

Peptide Hormones   Peptide hormones range from small peptides of only three amino acids to large proteins and glycoproteins. These water-soluble hormones dissolve easily for transport in the body's extracellular fluids. The half-life of activity for peptide hormones ranges in minutes;

Table 12.2	Storage, Synthesis, Release Mechanism, Transport Medium, Receptor Location and Receptor-Ligand Binding, and Target Organ Response for the Peptide, Steroid, and Amine Hormones			
			AMINE HORMONES	
	PEPTIDE HORMONES	**STEROID HORMONES**	**CATECHOLAMINES**	**THYROID HORMONES**
Examples	Insulin, glucagons, leptin, IGF-1	Androgens, DHEA, cortisol	Epinephrine, norepinephrine	Thyroxine (T_4)
Synthesis and storage	Made in advance; stored in secretory vesicles	Synthesized on demand from precursors	Made in advance; stored in secretory vesicles	Made in advance; precursor stored in secretory vesicles
Release from parent cell	Exocytosis[a]	Simple diffusion	Exocytosis	Simple diffusion
Transport medium	Dissolved in plasma	Bound to carrier proteins	Dissolved in plasma	Bound to carrier proteins
Lifespan (half-life[b])	Short	Long	Short	Long
Receptor location	On cell membrane	Cytoplasm or nucleus; some have membrane receptors	On cell membrane	Nucleus
Response to receptor-ligand binding[c]	Activation of second messenger systems; may activate genes	Activate genes for transcription and translation; may have nongenomic actions	Activation of second messenger systems	Activate genes for transcription and translation
General target response	Modification of existing proteins and induction of new protein synthesis	Induction of new protein synthesis	Modification of existing proteins	Induction of new protein synthesis

[a]Process in which intracellular vesicles fuse with the cell membrane and release their contents into the extracellular fluid.
[b]Amount of time required to reduce hormone concentration by one-half.
[c]A ligand (the molecule that binds to a receptor) binds to a membrane protein, which triggers endocytosis (process by which a cell brings molecules into the cytoplasm in vesicles formed from the cell membrane).

thus, if a peptide hormone's response requires maintenance beyond several minutes, the hormone secretion must continue. Most peptide hormones bind to surface membrane receptors and act through a second messenger. Tissues respond rapidly to peptide hormones compared with the response times of other hormones.

Steroid Hormones

Steroid Hormones   All steroid hormones have a similar chemical structure because of their derivation from cholesterol. But unlike peptide hormones made in diverse tissues, only the adrenal cortex, gonads, and placenta during pregnancy produce steroid hormones. These hormones diffuse easily across cell membranes, both out of the parent cell and into their target tissue. Steroid-secreting cells cannot store hormones; instead, they synthesize their hormones as needed. Steroid hormones move out of the secreting cell by simple diffusion. Steroid hormones are minimally soluble in plasma and other body fluids, so they bind to protein carrier molecules in the blood. To produce an effect on a target, the hormone must unbind from the protein.

Amine Hormones   Small molecules created from one or two amino acids comprise the amine hormones. The amine neurohormones catecholamines epinephrine and norepinephrine bind to cell membrane receptors in a manner similar to peptide hormones.

How Hormones Function

Most hormones do not directly affect cellular activity but rather combine with a specific receptor molecule on the cell surface. The cell then discharges a second chemical that initiates a cascade of cellular events. The binding hormone acts as **first messenger** to react with the enzyme **adenyl cyclase** in the plasma membrane to form **cyclic 3,5-adenosine monophosphate (cyclic-AMP)**. This compound then acts as "**second messenger**" or mediator to influence cellular function by initiating a predictable series of actions within the target cell by one of four mechanisms:

1. Changing the synthesis rate of intracellular proteins
2. Altering enzyme activity
3. Modifying cell membrane transport
4. Inducing secretory activity

A target cell's response to a hormone depends largely on the presence of specific protein receptors on its membrane or in its interior.

Three factors determine a hormone's plasma concentration:

1. Sum of synthesis and release by the host gland
2. Rate of receptor tissue uptake
3. Rate of removal from the blood by the liver and kidneys

In most cases, the hormone removal rate, which is usually measured in the urine, equals the rate of release.

Hormone Effects on Enzymes   *Alteration of enzymatic activity and enzyme-mediated membrane transport constitute the major mechanisms of hormone action.* Hormones affect enzyme activity in one of three ways:

1. Stimulate enzyme synthesis
2. Combine with the enzyme to change its shape through allosteric modulation, which increases or decreases the enzyme's ability to interact with a substrate
3. Activate many inactive enzyme forms to increase total enzyme activity

In addition to altering enzyme activity, hormones either facilitate or inhibit transport of substances into cells. Insulin, for example, promotes glucose uptake through the plasma membrane. In contrast, the hormone epinephrine inhibits a cell's glucose uptake.

Questions & Notes

List the 3 different types of hormones.

1.

2.

3.

Give one example of an amine hormone.

List the 4 ways hormones act at specific target cells.

1.

2.

3.

4.

List 2 ways hormones affect enzyme activity.

1.

2.

ⓘ For Your Information

HORMONE–RECEPTOR BINDING

Hormone–receptor binding serves as the first step in initiating hormone action. The extent of a target cell's activation by a hormone depends on three factors:

1. Hormone concentration in the blood
2. Number of target cell receptors for the hormone
3. Sensitivity or strength of the union between the hormone and receptor

Control of Hormone Secretion

Endocrine glands are stimulated in three ways: hormonal, humoral, or neural. Each of these stimulation methods function as a reflex pathway, singly or in combination, to ultimately trigger and regulate a specific hormone secretion. All reflex pathways exhibit similar components: stimulus, input signal, integration of the signal, output signal, and response. In endocrine reflexes, the output signal represents a hormone or neurohormone.

Figure 12.3 illustrates a negative feedback system that serves to turn off hormone release. In this example, an increase in blood glucose concentration after a meal initiates insulin secretion; insulin then travels in the blood to its target tissues to increase glucose uptake and metabolism. The resultant decrease in blood glucose concentration provides a negative feedback signal and turns off the reflex, ending further release of insulin. This illustration also shows insulin secretion triggered by input signals from the nervous system.

Hormonal Stimulation

Hormones often influence secretions of other hormones. For example, hormones

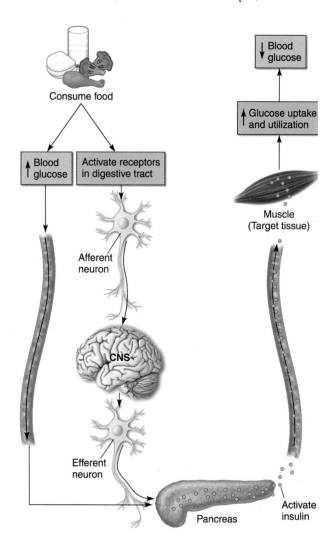

Figure 12.3 Multiple stimuli for insulin secretion. Insulin release is triggered by an increase in blood glucose levels or through nervous stimulation triggered by ingestion of a meal.

from the hypothalamic trophic-releasing and -inhibiting hormones (see **Table 12.1**) induce the discharge of most anterior pituitary hormones. The anterior pituitary hormones, in turn, stimulate other "target gland" endocrine organs to release their hormones into the circulation. Increased blood levels of these hormones provide feedback to inhibit release of anterior pituitary hormones; this ultimately inhibits target gland secretion.

Humoral Stimulation

Fluctuating blood levels of ions, nutrients, and bile stimulate hormone release. The term **humoral** denotes these stimuli to distinguish them from "fluid-borne" hormonal stimuli. An increase in the humoral agent blood glucose stimulates insulin release from the pancreas. Insulin promotes glucose entry so blood sugar levels decline to end the humoral initiative for insulin release.

Neural Stimulation

Nerve fibers affect hormone release. For example, during stress, sympathetic nervous system activation of the adrenal medulla initiates release of epinephrine and norepinephrine. In this case, the nervous system augments normal endocrine control to maintain homeostasis.

Neurohormones serve as chemical signals released into the blood by a neuron. The nervous system produces three major groups of neurohormones:

1. Catecholamines synthesized by modified neurons in the adrenal medulla
2. Hypothalamic neurohormones secreted from the posterior pituitary
3. Hypothalamic neurohormones that control hormone release from the anterior pituitary

Hormone–Hormone Interactions

Multiple hormones present at the same time control many cells and tissues. Three types of interactions of diverse hormones exist:

1. **Synergism:** Different hormones act together to augment the effect on specific tissues. For example, the pancreatic hormone glucagon in concert with cortisol and epinephrine acts synergistically to elevate blood glucose levels. When two or more hormones interact, the combined effect on the target often exceeds the additive effect of each hormone separately.
2. **Permissiveness:** One hormone cannot exert its full effect without the presence of a second hormone or a greater quantity of the first hormone. For example, thyroid hormone increases the number of receptors available for epinephrine at its target cells, thereby increasing epinephrine's effect at those cells.
3. **Antagonism:** Some hormones oppose the action of another hormone to diminish the first hormone's effectiveness. Glucagon and growth hormone (GH), for example, both raise blood glucose concentration to counter the glucose-lowering effect of insulin.

PATTERNS OF HORMONE RELEASE

Most hormones respond to peripheral stimuli on an as-needed basis, but others release at regular intervals during a 24-hour cycle, referred to as *diurnal variation*. Some secretory cycles span several weeks, and others follow daily cycles. These cycling patterns do not just pertain to one category of hormones.

Assessing pulsatile hormone release patterns reveals information not available from a single blood sample. Patterns of release and amplitude and frequency of discharge provide more meaningful information about hormone dynamics than a hormone's concentration examined at a single time period.

RESTING AND EXERCISE-INDUCED ENDOCRINE SECRETIONS

The following sections review important hormones, their functions during rest and exercise, and specific host–gland–hormone responses to exercise training.

ANTERIOR PITUITARY HORMONES

Figure 12.4 shows the **pituitary gland** (**hypophysis**), its secretions and various target glands, and their respective hormone secretions. The pituitary gland consists of distinct anterior and posterior lobes each with different hormone secretions. The gland attaches to the hypothalamus by neural elements that innervate the posterior pituitary. This nerve bundle (**hypophyseal stalk**) serves as a conduit for hormone movement from its site of synthesis in the

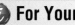

For Your Information

CAFFEINE STIMULATES LIPOLYSIS

Caffeine augments cyclic-AMP activity in fat cells; cyclic-AMP activates hormone-sensitive lipases to promote lipolysis and release free fatty acids into the plasma. Increased plasma free fatty acid levels stimulate fat oxidation, thus conserving liver and muscle glycogen.

For Your Information

TARGET CELL ACTIVATION

The activation of a target cell by hormone–receptor interaction depends on three factors:

1. Blood levels of the specific hormone
2. Relative number of target cell receptors for that hormone
3. Affinity or strength of the union between hormone and receptor

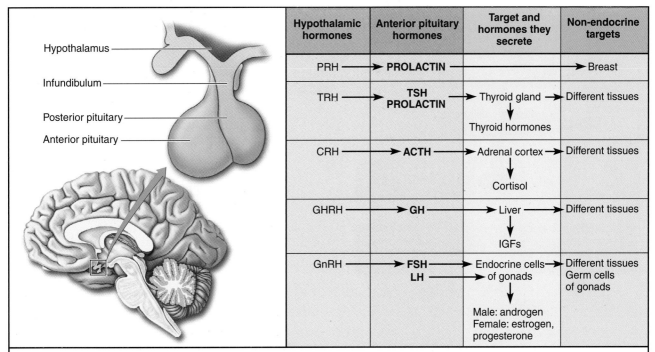

Figure 12.4 The pituitary gland, its secretions and various target glands and their hormone secretions.

hypothalamus to storage in the pituitary. Located beneath the base of the brain, the **anterior pituitary** secretes at least six different polypeptide hormones and influences the secretion of several others.

The **posterior pituitary**, an extension of hypothalamic neurons, secretes the hormones oxytocin, which acts on breast and uterus to stimulate milk production and induce labor and delivery, and vasopressin (**antidiuretic hormone [ADH]**), which acts on the kidneys to decrease urine output and control fluid balance.

Growth Hormone

Human growth hormone (GH or **somatotropin)** promotes cell division and proliferation throughout the body. This hormone facilitates protein synthesis in three ways:

1. Increasing amino acid transport through plasma membranes
2. Stimulating RNA formation
3. Activating cellular ribosomes that increase protein synthesis

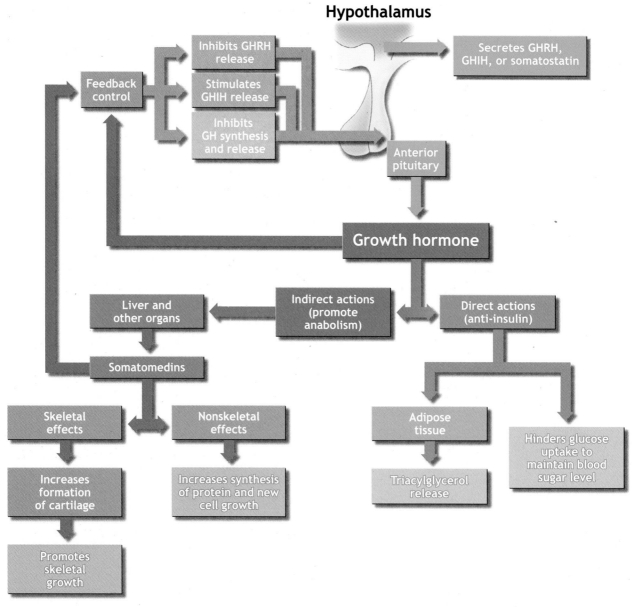

Figure 12.5 Overview of growth hormone (GH) actions. GH stimulates breakdown and release of triacylglycerols from adipose tissue and hinders cellular glucose uptake (anti-insulin effect) to maintain a relatively high blood glucose level. Somatomedins mediate the indirect anabolic effects of GH. Elevated GH levels and somatomedins provide feedback to promote GH-inhibiting hormone (GHIH) release and depress hypothalmic release of GH-releasing hormone (GHRH); this further inhibits GH release by the anterior pituitary gland.

GH release also depresses carbohydrate utilization while increasing fat use for energy. Insufficient GH secretion early in life blunts skeletal growth (*dwarfism*), and excess production produces extreme growth (*gigantism*). Excessive GH secretion after puberty causes continued soft tissue growth and bone thickening, a condition termed **acromegly**. Many of the growth-promoting effects of GH arise from intermediary chemical messengers on different target tissues rather than a direct action of GH itself. These peptide messengers, produced in the liver, are termed **somatomedins** or **insulin-like growth factors (IGFs)** because of their structural similarity to insulin. Two IGFs have been identified, IGF-1 and IGF-2; the liver directly releases them under the stimulatory effects of GH. These factors exert potent peripheral effects on motor units.

Hypothalamic secretion of GH-releasing hormone stimulates the anterior pituitary gland's production of GH. Another hormone, hypothalamic **somatostatin**, inhibits GH release. *Each primary pituitary hormone has its own hypothalamic releasing factor.* Anxiety, stress, and physical activity provide neural input to the hypothalamus, causing it to discharge its releasing hormones.

Exercise, Growth Hormone, and Tissue Synthesis

GH secretion increases a few minutes after exercise begins. Higher intensity exercise increases GH production and its total secretion. Moreover, GH secretion relates more closely to peak exercise intensity than exercise duration or total exercise volume. The exact stimulus for GH release with exercise remains unknown; neural factors most likely provide primary control.

One hypothesis maintains that exercise directly activates GH secretion that in turn stimulates anabolic processes. For example, exercise doubles GH pulse frequency and amplitude. Exercise also stimulates endogenous opiate release; these hormones facilitate GH discharge by inhibiting the liver's production of somatostatin, a hormone that blunts GH release.

Figure 12.5 illustrates the actions and regulation of GH. Elevated plasma GH stimulates triacylglycerol release from adipose tissue while inhibiting cellular glucose uptake, known as the anti-insulin effect. Inhibiting carbohydrate catabolism while maintaining blood glucose levels sustains prolonged exercise. Concurrently, GH promotes its anabolic, tissue-building effects mediated via somatomedins on diverse tissues that include bone and skeletal muscle. Elevated GH and somatomedins trigger the hypothalamus to release more GH-inhibiting hormone. This action depresses the release of GH-releasing hormone, thus inhibiting anterior pituitary release of GH.

Thyrotropin

Thyrotropin (thyroid-stimulating hormone [TSH]) maintains growth and thyroid gland development, including regulation of hormone output from thyroid cells. The thyroid gland plays an important role in controlling cellular metabolism. Physical activity usually increases anterior pituitary TSH output.

Corticotropin

The hypothalamus secretes corticotropin-releasing hormone (CRH) into the hypothalamic–hypophyseal portal system. CRH, transported to the anterior pituitary, stimulates the release of **corticotropin (adrenocorticotropic hormone [ACTH])**. ACTH in turn acts on the adrenal cortex to promote synthesis and release of cortisol, similar to how TSH controls thyroid secretions. ACTH directly enhances triacylglycerol mobilization from adipose tissue, increases the rate of gluconeogenesis, and stimulates protein catabolism. ACTH concentrations increase with exercise duration if the intensity exceeds 25% of aerobic capacity.

Questions & Notes

Name the true "master gland."

List the 3 factors that activate target cells by hormone-receptor interaction.

1.

2.

3.

List 2 factors that provide neural input to the hypothalamus causing it to discharge releasing hormones.

1.

2.

Does exercise increase or decrease TSH output.

For Your Information

THE TRUE MASTER GLAND

The early Greek physicians of antiquity, including Galen (131–201 AD), described the pituitary gland in their many treatises on health and disease. Galen mistakenly proposed that its role was to drain the phlegm from the brain to the nasopharynx. Over the next 19 centuries, the pituitary gland has been considered the body's master gland. In reality, the hypothalamus controls anterior pituitary activity, making it the true *master gland*.

Gonadotropic Hormones

The gonadotropic hormones include **follicle-stimulating hormone (FSH)** and **luteinizing hormone (LH)**. In women, FSH initiates follicle growth in the ovaries and stimulates ovarian secretion of estrogens, one type of female sex hormone. The combination of LH and FSH stimulates estrogen secretion and initiates rupture of the follicle to allow the ovum to pass through the fallopian tube for fertilization. In men, FSH stimulates germinal epithelial growth in the testes to promote sperm development. LH stimulates the testes to secrete the hormone testosterone.

The nature of gonadotropin release confounds interpretation of any exercise-associated alterations in FSH and LH. LH normally releases in a pulsatile manner so it becomes difficult to separate any specific exercise-related change from the normal secretory pattern. Anxiety affects LH levels via action of the "stress" hormone norepinephrine; thus, LH increases in anticipation of exercise and reaches its peak during recovery.

Prolactin

Prolactin (PRL) governs milk secretion from the mammary glands. PRL levels increase with higher exercise intensities and return toward baseline within 45 minutes of recovery. PRL plays an important role in female sexual function, making repeated exercise-induced PRL release inhibit the ovaries and disrupt the normal menstrual cycle, an effect often observed among athletic women. The significance of an increased PRL in men after acute maximal exercise remains unknown.

POSTERIOR PITUITARY HORMONES

Figure 12.4 also depicts the **posterior pituitary gland (neurohypophysis)** formed as an outgrowth of the hypothalamus. This gland stores two hormones, ADH or **vasopressin** and **oxytocin**. The posterior pituitary does not synthesize its hormones. Instead, it receives them from the hypothalamus for release to the general circulation via neural stimulation.

ADH primarily limits how much urine the kidneys produce. Oxytocin stimulates uterine muscle activity and milk ejection from the breasts during lactation; thus, oxytocin contributes importantly to birthing and nursing.

Physical activity provides a potent stimulus for ADH secretion. This secretion increases water reabsorption by the kidney tubules during and after exercise. ADH release stimulated by sweating preserves body fluids, particularly in hot weather exercise accompanied by dehydration. Excessive fluid intake inhibits ADH release, with urine volume increasing proportionately.

THYROID HORMONES

The butterfly-shaped thyroid gland, shown in **Figure 12.6**, weighs approximately 15 to 20 g and is located just

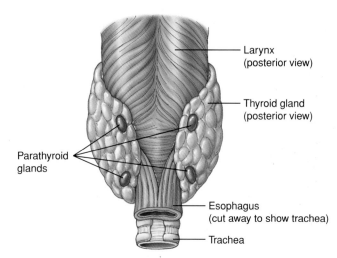

Figure 12.6 Thyroid gland located on both sides of the neck in the larynx region. Not visible externally under normal conditions.

below the larynx at the base of the throat. This larger endocrine gland has two distinct endocrine cell types that secrete **calcitonin**, a calcium-regulating hormone, and two protein-iodine bound hormones, **thyroxine (T_4)** and **triiodothyronine (T_3)**, often referred to as *major metabolic hormones*. TSH release by the anterior pituitary gland stimulates the thyroid gland to release its hormones.

Thyroid Hormones Affect Quality of Life

Thyroid hormones are not directly essential for life but they do affect its quality. In children, full expression of GH requires thyroid activity. Thyroid hormones provide essential stimulation for normal growth and development, especially of nerve tissue.

Hypersecretion of thyroid hormones (**hyperthyroidism**) has the following four effects:

1. Increases oxygen uptake and metabolic heat production during rest (heat intolerance is a common complaint)
2. Increases protein catabolism to cause subsequent muscle weakness and weight loss
3. Heightens reflex activity and psychological disturbances that range from irritability and insomnia to psychosis
4. Causes an abnormally rapid heart rate (tachycardia)

Hyposecretion of thyroid hormones (**hypothyroidism**) produces the following four effects:

1. Reduces the metabolic rate, leading to cold intolerance from reduced internal heat production
2. Decreases protein synthesis, resulting in brittle nails; thinning hair; and dry, thin skin
3. Depresses reflex activity, slows speech and thought processes, and causes feelings of fatigue; in infancy, causes cretinism marked by decreased mental capacity
4. Causes abnormally slow heart rate (bradycardia)

Blood levels of free T_4 not bound to plasma protein increase during exercise. This could result from core temperature increases with exercise that alter protein binding of several hormones, including T_4. The importance of these transient alterations in hormone levels remains unknown.

PARATHYROID HORMONE

Four small sections of tissue comprise the **parathyroid gland** within thyroid tissue (see **Fig. 12.6**). This gland secretes the calcium-regulating parathyroid peptide hormone (**parathyroid hormone [PTH]** or **parathormone**) to increase plasma calcium (Ca^{++}) concentration. PTH increases plasma Ca^{++} concentrations in three ways:

1. Mobilizes Ca^{++} from bone
2. Enhances renal Ca^{++} reabsorption
3. Indirectly increases intestinal Ca^{++} absorption by its influence on vitamin D_3

ADRENAL HORMONES

Figure 12.7 shows the flattened, caplike **adrenal glands** located just above each kidney. The glands form two distinct parts: the **adrenal medulla** in the inner portion and **adrenal cortex** in the outer portion. Each portion secretes a different type of hormone.

Adrenal Medulla Hormones

The adrenal medulla forms part of the sympathetic nervous system. It prolongs and augments sympathetic neural effects by secreting two hormones, **epinephrine** and **norepinephrine**, collectively termed **catecholamines**. Neural outflow from the hypothalamus directly influences adrenal medulla secretions (80% as epinephrine), which affect the heart, blood vessels, and glands in the same but slower way as direct sympathetic nervous system stimulation.

Questions & Notes

Name the 2 gonadotropic hormones.

1.

2.

Give one effect of thyroid hormone hypersecretion.

Give one effect of thyroid hormone hyposecretion.

Name the 2 parts of the adrenal glands.

1.

2.

What factor governs the quantity of adrenal medulla secretion?

List the two catecholamines.

1.

2.

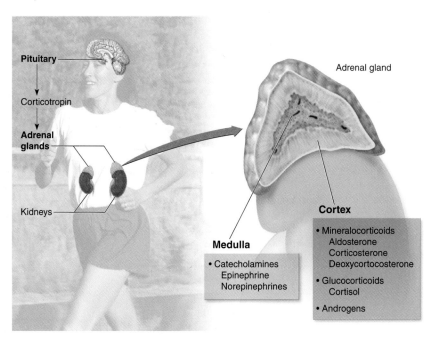

Figure 12.7 Adrenal gland and its secretions.

ⓘ For Your Information

DO NOT BLAME THE HORMONES

Depressed thyroid production blunts the basal metabolic rate (BMR), which usually leads to gains in body weight and body fat. However, fewer than 3% of obese persons show abnormal thyroid functions, so depressed thyroid activity cannot explain excessive body fat gain in more than 60% of adults in the U.S. population.

Exercise intensity directly governs quantity of adrenal medulla secretion. For example, norepinephrine levels increase two to six times throughout exercise gradations from light to maximum. Exercise duration also influences catecholamine response as revealed by the direct relationship between plasma epinephrine and norepinephrine levels and mileage run. Athletes involved in sprint–power training show greater sympathoadrenergic activation during maximal exercise than counterparts trained in aerobic exercise. This difference relates to the higher anaerobic contribution to maximal exercise energy output during sprint–power activities. Other factors that determine catecholamine response to exercise include age (greater catecholamine secretion in older subjects at an absolute exercise intensity) and gender (greater epinephrine secretion in men than women at the same relative exercise intensity).

Adrenal Cortex Hormones

The adrenal cortex secretes **adrenocortical hormones** in response to ACTH stimulation from the pituitary gland. These steroid hormones are categorized by function into one of three groups: **mineralocorticoids, glucocorticoids,**

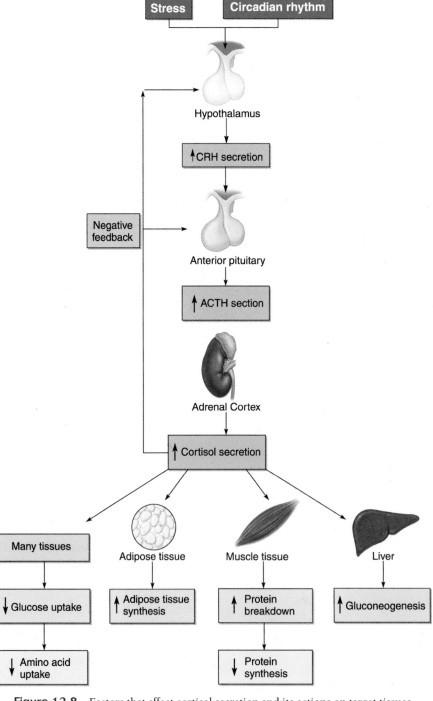

Figure 12.8 Factors that affect cortisol secretion and its actions on target tissues.

and **androgens**; each is produced in a different zone or layer of the adrenal cortex.

Mineralocorticoids

Mineralocorticoids regulate the mineral salts sodium and potassium in the extracellular fluid space. **Aldosterone**, the most physiologically important of these hormones, comprises almost 95% of all mineralocorticoids.

Aldosterone regulates sodium reabsorption in the kidneys' distal tubules. Increased aldosterone secretion moves sodium ions that also draw fluid from the renal filtrate back into the blood, with little sodium passing into the urine. Conservation of fluid via sodium reabsorption increases plasma volume, often with concomitants increase in cardiac output and arterial blood pressure. In contrast, sodium and fluid literally pour into the urine when aldosterone secretion ceases.

The kidneys exchange either a potassium or hydrogen ion for each reabsorbed sodium ion, enabling aldosterone to indirectly stabilize serum potassium and whole body pH. Mineral balance preserves nerve transmission and muscle function; neuromuscular activity would cease without proper regulation of sodium and potassium.

Outflow from the sympathetic nervous system during exercise constricts blood vessels to the kidneys. Reduced renal blood flow stimulates the kidneys to release the enzyme **renin** into the blood. Renin in turn stimulates the production of the protein **angiotensin**, a potent vasoconstrictor that also activates aldosterone secretion from the adrenal cortex. Aldosterone secretion increases progressively during exercise, with peak plasma levels as high as six times the resting value. The **renin–angiotensin mechanism** during rest controls aldosterone secretion in relation to changes in blood pressure in the kidneys' afferent arterioles.

Glucocorticoids

Figure 12.8 shows factors that affect **cortisol** (**hydrocortisone**) secretion, the major steroid glucocorticoid of the adrenal cortex, and its actions on target tissues. Cortisol secretes with a strong diurnal rhythm; secretion normally peaks in the morning and diminishes during the night. Cortisol secretion also increases with stress; thus, it is sometimes called the "stress hormone." Cortisol is considered a catabolic hormone because it counters hypoglycemia, making it essential for life. Animals whose adrenal glands have been removed die if they are exposed to significant environmental stress. Cortisol, required for full activity of glucagon and the catecholamines, exerts a *permissive effect* on those hormones.

Cortisol's six main effects include:

1. Promotes liver gluconeogenesis
2. Breaks down skeletal muscle proteins for gluconeogenic substrate
3. Enhances lipolysis (fat breakdown) during low energy intake and prolonged, moderate physical activity
4. Suppresses the immune system
5. Promotes negative calcium balance
6. Influences brain function, including mood changes and alterations in memory and learning

Physical activity varies cortisol response depending on exercise intensity and duration, fitness level, nutritional status, and even circadian rhythm. Cortisol output increases with exercise intensity. High cortisol levels occur in prolonged marathon running, long-duration cycling, and hiking. Plasma cortisol also increases at relatively low levels of sustained exercise and remains elevated for up to 2 hours in recovery.

Androgens

The adrenal glands and ovaries (in females) and testes (in males) produce sex steroid hormones collectively termed **androgens**. These endocrine-gland hormones promote sex-specific physical characteristics and initiate and maintain reproductive function. No distinctly "male" or "female"

Questions & Notes

Describe the response of norepinephrine during increasing levels of exercise from light to maximum.

Reduced renal blood flow stimulates the kidneys to release the enzyme _____ into the blood.

Name 3 tissues affected by cortisol's secretion.

1.

2.

3.

Cortisol secretion increases with _____.

List 3 main effects of cortisol.

1.

2.

3.

ⓘ For Your Information

A CAUSE OF HYPERTENSION

Chronic reduction in renal blood flow at rest, perhaps from abnormal sympathetic stimulation, activates the renin–angiotensin system. Hypertension occurs from the prolonged overresponse of this mechanism with resulting excess aldosterone output. High blood pressure associated with increased aldosterone production often occurs in obese teenagers, which relates to three factors:

1. Decreased salt sensitivity (hence increased water retention)
2. Increased sodium intake
3. Decreased sensitivity to the effects of insulin (hyperinsulinemia)

hormones exist but rather general differences in hormone concentrations between the sexes. Specifically, the ovaries provide the primary source of **estradiol** (**estrogen**) and luteal phase **progesterone**; the adrenal glands in males and females synthesize **dehydroepiandrosterone** (**DHEA**) and its sulfate, DHEAS. The testes produce **testosterone**, also secreted in small amounts by ovaries; conversely, testosterone converts to estrogen in peripheral tissues.

Plasma testosterone concentration in females, about one-tenth the level in males, increases with exercise (as do estradiol and progesterone). Resistance exercise and moderate aerobic exercise increase serum and free testosterone levels in untrained men after about 15 to 20 minutes. Testosterone decreases below resting values during longer duration, higher intensity aerobic exercise.

PANCREATIC HORMONES

The pancreas is about 14 cm long, weighs 60 g, and lies just below the stomach. **Figure 12.9** illustrates the location of the pancreas and its different endocrine cells. German microscopic anatomist and physician Paul Langerhans (1847–1888) first described the clusters of cells throughout the pancreas in his 1869 dissertation. These clusters, numbering close to 1 million, were named the **islets of Langerhans** to honor him. They contain four distinct cell types, each associated with a different peptide hormone. About three-quarters of the islet cells are β **cells** that produce **insulin** and a peptide called **amylin**; another 20%

are α **cells** that secrete **glucagon**. The remaining cells are **somatostatin**-secreting D cells and cells that produce **pancreatic polypeptide** (**PP**).

Insulin and glucagon act in antagonistic fashion to modulate plasma glucose levels. The blood usually contains both hormones; the ratio of the two hormones determines which hormone and its action dominates.

In the postabsorptive-fed condition, insulin dominates, and the body remains in a state of net anabolism. Ingested glucose provides substrate for energy metabolism; any excess is stored as glycogen or becomes synthesized to fat and protein. In the fasted state, in contrast, glucagon dominates to prevent low plasma glucose concentrations, called **hypoglycemia**.

Insulin Secretion

The following five factors influence insulin release following a meal:

1. **Increased blood glucose concentrations:** Plasma glucose concentrations greater than 100 mg·dL^{-1} represent the main stimulus to insulin secretion. Glucose absorbed from the small intestine travels in the bloodstream to the pancreas' β cells, where a transporter (glucose transporter 2 [GLUT2]) initiates insulin release.
2. **Increased blood amino acid concentrations:** Increased plasma amino acid concentration, which typically occurs after a meal, triggers insulin release.
3. **Gastrointestinal tract hormones:** Several hormones released from the intestinal tract after a meal travel

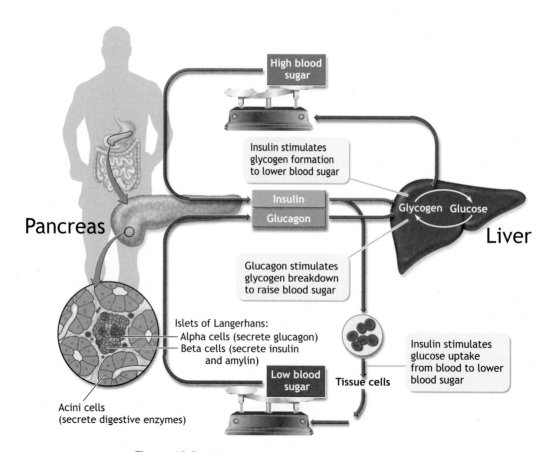

Figure 12.9 The pancreas, its secretions, and their actions.

in the circulation to the β cells to stimulate insulin release. The two most important of these hormones are glucagon-like peptide-1 (GLP-1) and glucose-dependent insulinotropic peptide (GIP). Both hormones trigger insulin release even before glucose reaches the β cells.

4. **Parasympathetic nervous system stimulation:** During and after a meal, an increase in parasympathetic stimulation of the intestinal region and pancreas directly promotes insulin release.
5. **Sympathetic nervous system stimulation:** Increased sympathetic activity inhibits insulin secretion. During stress, sympathetic input to the pancreas increases to inhibit insulin secretion and stimulate gluconeogenesis; this provides extra glucose fuel for the nervous system and skeletal musculature.

Insulin's Functions

Primary target tissues for insulin include the liver, adipose tissue, and skeletal muscle.

Insulin's major function regulates glucose metabolism by facilitating cellular glucose uptake in all tissues except the brain. Insulin exerts its action on glucose in the following four ways:

1. *Increases glucose transport into most, but not all, insulin-sensitive cells.* Adipose tissue and resting skeletal muscle do require insulin for glucose uptake during rest. Exercising skeletal muscle does *not* depend on insulin for its glucose uptake. When muscles become active, GLUT-4 transporters within cells activate without insulin stimulation to increase glucose uptake. The intracellular signal for this appears to be Ca^{++} and inorganic phosphate (P_i).
2. *Enhances cellular utilization and storage of glucose.* Insulin activates enzymes for glucose utilization (glycolysis) and glycogen and fat synthesis (glycogenesis and lipogenesis). Insulin simultaneously inhibits enzymes for glycogen breakdown (glycogenolysis), glucose synthesis (gluconeogenesis), and fat breakdown (lipolysis) to ensure that metabolism moves toward anabolism. Consuming more glucose than needed for energy metabolism causes the excess converts to glycogen or fatty acids.
3. *Enhances utilization of amino acids.* Insulin activates enzymes for protein synthesis and inhibits enzymes that promote protein breakdown.
4. *Promotes fat synthesis.* Insulin inhibits β-oxidation of fatty acids to promote conversion of excess glucose or amino acids into triacylglycerols via lipogenesis.

Figure 12.10 illustrates that the anabolic functions of insulin promote glycogen, protein, and fat synthesis. With insulin deficiency, the action of

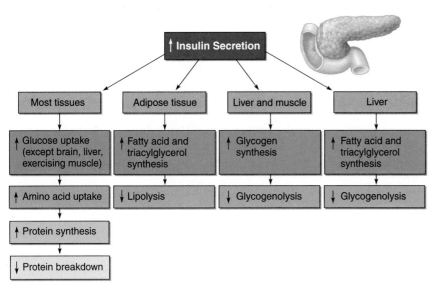

Figure 12.10 Increased insulin promotes glycogen, protein, and fat synthesis.

Questions & Notes

List 3 hormones secreted by the pancreas.

1.

2.

3.

Name 4 factors that influence insulin release following a meal.

1.

2.

3.

4.

List 3 functions of insulin.

1.

2.

3.

ⓘ For Your Information

GLUCOSE–INSULIN INTERACTION

Blood glucose levels within the pancreas directly control insulin secretion. Elevated blood glucose triggers insulin release. This in turn induces glucose entry into cells by lowering blood glucose, thus removing the stimulus for insulin release. In contrast, a decrease in blood glucose concentration dramatically lowers blood insulin levels to provide a favorable milieu to increase blood glucose. The interaction between glucose and insulin serves as a feedback mechanism to maintain blood glucose concentration within narrow limits. Rising levels of plasma amino acids also increase insulin secretion.

glucagon predominates and cells engage in catabolic activity.

Glucagon Secretion

The α cells of the islets of Langerhans secrete glucagon, the "insulin antagonist" hormone. In contrast to insulin, glucagon increases blood glucose levels and stimulates liver glycogenolysis and gluconeogenesis and lipid catabolism.

The blood glucose level regulates glucagon release. A decline in plasma glucose concentration below $100 \, \text{mg} \cdot \text{dL}^{-1}$ stimulates the α cells' release of glucagon, resulting in a near-instantaneous glucose release from the liver. Glucagon contributes to blood glucose regulation during endurance exercise and starvation; both conditions markedly decrease blood glucose and glycogen reserves.

Interestingly, plasma amino acids also stimulate glucagon release. This pathway prevents hypoglycemia after a person ingests a pure protein meal. If a meal contains protein without carbohydrate, amino acids in the food trigger insulin secretion. Even though no glucose has been absorbed, insulin-stimulated glucose uptake increases, and plasma glucose concentration decreases. Co-secretion of glucagon in this situation prevents hypoglycemia by stimulating hepatic glucose output. With amino acid ingestion, both glucose and amino acids become available to peripheral tissues.

Glucagon's Functions

Figure 12.11 shows that when glucagon action predominates, cells engage in catabolic activity. The liver represents glucagon's primary target tissue, stimulating glycogenolysis and gluconeogenesis to increase glucose output. During an overnight fast, 75% of the glucose produced by the liver comes from its glycogen stores, with the remaining 25% produced from gluconeogenic reactions. Glucagon also exerts a catabolic effect on adipose tissue throughout the body.

DIABETES MELLITUS

Diabetes mellitus consists of four subgroups of disorders that exhibit different pathophysiologies:

1. **Type 1 diabetes** results from the body's failure to produce insulin. Between 5% and 10% of Americans diagnosed with diabetes have the type 1 subgroup.
2. **Type 2 diabetes** refers to a relative insulin deficiency that results in hyperglycemia. Approximately 90% to 95% of Americans diagnosed with diabetes exhibit insulin resistance.
3. **Gestational diabetes** affects about 4% of all pregnant women or about 135,000 cases in the United States each year.
4. **Prediabetes** occurs when a person's blood glucose reaches higher-than-normal levels but not high enough for diagnosis as type 2 diabetes.

Clinicians have discontinued the former use of the terms **insulin-dependent diabetes mellitus** (IDDM; type 1) and **noninsulin-dependent diabetes mellitus** (NIDDM; type 2) because these diseases often require treatments that overlap and vary rather than reflect the underlying pathogenesis. For example, many people with type 2 diabetes require exogenous insulin to compensate for their relative insulin deficiency.

Diabetes Signs and Symptoms

Diabetes often progresses undiagnosed because many of its symptoms seem harmless. Importantly, early detection of the signs and symptoms of diabetes and subsequent treatment decrease the chance of developing the more serious complications of diabetes.

Twelve diabetes signs and symptoms include:

1. Elevated blood glucose (hyperglycemia)
2. Frequent urination (polyuria)
3. Excessive thirst (polydipsia)
4. Extreme hunger (polyphagia)
5. High levels of blood ketones from reliance on excessive fat catabolism
6. Unexplained weight loss
7. Increased fatigue
8. Irritability
9. Blurry vision
10. Numbness or tingling in the extremities (hands, feet)
11. Slow-healing wounds or sores
12. Abnormally high frequency of infection

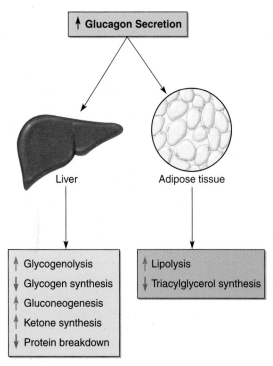

Figure 12.11 Glucagon secretion and its actions on target tissues.

The Genetics of Diabetes

A simple pattern of inherited characteristics does not fully explain the risk of contracting diabetes. Two factors predispose a person to diabetes: (1) individuals inherit a predisposition to the disease and (2) something in the environment triggers its activation.

Type 1 Diabetes

Most type 1 diabetics inherit risk factors from both parents, with inherited traits more common in whites than blacks or Asians. The most prominent "environmental triggers" include cold weather exposure (develops more often in winter than summer and more frequently in places with cold climates), viral infection, and early diet (less common in those who were breast-fed and in those who first ate solid foods at a later age). The development of type 1 diabetes seems to take many years.

Type 2 Diabetes

Type 2 diabetes has a stronger genetic basis than type 1, yet its occurrence also depends more on environmental factors. A family history of type 2 diabetes represents one of the strongest risk factors for the disease but *only* for people living a typical Western lifestyle consisting of a high-fat diet, low intake of complex carbohydrates and fiber, and too little exercise. Overfatness provides a considerable risk factor for type 2 diabetes. The ethnic groups in the United States with the highest risk for developing type 2 diabetes are African Americans, Mexican Americans, and Pima Indians. Three factors can produce high blood glucose levels in type 2 diabetes:

1. Inadequate insulin produced by the pancreas to control blood sugar known as **relative insulin deficiency**
2. Decreased insulin effects on peripheral tissue known as **insulin resistance**, particularly skeletal muscle
3. Combined effect of factors 1 and 2

A dysregulation in glycolytic and oxidative capacities of skeletal muscle also relates to insulin resistance in type 2 diabetes. The disease most likely results from the interaction of genes and lifestyle factors, including physical inactivity, weight gain (~80% of type 2 diabetics are obese), aging, and possibly a high-fat diet. These lifestyle factors contribute to the 70% increase in the disorder among persons in their 30s during the last decade of the 20th century and a 33% overall increase nationally. Also, the form of insulin resistance in type 2 diabetes has a strong

Questions & Notes

Name the "insulin antagonist" hormone.

Give the major function of glucagon.

Briefly describe the 2 types of diabetic disorders and give one fact about each.

1.

2.

For Your Information

A DISEASE OF EPIDEMIC PROPORTIONS

The current statistics regarding diabetes prevalence in the United States are staggering! Between 2003 and 2006, 25.9% of the United States population 20 years and older had diabetes; for those older than 60 years of age the prevalence was 34%. About 12.0 million, or 11.2%, of all men and 11.5 million, or 10.2%, of women age 20 years or older have diabetes. Nearly 15 million, or 9.8%, of non-Hispanic whites and 3.7 million, or 14.7%, of non-Hispanic blacks age 20 years or older have diabetes. The total number of Americans with diabetes jumped by more than 3 million between 2005 and 2007 to about 24 million, with another 57 million categorized as prediabetic with fasting blood sugar between 100 and 125 mg·dL^{-1}. Nearly one-third of newly diagnosed cases occur in children younger than 16 years, which has caused clinicians to label diabetes a "childhood disease." Experts estimate that up to 92% of type 2 diabetes can be changed by diet and lifestyle. Use the following Internet site to calculate your diabetes risk: *www.diabetes.org/ risk-test.jsp.*

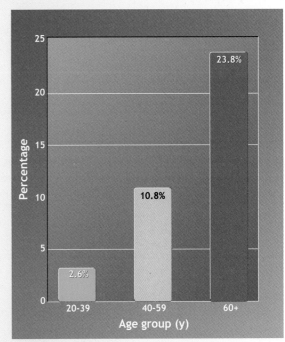

Prevalence of diagnosed and undiagnosed diabetes among people age 20 years or older, United States, 2007. Age 20 years or older: 23.5 million, or 10.7%, of all people in this age group have diabetes. Age 60 years or older: 12.2 million, or 23.8%, of all people in this age group have diabetes. (From 2004–2006 National Health Interview Survey estimates projected to the year 2007.)

genetic component. Diabetic-prone individuals possess a gene that directs synthesis of three mitogen-activated protein kinases that inhibits insulin's action in cellular glucose transport.

Tests for Diabetes

Several tests diagnose diabetes. The American Diabetes Association (*www.diabetes.org/home.jsp*) recommends the **fasting plasma glucose test (FPG)** rather than the popular oral glucose tolerance test. The latter evaluates blood sugar levels over a 2-hour interval after drinking a glucose-containing solution (see Close Up Box 12.1, *How to Detect Diabetes Mellitus*, below). The FPG test measures plasma glucose after an 8-hour fast.

The current value for suspected diabetes (FPG >126 mg·dL^{-1}) is lower than the previous standard of 140 mg·dL^{-1} and acknowledges that patients can be asymptomatic with microvascular complications (small blood vessel damage) with FPG values in the low to mid 120 mg·dL^{-1} range. The impaired range represents a transition between normal and diabetes at which the body no

---

BOX 12.1   CLOSE UP

How to Detect Diabetes Mellitus

Complications from diabetes mellitus can cause blindness, kidney failure, need for amputation, and birth defects. It also contributes to atherosclerosis and hypertension. About one-half of the people each year who learn they have diabetes go untreated.

Differences Between the Two Major Forms of Diabetes Mellitus

CONDITION	TYPE 1	TYPE 2
Other names	Type 1-IDDM	Type II-NIDDM
	Juvenile-onset	Adult-onset
	Ketosis-prone	Ketosis-resistant
	Brittle	Stable
Age of onset	<20 y (mean = 12 y)	>40 y; increasingly
	<40 y in some cases	prevalent in youth
Other condition	Viral infection	Obesity
Insulin required	Yes	Sometimes
Insulin receptors	Normal	Low or normal
Symptoms	Relatively severe	Relatively moderate
Prevalence in diabetic population	5 to 10%	90 to 95%

Key Blood Tests for Detecting Diabetes Mellitus

SUBSTANCE	NORMAL VALUES	DECISION LEVEL
Fasting plasma glucose (FPG); following 8-h fast	<110 mg·dL^{-1}	≤ 45 mg·dL^{-1}: indicates **hypoglycemia** and a prediabetic condition 110–125 mg·dL^{-1}: indicates **impaired range** >126 mg·dL^{-1}: indicates **suspected diabetes**
Total cholesterol	<200 mg·dL^{-1}	>240 mg·dL^{-1}: patients with diabetes often have elevated plasma cholesterol
Triacylglycerol	40–160 mg·dL^{-1}, males 35–135 mg·dL^{-1}, females	>250 mg·dL^{-1}: patients with diabetes often have elevated plasma triacylglycerols
Oral Glucose-Tolerance Test[a] Time = 0 Time = 60 min Time = 120 min	**Upper Limit of Normal** 115 mg·dL^{-1} 200 mg·dL^{-1} 140 mg·dL^{-1}	**Diabetic Values** >140 mg·dL^{-1} >200 mg·dL^{-1} >200 mg·dL^{-1}

[a]Previously preferred but an expensive, time consuming, and unpleasant test. Blood drawn following ingestion of a standard glucose load. Ordinarily, blood glucose rises initially and then returns to normal. In diabetes mellitus blood glucose remains elevated during the recovery period. Many variations exist in the timing of blood sampling and quantity of glucose ingested. A fasting plasma glucose (FPG) test is recommended.

longer responds properly to insulin or fails to secrete adequate amounts. These prediabetic individuals require close monitoring because they run a high risk of developing full-blown diabetes.

METABOLIC SYNDROME

Metabolic syndrome represents a multifaceted grouping of coronary artery disease risks often defined as having three or more of the criteria listed in Table 12.3. This "disease of modern civilization" affects millions of adults (more common in men than women) in Western industrialized countries. Disease occurrence relates to genetic, hormonal, and lifestyle factors that include obesity; physical inactivity; and nutrient excesses, including high intakes of saturated and trans fatty acids. The clustering of insulin resistance and hyperinsulinemia characterizes the metabolic syndrome. These individuals remain at higher risk for coronary artery disease and should receive special attention, diagnosis and treatment.

Psychosocial stress, socioeconomic disadvantage, and abnormal psychiatric traits also have been linked to the syndrome's pathogenesis.

ⓘ For Your Information

EXERCISE GUIDELINES FOR TYPE 1 DIABETICS

1. Ingest 15 to 30 g of carbohydrates for each 30 minutes of intense exercise.
2. Consume a carbohydrate snack after exercise.
3. Decrease insulin dose:
   a. Intermediate-acting insulin: Decrease the dose by 30 to 35% on the day of exercise.
   b. Intermediate- and short-acting insulin: Omit the dose if it precedes exercise.
   c. Multiple doses of short-acting insulin: Reduce the dose before exercise by 30% and supplement carbohydrate intake.
   d. Continuous subcutaneous insulin infusion: Eliminate mealtime bolus or insulin increment that precedes or follows exercise.
4. Avoid exercising for 1 hour those muscles receiving a short-acting insulin injection.
5. Avoid exercising in the late evening.

ⓘ For Your Information

COMBINING FIVE HEALTHY LIFESTYLE CHANGES THAT REDUCE DIABETES RISK

1. Engage in 30 to 60 minutes of daily exercise.
2. Keep alcohol consumption at the light to moderate level.
3. Do not smoke.
4. Keep body mass index less than 25 and waist size less than 34.6 inches for women and 36.2 inches for men.
5. Consume a healthy diet with above-average fiber intake, a positive ratio of polyunsaturated fat to saturated fat, low trans-fat, and foods with a relatively low glycemic index.

Instead of this:	Consume this:
Soft drinks, fruit drinks, fruit juice	Water, unsweetened coffee or tea
Saturated fat, trans fat (margarine, cream, pies, cake frostings, French fries)	Unsaturated fats (vegetable oils, nuts)
Refined grains and sweets	Whole grains
Red meats, especially processed meats (bacon, sausage, ham, hot dogs)	Seafood, poultry, beans, soy foods

Table 12.3 | Identifying the Metabolic Syndrome

RISK FACTOR	DEFINING LEVEL
Abdominal fatness (waist girth)[a]	
Men	>102 cm (>40 in)
Women	>88 cm (>35 in)
Triacylglycerols	≥150 mg/dL
High-density lipoprotein	
Men	<40 mg/dL
Women	<50 mg/dL
Blood pressure	≥130/≥85 mm Hg
Fasting glucose	≥110 mg/dL

[a]Overweight and overfatness are associated with insulin resistance and the metabolic syndrome. However, the presence of abnormal obesity is more highly correlated with the metabolic risk factors than an elevated body mass index (BMI). We recommend the simple measure of waist girth to identify the body weight component of the metabolic syndrome.

Questions & Notes

Give 2 risk factors that predispose a person to type 1 diabetes.

1.

2.

Give 2 risk factors that predispose a person to type 2 diabetes.

1.

2.

Such factors likely relate to a central neuroendocrine origin as enhanced activation of the hypothalamic–pituitary–adrenal axis.

DIABETES AND EXERCISE

Hypoglycemia during exercise represents the most common disturbance of glucose homeostasis in type 1 diabetes. During prolonged moderate exercise, hepatic glucose release does not keep pace with active muscle's increased glucose utilization. Reduced plasma glucose becomes severe in patients who require intensive insulin therapy throughout the day to normalize their glucose levels. Sedentary lifestyle and excessive body fat reduce exercise tolerance of type 1 and type 2 diabetics independent of blood glucose regulation.

Exercise Training Among Diabetics

The clinical use of exercise training to control glucose in type 1 diabetics remains complex despite the clear association between regular physical activity and improved insulin sensitivity by peripheral tissues. These individuals must exercise with caution because increased insulin sensitivity and fast delivery of injected insulin via rapid circulation accelerate glucose removal from plasma, which can induce serious hypoglycemia and diabetic shock.

As a consequence of obesity and possibly poor diet, many "normal" overweight men and women experience reduced glucose tolerance from a generalized insulin resistance; this triggers excessive insulin output from the pancreas and resulting hyperinsulinemia. For individuals who eventually develop type 2 diabetes, exercise training often reduces fasting plasma insulin levels and lowers insulin output, thus indicating improved insulin sensitivity.

Exercise Benefits for Type 2 Diabetics

Exercise training provides important nonpharmacologic therapy for individuals with type 2 diabetes. Refer to *http://journals.lww.com/acsm-msse/pages/collectiondetails.aspx?TopicalCollectionId=1* for the American College of Sports Medicine's position stand on physical activity and type 2 diabetes. Individuals at greatest risk for type 2 diabetes (obese, hypertensive, family history, sedentary lifestyle) gain the greatest benefit from exercise. Regular physical activity for people with type 2 diabetes improves glycemic control, cardiovascular function, body composition, and psychological profile and reduces a broad array of heart disease risks. Some patients with type 1 diabetes improve their control of blood glucose with lower daily insulin requirements with regular exercise, but the results are less consistent than for type 2 patients. Despite this limitation, people with type 1 and type 2 diabetes profit considerably from the benefits of regular exercise.

Glycemic Control   An acute bout of resistance or endurance training or both abruptly decrease plasma glucose levels in type 2 diabetics. Extending the duration of weekly physical activity by nearly 50% from 115 minutes to 170 minutes produces the greatest increase in insulin sensitivity. Improved glucose regulation with acute exercise may persist for hours to days because of the muscles' increased insulin sensitivity. Improved longer term glycemic control in physically active people with diabetes probably occurs from the cumulative effects of *each* acute exercise session rather than from changes in physical fitness per se. Consequently, patients with hyperinsulinemia show the greatest benefit from regular exercise, a response consistent with the notion that exercise reverses insulin resistance (i.e., increases insulin sensitivity). *Improved insulin sensitivity with regular physical activity provides type 2 diabetics with important "therapy" that ultimately lowers their insulin requirements. Improvements in blood glucose homeostasis with regular physical activity rapidly decrease when training ceases and completely dissipate within several weeks of inactivity.*

Cardiovascular Effects   Increases in disease state and mortality in type 2 diabetes occur from coronary heart disease, stroke, and peripheral vascular and nerve disease related to accelerated atherosclerosis and elevated blood glucose level. In this regard, regular physical activity favorably modifies plasma lipoproteins, hyperinsulinemia, hyperglycemia, some blood coagulation parameters, local vascularization, and blood pressure.

Weight Loss   Exercise without diet therapy only moderately reduces body weight among type 2 diabetics. A moderate effect should not be underestimated because small changes in body weight with exercise may not reflect the more favorable changes in overall body composition because an increase in lean tissue mass may accompany any body fat loss. For both diabetic and nondiabetic individuals, body fat loss occurs most effectively by combining diet *plus* exercise.

Psychological Benefits   Regular, moderate-intensity exercise for diabetics and nondiabetics decreases anxiety, improves mood and self-esteem, increases sense of well-being, and enhances overall quality of life.

Exercise Risks for Diabetics

The potential complications of exercise for diabetics can be minimized through proper patient screening before they begin an exercise program and careful monitoring during exercise. **Figure 12.12** lists some potential adverse effects of exercise for diabetics.

ENDURANCE TRAINING AND ENDOCRINE FUNCTION

Few studies have evaluated changes in hormonal response to systematic alterations in the frequency, intensity, and

Potential problems with exercise in type 2 diabetes	
System	**Potential Problem**
Systemic	• Retinal hemorrhage • Increased proteinuria • Acceleration of microvascular lesions
Cardiovascular	• Cardiac arrhythmias • Ischemic heart disease (often silent) • Excessive rise in blood pressure • Post-exercise orthostatic hypotension
Metabolic	• Increased hyperglycemia • Increased ketosis
Musculoskeletal	• Foot ulcers (in presence of neuropathy) • Orthopedic injury related to neuropathy • Accelerated degenerative joint disease • Eye injuries and retinal hemorrhage

Figure 12.12 Potential physical and physiologic problems for individuals with type 2 diabetes who begin an exercise program.

duration of exercise. Most of what we know about changes in hormonal dynamics with exercise training comes from studies in which hormone assessment occurred secondarily to other variables. Nevertheless, a picture has emerged of the integrated response of different hormones to exercise training, particularly with respect to fluid balance, energy modulation, glycemic control, cardiovascular changes, and growth and development. Table 12.4 lists selected endocrine hormones and their general responses to regular exercise. Because of complex interactions between endocrine secretions and central nervous system function, limited research exists concerning multiple hormone secretions and chronic exercise adaptations.

Endurance training generally decreases the magnitude of hormonal response to a standard exercise level. Exercise at a particular absolute intensity produces a lower hormonal response in trained subjects than in untrained counterparts. Adjusting exercise intensity to a percentage of each person's maximum capacity at the same relative intensity eliminates the training-related difference in hormonal response. With maximal exercise, trained subjects have a similar or slightly higher catecholamine and pituitary hormonal response than untrained subjects.

Anterior Pituitary Hormones

Growth Hormone and Long-Term Exercise Training Most research of GH involves responses to a single exercise session. Less information exists on GH levels during prolonged exercise training. Understanding the dynamics of GH secretions with chronic exercise takes on significance because of the causal relationship between GH availability and the maintenance of fat-free body mass (FFM) with aging and weight loss.

Figure 12.13 shows the effects of a run training program on 24-hour integrated serum GH concentrations in 21 healthy, eumenorrheic women. The study involved two training groups; one group ran at speeds corresponding to the lactate threshold (@LT), and the other group ran at speeds above lactate threshold (>LT). Nontraining subjects served as control subjects (C).

Both training groups completed similar weekly mileage. The distance covered during the first week equaled 5 miles; the weekly mileage gradually

Questions & Notes

Give the upper limit of fasting blood glucose that indicates type 1 diabetes.

List 3 benefits of exercise for type 2 diabetics.

1.

2.

3.

List 3 potential complications of exercise for type 1 diabetics.

1.

2.

3.

List 3 potential problems for type 2 diabetics who regularly exercise.

1.

2.

3.

For Your Information

COMMON CHARACTERISTICS OF THE METABOLIC SYNDROME

• Insulin resistance
• Glucose intolerance
• Dyslipidemia (high triacylglycerol, low high-density lipoprotein, high low-density lipoprotein levels)
• Stroke
• Upper-body obesity
• Type 2 diabetes mellitus
• Hypertension
• Coronary artery disease
• Reduced ability to dissolve blood clots

Table 12.4	Hormonal Response to Exercise Training
HORMONE	**TRAINING RESPONSE**
Hypothalamus-Pituitary Hormones	
GH	Resting values increased: trained tend to have less dramatic rise during exercise
TSH	No known training effect
ACTH	Trained persons have increased exercise values
PRL	Some evidence that training lowers resting values
FSH, LB, and Testosterone	Trained females have depressed values; testosterone levels may increase in males with long-term strength training
Posterior Pituitary Hormones	
Vasopressin (ADH)	Some evidence that training slightly reduces ADH at a given workload
Oxytocin	Limited human research available
Thyroid Hormones	
Thyroxine (T_4)	Reduced concentration of total T_3 and increased free thyroxine at rest
Trilodothyronine (T_3)	Increased turnover of T_3 and T_4 during exercise
Adrenal Hormones	
Aldosterone	No significant training adaptation
Cortisol	Trained exhibit slight elevations during exercise
Epinephrine	Decrease in secretion at rest and same absolute
Norepinephrine	exercise intensity after training
Pancreatic Hormones	
Insulin	Training increases sensitivity to insulin; normal decrease in insulin during exercise is greatly reduced
Glucagon	Smaller increase in glucose levels during exercise at both absolute and relative workloads
Kidney Hormones	
Renin (enzyme)	No apparent training effect
Angiotensin	

increased to 24 miles by week 20 and continued at this distance until week 40. Thereafter, the weekly mileage increased by 1.25 miles each additional 3 weeks. Subjects ran between 35 and 40 miles per week by the end of the study.

The year-long training program increased $\dot{V}O_{2max}$ by 9.9% for the @LT group and 11.8% for the >LT group. In addition, the @LT group increased exercise $\dot{V}O_2$ at lactate threshold ($\dot{V}O_2$–LT) by 21.5%, and the >LT group's $\dot{V}O_2$–LT increased by 28%. The control group did not change. No differences in body mass, percentage body fat, or body fat mass emerged among groups. FFM increased for both training groups.

For GH, the >LT group showed a marked 50% increase in integrated 24-hour resting GH concentration after training. GH concentrations remained unaffected by exercise training for the @LT and control groups. The researchers hypothesized that relatively strenuous exercise above the lactate threshold increased GH pulsatile secretion through the stimulating effect of endogenous opiates and cate-cholamines, while at the same time, such exercise inhibited somatostatin release.

Corticotropin (Adrenocorticotropic Hormone)

Corticotropin stimulates the adrenal cortex and increases fat mobilization for energy. Exercise training increases ACTH levels during physical activity. Enhanced fatty acid oxidation from ACTH spares muscle glycogen to benefit prolonged intense exercise performance.

Prolactin It remains unclear whether long-term training alters PRL other than the training-induced changes mediated by sympathetic activity or other multiple hormone interactions. It does appear that resting PRL levels of male runners average below values for sedentary nonrunners.

Follicle-Stimulating Hormone, Luteinizing Hormone, and Testosterone

Regular physical activity depresses reproductive hormone responses in women and men. Women with a history of exercise

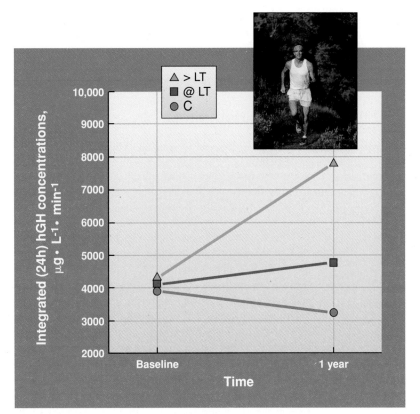

Figure 12.13 Integrated 24-hour human growth hormone (hGH) concentrations for subjects training at the lactate threshold (@LT), training above the lactate threshold (>LT), and non-training control subjects (C). Note the large (50%) increase in hGH concentrations for the >LT group compared with the @LT and C groups. (Data from Weltman, A., et al.: Endurance training amplifies the pulsatile release of growth hormone: effects of training intensity. *J. Appl. Physiol.*, 72:2188, 1992.)

Questions & Notes

Briefly describe the hormonal response to exercise training for the following hormones.

GH:

ADH:

Insulin:

Glucagon:

Thyroxine:

Cortisol:

Epinephrine:

Briefly describe differences in the effects of endurance training versus resistance training on testosterone levels.

participation have altered FSH and LH levels at different phases of the menstrual cycle. Alterations in these hormones often cause menstrual dysfunction. FSH levels decrease in trained women throughout an abbreviated anovulatory menstrual cycle, whereas LH and progesterone concentrations increase in the cycle's follicular phase. Factors other than acute and long-term exercise also can alter reproductive function in women athletes; these include weight loss, dietary changes, changes in lean-to-fat ratio, emotional stress of training and competition, and altered clearance rates of gonadal steroid hormones.

Endurance training in men affects pituitary–gonadal function, including testosterone and PRL concentrations. In comparisons of testosterone, LH, and FSH levels among 46 male runners (64 km average weekly distance) and 18 non-runners matched for age, stature, and body mass, the runners had depressed testosterone levels without a difference in LH and FSH compared with non-runners. Reduced testosterone concentration (both increased clearance and decreased production) in endurance-trained men parallels the sex steroid reductions in women who undergo endurance training and associated lower body fat levels. Because LH and FSH do not differ between trained and untrained persons, impaired gonadotropin release from the anterior pituitary does not explain reduced testosterone levels in the trained state. Resistance training presents a different picture because elite resistance-trained male athletes have elevated levels of serum testosterone, LH, and FSH.

Researchers studied the effects of a supraphysiologic dose of exogenous testosterone in healthy, untrained men randomly assigned to one of four groups: placebo with no exercise, testosterone with no exercise, placebo plus exercise, and testosterone plus exercise. The men received injections of 600 mg of testosterone or placebo weekly for 10 weeks. The exercise groups performed standardized weight lifting for the arms and legs three times weekly. Measurements before and after the treatment period included FFM (determined by underwater weighing), muscle size (determined by magnetic resonance imaging), and arms and leg strength (determined with bench-press and squatting exercises, respectively). For the no-exercise groups, men given testosterone experienced a 14% increase in arm muscle size compared with the placebo group and a 9% increase in arm strength. Similar results occurred for the lower body. Men assigned to testosterone and exercise showed greater increases in FFM and muscle size of the arms and legs compared with the testosterone with no exercise group. Neither mood nor behavior changed in any of the groups during training. These data support the conclusion that a supraphysiologic dose of testosterone, especially when combined with resistance training, increases FFM and muscle size and strength in healthy men.

Parathyroid Hormone Endurance training enhances exercise-related increases in PTH in young and elderly adults. The significance of a training-induced rise increase PTH for preserving bone mass with aging awaits further study.

Posterior Pituitary Hormones

Antidiuretic Hormone Maximal exhaustive exercise or prolonged submaximal exercise at the same relative intensity produces no difference in ADH response in trained and untrained individuals. ADH concentration decreases with training in response to submaximal exercise at the same absolute intensity.

Oxytocin Recent human research suggests that oxytocin (OT) in combination with arginine vasopressin (AVP) increase following prolonged high-intensity endurance exercise. These data allow for possible speclution that oxytocin and perhaps brain natriuetic peptide (BNP) may assist their companion hormones AVP and atrial natriuetic peptide (ANP) in the regulation of fluid balance during physical exertion.

Thyroid Hormones

Exercise training coordinates a pituitary–thyroid response that increases turnover of thyroid hormones, a response usually associated with excessive hormonal action that leads to hyperthyroidism. However, no evidence indicates that hyperthyroidism develops in highly trained individuals. BMR and resting core temperature remain normal with training. The increased T_4 turnover that accompanies chronic exercise occurs through a mechanism that differs from this hormone's normal dynamics.

Research with endurance-trained women reveals interesting responses for thyroid turnover. Training 48 km a week mildly depressed thyroid function as reflected by decreased T_3 and T_4 levels. In contrast, extending training distance to 80 km a week *increased* the levels of these hormones. The changes in body composition that accompany a high training volume may contribute to discrepancies in an exercise-induced change in thyroid function in women.

Adrenal Hormones

Aldosterone The renin–angiotensin–aldosterone system contributes to homeostatic control of body fluid volumes, electrolytes, and blood pressure, but exercise training does not affect resting levels of these compounds or their normal response to physical activity.

Cortisol Plasma cortisol levels increase less in trained than in sedentary subjects during the same (*absolute*) moderate exercise levels. Greater cortisol output among untrained individuals may partly result from heightened psychological stress experienced during exercise testing. Elevated cortisol levels promote fatty acid and protein catabolism to provide fuel for energy and substrates for tissue repair after exercise.

Epinephrine and Norepinephrine An important aspect of the catecholamine response to exercise and training involves the **sympathoadrenal response** rather than the typical adrenal gland response. **Figure 12.14** shows a large initial decrease in epinephrine and norepinephrine concentrations to a standard bout of intense exercise during the first 2 weeks of training. *Bradycardia and a smaller increase in blood pressure during submaximal exercise represent the most familiar sympathoadrenal adaptations to exercise training.* Both responses favorably lower myocardial oxygen demands to exercise and other stressors. Reduced catecholamine output most likely reflects the benefits of regular physical activity in diminishing the body's response to stressful situations.

For equivalent *relative* exercise intensities, a *higher* sympathoadrenal response occurs after aerobic training. More than likely, this training response reflects three factors requiring greater sympathetic nervous system activation from the increased exercise level:

1. Greater absolute demand for substrate use via glycogenolysis and lipolysis
2. Increased overall cardiovascular response via cardiac output
3. Larger muscle mass activation

Pancreatic Hormones

Insulin and Glucagon Endurance training maintains plasma insulin and glucagon levels in exercise similar to values at rest. *In essence, the trained state requires less insulin at any stage from rest through light to moderately intense physical activity.* This reduced hormonal response with exercise training occurs through two mechanisms:

1. Increased muscle and fat tissue sensitivity to insulin. Exercise training reduces the insulin requirement to regulate blood glucose. Improved insulin sensitivity most likely occurs from

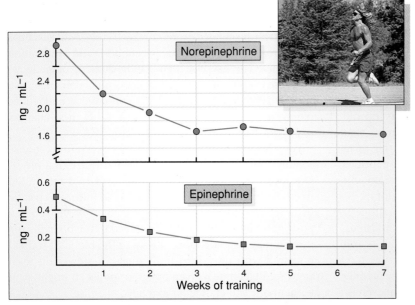

Figure 12.14 Week-by-week changes in plasma catecholamines during a 5-minute exercise bout at 243 watts for six male subjects. Training consisted of running and stationary cycling 6 days a week. Catecholamine levels decreased progressively during training, with the most rapid decline in the early training phase. (Data from Winder, W.W., et al.: Time course of sympathoadrenal adaptations to endurance exercise training in man. *J. Appl. Physiol.*, 45:370, 1978.)

improved insulin binding capacity to receptor sites on individual muscle fibers and adipocytes. Liver cells also increase their insulin sensitivity.
2. Increased percentage contribution of fat catabolism for fuel during submaximal exercise; decreased carbohydrate metabolism lowers the insulin requirement.

Resistance Training and Endocrine Function

The large variation among individuals in muscular strength and hypertrophy gains with similar programs of resistance training suggests considerable individual differences in endocrine dynamics with chronic muscle overload. Muscle remodeling with resistance training reflects a complex process that involves cell receptor interaction with specific hormones, which stimulates DNA synthesis of contractile proteins. The magnitude of the change links to the configuration of the exercise stimulus (e.g., frequency, intensity, volume, and mode) and more than likely a genetically influenced hormonal response. *In general, resistance training increases the frequency and amplitude of testosterone and GH secretion, thereby contributing to hypertrophic effects on muscle.*

Testosterone and GH represent two primary hormones in resistance training adaptations. Testosterone augments GH release and interacts with nervous system dynamics to increase muscle force production. The importance of these functions may exceed any direct anabolic effect of testosterone on muscle structure and function. A single session of resistance training generally elicits a short-term increase in serum testosterone and decrease in cortisol, with a greater response in men than women. Concurrently, catecholamine release from the adrenal medulla increases with the acute stress of high-force and high-power exercise protocols.

Resistance training in men increases the frequency and amplitude of testosterone and GH secretion, thereby creating a favorable hormonal environment for muscle growth. In contrast, most studies fail to demonstrate changes in testosterone and GH concentrations with such training in women. Gender differences in hormone output with resistance training may ultimately explain variations in responsiveness of muscle strength and size to prolonged muscular overload.

Questions & Notes

Name 2 hormones affected by resistance training adaptations.

1.

2.

Does resistance training increase or decrease growth hormone secretions?

Name the hormone thought to produce an "exercise high" response in some individuals.

List 3 opioid substances.

1.

2.

3.

Opioid Peptides and Exercise

Researchers in the 1970s isolated and purified two opioid pentapeptides, methionine and leucine enkephalin (Greek meaning "in the head"). These breakthrough discoveries provided the first direct evidence that endogenous substances behaved like opiates. By the early 1980s, researchers discovered groups of endogenous opioid compounds now generically termed "endorphins" that bind to families of receptors. By definition, the term *endorphin* characterizes a group of endogenous peptides whose pharmacologic action mimics those of opium and its analogs. Opioid substances include β-lipotrophin; β-endorphin; and dynorphin, the most potent opioid peptide. Endorphins regulate menstruation and modulate the response of GH, ACTH, PRL, catecholamines, and cortisol.

β-Endorphin and β-lipotrophin opioids generally increase with acute exercise. Plasma β-endorphin in exercis-ing men and women increase five times over resting levels, with higher values probably occurring within the brain. The most notable postulated exercise-related endorphin effect has been its role in triggering a state of euphoria and exhilaration (often refered to "**exercise high**") as the duration of moderate to intense exercise increases. The endorphin effect may also increase pain tolerance; improve appetite control; and reduce anxiety, tension, anger, and confusion. All of these changes are proposed benefits of regular exercise.

The effect of exercise training on endorphin response remains controversial. One could hypothesize that physical training increases an individual's sensitivity to opioid effects, so it takes less of the hormone to induce a specific effect. In this sense, regular exercise could be viewed as a "positive addiction." Opiates produced in the body during exercise may degrade more slowly in the blood of trained compared with untrained individuals. A slower disposal rate would facilitate a given opiate response; it might even augment one's tolerance for extended exercise.

SUMMARY

1. The endocrine system consists of a host organ, a hormone, and a target or receptor organ. Hormones exist as either steroids or amino acid (polypeptide) derivatives.

2. Hormones alter rates of cellular reactions by acting at specific receptor sites to enhance or inhibit enzyme function.

3. Hormone concentration in the blood depends on the amount of hormone synthesized, the amount released, the amount taken up by the target organ, and its rate of removal from the blood.

4. The anterior pituitary secretes at least six hormones: PRL, the gonadotropic hormones FSH and LH, corticotropin, thyrotropin, and GH. The anterior pituitary also releases endorphins.

5. GH promotes cell division and cellular proliferation; TSH controls the amount of hormone secreted by the thyroid gland; ACTH regulates the output of the hormones of the adrenal cortex; PRL affects reproduction and development of female secondary sex characteristics; and FSH and LH stimulate the ovaries to secrete estrogen and progesterone in women and testosterone in men.

6. The posterior pituitary gland secretes ADH to control water excretion by the kidneys. It also secretes oxytocin, which is important in birthing and milk secretion.

7. Thyroxine elevates the metabolic rate in all cells and increases carbohydrate and fat breakdown in energy metabolism.

8. The inner medulla and outer cortex components of the adrenal gland secrete two different types of hormones. The medulla secretes the catecholamines epinephrine and norepinephrine. The adrenal cortex secretes mineralocorticoids that regulate extracellular sodium and potassium, glucocorticoids that stimulate gluconeogenesis and serve as an insulin antagonist, and androgens (control secondary sex characteristics).

9. Insulin secreted by the pancreas' β cells increases glucose transport into cells to control the body's rate of carbohydrate metabolism. The α cells of the pancreas secrete glucagon, an insulin antagonist that increases blood sugar.

10. Type 1 diabetes causes insulin deficiency by destroying the pancreas' insulin-producing β cells. Type 2 diabetes generally occurs in overweight, sedentary, middle-aged individuals with a family history of the disease. It arises mainly from insulin resistance (body tissues require greater than normal insulin for glucose regulation). Eventually, even a large insulin output fails to properly regulate blood sugar.

11. The increase in type 2 diabetes in children and adults has reached epidemic proportions worldwide. More than one-third of all new cases occur in children younger than age 16 years.

12. Exercise training exerts differential effects on resting and exercise-induced hormone production and release. Training elevates hormone response during exercise for ACTH and cortisol and depresses GH, PRL, FSH, LH, testosterone, ADH, T_4, and insulin; no known training response occurs for aldosterone and angiotensin.

13. Exercise-induced elevation of β-endorphins coincides with euphoria, increased pain tolerance, the "exercise high," and menstrual dysfunction.

THOUGHT QUESTIONS

1. Visit a local health food store and list the supplements that claim to enhance exercise performance. Identify the ingredients and their alleged effects. Which supplements purport to simulate hormonal release? Based on your knowledge of hormonal regulation and function, can any of these products deliver on their claims?

2. Discuss how hormones act as silent messengers to integrate the body as a unit.

3. Hormones play crucial roles in normal growth and development and physiologic function. Give specific examples of why *more* is not necessarily *better* regarding these chemicals.

SELECTED REFERENCES

The Action to Control Cardiovascular Risk in Diabetes Study Group: Effects of intensive glucose lowering in type 2 diabetes. *N. Engl. J. Med*, 358:2545, 2008.

Ahtiainen, J.P., et al.: Acute hormonal responses to heavy resistance exercise in strength athletes versus nonathletes. *Can. J. Appl. Physiol.*, 29:527, 2004.

American College of Sports Medicine: Position stand. The recommended quantity and quality of exercise for developing and maintaining cardiorespiratory and muscular fitness, and flexibility in healthy adults. *Med. Sci. Sports Exerc.*, 30:975, 1998.

American College of Sports Medicine: Position stand. Exercise and type 2 diabetes. *Med. Sci. Sports Exerc.*, 32:1345;2000.

Baylor, L.S., Hackney, A.C.: Resting thyroid and liptin changes following intense, prolonged exercise training. *Eur. J. Appl. Physiol.*, 88:480, 2003.

Bertoli, A., et al.: Lipid profile, BMI, body fat distribution, and aerobic fitness in men with metabolic syndrome. *Acta. Diabetol.*, 40(Suppl 1):S130, 2003.

Boecker, H., et al.: The runner's high: Opioidergic mechanisms in the human brain. *Cereb. Cortex.*, 18:2523, 2008.

Bruce, C.R., Hawley, J.A.: Improvements in insulin resistance with aerobic exercise training: A lipocentric approach. *Med. Sci. Sports Exerc.*, 36:1196, 2004.

Caruso, J.F., et al.: Blood lactate and hormonal responses to prototype flywheel ergometer workouts. *J. Strength Cond. Res.*, 24:749, 2010.

Charro, M.A., et al.: Hormonal, metabolic and perceptual responses to different resistance training systems. *J. Sports Med. Phys. Fitness.*, 50:229, 2010.

Chwalbinska-Moneta, J., et al.: Early effects of short-term endurance training on hormonal responses to graded exercise. *J. Physiol. Pharmacol.*, 56:87, 2005.

Cox, A.J., et al.: Cytokine responses to treadmill running in healthy and illness-prone athletes. *Med. Sci. Sports Exerc.*, 39:1918, 2007.

Daly, W., et al.: Relationship between stress hormones and testosterone with prolonged endurance exercise. *Eur. J. Appl. Physiol.*, 93:375, 2005.

Di Luigi, L., et al.: Heredity and pituitary response to exercise-related stress in trained men. *Int. J. Sports Med.*, 24:551, 2003.

Ford, E.S., et al.: Prevalence of the metabolic syndrome among US adults: Findings from the third National Health and Nutrition Examination Survey. *JAMA.*, 287:356, 2002.

Gerson, L.S., Braun, B.: Effect of high cardiorespiratory fitness and high body fat on insulin resistance. *Med. Sci. Sports Exerc.*, 38:1709, 2006.

Gleeson, M.: Immune function in sport and exercise [invited review]. *J. Appl. Physiol.*, 103:963, 2007.

Goto, K., et al.: The impact of metabolic stress on hormonal responses and muscular adaptations. *Med. Sci. Sports Exerc.*, 37:955, 2005.

Hawley, J.A., Zierath, J.R.: *Physical Activity and Type 2 Diabetes.* Champaign IL: Human Kinetics, 2008.

Healy, M.L., et al.: High dose growth hormone exerts an anabolic effect at rest and during exercise in endurance-trained athletes. *J. Clin. Endocrinol. Metab.*, 88:5221, 2003.

Hew-Butler T., et al.: Acute changes in endocrine and fluid balance markers during high-intensity, steady-state, and prolonged endurance running: unexpected increases in oxytocin and brain natriuretic peptide during exercise. *Eur. J. Endocrinol.*, 15:729, 2008.

Holmes, B., Dohm, G.L.: Regulation of GLUT 4 gene expression during exercise. *Med. Sci. Sports Exerc.*, 36:1202, 2004.

Houmard, J.A., et al.: Effect of the volume and intensity of exercise training on insulin sensitivity. *J. Appl. Physiol.* 96:101, 2004.

Huang, W.S., et al.: Effect of treadmill exercise on circulating thyroid hormone measurements. *Med. Princ. Pract.*, 13:15, 2004.

Ivy, J.L.: Muscle insulin resistance amended with exercise training: Role of GLUT4 expression. *Med. Sci. Sports Exerc.*, 36:1207, 2004.

Izquierdo, M., et al.: Maximal strength and power, muscle mass, endurance and serum hormones in weightlifters and road cyclists. *J. Sports Sci.*, 22:465, 2004.

Jurca, R., et al.: Associations of muscle strength and aerobic fitness with metabolic syndrome in men. *Med. Sci. Sports Exerc.*, 36:1301, 2004.

Kasa-Vubu, J.Z., et al.: Differences in endocrine function with varying fitness capacity in postpubertal females across the weight spectrum. *Arch. Pediatr. Adolesc. Med.*, 158:333, 2004.

Kraemer, W.J., et al.: Changes in exercise performance and hormonal concentrations over a big ten soccer season in starters and nonstarters. *J. Strength Cond. Res.*, 18:121, 2004.

Kraemer, W.J., et al.: Cortisol supplementation reduces serum cortisol responses to physical stress. *Metabolism*, 54:657, 2005.

Kraemer, W.J., et al.: Influence of muscle strength and total work on exercise-induced plasma growth hormone isoforms in women. *J. Sci. Med. Sport*, 6:295, 2003.

Kraemer, W.J., Ratamess, N.A.: Hormonal responses and adaptations to resistance exercise and training. *Sports Med.*, 35:339, 2005.

Kriska, A.M., et al.: Physical activity and the prevention of type II diabetes. *Curr. Sports Med. Rep.*, 7:182, 2008.

Lane, A.R., et al.: Influence of dietary carbohydrate intake on the free testosterone: cortisol ratio responses to short-term intensive exercise training. *Eur. J. Appl. Physiol.*, 108:1125, 2010.

Lakka, T.M., et al.: Sedentary lifestyle, poor cardiorespiratory fitness, and the metabolic syndrome. *Med. Sci. Sports Exerc.*, 35:1279, 2003.

Malecki, M.T.: Genetics of type 2 diabetes mellitus. *Diabetes Res. Clin. Pract.*, 68(Suppl 1):S10, 2005.

Marliss, E.B., et al.: Gender differences in glucoregulatory responses to intense exercise. *J. Appl. Physiol.*, 88:457, 2000.

Mârtins, A.S., et al.: Hypertension and exercise training differentially affect oxytocin and oxytocin receptor expression in the brain. *Hypertension.*, 46:1004, 2005.

Mäestu, J., et al.: Anabolic and catabolic hormones and energy balance of the male bodybuilders during the preparation for the competition. *J. Strength Cond. Res.*, 24:1074, 2010.

Michelini, L.C.: Oxytocin in the NTS. A new modulator of cardiovascular control during exercise. *Ann. N.Y. Acad. Sci.* 940:206, 2001.

Mikulski, T., et al.: Metabolic and hormonal responses to body carbohydrate store depletion followed by high or low carbohydrate meal in sedentary and physically active subjects. *J. Physiol Pharmacol.*, 61:193, 2010.

McMurray, R.G., Hackney, A.C.: Interactions of metabolic hormones, adipose tissue and exercise. *Sports Med.*, 35:393, 2005.

Neville, V., et al.: Salivary IgA as a risk factor for upper respiratory infections in elite professional athletes. *Med. Sci. Sports Exerc.*, 40:1228, 2008.

Nieman, D.C., et al.: Influence of carbohydrate ingestion on immune changes after 2 h of intensive resistance training. *J. Appl. Physiol.*, 96:1293, 2004.

Peres, S.B., et al.: Endurance exercise training increases insulin responsiveness in isolated adipocytes through IRS/PI3-kinase/Akt pathway. *J. Appl. Physiol.*, 98:1037, 2005.

Permutt, M.A., et al.: Genetic epidemiology of diabetes. *J. Clin. Invest.*, 115:1431, 2005.

Ponjee, G.A.E., et al.: Androgen turnover during marathon running. *Med. Sci. Sports Exerc.*, 26:1274, 1994.

Praet, S.E., van Loon, L.J.: Optimizing the therapeutic benefits of exercise in Type 2 diabetes. *J. Appl. Physiol.*, 103:1113, 2007.

Rahimi, R., et al.: Effects of very short rest periods on hormonal responses to resistance exercise in men. *J. Strength Cond. Res.*, 24:1851, 2010.

Ratamess, N.A., et al.: Androgen receptor content following heavy resistance exercise in men. *J. Steroid Biochem. Mol. Biol.*, 93:35, 2005.

Roberts, C.K., Barnard, R.J.: Effects of exercise and diet on chronic disease. *J. Appl. Physiol.*, 98:3, 2005.

Rubin, M.R., et al.: High-affinity growth hormone binding protein and acute heavy resistance exercise. *Med. Sci. Sports Exerc.*, 37:395, 2005.

Seo, D.I., et al.: 12 weeks of combined exercise is better than aerobic exercise for increasing growth hormone in middle-aged women. *Int. J. Sport Nutr. Exerc. Metab.*, 20:21, 2010.

Scharhag, J., et al.: Effects of graded carbohydrate supplementation on the immune response in cycling. *Med. Sci. Sports Exerc.*, 38:286, 2006.

Sillanpää, E., et al.: Serum basal hormone concentrations, nutrition and physical fitness during strength and/or endurance training in 39–64-year-old women. *Int. J. Sports Med.*, 31:110, 2010.

Storer, T.W., et al.: Testosterone dose-dependently increases maximal voluntary strength and leg power, but does not affect fatigability or specific tension. *J. Clin. Endocrinol. Metab.*, 88:1478, 2003.

Teran-Garcia, M., et al.: Endurance training-induced changes in insulin sensitivity and gene expression. *Am. J. Physiol. Endocrinol. Metab.*, 288:E1168, 2005.

Tremblay, M.S., et al.: Effect of training status and exercise mode on endogenous steroid hormones in men. *J. Appl. Physiol.*, 96:531, 2004.

Vaananen, I., et al.: Hormonal responses to 100 km cross-country skiing during 2 days. *J. Sports Med. Phys. Fitness*, 44:309, 2004.

Volek, J.S.: Influence of nutrition on responses to resistance training. *Med. Sci. Sports. Exerc.*, 36:689, 2004.

Weinstein, A.R., Sesso, H.D.: Joint effects of physical activity and body weight on diabetes and cardiovascular disease. *Exerc. Sport Sci. Rev.*, 34:10, 2006.

Weiss, E.P., et al.: Endurance training-induced changes in the insulin response to oral glucose are associated with the peroxisome proliferator-activated receptor-gamma2 Pro12Ala genotype in men but not in women. *Metabolism*, 54:97, 2005.

Weltman, A., et al.: Effects of continuous versus intermittent exercise, obesity, and gender on growth hormone secretion. *J. Clin. Endocrinol. Metab.*, 93:4711, 2008.

Wesche, M.F., Wiersinga, W.M.: Relation between lean body mass and thyroid volume in competition rowers before and during intensive physical training. *Horm. Metab. Res.*, 33:423, 2001.

Wideman, L., et al.: The impact of sex and exercise duration on growth hormone secretion. *J. Appl. Physiol.*, 101:1641, 2006.

Williams, P.T. Reduced diabetic, hypertensive, and cholesterol medication use with walking. *Med. Sci. Sports Exerc.*, 40:433, 2008.

Yang, X., et al.: The longitudinal effects of physical activity history on metabolic syndrome. *Med. Sci. Sports Exerc.*, 40:1424, 2008.

Exercise Training and Adaptations

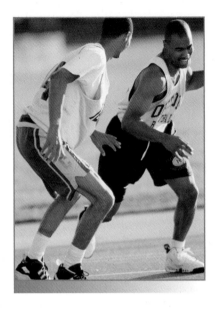

Training for sports often entails more art than science. Individual achievements or win–loss records rather than scientific inquiry and discovery frequently gauge the success of diverse conditioning programs. For example, basketball and soccer coaches frequently place considerable importance on developing aerobic capacity yet may not devote enough time to vigorous anaerobic training. These sports require a relatively steady release of aerobic energy, yet crucial game situations frequently demand maximal effort. A poorly trained anaerobic energy transfer system can prevent a player from performing at full potential.

Training the anaerobic capacity of endurance athletes, on the other hand, proves wasteful because of the minimal contribution of anaerobic energy transfer to successful performance. Instead, endurance activities demand a highly conditioned heart and vascular system capable of delivering large quantities of blood to specifically trained muscles with a high capacity to generate adenosine triphosphate aerobically. At the other extreme, one's aerobic metabolic capacity contributes little to overall success in sprint activities and sports such as football. In these sports, performance largely depends on muscular strength and power, which require energy generated in reactions *without* oxygen.

Developing a training program to achieve optimum exercise and sports performance requires a clear understanding of energy transfer and how specific training affects energy delivery and utilization systems.

Chapters 13 and 14 focus on training for aerobic and anaerobic power and muscular strength, the physiologic consequences of such training, and important factors that affect training success. Chapter 15 examines how different environmental conditions and special aids affect physiologic function and exercise performance.

The test of a first-rate intelligence is the ability to hold two opposed ideas in mind at the same time and still retain the ability to function.

— F. Scott Fitzgerald

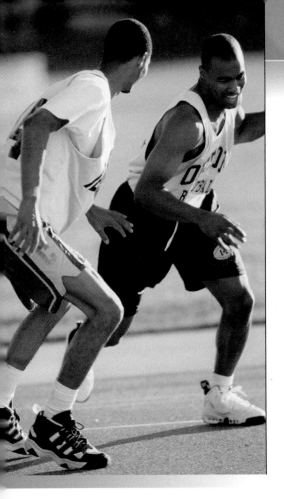

THE HENLEY COLLEGE LIBRARY

Chapter

13

Training the Anaerobic and Aerobic Energy Systems

CHAPTER OBJECTIVES

- Define each of the following four principles of exercise training: *overload*, *specificity*, *individual differences*, and *reversibility*.

- Discuss the overload principle for training the intramuscular high-energy phosphates and glycolytic systems. Outline the specific adaptations in each system with exercise training.

- Describe how the following five factors affect an aerobic training program: initial fitness level, genetics, training frequency, training duration, and training intensity.

- List five cardiovascular and pulmonary adaptations to aerobic training.

- Explain how exercise heart rate can establish the appropriate exercise intensity for aerobic training.

- Define the *training-sensitive zone*.

- Outline a typical exercise training session for aerobic fitness improvement.

- Explain the need to adjust the training-sensitive zone for swimming and other modes of upper-body exercise.

- Explain the influence of age on maximum heart rate and the training-sensitive zone.

- Contrast continuous versus intermittent aerobic exercise training, including advantages and disadvantages of each.

- Outline five potential benefits and risks of exercising during pregnancy.

TRAINING MUST FOCUS ON ENERGY REQUIREMENTS

Many forms of physical activity require rapid bursts of power during which energy requirements far exceed the body's oxygen delivery capacity. Even with available oxygen, cellular energy transfer from aerobic reactions progresses too slowly to match energy demands. This means that rapid anaerobic energy transfer capacity determines how fast a running back plows through the line in American football, a volleyball player spikes the ball over the net, and a softball player beats out an infield hit. Even longer duration basketball, tennis, field hockey, lacrosse, ice hockey, and soccer involve sprinting, dashing, darting, and stop-and-go movements, during which the capacity to generate short bursts of anaerobic power plays an important role.

At the other extreme, success in endurance activities necessitates a highly trained aerobic energy system. This requires a cardiovascular system capable of delivering large quantities of blood to active tissues for an extended time and a musculature with high capacity to process oxygen for the aerobic resynthesis of adenosine triphosphate (ATP).

ENERGY FOR EXERCISE: KNOWING WHAT TO TRAIN FOR

Stimulating structural and functional adaptations to improve performance in specific physical tasks remains a major objective of exercise training. Training for a particular sport or performance goal requires careful evaluation of the activity's energy components. This forms the basis to effectively select the appropriate energy transfer system to achieve specific training objectives.

Recall that three energy systems (ATP–phosphocreatine [PCr] system, lactic acid [glycolytic] system, and aerobic system) operate concurrently. Their contributions to total energy requirement can differ markedly depending on exercise duration and intensity, including the participant's fitness level.

A maximum burst of effort for a tennis serve, golf swing, front flip in gymnastics, and even a 60- or 100-m sprint requires immediate energy transfer. This occurs anaerobically, almost exclusively from the intramuscular high-energy phosphates ATP and PCr. In performances lasting up to 90 seconds in duration (e.g., 100-m swim or 440-m run), anaerobic energy transfer reactions still predominate. In this case, the initial glycolytic phase of carbohydrate breakdown with subsequent lactate formation provides the primary energy source. One's capacity and tolerance for lactate accumulation determine the magnitude of energy generated from anaerobic sources. Training for anaerobic-type activities must reach sufficient intensity and duration to overload the glycolytic energy transfer system.

Wrestling, boxing, ice hockey, a 200-m swim, a 1500-m run, or a full-court press in basketball all require rapid anaerobic energy transfer, with important contributions from aerobic energy metabolism. As exercise intensity diminishes somewhat and duration extends between 2 to 4 minutes, reliance on energy from anaerobic metabolism decreases, but energy release from oxygen-consuming reactions predominates. Beyond 4 minutes, exercise becomes progressively more dependent on aerobic metabolism; energy from aerobic reactions almost exclusively powers a marathon run, long-distance swim, and 25-mile continuous bicycle ride.

GENERAL TRAINING PRINCIPLES

Effective physiologic conditioning requires adherence to carefully planned and executed physical activity. Attention focuses on appropriate competition and the frequency and length of workouts, type of training, and the speed, intensity, duration, and repetition of the activity. These factors vary depending on the performance goal. Several general principles of physiologic conditioning underlie performance classifications based on intensity and duration of activity shown in **Figure 13.1**. *The basic approach to physiologic conditioning applies similarly to men and women within a broad age range—both respond and adapt to training in essentially the same way.*

Overload Principle

The regular application of a specific **exercise overload** enhances physiologic function to produce a training response. Exercising at intensities greater than normal induces a variety of highly specific adaptations that enable the body to function more efficiently. Achieving the appropriate overload requires manipulating combinations of training frequency, intensity, and duration, with focus on exercise mode. We discuss these factors later in this chapter.

The concept of overload applies to the athlete, sedentary, disabled, and even cardiac patient. An increasing number of people in the latter group have applied appropriate exercise rehabilitation to walk, jog, and eventually participate in marathons and ultraendurance events.

Specificity Principle

Exercise training specificity refers to adaptations in metabolic and physiologic systems that depend on the type of overload imposed and muscle mass activated. In a broad sense, an exercise stress as strength-power training develops specific strength-power adaptations; likewise, regular aerobic exercise elicits specific endurance-training adaptations with essentially no transfer effects between strength-power training and aerobic training. The specificity principle also encompasses activities with *identical* metabolic components. For example, aerobic fitness for swimming, bicycling, running, or rowing improves most effectively when the exerciser trains the specific muscles

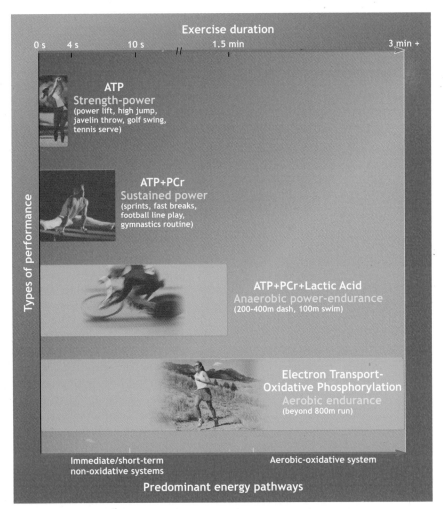

Figure 13.1 Classification of physical activity based on duration of all-out exercise and corresponding predominant intracellular energy pathways.

required for the activity. In essence, specific exercise elicits specific adaptations, creating specific training effects referred to as the **SAID principle**—**specific adaptations to imposed demands**.

Individual Differences Principle

All individuals do not respond similarly to a given training stimulus. Many factors contribute to variations in training responses among individuals, including relative fitness level at the start of training. People vary in initial fitness and state of training at the start of a conditioning program and thus respond differently to the same training stimulus. Insisting that all performers on a team or even those in the same event train the same way and at the same relative or absolute exercise intensity does not optimize training because it does not recognize **individual differences** in training responsiveness. Rather, training programs must meet individual needs and capacities. Coaches and trainers should recognize how athletes and trainees respond to a given exercise stimulus and adjust the exercise prescription based on that response.

Reversibility Principle

The **reversibility** of training effects, referred to as detraining, occurs relatively rapidly when a person quits his or her exercise training regimen. After only a week or two of detraining, measurable reductions occur in physiologic function and exercise capacity, with a total loss of training improvements occurring within several months. **Figure 13.2** shows average percentage change reported

Questions & Notes

Give an example of a sporting event or physical activity that relies on each of the 3 energy systems.

ATP-PCr system:

Glycolytic system:

Aerobic system:

List the 4 training principles.

1.

2.

3.

4

List 4 variables for manipulation to achieve exercise overload.

1.

2.

3.

4.

Give one example of exercise training specificity.

BOX 13.1 CLOSE UP

An Example of Exercise Training Specificity

In an experiment in one of our laboratories on aerobic training specificity, 15 men swam 1 hour a day 3 days a week for 10 weeks at heart rates between 85% and 95% of maximum heart rate (HR_{max}). $\dot{V}O_{2max}$ was measured during treadmill running and tethered swimming before and after training. Because vigorous swim training overloads the central circulation (as reflected by high exercise heart rates), we anticipated at least some transfer in aerobic power improvements from swim training to running. This did not occur; an almost total specificity accompanied the $\dot{V}O_{2max}$ improvement with swim training.

The accompanying figure illustrates that swim training improved $\dot{V}O_{2max}$ by 11% when measured during swimming but only by 1.5% when measured during run-

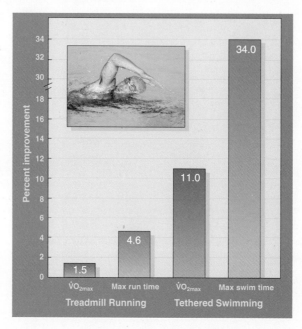

ning. If only treadmill running had been used to evaluate swim training effects, we would mistakenly have concluded that there was *no training effect*. For maximum performance during testing, subjects improved 34% in swim time to exhaustion but only 4.6% in run time on the treadmill test.

These findings and other research studies strongly indicate that training for specific aerobic activities must provide an appropriate general level of cardiovascular stress *and* overload the *specific muscles* required by the activity. Little improvement results when a dissimilar exercise measures aerobic capacity or exercise performance. In contrast, considerable improvements emerge when the exercise training mode evaluates aerobic adaptations.

---

from several studies for the decrease in physiologic and metabolic variables with detraining including bed rest.

In one experiment, $\dot{V}O_{2max}$ decreased 25% in five subjects confined to bed for 20 consecutive days; a similar decrease in maximal stroke volume and cardiac output accompanied the loss of aerobic capacity (~1% per day). Capillary number within trained muscle also decreased 14% to 25% over the detraining period.

The above results clearly highlight the transient and reversible nature of exercise training improvements, even among high-performance athletes. For this reason, athletes typically begin a reconditioning program several months before the start of the competitive season, or they maintain some moderate level of off-season, sport-specific exercise to slow down the rate of deconditioning.

ADAPTATIONS TO EXERCISE TRAINING

Individual differences in improvement generally represent the rule rather than the exception, particularly among children and older adults. Among individuals in the same exercise-training program, one person might show 10 times more improvement than another. Such variation in results is common; simply stated—some individuals respond more readily than do others to an identical training stimulus.

The concept of **responders** and **nonresponders** emerged from training data collected on identical twins. For example, in one study, 10 pairs of identical twins separated at birth and reared in different environments completed the same 20-week endurance-training program. The results showed a strong genetic component for improvements in cardiovascular and metabolic variables. Both members of the twin pair showed nearly the same training response; a large improvement in one twin mirrored similar improvement in the other and vice versa. In the mid-1960s, the renowned Swedish physiologist Dr. Per-Olof Åstrand (Chapter 1) prophetically commented concerning the yet to be quantified role of genetics in exercise performance: "To be an Olympic-caliber performer, you must choose your parents wisely." Future research in molecular genetics may someday uncover a practical means to identify responders and nonresponders and individualize conditioning programs to optimize overall improvements for each.

Anaerobic System Changes

Figure 13.3 presents a generalized summary of the metabolic adaptations in anaerobic function that accompany strenuous physical training that requires considerable overload of the anaerobic energy transfer systems. Changes in anaerobic power and capacity occur *without* concomitant increases in aerobic functions. Adaptations with sprint-power training include:

1. *Increased levels of anaerobic substrates.* Muscle biopsies taken before and after resistance training reveal increases in the trained muscle's resting levels of ATP, PCr, free creatine, and glycogen, accompanied by an improvement in muscular strength. Other studies show higher levels of ATP and total creatine content in the trained muscles of sprint runners and track speed cyclists compared with distance runners and road racers.

2. *Increased quantity and activity of key enzymes that control the anaerobic phase of glucose catabolism.* The most dramatic increases in anaerobic enzyme function and fiber size occur in fast-twitch muscle fibers. These changes do not reach the magnitude observed for oxidative enzymes with aerobic training.

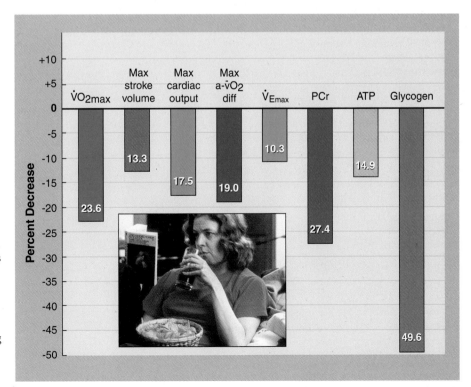

Figure 13.2 Average changes in physiologic and metabolic variables with different durations of detraining. Based on data from six studies. Values are as follows: $\dot{V}O_{2max}$ in $L \cdot min^{-1}$; stroke volume in $mL \cdot b^{-1}$; cardiac output in $L \cdot min^{-1}$; $a\text{-}\bar{v}O_2$ diff = arteriovenous oxygen differences in $mL \cdot dL^{-1}$; $\dot{V}_{Emax}$ = maximum minute ventilation in $L \cdot min^{-1}$; PCr in $mmol \cdot g$ wet muscle^{-1}; ATP in $mmol \cdot g$ wet muscle^{-1}; and glycogen in $mmol \cdot g$ wet muscle^{-1}.

*Q*uestions & Notes

Describe the individual difference principle.

Describe the reversibility principle.

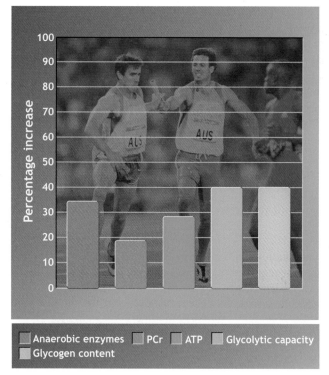

Anaerobic enzymes ☐ PCr ☐ ATP ☐ Glycolytic capacity
☐ Glycogen content

Figure 13.3 Generalized potential for increases in anaerobic energy metabolism of skeletal muscle with intense training.

3. *Increased capacity to generate high levels of blood lactate during all-out exercise.* Enhanced lactate-producing capacity probably results from a training-induced increased levels of glycogen and glycolytic enzymes and improved motivation and "pain" tolerance to fatiguing exercise.

Improved Buffering Capacity? Individuals who engage in anaerobic training tolerate higher blood lactate levels and lower pH values than untrained counterparts. This raises speculation that anaerobic training improves the body's capacity for acid–base regulation, perhaps by enhancing chemical buffers or alkaline reserve. Research has yet to demonstrate that exercise training augments buffering capacity. Motivational factors probably improve training-induced tolerance to elevated plasma acidity.

Aerobic System Changes

Table 13.1 summarizes important metabolic and physiologic differences when comparing typical values of healthy untrained individuals and endurance athletes. Aerobic adaptations to training generally occur independent of gender and age. They also take place in medically cleared individuals with cancer, coronary heart disease, diabetes, hypertension, and obstructive pulmonary disease (see Chapter 17).

Table 13.1	**Typical Metabolic and Physiologic Values for Healthy Endurance-Trained and Untrained Men[a]**		
VARIABLE	**UNTRAINED**	**TRAINED**	**PERCENTAGE DIFFERENCE[b]**
Glycogen, mmol·g wet muscle^{-1}	85.0	120	41
Number of mitochondria, mmol^3	0.59	11.20	103
Mitochondrial volume, % muscle cell	2.15	8.00	272
Resting ATP, mmol·g wet muscle^{-1}	3.0	6.0	100
Resting PCr, mmol·g wet muscle^{-1}	11.0	18.0	64
Resting creatine, mmol·g wet muscle^{-1}	10.7	14.5	35
Glycolytic enzymes			
Phosphofructokinase, mmol·g wet muscle^{-1}	50.0	50.0	0
Phosphorylase, mmol·g wet muscle^{-1}	4–6	6–9	60
Aerobic enzymes			
Succinate dehydrogenase, mmol·kg wet muscle^{-1}	5–10	15–20	133
Max lactate, mmol·kg wet muscle^{-1}	110	150	36
Muscle fibers			
Fast twitch, %	50	20–30	−50
Slow twitch, %	50	60	20
Max stroke volume, mL·b^{-1}	120	180	50
Max cardiac output, L·min^{-1}	20	30–40	75
Resting heart rate, b·min^{-1}	70	40	−43
HR$_{max}$, b·mm^{-1}	190	180	−5
Max a-$\bar{v}O_2$ diff, mL·100 mL^{-1}	14.5	16.0	10
$\dot{V}O_{2max}$, mL·kg^{-1}·min^{-1}	30–40	65–80	107
Heart volume, L	7.5	9.5	27
Blood volume, L	4.7	6.0	28
$\dot{V}_{Emax}$, L·min^{-1}	110	190	73
Percent body fat, %	15	11	−27

[a]In some cases, we list approximate values. In all cases, the trained values represent data from endurance athletes. We advise caution in assuming that the percentage differences between trained and untrained men necessarily result from training because genetic differences between individuals probably exert a strong influence on many of these factors.
[b]Computed as the percentage that the value for the trained differs from the corresponding value for the untrained.

Metabolic Adaptations   Aerobic exercise training induces intracellular changes that enhance a muscle fiber's capacity to aerobically generate ATP.

Metabolic Machinery   An increase in mitochondrial size and number in aerobically trained skeletal muscle improves its capacity to generate ATP by oxidative phosphorylation.

Enzymes   A twofold increase in the level of aerobic system enzymes complements the increase in mitochondrial size and number and coincides with increased mitochondrial capacity to generate ATP. These adaptations likely allow the trained person to sustain a high percentage of aerobic capacity during prolonged exercise without accumulating blood lactate (i.e., achieve a higher blood lactate threshold [LT]).

Fat Catabolism   Regular aerobic exercise profoundly improves ability to oxidize fatty acids, particularly triacylglycerols stored within active muscle during steady-rate exercise (**Fig. 13.4**). Lipolysis increases from greater blood flow within trained muscle and a higher quantity of fat-mobilizing enzymes from adipocytes and fat-metabolizing within muscle fibers enzymes. This allows the endurance athlete to exercise at a higher absolute level of submaximal exercise before experiencing the fatiguing effects of glycogen depletion compared with an untrained person.

Carbohydrate Catabolism   Aerobically trained muscle exhibits an enhanced capacity to oxidize carbohydrate. Consequently, a considerable quantity of pyruvate moves through the aerobic energy pathways during intense endurance exercise. A trained muscle's greater mitochondrial oxidative capacity and increased glycogen storage contribute to the enhanced capacity for carbohydrate breakdown. Increased carbohydrate catabolism during intense aerobic exercise serves two important functions:

1. Provides a considerably faster aerobic energy transfer than from fat breakdown
2. Liberates about 6% more energy than fat per quantity of oxygen consumed

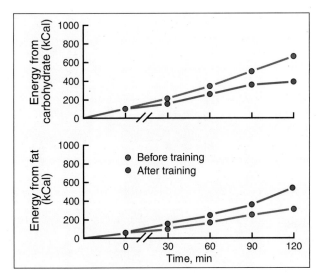

Figure 13.4   Training enhances fat burning during submaximal exercise. This carbohydrate-sparing results from a facilitated release of fatty acids from adipose tissue depots, an increased intramuscular fat content, and enhanced mitochondrial fat oxidation capacity in endurance-trained muscle. (Data from Hurley, B.F., et al.: Muscle triglyceride utilization during exercise: Effect of training. *J. Appl. Physiol.*, 60:562, 1986.)

Questions & Notes

List 5 specific metabolic adaptations to aerobic training.

1.

2.

3.

4.

5.

Explain the advantage for endurance performance of training induced increased Lipolysis.

Give 2 reasons why endurance training reduces total carbohydrate catabolism during submaximal exercise.

1.

2.

For Your Information

IMPORTANT CONTRIBUTORS TO AEROBIC EFFECTS

Endurance training causes the heart's stroke volume to *increase* during rest and exercise regardless of age or gender. Four factors produce this change:

1. Increased internal left ventricular volume consequent to the training-induced plasma volume expansion and mass
2. Reduced stiffness in coronary and other major arterial blood vessels
3. Increased diastolic filling time (from training-induced bradycardia)
4. Possibly improved intrinsic cardiac contractile function

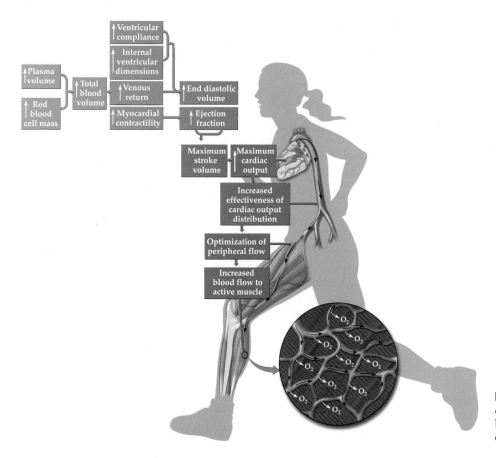

Figure 13.5 Adaptations in cardiovascular function with aerobic exercise training that increase oxygen delivery to active muscles.

Muscle Fiber Type and Size Endurance training produces aerobic metabolic adaptations in *both* muscle fiber types. This enhances each fiber's existing aerobic capacity and LT level without modifying the muscle fiber type. Selective hypertrophy also occurs in different muscle fiber types in specific overload training. Highly trained endurance athletes have larger slow- than fast-twitch fibers in the same muscle. Conversely, for athletes trained in anaerobic-power activities, fast-twitch fibers occupy more of the muscles' cross-sectional area. As might be expected, slow-twitch muscle fibers with high capacity to generate ATP aerobically contain relatively large quantities of the iron-containing globular protein myoglobin, which facilitates oxygen transfer to mitochondria.

Cardiovascular Adaptations **Figure 13.5** summarizes important adaptations in cardiovascular function with aerobic exercise training. Such training produces dimensional and functional cardiovascular adaptations because of the intimate linkage of the cardiovascular system to aerobic processes.

Heart Size Long-term aerobic training generally increases the heart's mass and volume with greater left ventricular end-diastolic volumes during rest and exercise. This enlargement, characterized by increased size of the left ventricular cavity (**eccentric hypertrophy**) and modest thickening of its walls (**concentric hypertrophy**), improves the heart's stroke volume. With reduced training intensity, or when training ceases, myocardial structure returns to control levels.

Myocardial overload stimulates greater cellular protein synthesis, with concomitant reductions in protein breakdown. Accelerated protein synthesis occurs largely from an increase in the trained myocardium's RNA content. Individual myofibrils thicken, and the number of these

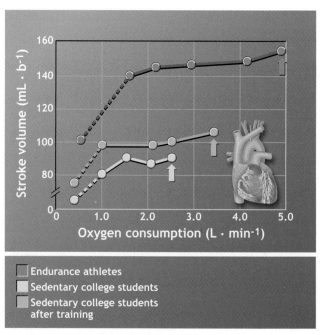

Figure 13.6 Typical response for stroke volume in relation to oxygen uptake during upright exercise in endurance athletes and sedentary adults before and after 2 months of aerobic training (*arrows* indicate maximal values).

contractile filaments concurrently increases.

Plasma Volume Only four training sessions increase plasma volume up to 20%. This adaptation enhances circulatory and thermoregulatory dynamics and facilitates oxygen delivery to muscle during exercise. The rapid increase in plasma volume with aerobic training also contributes to training-induced eccentric hypertrophy with concomitant increases in stroke volume.

Stroke Volume **Figure 13.6** illustrates the typical stroke volume response for two groups of men during upright exercise of increasing intensity. One group of endurance athletes trained for several years; sedentary, healthy adults comprised the other group. Graded treadmill exercise evaluated the sedentary adults' responses before and after a 2-month training program to improve aerobic fitness.

These data reveal important (and representative) findings concerning aerobic training adaptations:

1. An endurance athlete's heart has a considerably larger stroke volume at rest and during exercise than an untrained person of similar age.
2. For trained and untrained individuals, the greatest increase in stroke volume in upright exercise occurs in the transition from rest to moderate exercise. Further increases in exercise intensity increase stroke volume only minimally.
3. The heart's stroke volume achieves near-maximum values at 40% to 50% of $\dot{V}O_{2max}$; in young adults, this usually represents a heart rate between 120 and 140 bpm.
4. For untrained individuals, only a small stroke volume increase occurs in the transition from rest to exercise. For them, acceleration in heart rate produces the major increase in cardiac output. For trained endurance athletes, *both* heart rate and stroke volume increases augment cardiac output, with stroke volume increasing 50% to 60% above resting values.

For Your Information

THE ALASKAN SLED DOG: A PHYSIOLOGIC CHALLENGE TO HUMAN EXERCISE CAPACITY

Prime candidates for the greatest athletes of any species in any sport with sheer capacity for prolonged exercise are multibreed dogs with a little Siberian husky in the mix—the dogs who pull sleds in the Iditarod race across Alaska. Consider the following:

- A $\dot{V}O_{2max}$ of about 200 mL·kg^{-1}·min^{-1} compared to the value of a highly trained human challenger of 80 mL·kg^{-1}·min^{-1}.
- Ability to run up to 100 miles a day at 50% of $\dot{V}O_{2max}$ for 8 consecutive days.
- Ability to maintain a sub-4-minute mile pace for up to 70 miles as part of a team of dogs pulling a sled.
- Ability to maintain relatively large blood flow to vital organs such as the gastrointestinal tract and splanchnic (liver) region while performing intense endurance exercise.
- Response to just several months of regular exercise with a 50% increase heart size.
- Muscle cells that possess nearly 70% more mitochondria than do humans.
- Ability to dissipate metabolic heat through the tongue, paws, and nose without relying on evaporative cooling via the sweat mechanism, thus conserving fluid and vital electrolytes.
- Superb fat-burning "machines" with predominant reliance on cooler burning, energy-dense fat as an energy substrate source compared with the heavy reliance of humans on the limited supply of blood glucose and stored glycogen.

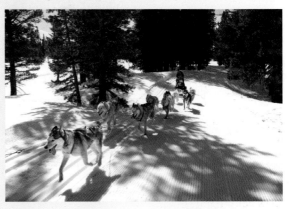

References

McKenzie, E., et al.: Recovery of muscle glycogen concentrations in sled dogs during prolonged exercise. *Med Sci Sports Exer.*, 37:1307, 2005.

McKenzie, E., et al.: Hypogammaglobulinemia in racing Alaskan sled dogs. *J. Vet. Intern. Med.*, 24:97, 2010.

For Your Information

SIX POTENTIAL PSYCHOLOGIC BENEFITS FROM REGULAR EXERCISE

1. Reduced state of anxiety (i.e., the level of anxiety at the time of measurement)
2. Decreased mild to moderate depression
3. Reduced neuroticism (long-term exercise effect)
4. Adjunct to professional treatment of severe depression
5. Improvement in mood, self-esteem, and self-concept
6. Reduction in various indices of stress

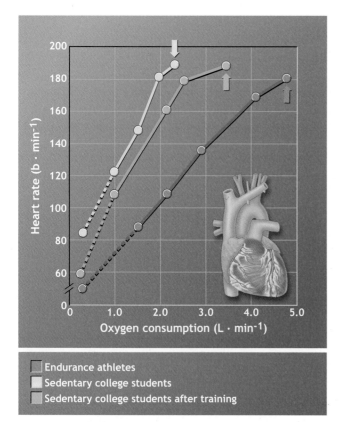

☐ Endurance athletes
■ Sedentary college students
■ Sedentary college students after training

Figure 13.7 Typical response for heart rate in relation to oxygen uptake during upright exercise in endurance athletes and sedentary adults before and after 2 months of aerobic training; (*arrows* indicate maximal values).

5. For previously sedentary subjects, 2 months of aerobic training substantially increases stroke volume, but these values remain well below the average of elite athletes. The precise reason for this difference remains unknown. More than likely, prolonged intense training, genetics, or a combination of both factors contributes to the differences.

Heart Rate   A proportionate reduction in heart rate during submaximal exercise accompanies the large stroke volume of elite endurance athletes and stroke volume increase of sedentary individuals with aerobic training. **Figure 13.7** illustrates this training effect for the relationship between heart rate and oxygen uptake for endurance athletes and sedentary adults before and after training.

A linear relationship between heart rate and oxygen uptake exists for both groups throughout the major portion of the exercise range. As exercise intensity increases, the heart rates of the athletes accelerate to a lesser extent than untrained adults; the *slope* or rate of change in the lines differ considerably. Consequently, the athlete (or trained adult) with an efficient cardiovascular response to exercise achieves a higher oxygen uptake before reaching a particular submaximal heart rate than a sedentary adult. At an oxygen uptake of 2.0 L·min^{-1}, the athletes' heart rate averages 70 b·min^{-1} lower than the heart rate of the sedentary counterparts. After the sedentary adults trained for 2 months, the

difference in submaximal heart rate decreases to 40 b·min^{-1}. In each instance, cardiac output remains about the same. This means that larger stroke volumes account for the lower exercise heart rates. If the heart pumps a large quantity of blood with each beat, then adequate delivery of blood (oxygen) to the active muscles requires only a small heart rate increase and vice versa for a heart with a relatively small stroke volume.

Cardiac Output   *An increase in maximum cardiac output represents the most significant change in cardiovascular function with aerobic training* (**Fig. 13.8**). Maximum heart rate may decrease slightly with training, so the heart's increased outflow capacity results directly from the heart's improved stroke volume.

Aerobic training, while improving the maximal cardiac output, reduces the heart's minute volume during moderate exercise. In one study, the average cardiac output of young men after 16 weeks of aerobic training decreased 1.1 and 1.5 L·min^{-1} at a specific submaximal oxygen consumption. As expected, maximal cardiac output increased 8% from 22.4 to 24.2 L·min^{-1}. With reduced submaximal cardiac output, a corresponding increase in oxygen extraction in the active muscles (increased a-$\bar{v}O_2$ difference) matches the exercise oxygen requirement. A training-induced reduction in submaximal cardiac output reflects two factors:

1. More effective distribution of blood flow
2. Trained muscles' increased capacity to generate ATP aerobically at a lower tissue PO_2

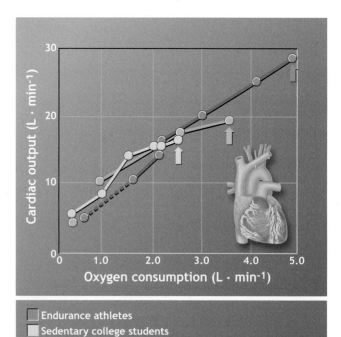

☐ Endurance athletes
■ Sedentary college students
■ Sedentary college students after training

Figure 13.8 Typical response for cardiac output to oxygen uptake during upright exercise in endurance athletes and sedentary adults before and after 2 months of aerobic training (*arrows* indicate maximal values).

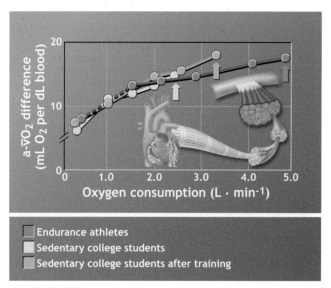

Figure 13.9 Typical response for a-v̄O₂ difference to oxygen uptake during upright exercise in endurance athletes and sedentary adults and after 2 months of aerobic training (*arrows* indicate maximal values).

Oxygen Extraction Aerobic training increases the maximum quantity of oxygen extracted from arterial blood during exercise. A more effective distribution of cardiac output to working muscles and enhanced capacity of muscle fibers to metabolize oxygen produce the increase in a-v̄O₂ difference.

Figure 13.9 compares the relationship between oxygen extraction and exercise intensity for trained athletes and untrained adults. For adults, the a-v̄O₂ difference increases steadily during light and moderate exercise to a maximum of 15 mL of oxygen per dL of blood. After 55 days of training, the adults' maximum oxygen extraction increased 13% to 17 mL of oxygen per dL. This means that during intense exercise, arterial blood released approximately 85% of its oxygen content. Actually, the active muscles extract even more oxygen because the a-v̄O₂ difference reflects an average based on sampling of mixed-venous blood. This sample contains blood returning from tissues that use much less oxygen during exercise than active muscle (e.g., skin, kidneys, non-active musculature). The posttraining value for maximal a-v̄O₂ difference for the previously untrained adults equals the value of the endurance athletes. Obviously, the adults' lower cardiac output capacity explains the large difference in V̇O₂max that still differentiates athletes and lesser trained counterparts (see **Fig. 13.8**).

ⓘ For Your Information

PROLONGED RECOVERY

Considerable recovery time occurs with intense exercise that elevates core temperature, disrupts internal equilibrium, and elevates blood lactate. For this reason, intervals of anaerobic training should be applied at the end of a workout. Otherwise, fatigue from training carries over and perhaps hinders the ability to perform subsequent aerobic training.

ⓘ For Your Information

10,000 STEPS A DAY: A PRACTICAL GOAL FOR SEDENTARY AMERICANS

Walking represents "big muscle" low-impact physical activity performed with minimal equipment and at little expense. The typical American achieves between 1000 and 3000 steps daily. A walking goal of 10,000 steps a day—the approximate equivalent of walking 5 miles—falls in line with most recommendations for physical activity to reduce disease risk and capture the benefits of a healthier lifestyle. Commercially available pedometers easily monitor and log daily steps. Positive feedback provides motivation to continue with the walking program. For an added fitness bonus, intersperse regular walking pace with 2- to 3-minute intervals of more brisk walking at a pace the participant rates as feeling "somewhat hard." For a walking program targeted toward weight loss, gradually increasing walking speed and number of daily steps to the 15,000-step range provides the necessary additional calorie-burning effects.

𝒬uestions & Notes

Explain the most significant change in cardiovascular function with aerobic training.

Does oxygen extraction increase or decrease during maximal exercise after aerobic training?

| Table 13.2 | Measures of Blood Pressure During Rest and Submaximal Exercise Before and After 4 to 6 Weeks of Aerobic Training in Seven Middle-Aged Patients with Coronary Heart Disease[a] | | | | | |

| | REST | | | SUBMAXIMAL EXERCISE | | |
| | MEAN VALUE | | DIFFERENCE (%) | MEAN VALUE | | DIFFERENCE (%) |
MEASURE[b]	BEFORE	AFTER		BEFORE	AFTER	
Systolic blood pressure (mm Hg)	139	133	−4.3	173	155	−10.4
Diastolic blood pressure (mm Hg)	78	73	−6.4	92	79	−14.1
Mean arterial blood pressure (mm Hg)	97	92	−5.2	127	109	−14.3

[a] Modified from Clausen, J.P., et al.: Physical training in the management of coronary artery disease. *Circulation*, 40:143, 1969.
[b] Blood pressure measured directly by a pressure transducer inserted into the brachial artery.

Blood Flow and Distribution Three factors explain why aerobic training causes large increases in muscle blood flow during maximal exercise:

1. Improvements in maximum cardiac output
2. Redistribution (shunting) of blood from non-active areas that temporarily compromise blood flow in all-out exercise effort
3. Increased capillarization within the trained muscle tissues

Blood Pressure Aerobic exercise training decreases systolic and diastolic blood pressures during rest and submaximal exercise. The most apparent effect occurs for systolic pressure, particularly for hypertensive subjects. Table 13.2 shows that the average resting systolic pressure of seven middle-aged male patients decreased from 139 to 133 mm Hg after 4 to 6 weeks of interval training. Systolic pressure in submaximal exercise declined from 173 to 155 mm Hg, and diastolic pressure decreased from 92 to 79 mm Hg. *Regular aerobic exercise for previously sedentary adult men and women of all ages reduces systolic blood pressure approximately 6 to 10 mm Hg.*

A training-induced reduction in sympathetic nervous system hormones (catecholamines) contributes to the lowering effect of regular exercise on blood pressure, perhaps via a reduction in peripheral vascular resistance to blood flow. Exercise training also facilitates the kidneys' elimination of sodium, which subsequently reduces fluid volume and blood pressure. *Regular aerobic exercise represents a prudent first line of defense in most therapeutic programs to manage borderline hypertension.* More severe elevations in blood pressure require combinations of diet, weight loss, exercise, and ultimately, pharmacologic intervention.

Pulmonary Adaptations

Aerobic training induces alterations in pulmonary dynamics during exercise. Such changes contribute to a more effective ventilatory response to the stress of physical activity.

Maximal Exercise Improvements in maximal oxygen uptake with training increase maximal exercise minute ventilation. This adaptation makes sense physiologically because improved aerobic capacity reflects larger oxygen utilization and the need to eliminate greater quantities of carbon dioxide by increased alveolar ventilation.

Submaximal Exercise Exercise training improves the ability to sustain high levels of submaximal ventilation. For example, 20 weeks of regular run training increased the endurance of ventilatory muscles by 16% in healthy adult men and women. Less lactate accumulated during submaximal breathing exercise, probably from the increase in aerobic enzyme levels in the ventilatory musculature. Enhanced ventilatory endurance reduces the feeling of breathlessness and pulmonary discomfort frequently experienced by untrained persons who perform prolonged submaximal exercise.

Only 4 weeks of training considerably *reduces* the ventilatory equivalent for oxygen ($\dot{V}_E/\dot{V}O_2$) in submaximal exercise. Consequently, a particular level of submaximal oxygen uptake requires breathing less air; this reduces the percentage of the total oxygen cost of exercise attributable to breathing. Enhanced ventilatory economy contributes to endurance performance in two ways:

1. Reduces the fatiguing effects of exercise on ventilatory musculature
2. Frees oxygen from respiratory muscles for use by nonrespiratory active muscles

The precise mechanism for the reduced ventilatory equivalent during submaximal exercise after training remains unresolved. The decrease consistently occurs in adolescents and adults. In general, tidal volume increases, breathing frequency decreases, and air remains in the lungs for a longer time interval between breaths. Slower breathing increases the amount of oxygen the alveoli extracts from the inspired air volume. For example, whereas the exhaled air of trained individuals contains only 14% to 15% oxygen during submaximal exercise, an untrained person's expired air contains about 17% oxygen at the same exercise intensity. This means the untrained person must ventilate proportionately more air to achieve the same submaximal oxygen uptake.

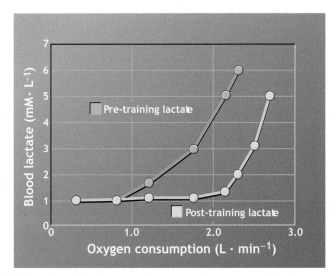

Figure 13.10 Generalized response for pre- and posttraining lactate accumulation during graded exercise. (Plots based on data from the Applied Physiology Laboratory, University of Michigan, Ann Arbor, MI.)

Blood Lactate Concentration **Figure 13.10** illustrates the generalized effect of endurance training in lowering blood lactate levels and extending exercise duration before onset of blood lactate accumulation (OBLA) during exercise of increasing intensity. The explanation underlying this effect centers on three possibilities related to central and peripheral adaptations to training discussed in this chapter:

1. Decreased rate of lactate formation during exercise
2. Increased rate of lactate clearance (removal) during exercise
3. Combined effects of decreased lactate clearance and increased lactate removal

More than likely, the combination of both factors exerts the influence.

Body Composition Changes For overfat or borderline overfat people, regular aerobic exercise reduces body mass and body fat. Increases in fat-free body mass also accompany a regular program of resistance training. Exercise only, or exercise combined with calorie restriction, reduces body fat more than fat lost with only dieting because exercise conserves the body's lean tissue mass.

Temperature Regulation Well-hydrated, aerobically trained individuals exercise more comfortably in hot environments because of a larger plasma volume and more-responsive thermoregulatory mechanisms. Trained men and women dissipate heat faster and more effectively than untrained persons. For trained individuals, the metabolic heat generated by exercise poses less of a detriment to exercise performance and overall safety.

Endurance Performance Changes Enhanced endurance accompanies the physiologic adaptations with training. **Figure 13.11** depicts the results for cycling performance after training performed 4 days per week for 40 to 60 minutes for 10 weeks at an intensity of 85% $\dot{V}O_{2max}$. The performance test required subjects to attempt to maintain a constant work rate of 265 watts for 8 minutes. Training produced less drop-off in power output during the prescribed 8-minute exercise test.

Psychologic Benefits Regular exercise, either aerobic or resistance training produces psychologic benefits regardless of age. Adaptations often occur to a degree equal to that achieved with other therapeutic interventions.

Questions & Notes

List 3 factor that explain why aerobic training causes large increases in muscle blood flow during maximal exercise.

1.

2.

3.

Briefly describe the effects of endurance training on the blood pressure response at rest and during submaximal exercise.

Rest:

Submax Exercise:

Give the major benefit of improved pulmonary adaptations with exercise training.

List 2 factors to explain why endurance training lowers blood lactate levels during exercise of progressively increasing intensity.

1.

2.

Give one change in body composition resulting from aerobic training.

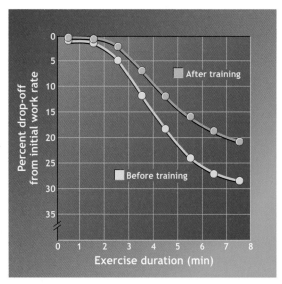

Figure 13.11 Percentage drop-off from initial exercise intensity before and after 10 weeks of endurance cycling training. (From the Applied Physiology Laboratory, University of Michigan, Ann Arbor, MI.)

FACTORS AFFECTING THE AEROBIC TRAINING RESPONSE

Two major goals of aerobic training include:

1. Enhance central circulatory capacity to deliver oxygen
2. Increase active muscles' capacity to consume oxygen

The several factors that influence outcomes of aerobic training include initial level of cardiovascular fitness and training frequency, training duration, and training intensity. The Close Up Box 13.2: *American College of Sports Medicine and American Heart Association Updated Fitness Guidelines and Recommendations* provides up to date guidelines on the types and amounts of physical activity for healthy adults and for the elderly.

Initial Level of Cardiorespiratory Fitness

The initial level of cardiorespiratory fitness affects the magnitude of training improvement. Considerable improvement occurs when initial fitness remains low; conversely,

BOX 13.2 CLOSE UP

American College of Sports Medicine and American Heart Association Updated Fitness Guidelines and Recommendations

The American College of Sports Medicine (ACSM; www.acsm.org) and American Heart Association (AHA; www.aha.org) have jointly published guidelines for a "well-rounded training program" for adults ages 18 to 65 years. This was done to update and clarify previous recommendations on the types and amounts of physical activity needed by healthy adults to improve and maintain health (**Table 1**). For example, a combined program

of aerobic training and resistance training increases muscular strength and aerobic power, decreases body fat, and increases basal metabolic rate. In contrast, singular-focus programs of either resistance *only* or aerobic training *only* produce singularly larger but more limited overall effects. For elderly individuals (**Table 2**), emphasis focuses on exercises to increase joint flexibility and improve balance to reduce injury risk from slips and falls.

Table 1   Physical Activity Recommendations by the American College of Sports Medicine and the American Heart Association for Healthy Adults Ages 18 to 65 Years

1. To promote and maintain good health, adults aged 18-65 yr should maintain a physically active lifestyle.
2. They should perform moderate-intensity aerobic (endurance) physical activity for a minimum of 30 min on 5 days each week or vigorous-intensity aerobic activity for a minimum of 20 min on three days each week.
3. Combinations of moderate- and vigorous-intensity activity can be performed to meet this recommendation. For example, a person can meet the recommendation by walking briskly for 30 min twice during the week and then jogging for 20 min on 2 other days.
4. These moderate- or vigorous-intensity activities are in addition to the light-intensity activities frequently performed during daily life (e.g., self care, washing dishes, using light tools at a desk) or activities of very short duration (e.g., taking out trash, walking to parking lot at store or office).
5. Moderate-intensity aerobic activity, which is generally equivalent to a brisk walk and noticeably accelerates the heart rate, can be accumulated toward the 30-min minimum by performing bouts each lasting 10 or more minutes.
6. Vigorous-intensity activity is exemplified by jogging and causes rapid breathing and a substantial increase in heart rate.
7. In addition, at least twice each week adults will benefit by performing activities using the major muscles of the body that maintain or increase muscular strength and endurance.
8. Because of the dose-response relation between physical activity and health, persons who wish to further improve their personal fitness, reduce their risk for chronic diseases and disabilities, or prevent unhealthy weight gain will likely benefit by exceeding the minimum recommended amount of physical activity.

From Haskell W.L., et al.: Physical activity and public health: Updated recommendation for adults from the American College of Sports Medicine and the American Heart Association. *Med. Sci. Sports Exerc.,* 39:1423, 2007.

Table 2 Physical Activity Recommendations by the American College of Sports Medicine and the American Heart Association for Older Adults (>65 Years)

1. To promote and maintain good health, older adults should maintain a physically active lifestyle.
2. They should perform moderate-intensity aerobic physical activity for a minimum of 30 min on 5 days each week or vigorous-intensity aerobic activity for a minimum of 20 min on three days each week. Moderate-intensity aerobic activity involves a moderate level of effort relative to an individual's aerobic fitness. On a 10-point scale, where sitting is 0 and all-out effort is 10, moderate-intensity activity is a 5 or 6 and produces noticeable increases in heart rate and breathing. On the same scale , vigorous-intensity activity is a 7 or 8 and produces large increases in heart rate and breathing. For example, given the heterogeneity of fitness levels in older adults, for some older adults a moderate-intensity walk is a slow walk, and for others it is a brisk walk.
3. Combinations of moderate- and vigorous-intensity activity can be performed to meet this recommendation. These moderate- or vigorous-intensity activities are in addition to the light intensity activities frequently performed during daily life (e.g., self care, washing dishes) or moderate-intensity activities lasting 10 min or less (e.g., taking out trash, walking to parking lot at store or office).
4. In addition, at least twice each week older adults should perform muscle strengthening activities using the major muscles of the body that maintain or increase muscular strength and endurance. It is recommended that 8–10 exercises be performed on at least two nonconsecutive days per week using the major muscle groups. To maximize strength development, a resistance (weight) should be used that allows 10–15 repetitions for each exercise. The level of effort for muscle-strengthening activities should be moderate to high.
5. Because of the dose-response relationship between physical activities and health, older persons who wish to further improve their personal fitness, reduce their risk for chronic diseases and disabilities, or prevent unhealthy weight gain will likely benefit by exceeding the minimum recommended amount of physical activity.
6. To maintain the flexibility necessary for regular physical activity and daily life, older adults should perform activities that maintain or increase flexibility on at least 2 days each week for at least 10 min each day.
7. To reduce risk of injury from falls, community-dwelling older adults with substantial risk of falls should perform exercises that maintain or improve balance.
8. Older adults with one or more medical conditions for which physical activity is therapeutic should perform physical activity in a manner that effectively and safely treats the condition(s).
9. Older adults should have a plan for obtaining sufficient physical activity that addresses each recommended type of activity. Those with chronic conditions for which activity is therapeutic should have a single plan that integrates prevention and treatment. For older adults who are not active at recommended levels, plans should include a gradual (or stepwise) approach to increase physical activity over time. Many months of activity at less than recommended levels is appropriate for some older adults (e.g., those with low fitness) as they increase activity in a stepwise manner. Older adults should also be encouraged to self-monitor their physical activity on a regular basis and to reevaluate plans as their abilities improve or as their health status changes.

From Nelson M.E. et al.: Physical activity and public health in older adults: Recommendation from the American College of Sports Medicine and the American Heart Association. *Med. Sci. Sports. Exerc.*, 39:1435, 2006.

---

an exceptionally high level of initial fitness leaves little room for improvement. For example, a 5% improvement in physiologic function for an elite athlete can be more significant than a 25% increase for a sedentary person. As a general guideline, aerobic fitness improvements range between 5% and 25% with endurance training. Some of this improvement occurs within the first week of training.

Training Frequency

Exercising at least 3 days a week generally initiates adaptive aerobic system changes. Several research studies report improvements when training only once per week. Those subjects, however, had been sedentary; thus, for them, any form of overload stimulates improvement. *In general, a training response occurs with exercise performed at least three times weekly for at least 6 weeks.* Interestingly, several studies show that training four or five times a week generated only *slightly* greater physiologic improvements compared with thrice-weekly exercise. For the average person, the small improvement in physiologic

ⓘ For Your Information

DIFFERENCES IN MAXIMAL PHYSIOLOGIC RESPONSE TO ACUTE EXERCISE IN CHILDREN RELATIVE TO ADULTS

Variable	Responses
Oxygen uptake ($\dot{V}O_2$, L·min^{-1})	Lower
Oxygen uptake ($\dot{V}O_2$, mL·kg^{-1}·min^{-1})	Higher
Heart rate	Higher
Cardiac output	Lower
Stroke volume	Lower
Systolic blood pressure	Lower
Diastolic blood pressure	Lower
Respiratory rate	Higher
Tidal volume	Lower
Minute ventilation ($\dot{V}E$)	Lower
Respiratory exchange ratio	Lower

From *ACSM's Guideline for Exercise Testing and Prescription*, 8th ed. Philadelphia: Lippincott Williams & Wilkins, 2010.

function as measured by $\dot{V}O_{2max}$ may not warrant the extra 1- or 2-day time investment in training. In contrast, the extra caloric expenditure from daily exercise justifies more frequent and longer duration of exercise targeted for weight control. Individuals should exercise on most days of the week to derive maximum health benefits. Chapter 17 discusses the health benefits of regular physical activity.

Training Duration

A common inquiry about exercise participation concerns the duration of daily workouts. For example, does 10 minutes of jogging provide twice the benefits of 5 minutes? Would a 2- or 3-minute run repeated eight to ten times provide greater training benefits than a continuous 20- to 30-minute run at a similar intensity? Precise answers to these questions remain elusive because of an incomplete understanding of the mechanisms that underly aerobic fitness improvements and the proper criteria for evaluating such changes. Aerobic capacity improves from both continuous and more intense intermittent exercise overload. In general, performing less exhaustive, moderate-paced exercise for at least 30 minutes each session establishes a realistic exercise duration recommendation for the average person. In contrast, most competitive endurance athletes devote several hours each training session to activities that enhance the aerobic system's functional capacity.

As for training volume, more does not necessarily produce greater results. In a study of collegiate swimmers, one group trained for 1.5 hours daily, and another group performed two 1.5-hour exercise sessions each day. Despite one group exercising at twice the daily exercise volume, no differences in the improvement in swimming power, endurance, or performance time emerged between groups. About 60 minutes of daily physical activity provides optimal health benefits and sets the lower limit for exercise duration to achieve weight loss.

Training Intensity

Exercise intensity represents the most critical factor for successful aerobic training. Intensity generally reflects the activity's energy requirements per unit time and specific energy systems activated in relation to an individual's energy-generating capacity. One can express exercise intensity in one of six ways:

1. Calories expended per unit time
2. Exercise level or power output
3. Level of exercise below, at, or above the blood LT
4. Percentage of $\dot{V}O_{2max}$
5. Heart rate or percentage of maximum heart rate
6. Multiples of resting metabolic rate (METs)

By far, monitoring exercise heart rate provides the most practical way to assess exercise strenuousness. Researchers frequently use heart rate to structure a training program and evaluate the effectiveness of various training intensities. For college-age men and women, exercise must reach an intensity to raise heart rate to at least 130 to 140 b·min^{-1}. This equals about 50% to 55% of $\dot{V}O_{2max}$ or 70% HR$_{max}$. Generally, this exercise intensity represents the *minimal threshold stimulus* for cardiovascular improvement. More intense exercise proves even more effective. Conversely, extending exercise duration induces fitness improvement in untrained persons if intensity of effort does not meet the threshold level.

Overly Strenuous Exercise Not Required An exercise heart rate at 70% HR$_{max}$ represents only moderate exercise that can continue for a long duration with little or no physiologic discomfort. The term **conversational exercise** describes this training level (i.e., sufficiently intense to stimulate a training effect yet not so strenuous it limits a person from talking during the workout).

Figure 13.12 shows that aerobic fitness improvements gradually decreases heart rate at a given level of submaximal

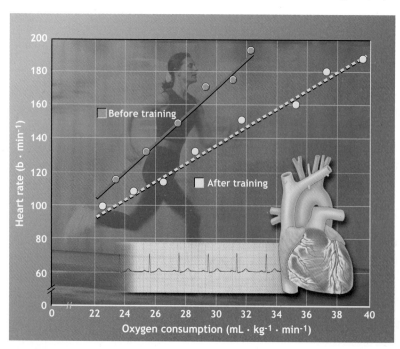

Figure 13.12 Improvements in heart rate response to oxygen uptake with aerobic training. Reduced submaximal exercise heart rate with training usually reflects an enhanced stroke volume of the heart.

exercise or oxygen uptake. Consequently, the absolute exercise level (running or swimming speed, power output on a cycle ergometer) must increase accordingly to achieve the desired target heart rate. A person who began training by slow walking now walks more briskly; eventually, periods of the workout include jogging. Ultimately, exercising at the training heart rate requires continuous running.

A minimal threshold intensity exists below which a training effect does not occur; a ceiling may also exist where higher intensity exercise produces no further gains. The lower and upper limits of the training-sensitive zone depend on the participant's age, initial fitness level, and state of training. For people with relatively poor aerobic fitness including older men and women, the training threshold approaches 60% to 65% HR_{max}, which corresponds to about 45% $\dot{V}O_{2max}$; more fit individuals generally require a higher threshold level. The ceiling for training intensity remains unknown, although 90% HR_{max} probably represents the upper limit. Above this level, increases in exercise intensity primarily overload the anaerobic system for energy transfer. Close Up Box 13.4: *Predicting Maximum Heart Rate and the Training-Sensitive Zone,* page 430 discusses common methods for using heart rate to establish the appropriate exercise level for aerobic training.

How Long Before Improvement Occurs?

Positive adaptations in cardiorespiratory fitness and aerobic capacity with training generally occur within several weeks after beginning an exercise program. **Figure 13.13** shows absolute and percentage improvements in $\dot{V}O_{2max}$ for men who trained 6 days a week for 10 weeks. Training consisted of 30 minutes of bicycling 3 days a week combined with running for up to 40 minutes on alternate days. This produced a continuous week-by-week improvement in aerobic capacity. Adaptive

Questions & Notes

List 4 factors that affect magnitude of the aerobic training response.

  1.

  2.

  3.

  4.

Give the generally expected range for percentage improvement in $\dot{V}O_{2max}$ with training.

List 5 ways to express exercise intensity.

  1.

  2.

  3.

  4.

  5.

Describe the best practical way to estimate the strenuousness of physical activity.

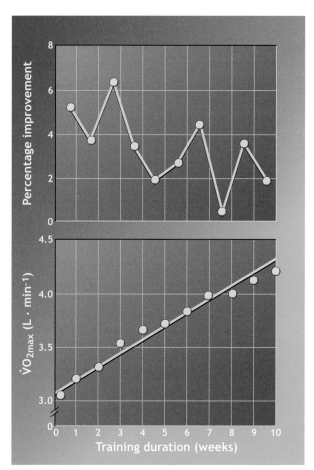

Figure 13.13   Continuous improvements in $\dot{V}O_{2max}$ during 10 weeks of intense aerobic training. (From Hickson, R.C., et al.: Linear increases in aerobic power induced by a program of endurance exercise. *J. Appl. Physiol.,* 42:373, 1977.)

BOX 13.3 CLOSE UP

Cardiovascular Fitness Categories Using $\dot{V}O_{2max}$

The $\dot{V}O_{2max}$ test represents the most often cited criterion of cardiorespiratory fitness. Current practice evaluates the $\dot{V}O_{2max}$ score against **criterion-referenced standards** rather than norm-referenced standards. Criterion-referenced standards establish a *minimum* $\dot{V}O_{2max}$ consistent with good health similar to blood pressure and cholesterol standards, independent of the score's percentile ranking within a particular normative data set. The accompanying table presents a five-part classification scheme for $\dot{V}O_{2max}$ for

men and women of different ages. The poor category for each age group represents the lower limit of cardiorespiratory fitness below which probably places the individual at increased risk for cardiovascular disease.

The highest $\dot{V}O_{2max}$ values are generally achieved by individuals who regularly engage in distance running, swimming, bicycling, and cross-country skiing. These individuals have almost double the $\dot{V}O_{2max}$ of sedentary individuals.

Cardiovascular Fitness Classifications Based on $\dot{V}O_{2max}$ ($mL \cdot kg^{-1} \cdot min^{-1}$)

GENDER	AGE	POOR	FAIR	AVERAGE	GOOD	EXCELLENT
Men	≤29	≤24.9	25–33.9	34–43.9	44–52.9	≥53
	30–39	≤22.9	23–30.9	31–41.9	42–49,9	≥50
	40–49	≤19.9	20–26.9	27–38.9	39–44.9	≥45
	50–59	≤17.9	18–24.9	25–37.9	38–42.9	≥43
	60–69	≤15.9	16–22.9	23–35.9	36–40.9	≥41
Women	≤29	≤23.9	24–30.9	31–38.9	39–48.9	≥49
	30–39	≤19.9	20–27.9	28–36.9	37–44.9	≥45
	40–49	≤16:9	17–24.9	25–34.9	35–41.9	≥42
	50–59	≤14.9	15–21.9	22–33.9	34–39.9	≥40
	50–69	≤12.9	13–20.9	21–32.9	33–36.9	≥37

responses to training eventually level off as a person reaches the genetically determined maximum.

Trainability and Genes

The limits for developing fitness capacity link closely to natural endowment. For two individuals in the same exercise program, one might show 10 times more improvement than the other. Genetics research indicates a genotype dependency for much of one's sensitivity in responding to maximal aerobic and anaerobic power training, including adaptations of most muscle enzymes. Genetic makeup plays such a predominant role in training responsiveness that it makes it almost impossible to predict a specific individual's response to a given training stimulus.

Maintenance of Aerobic Fitness Gains

An important question concerns optimal exercise frequency, duration, and intensity to *maintain* aerobic improvements with training. In one study, healthy young adults increased $\dot{V}O_{2max}$ 25% with 10 weeks of interval training by bicycling and running for 40 minutes 6 days a week. They then joined one of two groups that continued to exercise for an additional 15 weeks at the same intensity and duration but at a reduced frequency of either 4 or 2 days a week. Both groups maintained their gains in aerobic capacity despite up to two-thirds reduction in training frequency.

Aerobic capacity improvement involves somewhat different training requirements than its maintenance. With intensity held constant, the frequency and duration of exercise required to maintain a certain level of aerobic fitness remain considerably lower than required for its improvement. A small decline in exercise intensity, in contrast, reduces $\dot{V}O_{2max}$. *This indicates that exercise intensity plays a principal role in maintaining the increase in maximal aerobic power achieved through training.*

Fitness components other than $\dot{V}O_{2max}$ more readily show adverse effects of reduced exercise training volume. Well-trained endurance athletes who normally trained 6 to 10 hours a week reduced weekly training to one 35-minute session; this did not decrease their $\dot{V}O_{2max}$ over a 4-week period. However, endurance capacity at 75% $\dot{V}O_{2max}$ considerably decreased and was related to reduced pre-exercise glycogen stores and a diminished level of fat oxidation during exercise. *These findings indicate that a single measure such as $\dot{V}O_{2max}$ cannot adequately evaluate all of the important factors that affect adaptations to training and detraining.*

Tapering for Peak Performance

In most instances, little improvement occurs in the aerobic systems during the competitive season. At best, athletes strive to prevent physiologic and performance deteriorations during this period. Before major competition, athletes often reduce or **taper** training intensity, volume, or both, believing that such adjustments produce peak performance. The taper period and exact alterations in training vary by sport.

No clear answers exist about optimum taper duration or training modification. *From a physiologic perspective, 4 to 7 days probably provides sufficient time to achieve maximum muscle and liver glycogen replenishment and optimal nutritional support and restoration, minimize residual muscle soreness, and speed healing of minor injuries.*

FORMULATING AN AEROBIC TRAINING PROGRAM

This section presents guidelines for initiating aerobic training and describes a method to gauge and adjust training intensity. We also discuss advantages and possible limitations of aerobic training through intermittent and continuous procedures.

General Guidelines

Regardless of present physiologic fitness, some basic guidelines based on both research and common sense provide important structure when initiating an aerobic exercise training program:

- **Start slowly.** Injuries occur when a person initiates vigorous activity after years of sedentary living. Minor muscle aches and joint pain normally follow the start of an exercise program, particularly with eccentric muscle actions (see Chapter 14). Severe muscular discomfort and excessive cardiovascular strain offer no additional training benefits; excessive fatigue frequently discourages beginners from continuing a regular exercise program.
- **Allow a warm-up period.** Mild stretching and aerobic exercise (e.g., running in place, jogging on a treadmill, skipping rope, rowing, calisthenics, or stationary cycling) for 5 to 10 minutes provides an adequate muscular and cardiovascular warm-up immediately before the aerobic workout phase. Rhythmic, moderate exercise at a heart rate between 50% to 60% of maximum also adjusts coronary blood flow for more favorable myocardial oxygenation.
- **Allow a cool-down period.** After the training phase of exercise, slow down gradually before stopping to allow metabolism to progress to resting levels. More importantly, a gradual cool down prevents blood from pooling in the large veins of the previously exercised muscles. Venous pooling could decrease blood pressure and reduce blood flow to the heart and brain. This produces dizziness, nausea, and sometimes fainting. Reduced blood to the myocardium often precipitates a series of irregular heart beats that could trigger a catastrophic cardiac episode.

Guidelines for Children

Children are not small adults. Children's physical activity programs should be general in nature compared with specific formulations used for adults. Guidelines from the National Association for Sport and Physical Education (*www.aahperd.org/Naspe/*) recommend the following:

1. Accumulate more than 60 minutes and up to several hours daily of age- and developmentally appropriate activities for elementary school children.
2. Some of the child's physical activity each day should be in blocks lasting 15 minutes or longer and include large muscle, rhythmic moderate to vigorous aerobic activity performed intermittently with brief rest and recovery periods.
3. Extended periods of inactivity are *not* appropriate for normal, healthy children.

Questions & Notes

Name the principle exercise training variable to maintain a training-induced increase in $\dot{V}O_{2max}$.

List 3 general guidelines for initiating a general fitness program.

1.

2.

3.

About how long would you recommend for optimum tapering?

Are children just "small adults" with respect to exercise training guidelines? Discuss.

4. Elementary school children should participate in a variety of physical activities of various levels of intensities.

Cardiorespiratory Fitness Standards for Children

A valid method to evaluate cardiorespiratory fitness in children uses time to complete a 1-mile walk–run. Table 13.3 presents standards (upper and lower end) for the Healthy Fitness Zone consistent with good health for $\dot{V}O_{2max}$ and 1-mile times for different age children.

Setting fitness standards for children requires careful attention. The $\dot{V}O_{2max}$ expressed in $mL \cdot kg^{-1} \cdot min^{-1}$ remains relatively stable or decreases slightly between ages 5 and 19 years; however, walk–run performance almost doubles from growth and development and improved exercise economy during this period (a 12-year-old child runs a mile twice as fast as a 5-year-old child). Also, $\dot{V}O_{2max}$ improves only slightly for children who undergo aerobic training, but exercise performance increases considerably. This raises the question of whether aerobic capacity or exercise performance represents the "best" expression of cardiorespiratory fitness in children and its improvement with training.

Applying a single mathematical equation to predict $\dot{V}O_{2max}$ based on a walk–run test in children poses problems because of continually increasing levels of running economy as a child ages. Variations in exercise economy alter the relationship between aerobic fitness and running performance through all stages of growth and development.

ESTABLISHING TRAINING INTENSITY

What represents a considerable aerobic exercise stress for a sedentary person falls below an elite athlete's threshold training intensity. Consequently, exercise intensity must be assessed relative to the stress it places on a person's aerobic system. Within this framework, one could justifiably maintain that three individuals performing their best marathon times of 2.5, 3.0, and 4.0 hours experience equivalent levels of physiologic stress despite large variations in running speed.

Train at Percentage of $\dot{V}O_{2max}$

An individual can train at a percentage of $\dot{V}O_{2max}$ determined directly in the laboratory or estimated from exercise intensity. For example, if running at 5.5 mph requires an oxygen uptake of 33 $mL \cdot kg^{-1} \cdot min^{-1}$ and $\dot{V}O_{2max}$ equals 60 $mL \cdot kg^{-1} \cdot min^{-1}$, the exercise represents a stress of 55% of aerobic capacity. For another individual with a lower $\dot{V}O_{2max}$ of 40 $mL \cdot kg^{-1} \cdot min^{-1}$, the oxygen cost of running at 5.5 mph still requires 33 $mL \cdot kg^{-1} \cdot min^{-1}$, yet this person must exercise at 83% of maximum. To provide a similar overload (intensity) of 83% of $\dot{V}O_{2max}$ for the first jogger, the pace must increase to a speed requiring 48 mL O_2 $mL \cdot kg^{-1} \cdot min^{-1}$ or 8.6 mph.

Train at Percentage of Maximum Heart Rate

Assessing exercise intensity accurately by direct measurement of oxygen uptake requires laboratory measurements. A more practical alternative uses heart rate to classify exercise by intensity (strenuousness) and individualizes aerobic training to keep pace as fitness improves. This approach applies the well-established relationship between percentage $\dot{V}O_{2max}$ and percentage HR_{max}.

The error in estimating percentage $\dot{V}O_{2max}$ from percentage HR_{max}, or vice versa, averages about ±8%. From this intrinsic relationship, one need only monitor exercise heart rate to estimate percentage $\dot{V}O_{2max}$. *The relationship between percentage $\dot{V}O_{2max}$ and percentage HR_{max} remains the same for arm or leg exercise among healthy subjects, normal weight and obese groups, cardiac patients, and people with spinal cord injuries.* Importantly, a lower HR_{max} occurs in upper-body arm compared with lower body leg exercise; one must consider this difference in formulating the exercise prescription for different exercise modes (see Close Up on p. 430).

Table 13.3	Standards for the Healthy Fitness Zone for 1-Mile Walk–Run Times and $\dot{V}O_{2max}$[a] for Children Ages 10 to 17 Years			
	1-Mile Run Time (min:s)		$\dot{V}O_{2max}$ (mL·kg⁻¹·min⁻¹)	
AGE	BOYS[b]	GIRLS[b]	BOYS[b]	GIRLS[b]
10	11:30–9:00	12:30–9:30	42–52	39–47
11	11:00–8:30	12:00–9:00	42–52	38–46
12	10:30–8:00	12:00–9:00	42–52	37–45
13	10:00–7:30	11:30–9:00	42–52	36–44
14	9:30–7:00	11:00–8:30	42–52	35–43
15	9:00–7:00	10:30–8:00	42–52	35–43
16	8:30–7:00	10:00–8:00	42–52	35–43
17	8:30–7:00	10:00–8:00	42–52	35–43

[a]$\dot{V}O_{2max}$, maximal oxygen consumption.
[b]Number on left is the lower end of Healthy Fitness Zone; number on right is the upper end of Health Fitness Zone.
From The Cooper Institute: *FITNESSGRAM/ACTIVITYGRAM Test Administration Manual* 4th ed. . Champaign, IL: Human Kinetics, 2007.

To train at a percentage of HR_{max} requires knowledge of the heart rate in near-maximal exercise. Three or 4 minutes of all-out running or swimming elicits HR_{max} values. Such intense exercise requires considerable motivation and endangers those predisposed to coronary heart disease. For this reason, predicting HR_{max} has become standard practice. The following presents the most common formula to estimate maximum heart rate:

$$HR_{max} = 220 - \text{Age in years}$$

More recent research suggests substantial individual differences using this method when applied to all individuals. New formulae predict HR_{max} results with less error. Close Up Box 13.4 presents the formulae and common heart rate methods to establish individual training levels.

Effectiveness of Less Intense Exercise   The recommendation to train at 70% of HR_{max} as the threshold for aerobic improvement represents a *general guideline* for a comfortable yet effective exercise intensity. Twenty to 30 minutes of continuous exercise at the 70% level stimulates a training effect; exercise at a lower intensity of 60% to 65% HR_{max} for 45 minutes also proves beneficial. *In general, longer exercise duration offsets lower exercise intensity, particularly for older and less fit individuals.* Regardless of exercise level, more is not necessarily better because excessive exercise increases the chance for sustaining bone, joint, and muscle injuries.

Train at Perception of Effort

In addition to oxygen consumption, heart rate, and blood lactate as indicators of exercise intensity, one also can use the **rating of perceived exertion (RPE)**. With this psychophysiologic approach, the exerciser rates on a numerical scale (sometimes called the Borg scale after researcher Gunnar Borg who developed the first of these scaling systems) perceived feelings relative to exertion level. Monitoring and adjusting RPE during exercise provides an effective strategy to prescribe exercise based on an individual's perception of effort that coincides with objective measures of physiologic or metabolic strain ($\%HR_{max}$, $\%\dot{V}O_{2max}$, blood lactate concentration). Exercise levels corresponding to higher levels of energy expenditure and physiologic strain produce higher RPE ratings. For example, an RPE of 13 or 14 (exercise that feels "somewhat hard"; **Fig. 13.14**) coincides

Questions & Notes

Write 2 formulae to predict maximum heart rate from age. (Hint: see close-up Box 13.4)

1.

2.

What is the recommended % HR_{max} training level for sedentary individuals starting an exercise program?

RPE Scale		Equivalent % HR_{max}	Equivalent % $\dot{V}O_{2max}$
6			
7	Very, very light		
8			
9	Very light		
10			
11	Fairly light	52-66	31-50
12			
13	Somewhat hard	61-85	51-75
14			
15	Hard	86-91	76-85
16			
17	Very hard	92	85
18			
19	Very, very hard		

Figure 13.14   The Borg scale and accompanying estimates of relative exercise intensity for obtaining the rating of perceived exertion (RPE) during exercise. (Modified from Borg, G.A.: Psychological basis of physical exertion. *Med. Sci. Sports Exerc.*, 14:377, 1982.)

i For Your Information

REGULAR DOSES OF AEROBIC EXERCISE COMBAT OBESITY

Sixty minutes of moderate daily exercise (low-impact walking or aerobic dancing, swimming, stationary cycling) reduces excess body fat. Exercise can be divided into 10-, 20-, or 30-minute sessions, as long as the daily total equals 60 minutes or more. For an individual who weighs 216 pounds, the caloric expenditure during slow walking equals 7.8 kCal each minute (470 kCal per hour). Over 1 month, total exercise calories would accumulate to 14,100 kCal (470 kCal × 30 days), the equivalent of 4.0 lb of body fat. In 1 year, as long as caloric intake remains constant, fat loss (without dieting) would amount to nearly 50 pounds.

BOX 13.4 CLOSE UP

Predicting Maximum Heart Rate and the Training-Sensitive Zone

Percentage of maximum HR predicts exercise intensity (an activity's relative energy requirements).

HR_{max} in beats per min (bpm) can be predicted by age, independent of gender and physical activity status. For *nonfat* men and women, HR_{max} predicts as:

$$HR_{max} = 208 - 0.7 \times (Age, y)$$

Example
Calculate the HR_{max} for a 20-year-old man.

$$HR_{max} = 208 - 0.7 \times (Age, y)$$
$$= 194 \text{ bpm}$$

PREDICTING HR_{max} FOR MEN AND WOMEN WITH ≥30% BODY FAT

For overfat men and women with percentage body fat levels 30% or above, HR_{max} predicts as:

$$HR_{max} = 200 - 0.5 \times (Age, y)$$

Example
Calculate the HR_{max} for a 25-year-old woman with a percentage body fat of 32%.

$$HR_{max} = 200 - 0.5 \times (Age, y)$$
$$= 188 \text{ bpm}$$

COMPUTING LOWER- AND UPPER-LIMIT TRAINING HEART RATES

For men and women younger than 60 years of age, the minimal or lower-limit target threshold heart rate (LL_{THR}) stimulus for cardiovascular improvement ranges between 60% and 70% of HR_{max}, representing about 50% to 60% of $\dot{V}O_{2max}$. The **upper-limit target heart rate (UL_{THR})** equals about 90% of HR_{max}, representing about 85% to 90% of $\dot{V}O_{2max}$. In individuals older than 60 years of age, LL_{THR} equals 60%, and UL_{THR} equals 75% of HR_{max}.

Method 1: Percentage Method
This method calculates the lower- and upper-limit target heart rates as a simple percentage of age-predicted HR_{max}.

1. Calculate LL_{THR} as:

$$LL_{THR} = \text{Predicted } HR_{max} \times$$
$$\text{Lower-limit percentage for age}$$

where the lower-limit percentage = 70% for men and women age 60 years and younger and 60% for men and women older than age 60 years.

2. Calculate UL_{THR} as:

$$UL_{THR} = \text{Predicted } HR_{max} \times$$
$$\text{Upper-limit percentage for age}$$

where the upper-limit percentage = 90% for men and women 60 years and younger and 80% for men and women older than age 60 years.

Example
Data: Male, age 55 years.

1. Calculate predicted HR_{max}

$$HR_{max} = 208 - 0.7 \times (Age, y) = 170 \text{ bpm}$$
$$LL_{THR} = 170 \times \text{Lower-limit percentage for age}$$
$$= 170 \times 0.70$$
$$= 119 \text{ bpm}$$

2. Calculate UL_{THR}

$$UL_{THR} = HR_{max} \times \text{Upper-limit percentage for age}$$
$$= 170 \times 0.90$$
$$= 153 \text{ bpm}$$

Method 2: Karvonen Method (Heart Rate Reserve)
An alternate, equally effective method calculates the lower- and upper-threshold HR levels at a percentage of the difference between resting and maximum HR, termed **heart rate reserve (HRR**; also referred to as the **Karvonen method** named after the Finnish physiologist who introduced this method). Karvonen's method produces somewhat higher values compared with heart rate computed as percentage of HR_{max}. The Karvonen method uses about 50% of HRR as the LL_{THR} and 85% of HRR as UL_{THR}.

1. Calculate predicted HR_{max}:

$$HR_{max} = 208 - 0.7 \times Age, y$$

2. Calculate LL_{THR}:

$$LL_{THR} = [(HR_{max} - HR_{rest}) \times 0.50] + HR_{rest}$$

3. Calculate UL_{THR}:

$$UL_{THR} = [(HR_{max} - HR_{rest}) \times 0.85] + HR_{rest}$$

Example
Data: Male, age 55 years, $HR_{rest} = 60 \text{ b·min}^{-1}$.

1. Calculate predicted HR_{max}:

$$HR_{max} = 208 - 0.7 \times Age, y$$
$$= 170 \text{ bpm}$$

2. Calculate LL_{THR}:

$$LL_{THR} = [(HR_{max} - HR_{rest}) \times 0.50] + HR_{rest}$$
$$= [(170 - 60) \times 0.50] + 60$$
$$= 115 \text{ bpm}$$

3. Calculate UL_{THR}:

$$UL_{THR} = [(HR_{max} - HR_{rest}) \times 0.85] + HR_{rest}$$
$$= [(170 - 60) \times 0.85] + 60$$
$$= 154 \text{ bpm}$$

Adjust for Swimming and Other Upper-Body Exercises

In trained and untrained subjects, swimming HR_{max} averages about 13 bpm lower than in running. The smaller arm muscle mass activated during swimming probably causes this difference. Consequently, HR_{max} must be adjusted downward for swimming or other upper-body exercise. Subtract 13 bpm from the age-predicted HR_{max} values to calculate training heart rate during swimming. For example, a 25-year-old person wanting to swim at 80% of HR_{max} should select a swimming speed that produces an exercise heart rate (percentage method) of about 142 bpm $(0.80 \times [191 - 13])$.

Method 3: Perhaps a Modification Required

Recent evidence from a longitudinal study of 132 persons measured an average seven times over 9 years indicates a bias in the widely used 220 – Age prediction of HR_{max}. The bias *overestimates* this measure in men and women younger than age 40 years and *underestimates* it in persons older than 40 years (see accompanying figure). This modified prediction equation (with a 5 to 8 bpm standard deviation), is independent of gender, body mass index, and resting heart rate:

$$HR_{max} = 206.9 - 0.67 \times Age \text{ (y)}$$

For example, use the above equation to estimate maximum heart rate for a 30-year-old man or woman:

$$HR_{max} = 206.9 - (0.67 \times 30)$$
$$= 206.9 - 20.1$$
$$= 187 \text{ b} \cdot \text{min}^{-1}$$

These prediction formulas associate with a plus/minus error and should be used with caution. Each formula represents a convenient rule of thumb but should not determine a specific person's maximum heart rate. For example, within normal variation limits and using the 220 – Age formula, a maximum heart rate of 95% (± 2 standard deviations) for 40-year-old men and women ranges between 160 and 200 b·min^{-1}.

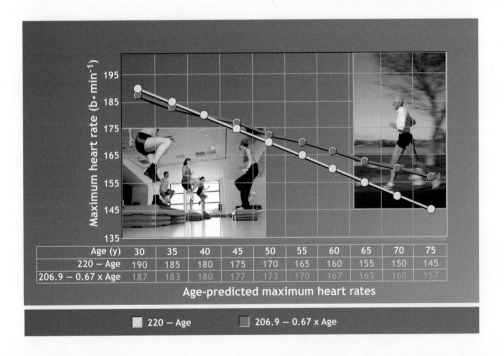

Age (y)	30	35	40	45	50	55	60	65	70	75
220 – Age	190	185	180	175	170	165	160	155	150	145
206.9 – 0.67 x Age	187	183	180	177	173	170	167	163	160	157

Age-predicted maximum heart rates

■ 220 – Age   □ 206.9 – 0.67 x Age

REFERENCES

Davis, J.A., Convertino, V.A.: A comparison of heart rate methods for predicting endurance training intensity. *Med. Sci. Sports Exerc.*, 7:295, 1975.

Gellish, R.L., et al.: Longitudinal modeling of the relationship between age and maximal heart rate. *Med. Sci. Sports Exerc.*, 39:822, 2007.

Karvonen, M., et al.: The effects of training on heart rate. A longitudinal study. *Ann. Med. Exp. Biol. Fenn.*, 35:307, 1957.

Miller, W.C., et al.: Predicting max HR and the HR-$\dot{V}O_2$ relationship for exercise prescription in obesity. *Med. Sci. Sports Exerc.*, 25:1077, 1993.

Tanaka, H., et al.: Age-predicted maximal heart rate revisited. *J. Am. Coll. Cardiol.*, 37:153, 2001.

with about 70% HR_{max} during cycle ergometer and treadmill exercise; an RPE between 11 and 12 corresponds to exercise at LT for trained and untrained individuals. Individuals learn quickly to exercise at a specific RPE. In this sense, the axiom "listen to your body" becomes apropos.

Train at the Lactate Threshold

Exercising at or slightly above the LT provides effective aerobic training, with the higher exercise levels producing the greatest benefits, particularly for fit individuals. **Figure 13.15** illustrates how to determine the appropriate exercise level by plotting exercise intensity (e.g., running speed) versus blood lactate level. In this example, the running speed that produced a blood lactate concentration at the 4-mM level (OBLA) represented the recommended training intensity. Many coaches use 4-mM blood lactate level as the optimal aerobic training intensity, yet no convincing evidence exists to justify this particular blood lactate level as "ideal." Regardless of the specific blood lactate level chosen for endurance training, the blood lactate–exercise intensity relationship should be evaluated periodically, with exercise intensity adjusted to meet aerobic fitness improvements. If regular blood lactate measurement proves impractical, exercise heart rate at the initial lactate determination remains a convenient and relatively stable marker for setting the appropriate predetermined exercise intensity. This is because no systematic training-induced change occurs in the heart rate–blood lactate relationship during incremental exercise.

One important distinction between the use of %HR_{max} and LT to establish training intensity rests with the physiologic dynamics each method reflects. The %HR_{max} method establishes a level of exercise stress to overload the central circulation (e.g., stroke volume, cardiac output). The LT method places emphasis on the peripheral vasculature and active muscles to sustain steady-rate aerobic metabolism.

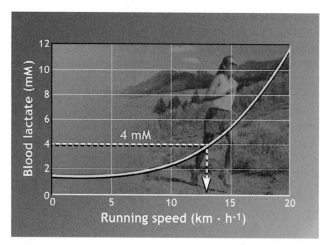

Figure 13.15 Blood lactate concentration in relation to running speed for one subject. At a lactate level of 4.0 mM, the corresponding running speed was approximately 13 km·h⁻¹. This speed establishes the subject's initial training intensity.

METHODS OF TRAINING

Performance improvements occur in almost all athletic competitions each year. These advances generally relate to increased opportunities for participation; individuals with "natural endowment" more likely become exposed to particular sports. Also, improved nutrition and health care, better equipment, and more systematic and scientific approaches to athletic training contribute to superior performance. The following sections present general guidelines for anaerobic and aerobic training.

Anaerobic Training

The capacity to perform all-out exercise for up to 60 seconds largely depends on ATP generated by the immediate and short-term anaerobic systems for energy transfer (see **Fig. 13.1**).

The Intramuscular High-Energy Phosphates
Football, weight lifting, and other brief, sprint-power sport activities rely exclusively on energy derived from ATP and PCr, the muscles' high-energy phosphates. Engaging specific muscles in repeated 5- to 10-second maximum bursts of effort overloads the phosphagen pool. The intramuscular high-energy phosphates supply energy for intense but brief exercise, so little lactate accumulates, and recovery progresses rapidly. Thus, exercise can begin again after about a 30-second rest. Brief, all-out exercise interspersed with recovery represents a specific application of interval training for anaerobic conditioning.

The activities selected to enhance ATP–PCr energy transfer capacity must engage the specific muscles at the movement speed and power output for which the athlete desires improved anaerobic power (*specificity principle*). Not only does this enhance the metabolic capacity of the specifically trained muscle fibers, but it also facilitates recruitment and modulation of firing sequence of the appropriate motor units activated in the movement.

Lactate-Generating Capacity As the duration of maximal effort extends beyond 10 seconds, dependence on anaerobic energy from the intramuscular high-energy phosphates decreases, with a proportionate increase in anaerobic energy transfer from anaerobic glycolysis. To improve energy transfer capacity by the short-term lactic acid energy system, training must overload this aspect of energy metabolism.

Anaerobic training requires extreme physiologic demands and considerable motivation. Repeated bouts of up to 1-minute maximum exercise stopped 30 seconds before subjective feelings of exhaustion cause blood lactate to increase to near-maximum levels. The individual repeats each exercise bout after 3 to 5 minutes of recovery. Repetition of exercise causes "lactate stacking," which results in a higher blood lactate level than with just one bout of exhaustive effort. As with all training regimens, one must exercise the specific muscle groups that require enhanced lactate-producing capacity.

BOX 13.5 CLOSE UP

Determine 10,000-M Running Pace from Lactate Threshold

Physiologic measurements during exercise help to (1) pinpoint strengths and weaknesses about an individual's performance capacity and potential and (2) optimize training intensity for the most effective outcome. For example, research indicates that athletes run 10,000 m at a pace approximately 5 m·min^{-1} faster than the running speed associated with their LT. Knowledge of the exercise intensity associated with LT should provide the athlete and coach with a realistic performance expectation based on an individualized assessment of the aerobic metabolic response to exercise. This information puts into a biologic perspective for both the coach and the athlete an answer to the questions: "How fast can I perform this event?" and "What training pace is best for me?"

TESTING

Step 1. Determine the LT (see Chapter 9; if blood lactate cannot be directly measured, use the ventilatory threshold method discussed in Chapter 9). **Figure 1** shows the relationship between blood lactate and oxygen uptake during graded treadmill exercise, with LT indicated by the *arrow*. In this example, LT occurred at a $\dot{V}O_2$ of 43.5 mL·kg^{-1}·min^{-1}.

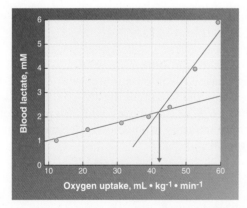

Figure 1 Determination of LT from measures of blood lactate and $\dot{V}O_2$ during graded trademill exercise.

Step 2. Determine the relationship between $\dot{V}O_2$ (mL·kg^{-1}·min^{-1}; either actual or estimated) and running speed (m·min^{-1}). The subject runs on a treadmill for 5 minutes at each of six different submaximal speeds. Construct a graph relating $\dot{V}O_2$ versus running speed (**Fig. 2**). Draw a best-fit line through the plotted points.

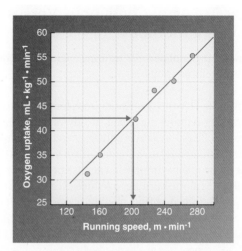

Figure 2 Oxygen uptake related to running speed during treadmill exercise at progressively faster running speeds.

Step 3. Convert the $\dot{V}O_2$ at LT (43.5 mL·kg^{-1}·min^{-1}; **Fig. 1**) to a running speed using the best-fit line presented in **Figure 2**. Draw a horizontal line from the oxygen uptake value on the y-axis until it intersects the line of best fit; from this intersection, draw a perpendicular line to the x-axis that indicates running speed. The *arrow* shows the corresponding speed (m·min^{-1}) as 204 m·min^{-1}.

COMPUTING EXPECTED PERFORMANCE

Assume an athlete exceeds by 5 m·min^{-1} his or her running speed at LT during training (and competition) for 10,000 m (and other endurance events); the projected average running speed for this person equals 209 m·min^{-1} (204 m·min^{-1} + 5 m·min^{-1}).

DETERMINE THE PROJECTED RACE TIME FOR THE 10,000-M RUN

Use the data from Figures 1 and 2 to estimate the time for a 10,000-m race.

$$\begin{aligned}
\text{Estimated time} &= \text{Distance} \div \text{Speed} \\
&= 10,000 \text{ m} \div 209 \text{ m·min}^{-1} \\
&= 47.85 \text{ min } (47 \text{ min:}51 \text{ s})
\end{aligned}$$

This analysis based on LT measurements indicates that the athlete should complete the 10,000-m run in 47 minutes and 51 seconds. It also represents a realistic estimate of an appropriate training intensity to achieve the performance goal.

A backstroke swimmer should train by swimming the backstroke; a cyclist should bicycle; and basketball, hockey, or soccer players should perform movements and direction changes similar to those required by the sport.

Aerobic Training: Continuous Versus Intermittent Methods

Two general types of aerobic training include continuous and intermittent methods.

Continuous Training

Continuous **long slow distance (LSD)** training requires sustained, steady-rate aerobic exercise. Because of its submaximal nature, exercise continues for considerable time in relative comfort. This makes LSD training ideal for people beginning an exercise program or wanting to enhance calorie burning to reduce excess body fat. *The greatest health-related benefits of exercise emerge when a person moves from a sedentary lifestyle to one that incorporates only a moderate level of continuous aerobic exercise.* LSD training generally progresses at the relatively comfortable threshold intensity of 70% HR_{max}. It can also remain effective at the more intense 85% or 90% level.

Endurance athletes overload the cardiovascular and energy transfer systems using continuous exercise training at nearly the same intensity as competition. This specifically activates slow-twitch muscle fibers in sustained exercise. A champion middle-distance runner may run 5 miles continuously in 25 minutes during workouts at a heart rate of 180 b·min^{-1}; this pace does not exhaust the athlete but still nearly duplicates race conditions. By finishing each exercise session with several all-out sprints stopped 30 to 40 seconds before exhaustion, the athlete also trains the short-term anaerobic energy system (glycolysis) that contributes to race performance, particularly at the finish. A marathon runner trains at a slightly slower pace than a middle-distance athlete to simulate the intensity, distance, and energy requirements of competition.

Interval Training

Periods of intense activity interspersed with moderate to low energy expenditure characterize many sport and life activities. **Interval exercise training** simulates this variation in energy transfer intensity through specific spacing of exercise and rest periods. With this approach, a person trains at an inordinately high exercise intensity with minimal fatigue that would normally prove exhausting if done continuously. Rest-to-exercise intervals vary from a few seconds to several minutes depending on the energy system(s) overloaded. Four factors formulate the interval training prescription:

1. Intensity of exercise interval
2. Duration of exercise interval
3. Duration of recovery interval
4. Repetitions of exercise-recovery interval

BOX 13.6 CLOSE UP

A Typical Aerobic Exercise Session

The accompanying figure illustrates a typical aerobic training session for a 50-year-old woman. The session begins with a 5- to 10-minute warm-up period of light to moderate walking or jogging in place with a heart rate at about 120 bpm. This continues with the conditioning phase (30- to 60-minute) with exercise heart rates within 70% to 85% of the age-predicted maximal heart rate. A 5- to 10-minute cool-down period follows as exercise intensity exponentially declines toward the resting level.

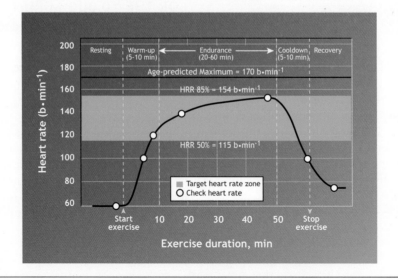

Table 13.4	Guidelines for Determining Interval-Training Exercise Intensities for Running and Swimming Different Distances[a]	
INTERVAL TRAINING DISTANCES (YARDS)		**WORK RATE FOR EACH EXERCISE INTERVAL OR REPEAT**
Run	**Swim**	
55	15	1.5 ⎫ seconds *slower* than best
110	25	3.0 ⎬ times from a running or swimming start for each
220	55	5.0 ⎭ for each distance
440	110	1 to 4 seconds *faster* than the average run or 110-yd swim time recorded during a 1-mile run or 440-yd swim
660–1320	165–320	3 to 4 seconds *slower* than the average 440-yd run or 100-yard swim time recorded during a 1-mile run or 440-yd swim

[a]From Fox, E. L., Matthews, D.K.: *Interval Training*, Philadelphia: W. B. Saunders, 1974.

Running continuously at a 4-minute mile pace exhausts most people within a minute because of rapid lactate accumulation. Running at this speed for only 15 seconds followed by a 30-second rest period enables a person to accomplish 4 minutes of running at this near-record pace. This does not equate to a 4-minute mile, but during 4 minutes of running the person covers a 1-mile distance even though the combined exercise and rest intervals require 11 minutes 30 seconds.

Rationale for Interval Training   A sound rationale forms the basis for interval training. In the example of a continuous run by an average person at a 4-minute mile pace, the predominant energy for exercise comes from the short-term anaerobic energy pathway with rapid lactate accumulation. The individual becomes exhausted within 60 to 90 seconds. In contrast, running at this speed for 15-second intervals or less places significant demands on the immediate energy system (intramuscular ATP and PCr) with little lactate accumulation. Repetitively linking specific exercise and rest intervals as part of interval training eventually places considerable demand on aerobic energy metabolism.

In interval training, as with other forms of physiologic conditioning, exercise intensity must overload the specific energy system(s) desired for improvement through sport-specific muscle activation. Table 13.4 outlines a practical method for determining exercise intensity for interval training in running and swimming.

No one method has proved superior for either continuous or interval training to improve aerobic fitness. Both methods probably can be applied interchangeably. Importantly, continuous LSD training gives the endurance athlete a more "task-specific" cardiovascular and metabolic overload that more closely mimics the duration and intensity of race conditions. Likewise, sprint and middle-distance athletes benefit from the intense metabolic demands and specific neuromuscular and fiber-type activation that interval training provides.

Formulating the Exercise:Relief Interval

Exercise Interval

- Add 1.5 to 5 s to the exerciser's "best time" for training distances between 60 and 220 yd for running and 15 and 55 yd for swimming. If a person covers 60 yd from a running start in 8 s, the exercise duration for each repeat equals 8 + 1.5 or 9.5 s. Add 3 s to the best running time for interval training distances of 110 yd and 5 s to a distance of 220 yd. This particular

Questions & Notes

List 2 general types of aerobic training.

1.

2.

List 2 factors used to formulate an interval training prescription.

1.

2.

Explain the rationale for interval training.

Which types of athletes are most likely to benefit from interval training?

application of interval training most effectively trains the intramuscular high-energy phosphate component of the anaerobic energy system.

- For training distances of 440 yd running or 110 yd swimming, determine the exercise rate by subtracting 1 to 4 s from the average 440-yd portion of a mile run or 110-yd portion of a 440-yd swim. If a person runs a 7-minute mile (averaging 105 s per 440 yd), the interval time for each 440-yd repeat ranges between 104 s ($105 - 1$) and 101 s ($105 - 4$).
- For run training intervals beyond 440 yd (and swim intervals beyond 110 yd) add 3 to 4 s to the average 440-yard portion of a mile run or 110-yard portion of a 440-yard swim. In running an 880-yard interval, the 7-minute miler runs each interval in about 216 s ($[105 + 3] \times 2 = 216$).

Relief Interval

- The relief (recovery) interval occurs either passively (rest:relief) or actively (exercise:relief). Recovery duration represents a multiple of the exercise interval. A 1:3 ratio overloads the immediate energy system. For a sprinter who runs 10-s intervals, the relief interval equals 30 s. For training the short-term glycolytic energy system, the relief interval doubles (ratio of 1:2). In this case, a 2-min recovery follows a 1-min run or swim. These specified ratios for the exercise to relief interval for training allow sufficient restoration of high-energy phosphates and lactate removal so subsequent exercise proceeds with undue fatigue.
- For training the long-term aerobic energy system, the exercise:relief interval usually equals 1:1 or 1:1.5. During a 60- to 90-s exercise interval, for example, oxygen uptake increases rapidly to a high level. Although some lactate accumulates during this relatively intense exercise, the duration remains brief enough to prevent exhaustion. A 1- to 2-min recovery permits exercise to begin again before oxygen uptake returns to its pre-exercise level. Consecutive repeat exercise:relief intervals ensures that cardiovascular response and aerobic metabolism eventually maintain near-maximal levels throughout exercise and recovery. Performing continuously at this exercise intensity exhausts the person within several minutes, and training would cease.

Fartlek Training

Fartlek training, developed in 1937 by Gösta Holmér (1891–1983), means "speed play." Holmér, the Swedish National Track coach, based his training system after the incomparable Finnish world champion runner and multiple Olympic gold medal winner Paavo Nurmi (*www.urheilumuseo.org/paavonurmi/pnhome.htm*). During that era, this relatively unscientific blending of interval and continuous training introduced to the United States in the early 1940s had particular application to exercise out-of-doors over natural terrain. The system used alternate running at fast and slow speeds over both level and hilly landscape.

Fartlek training workouts do not require systematic manipulation of exercise and relief intervals in contrast to the precise exercise-interval training prescription. In fartlek, the performer determines the training schema based on "how it feels" at the time, in a way similar to gauging exercise intensity based on one's rating of perceived exertion. If used properly, this method will overload one or all of the energy systems. Fartlek training provides an ideal means of general conditioning and off-season training, but it lacks the systematic quantified approaches of interval and continuous training.

THE OVERTRAINING SYNDROME

Ten percent to 20% of athletes experience the syndrome of **overtraining** or "staleness." As a result of complex interactions among biologic and psychologic influences, an athlete can fail to endure and adapt to training so that normal exercise performance deteriorates and the individual encounters increasing difficulty fully recovering from a workout. This takes on crucial importance for elite athletes for whom performance decrements of less than 1% can cause a gold medalist to fail to qualify for competition. Stated somewhat differently, a 1% *improvement* in performance will make the difference between a gold and silver medal or no medal at all.

Two clinical forms of overtraining exist:

1. The less common **sympathetic form** characterized by increased sympathetic activity during rest, and generally typified by hyperexcitability, restlessness, and impaired exercise performance. This form of overtraining may reflect excessive psychological or emotional stress that accompanies the interaction among training, competition, and responsibilities of normal living.
2. The more common **parasympathetic form** is characterized by predominance of vagal activity during rest and exercise. More properly termed **overreaching** in the early stages within as few as 10 days, the syndrome is qualitatively similar in symptoms to the full-blown parasympathetic overtraining syndrome but of shorter duration. Overreaching generally results from excessive and protracted exercise overload with inadequate recovery and rest. Initially, maintenance of exercise performance requires greater effort, which eventually leads to performance deterioration in training and competition. Short-term rest intervention of a few days up to several weeks usually restores full function. Untreated overreaching eventually progresses to the overtraining syndrome.

Symptoms of Overtraining and Staleness

The eight most common overtraining characteristics include:

1. Unexplained and persistently poor athletic performance and high fatigue ratings
2. Prolonged recovery from typical training sessions or competitive events

3. Disturbed mood states characterized by general fatigue, apathy, depression, irritability, and loss of competitive drive
4. Persistent feelings of muscle soreness and stiffness in muscles and joints
5. Elevated resting pulse and increased susceptibility to upper respiratory tract infections (altered immune function) and gastrointestinal disturbances
6. Insomnia
7. Loss of appetite, weight loss, and inability to maintain proper body weight for competition
8. Overuse injuries

No simple, reliable method can diagnose overtraining in its earliest stages. The best indications include deterioration in physical performance and alterations in mood rather than changes in immune function.

EXERCISE TRAINING DURING PREGNANCY

During pregnancy, walking, swimming, and aerobics are the most popular physical activities. Older mothers, women who have delivered more than one child or had previous children, and those with unfavorable reproductive histories are less likely to exercise during pregnancy.

Energy Cost and Physiologic Demands of Exercise

Cardiovascular responses during exercise in pregnancy follow normal patterns. An uncomplicated pregnancy offers no greater physiologic strain to the mother during moderate exercise other than provided by the additional weight gain and the possible encumbrance of fetal tissue. Increases in maternal body mass add considerably to exercise effort in weight-bearing walking, jogging, and stair climbing.

Fetal Blood Supply

Any factor that might compromise fetal blood supply raises concern regarding exercise during pregnancy. Studies of uterine blood flow during exercise in various mammalian species indicate that healthy animals maintain adequate oxygen supply to the developing fetus during moderate to intense maternal exercise.

Exercise probably diverts some blood from the uterus and visceral organs for preferential distribution to active muscles; as such, intense exercise could pose a hazard to a fetus with restricted placental blood flow. In addition, elevated maternal core temperature hinders heat dissipation from the fetus through the placenta. Maternal hyperthermia negatively affects fetal development (e.g., increased risk for neural tube defect) early in pregnancy. During warm weather, exercise should take place in the cool part of the day and for shorter intervals while maintaining regular fluid intake.

Current medical opinion maintains that 30 or 40 minutes of moderate aerobic exercise by a previously active, healthy, low-risk woman during an uncomplicated pregnancy does not compromise fetal oxygen supply, acid–base status, or produce other adverse effects to the mother or fetus. Performed regularly, moderate exercise maintains cardiovascular fitness with the added benefit of producing a beneficial training effect.

Pregnancy Course and Outcome

No overall consensus previously existed on whether regular exercise enhanced the course of pregnancy, including labor, delivery, and outcome. Current data now support a recommendation for regular, moderate physical activity during pregnancy, even after the first trimester. In many ways, maternal physiologic

Questions & Notes

Briefly explain Fartlek training.

Describe the 2 clinical forms of overtraining.

1.

2.

List 3 common symptoms of the overtraining syndrome.

1.

2.

3.

List 3 contraindications for exercising during pregnancy.

1.

2.

3.

responses and adaptations to exercise beneficially interact with physiologic changes in pregnancy.

Regular aerobic exercise throughout pregnancy accomplishes the following:

1. Reduces birth weight
2. Reduces birth weight percentile
3. Reduces the offspring's calculated percentage body fat and fat mass

Follow-up studies of children whose mothers regularly exercised during the second and third trimesters indicated these children maintained similar height and head girth but weighed less and had significantly lower sum of five skinfolds and lower upper-arm fat than children of sedentary women during pregnancy. The offspring of active mothers had higher scores on intelligence tests, including superior oral language skills. Benefits to fetal neurologic development and increased mental capacity have been linked to one or more of the following for providing the "stimulus" for positive benefits associated with regular exercise during pregnancy: intermittent stress, vibration, sound, motion, and accelerated heartbeat. *The offspring of exercising women did not show evidence of a comparative deficit in any area examined.* These findings should reassure active women who chose to continue exercising during an uncomplicated pregnancy.

Fourteen Contraindications for Exercising During Pregnancy

1. Pregnancy-induced hypertension
2. Preterm rupture of membranes
3. Preterm labor during the prior or current pregnancy
4. Incompetent cervix
5. Persistent second to third trimester bleeding
6. Intrauterine growth retardation
7. Type 1 diabetes
8. History of two or more spontaneous abortions
9. Multiple pregnancy
10. Smoking
11. Excessive alcohol intake
12. History of premature labor
13. Anemia
14. Excessive obesity

 SUMMARY

1. Activation of a specific energy transfer system in exercise provides a way to classify diverse physical activities. Effective training allocates appropriate time to overload the energy system(s) involved in the activity.

2. Exercise intensity and duration largely determine the degree of anaerobic and aerobic energy transfer during physical activity.

3. During sprint-power activities, primary energy transfer involves the immediate and short-term energy systems.

4. The long-term aerobic system becomes progressively more important in activities longer than 2 minutes' duration.

5. Proper exercise training recognizes four principles for producing and maintaining optimum improvements: overload, specificity, individual differences, and reversibility.

6. Anaerobic training increases resting intramuscular anaerobic substrates and key glycolytic enzymes that typically increase all-out, sprint-power exercise performance.

7. Aerobic training must overload both circulatory function and metabolic capacity of specific muscles. Peripheral adaptations in active tissues exert a substantial benefit to exercise performance.

8. The four major factors that affect aerobic training improvement include initial fitness level, frequency of training, duration of exercise, and exercise intensity. Exercise intensity exerts the most profound influence.

9. Aerobic training adaptations to generate ATP aerobically include (1) increases in mitochondrial size and number, (2) improved activity of aerobic enzymes, (3) greater capillarization of trained muscle, and (4) enhanced oxidation of fats during submaximal exercise.

10. Functional and dimensional changes in the cardiovascular system induced by aerobic training include (1) decrease in resting and submaximal exercise heart rate, (2) enlarged left ventricular cavity, (3) enhanced stroke volume and cardiac output, and (4) expanded a-$\bar{v}O_2$ difference.

11. Two ways establish training intensity: (1) on an absolute basis (standard exercise load or oxygen uptake) or (2) on a relative basis geared to an individual's physiologic response (%$\dot{V}O_{2max}$ or %HR_{max}).

12. The most effective methods to prescribe exercise are based on (1) percentage of HR_{max} ($\geq$65% to 70% age-predicted HR_{max}), (2) percentage of heart rate reserve, or (3) rating of perceived exertion.

13. HR_{max} averages about 13 bpm lower in upper-body exercise (arm-cranking, swimming) than in lower-body exercise (walking, running, cycling, stair stepping).

14. Three days minimum per week represents an effective frequency for aerobic training.

15. When intensity, duration, and frequency remain constant, similar training improvements emerge regardless of training mode provided the evaluation test uses the training exercise.

16. If exercise intensity remains at the training level, exercise frequency and duration can decrease by two-thirds without compromising gains in $\dot{V}O_{2max}$.

17. Prolonged and intense training can lead to overtraining or staleness with associated alterations in neuroendocrine and immune functions. The syndrome includes chronic fatigue, poor exercise performance, frequent infections, and general loss of interest in training.

18. Moderate aerobic exercise by a previously active and healthy, low-risk woman during an uncomplicated pregnancy does not compromise fetal well-being or produce adverse maternal effects.

THOUGHT QUESTIONS

1. Discuss whether regular physical activity benefits a person, even if exercise remains insufficient to stimulate a training effect.

2. Your personal training client insists that a single mode of cross-training exercise improves aerobic fitness for all physical activities that require a high level of aerobic fitness. Give your opinion regarding the effectiveness of single-mode cross-training exercise.

3. Respond to the question, "How long will it take me to get in shape once I begin an exercise program?"

4. What information do you need to develop a program to effectively improve and evaluate aerobic capacity for the specific physical job performance requirements for firefighters, police officers, and oilfield workers?

SELECTED REFERENCES

Albertus, Y., et al.: Effect of distance feedback on pacing strategy and perceived exertion during cycling. *Med. Sci. Sports Exerc.*, 37:461, 2005.

American College of Sports Medicine: *Guidelines for Exercise Testing and Prescription*, 8th ed. Baltimore: Lippincott, Williams & Wilkins, 2010.

American College of Sports Medicine: Position stand on the recommended quantity and quality of exercise for developing and maintaining cardiorespiratory and muscular fitness, and flexibility in healthy adults. *Med. Sci. Sports Exerc.*, 30:975, 1998.

Bautmans, I., et al.: Biochemical changes in response to intensive resistance exercise training in the elderly. *Gerontology*, 51:253, 2005.

Borg-Stein, J., et al.: Musculoskeletal aspects of pregnancy. *Am. J. Phys. Med. Rehabil.*, 84:180, 2005.

Borg, G.A.: Psychological basis of physical exertion. *Med. Sci. Sports Exerc.*, 14:377, 1982.

Bosquet, L., et al.: Effects of tapering on performance: A meta-analysis. *Med. Sci. Sports Exerc.*, 39:1358, 2006.

Boule, N.G., et al.: HERITAGE Family Study. Effects of exercise training on glucose homeostasis: the HERITAGE Family Study. *Diabetes Care*, 28:108, 2005.

Boule, N.G., et al.: Physical fitness and the metabolic syndrome in adults from the Quebec Family Study. *Can. J. Appl. Physiol.*, 30:140, 2005.

Church, T.S., et al.: Effects of different doses of physical activity on cardiorespiratory fitness among sedentary, overweight or obese postmenopausal women with elevated blood pressure: A randomized controlled trial. *JAMA.*, 2007;297:2081.

Colado, J.C., García-Massó, X.: Technique and safety aspects of resistance exercises: A systematic review of the literature. *Phys. Sportsmed.*, 37(2):104, 2009.

Coyle, E.F.: Improved muscular efficiency displayed as Tour de France champion matures. *J. Appl. Physiol.*, 98:2191, 2005.

Coyle, E.F.: Very intense exercise-training is extremely potent and time efficient: A reminder. *J. Appl. Physiol.*, 98:1983, 2005.

Dempsey, J.C., et al.: No need for a pregnant pause: physical activity may reduce the occurrence of gestational diabetes mellitus and preeclampsia. *Exerc. Sport Sci. Rev.*, 33:141, 2005.

Denadai, B.S., Higino, W.P.: Effect of the passive recovery period on the lactate minimum speed in sprinters and endurance runners. *J. Sci. Med. Sport*, 7:488, 2004.

Dolezal, B.A., Potteiger, J.A.: Concurrent resistance and endurance training influence basal metabolic rate in nondieting individuals. *J. Appl. Physiol.*, 85:695, 1998.

Duffield, R., et al.: Energy system contribution to 400-metre and 800-metre track running. *J. Sports Sci.*, 23:299, 2005.

Eston, R.G., et al.: The validity of predicting maximal oxygen uptake from a perceptually-regulated graded exercise test. *Eur. J. Appl. Physiol.*, 94:221, 2005.

Faulkner, J.A., et al.: Age-related changes in the structure and function of skeletal muscles. *Clin. Exp. Pharmacol Physiol.*, 34:109, 2007.

Flerreira, I., et al.: Longitudinal changes in $\dot{V}O_{2max}$: associations with carotid IMT and arterial stiffness. *Med. Sci. Sports Exerc.*, 35:1670, 2003.

García-Pallarés, J., et al.: Physiological effects of tapering and detraining in world-class kayakers. *Med. Sci. Sports Exerc.*, 42: 1209, 2010.

Gaston, A., Prapavessis, H.: Maternal-fetal disease information as a source of exercise motivation during pregnancy. *Health Psychol.*; 28:726, 2009.

Gavard, J.A., Artal, R.: Effect of exercise on pregnancy outcome. *Clin. Obstet. Gynecol.*, 51:467, 2008.

Gellish, R.L., et al.: Longitudinal modeling of the relationship between age and maximal heart rate. *Med. Sci. Sports Exerc.*, 39:822, 2007.

Gibala, M.J., McGee, S.L.: Metabolic adaptations to short-term high-intensity interval training: A little pain for a lot of gain? *Exerc. Sport Sci. Rev.*, 36:58, 2008.

Glowacki, S.P., et al.: Effects of resistance, endurance, and concurrent exercise on training outcomes in men. *Med. Sci. Sports Exerc.*, 36:2119, 2004.

Gomez-Cabrera, M.C., Viña, J., Ji, L.L.:Interplay of oxidants and antioxidants during exercise: implications for muscle health. *Phys. Sportsmed.*, 37(4):116, 2009.

González-Alonso, J.: Point: Counterpoint: Stroke volume does/does not decline during exercise at maximal effort in healthy individuals. *J. Appl. Physiol.*, 104:275, 2008.

Green, J.G., et al.: Active recovery strategies and handgrip performance in trained vs. untrained climbers. *J. Strength Cond. Res.*, 24:494, 2010.

Gurd, B.J., et al.: High-intensity interval training increases SIRT1 activity in human skeletal muscle. *Appl. Physiol. Nutr. Metab.*, 35:350, 2010.

Hagberg, J.M., et al.: Specific genetic markers of endurance performance and $\dot{V}O_{2max}$. *Exer. Sport Sci. Rev.*, 29:15, 2001.

Hartmann, U., Mester, J.: Training and overtraining markers in selected sport events. *Med. Sci. Sports Exerc.*, 32:209, 2000.

Haskell, W.L., et al.: Physical activity and public health: Updated recommendation for adults from the American College of Sports Medicine and the American Heart Association. *Med. Sci. Sports Exerc.*, 39:1423, 2007.

Helgerud, J., et al.: Aerobic high-intensity intervals improve $\dot{V}O_{2max}$ more than moderate training. *Med. Sci. Sports Exerc.*, 39:665, 2007.

Holloszy, J.O., Coyle, E.F.: Adaptations of skeletal muscle to endurance exercise and their metabolic consequences. *J. Appl. Physiol.*, 56:831, 1984.

Holloszy, J.O.: Metabolic consequences of endurance training. In: *Exercise, Nutrition, and Energy Metabolism*. Horton, E.S. and Terjung, R.L. (eds.). New York: Macmillan, 1988.

Jougla, A., et al.: Effects of active vs. passive recovery on repeated rugby-specific exercises. *J. Sci. Med. Sport*, 13:350, 2010.

Juhl, M., et al.: Physical exercise during pregnancy and the risk of preterm birth: a study within the Danish National Birth Cohort. *Am. J. Epidemiol.*, 1;167:859, 2008.

Kang, J., et al.: Metabolic and perceptual responses during spinning cycle exercise. *Med. Sci. Sports Exerc.*, 37:853, 2005.

Kardel, K.R.: Effects of intense training during and after pregnancy in top-level athletes. *Scand. J. Med. Sci. Sports*, 15:79, 2005.

Keytel, L.R., et al.: Prediction of energy expenditure from heart rate monitoring during submaximal exercise. *J. Sports Sci.*, 23:289, 2005.

Klika, R.J., Callahan, K.E., Drum, S.N.: Individualized 12-week exercise training programs enhance aerobic capacity of cancer survivors. *Phys., Sportsmed.*, 37(3):68, 2009.

Kraemer, W.J., et al.: Effects of concurrent resistance and aerobic training on load-bearing performance and the Army physical fitness test. *Mil. Med.*, 169:994, 2004.

Lee, C.M., et al.: Influence of short-term endurance exercise training on heart rate variability. *Med. Sci. Sports Exerc.*, 35:961, 2003.

Lee, I-M., et al.: Physical activity and coronary heart disease in women: is "no pain no gain" passé? *JAMA.*, 285:1447, 2001.

Luden, N., et al.: Myocellular basis for tapering in competitive distance runners. *J. Appl. Physiol.*, 108:1501, 2010.

Manzi, V., et al.: Profile of weekly training load in elite male professional basketball players. *J. Strength Cond. Res.*, 24:1399, 2010.

Mayo, M.J., et al.: Exercise-induced weight loss preferentially reduces abdominal fat. *Med. Sci. Sports Exerc.*, 35:207, 2003.

Menzies, P., et al.: Blood lactate clearance during active recovery after an intense running bout depends on the intensity of the active recovery. *J. Sports Sci.*, 28:975, 2010.

Messonnier, L., et al.: Are the effects of training on fat metabolism involved in the improvement of performance during high-intensity exercise? *Eur. J. Appl. Physiol.*, 94:434, 2005.

Meyer, T., et al.: A conceptual framework for performance diagnosis and training prescription from submaximal gas exchange parameters—theory and application. *Int. J. Sports Med.*, 26(Suppl 1):S38, 2005.

Morris, S.N., Johnson, N.R.: Exercise during pregnancy: a critical appraisal of the literature. *J. Reprod. Med.*, 50:181, 2005.

Mourtzakis, M., et al.: Hemodynamics and O_2 uptake during maximal knee extension exercise in untrained and trained human quadriceps muscle. *J. Appl. Physiol.*, 97:1796, 2004.

Mujika, I., Padilla, S.: Scientific basis for precompetition tapering strategies. *Med. Sci. Sports Exerc.*, 34:1182, 2003.

Murtagh, E.M., et al.: The effects of 60 minutes of brisk walking per week, accumulated in two different patterns, on cardiovascular risk. *Prev. Med.*, 41:92, 2005.

Nelson, M.E., et al.: Physicl activity and public health in older adults: Recommendation from the American College of Sports Medicine and the American Heart Association. *Med. Sci. Sports Exerc.*, 39:1435, 2006.

Pena, K.E., Stopka, C.B., et al.: Effects of low-intensity exercise on patients with peripheral artery disease. *Phys. Sportsmed.*, 3 7(1):106, 2009.

Persinger, R.C., et al.: Consistency of the talk test for exercise prescription. *Med. Sci. Sports Exerc.*, 36:1632, 2004.

Poudevigne, M.S., O'Connor, P.J.: Physical activity and mood during pregnancy. *Med. Sci. Sports Exerc.*, 2005;37:1374.

Ramírez-Vélez, R., et al.: Clinical trial to assess the effect of physical exercise on endothelial function and insulin resistance in pregnant women. *Trials.*, 17;104, 2009.

Rankinen, T., et al.: The human gene map for performance and health-related fitness phenotypes: The 2003 update. *Med. Sci. Sports Exerc.*, 36:1451, 2004.

Ricardo, D.R., et al.: Initial and final exercise heart rate transients: Influence of gender, aerobic fitness, and clinical status. *Chest*, 127:318, 2005.

Robergs, R.A., et al.: Biochemistry of exercise-induced metabolic acidosis. *Am. J. Physiol. Regul. Integr. Comp. Physiol.*, 287:R502, 2004.

Tanasescu, M., et al.: Exercise type and intensity in relation to coronary heart disease in men. *JAMA.*, 288:1994, 2002.

Tinken, T.M., et al: Shear stress mediates endothelial adaptations to exercise training in humans. *Hypertension.*, 55:312, 2010.

Trinity, J.D., et al.: Maximal mechanical power during a taper in elite swimmers. *Med. Sci. Sports Exerc.*, 38:1643, 2006.

Venables, M.C., Jeukendrup, A.E.: Endurance training and obesity: Effect on substrate metabolism and insulin sensitivity. *Med. Sci. Sports Exerc.*, 40:495, 2008.

Vollaard, N.B., et al.: Exercise-induced oxidative stress in overload training and tapering. *Med. Sci. Sports Exerc.*, 38:1335, 2006.

Walter, A.A., et al.: Six weeks of high-intensity interval training with and without beta-alanine supplementation for improving cardiovascular fitness in women. *J. Strength Cond. Res.*, 24: 1199, 2010.

Walther, C., et al.: The effect of exercise training on endothelial function in cardiovascular disease in humans. *Exerc. Sport Sci. Rev.*, 32:129, 2004.

Warburton, D.E.R., Gledhill, N.: Counterpoint: Stroke volume does not decline during exercise at maximal effort in healthy individuals. *J. Appl. Physiol.*, 104:276, 2008.

Warner, S.O., et al.: The effects of resistance training on metabolic health with weight regain. *J. Clin. Hypertens.*, 12:64, 2010.

Weltman, A., et al.: Exercise training at and above lactate threshold in previously untrained women. *Int. J. Sports Med.*, 13:257, 1992.

Weltman, A., et al.: Repeated bouts of exercise alter the blood lactate-RPE relation. *Med. Sci. Sports Exerc.*, 30:1113, 1998.

Westcott, W.L., et al.: Prescribing physical activity: Applying the ACSM protocols for exercise type, intensity, and duration across 3 training frequencies. *Phys. Sportsmed.*, 37(2):51, 2009.

Wiltshire, E.V., et al.: Massage impairs postexercise muscle blood flow and "lactic acid" removal. *Med. Sci. Sports Exerc.*, 42:1062, 2010.

Zaryski, C., Smith, D.J.: Training principles and issues for ultra-endurance athletes. *Curr. Sports Med. Rep.*, 4:165, 2005.

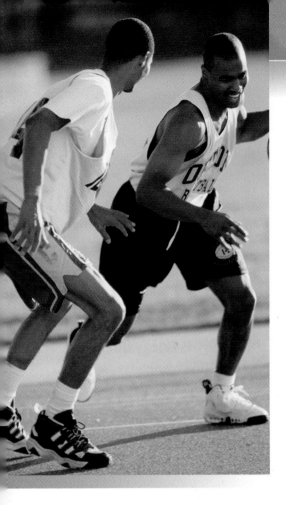

14

Training Muscles to Become Stronger

CHAPTER OBJECTIVES

- Describe the following four methods to assess muscular strength: cable tensiometry, dynamometry, one-repetition maximum (1-RM), and computer-assisted isokinetic dynamometry.

- Outline the procedure to assess 1-RM for bench press and leg press.

- Explain how to ensure test standardization and fairness when evaluating muscular strength.

- Compare absolute and relative upper- and lower-body muscular strength in men and women.

- Define *concentric*, *eccentric*, and *isometric* muscle actions, including examples of each.

- Recommend the appropriate frequency, overload, and sets and repetitions for dynamic exercise resistance training.

- Explain the specificity of training response for muscular strength related to enhanced performance in sports and occupational tasks.

- Compare isokinetic resistance training with conventional dynamic and static resistance training.

- Describe the rationale for plyometric training to improve muscular strength and power and give examples of exercises for these purposes.

- Indicate how psychological and muscular factors influence maximum strength capacity.

- Outline the major physiologic adaptations to resistance training.

- Develop a circuit resistance training program to improve muscular strength and aerobic fitness simultaneously.

- Describe tests to assess muscular endurance for the abdominals and chest–shoulder areas.

- Describe delayed-onset muscle soreness (DOMS) related to (1) type of exercise most frequently associated with DOMS, (2) best way to minimize DOMS effects when beginning a training program, and (3) cellular factors related to DOMS.

| Part 1 | Muscular Strength
Measurement and
Improvement |
| --- | --- |

Lifting weights began as a spectator sport in the United States and Europe in the early 1840s practiced by "strongmen" showcasing their prowess in traveling carnivals and sideshows. Much of the "science" of strength development at that time can be attributed to Pehr Henrik Ling remembered as the father of Swedish gymnastics who in 1813 founded the current Swedish School of Sport and Health Sciences under the name of the Royal Central Institute of Gymnastics, Stockholm and his son Hylmar (1820–1886), both influential writers and practitioners during the genesis of early movement science education and methodology. Their many disciples became experts in physical education in Sweden and Europe, and their influential techniques of strength development migrated to the British Isles and eventually the United States. Teachers were trained not only as physical education instructors in the schools but also for government work as military gymnastics instructors and physiotherapists.

Figure 14.1 shows examples of late 19th century "strength and exercise machines" popularized by Swedish physician Gustav Zander, MD (1835–1920), which were strongly influenced by the Lings' Swedish Gymnastic movement. Zander's methods for treating patients and the common person included standard gymnastic exercise regimens, mostly calistenics, balance, and core trunk and limb. Included were workouts on his mechanical exercise machines that served double duty for general strength development and "mechanical gymnastic treatments" for morbid disorders and diseases of the heart, nerves, respiratory and abdominal organs, obesity, gout, and rheumatism of the articulations including scoliosis. Dr. Zander's many successful treatment clinics in the 1890s that featured his machines opened up a new vista and attitude toward self-enhancement through exercise for fitness and health. During this period in the United States, measuring muscular strength became popular to evaluate physical fitness and body development, particularly in schools, colleges, physiotherapy centers, and local gymnasia and exercise training centers.

In 1897 at a meeting of American College Gymnasium Directors, strength contests were established to determine overall body strength based on back, leg, arm, and chest strength. The first six colleges to participate were Amherst College, Columbia University, Harvard University, The University of Minnesota, Dickinson College, and Wesleyan College. The overall winner of the competition was Harvard followed closely by Columbia. By the mid-1900s, physical culture specialists, body builders, competitive weight lifters, field-event athletes, and some wrestlers used traditional weight lifting exercises, not the passive methods of massage and electrical vibration that also flourished during this time. Research in the late 1950s and early 1960s dispelled the myth that traditional muscle-strengthening exercises reduces movement speed or range of joint motion. Instead, the opposite usually occurred; elite weight lifters, body builders, and "muscle men" had exceptional joint flexibility without limitations in general limb movement speed. For untrained healthy individuals, heavy-resistance exercises increased the speed and power of muscular effort without impairing subsequent sports performance.

The following sections explore the underlying rationale for strength training, including acute and chronic physiologic adjustments as muscles become stronger with training.

FOUNDATIONS FOR STUDYING MUSCULAR STRENGTH

The inclusion of strength development programs as part of athletic training regimens is not new; it prepared men for warfare in ancient China, Japan, India, Greece, and Rome. When the ancient Olympic games first began in 776 BC, athletes trained nearly year-round and incorporated muscle-strengthening exercises into their training regimens.

The scientific foundations for strength training for athletes began with the Chinese in 3600 BC. During the Chou dynasty (1122–249 BC) conscripts had to pass weight-lifting tests before becoming soldiers. Weight training also took place in ancient Egypt and India; sculptures and illustrations depict athletes training with heavy stone weights. Women practiced weight training; wall mosaics recovered from Roman villas showed young women exercising with handheld weights. During the "Age of Strength" in the 6th century, weight-lifting competitions often took place between soldiers and athletes. Galen, the famous early Greek physician (see Chapter 1), referred to exercising with weights (halters) in his insightful treatise, *The Preservation of Health*.

OBJECTIVES OF RESISTANCE TRAINING

Resistance training and strength development, besides having a theoretical basis, apply to six main areas:

1. Weight lifting and power lifting competition (who is strongest?)
2. Body building (maximize muscular development for aesthetic goals)
3. General strength training (fitness and health enhancement)
4. Physical therapy (rehabilitation from injury or disease)

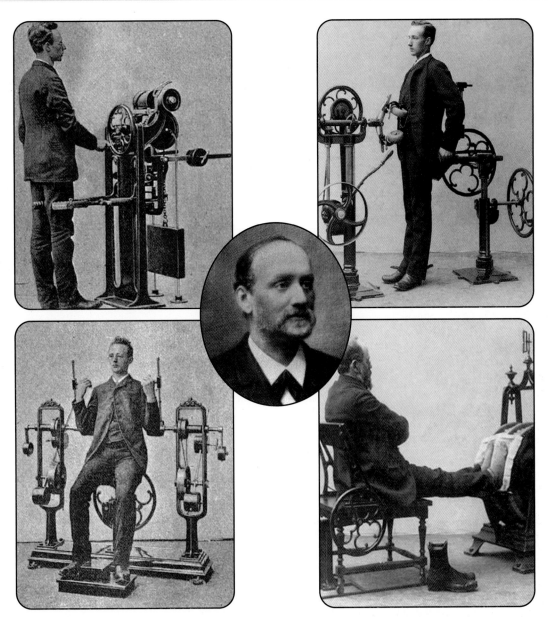

Figure 14.1   Four examples of late 19th century "strength machines" popularized by Swedish physician Gustav Zander, MD (1835–1920), who produced 27 mechanical apparatuses that became prototypes of common equipment now ubiquitous in physical fitness gyms and training centers worldwide. Perhaps serendipitously (or not), the successful Nautilus line of exercise equipment was remarkably similar in design to many of Zander's machines (*www.studioumanyc.com/zander.html*). Zander and his followers believed their complex mechanized machines using pulleys and counterbalances that emphasized "progressive exertion" to control the body's muscles to build strength could play a decisive role to create more positive health outcomes than bloodletting, purging, or strenuous acrobatics and non–physician-approved allopathic "cures" of the time. Zander marketed his steam-powered machines as a "preventative against the evils engendered by a sedentary life and the seclusion of the office." At the turn of the twentieth century, Zander machines were showcased at elite east coast health spas, at the Massachusetts General Hospital outpatient department beginning in 1904, and at private clinics near Central Park in New York City. While strapped into the apparatus, the motor provided the power to passively exercise the joints and muscles throughout their range of motion. Each machine was designed to exercise a different body region. Zander's mechanized machines disappeared after the Great Depression, replaced by smaller, more compact equipment that evolved over the next 75 years into modern strength and fitness training "active machines." (Photos from Levertin, A.: *Dr. G. Zanders Medico-Mechanical Gymnastics. It's Method, Importance and Application*. Stockholm: P.A. Norstead & Sonner, 1893.)

5. Sport-specific resistance training (maximize sport performance)
6. Muscle physiology (understanding structure and function)

RESISTANCE TRAINING VOCABULARY

Many terms and jargon abound in the area of resistance training, yet certain terms consistently appear in the research literature and popular writings about resistance training methods and outcomes. Table 14.1 defines common resistance training terms.

TYPES OF MUSCLE ACTION

The three types of muscle action include:

1. **Concentric action** represents the most common form of muscle action; it occurs in dynamic activities during which muscles shorten and produce tension through the range of motion. **Figure 14.2A** illustrates a concentric muscle action by raising a dumbbell from the extended to flexed elbow position.
2. **Eccentric action** (also called *lengthening or plyometrics*) occurs when external resistance

Table 14.1	Definition of Selected Terms Appearing in the Resistance Training Literature
1. Cheating	Breaking from strict form when performing an exercise (e.g., rather than maintaining an erect upper body when performing a standing arm curl, a slight body swing at the start the movement allows the person to lift a heavier weight or the same weight more times). Cheating increases the risk of injury if performed improperly.
2. Circuit resistance training (CRT)	Series of resistance training exercises performed in sequence with minimal rest between exercises. More frequent repetitions with less resistance (usually 40% to 50% of 1-RM) stimulate the cardiovascular system to produce an aerobic training effect.
3. Concentric action	Muscle shortening during force application.
4. Dynamic constant external resistance (DCER) training	Resistance training in which external resistance or weight does not change; joint flexion and extension occur with each repetition. Formerly (but incorrectly) referred to as "isotonic" exercise.
5. Eccentric action	Muscle lengthening occurs during force application.
6. Exercise intensity	Muscle force expressed as a percentage of muscle's maximum force-generating capacity or some level of maximum.
7. Isokinetic action	Muscle action performed at constant angular limb velocity.
8. Isometric action	Muscle action without noticeable change in muscle length.
9. Maximal voluntary muscle action (MVMA)	Maximal force generated in one repetition (1-RM), or performing a series of submaximal actions to momentary failure.
10. Muscular endurance	Sustaining maximum (or submaximum) force; often determined by assessing maximum number of exercise repetitions at a percentage of maximum strength.
11. Overload	A muscle acting against a resistance normally not encountered (unaccustomed stress).
12. Periodization	Variation in training volume and intensity over a specified time period; the goal is to prevent staleness while peaking physiologically for competition.
13. Plyometrics	Resistance training involving eccentric-to-concentric actions performed quickly so a muscle stretches slightly before the concentric action, using the stretch reflex to augment the muscle's force-generating capacity.
14. Power	Rate of performing work (Force × Distance ÷ Time, or Force × Velocity). Power applied to weight lifting relates to the mass lifted times the vertical distance it moves divided by the time to complete the movement. If 100 lb moves vertically 3 feet in 1 second, then the power generated = 100 lb × 3 ft ÷ 1 s or 300 ft-lb·s^{-1}.
15. Progressive overload	Incrementally increasing the stress placed on a muscle to produce greater force or greater endurance.
16. Range of motion (ROM)	Maximum ROM through an arc of a joint.
17. Repetition	One complete exercise movement, usually consisting of concentric and eccentric muscle actions or one complete isometric muscle action.
18. Repetition maximum (RM)	Greatest force generated for one repetition of a movement (1-RM) or predetermined number of repetitions (e.g., 5- or 10-RM).
19. Set	Pre-established number of repetitions performed.
20. Sticking point	Region in an exercise movement (against a set resistance) that provides the greatest difficulty to complete the movement.
21. Strength	Maximum force-generating capacity of a muscle or group of muscles.
22. Suspension training	Leveraging a person's body weight during exercise (without reliance on externally fixed weights, pulleys, or cams) by increasing or decreasing the suspension coordinates—the height of ropes, pulleys, slings, or bungee cords—relative to the suspension point.
23. Torque	Force that produces a turning, twisting, or rotary movement in any plane about an axis (i.e., movement of bones about a joint); commonly expressed in newton-meters (Nm).
24. Training volume	Total work performed in a single training session.
25. Variable resistance training	Training with equipment that uses a lever arm, cam, hydraulic system, or pulley to alter the resistance to match the increases and decreases in a muscle's capacity throughout a joint's ROM.

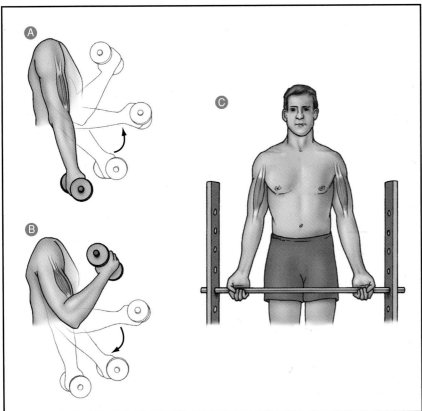

Figure 14.2 Muscular force during concentric (shortening) (**A**), eccentric (lengthening) (**B**), and isometric (static) (**C**) actions.

exceeds muscle force, and muscle lengthens as tension develops. **Figure 14.2B** shows a weight slowly lowered against the force of gravity. The sarcomeres in the activated muscle fibers of the upper-arm muscles lengthen in an eccentric action to prevent the dumbbell from crashing to the surface. In weight lifting, muscles frequently act eccentrically as the weight slowly returns to the starting position to begin the next concentric (shortening) muscle action. Eccentric action during this "recovery" phase adds to the total work and effectiveness of the exercise repetition.

The term *isotonic*, derived from the Greek word *isotonos* (*iso* meaning the same or equal, *tonos* meaning tension or strain), commonly refers to concentric and eccentric muscle actions because movement occurs. This term lacks precision when applied to muscle actions that involve movement because the muscle's effective force-generating capacity continually varies as the joint angle changes throughout the ROM.

3. **Isometric action** (also called *static* or *stationary*) occurs when a muscle generates force and attempts to shorten but cannot overcome the external resistance as shown in **Figure 14.2C** during muscular action against an immovable bar in an isometric rack. From a physics standpoint, this type of muscle action does not produce external work. An isometric action can generate considerable force despite the lack of noticeable lengthening or shortening of muscle and subsequent joint movement.

Dynamic constant external resistance (**DCER**) refers to resistance training during which external resistance or weight does not change, but raising (concentric) and lowering (eccentric) phases occur during each repetition. *DCER implies that the external weight or resistance remains constant throughout the movement.*

Questions & Notes

List 2 objectives of resistance training.

1.

2.

List the 3 types of muscle actions.

1.

2.

3.

Define the following terms:

Eccentric:

Concentric:

Muscular endurance:

Torque:

Define 1-RM maximum.

MEASUREMENT OF MUSCULAR STRENGTH

Different methods commonly assess isometric and concentric/eccentric **muscular strength** (defined as the maximum force, tension, or torque generated by a muscle or muscle groups).

Isometric Muscle Testing

With **isometric** testing, muscle force is measured at a specific joint angle. **Figure 14.3** shows three different isometric testing devices. In **Figure 14-3A, a** cable tensiometer assesses static muscular force during knee extension. Increased force on the cable depresses a riser over which the cable passes; this deflects the pointer and indicates the amount of force applied. The application of the tensiometer for strength measurements differs considerably from its original use for measuring tension on steel cables linking various parts of an airplane.

Figures 14.3B and **C** display hand-grip and back-lift **dynamometers** to assess static strength. Both devices operate on the principle of compression. Application of

external force to the dynamometer compresses a steel spring and moves a pointer. By knowing how much force must move the pointer a given distance, one can determine how much external "static" force has been applied to the dynamometer.

Computer-assisted devices (see next section) are also used to assess isometric muscle force.

Eccentric/Concentric Muscle Strength Testing

One-Repetition Maximum The **one-repetition maximum** (**1-RM**) technique refers to a dynamic method to assess eccentric/concentric. To test 1-RM for single or multiple muscle groups, choose the initial weight close to but below maximum lifting capacity (see Close Up Box 14.1, *How to Assess and Evaluate One-Repetition Maximum for Bench Press and Leg Press* on page 450). Weight is progressively added on subsequent attempts until the person reaches maximum lift capacity. The weight increments range between 1 to 5 kg depending on the muscle group evaluated. Rest intervals of 1 to 5 minutes provide sufficient recuperation before attempting a lift at the next heavier weight.

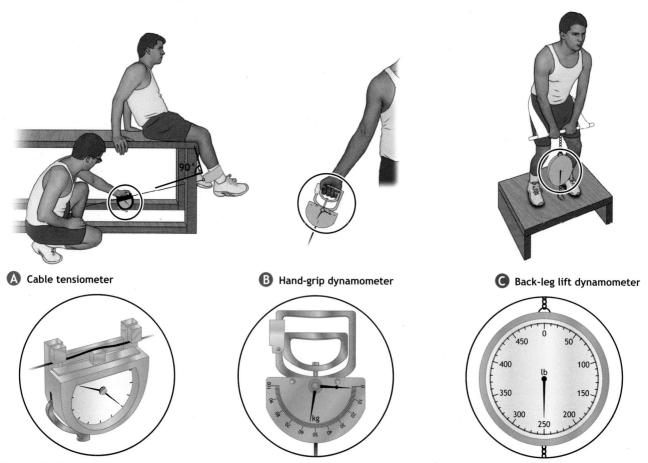

A Cable tensiometer   **B** Hand-grip dynamometer   **C** Back-leg lift dynamometer

Figure 14.3 Measurement of static strength by cable tensiometer (**A**), hand-grip dynamometer (**B**), and (**C**) back-leg lift dynamometer (**C**).

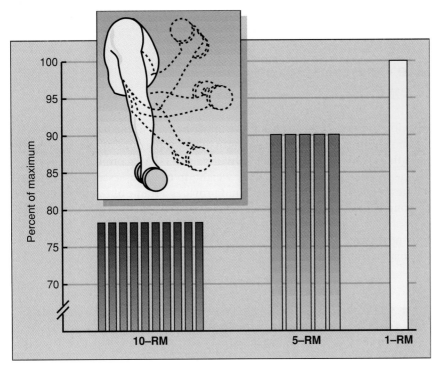

Figure 14.4 Three methods for assessing force-generating capacity in a dynamic movement.

*Q*uestions & Notes

Define muscular strength.

List 2 methods to assess isometric strength.

  1.

  2.

What is the optimum weight increment when using the 1-RM method to test muscle strength.

Describe the relationship between muscular endurance and percentage of 1-RM lifted.

In addition to the 1-RM method, **Figure 14.4** illustrates two submaximal methods and the percentage of maximum each represents to evaluate a muscle's force- and power-generating capacity. In these tests, the greatest amount of weight lifted five or 10 times becomes the repetition maximum to assess strength. The measurement procedure in these cases assesses 5-RM (generally 90% of maximum) or 10-RM (~78% of maximum). The 5- and 10-RM methods provide appropriate markers of muscular strength for testing children and older adults in whom maximal lifting may be contraindicated.

Estimating 1-RM Strength Using Submaximum Repetitions-to-Fatigue Test Scores
A strong inverse relationship exists between muscular endurance (number of repetitions-to-fatigue using a submaximum resistance) and percentage of 1-RM lifted; that is, the heavier the load, the fewer number of repetitions performed (see Load-Repetition Relationship in Table in Close Up Box 14.2: *How to Assign Load (Resistance) and Repetition Number to Achieve Different Training Goals*, on page 454). When 1-RM testing is unwarranted or ill-advised (i.e., in preadolescents, elderly people, individuals wth cardiovascular disease or physical limitations, poorly conditioned individuals), 1-RM strength can be predicted using repetitions-to-fatigue with a submaximum weight. The two equations shown differ because resistance training alters the relationship between a submaximal performance (7- to 10-RM) and maximal lift capacity (1-RM). Generally, the weight that one can lift for 7- to 10-RM represents about 68% of the 1-RM score for the untrained person and 79% of the new 1-RM after training.

ⓘ For Your Information

FIVE QUESTIONS TO ANSWER BEFORE INITIATING RESISTANCE TRAINING FOR CHILDREN

1. Is the child psychologically and physically ready to participate?
2. Does the child understand proper lifting techniques for each exercise?
3. Does the child understand the safety needs?
4. Does the equipment fit the child?
5. Does the child have a balanced overall physical activity program?

$$\text{Untrained: 1-RM (kg)} = 1.554 \times \text{7- to 10-RM weight (kg)} - 5.181$$

$$\text{Trained: 1-RM (kg)} = 1.172 \times \text{7- to 10-RM weight (kg)} + 7.704$$

BOX 14.1 CLOSE UP

How to Assess and Evaluate One-Repetition Maximum for Bench and Leg Press

The maximum weight (resistance) lifted with proper form for 1-RM for a particular muscle action measures maximum eccentric/concentric muscle strength. A trial-and-error approach determines the 1-RM strength value. After each successful single lift (rest 2–3 minutes between attempts), the weight increases by 5 to 10 pounds until achieving the maximum weight lifted.

The 1-RM bench press (illustrated on the next page) assesses maximum muscular strength of the major mus-cle groups of the upper body, and the leg press assesses maximum strength of major portions of the lower-body musculature. Dividing the 1-RM score by body weight (1-RM, ÷ Body weight, lb or kg) assesses relative mus-cular strength and provides a frame of reference to eval-uate different body weight comparisons (see table below).

Reference Values for 1-RM Bench Press and Leg Press Expressed Relative to Body Weight[a]

	AGE, y			
RATING	20–29	30–39	40–49	50–59
Men				
Excellent				
Bench Press	>1.26	>1.08	>0.97	>0.86
Leg Press	>2.08	>1.88	>1.76	>1.66
Good				
Bench Press	1.17–1.25	1.01–1.07	0.91–0.96	0.81–0.85
Leg Press	2.00–2.07	1.80–1.87	1.70–1.75	1.60–1.65
Average				
Bench Press	0.97–1.16	0.86–1.00	0.78–0.90	0.70–0.80
Leg Press	1.83–1.99	1.63–1.79	1.56–1.69	1.46–1.59
Fair				
Bench Press	0.88–0.96	0.79–0.85	0.72–0.77	0.65–0.69
Leg Press	1.65–1.82	1.55–1.62	1.50–1.55	1.40–1.45
Poor				
Bench Press	<0.87	<0.78	<0.71	<0.60
Leg Press	<1.64	<1.54	<1.49	<1.39
Women				
Excellent				
Bench Press	>0.78	>0.66	>0.61	>0.54
Leg Press	>1.63	>1.42	>1.32	>1.26
Good				
Bench Press	0.72–0.77	0.62–0.65	0.57–0.60	0.51–0.53
Leg Press	1.54–1.62	1.35–1.41	1.26–1.31	1.13–1.25
Average				
Bench Press	0.59–0.71	0.53–0.61	0.48–0.56	0.43–0.50
Leg Press	1.35–1.53	1.20–1.34	1.12–1.25	0.99–1.12
Fair				
Bench Press	0.53–0.58	0.49–0.52	0.44–0.47	0.40–0.42
Leg Press	1.25–1.34	1.13–1.19	1.06–1.11	0.86–0.98
Poor				
Bench Press	<0.52	<0.48	<0.43	<0.39
Leg Press	<1.25	<1.12	<1.05	<0.85

Adapted from: Cooper Institute for Aerobics Research, 1997.
[a]Score = 1-RM, lb ÷ Body weight, lb.

Procedures for Bench Press Test

MUSCLE GROUPS	EQUIPMENT	STARTING POSITION	MOVEMENT
Shoulder flexors and adductors; elbow extensors	Barbell or bench press station on a single- or multistation resistance machine	Overhand (pronated) grip, slightly wider than shoulder width apart. Lay supine on a bench with the feet on the floor straddling the bench. Signal a spotter to position the bar at arms' length above the chest with the arms extended.	Downward movement: lower the bar until it touches the chest. Upward movement: push the bar up to full elbow extension while maintaining body position without arching the back. The spotter maintains grip on the bar throughout the movement without offering assistance; also helps to place the bar on the supports.

Procedures for Leg Press Test

MUSCLE GROUPS	EQUIPMENT	STARTING POSITION	MOVEMENT
Knee extensors and hip extensors.	Leg press on a single- or multistation resistance machine.	1. Sit with the legs parallel and the feet on the machine's foot rests. 2. Grasp the seat's handle.	1. Forward movement: push the foot rests steadily forward; do not forcefully lock out the knees during extension. 2. Backward movement: move the footrests slowly back to the starting position.

A = beginning; B = forward; C = and return.

For example, estimate 1-RM bench press score for a trained person whose 10-RM bench press equals 70 kg as follows:

$$1\text{-RM (kg)} = 1.172 \times 70 \text{ kg} + 7.704 = 89.7 \text{ kg}$$

Testing Protocol   Determine the maximum number of repetitions-to-fatigue a person can achieve at a given weight lifted. Use this number to predict the 1-RM. (Refer to the Close Up Box 14.2, *How To Assign Load [Resistance] and Repetition Number to Achieve Different Training Goals* for procedures to determine the maximum number of repetitions on page 454.) Use the data in Table 14.2 derived from several sources to determine 1-RM in these three steps:

1. Read across the Max Reps (RM) row and find the number of repetitions completed.
2. Read down the column to the load lifted (weight completed, in lb).
3. Read across the row to the far left to find the estimated 1-RM.

An example follows for an individual who performs a 5-RM test and lifts 174 lb.

1. Read across the Max Reps (RM) row and find the number 5 (number of repetitions-to-fatigue).

Table 14.2 — Estimating 1-RM from Submaximum Load (Weight) and Number of Repetitions

To use the table (1) read across the Max Reps (RM) row and find the number of repetitions completed; (2) read down the column to the load (weight completed, lb) lifted; (3) read across the row to the far left to find the estimated 1-RM.

MAX REPS (RM)	1	2	3	4	5	6	7	8	9	10	12	15
%1-RM	100	95	93	90	87	85	83	80	77	75	67	65
Load lifted (weight completed, lb) 10	10	10	9	9	9	9	8	8	8	8	7	7
20	20	9	19	18	17	17	17	16	15	15	13	13
30	30	9	28	27	26	26	25	24	23	23	20	20
40	40	38	37	36	35	34	33	32	31	30	27	26
50	50	48	47	45	44	43	42	40	39	38	34	33
60	60	57	56	54	52	51	50	48	46	45	40	39
70	70	67	65	63	61	60	58	56	54	53	47	46
80	80	76	74	72	70	68	66	64	62	60	54	52
90	90	86	84	81	78	77	75	72	69	68	60	59
100	100	95	93	90	87	85	83	80	77	75	67	65
110	110	105	102	99	96	94	91	88	85	83	74	72
120	120	114	112	108	104	102	100	96	92	90	80	78
130	130	124	121	117	113	111	108	104	100	98	87	85
140	140	133	130	126	122	119	116	112	108	105	94	91
150	150	143	140	135	131	128	125	120	116	113	101	98
160	160	152	149	144	139	136	133	128	123	120	107	104
170	170	162	158	153	148	145	141	136	131	128	114	111
180	180	171	167	162	157	153	149	144	139	135	121	117
190	190	181	177	171	165	162	158	152	146	143	127	124
200	200	190	186	180	174	170	166	160	154	150	134	130
210	210	200	195	189	183	179	174	168	162	158	141	137
220	220	209	205	198	191	187	183	176	169	165	147	143
230	230	219	214	207	200	196	191	184	177	173	154	150
240	240	228	223	216	209	204	199	192	185	180	161	156
250	250	238	233	225	218	213	208	200	193	188	168	163
260	260	247	242	234	226	221	206	208	200	195	174	169
270	270	257	251	243	235	230	224	216	208	203	181	176
280	280	266	260	252	244	238	232	224	216	210	188	182
290	290	276	270	261	252	247	241	232	223	218	194	189
300	300	285	279	270	261	255	249	240-	231	225	201	195
310	310	295	288	279	270	264	257	248	239	233	208	202
320	320	304	298	288	278	272	266	256	246	240	214	208
330	330	314	307	297	287	281	274	264	254	248	221	215
340	340	323	316	306	296	289	282	272	262	255	228	221
350	350	333	326	315	305	298	291	280	270	263	235	228
360	360	342	335	324	313	306	299	288	277	270	241	234
370	370	352	344	333	322	315	307	296	285	278	248	241
380	380	361	353	342	331	323	315	304	293	285	255	247
390	390	371	363	351	339	332	324	312	300	293	261	254
400	400	380	372	360	348	340	332	320	308	300	268	260

From Baechle, T.R., et al.: Resistance Training. In: *Essentials of Strength Training and Conditioning.* 2nd Ed. Champaign, IL: Human Kinetics Press, 2000.

2. Read down the column to the number 174 (the load lifted in lb).
3. Read across the row to the far left and find the estimated 1-RM (in this example, 200 lb).

The data in Table 14.2 also estimate the load (weight in lb) at a given percentage of 1-RM. For example, find the 1-RM load in column 1 (e.g., 120 lb); go across to the desired percentage in row 2 (%1-RM; 80%) and find the weight (in lb) corresponding to that percentage in the intersecting cell (in this example, 96 lb).

Computer-Assisted Electromechanical and Isokinetic Determinations

Microprocessor technology integrated with exercise equipment quantifies muscular force and power during a variety of movements. Modern instrumentation measures force, acceleration, and velocity of body segments in various movement patterns. Force platforms measure external application of muscular force by limbs during jumping. Other electromechanical devices measure forces generated during all movement phases of cycling, rowing, supine bench press, seated and upright leg press, as well as exercises for other trunk, arm, and leg movements.

An **isokinetic dynamometer**, an electromechanical accommodating resistance instrument with a speed-controlling mechanism, accelerates to a preset, constant velocity with applied force regardless of the force exerted on the movement arm. When this velocity is attained, the isokinetic loading mechanism adjusts automatically to provide a counterforce to variations in force generated by muscle as movement continues throughout the "strength curve." *Thus, maximum force or any percentage of maximum effort generates throughout the full ROM at a preestablished velocity of limb movement.* This allows training and measurement along a continuum from high-velocity (low-force) to low-velocity (high-force) conditions. A microprocessor within the dynamometer continuously monitors the immediate level of applied force. An electronic integrator in series with a monitor displays the average or peak force generated during any interval for almost instantaneous feedback about performance (e.g., force, torque, work).

The interface of microprocessor technology with mechanical devices provides the sport and exercise scientist with valuable data to evaluate, test, train, and rehabilitate individuals. The argument in support of isokinetic strength measurement maintains that muscle strength dynamics involve considerably more than *just* the final outcome of 1-RM. For example, two individuals with identical 1-RM scores could exhibit dissimilar force curves throughout the movement. Individual differences in force dynamics (e.g., time to peak tension) throughout the full ROM may reflect an entirely different underlying neuromuscular physiology that 1-RM cannot assess.

STRENGTH TESTING CONSIDERATIONS

Seven important considerations exist for muscle strength testing regardless of the measurement method:

1. Provide standardize instructions before testing.
2. Ensure uniformity in the duration and intensity of the warm–up.
3. Provide adequate practice before testing to minimize "learning" that could compromise initial results.
4. Ensure consistency among subjects in the angle of limb measurement or body position on the test device.
5. Predetermine a minimum number of trials (repetitions) to establish a criterion strength score. For example, if administering five repetitions of

*Q*uestions & Notes

List the 4 major training goals.

1.

2.

3.

4.

To achieve maximum strength goals, what is the recommended number of training repetitions?

List 3 important considerations for muscle strength training.

1.

2.

3.

Describe an isokinetic dynamometer.

a test, what score represents the individual's strength score? Is the highest score best, or should one use the average? In most cases, an average of several trials provides a more representative (reliable) strength or power score than a single measure.

6. Select test measures with high test score reproducibility. This crucial but often overlooked aspect of testing evaluates the variability of the subject's responses on repeated efforts. A lack of test score consistency (unreliability) can mask an individual's representative performance on the measure

or change in performance when evaluating strength improvement.

7. Recognize individual differences in body size and composition when evaluating strength scores among individuals and groups.

TRAINING MUSCLES TO BECOME STRONGER

A muscle strengthens when trained near its current maximal force-generating capacity. Standard weight-lifting equip-

---

BOX 14.2 CLOSE UP

How to Assign Load (Resistance) and Repetition Number to Achieve Different Training Goals

Assigning combinations of load (resistance) and repetition number (reps) constitutes the most important aspects of establishing a resistance training program. Research and practical experience indicate that resistances producing a maximum of 6 or fewer reps elicits the greatest increase in strength and maximal power output. Resistances that produce 10 to 15 or even 20 and above repetitions greatly impact muscular endurance development. This knowledge makes it possible to specifically train for a desired type of muscular performance.

IDENTIFYING TRAINING GOALS

Age, physical maturity, training history, and psychological and physical tolerance should formulate training goals or program design. Training goals center around four major objectives:

1. **Strength development** of specific muscle groups (i.e., upper or lower body, abdomen, back) for purposes relating to sports or job performance
2. **Power development** for specific sports performance (i.e., running back in football, basketball rebounder, high jumper, shot putter)
3. **Hypertrophic development** for appearance or to alter body size (i.e., weight gain) and to improve overall muscular strength
4. **Muscle endurance development** related to enhanced job or sports performance

ASSIGNING LOAD AND REPETITION

The accompanying Table recommends specific repetition maximums (RM) and load expressed as a percentage of 1-RM (%1-RM).

The following five-step sequence to determine loads and repetition number for individualized training makes use of data from **Table 14.2**:

Load: Repetition Continuum for Specific Training Goals		
TRAINING GOAL	**LOAD (% 1-RM)**	**GOAL REPETITIONS**
Strength	≥85	≤6
High power	80–90	1–2
Low power	75–85	3–5
Hypertrophy	67–85	6–12
Endurance	≤67	≥12

From Baechle, T.R., et al.: Resistance training. In: Baechle, T.R., Earle, R.W. (eds.). *Essentials of Strength Training and Conditioning,* 2nd ed. Champaign, IL: Human Kinetics Press, 2000.

1. Determine the 1-RM in kg or lb as follows:
   a. Warm-up using five to seven reps with light resistance.
   b. Rest for 1–2 minutes; perform slow stretching.
   c. Increase the load by 10–20 lb (4–9 kg) or 8% to 10% for upper-body exercise and by 30 to 40 lb (14–18 kg) or 10% to 20% for lower-body exercise. Complete three to 10 reps; stop at 10 reps.
   d. Rest for 1 to 2 minutes; perform slow stretching.
   e. Increase load above previous level (step c above), attempting to approach "near" maximum; increase 10–20 lb (4–9 kg) or 8% to 10% for upper-body exercise and 30 to 40 lb (14–18 kg) or 10% to 20% for lower-body exercise; complete as many reps as possible (at this load, maximum reps will probably range between two and six).
   f. Rest for 2 to 3 minutes; perform slow stretching.

g. Increase the load above previous level (step e above), attempting to approach "near" maximum; increase 10 to 20 lb (4–9 kg) or 8% to 10% for upper-body exercise and 30 to 40 lb (14–18 kg) or 10% to 20% for lower-body exercise. Complete as many reps as possible (at this load repetitions will probably range between one and four).

h. Rest for 2 to 3 minutes; perform slow stretching.

i. If the previous load produced 1-RM or more, rest 2 to 3 minutes (perform slow stretching). Increase the load 5 to 10 lb (2–4 kg) or 1% to 5% and attempt again. If the previous load could not be completed one time, rest for 2 to 3 minutes (perform slow stretching) and decrease the load by 5 to 10 lb (2–4 kg) or 1% to 5% for upper-body exercise and by 10 to 20 lb (4–9 kg) for lower-body exercise; attempt the lift again, trying to achieve the 1-RM.

2. Determine training goal(s) (e.g., strength, power, hypertrophy, endurance).

3. Determine the appropriate *repetition number* for the specific training goal (see **Table 14.2**).

4. Determine the specific %1-RM based on the repetition number (see **Table 14.2**).

5. Determine the training load (weight).

   a. Multiply the 1-RM load by the %1-RM (expressed as a decimal) selected for training

Examples

With a training goal to achieve muscle hypertrophy, and 1-RM of 200 lb, follow the five-step procedure outlined previously to determine load and repetition number:

1. Determine the 1-RM.

   1-RM = 200 lb

2. Determine the training goal.

   Muscle hypertrophy

3. Determine the appropriate repetition number for the specific training goal (see Table).

   The repetition number is six to 12; use eight.

4. Determine the specific %1-RM based on the repetition number (see **Table 14.2**).

   For goal repetitions six to 12, the %1-RM is 67% to 85%; use 75%.

5. Determine the training load (weight); multiply the 1-RM load by the %1-RM (expressed as a decimal) selected for training.

   Training load = 200 × 0.75 = 150 lb

This person would train using 8 reps with a weight of 150 lb. Retest the 1-RM as improvement progresses every 2 weeks or so to adjust the training load.

REFERENCES

Baechle, T.R., Earle, R.W. (eds.): *Essentials of Strength Training and Conditioning*, 3rd ed. Champaign, IL: Human Kinetics Press, 2008.

Fleck, S.J., Kraemer, W.J.: *Designing Resistance Training Programs*, 3rd Ed. Champaign, IL: Human Kinetics Press, 2004.

Kraemer, W.J., an Koziris, L.P.: Muscle strength training: Techniques and considerations. *Phys. Ther. Pract.*, 2:54, 1992.

ment, pulleys, slings, springs, immovable bars, resistance bands, and a variety of isokinetic and hydraulic devices provide effective muscle overload. Certain exercise methods lend themselves to precise and systematic overload applications. **Progressive-resistance weight training**, **isometric training**, and **isokinetic training** represent three common exercise systems to train muscles to become stronger. Strengthening muscles requires adherence to exercise training principles and specific guidelines.

Overload (Intensity)

Resistance training applies the **overload principle** with weights (dumbbells or barbells); immovable bars; straps; pulleys; suspension and bungee cords; springs; and oil, air, and water hydraulic devices. *In each case, the muscle responds to the intensity of the overload (level of tension placed on muscle) rather than the form of overload.*

The amount of overload reflects a percentage of the maximum strength (1-RM) of a nonfatigued muscle or muscle group. Performing a **voluntary maximal muscle action** means a muscle must exert as much force as its *present* capacity

*Q*uestions & Notes

Explain the overload principle.

allows. A partially fatigued muscle cannot generate the same force as a nonfatigued muscle. The last repetition to momentary failure in a set denotes a voluntary maximal muscle action. Muscular overload in resistance training usually requires such voluntary maximal muscle actions.

Three approaches either singularly or in combination apply muscular overload in resistance training:

1. Increase load or resistance
2. Increase number of repetitions
3. Increase speed of muscle action

The degree of muscular overload, often called training intensity, represents the most important factor in strength development; it requires training above a minimum threshold level to induce a training response. *Minimal intensity for muscular overload occurs between 60% and 70% of 1-RM.* This means that performing a large number of repetitions with light resistance at a low percentage of 1-RM produces only minimal strength improvements.

Force–Velocity Relationship

Different physical activities require different amounts of strength (force) and power. Absolute or peak force generated in a movement depends on the speed of muscle lengthening and shortening. **Figure 14.5** shows the **force–velocity relationship** for concentric and eccentric muscle actions. Muscles shorten (and lengthen) at different maximum velocities (horizontal axis of graph) depending on the load placed on them. As the load increases, maximum shortening velocity decreases. Conversely, a muscle's

force-generating capacity (vertical axis of graph) rapidly declines with increased shortening velocity. This explains the difficulty attempting to move a heavy weight rapidly.

A shortening (concentric) action becomes a lengthening (eccentric) action when the external load exceeds a muscle's maximum isometric force capacity (noted as point 0 on the horizontal axis). In contrast to a concentric muscle action, rapid eccentric actions generate the greatest force. This may explain the relatively greater muscle damage and delayed muscle soreness that accompany a bout of eccentric exercise. Force at zero velocity of shortening (isometric action) exceeds all forces generated with concentric/eccentric muscle actions. Muscle fiber type also influences the force–velocity relationships; fast-twitch muscle fibers produce greater muscle force at fast movement speeds than slow-twitch fibers because they possess higher ATPase activity, which accelerates adenosine triphosphate breakdown. Athletes who possess a high percentage of fast-twitch fibers have a distinct performance advantage in power-type physical activities.

Power–Velocity Relationship

Figure 14.6 shows an inverted U relationship between a muscle's maximal power output and speed of limb movement during concentric muscle action. Peak power rapidly increases with increasing velocity to a **peak velocity region**. Thereafter, maximal power output decreases because of reduced maximum force at faster movement speeds. *Each muscle group has an optimum movement speed to produce maximum power.* Similar to the force–velocity

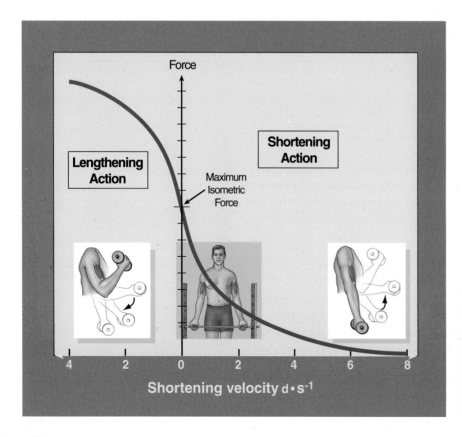

Figure 14.5 Maximum force–velocity relationship for shortening and lengthening muscle actions. Rapid shortening velocities (degrees per second, $d \cdot s^{-1}$) generate the least maximum force. Shortening velocity becomes zero (maximum isometric force) when the curve crosses the y-axis. Force-generating capacity increases to its highest as the muscle lengthens at rapid velocities.

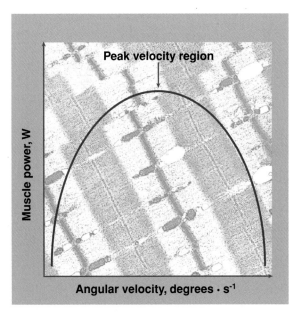

Figure 14.6 Power–velocity inverted U relationship. Power (work per unit time) increases as a function of movement velocity up to a peak velocity region. Thereafter, power decreases with further increases in angular velocity.

relationship, greater peak power occurs in fast-twitch fibers than in slow-twitch fibers at any movement velocity.

Load–Repetition Relationship

The total work accomplished by muscle action depends on the load (resistance) placed on the muscle. One can perform high repetitions with light loads but only few repetitions with near-maximal loads. **Figure 14.7A** shows this relationship for the full range of percentages of 1-RM. The area from 60% to 100% 1-RM represents the **strength training zone**, the training stimulus that optimizes strength improvement.

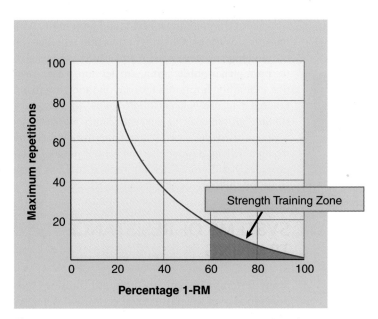

Figure 14.7 Relationship between maximum number of repetitions to failure and load at 20% to 100% 1-RM. (From Siff, M.C., Verkhoshansky, Y.V.: *Supertraining: Special Strength Training for Sporting Excellence.* Perry, OH: Strength Coach, Inc., 1997.)

Questions & Notes

List 3 approaches to apply overload in resistance training.

   1.

   2.

   3.

Describe the force-velocity relationship.

Describe the power-velocity relationship.

Describe the load-repetition relationship.

GENDER DIFFERENCES IN MUSCULAR STRENGTH

Two strength-testing approaches determine whether true gender differences exist in muscular strength:

1. Assess absolute strength (total force exerted).
2. Assess relative strength (force exerted related to body mass, fat-free body mass [FFM], or muscle cross-sectional area).

Absolute Muscle Strength

Comparisons of muscular strength on an *absolute* score basis (i.e., total force in lb or kg) indicate that men possess considerably greater strength than women for all muscle groups tested. Women score about 50% lower than men for upper-body strength and about 30% lower for leg strength. This gender disparity exists independent of the measuring device and generally coincides with gender-related difference in muscle mass distribution. Exceptions usually emerge for strength-trained female track-and-field athletes and body builders who have strength trained for years.

Table 14.3 shows the strength ratios for different muscle groups (Female strength score ÷ Male strength score). These data represent averages from the research literature based on strength scores of men and women for concentric and eccentric muscle actions. Overall, the typical woman's total body strength represents 64% of the typical man's strength; for upper-body strength, women average 56% of the men's score, and lower-body strength averages 72% of values achieved by men.

Relative Muscle Strength

Human skeletal muscle fibers in vitro (outside of the body) generate 16 to 30 Newtons (N) maximal force per square centimeter of **muscle cross-sectional area** (MCSA) regardless of gender. In the body (in vivo), force-output capacity varies depending on the bony lever's arrangement and muscle architecture.

The results of a classic study depicted in **Figure 14.8** compared arm flexor strength of men and women related to MCSA. The strong linear, positive relationship ($r = 0.95$) suggests that individuals with larger MCSA generate the greatest muscular force, and those with the smaller MCSA generate the lowest force. This is true for the entire range of force outputs from the lowest to highest scores. The *inset graph* shows equality in strength between genders when expressing arm flexor strength per unit MCSA. See the accompanying Close Up Box 14.3: *Determining Upper-Arm Muscle and Fat Areas,* on page 462 for how to determine MCSA.

Relative strength computes using one of three variables:

1. Body mass (strength score in lb or kg ÷ body mass in lb or kg)
2. Segmental or total FFM (strength score in lb or kg ÷ FFM in lb or kg)
3. MCSA (strength score in lb or kg ÷ MCSA)

A relative score increases the "fairness" when comparing two individuals' strength performances (or the same person assessed before, during, and after a training regimen or weight-loss program).

RESISTANCE TRAINING FOR CHILDREN

Resistance training for children has gained popularity over the past 2 decades, yet its benefits and possible risks remain fertile ground for further research. Incomplete skeletal development in young children and adolescents raises concern about the potential for bone and joint injury with heavy muscular overload. One might question whether resistance training improves strength at a relatively young age because the hormonal profile continues to develop, particularly for the tissue-building hormones testosterone and growth hormone. *Limited evidence indicates that closely supervised resistance training programs using concentric-only muscle actions with high repetitions and low resistance improve children's muscular strength without adverse effect on bone or muscle.* Table 14.4 provides basic guidelines for resistance exercise progressions for children at different ages.

SYSTEMS OF RESISTANCE TRAINING

Many different systems of "strength training" have been developed over the past several centuries. When we think of more modern methods to develop muscular strength, we usually think of some variation of free weights or barbells. For historical perspective, the Ling system referred to previously on page 444 devised systems of progressive

	Ratio of Female Strength to Male Strength for Different Muscle Groups[a]	
Table 14.3		

MUSCLE GROUP	STRENGTH RATIO (FEMALE ÷ MALE)
Elbow flexors	0.55
Elbow extensors	0.48
Knee flexors	0.69
Knee extensors	0.68
Shoulder flexors	0.55
Trunk extensors and flexors	0.60
Hip extensors and flexors	0.80
Finger flexors	0.60

[a]Data represent an average of values in the literature that reported female:male data. The ratios were obtained by dividing the female mean strength for a given muscle(s) by the mean male strength score. These data can be used to (1) evaluate performance of women relative to men, (2) select first approximations of suitable loads for women based on data for men, or (3) approximate data for men if only data for women are available.

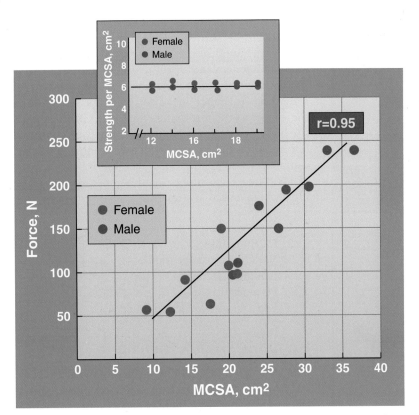

Figure 14.8 Plot of force (Newtons, N) versus muscle cross-sectional area (MCSA, cm²). Data represent elbow flexion. The inset figure shows the strength per unit MCSA. (Data from Miller, J.D., et al.: Gender differences in strength and muscle fiber characteristics. *Eur. J. Appl. Physiol.*, 66:254, 1992 and Ikai, M., Fukunaga, R.: Calculation of muscle strength per unit cross-sectional area of human muscle by means of ultrasonic measurements. *Arbeitsphysiologie*, 26:26, 1968.)

exercises to strengthen total body musculature. The method of progressive sling suspension training shown in the top panel of **Figure 14.9** was pioneered in Sweden beginning in the 1840s. Between 1914 and 1918 more advanced suspension and sling exercise and training methods shown in the *middle panel* were developed by physiotherapists working in English hospitals and

Table 14.4	Guidelines for Resistance Exercise for Children[a]

AGE, y	GUIDELINES
5–7	Introduce child to basic exercises with little or no weight; develop the concept of a training session; teach exercise techniques; progress from body weight calisthenics, partner exercises, and lightly resisted exercises; keep volume low
8–10	Gradually increase the exercise number; practice exercise techniques for all lifts; start gradual progressive loading of exercises; keep exercises simple; increase volume slowly; carefully monitor tolerance to exercise stress
11–13	Teach all basic exercise techniques; continue progressive loading of each exercise; emphasize exercise technique; introduce more advanced exercises with little or no resistance
14–15	Progress to more advanced resistance exercise programs; add sport-specific components; emphasize exercise techniques; increase volume
16+	Entry level into adult programs after the person masters all background experience

[a]Note: If a child at a particular age level has no previous experience, progression must start at previous levels and move to more advanced levels as exercise tolerance, skill, and understanding permit.
From Kraemer, W.J., Fleck S.J.: *Designing Resistance Training Programs.* Champaign, IL: Human Kinetics, 1997.

Questions & Notes

List the 2 approaches to determine gender differences in strength.

1.

2.

On an absolute basis, compared to males, how much less strength do women score for the upper band lower body.

Upper:

Lower:

List the 3 ways to express relative muscle strength.

1.

2.

3.

Describe the relationship been force and muscle cross-sectional area.

List to "general" guidelines for resistance exercise for children between 7 to 10 y.

1.

2.

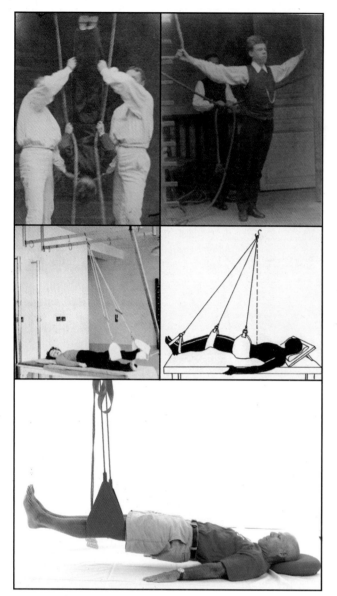

Figure 14.9 Different systems of sling suspension progressive exercise to strengthen total body musculature. **Top.** Progressive rope and sling suspension remedial exercise regimens pioneered in Sweden beginning in the 1840s. **Middle.** Sling suspension and reciprocal weight and pulley exercise training methods pioneered in the British Isles in the 1920s to 1950s by Olive Frances Guthrie Smith (1883–1956) and colleagues first published with A.E. Porritt in 1931 (Smith, O.F.G.S., Porritt, A.E.: A method of exciting incipient movement in weakened and paralyzed muscles. *Br. Med. J.* 1:54, 1931). **Bottom.** Norwegian suspension training techniques developed in the 1990s that emphasized unstable, closed kinetic chain exercise for physical therapy applications, strength development, and general and specific fitness training. Suspension training uses a person's body weight without reliance on externally fixed weights, pulleys, or cams by increasing or decreasing the suspension coordinates—the height of ropes, pulleys, slings, or bungee cords—relative to the suspension point.

rehabilitation facilities during and after World War I. Norwegian sling suspension training methods developed in the early 1990s (*bottom panel*) also complemented physical therapy applications and supports strength development and general and specific fitness training. The sling suspension methodologies leverage the person's body weight as resistance increases or decreases by altering the suspension coordinates, the height of the slings, or the body position relative to the suspension point without reliance on externally fixed weights, pulleys, or cams.

Six different but interrelated popular systems of training develop muscular strength:

1. Isometric training
2. DCER training
3. Variable resistance training
4. Isokinetic training
5. Plyometric training
6. Body weight–loaded training

Isometric (Static) Training

Isometric strength training gained popularity between 1955 and 1965. Research in Germany during this time showed a 5% per week increase in isometric strength from only one daily, two-thirds maximum isometric action for 6 seconds in duration. Repeating this action five to 10 times increased isometric strength. Strength gains from this simple exercise seemed beyond belief, and subsequent research demonstrated that isometric strength gains progressed at a slower rate. Research also showed that gains in strength from isometrics related to repetitions, duration of muscle action, and training frequency.

Research since 1965 has revealed the following regarding isometric training:

1. Maximal voluntary isometric actions (100% of maximum) produce greater gains in isometric strength than submaximal isometric actions.
2. Duration of muscle activation directly relates to increases in isometric strength.
3. One daily isometric action does not increase isometric strength as effectively as repeated actions.
4. An optimal isometric training program consists of daily repeated isometric actions.
5. Isometric training does not provide a consistent stimulus for muscular hypertrophy.
6. Gains in isometric strength occur predominantly at the joint angle used in training.

Limitations of Isometrics A drawback to isometric training involves difficulty in monitoring exercise intensity and training results. Because no movement occurs, it becomes difficult to determine objectively if the person's strength actually improves and whether the person applies an appropriate overload force during training.

Benefits of Isometrics Isometric exercise effectively improves the strength of a particular muscle or group of muscles when the applied isometric force covers four or five joint angles through the ROM. Isometric training works well in orthopedic and physical therapy applications that isolate strengthening movements during rehabilitation. Isometric measurement pinpoints an area of muscle weakness, and isometric training strengthens muscles at the appropriate joint angle in the ROM.

Dynamic Constant External Resistance (DCER) Training

This popular system of resistance training involves lifting (concentric) and lowering (eccentric) phases with each repetition using weight plates (barbells and dumbbells) or exercise machines that feature different applications of muscle overload.

Progressive Resistance Exercise

Researchers in rehabilitation medicine after World War II devised a method of resistance training to improve the force-generating capacity of previously injured muscles. Their method involved three sets of exercise, each consisting of 10 repetitions done consecutively without rest. The first set involved one-half the maximum weight lifted 10 times or one-half 10-RM; the second set used three-quarters 10-RM; the final set required maximum weight for 10 repetitions or 10-RM. As patients became stronger, the resistance increased periodically to match strength improvements. This technique of **progressive resistance exercise** (**PRE**), a practical application of the overload principle, forms the basis for most popular resistance training programs.

Variations of Progressive Resistance Exercise Research has varied PRE to determine an optimal number of sets and repetitions and frequency and relative intensity of training to improve strength. The following summarizes 13 general findings from research studies on the optimal number of sets and repetitions, including frequency and relative intensity of PRE training for optimal strength improvement:

1. Eight- to 12-RM proves effective in novice training, and 1- to 12-RM effectively loads for intermediate training. This can then increase to heavy loading using 1- to 6-RM.
2. Rest for 3 minutes between sets of an exercise at moderate movement velocity (1 to 2 s of concentric; 1 to 2 s of eccentric).
3. For PRE at a specific RM load, increase the load 2% to 10% when the individual performs 1 to 2 repetitions above the current workload.
4. Performing one exercise set induces only slightly less strength improvement in recreational weight lifters than performing two or three sets. For those who desire to maximize muscle strength and size gains, higher volume, multiple-set paradigms emphasizing 6- to 12-RM at moderate velocity with 1- to 2-minute rests between sets prove most effective.
5. Single-set programs generally produce most of the health and fitness benefits of multiple-set programs. These "lower volume" programs also produce greater compliance and reduce financial cost and time commitment.
6. Novices and intermediates train 2 to 3 days a week, whereas the advanced typically train 3 to 4 days a week and sometimes more. Such a generalization is not without a potential downside. High training frequency extends the transient activation of inflammatory signaling cascades, comcomitant with persistent suppression of key mediators of anabloic responses, which could blunt the training response.
7. Training twice every second day produces overall superior results compared with daily training. This may occur from the effects of low muscle glycogen content (with training twice every second day) on enhanced transcription of genes involved in training adaptations.

Questions & Notes

List the 6 different systems for developing muscular strength.

1.

2.

3.

4.

5.

6.

List 2 positive aspects of isometric strength training.

1.

2.

Which system of strength training centers on concentric and ecentric muscle action?

Describe the basis of PRE training.

8. If training includes multiple exercises, 4 or 5 days per week may produce less improvement than training 2 or 3 days per week because near-daily training of the same muscles impairs muscle recuperation between training sessions. Inadequate recovery retards progress in neuromuscular and structural adaptations and strength development.

9. A fast rate of moving a given resistance generates more strength improvement than moving at a slower rate. Neither free weights (barbells, weight plates, dumbbells) nor an array of exercise machines shows inherent superiority for developing muscle strength.

10. Exercise should sequence to optimize workout quality by engaging large before small muscle groups, multiple-joint exercises before single-joint exercises, and higher intensity exercise before lower intensity exercise.

11. Combined resistance-training concentric and eccentric muscle actions augment effectiveness; include both single- and multiple-joint exercises to potentiate a muscle's strength and fiber size.

BOX 14.3 CLOSE UP

Determining Upper-Arm Muscle and Fat Areas

Girth measurements include bone surrounded by a mass of muscle tissue ringed by a layer of subcutaneous fat (**Fig. 1**). Muscle represents the largest component of the girth (except in obese and elderly individuals), so girth indicates one's relative muscularity. Estimating limb muscle area assumes similarity between a limb and a cylinder, with subcutaneous fat evenly distributed around the cylinder (**Fig. 1**).

MEASUREMENTS

Determine the following:

1. Upper-arm girth (relaxed triceps; G_{arm}): Measure with arm extended relaxed at the side (or parallel to the ground in an abducted position). Measure girth (cm) midway between the acromial and olecranon process (**Fig. 2**).

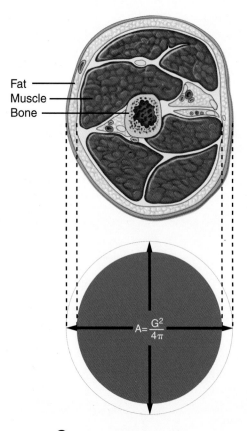

Fat
Muscle
Bone

$$A = \frac{G^2}{4\pi}$$

Ⓐ Upper-arm composition and area

Figure 1 Upper-arm composition and area.

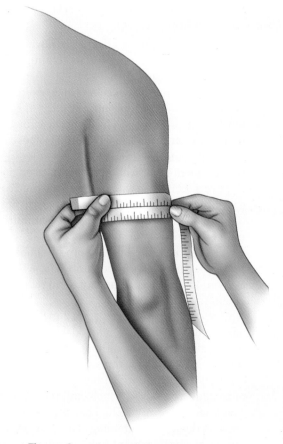

Figure 2 Relaxed triceps arm girth, cm.

2. Triceps skinfold (Sf_{tri}): Measure in decimeters (dm; mm × 10) on the back of the arm, over the triceps muscle, as a vertical fold at the same level as the relaxed arm girth (**Fig. 3**).

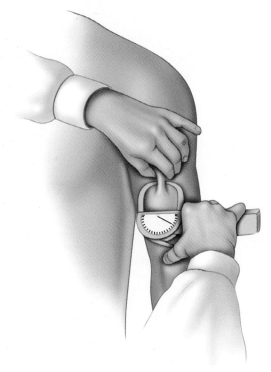

Figure 3 Triceps skinfold, mm.

EXAMPLE

Data

Upper-arm girth (G_{arm}) in cm, 30.0; triceps skinfold (Sf_{tri}) in dm, (25 mm).

COMPUTATIONS

1. Arm muscle girth, cm = $G_{arm} - (\pi Sf_{tri})$
   $$= 30.0 \text{ cm} - (\pi 2.5 \text{ dm})$$
   $$= 30.0 - 7.854$$
   $$= 22.1 \text{ cm}$$

2. Arm muscle area, cm^2 = $[G_{arm} - (\pi Sf_{tri})] \div 4\pi$
   $$= (30.0 \text{ cm}) - (\pi 2.5 \text{ dm})^2 \div 4\pi$$
   $$= 488.4 \div 12.566$$
   $$= 38.9 \text{ cm}^2$$

3. Arm area (A), cm^2 = $(G_{arm})^2 \div 4\pi$
   $$= (30.0 \text{ cm})^2 \div 4\pi$$
   $$= 900 \div 12.566$$
   $$= 71.6 \text{ cm}^2$$

4. Arm fat area, cm^2 = Arm area − Arm muscle area
   $$= 71.6 \text{ cm}^2 - 38.9 \text{ cm}^2$$
   $$= 32.7 \text{ cm}^2$$

5. Arm fat index, % fat area
   $$= (\text{Arm fat area} \div \text{Arm area}) \times 100$$
   $$= (32.7 \text{ cm}^2 \div 71.6 \text{ cm}^2) \times 100$$
   $$= 45.7\%$$

12. Overload training that includes eccentric muscle actions preserves strength gains better during a maintenance phase than concentric-only training.
13. Power training should apply the strategy to improve muscular strength plus include lighter loads (30%–60% of 1 RM) performed at fast contraction velocity. Use 2- to 3-minute rest periods between sets. Emphasize multiple-joint exercises that activate large muscle groups.

The American College of Sports Medicine has published a position stand on progression models in resistance training for healthy adults that can be downloaded free as a PDF (*http://journals.lww.com/acsm-msse/Fulltext/2009/03000/ Progression_Models_in_Resistance_Training_for.26.aspx*).

Responses of Men and Women to Dynamic Constant External Resistance Training

Figure 14.10 shows strength changes for men and women with DCER training. These data represent an average from 12 experiments. Women achieved a higher percentage improvement than men, although considerable overlap existed. These findings indicate a relative *equality* in trainability between women and men, at least with short-duration resistance training.

Variable Resistance Training

A limitation of typical DCER weight-lifting exercise involves failure of muscles to generate maximum force through all movement phases. **Variable resistance training equipment** alters external resistance to movement by use of a lever arm, irregularly shaped metal cam, air, hydraulics, or a pulley to match

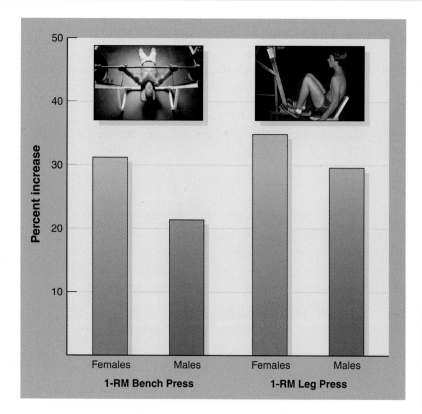

Figure 14.10 Percentage increase in one-repetition maximum (1-RM) bench press and leg press of women and men in response to resistance training. Values represent an average of 12 studies using dynamic constant external resistance (DCER) training for a minimum of 9 weeks duration 3 days per week with 2 or more sets per session.

increases and decreases in force capacity related to joint angle (lever characteristics) throughout a ROM. This adjustment, based on average physical dimensions of a population, theoretically should facilitate strength gains because it allows near-maximal force production throughout the full ROM.

Biomechanical research shows that a single cam device cannot possibly compensate fully for individual differences in mechanics in force applications during all phases of a particular movement. Variations in limb length, point of attachment of muscle tendons to bone, body size, and muscle force output at different joint angles all affect maximum force generated throughout a ROM. Variable resistance devices improve strength comparable to other weight-lifting (resistance) equipment.

Musculoskeletal Conditions and the Lower Back

According to the Bone and Joint Decade Monitor Project and the World Health Organization (WHO) (*www.ota.org/downloads/bjdExecSum.pdf*), the total costs in the United States related to musculoskeletal conditions exceeds $250 billion yearly. Of this amount, direct costs account for $88.7 billion. Thirty-eight percent was spent on hospital admissions, 21% on nursing home admissions, 17% on physician visits, and 5% on administrative costs. Indirect costs account for 58% of the total ($126.2 billion), which include lost wages through morbidity or premature mortality. Musculoskeletal diseases include approximately 150 different diseases and syndromes typically associated with pain or inflammation.

Back injuries account for one-fourth of all work-related injuries and one-third of all compensation costs, which, according to the Bureau of Labor Statistics (*www.bls.gov*), cost the government about $90 billion yearly in related health costs. Most cases result from on-the-job injuries, particularly in men in lumber and building retailing (highest risk) and construction (most cases); major-risk industries for women include nursing and work in personal care centers (highest risk) and hospitals (most cases). Work in grocery stores and agricultural crop production rank among the top 10 occupations for lower back injury for men and women. Estimates indicate that at least 32 million adult Americans frequently experience lower back pain, the primary cause for workplace disability. Workplace disability from injuries to the lower back region also occurs in common tasks such as refuse collection and other manual handling and lifting tasks.

Muscular weakness, particularly in the abdominal and lower lumbar back regions, lumbar spine instability, and poor joint flexibility in the back and legs represent primary external factors related to *low-back pain syndrome*.

Prevention of and rehabilitation from chronic low-back strain commonly use muscle-strengthening and joint-flexibility exercises. Continuing normal activities of daily living (within limits dictated by pain tolerance) yields more rapid recovery from acute back pain than bed rest. Maintaining normal physical activity facilitates greater recovery than specific back-mobilizing exercises performed after pain onset. Prudent use of resistance-type training isolates and strengthens the abdomen and lower lumbar extensor muscles that support and protect the spine through its full ROM. Patients with low-back pain who strengthen their lumbar extensors and pelvic stabilizer muscles experience fewer acute and chronic symptoms, improved muscular strength and endurance, and increased ROM.

Resistance-training exercise poses a dilemma for those with low-back syndrome. Improper performance of a typical resistance-exercise movement (with a relatively heavy load and the hips thrust forward with an arched back) creates considerable compressive force on the lower spine. For example, pressing and curling exercises with back hyperextension create unusually high shearing stress on the lumbar vertebrae, often triggering low-back pain accompanied by regional muscle instability.

Compressive forces with heavy lifting also can hasten damage to the disks that cushion the vertebrae. Performing half squats with barbell loads from 0.8 to 1.6 times body mass produces compressive loads on the L3–L4 segment of the spine equivalent to six to 10 times body mass. A person who weighs 90 kg and squats with 144 kg can create peak compressive forces in excess of 1367 kg (13,334 N)! A sudden amplification of compressive force can precipitate anterior disk prolapse; a lower-intensity but sustained compressive force that produces fatigue can increase posterior bulging of the lamellas in the posterior annulus. In national-level male and female power lifters, average compressive loads on L4–L5 reached 1757 kg (17,192 N). At the practical level during sports training with resistance methods (i.e., functional training with free weights), one should not sacrifice proper execution of an exercise to lift a heavier load or "squeeze out" additional repetitions. The extra weight lifted through improper technique does not facilitate muscle strengthening; instead, improper body alignment or unwarranted muscle substitution during force production can trigger debilitating injury in which surgery unfortunately becomes the option of choice. This fact should encourage proper strengthening of "core" abdominal and lower back muscles to avoid either prolonged reliance on pain-relieving drugs or potentially debilitating surgical alternatives.

Weight-Lifting Belts Reduce Intraabdominal Pressure

Wearing a relatively stiff weight-lifting belt during heavy lifts (squats, dead lifts, clean-and-jerk maneuvers) reduces intraabdominal pressure compared with lifting without a belt. The belt reduces potentially injurious compressive forces on spinal disks during near-maximal lifting, including most Olympic and power-lifting events and associated training. In one study, nine experienced weightlifters lifted barbells up to 75% body weight under three conditions: (1) while inhaling and wearing a belt, (2) while inhaling and not wearing a belt, and (3) while exhaling and wearing a belt. Measurements included intraabdominal pressure, trunk muscle electromyography (EMG), ground reaction forces, and kinematics. The belt reduced compression forces by about 10%, but only when the weight lifter inhaled before lifting. The authors concluded that wearing a tight and stiff-back belt while inhaling before lifting reduces spinal loading during the lift.

Questions & Notes

Describe 3 findings of the Bone and Joint Decade monitor perfect.

1.

2.

3.

Describe the major limitation of DCER exercises.

Which type of resistance exercises are particularly bad for those susceptible to back pain?

Describe the major benefit of using weight-lifting belts.

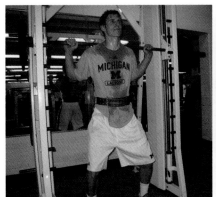
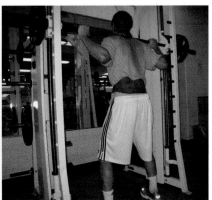

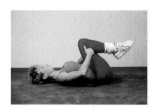

(A) Knees-to-chest stretch: Lie supine and pull knees into chest while keeping lower back flat on the surface.

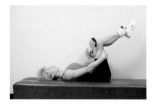

(B) Cross-leg strech: Cross legs like sitting male. Cross legs and pull 90°-flexed knee toward chest.

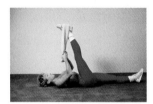

(C) Hamstring stretch: Wrap strap over foot, keeping lower back flat; pull leg upward toward head.

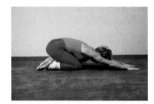

(D) Allah stretch: Sit with buttocks on bilateral heels; move hands as far forward along the surface as possible.

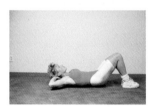

(E) Bent-knee sit-up: Keep hands low on neck (or across chest) with head positioned over the shoulders. Roll up slowly, engaging one row of abdominals at a time. Raise the shoulders 4 to 6 inches off the surface.

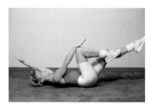

(F) Dying bug: Flex the pelvis to flatten the lower back against the surface. Over one side, bring an extended arm and flexed knee together. The opposing side should extend a straight arm overhead and straight leg backward. Maintain pelvic flexion while exchanging opposing arms and legs in this position.

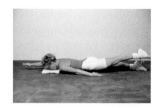

(G) Dry-land swimming: Lying prone with pelvic flextion, alternate lifting opposite arm and legs.

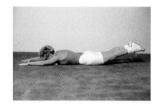

(H) Both legs up: Lying prone with pelvic flexion, lift both legs simultaneously while keeping the head on the floor.

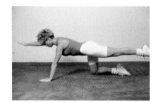

(I) Pointer (bird dog): Start with hands and knees on the floor. Flex pelvis into counter position. Exchange pointing opposite arm and leg while keeping the torso level.

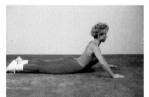

(J) Upper body up: Lying prone with pelvic flexion and arms outstretched or behind the back, lift the upper torso while keeping the legs on the floor.

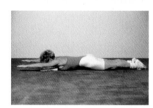

(K) Prone cobra push-up: Keep the pelvis on the floor while pressing up with the arms, causing lower back extension.

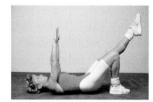

(L) Leg pointer: Lie supine on the floor and flex the pelvis with the lower abdominals to flatten the lower back into the surface. Extend one arm upward and one leg outward while keeping the quadriceps level.

Figure 14.11 Examples of 12 general exercises to strengthen the abdomen and lower back and increase hamstring and lower back flexibility. (Photos courtesy of Dr. Bob Swanson, Santa Barbara Back and Neck Care Center. Santa Barbara, CA.)

A person who normally trains wearing a belt should generally refrain from lifting without one. Further recommendations include performing at least some submaximal resistance training without a belt to strengthen the deep abdominal and pelvic-stabilizing muscles. This also develops the proper pattern of muscle recruitment to generate high intraabdominal pressures when not wearing a belt.

Wearing a back belt to ameliorate low-back injuries in the workplace does not provide a clear-cut biomechanical advantage. A 2-year prospective study of nearly 14,000 material-handling employees in 30 states evaluated the effectiveness of using back belts to reduce back injury worker's compensation claims and reports of low-back pain. Neither frequent back belt use (usually once a day and once or twice a week) nor a store policy that required the use of these belts reduced injury or reports of low-back pain. Researchers worldwide continue to probe for answers about the cause of low-back pain syndrome and how to minimize its severity and reduce its occurrence.

General Back Exercises

Figure 14.11 illustrates 12 exercises that provide general strengthening of the abdomen, pelvic region, and lower back and improve hamstring and lower-back flexibility for individuals with no apparent lower back and spinal injuries. Symptomatic individuals (including athletes) require specific back exercises.

Isokinetic Training

Isokinetic resistance training differs markedly from isometric, DCER, and variable resistance methods. Isokinetic training uses a muscle action performed at constant angular limb velocity. Unlike dynamic resistance exercise, isokinetic exercise does not require a specified initial resistance; rather, the isokinetic device controls movement velocity. The muscles exert maximal forces throughout the ROM while shortening (concentric action) at a specific velocity. Advocates of isokinetic training argue that exerting maximal force throughout the full ROM optimizes strength development. Also, concentric-only actions minimize the potential for muscle and joint injury and pain.

Experiments with Isokinetic Exercise and Training

Experiments using isokinetic exercise explored the force–velocity relationship in various exercises and related this to the muscle's fiber-type composition. **Figure 14.12** displays the progressive decline in concentric peak torque output with increasing angular velocity of the knee extensor muscles in two groups that differed in sports training and muscle fiber composition. For movement at

Questions & Notes

Describe isokinetic training.

Describe the major difference between isokinetic and DCER training.

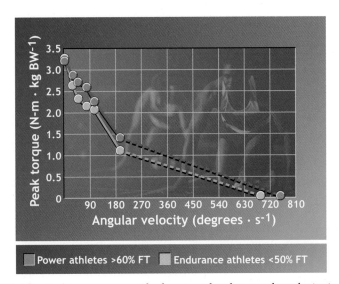

Figure 14.12 Peak torque per unit body mass related to angular velocity in two groups of athletes with different muscle fiber compositions. The torque–velocity curves were extrapolated (*dashed line*) to an estimated maximal velocity for knee extension. (Data from Throstensson, A.: Muscle strength, fiber types, and enzyme activities in man. *Acta. Physiol. Scand.*, (suppl):443, 1976.)

$180°·s^{-1}$, power athletes, (elite Swedish track and field sprinters and jumpers) achieved higher torque per kilogram of body mass than competition walkers and cross-country runners (endurance athletes). At this angular velocity, maximal torque equaled about 55% of maximal isometric force ($0°·s^{-1}$). The athletes' muscle fiber composition distinguishes the two curves in **Figure 14.12**. At zero velocity shortening (isometric action), the same peak force (per unit body mass) occurred for athletes with relatively high (power athletes) or low (endurance athletes) percentages of fast-twitch muscle fibers; this indicated that maximal isometric knee extension activated both fast- and slow-twitch motor units. Increasing movement velocity produced greater torque by individuals with a higher percentage of fast-twitch fibers. More than likely, fast-twitch muscle fibers favor performance in power activities where

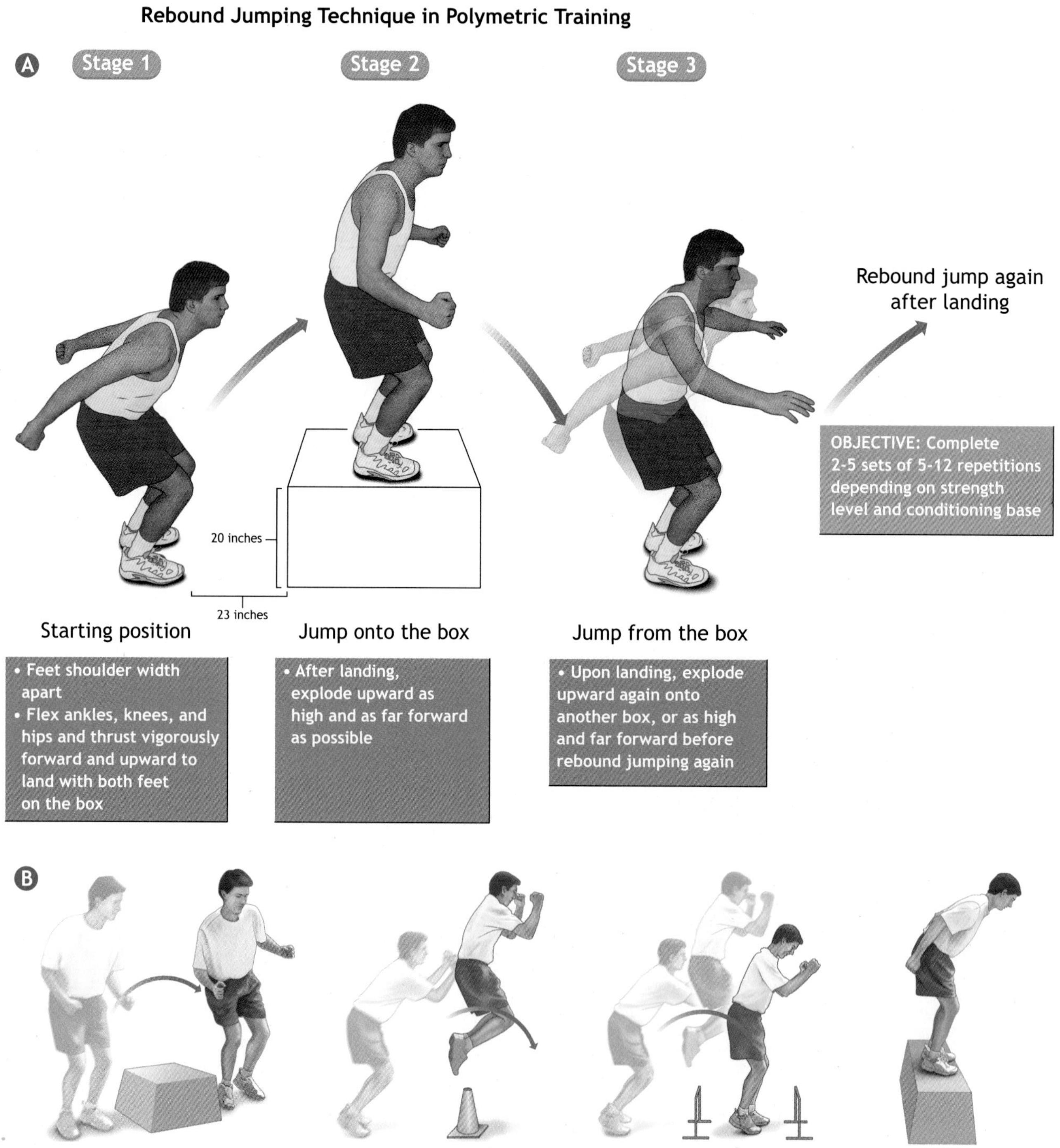

Rebound Jumping Technique in Polymetric Training

A Stage 1 Stage 2 Stage 3

Rebound jump again after landing

20 inches

23 inches

Starting position
- Feet shoulder width apart
- Flex ankles, knees, and hips and thrust vigorously forward and upward to land with both feet on the box

Jump onto the box
- After landing, explode upward as high and as far forward as possible

Jump from the box
- Upon landing, explode upward again onto another box, or as high and far forward before rebound jumping again

OBJECTIVE: Complete 2-5 sets of 5-12 repetitions depending on strength level and conditioning base

B

Figure 14.13 (A) Rebound jumping technique in plyometric training. (B) Four examples of plyometric exercise drills: 1. box jump, 2. cone hop, 3. hurdle hop, and 4. long jump from a box. (Examples courtesy of Dr. Thomas D. Fahey, California State University at Chico, Chico, CA.)

during which torque generation at rapid movement velocities often dictates success.

Plyometric Training

For sports that require powerful, propulsive movements—football, volleyball, sprinting, high jump, long jump, and basketball—athletes apply a special form of exercise training termed **plyometrics** or *explosive jump training*. Plyometric exercise requires various jumps in place or rebound jumping (drop jumping from a preset height) to mobilize the inherent stretch–recoil characteristics of skeletal muscle and its modulation via the stretch or myotatic reflex.

Stated somewhat differently, plyometric exercise involves rapid stretching followed by shortening of a muscle group during a dynamic movement. Stretching produces a stretch reflex and elastic recoil within muscle. When combined with a vigorous muscle contraction, plyometric actions should greatly increase the force that overloads the muscles, thereby facilitating increases in strength and power. Plyometric exercises range in difficulty from calf jumps off the ground with a rebound jump to multiple one-leg jumps to and from boxes ranging in height from 1 foot to 6 feet. Four examples of plyometric exercise drills are illustrated in **Figure 14.13**. The basic principle for all jumping and plyometric exercises is to absorb the shock with the arms or legs and then immediately contract the muscles. For example, when doing a series of squat jumps, the person should jump again as quickly into the air as possible after landing while at the same time, if possible, thrusting both heels up toward the buttocks. Quicker jumps provide greater overload to the muscles. In essence, "fast" plyometric exercise "trains" the nervous system to react quickly to activate muscles rapidly.

Plyometric maneuvers avoid the disadvantage of having to decelerate a mass in the latter part of the joint ROM during a fast movement; this provides for maximal power production. **Figure 14.14** compares a traditional bench press movement to achieve maximal power output with a ballistic bench throw that attempts to maximize power output by projecting the barbell from the hands. The results were unequivocal. During a bench press, deceleration begins at about 60% of the bar position relative to the total concentric movement distance (*purple line*). In contrast, velocity during the bench throw (*yellow line*)

$\mathcal{Q}$uestions & Notes

Describe plyometric training.

Describe the major disadvantage of plyometric training.

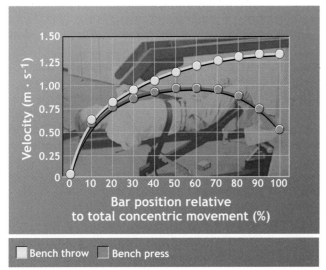

Figure 14.14 Mean bar velocity in relation to total concentric bar movement for bench throw and traditional bench press performed rapidly. (Data from Newton, R.U., et al.: Kinematics, kinetics, and muscle activation during explosive upper body movements. *J. Appl. Biomech.*,12:31, 1996.)

 For Your Information

HOLD THAT STRETCH!

Stretching with fast, bouncing, jerky movements that use the body's momentum can strain or tear muscles and create a reflex action that resists the muscle stretch.

continues to increase throughout the ROM and remains higher at all bar positions after movement begins. This translates into greater average force, average power, and peak power outputs. Achieving a faster average and peak velocity throughout the ROM produces greater power output and muscle activation (assessed by EMG) than the traditional weight-lifting exercise movement. The throw condition produced greater muscle activity for the pectoralis major (+19%), anterior deltoid (+34%), triceps brachii (+44%), and biceps brachii (+27%).

Allowing the athlete to develop greater power at the end of the movement more closely simulates the projection phase of throwing a ball or implement, maximal effort jumping movements, or impact in striking movements. In this form of training, called **ballistic resistance training**, the person moves the weight or projectile as fast as possible while trying to produce maximal force before releasing it. Sports performance examples include the shot put, overhead soccer throw, javelin and discuss throws, push away from the pole vigorously in the pole vault, takeoff jump for a volleyball spike, positioning and jumping for a basketball rebound, multiple punches in boxing, and takeoff in the high jump.

Plyometric exercise overloads a muscle to provide forcible and rapid stretch (eccentric or stretch phase) immediately before the concentric or shortening phase of action. The **stretch–shortening cycle (SSC)** represents an important concept that describes how skeletal muscles function efficiently in unrestricted human locomotor activities. When the muscle spindles of the gastrocnemius muscle suddenly become stretched, their sensory receptors fire with the impulses traveling through the dorsal root into the spinal cord (to activate the anterior motoneuron) and trigger the stretch reflex (see Chapter 11), the timing of which relies on the speed of movement. The sequence of stretching and shortening muscle fibers (as in the contact phase of running) serves a fundamental purpose—to enhance the final push-off phase. In many sports situations, the rapid lengthening phase in the SSC produces a more powerful subsequent movement.

From a practical standpoint, a plyometric drill uses body mass and gravity for the important rapid prestretch or "cocking" phase of the SCC to activate the muscles' natural elastic recoil elements. Prior stretch augments the subsequent concentric muscle action in the opposite direction. Forcibly dropping the arms to the side before vertical jumping produces an eccentric prestretch of the quadriceps muscle group and exemplifies a natural plyometric movement. Lower-body plyometric drills include a standing jump, multiple jumps, repetitive jumping in place, depth jumps or drop jumping from a height of about 1 m, single- and double-leg jumps, and various modifications. Proponents believe that repetitive plyometric actions serves as neuromuscular training to enhance the power output of specific muscles and sport-specific power performances as in jumping. A position paper from the National Strength and Conditioning Association *(www.nsca-lift.org)* suggests that athletes first achieve lifts of 1.5 times body

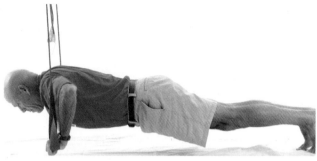

Figure 14.15 Example of a push-up exercise using the Norwegian suspension training apparatus; the individual performs the down and up phases of the pushup movement while countering instability of the dual suspended ropes. The idea is to maintain stability and balance during the push-up, similar to a conventional push-up with the hands supported on a solid surface. Placing both feet on a single balance cushion or each foot on a separate cushion increases the instability during the movement. (Photo courtesy of Redcord, Inc. Staubø, Norway.)

weight in the squat exercise before initiating high-intensity plyometric training. This practical guideline requires validation.

Body Weight–Loaded Training

Body weight–loaded training or closed-kinetic chain exercise to enhance sports performance has gained popularity and research support, including such training in job-related functions and treatment of pelvic pain after pregnancy.

In an example of body weight–supported push-up exercise (**Fig. 14.15**), the arms in the slings not the contact surface of the floor, bear the person's body weight. This example of body weight loading using slings to activate both agonists and antagonist muscles about a joint, including additional muscle groups along the kinetic chain. **Suspension training** introduces the added component of instability to further challenge trunk and back muscle neuromuscular control. The role of adding such *perturbation* during relatively simple or complex movements may play a key role in "training" the intricate signaling patterns that control the basics of human movement.

Recent studies using body weight–loaded training with suspension slings for soccer, golf, handball, and softball show improvements in functionally related sport movements that range from 3% to 5% in velocity of limb movement, increased golf club head velocity and hence distance, and improved static and dynamic balance and shoulder stabilization.

Concept of Core Training
The last decade has seen a resurgence of "**core training**"—also referred to as lumbar stabilization, core strengthening, dynamic stabilization, neutral spine control, trunk stabilization, abdominal strength, core "pillar" training, and core-functional strength training.

The concept considers the core as a four-sided muscular frame with abdominal muscles in front, the paraspinals and gluteals in back, the diaphragm at the top, and the pelvic floor and hip girdle musculature framing the bottom. The "core" does not simply refer to muscles that cross the midsection of the body to form "six-pack" abdominals commonly portrayed in magazine advertisements. The core region includes 29 pairs of muscles that hold the trunk steady, in addition to balancing and stabilizing the bony structures of the spine, pelvis, thorax, and other structures activated during most movements. The totality of these spine-frame structures without adequate "strength and balance" would become mechanically unstable. A properly functioning core provides appropriate distribution of forces along the muscle–joint–bone axis, optimal control and efficiency of movement; adequate absorption of ground-impact forces; and absence of excessive compressive, translational, and shearing forces on joints along the kinetic chain that must support the body weight.

SPECIFICITY OF STRENGTH-TRAINING RESPONSE

An isometrically trained muscle shows greatest strength improvement when measured isometrically; similarly, a dynamically trained muscle tests best when evaluated in resistance activities that require movement. Isometric strength developed at or near one joint angle does not readily transfer to other angles or body positions that must rely on the same muscles. In contrast, muscles trained dynamically through movement over a limited ROM show the greatest strength improvement when measured in that ROM. Even *body position specificity* exists; muscular strength of ankle plantar and dorsiflexors developed in the standing position with concentric and eccentric muscle actions showed no transfer with the same muscles evaluated in the supine position. Resistance training specificity makes sense because strength improvement blends adaptations in two factors:

1. The muscle fiber and connective tissue harness itself
2. Neural organization and excitability of motor units that power discrete patterns of voluntary movement

Likewise, a muscle's maximal force output depends on neural factors that effectively recruit and synchronize firing of motor units, not *just* the intrinsic factors of muscle fiber type and cross-sectional area.

A 3-month study of young adult men and women emphasized the highly specific nature of resistance-training adaptations. One group trained the hand's adductor pollicis muscle isometrically with 10 daily actions of 5 seconds' duration at a frequency of 1 per minute. The other group trained the same muscle dynamically with 10 daily 10-repetition bouts of weight movement at one-third maximal strength. The untrained muscle served as the control. To eliminate any training influence from psychologic factors and central nervous system (CNS) adaptations, a supermaximal electrical stimulation applied to the motor nerve evaluated the force capacity of the trained muscle. The results were clear—both training groups improved maximal force capacity and peak rate of force development. The improvement in maximal force for the isometrically trained group nearly doubled the improvement for the dynamically trained group. Conversely, improvement in speed of force development averaged about 70% greater in the group trained with dynamic muscle actions. Such findings provide strong evidence that resistance training per se does not induce all-inclusive (*general*) adaptations in muscle structure and function. Rather, a muscle's contractile properties, such as maximal force, velocity of shortening, and rate of tension development, improve in a manner that is *highly specific* to the muscle action in training. Both static and dynamic training methods produce strength increases, yet no one system rates consistently superior to the other in how best to train and assess muscle function.

Questions & Notes

Describe the stretch-shortening cycle and why it is important.

Explain the difference between body-weight loaded training and traditional resistance training.

Describe the body "core".

Explain strength-training specificity.

The crucial consideration concerns the intended purpose of newly acquired strength.

Practical Implications

The complex interaction between nervous and muscular systems helps explain why leg muscles strengthened in squats or deep knee bends fail to show equivalent improved force capability in other leg movements such as jumping or leg extension. Low relationships emerge between dynamic measures of leg extension force at any speed and vertical jumping height. A muscle group strengthened and enlarged by dynamic resistance training does not demonstrate equal improvement in force capacity when measured isometrically or isokinetically. Consequently, strengthening muscles for a specific athletic or occupational activity (e.g., golf, tennis, rowing, swimming, football, firefighting, package handling) demands more than just identifying and overloading the muscles in the movement; it also requires neuromuscular training specifically in the important movements that necessitate improved strength. *A more appropriate name for this type of training is* **functional strength training** *or* **functional resistance movement training.** Increasing leg muscle "strength" through general weight lifting may not necessarily improve performance in a variety of subsequent leg movements. *Newly acquired strength seldom transfers fully to other types of strength movements, even those that activate the same muscles.* A standard program of weight training for leg extension increased leg extension strength by 227%. Evaluating leg extension peak torque of the same leg with an isokinetic dynamometer detected only a 10% to 17% improvement! *To improve a specific physical performance through resistance training, it is important to train the muscle(s) in movements that mimic the movement requiring force–capacity improvement, with a focus on force, velocity, and power requirements rather than simply an isolated joint or muscle action.* To train a specific muscle or group of muscles, the coach and athlete must carefully assess the muscle group(s) involved in a particular movement. Performing triceps extensions with weights would not seem appropriate to train the specific upper arm musculature involved in the skilled movements required in the shot put or rapid downswing in the golf swing even though both skills require triceps activation. *Training should develop maximum force-generating capacity for those muscle groups throughout the ROM at a movement pattern and speed that closely mimics actual sports performance.* Isometric training cannot accomplish this goal because no limb movement occurs; isokinetic actions provide maximal overload potential at diverse movement velocities because movement speed with electromechanical dynamometers can approach $400°·s^{-1}$. Even moving at this relatively "fast" speed does not mimic movement velocity during some sports in which limb velocity approaches $2000°·s^{-1}$. For example, arm velocity measured about the elbow joint during a baseball pitch routinely exceeds 600 to $700°·s^{-1}$, and leg velocity during a football, rugby, or soccer kick nearly doubles the speed of the fastest electromechanical measuring and "strength" training equipment.

PERIODIZATION

In 1972, Russian scientist Leonid Matveyev introduced the concept of strength-training **periodization**. This concept has since become incorporated into the training regimens of novice and champion athletes. Conceptually, periodization varies training intensity and volume to ensure that peak performance coincides with major competition. Periodization subdivides a specific resistance-training period such as 1 year (macrocycle) into smaller periods or phases (mesocycles), with each mesocycle again separated into weekly microcycles. In essence, the training model progressively decreases training volume and increases intensity as the program duration progresses to maximize newly acquired improvements in muscular strength and power. Fractionating the macrocycle into components allows manipulation of training intensity, volume, frequency, sets, repetitions, and rest periods to prevent overtraining. It also provides a way to alter workout variety. Periodization variation can reduce negative overtraining or "staleness" effects so athletes achieve peak performance at competition. **Figure 14.16** (*top*) depicts the generalized design for periodization and a typical macrocycle's four distinct phases. As competition approaches, training volume gradually decreases, and training intensity concurrently increases. The four phases of periodization include:

1. The **preparation phase** emphasizes modest strength development with *high-volume* (3–5 sets; 8–12 reps), *low-intensity* workouts (50%–80% 1-RM plus flexibility and aerobic and anaerobic training).
2. The **first transition phase** emphasizes strength development with workouts of *moderate volume* (3–5 sets; 5–6 reps) and *moderate intensity* (80%–90% 1-RM plus flexibility and interval aerobic training).
3. The **competition phase** lets the participant peak for competition. Selective strength development is emphasized with *low-volume, high-intensity* workouts (3–5 sets; 2–4 reps at 90%–95% 1-RM) plus short periods of interval training that emphasize sport-specific exercises.
4. The **second transition phase** (**active recovery**) emphasizes recreational activities and low-intensity workouts that incorporate different exercise modes. For the next competition, the athlete repeats the periodization cycle.

Periodization structures an inverse relation between training volume and training intensity through the competition phase; it then decreases both aspects during the second transition or recuperation period. Note the increase in time devoted to technique training as competition approaches,

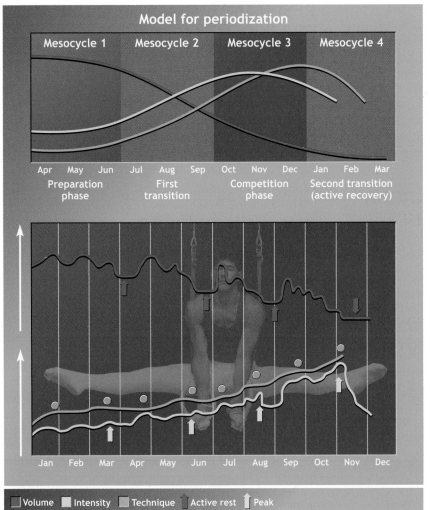

Describe functional strength.

List the 4 phases of periodization.

1.

2.

3.

4.

During the competition phase, describe the relationship between training volume and training intensity.

Figure 14.16 **Top.** Periodization subdivides a macrocycle into distinct phases or mesocycles. These in turn separate into weekly microcycles. The general plan provides modifications, but mesocycles typically include four parts: (1) preparation phase, (2) first transition phase, (3) competition phase, and (4) a second transition or active recovery phase. **Bottom.** Example of periodization for an elite athlete (gymnast) preparing for competition. Competitions took place throughout the yearly training program, so periodization focused on achieving peak performance at the end of each macrocycle. Periodization places training into context for intensity, duration, and frequency of strength–power workouts. The major purpose of this focus attempts to avoid overtraining (staleness), minimize injury potential, and reduce training monotony while progressing toward peak competition performance (*filled green circles*).

with training volume at the periodization cycle's lowest point. The *bottom* of **Figure 14.16** illustrates how training volume and intensity interact within a mesocycle for an athlete in a specific sport.

Sport-specific training principles usually apply in periodization to design a training regimen based on a sport's distinct *strength*, *power*, and *endurance* requirements. A detailed analysis of metabolic and technical requirements of the sport also frames the training paradigm.

Sport-Specific Training Principles

Sport-specific training principles apply in periodization as the coach (and athlete) design training based on the sport's particular strength, power, and endurance requirements. A detailed analysis of metabolic and technical requirements of the sport also frames the training paradigm. The concept of periodization makes intuitive sense, yet few if any studies present conclusive evidence for this training approach. Confounding factors include difficulty controlling for differences in training intensity, training volume, and the participants' fitness capacities. One critical review of periodized strength training concluded that it produced greater improvements in muscular strength, body mass, lean body mass, and percentage body fat than nonperiodized multi- and single-set training programs.

PRACTICAL RECOMMENDATIONS FOR INITIATING A RESISTANCE-TRAINING PROGRAM

1. Avoid maximum lifts in the beginning stages of resistance training. Excessive resistance contributes little to strength development and greatly increases the risk of muscle or joint injury. A load equal to 60% to 80% of a muscle's force-generating capacity sufficiently stimulates increase in muscular strength. This load generally allows completion of about 10 repetitions of a particular movement.
2. Use lighter resistance to perform more repetitions at the start of training. Novices should initially attempt 12 to 15 repetitions. This regimen does not place excessive strain on the musculoskeletal system during the early phase of the program. Use a heavier load if 12 repetitions feel too easy. The resistance is too heavy if the exerciser cannot complete 12 repetitions. This trial-and-error process may take several exercise sessions to establish the proper starting weight.
3. After several weeks of training, when the muscles adapt and the exerciser learns the correct movements, decrease the repetitions to between 6 and 8.
4. Add more resistance after reaching the target number of repetitions. This regimen represents progressive resistance training; as muscles become stronger, resistance increases with the lifting of a heavier load.
5. The exercise sequence should proceed from larger to smaller muscle groups to avoid premature fatigue of the smaller group.

RESISTANCE-TRAINING GUIDELINES FOR SEDENTARY ADULTS, ELDERLY INDIVIDUALS, AND CARDIAC PATIENTS

Currently, the ACSM (*www.acsm.org*), American Heart Association (*www.aha.org*), Centers for Disease Control and Prevention (*www.cdc.gov*), American Association of Cardiovascular and Pulmonary Rehabilitation (*www.aacvpr.org*), and the U.S. Surgeon General's Office (*www.surgeongeneral.gov*) consider regular resistance exercise an important component of a comprehensive, health-related physical fitness program. Resistance training goals for competitive athletes focus on optimizing muscular strength, power, and muscular hypertrophy "with high-intensity" 1- to 6-RM training loads. In contrast, goals for most middle-aged and older adults focus on maintenance (and possible increase) of muscle and bone mass and muscular strength and muscular endurance to enhance the overall health and physical-fitness profile. Adequate muscular strength in midlife maintains a margin of safety above the necessary threshold required to prevent injury in later life.

The resistance-training program recommended for middle-aged and older men and women classifies as "moderate intensity." In contrast to the multiple-set, heavy-resistance approach used by younger athletes, the program uses single sets of different exercises performed between 8- and 15-RM a minimum of twice weekly.

Resistance Training Plus Aerobic Training Equals Less Strength Improvement

Concurrent resistance and aerobic training programs produce less muscular strength and power improvement than training for strength only. This partly explains why power athletes and body builders refrain from endurance activities while participating in resistance training. More than likely, the added energy (and perhaps protein) demands of intense endurance training impose a limit on a muscle's growth and metabolic responsiveness to resistance training. Also, an acute, short-term bout of intense endurance exercise inhibits performance in subsequent muscular strength activities.

 SUMMARY

1. The four common methods to measure muscular strength include: tensiometry; dynamometry; 1-RM testing with weights; and computer-assisted force and work-output determinations, including isokinetic measurement.

2. Substantial physiologic and performance specificity in the response to training cast doubt on the appropriateness of general fitness measures, including strength tests, to determine the success in specific physical tasks or occupations.

3. Human skeletal muscle theoretically generates a maximum of 16 to 30 N of maximum force per cm² of muscle cross-section regardless of gender.

4. On an absolute basis, men outperform women on tests of strength because of men's larger quantity of muscle mass. These differences are greatest in upper-body muscular strength.

5. Muscles become stronger with overload training that increases the load, increases the speed of muscle action, or combines both increases in load and speed.

6. Strength gains occur when the overload represents at least 60% to 80% of a muscle's maximum force-generating capacity.

7. Closely supervised resistance training for children using moderate levels of concentric exercise improves muscular strength with no adverse effects on bone or muscle.

8. Three major exercise systems develop muscular strength: dynamic constant external resistance training, isometric training, and isokinetic training. Each system produces highly specific strength gains that relate directly to the training mode.

9. Resistance training exercises performed incorrectly with excessive hyperextension or back arch create shearing forces that produce undesirable muscle strain or spinal pressure and trigger low-back pain.

10. Isokinetic training generates maximum force throughout the full ROM at different limb movement velocities. This training method applies resistance training to enhance specific sports performance.

11. Plyometric training incorporates the inherent stretch–recoil characteristics of the neuromuscular system to develop specific muscular power.

12. Body weight loading with suspension training activates both agonists and antagonist muscles about a joint, including additional muscle groups along the kinetic chain.

13. Suspension training introduces the added component of instability to further challenge trunk and back muscle neuromuscular control.

14. Periodization divides a distinct period or macrocycle of resistance training into smaller training mesocycles; these subdivide into weekly microcycles. Compartmentalization of training minimizes staleness and overtraining effects to maximize peak performance that coincides with competition.

15. Resistance training for competitive athletes optimizes muscular strength, power, and hypertrophy.

16. Functional movement training via body weight–supported exercise offers a unique approach to sports training.

17. Resistance training goals for middle-aged and older adults aim to modestly improve muscular strength and endurance, maintain muscle and bone mass, and enhance overall health and fitness.

18. The specificity of physiologic and performance measures and their response to training casts doubt on the efficacy of general fitness measures to predict ability to perform specific tasks or occupations.

19. Resistance training for specific sports should develop maximum force-generating capacity throughout a muscle's ROM at a speed that closely mimics the actual performance.

20. Concurrent training for muscular strength and aerobic capacity inhibits the magnitude of strength improvement compared with training only for muscular strength.

THOUGHT QUESTIONS

1. Explain why athletes have spotters apply external force to the bar in the early phase of a bench press with weight to increase difficulty and then provide assistance toward its completion.

2. Based on your knowledge of gender-related differences in muscular strength, devise a physical test that (1) minimizes and (2) maximizes performance differences between men and women.

3. If a man and a woman of the same age and body weight could be matched for MCSA of the upper arms and shoulders and they both performed a 1-RM seated press, who would achieve the higher press score, the man or the woman?

4. Discuss the statement: "There is no one best system of resistance training."

Part 2 | Adaptations to Resistance Training

Resistance training produces both acute responses and chronic adaptations. *An **acute response** refers to immediate changes in muscle or other cells, tissues, or systems during or immediately after a single exercise bout.* For example, energy stores and cardiovascular dynamics change in response to specific muscle actions. Repeated exposure to a stimulus produces a longer lasting change that influences the acute response over time (e.g., less disruption in cellular integrity [muscle damage] with a given level of exercise). *Adaptation refers to how the body adjusts to a repeated (chronic) stimulus.*

Knowing the acute and chronic responses to resistance training facilitates exercise prescription and program design. Adaptations to repeated muscular overload ultimately determine a training program's effectiveness. The time course of adaptations varies among individuals and depends on the nature and magnitude of prior adaptations. Also, a resistance-training program must consider the expression of individual differences in adaptation (training responsiveness).

Adaptations to resistance training occur from the cellular to systemic levels. **Figure 14.17** displays six factors that impact muscle mass development and maintenance. More than likely, genetic factors strongly influence the effect of each factor on the ultimate training outcome. Resistance training contributes little to tissue growth without appropriate nutrition. Similarly, training outcome depends on specific hormones and patterns of nervous system activation. Without muscular overload, each of the other factors cannot work synergistically to increase muscle mass and muscle strength.

NEURAL ADAPTATIONS

Well-documented changes from overload training occur in the gross structural and microscopic architecture within muscle tissue. **Figure 14.18** showcases the relative roles of neural and muscular adaptations in strength improvement with resistance training. Note that neural adaptations predominate in the early phase of training (this phase encompasses the duration of most research studies). Hypertrophy-induced adaptations place the upper limit on longer term training improvements. This tempts many athletes to use anabolic steroids or human growth hormone (*dashed line*) to induce continual hypertrophy if training alone fails to stimulate further muscle growth.

A classic series of experiments illustrates the importance of psychologic factors in expressing muscular strength in humans. The researchers measured arm strength in college-age men under five conditions: (1) normal conditions, (2) immediately after a loud noise, (3) while the subject screamed loudly at the time of exertion, (4) under the influence of alcohol and amphetamines ("pep pills"), (5) and under hypnosis (told they possessed considerable strength and should not fear injury). Each of the alterations generally increased strength above normal levels; hypnosis, the most "mental" of all treatments, produced the greatest increments.

The investigators theorized that temporary modifications in CNS function accounted for strength improvements under the various conditions. They argued that most persons normally operate at a level of neural inhibition, perhaps via protective reflex mechanisms that constrain the expression of strength capacity. Three factors—muscle cross-section, fiber type, and mechanical arrangement of bone and muscle—explain strength capacity.

Neuromuscular inhibition can come from unpleasant past experiences with exercise, an overly protective home environment, or fear or avoidance of injury. Regardless of the reason, individuals typically cannot express their maximum strength capacity. Increased neurologic arousal may account for "unexplainable" feats of strength and power during highly charged emergency and rescue situations (e.g., a relatively small person lifting an extremely heavy object off an injured person). In athletics, the excitement of intense competition or the influence of disinhibitory drugs or hypnotic suggestion can induce a "supermaximal"

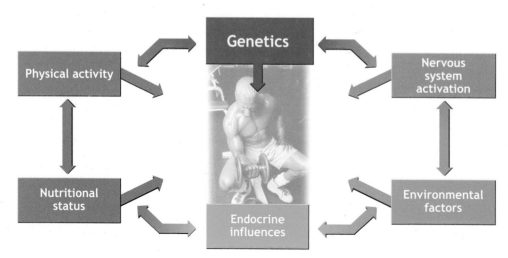

Figure 14.17 Interaction of six factors that develop and maintain muscle mass.

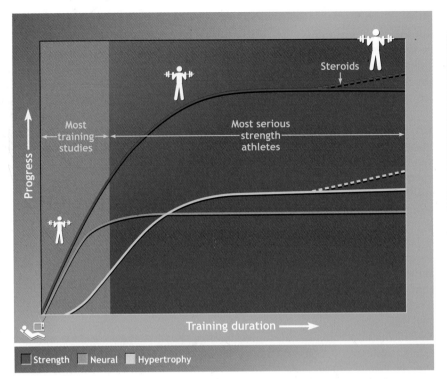

Figure 14.18 Relative roles of neural and muscular adaptations in strength improvement with resistance training. Neural adaptations predominate in the early phase of training and hypertrophy-induced adaptations place the upper limit on longer term training improvements. This tempts many athletes to use anabolic steroids or human growth hormone (*dashed line*) to induce continual hypertrophy. (From Sale, D.G.: Neural adaptation to resistance training. *Med. Sci. Sports Exerc.*, 20:135, 1988.)

Questions & Notes

List 4 factors that impact development and maintenance of muscle mass.

1.

2.

3.

4.

List 2 factors that determine a person's muscular strength capacity.

1.

2.

ⓘ For Your Information

NEURAL ADAPTATIONS ARE IMPORTANT

Three factors enhance neural adaptations with resistance training:

1. Increased CNS activation
2. Improved motor unit synchronization
3. Lowered neural inhibitory reflexes

performance from greatly reduced neural inhibition and optimal motoneuron recruitment. Rapid improvements in muscular strength during the first few weeks of strength training largely result from a "learning" phenomenon, or a lessening of fear and psychological inhibition, as the novice becomes more practiced with the specific strength activity (e.g., proper form in bench press or squat exercise).

Highly trained athletes often create an almost self-hypnotic state by intensely concentrating, or "psyching," before competition. It sometimes takes years of training to perfect the "block out" of extraneous stimuli (e.g., crowd noise) so the muscle action ties in directly to performance. This practice has been perfected in power-lifting competition where success depends on precise, coordinated movements *with* maximal muscle tension output. Enhanced arousal level and accompanying neural disinhibition, or facilitation can fully activate muscle groups.

ⓘ For Your Information

NEURAL AND MUSCULAR FACTORS DETERMINE STRENGTH

Generalized response curve for gains in muscle strength with resistance training occur from both neural (*orange*) or muscular (*yellow*) factors. During a typical 8-week training interval, neural factors account for approximately 90% of the "strength" gains over the first 2 weeks of workouts. In the subsequent 2 weeks, between 40 and 50% of the strength improvement still relates to nervous system adaptation (in the higher centers and local muscle levels). Thereafter, muscle fiber adaptations become progressively more important to strength improvement. Experiments of this type generally assess the neural contributions from integrated surface EMG recordings of the muscle groups trained or other aspects of neural control involved in timing and coordination patterning.

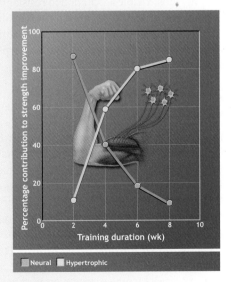

Motor Unit Activation: Size Principle Recruitment of motor units occurs in sequence from low to high thresholds and thus from low to high muscle force output. An increased rate of motor unit firing also increases a muscle's force output. These two factors—recruitment of motor units and increase in their firing rate—produce a continuum of voluntary force output from muscle.

Type II motor units have a high twitch force; they become activated in activities requiring significant force. In contrast, type I motor units activate under requirements that generate less force. Individuals unaccustomed to intense physical demands probably cannot voluntarily recruit all their higher threshold type II motor units; thus, they cannot maximally tap their muscle's true strength potential. An adaptation to resistance training develops how well an untrained person recruits more motor units to achieve a maximal muscle action. Increased synchronization of motor unit firing provides another neural adjustment to increase force production with training. Greater synchronization causes more motor units to fire simultaneously.

In experienced weight lifters, neural components also contribute to strength improvements. In one study, minimal changes took place in muscle fiber size, yet 2 years of training increased absolute strength and power. EMG analysis revealed enhanced voluntary activation of muscle over the training period. This suggests that neural components contribute significantly to strength improvements.

MUSCLE ADAPTATIONS

As previously pointed out, psychological inhibitions and learning factors greatly modify muscular strength, yet the anatomic and intrinsic physiologic factors within the muscle determine the ultimate limit of strength development. Gross and ultrastructural changes in muscle with chronic resistance training generally produce adaptations in the contractile apparatus accompanied by substantial gains in muscular strength and power. Increase in muscle external size represents the most visible adaptation to resistance training. **Muscle fiber hypertrophy** (increased muscle fiber size) usually explains increases in gross muscle size, although increased muscle fiber number, termed **fiber hyperplasia** provides a controversial complementary hypothesis.

Muscle Fiber Hypertrophy

An increase in muscular tension (force) with exercise training provides the primary stimulus to initiate the process of skeletal muscle growth or hypertrophy. Changes in muscle size become detectable as early as 3 weeks of training, and the remodeling of muscle architecture precedes gains in muscle cross-sectional area. *Muscle hypertrophy with resistance training represents a fundamental biologic adaptation.* The extraordinarily large muscle size and well-defined "ripped" musculature of weight lifters and body builders results from enlargement of muscle cells, mainly

the fast-twitch, type II fibers. Growth takes place from one or more of the following four adaptations:

1. Increased amounts of contractile proteins (actin and myosin)
2. Increased number and size of myofibrils per muscle fiber
3. Increased amounts of connective, tendinous, and ligamentous tissues
4. Increased quantity of enzymes and stored nutrients

Not all muscle fibers undergo the same degree of enlargement with resistance training. *Muscle growth depends on muscle fiber type activation and their recruitment pattern.* As discussed previously, improving muscular strength and power does not necessarily require muscle fiber hypertrophy because important neurologic factors initially affect the expression of human strength. The later, slower occurring strength improvements generally coincide with noticeable alterations in a muscle's subcellular molecular

Table 14.5	Physiologic Adaptations to Resistance Training
SYSTEM/VARIABLE	**RESPONSE**
Muscle Fibers	
Number	Equivocal
Size	Increase
Type	Unknown
Capillary Density	
In bodybuilders	No change
In powerlifters	Decrease
Mitochondria	
Volume	Decrease
Density	Decrease
Twitch Contraction Time	
Enzymes	Decrease
Creatine phosphokinase	Increase
Myokinase	Increase
Enzymes of Glycolysis	
Phosphofructokinase	Increase
Lactate dehydrogenase	No change
Aerobic Metabolism Enzymes	
Carbohydrate	Increase
Triacylglycerol	Not known
Intramuscular Fuel Stores	
Adenosine triphosphate	Increase
Phosphocreatine	Increase
Glycogen	Increase
Triacylglycerols	Not known
$\dot{V}O_{2max}$	
Circuit resistance training	Increase
Heavy resistance training	No change
Connective Tissue	
Ligament strength	Increase
Tendon strength	Increase
Collagen content of muscle	No change
Bone	
Mineral content	Increase
Cross-sectional area	No change
Resistance to fracture	Increase

Modified from Fleck, S.J., and Kramer, W.J.: Resistance training: Physiological responses and adaptations (Part 2 of 4). *Phys. Sports Med.,* 16:108, 1988.

architecture. As training continues, contractile proteins increase in conjunction with enlarged muscle fiber cross-sectional area. *Overload training enlarges muscle fibers with subsequent muscle growth.* The fast-twitch fibers of weight lifters average about 45% larger than fibers of healthy sedentary persons and endurance athletes. The hypertrophic process couples directly to increased mononuclear number and synthesis of cellular components, particularly protein filaments (myosin heavy chain and actin) that constitute the contractile elements. Skeletal muscle *remodels* its internal architecture, potentially reconfiguring external orientation and hence its shape. **Table 14.5** lists important cellular and physiologic adaptations in muscle to resistance training.

Significant Metabolic Adaptations Occur

Success at elite levels of sport performance undoubtedly requires a particular muscle fiber distribution. The relatively fixed nature of muscle fiber type suggests an obvious genetic predisposition for exceptional, world-class level performance. Considerable plasticity exists for metabolic potential because specific training enhances the anaerobic and aerobic energy transfer capacity of both fiber types. The heightened oxidative capacity of fast-twitch fibers with endurance training brings them to a level nearly equal to the aerobic capacity of the slow-twitch fibers of untrained counterparts. Age presents no barrier to training adaptations of muscle fibers. With an adequate training stimulus, skeletal muscle fiber size, capillarization, and glycolytic and respiratory enzymes of older men and women adapt to both endurance and resistance training similar to younger persons.

Endurance training induces some intraconversion of contractile and neural characteristics of type II fibers. The well-documented increase in mitochondrial size and number and corresponding increase in the total quantity of citric acid cycle and electron transport enzymes accompany these fiber subdivision adaptations. Only specifically trained muscle fibers adapt to regular exercise; this explains why well-trained athletes who change to a sport demanding use of primarily different muscle groups or different portions of the same muscle often feel untrained for the new activity. Within this framework, swimmers or canoeists with well-trained upper-body musculature do not necessarily transfer their upper body fitness to a running sport that relies predominantly on a highly conditioned lower-body musculature with its specifically-trained fiber type distribution.

Muscle Remodeling: Can Fiber Type Be Changed?

Skeletal muscle represents dynamic tissue whose cells do not remain as fixed populations of cells throughout life. Rather, muscle fibers undergo regeneration and remodeling in response to diverse functional demands like resistance or endurance training to alter their phenotypic profile. Activation of muscle via specific types and intensities of long-term use stimulates otherwise dormant myogenic stem cells (**satellite cells**) beneath a muscle fiber's basement membrane to proliferate and differentiate to form new fibers. Fusion of satellite cell nuclei and their incorporation into existing muscle fibers probably enables the fiber to synthesize more proteins to form additional myofibrils. This most likely contributes directly to muscular hypertrophy with chronic overload and may stimulate transformation of existing fibers from one type to another. A variety of extracellular signal molecules, primarily peptide growth factors (e.g., insulin-like growth factor [IGF], fibroblast growth factors, transforming growth factors, and hepatocyte growth factor), governs satellite cell activity and possibly exercise-induced muscle fiber proliferation and differentiation.

Studies with humans and animals support the concept that skeletal muscle adapts to altered functional demands. *Muscle fiber-type transformation may occur with specific exercise training.* In one study, four athletes trained anaerobically for 11 weeks followed by 18 weeks of aerobic training. Anaerobic training increased the percentage of type II fibers and decreased the percentage of type I fibers; the opposite occurred during the aerobic training phase. Similarly, 4 to

Questions & Notes

Briefly describe the size principle of motor unit recruitment.

List 3 adaptations in muscle that influence muscle growth.

1.

2.

3.

Indicate (with an up or down arrow) the specific physiologic adaptations to resistance training that occur for the following variables:

Muscle fiber size:

Mitochondria volume:

Mitochondria density:

Twitch contraction time:

Connective tissue ligament strength:

Bone mineral content:

Give one reasonable explanation for muscle hypertrophy.

Explain if resistance training induced muscle remodeling occurs.

6 weeks of sprint training increased the percentage of type II with a commensurate decrease in type I fiber percentage. Increasing the daily training duration also increases the fast- to slow-twitch shift in myosin heavy-chain phenotype in rat hindlimb muscles. Specific training (and perhaps inactivity) may convert different physiologic characteristics of type I to type II fibers and within type II (and vice versa). Available evidence does not permit definitive statements concerning the fixed nature of a muscle's fiber composition. *The genetic code more than likely exerts the greatest influence on fiber-type distribution.* The major direction of a muscle's fiber composition probably becomes fixed before birth or during the first few years of life.

Favorable Response of Middle-Aged and Elderly Individuals

Muscles and tendons, which are highly adaptable tissues, respond favorably to chronic changes in loading independent of age or gender. As such, men and women experience considerable physiologic and performance adaptations with resistance training, independent of aging effects. A study of five older healthy men (average age, 68 y) clearly demonstrates the remarkable plasticity of human skeletal muscle among middle-aged individuals. The men trained for 12 weeks using heavy-resistance, isokinetic, and free-weight exercises. Training increased muscle volume and cross-sectional area of the biceps brachii (14%) and brachialis (26%), and hypertrophy increased by 37.2% in the type II muscle fibers. Increases of 46.0% in peak torque and 29% in total work output accompanied these cellular adaptations (**Fig. 14.19**).

Equally impressive training responses occur for elderly persons. One hundred nursing home residents (average age, 87.1 y) trained for 10 weeks with high-intensity resistance training. For the 63 women and 37 men who participated, muscle strength increased an average of 113%. Strength increases also paralleled improved function, reflected by an 11.8% increase in normal gait velocity and 28.4% increase in stair-climbing speed; thigh muscle cross-sectional area increased by about 3%. Other studies also have verified the benefits of functional strength training to improve *activities of daily living (ADLs)*, including countering the devastating medical consequences of slips and falls in elderly people.

Changes in Muscle Fiber-Type Composition with Resistance Training

Research has evaluated the effects of resistance exercise training on muscle fiber size and composition for leg extensor muscles. Biopsy specimens from vastus lateralis muscle before and after resistance training showed no change in percentage distribution of fast- and slow-twitch muscle fibers indicated by changes in myofibrillar ATPase.

Metabolic characteristics of specific fibers and fiber subdivisions undergo modification within 4 to 8 weeks of resistance training. This occurs despite the lack of dramatic changes in inherent muscle fiber types with chronic exercise. Remodeling of type II fibers denotes one of the more prominent and rapid resistance training adaptations.

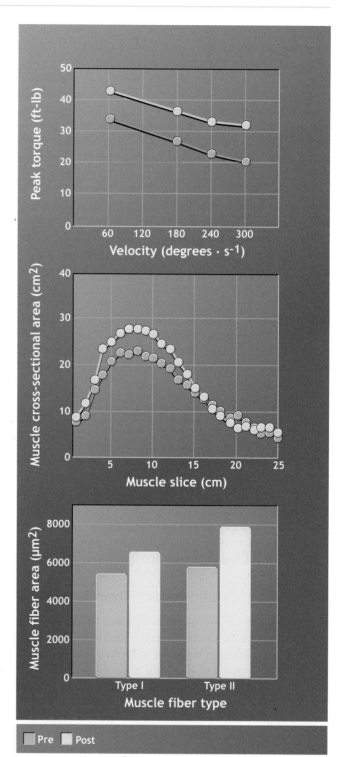

Figure 14.19 Plasticity of aging muscle. Data from five older men before (*orange*) and after (*yellow*) 12 weeks of heavy-resistance training. **Top.** Peak torque of elbow flexors. **Middle.** Plot of flexor cross-sectional area computed from magnetic resonance imaging scans from proximal (*right*) to distal (*left*) end of muscle. **Bottom.** Average for type I and type II fiber areas. (From Roman, W.J., et al.: Adaptations in the elbow flexors of elderly males after heavy-resistance training. *J. Appl. Physiol.*, 74:750, 1993.)

*Muscle Fiber Hypertrophy and Testos-
terone Levels*   Popular dogma maintains
that the chief male sex hormone, testosterone, facilitates muscle hypertrophy with
resistance training. Variation in testosterone levels may explain individual differences in muscular enlargement with
resistance training and the smaller hypertrophic response of women to similar muscular overload. *Essentially no correlation
exists between plasma testosterone levels and
body composition and muscular strength in
men and women.* Individuals with high muscle strength or FFM can have high, intermediate, or low testosterone levels. Acute
increases in sex hormone release occurs
after a single bout of maximal resistance
training (or any maximal effort exercise),
the effect remains transient and probably of
little consequence to muscle development
or training responsiveness.

ⓘ For Your Information

How athletes integrate
five crucial components
involved in fitness or
physical training that
contribute to the window
for explosive power
development.

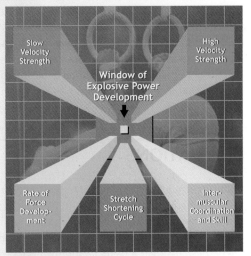

(Adapted with permission from Kraemer, W.J.,
Newton, R.U.: Training for muscular power.
Phys. Med. Rehabil. Clin., 11:341, 2000.)

Muscle Fiber Hypertrophy: Male Versus Female   Computed tomography
scans to evaluate muscle cross-sectional area show that men and women experience *similar* hypertrophic responses to resistance training. Men achieve a
greater absolute increase in muscle size because of a larger initial total muscle
mass but without a difference in muscle enlargement on a percentage basis
compared with women of similar training status.

Other comparisons between elite male and female bodybuilders verify these
observations. *Limited data from short-term studies indicate that women can use
conventional resistance training methods to gain muscle strength and size on a similar percentage basis as men.*

Muscle Fiber Hyperplasia

A common question concerns whether resistance training produces hyperplasia
or increased number of muscle cells. If this does occur, to what extent does it
contribute to muscle enlargement? Chronic overload of skeletal muscle in various animal species develops new muscle fibers from satellite cells between the
basement layer and plasma membrane or by longitudinal splitting. Under conditions of stress, neuromuscular disease, and muscle injury, the normally dormant satellite cells develop into new muscle fibers. With longitudinal splitting,
a relatively large muscle fiber splits into two or more smaller individual daugh-
ter cells through lateral budding. These fibers function more efficiently than the
large single fiber from which they originated.

Generalizing findings from research on animals to humans poses a problem.
The massive cellular hypertrophy in humans with resistance training does not
occur in many animal species. In cats, for example, muscle fiber hyperplasia
reflects the primary compensatory adjustment to muscular overload.

Some evidence supporting hyperplasia in humans does exist. Autopsy data from
young, healthy men who died accidentally show that muscle fiber counts of the
larger and stronger leg (the leg opposite the dominant hand) contained 10%
more muscle fibers than the smaller leg. Cross-sectional studies of body
builders with large limb circumferences and muscle mass failed to show that
they possessed above-normal-size individual muscle fibers. The possibility does
exist that some of the body builders inherited an initially large number of small
muscle fibers that then "hypertrophied" to normal size with resistance training,
yet the findings suggest the likelihood of hyperplasia with certain forms of

Questions & Notes

*Briefly describe the possible role of testos-
terone in the hypertrophic response to
resistance training.*

Describe muscle fiber hyperplasia.

*Do women respond similarly to resistance
training as men?*

ⓘ For Your Information

MUSCULAR STRENGTH AND PUBERTY

Until puberty, boys maintain about
10% greater muscle strength than girls.
After age 12 years, boys continue to
increase in strength, but strength
plateaus in girls. Gender-related
changes in body composition account
for much of the strength difference.

resistance training. Muscle fibers may adapt differently to high-volume, high-intensity training used by body builders than to the typical low-repetition, heavy-load system favored by strength and power athletes. *Even if other human studies replicate training-induced hyperplasia and even if the response reflects a positive adjustment, hypertrophy represents the most important contribution to increased muscle size from overload training in humans.*

CONNECTIVE TISSUE AND BONE ADAPTATIONS

Ligaments, tendons, and bone correspondingly strengthen as muscle strength and size increase. Increases in ligament and tendon strength generally parallel the rate of muscle fiber adaptation. In contrast, changes in bone improve more slowly, perhaps over a 6- to 12-month period. Connective tissue proliferates around individual muscle fibers to thicken and strengthen the muscle's connective tissue strutures. Such adaptations from resistance training help to protect joints and muscles from injury and justify resistance exercise for preventive and rehabilitative strategies. Resistance training also positively affects bone dynamics in young individuals. Elite 14- to 17-year-old Junior Olympic weight lifters, for example, have higher bone densities in the hip and femur regions than age-matched control subjects or adults.

CARDIOVASCULAR ADAPTATIONS

Training volume and intensity influence the impact of resistance training on cardiovascular system adaptations (Table 14.6).

Subtle yet important differences exist between myocardial enlargement from resistance training (**physiologic hypertrophy**) and enlargement from chronic hypertension (**pathologic hypertrophy**). In pathologic conditions, ventricular wall thickness increases beyond normal limits for age and gender independent of the assessment method and evaluative criteria. Dilation and weakening of the left ventricle, a frequent response to chronic hypertension (and subsequent heart failure), do not accompany the compensatory increase in myocardial wall thickness that occurs with resistance training. The hearts of champion resistance-trained athletes usually exceed the size of untrained counterparts, but heart size generally falls within the upper range of normal limits related to body size or cardiac function variables.

Resistance exercise more acutely increases blood pressure than lower intensity dynamic movements but does *not* produce any long-term increase in resting blood pressure. Weight lifters and body builders with hypertension probably have pre-existing essential hypertension (no medical cause can explain it), experience chronic overtraining syndrome, use anabolic steroids, or possess an undesirable level of body fat or other hypertension risks established for the general population.

Table 14.6	Cardiovascular Adaptations to Resistance Training	
VARIABLE		**ADAPTATION**
Rest		
Heart rate		No change
Blood pressure		
Diastolic		Decrease or no change
Systolic		Decrease or no change
Rate-pressure product (HR $\times$ SBP)		Decrease or no change
Stroke volume		Increase or no change
Cardiac function		Increase or no change
Left ventricular wall thickness		Increase
Right ventricular wall thickness		No change
Left ventricular chamber volume		No change
Right ventricular chamber volume		No change
Left ventricular mass		Increase
Lipid profile		
Total cholesterol		Decrease
HDL-C		Increase or no change
LDL-C		Decrease or no change
During exercise		
Heart rate		No change
Blood pressure		
Diastolic		Decrease
Systolic		Decrease
Rate-pressure product		Decrease
Stroke volume		Increase or no change
Cardiac output		Increase or no change
$\dot{V}O_{2peak}$		Increase or no change

Metabolic Stress of Resistance Training

Metabolic and cardiovascular evaluations indicate that traditional resistance training methods offer little benefit for aerobic fitness or weight control or for significantly modifying risk factors related to cardiovascular disease. Oxygen uptake for both isometric and typical weight-lifting exercises classify as "light to moderate" for energy expenditure even though participants report considerable muscular stress. A person can perform 15 or 20 different resistance exercises during a 1-hour training session, yet the net total time to perform exercise usually lasts no longer than 6 or 7 minutes. This relatively brief activity period (with only moderate energy expenditure) reinforces that traditional resistance training programs would not improve endurance capacity in sports with a large running component such as soccer or basketball. Resistance training exercises also serve only limited value as the primary activities in a weight-loss program because of the relatively low total energy expenditure during "typical" training sessions.

Circuit Resistance Training: Increased Energy Expenditure

Modifying standard resistance training by de-emphasizing heavy overload and emphasizing more repititions with lighter weights increases exercise caloric expenditure and workout volume to improve more than one aspect of physical fitness. Research has focused on the energy cost and cardiorespiratory demands of **circuit resistance training** (CRT). In CRT, a pre-established exercise-rest sequence usually consists of eight to 15 different

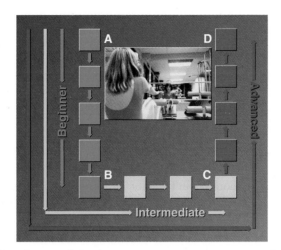

Figure 14.20 A basic multilevel exercise circuit. Beginners can work twice through the circuit from A to B. After several weeks, they progress three times through this portion of the circuit. Finally, they increase the number of circuit revolutions up to six, depending on the number of stations. At the intermediate level, several stations are added, and participants proceed three to six times through circuits A to C. Progression is built into each circuit by increasing the number of stations (A to D) or exercise load, repetitions, and duration.

exercise stations, with 15 to 20 repetitions performed for each exercise. *Exercise resistance requires between 40% and 50% of 1-RM.* After a 15- to 30-second rest interval, participants move to succeeding exercise stations to complete the circuit. **Figure 14.20** outlines the sequence of progression through a multilevel, five- to 12-station circuit.

In one experiment, net energy expended (excluding resting metabolism) equaled 129 kCal for men and 95 kCal for women over the total exercise period. Heart rate averaged 142 b·min^{-1} (72% HR$_{max}$; 40% $\dot{V}O_{2max}$) for men and 158 b·min^{-1} (82% HR$_{max}$; 45% $\dot{V}O_{2max}$) for women.

CRT provides an alternative for fitness enthusiasts who desire a general conditioning program that improves both muscular strength and aerobic capacity. It also can supplement an off-season fitness program for sports that require a high level of muscular strength, power, and endurance.

Table 14.7 presents energy expenditure data for different types of resistance-type exercises compared with walking on the level. Isokinetic CRT procedures produced the highest energy expenditures.

Table 14.7	Energy Expenditure for Different Modes of Resistance Exercise Compared with Walking[a]		
MODE	**GENDER**	**kJ·min^{-1}**	**kCal·min^{-1}**
Nautilus, circuit	M	29.7	7.1
	F	24.3	5.8
Nautilus, circuit	M	22.6	5.4
Universal, circuit	M	33.1	7.9
	F	28.5	6.8
Isokinetic, slow	M	40.2	9.6
Isokinetic, fast	M	41.4	9.9
Isometric and free weight	M	25.1	6.0
Hydra-Fitness, circuit	M	37.7	9.0
Walking on level	M	22.6	5.4

[a]Based on a body weight of 68 kg.
Data from Katch, F.I., et al.: Evaluation of acute cardiorespiratory responses to hydraulic resistance exercise. *Med. Sci. Sports Exerc.,* 17:168, 1985.

Questions & Notes

List 3 cardiovascular adaptations resulting from resistance training.

1.

2.

3.

Discuss the differences between physiologic and pathologic myocardial hypertrophy.

Describe the basis of circuit resistance training.

Which type or CRT program produces the greatest energy expenditure?

BOX 14.4 CLOSE UP

How to Assess Muscular Endurance

Muscular endurance represents how well a muscle or muscle group exerts submaximum force repeatedly within a given time period, or the duration a given muscle action can sustain a percentage of its 1-RM either dynamically or isometrically. The number of total repetitions of a muscle action in a given time (e.g., number of curl-ups, sit-ups, or push-ups within 1 minute or while maintaining a given cadence) provides a common yardstick for expressing muscular endurance. Muscular endurance depends somewhat on a muscle's maximum strength but little on cardiorespiratory fitness because components of aerobic fitness represent separate physiological (and fitness) entities. To test muscular endurance using free weights, the weight lifted should coincide with either a percentage of body weight (**Table 1**) or a percentage of 1-RM, so total repetition number averages between 15 and 20.

Two of the more popular muscular endurance tests do not require weights to assess endurance of the abdominal (curl-up) and upper-body (push-up) musculatures.

CURL-UP MUSCULAR ENDURANCE TEST

Initial Position
The individual lies supine with knees flexed and feet about 1 foot from the buttocks. The arms extend forward with fingers palm down on the thighs pointing toward the knees (**Fig. 1A**). The tester kneels behind the person with hands cupped (about 2 inches off the floor) under the individual's head.

Movement
The person curls up slowly, sliding the fingers up the legs until the fingertips touch the patellae (knee caps; **Fig. 1B**) followed by slowly returning to the starting position with the back of the head touching the tester's hands. To reduce lower back strain, minimize rectus femoris involvement and emphasize abdominal muscle action; no assistance should anchor or support the feet.

Table 1	Recommended Percentage of Body Weight Lifted in Different Resistance Exercise Movements to Assess Muscular Endurance	
	PERCENTAGE OF BODY WEIGHT	
EXERCISE	**MEN**	**WOMEN**
Arm curl	0.33	0.25
Bench press	0.66	0.50
Lateral pull-down	0.66	0.50
Triceps extension	0.33	0.33
Leg extension	0.50	0.50
Leg curl	0.33	0.33

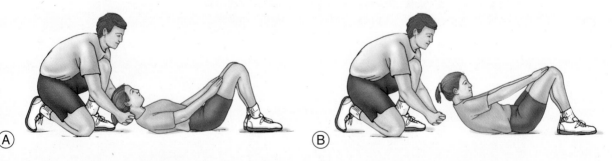

(A)   (B)

Figure 1 Start (**A**) and finish (**B**) positions for the curl-up test.

The Test and Standards

Required curl-up rate equals 20 repetitions per minute (3 s per curl-up; metronome set at 40 b·min^{-1}, or 2 beats per curl-up and recovery). Individuals perform as many curl-ups as possible at a cadence (which must be maintained) to a maximum of 75. Table 2 presents standards for evaluating scores on the curl-up test.

PUSH-UP MUSCULAR ENDURANCE TEST

The push-up muscular endurance test can be performed in one of two ways: (1) full-body push-up and (2) modified push-up that reduces the body mass above the arms, chest, and shoulders. The modified push-up serves as an alternative to assess individual differences in upper-body strength for women because they possess considerably less relative strength in upper-body musculature compared with men.

Initial Position

Full-Body Push-up: The person assumes a relatively stiff prone position from head to ankles, keeping the hands shoulder width apart and the arms fully extended (**Fig. 2A**).

Modified Push-up: The person assumes the bent-knee position with hips and buttocks pressing downward in line with the neck and shoulders (**Fig. 2B**).

Table 2 Test Standards to Assess Curl-up Performance			
	NUMBER OF CURL-UPS COMPLETED		
	AGE, y		
RATING	**<35**	**35–44**	**>45**
Excellent			
Men	60	50	40
Women	50	40	30
Good			
Men	45	40	25
Women	40	25	15
Fair			
Men	30	25	15
Women	25	15	10
Poor			
Men	15	10	5
Women	10	6	4

From Faulkner, R.A., et al.: A partial curl-up protocol for adults based on an analysis of two procedures. *Can. J. Sport Sci.*, 14:135, 1989 and Sparling, P.B., et al.: Development of a cadence curl-up for college students. *Res. Q. Exerc. Sport.*, 68:309, 1997.

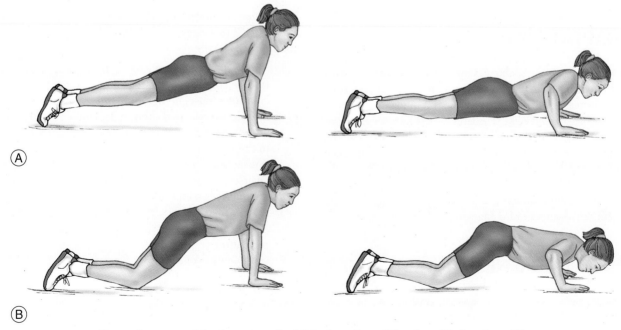

Figure 2 Start and finish positions for full-body push-up (**A**) and modified push-up (**B**).

(continued)

BOX 14.4 CLOSE UP

How to Assess Muscular Endurance (Continued)

Movement

Full-Body Push-up and Modified Push-up: The body lowers until the elbows reach 90° of flexion; the return action requires pushing up until the arms fully extend. The push-up action should proceed in a continuous motion without rest pauses between flexion–extension movements.

Standards

Table 3 presents standards for scoring the full body push-up (men) and modified push-up (women) tests.

Table 3 Test Standards to Assess Push-up Performance of Men (Full-Body Push-up) and Women (Modified Push-up)					
NUMBER OF PUSH-UPS COMPLETED					
	AGE, y				
RATING	20–29	30–39	40–49	50–59	60+
Full-body push-up					
Excellent	>54	>44	>39	>34	>29
Good	45–54	35–44	30–39	25–34	20–29
Average	35–44	25–34	20–29	15–24	10–19
Fair	20–34	15–24	12–19	8–14	5–9
Poor	<20	<15	<12	<8	<5
Modified push-up					
Excellent	>48	>39	>34	>29	>19
Good	34–48	25–39	20–34	15–29	5–19
Average	17–33	12–24	8–19	6–14	3–4
Fair	6–16	4–11	3–7	2–5	1–2
Poor	<6	<4	<3	<2	<1

From Pollock, M.L., et al.: *Health and Fitness Through Physical Activity*. New York: John Wiley & Sons, 1984.

BODY COMPOSITION ADAPTATIONS

Table 14.8 displays changes in body composition with DCER training from different experiments. For the most part, small decreases occur in body fat, with minimal increases in total body mass and FFM. The largest FFM increases amount to about 3 kg (6.6 lb) over 10 weeks, or about 0.3 kg weekly, with results about the same for men and women. Adherence to a reduced daily intake of calories can accelerate the weight loss. Body composition data for other dynamic strength training systems show similar results. No one resistance training system proves superior for changing body composition.

MUSCLE SORENESS AND STIFFNESS

Most people experience soreness and stiffness in the exercised joints and muscles after an extended layoff from exercise. Temporary soreness may persist for several hours immediately after unaccustomed exercise, but a residual delayed-onset muscle soreness (DOMS) appears later and can last for 3 or 4 days. Any of the following seven factors can produce DOMS:

1. Minute tears in muscle tissue or damage to its contractile components with accompanying release of creatine kinase, myoglobin, and troponin I (the muscle-specific marker of muscle fiber damage)
2. Osmotic pressure changes that cause fluid retention in the surrounding tissues
3. Muscle spasms
4. Overstretching and perhaps tearing of portions of the muscle's connective tissue harness
5. Acute inflammation
6. Alteration in the cells' mechanism for calcium regulation
7. Combination of the above factors

Eccentric Actions Produce Muscle Soreness

The precise cause of muscle soreness remains unknown. The degree of discomfort and muscle disturbance depends largely on the intensity and duration of effort and type of exercise performed. The magnitude of active strain imposed on a muscle fiber precipitates muscle damage and soreness. Eccentric and, to some extent, isometric muscle actions generally trigger the greatest postexercise discomfort, magnified among older individuals. Existing muscle damage or soreness from previous exercise does not exacerbate subsequent muscle damage or impair the regenerative process.

Cell Damage

The first bout of repetitive, unaccustomed physical activity disrupts the integrity of the cells' internal environment. This can produce microlesions and temporary ultrastructural damage in a pool of stress-susceptible or degenerating muscle fibers. Damage becomes more extensive several days after exercise than in the immediate postexercise period. A single bout of moderate concentric exercise provides a prophylactic effect on muscle soreness from subsequent high-force eccentric exercise, with the beneficial effect lasting up to 6 weeks. *Such results support the wisdom of initiating a training program with repetitive, moderate concentric exercise to protect against the muscle soreness that occurs after exercise with an eccentric component.*

Altered Sarcoplasmic Reticulum

Four factors produce major alterations in sarcoplasmic reticulum structure and function with unaccustomed exercise:

1. Changes in pH
2. Changes in intramuscular high-energy phosphates
3. Changes in ionic balance
4. Changes in temperature

These effects depress the rates of Ca^{2+} uptake and release and increase free Ca^{2+} concentration as the mineral rapidly moves into the cytosol of the damaged fibers. Intracellular Ca^{2+} overload contributes to the autolytic process within damaged muscle fibers that degrades the contractile and noncontractile structures.

Current Delayed-Onset Muscle Soreness Model

Figure 14.21 diagrams the probable steps in the development of DOMS that ultimately leads to an inflammatory process and subsequent recuperation.

Questions & Notes

Define DOMS.

When does DOMS usually develop following exercise?

List 4 factors that produce DOMS.

1.

2.

3.

4.

Name the type of muscle overload that produces the greatest level of DOMS.

Are changes in body composition resulting from DCER training the same for males and females?

			BODY COMPOSITION CHANGES		
GENDER	TRAINING DURATION, wk	# OF EXERCISES	BODY MASS, kg	FFM, kg	% BODY FAT
F	10	10	0.1	1.3	−1.8
M	20	10	0.7	1.7	−1.5
M	9	5	0.5	1.4	−1.0
F	24	4	−0.04	1.0	−2.1
F	9	11	0.4	1.5	−1.3
M	8	10	1.0	3.1	−2.9
M	10	11	1.7	2.4	−9.1
F	10	8	−0.1	1.1	−1.9
M	10	8	0.3	1.2	−1.3
M	20	10	0.5	1.8	−1.7

Table 14.8 Body Composition Changes with Resistance Training[a]

[a]Data from different studies in the literature. F = female; M = male; FFM = fat-free mass.

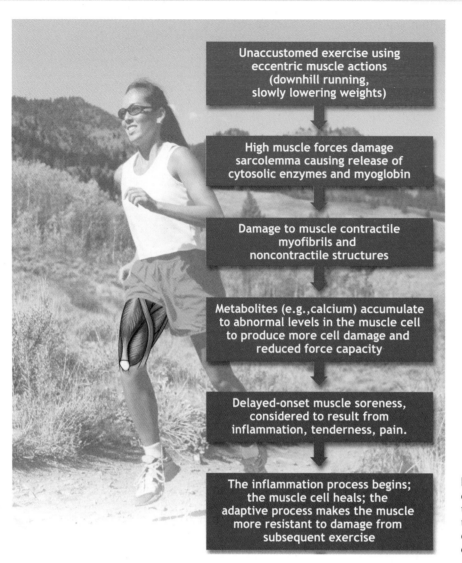

Figure 14.21 Proposed sequence for delayed-onset muscle soreness after unaccustomed exercise. Cellular adaptations to short-term exercise provide enhanced resistance to subsequent damage and pain.

SUMMARY

1. Genetic, exercise, nutritional, hormonal, environmental, and neural factors interact to regulate skeletal muscle mass and corresponding strength development.

2. Physiologic factors that include muscle fiber size and type and anatomic-lever arrangement of bone and muscle ultimately determine an individual's muscular strength. Neural influences from the CNS that activate prime movers in a specific movement greatly affect one's ability to express this strength.

3. Muscular strength increases with resistance training from improved capacity for neuromuscular activation and alterations in a muscle fiber's contractile elements.

4. As overloaded muscles become stronger, individual fibers normally grow larger (hypertrophy). Total muscle enlargement involves increased protein synthesis within the fiber's contractile elements and proliferation of cells that thicken and strengthen the muscle's connective tissue harness.

5. Muscle fiber hypertrophy involves structural changes within the contractile mechanism of individual fibers particularly fast-twitch fibers and increases intramuscular anaerobic energy stores.

6. Intense resistance training does not induce cellular component adaptations to enhance aerobic energy transfer.

7. Women and men improve strength and muscle size to about the same relative percentage with resistance training.

8. Conventional resistance-training exercises contribute little to enhance cardiovascular-aerobic fitness. Most resistance training programs without dietary constraint do not reduce body fat significantly because of the relatively low energy cost.

9. CRT using lower resistance and higher repetitions combines the muscle-training benefits of resistance

exercise with cardiovascular, calorie-burning benefits of intense continuous exercise.

10. Eccentric muscle actions produce more DOMS compared with concentric only and isometric exercise.

11. Muscle tears and connective tissue damage (ultimate leading to an inflamatory process) cause DOMS.

THOUGHT QUESTIONS

1. How would you apply the principle of specificity to (1) evaluate current muscular strength and power and (2) improve muscular performance for a football lineman?

2. Outline the steps in designing a resistance-training program for sedentary, middle-age men and women.

3. Outline tests to evaluate muscular performance to best reflect the force–power requirements for firefighters.

4. Respond to a friend who comments: "I run and work out with free weights regularly, yet every spring my muscles are sore a day or two after a few hours of yard work."

SELECTED REFERENCES

Adamson, M., et al.: Unilateral arm strength training improves contralateral peak force and rate of force development. *Eur. J. Appl. Physiol.*, 103:553, 2008.

Alcaraz, P.E., et al.: Physical performance and cardiovascular responses to an acute bout of heavy resistance circuit training versus traditional strength training. *J. Strength Cond. Res.*, 22:667, 2008.

Allison, G.T., et al.: Feedforward responses of transversus abdominis are directionally specific and act asymmetrically: Implications for core stability theories. *J. Orthop. Sports Phys. Ther.*, 38:228, 2008.

Andersen, L.L., et al.: Neuromuscular adaptations to detraining following resistance training in previously untrained subjects. *Eur. J. Appl. Physiol.*, 93:511, 2005.

Andersen, L.L., et al.: The effect of resistance training combined with timed ingestion of protein on muscle fiber size and muscle strength. *Metabolism*, 54:151, 2005.

Arts, M.P., et al.: The Hague Spine Intervention Prognostic Study (SIPS) Group. Management of sciatica due to lumbar disc herniation in the Netherlands: a survey among spine surgeons. *J. Neurosurg. Spine*, 9:32, 2008.

Azegami, M., et al.: Effect of single and multi-joint lower extremity muscle strength on the functional capacity and ADL/IADL status in Japanese community-dwelling older adults. *Nurs. Health Sci.*, 9:168, 2007.

Baker, D., Newton, R.U.: Acute effect on power output of alternating an agonist and antagonist muscle exercise during complex training. *J. Strength Cond. Res.*, 19:202, 2005.

Beck, T.W., et al.: Effects of a protease supplement on eccentric exercise-induced markers of delayed-onset muscle soreness and muscle damage. *J. Strength Cond. Res.*, 21:661, 2007.

Ben Sira, D., et al.: Effect of different sprint training regimes on the oxygen delivery-extraction in elite sprinters. *J. Sports Med. Phys. Fitness*, 50:121, 2010.

Black, C.D., et al.: High specific torque is related to lengthening contraction-induced skeletal muscle injury. *J. Appl. Physiol.*, 104:639, 2008.

Bodine, S.C.: mTOR signaling and the molecular adaptation to resistance exercise. *Med. Sci. Sports Exerc.*, 38:1950, 2007.

Bohannon, R.W.: Hand-grip dynamometry predicts future outcomes in aging adults. *J. Geriatr. Phys. Ther.*, 31:3, 2008.

Brocherie, F., et al.: Electrostimulation training effects on the physical performance of ice hockey players. *Med. Sci. Sports Exerc.*, 37:455, 2005.

Buford, T.W., et al.: A comparison of periodization models during nine weeks with equated volume and intensity for strength. *J. Strength Cond. Res.*, 21:1245, 2007.

Caserotti, P., et al.: Changes in power and force generation during coupled eccentric-concentric versus concentric muscle contraction with training and aging. *Eur. J. Appl. Physiol.*, 103:151, 2008.

Castagna, C., et al.: Aerobic and explosive power performance of elite Italian regional-level basketball players. *J. Strength Cond. Res.*, 23:1982, 2009.

Chatzinikolaou, A., et al.: Time course of changes in performance and inflammatory responses after acute plyometric exercise. *J. Strength Cond. Res.*, 24:1389, 2010.

Cockbum, E., et at.: Effect of milk-based carbohydrate-protein supplement timing on the attenuation of exercise-induced muscle damage. *Appl. Physiol. Nutr. Metab.*, 35:270, 2010.

Coeffey, V.G., et al.: Effect of high-frequency resistance exercise on adaptive responses in skeletal muscle. *Med. Sci. Sports Exerc.*, 39:2135, 2007.

Colado, J.C., Triplett, N.T.: Effects of a short-term resistance program using elastic bands versus weight machines for sedentary middle-aged women. *J. Strength Cond. Res.*, 22:1441, 2008.

Cronin, N.J., et al.: Effects of contraction intensity on muscle fascicle and stretch reflex behavior in the human triceps surae. *J. Appl. Physiol.*, 105:226, 2008.

Cronin, J., Crewther, B.: Training volume and strength and power development. *J. Sci. Med. Sport*, 7:144, 2004.

Cronin, J.B., Hansen, K.T.: Strength and power predictors of sports speed. *J. Strength Cond. Res.*, 19:349, 2005.

Crowther, R.G., et al.: Kinematic responses to plyometric exercises conducted on compliant and noncompliant surfaces. *J. Strength Cond. Res.*, 21:460, 2007.

Curtis, D., et al.: The efficacy of frequency specific microcurrent therapy on delayed onset muscle soreness. *J. Body Mov. Ther.*, 14:272, 2010.

Daly, R.M., et al.: Muscle determinants of bone mass, geometry and strength in prepubertal girls. *Med. Sci. Sports Exerc.*, 40:1135, 2008.

de Villarreal, E.S., et al.: Determining variables of plyometric training for improving vertical jump height performance: a meta-analysis. *J. Strength Cond. Res.*, 23:495, 2009.

de Vos, N.J., et al.: Optimal load for increasing muscle power during explosive resistance training in older adults. *J. Gerontol. A. Biol. Sci. Med. Sci.*, 60:638, 2005.

DeLorme, T.L., Watkins, A.L.: *Progressive Resistance Exercise.* New York: Appleton-Century-Crofts, 1951.

Elvested, P., et al.: The effects of a worksite neuromuscular activation program on sick leave: a pilot study. *Med. Sci. Sports Exerc.*, 40(suppl):S434, 2008.

Falla, D., Farina, D.: Neural and muscular factors associated with motor impairment in neck pain. *Curr. Rheumatol. Rep.*, 9:497, 2007.

Flanagan, E.P., et al.: Reliability of the reactive strength index and time to stabilization during depth jumps. *J. Strength Cond. Res.*, 5:1677, 2008.

Gotshalk, L.A., et al.: Cardiovascular responses to a high-volume continuous circuit resistance training protocol. *J. Strength Cond. Res.*, 18:760, 2004.

Graves, J.E., et al.: Specificity of limited range of motion variable resistance training. *Med. Sci. Sports Exerc.*, 21:84, 1989.

Hackney, K.J., et al.: Resting energy expenditure and delayed-onset muscle soreness after full-body resistance training with an eccentric concentration. *J. Strength Cond. Res.*, 22:1602, 2008.

Hakkinen, A., et al.: Effects of home strength training and stretching versus stretching alone after lumbar disk surgery: A randomized study with a 1-year follow-up. *Arch. Phys. Med. Rehabil.*, 86:865, 2005.

Hartmann, H., et al.: Effects of different periodization models on rate of force development and power ability of the upper extremity. *J. Strength Cond. Res.*, 23:1921, 2009.

Haswell, K., et al.: Clinical decision rules for identification of low back pain patients with neurologic involvement in primary care. *Spine.* 1;33:68, 2008.

Hedayatpour, N., et al.: Sensory and electromyographic mapping during delayed-onset muscle soreness. *Med. Sci. Sports Exerc.*, 40:326, 2008.

Henwood, T.R., Taaffe, D.R.: Improved physical performance in older adults undertaking a short-term programme of high-velocity resistance training. *Gerontology*, 51:108, 2005.

Hubal M.J., et al.: Mechanisms of variability in strength loss after muscle-lengthening actions. *Med. Sci. Sports Exerc.*, 39:461, 2007.

Iguchi, M., Shields RK. Quadriceps low-frequency fatigue and muscle pain are contraction-type-dependent. *Muscle Nerve.*, 42:230, 2010.

Ikai, M., Steinhaus, A.H.: Some factors modifying the expression of human strength. *J. Appl. Physiol.*, 16:157, 1961.

Impellizzeri, F.M., et al.: Effect of plyometric training on sand versus grass on muscle soreness and jumping and sprinting ability in soccer players. *Br. J. Sports Med.*, 42:42, 2008.

Ishikawa, M., Komi, P.V.: Muscle fascicle and tendon behavior during human locomotion revisited. *Exerc. Sport Sci. Rev.*, 36:193, 2008.

Ispirlidis, I., et al.: Time-course of changes in inflammatory and performance responses following a soccer game. *Clin. J. Sport Med.*, 18:423, 2008.

Issurin, V.: Block periodization versus traditional training theory: a review. *J. Sports Med. Phys. Fitness.*, 48:65, 2008.

Jensen, I., Harms-Ringdahl, K.: Strategies for prevention and management of musculoskeletal conditions. Neck pain. *Best Pract. Res. Clin. Rheumatol.*, 21:93, 2007.

Katch, V.L.: The lumbopelvic system: Anatomy, physiology, motor control, instability and description of a unique treatment modality. In: Donatell, R.A., Wooden, M.J. (eds.). *Orthopaedic Physical Therapy*, 4th ed. St. Louis: Churchill Livingston Elsevier, 2010.

Kemmler, W.K., et al.: Effects of single- vs. multiple-set resistance training on maximum strength and body composition in trained postmenopausal women. *J. Strength Cond. Res.*, 18:689, 2004.

Kubo, K., et al.: Effects of plyometric and weight training on muscle-tendon complex and jump performance. *Med. Sci. Sports Exerc.*, 39:1801, 2007.

Lamon, S., et al.: Regulation of STARS and its downstream targets suggest a novel pathway involved in human skeletal muscle hypertrophy and atrophy. *J. Physiol.*, 15;587(Pt 8):1795, 2009.

Leukel, C., et al.: Influence of falling height on the excitability of the soleus H-reflex during drop-jumps. *Acta. Physiol. (Oxf).* 192:569, 2008.

Lieber, R.L.: *Skeletal Muscle Structure, Function, and Plasticity: The Physiological Basis of Rehabilitation*, 3rd ed. Baltimore: Lippincott, Williams & Wilkins, 2010.

Lin, J.D., et al.: The effects of different stretch amplitudes on electromyographic activity during drop jumps. *J. Strength Cond. Res.*, 22:32, 2008.

Lund, H., et al.: Learning effect of isokinetic measurements in healthy subjects, and reliability and comparability of Biodex and Lido dynamometers. *Clin. Physiol. Funct. Imaging*, 25:75, 2005.

Mandroukas, A., et al.: Deltoid muscle fiber characteristics in adolescent and adult wrestlers. *J. Sports Med. Phys. Fitness.*, 50:113, 2010.

McCaulley, G.O., et al.: Mechanical efficiency during repetitive vertical jumping. *Eur. J. Appl. Physiol.*, 101:115, 2007.

McCurdy, K.W., et al.: The effects of short-term unilateral and bilateral lower-body resistance training on measures of strength and power. *J. Strength Cond. Res.*, 19:9, 2005.

McGill, S.: *Low Back Disorders: Evidence-Based Prevention and Rehabilitation*. Champaign, IL: Human Kinetics, Inc., 2007.

Miyaguchi, K., Demura, S.: Relationships between stretch-shortening cycle performance and maximum muscle strength. *J. Strength Cond. Res.*, 22:19, 2008.

Mjolsnes, R., et al.: A 10-week randomized trial comparing eccentric vs. concentric hamstring strength training in well-trained soccer players. *Scand. J. Med. Sci. Sports*, 14:311, 2004.

Molski, M.: Two-wave model of the muscle contraction. *Biosystems.*, 96:136, 2009.

Narici, M.V., Maganaris, C.N.: Plasticity of the muscle-tendon complex with disuse and aging. *Exerc. Sport Sci. Rev.*, 35:126, 2007.

Nosaka, K., et al.: Partial protection against muscle damage by eccentric actions at short muscle lengths. *Med. Sci. Sports Exerc.*, 37:746, 2005.

Nunan, D., et al.: Exercise-induced muscle damage is not attenuated by beta-hydroxy-beta-methylbutyrate and alpha-ketoisocaproic acid supplementation. *J. Strength Cond. Res.*, 24:531, 2010.

Petrella, J.K., et al.: Age differences in knee extension power, contractile velocity, and fatigability. *J. Appl. Physiol.*, 98:211, 2005.

Prestes, J., et al.: Comparison between linear and daily undulating periodized resistance training to increase strength. *J. Strength Cond. Res.*;23:2437, 2009.

Prokopy, M., et al.: Closed–kinetic chain upper-body training improves throwing performance of NCAA Division I softball players. *J. Strength Cond. Res.*, 22:1790, 2009.

Reeves, N.D., et al.: Plasticity of dynamic muscle performance with strength training in elderly humans. *Muscle Nerve*, 31:355, 2005.

Regueme, S.C., et al.: Delayed influence of stretch-shortening cycle fatigue on large ankle joint position coded with static positional signals. *Scand. J. Med. Sci. Sports*, 18:373, 2008.

Sangnier, S., Tourny-Chollet, C.: Study of the fatigue curve in quadriceps and hamstrings of soccer players during isokinetic endurance testing. *J. Strength Cond. Res.*, 22:1458, 2008.

Santana, J.C., et al.: A kinetic and electromyographic comparison of the standing cable press and bench press. *J. Strength Cond. Res.*, 21:1271, 2007.

Seeman, E. Structural basis of growth-related gain and age-related loss of bone strength. *Rheumatology (Oxford).* 47(suppl 4):iv2, 2008.

Seger, J.Y., Thorstensson, A.: Effects of eccentric versus concentric training on thigh muscle strength and EMG. *Int. J. Sports Med.*, 26:45, 2005.

Seiler, S., Sæterbakken, A.: A unique core stability training program improves throwing velocity in female high school athletes. *Med. Sci. Sports Exerc.*, 40(suppl):S248, 2008.

Seyennes, O.R., et al.: Early skeletal muscle hypertrophy and architectural changes in response to high-intensity resistance training. *J. Appl. Physiol.*, 102:373, 2007.

Shaw, W.S., et al.: Patient clusters in acute, work-related back pain based on patterns of disability risk factors. *J. Occup. Environ. Med.*, 49:185, 2007.

Shepstone, T.N., et al.: Short-term high- vs low-velocity isokinetic lengthening training results in greater hypertrophy of the elbow flexors in young men. *Scand. J. Med. Sci. Sports*, 15:135, 2005.

Shimano, T., et al.: Relationship between the number of repetitions and selected percentages of one repetition maximum in free weight exercises in trained and untrained men. *J. Strength Cond. Res.*, 20:819, 2006.

Shimomura, Y., et al.: Branched-chain amino acid supplementation before squat exercise and delayed-onset muscle soreness. *Int. J. Sport Nutr. Exerc. Metab.*, 20:236. 2010.

Signorile, J.F., et al.: Early plateaus of power and torque gains during high- and low-speed resistance training of older women. *J. Appl. Physiol.*, 98:1213, 2005.

Spiering, B.A., et al.: Resistance exercise biology: manipulation of resistance exercise programme variables determines the responses of cellular and molecular signaling pathways. *Sports Med.*, 38:527, 2008.

Storch, E.K., Kruszynski, D.M.: From rehabilitation to optimal function: Role of clinical exercise therapy. *Curr. Opin. Crit. Care.*, 14:451, 2008.

Symons, T.B., et al.: Effects of maximal isometric and isokinetic resistance training on strength and functional mobility in older adults. *J. Gerontol. A. Biol. Sci. Med. Sci.*, 60:777, 2005.

Thomas, G.A., et al.: Maximal power at different percentages of one repetition maximum: Influence of resistance and gender. *J. Strength Cond. Res.*, 21:336, 2007.

Thomas, K., et al.: The effect of two plyometric training techniques on muscular power and agility in youth soccer players. *J. Strength Cond. Res.*, 23:332, 2009.

Twist, C., et al.: The effects of plyometric exercise on unilateral balance performance. *J. Sports Sci.*, 10:1073, 2008.

Verghese, J., et al.: Self-reported difficulty in climbing up or down stairs in nondisabled elderly. *Arch. Phys. Med. Rehabil.*, 89:100, 2008.

Vikne, J., et al.: A randomized study of new sling exercise treatment vs traditional physiotherapy for patients with chronic whiplash-associated disorders with unsettled compensation claims. *J. Rehabil. Med.*, 39:252, 2007.

Walts, C.T., et al.: Do sex or race differences influence strength training effects on muscle or fat? *Med. Sci. Sports Exerc.*, 40:229, 2008.

Wenke, J.C., et al.: Mouse plantar flexor muscle size and strength after inactivity and training. *Aviat. Space Environ. Med.*, 81:632, 2010.

Wilson, J.M., Flanagan, E.P.: The role of elastic energy in activities with high force and power requirements: a brief review. *J. Strength Cond. Res.*, 5:1705, 2008.

Wood, L.E., et al.: Elbow flexion and extension strength relative to body or muscle size in children. *Med. Sci. Sports Exerc.*, 36:1977, 2004.

Zammit, P.S.: All muscle satellite cells are equal, but are some more equal than others? *J. Cell Sci.*, 121:2975, 2008.

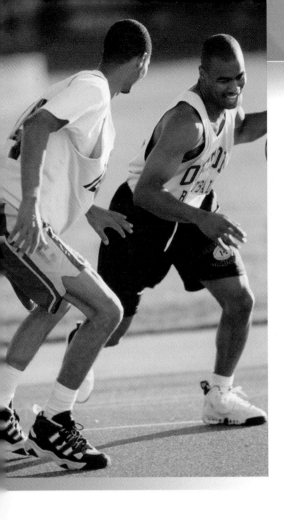

Factors Affecting Physiologic Function
The Environment and Special Aids to Performance

CHAPTER OBJECTIVES

- Explain the statement: The hypothalamus plays the most important role in regulating thermal balance.

- Name four physical factors that contribute to heat exchange during rest and exercise.

- Describe how the circulatory system serves as a "workhorse" for thermoregulation.

- List desirable clothing characteristics during exercise in cold and warm weather.

- Describe how cardiac output, heart rate, and stroke volume respond during submaximal and maximal exercise with environmental heat stress.

- Describe circulatory adjustments that maintain blood pressure during hot-weather exercise.

- Quantify fluid loss during hot-weather exercise.

- Identify the physiologic consequences of dehydration.

- Explain how acclimatization, training, age, gender, and body fat modify heat tolerance during exercise.

- Identify factors that comprise the heat stress index.

- Explain the purpose of the wind-chill index.

- Describe the physiologic adjustments to cold stress.

- Outline the effects of increasingly higher altitudes on (1) partial pressure of oxygen in ambient air, (2) saturation of hemoglobin with oxygen in the pulmonary capillaries, and (3) $\dot{V}O_{2max}$ (maximal oxygen consumption).

- Describe immediate and long-term physiologic adjustments to altitude exposure.

- Outline three approaches for creating an altitude environment at sea level so an athlete can spend sufficient time to stimulate an acclimatization response.

- Describe the typical time course for red blood cell reinfusion and mechanism for its ergogenic effect on endurance performance and aerobic capacity.

- Discuss the medical use of erythropoietin and its potential dangers for healthy athletes.

- Contrast "general warm-up" and "specific warm-up."

- Identify potential cardiovascular benefits of moderate warm-up immediately before extreme physical effort.

- Provide a rationale for breathing a hyperoxic gas mixture to enhance exercise performance and quantify its potential to increase tissue oxygen availability.

This chapter discusses specific problems encountered during exercise in hot and cold environments and at high altitude. We present this information within the framework of the immediate physiologic adjustments and longer term adaptations as the body strives to maintain internal consistency despite an environmental challenge. We also explore three common ergogenic interventions—blood doping, warm-up, and hyperoxic gas—to improve physiologic function, exercise capacity, and athletic performance.

| Part 1 | Mechanisms of Thermoregulation |

THERMOREGULATION

Normal body temperature fluctuates several degrees during the day in response to physical activity, emotions, and ambient temperature variations, with oral temperature averaging about 1.0°F (0.56°C) less than rectal temperature. Body temperature also exhibits diurnal fluctuations; the lowest temperatures occur during sleep, and slightly higher temperatures persist when awake, even when the person remains relaxed in bed.

Thermoregulation plays such an important role in the body's homeostatic balance that the price of failure often is death. A person can tolerate a drop in core temperature of 18°F (10°C) but only an increase of 5°C (9°F). Over the past 30 years, more than 100 football players and collegiate wrestlers have died from excessive heat stress during practice or competition. Heat injury also commonly occurs during military training and operations and longer duration athletic events, as it often does in industry (mining) and farming (migrant pickers).

Understanding thermoregulation and the most effective ways to support temperature control mechanisms can dramatically reduce heat-related tragedies. Coaches, athletes, and race and event organizers must reduce factors that promote heat gain and dehydration. Concern should also focus on the most effective behavioral approaches like prudent scheduling of events; acclimatization; proper clothing; and fluid and electrolyte replacement before, during, and after exercise to blunt the potential for negative effects on performance and safety.

THERMAL BALANCE

Figure 15.1 lists factors that contribute to heat gain and heat loss as the body attempts to maintain thermal neutrality. This balance results from integrative mechanisms that accompllish the following:

1. Alter heat transfer to the periphery (**shell**)
2. Regulate evaporative cooling
3. Vary the rate of heat production

The temperature of the deeper tissues or **core** rises quickly when heat gain exceeds heat loss during vigorous exercise in a warm environment. In the cold, in contrast, heat loss begins to exceed heat production, and core temperature plummets.

Body Temperature Measurement

A thermal gradient exists within the body, with core body temperature (T_{core}) the highest and shell temperature ($\bar{T}_{skin}$) the lowest. Mean body temperature ($\bar{T}_{body}$) represents an average of skin and internal temperatures. Common sites to estimate average core temperature ($\bar{T}_{core}$) include the rectum, eardrum (tympanic temperature), and esophagus (esophageal temperature). Temperature sensors (thermistors) placed at various skin locations estimate T_{skin}. Mean skin temperature ($\bar{T}_{skin}$) denotes the weighted average of different skin temperatures that reflect the portion of the body's surface each site represents (e.g., arm, trunk, leg, head). $\bar{T}_{body}$ computes as follows:

$$\bar{T}_{body} = (0.6 \times \bar{T}_{core}) + (0.4 \times \bar{T}_{skin})$$

The relative proportion of the body's average temperature represented by the core equals 0.6 (60%) and 0.4 (40%) for the skin.

HYPOTHALAMIC REGULATION OF BODY TEMPERATURE

The hypothalamus contains the central coordinating center for temperature regulation. This group of specialized neurons at the floor of the brain serves as a thermostat to carefully regulate temperature within a narrow range of 37°C ± 1°C (98.6°F ± 1.8°F). Unlike a home thermostat, however, the hypothalamus cannot turn off the heat; it only initiates responses to protect the body when core temperature changes from its "norm" because of heat gain or heat loss. Temperature-regulating mechanisms become activated in two ways:

1. Thermal receptors in the skin provide peripheral input to the hypothalamic central control center
2. Temperature changes in blood that perfuses the hypothalamus directly stimulate the hypothalamic control center

The hypothalamic regulatory center plays the most important role in maintaining thermal balance. Cells in the anterior hypothalamus directly detect changes in blood temperature in addition to receiving peripheral input. Cells then activate either the posterior hypothalamus to initiate coordinated responses for heat conservation or the anterior hypothalamus for heat loss. Peripheral receptors in the skin primarily detect cold; the hypothalamus monitors body warmth by the temperature of the blood that perfuses this area. **Table 15.1** summarizes the mechanisms that

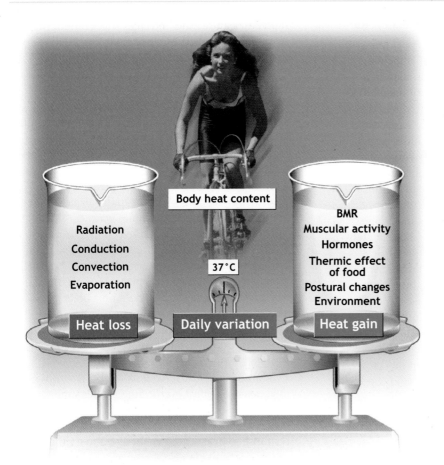

Figure 15.1 Factors that contribute to heat gain and heat loss as the body regulates core temperature at approximately 98.6°F (37°C).

regulate body temperature; each responds in a graded manner, increasing or decreasing as required for themoregulation.

REGULATING BODY TEMPERATURE DURING COLD AND HEAT EXPOSURE

Cold Stress

In extreme cold, excessive heat loss occurs at rest. This increases the body's heat production and slows heat loss as physiologic adjustments combat the decrease in core temperature.

Table 15.1	Mechanisms for Temperature Regulation
Stimulated by Cold	**Mechanism**
Decreases heat loss	Vasoconstriction of skin vessels; postural reduction of surface area (curling up)
Increases heat production	Shivering and increased voluntary activity; increased thyroxine and epinephrine secretion
Stimulated by Heat	
Increases heat loss	Vasodilation of subcutaneous skin vessels; sweating
Decreases heat production	Decreased muscle tone and voluntary activity; decreased thyroxine and epinephrine secretion

Questions & Notes

Give the average difference between oral and rectal temperature.

List 3 factors that contribute to body heat gain.

　1.

　2.

　3.

List 3 factors that result in body heat loss.

　1.

　2.

　3.

Define mean body temperature.

Name the central coordinating center for temperature regulation.

ⓘ For Your Information

ORAL TEMPERATURE DOES NOT MEASURE CORE TEMPERATURE

Oral temperature does not accurately measure deep body (core) temperature after strenuous exercise. For example, large and consistent differences occurred between oral and rectal temperatures after a 14-mile race in a tropical climate; whereas the rectal temperature averaged 103.5°F (39.7°C), oral temperature remained a normal 98.6°F (37°C). This discrepancy partly results from evaporative cooling of the mouth and airways from relatively high ventilatory volumes during and immediately after intense exercise.

Three integrated factors regulate body temperature during cold exposure:

1. **Vascular adjustments:** Circulatory adjustments "fine tune" temperature regulation. Stimulation of cutaneous cold receptors constricts peripheral blood vessels. Vasoconstriction immediately reduces the flow of warm blood to the body's cooler surface and redirects it to the warmer core that includes cranial, thoracic, and abdominal cavities and portions of the muscle mass. Consequently, skin temperature decreases toward ambient temperature to optimize the insulatory benefits of skin and subcutaneous fat.

2. **Muscular activity:** Shivering generates metabolic heat (maximum of three to five times resting metabolism), but physical activity provides the greatest contribution in defending against cold. Exercise energy metabolism can sustain a constant core temperature when air temperatures decrease to −30°C (−22°F) without the need for heavy clothing.

3. **Hormonal output:** Increased release of the "calorigenic" hormones epinephrine and norepinephrine by the adrenal medulla partially account for increased basal heat production during cold exposure. Prolonged cold stress also increases the thyroid galnd's release of thyroxine to elevate resting metabolism.

Heat Stress

Thermoregulatory mechanisms primarily protect against overheating. Thwarting excessive body heat buildup becomes important during sustained intense exercise when metabolic rate often increases 20 to 25 times the resting level—heat production that could increase core temperature by 1.8°F (1°C) every 5 minutes. Here, competition exists between mechanisms that maintain a large muscle blood flow and mechanisms that regulate body temperature. **Figure 15.2** illustrates the following four potential avenues for heat exchange when exercising:

1. **Radiation:** Objects continually emit electromagnetic heat waves. Because the body is usually warmer than the environment, the net exchange of radiant heat energy occurs from the body through the air to solid, cooler objects in the environment. Despite subfreezing temperatures, a person can remain warm by absorbing sufficient radiant heat energy from direct sunlight or reflected from the snow, sand, or water. The body absorbs radiant heat energy when the temperature of objects in the environment exceeds skin temperature, making evaporative cooling the only avenue for heat loss.

2. **Conduction:** Heat loss by conduction directly transfers heat through a liquid, solid, or gas from one molecule to another. Circulation transports most of the body heat to the shell, but a small amount continually moves by conduction directly through the warmer deep tissues to the cooler surface. Conductive heat loss then warms air molecules and cooler surfaces that contact the skin. The rate of conductive heat loss depends on the temperature gradient between the skin and surrounding surfaces and their thermal qualities. For example, when hiking outdoors in the heat, some relief can come from lying on a cool rock shielded from the sun. Conductance between the rock's colder surface and the hiker's warmer surface facilitates body heat loss until the rock warms to body temperature.

3. **Convection:** The effectiveness of heat loss by conduction depends on how rapidly air near the body exchanges after it becomes warmed. With little or no air movement (convection), air next to the skin warms and acts as a zone of insulation, minimizing further conductive heat loss. Conversely, if cooler air continuously replaces warmer air surrounding the body, as it does on a breezy day, in a room with a fan, or during running, heat loss increases because convective currents carry the heat away. For example, air currents at 4 mph cool twice as effectively as air moving at 1 mph.

4. **Evaporation:** *Evaporation provides the major physiologic defense against overheating.* Water vaporization from the respiratory passages and skin surface continually transfers heat to the environment. In response to heat stress, the body's 2 to 4 million sweat (eccrine) glands secrete large quantities of hypotonic saline solution (0.2%–0.4% NaCl). Cooling occurs when sweat reaches the skin and fluid evaporates. The cooled skin then cools the blood shunted from the interior to the surface. Along with heat loss through sweating, approximately 350 mL of water seeps through the skin (insensible perspiration) each day and evaporates to the environment. Also, 300 mL of water vaporizes daily from respiratory passages' moist mucous membranes. In cold weather, respiratory tract evaporation appears as "foggy breath."

Evaporative Heat Loss at High Ambient Temperatures
Increased ambient temperature reduces effectiveness of heat loss by conduction, convection, and radiation. When ambient temperature exceeds body temperature, these three mechanisms of thermal transfer actually contribute to heat gain. When this occurs, or when conduction, convection, and radiation cannot adequately dissipate a large metabolic heat load, sweat evaporation and water vaporization from the respiratory tract provide the *only* avenue for dissipating heat. For someone relaxing in a hot, humid environment, the normal 2-L daily fluid requirement doubles or even triples from evaporative fluid loss.

Heat Loss in High Humidity
Sweat evaporation from the skin depends on three factors:

1. Surface exposed to the environment
2. Temperature and relative humidity of ambient air
3. Convective air currents around the body

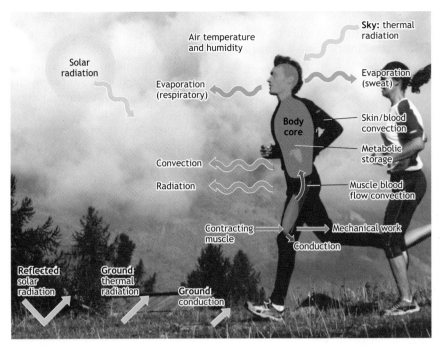

Figure 15.2 Heat production within active muscle and its transfer from the core to the skin. Under appropriate environmental conditions, excess body heat dissipates to the environment to regulate core temperature within a narrow range. (Modified from Gisolfi, C.V., Wenger, C.B.: Temperature regulation during exercise: old concepts, new ideas. *Exerc. Sport Sci. Rev.,* 12:339, 1984.)

Relative humidity exerts the greatest impact on the effectiveness of evaporative heat loss. Relative humidity describes the ratio of water in ambient air to its total capacity for moisture at a particular ambient temperature, expressed as a percentage. For example, 40% relative humidity means that ambient air contains only 40% of the air's moisture-carrying capacity at a specific temperature.

With high humidity, ambient air's vapor pressure approaches that of moist skin (~40 mm Hg). When this happens, evaporation decreases even though large quantities of sweat bead on the skin and eventually roll off. This response represents a useless water loss that can precipitate dehydration and overheating. Continually drying skin with a towel before sweat evaporates also hinders evaporative cooling. *Sweat does not cool the skin; rather, skin cooling occurs when sweat evaporates.* Individuals can tolerate relatively high environmental temperatures when humidity remains low. For this reason, hot, dry desert climates are more thermally "comforting" than cooler but more humid tropical climates.

INTEGRATION OF HEAT-DISSIPATING MECHANISMS

Heat dissipation involves the integration of three physiologic mechanisms: circulation, evaporation, and hormonal adjustments.

Circulation

The circulatory system serves as "workhorse" for thermal balance. At rest in hot weather, heart rate and cardiac output increase, and superficial arterial and venous blood vessels dilate to divert warm blood to the body's cooler outer shell. Peripheral vasodilation causes a flushed or reddened face on a hot day or

Questions & Notes

List 3 factors that regulate body temperature during cold exposure.

1.

2.

3.

List 4 ways the body loses heat.

1.

2.

3.

4.

List 3 factors that influence sweat evaporation from the skin.

1.

2.

3.

Give the main environmental factor that affects the magnitude of evaporative heat loss.

during vigorous exercise. With extreme heat stress, 15% to 25% of cardiac output passes through the skin, greatly increasing thermal conductance of peripheral tissues. This favors radiative heat loss to the environment, mostly from the hands, forehead, forearms, ears, and tibial region.

Evaporation

Sweating begins several seconds after initiation of vigorous exercise. After about 30 minutes, it reaches equilibrium that directly relates to exercise load. A large cutaneous blood flow coupled with evaporative cooling usually produces an effective thermal defense. Cooled peripheral blood then returns to deeper tissues to acquire additional heat on its return to the heart.

Hormonal Adjustments

Heat stress initiates hormonal adjustments to conserve body salts (electrolytes) and fluid lost in sweat. In response to a thermal challenge, the pituitary gland releases **vasopressin (antidiuretic hormone [ADH])**. *ADH stimulates water reabsorption from the kidney tubules to form concentrated urine during heat stress.* Concurrently, with even a single bout of exercise or repeated days of exercise in hot weather, the adrenal cortex releases the sodium-conserving hormone **aldosterone** to increase the renal tubules' reabsorption of sodium. Aldosterone also acts on sweat glands to reduce sweat's osmolality to further conserve electrolytes.

EFFECTS OF CLOTHING ON THERMOREGULATION

Clothing insulates the body from its surroundings. It reduces radiant heat gain in a hot environment or retards conductive and convective heat loss in the cold.

Cold-Weather Clothing

The mesh of the clothing's fibers traps air and warms it to insulate from the cold. This establishes a barrier to heat loss because cloth and air both conduct heat poorly. A thicker zone of trapped air next to the skin provides more effective insulation. Several layers of light clothing or garments lined with animal fur, feathers, or synthetic fabrics with numerous layers of trapped air insulate better than a single bulky layer of winter clothing.

The ideal winter garment in cold, dry weather blocks air movement but also allows water vapor from sweating to escape through clothing for subsequent evaporation. Wool or synthetics like polypropylene and such derivitive "wicking" fabrics as "coolmax" and "drylite" that insulate well and dry quickly serve this purpose. When clothing becomes wet, either through external moisture or condensation from sweating, it loses nearly 90% of its insulating properties. Wet clothing facilitates heat transfer from the body because water conducts heat faster than air.

When working or exercising in cold air, the adequacy of insulation does not usually present a problem; rather, the key factor involves dissipation of metabolic heat and sweat through a thick air–clothing barrier. Cross-country skiers alleviate this dilemma by removing layers of clothing as the body warms. This maintains core temperature without reliance on evaporative cooling.

Warm-Weather Clothing

Dry clothing, no matter how lightweight, *retards* heat exchange more than the same clothing soaking wet. The common practice of switching from a soaked garment to a dry tennis, basketball, or football uniform in hot weather makes little sense for temperature regulation because evaporative heat loss occurs only when clothing becomes wet throughout. A dry uniform simply prolongs the time between evaporative heat loss from sweating and its cooling effects.

Different materials absorb water at different rates. Cottons and linens, for example, readily absorb moisture. In contrast, heavy sweatshirts and rubber or plastic garments produce high relative humidity close to the skin, thus retarding sweat evaporation and cooling. Individuals should wear loose-fitting clothing to permit free convection of air between the skin and environment to promote evaporation from the skin. Moisture-wicking fabrics adhere closely to the skin to optimally transfer heat and moisture from the skin to the environment, particularly during intense exercise in hot weather. These fabrics wick moisture away from the skin. They also offer benefits during exercise in cold environments because dry clothing (in contrast to sweat-drenched clothing) greatly reduces hypothermia risk. Color also plays an important role; dark colors absorb light rays and add to radiant heat gain, lighter color clothing reflects heat rays.

Football Uniforms *Of all athletic uniforms and equipment, football clothing plus pads plus helmet presents the greatest barrier to heat dissipation.* The 6 or 7 kg of equipment, carried over a relatively hot artificial playing surface, also adds considerably to the total metabolic load.

Wearing football gear while exercising produces higher rectal and skin temperatures during exercise and recovery than other exercise conditions. Skin temperature directly beneath padding averages only 1°C less than rectal temperature. This indicates that subcutaneous blood in these areas cooled only about one-fifth as much as blood near the skin surface directly exposed to the environment. Rectal temperature remains elevated in recovery with uniforms, making a rest period of limited value in normalizing thermal status unless the athlete removes the uniform.

SUMMARY

1. Humans tolerate only relatively small variations in internal (core) temperature. Exposure to heat or cold stress initiates thermoregulatory responses that either generate or conserve heat at low ambient temperatures and dissipate heat at high temperatures.

2. The hypothalamus serves as the "thermostat" for temperature regulation. This coordination center initiates regulatory adjustments from peripheral thermal receptors in the skin and changes in hypothalamic blood temperature.

3. Heat conservation in cold stress occurs by vascular adjustments that shunt blood from the cooler periphery to the warmer deep tissues of the body's core. If this proves ineffective, shivering increases metabolic heat. Thermogenic hormones initiate an additional small but prolonged increase in resting metabolism.

4. Heat stress causes warm blood to divert from the body's core to the shell. Heat loss occurs by radiation, conduction, convection, and evaporation. Evaporation provides the major physiologic defense against overheating at high ambient temperatures and during exercise.

5. Humid environments dramatically decrease the effectiveness of evaporative heat loss. This makes a physically active person particularly vulnerable to a dangerous state of dehydration and a spiraling core temperature.

6. Ideal warm-weather clothing includes lightweight, loose-fitting, and light-colored clothes. Even when wearing ideal clothing, heat loss slows until evaporative cooling achieves optimal levels.

7. Several layers of light clothing provide a thick zone of trapped air near the skin for more effective insulation than a single thick layer of clothing. Wet clothing decreases insulation making heat flow readily from the body.

 THOUGHT QUESTIONS

1. What mechanism might explain how improved aerobic fitness increases exercise tolerance in a warm, humid environment?

2. From the standpoint of survival, discuss why the body's physiology is more geared to regulate temperature in heat stress than in cold stress.

3. Describe the ideal personal physical and physiologic characteristics that minimize heat injury risk in exercise during environmental heat stress.

4. How should a person dress who wishes to play 90 minutes of outdoor paddle tennis at 20°F (26.7°C)?

Part 2	Exercise, the Environment, and Thermoregulation

EXERCISE IN THE HEAT

Cardiovascular adjustments and evaporative cooling facilitate metabolic heat dissipation during exercise, particularly in hot weather. A trade-off occurs because fluid loss in thermoregulation (sweating) often creates a relative state of dehydration. Excessive sweating leads to more serious fluid loss that reduces plasma volume. The extreme end result involves circulatory failure with core temperature increasing to lethal levels.

Circulatory Adjustments

Two competitive cardiovascular demands exist when exercising in hot weather:

1. Oxygen delivery to active muscles must increase to sustain exercise energy metabolism.

Questions & Notes

Name the hormone released from the pituitary gland in response to a thermal challenge.

Describe the ideal winter garment for cold, dry climates.

2. Peripheral blood flow to the skin must increase to transport metabolic heat from exercise for dissipation at the body's surface; this blood no longer remains available to active muscles.

Cardiac output remains similar during submaximal exercise in hot and cold environments, but the heart's stroke volume becomes smaller when exercising in the heat. In fact, stroke volume decreases in proportion to fluid deficit created during exercise. This produces *higher* heart rates at all submaximal exercise levels. Maximal cardiac output and aerobic capacity decrease during exercise in the heat because the compensatory increase in heart rate does not offset the decrease in stroke volume.

Vascular Constriction and Dilation Adequate skin and muscle blood flow during heat stress occurs at the expense of other tissues that temporarily compromise their blood supply. For example, compensatory constriction of the splanchnic vascular bed and renal tissues rapidly counters vasodilation of the subcutaneous vessels. A prolonged reduction in blood flow to visceral tissues contributes to liver and renal complications sometimes noted with exertional heat stress.

Maintaining Blood Pressure Arterial blood pressure remains stable during exercise in the heat because visceral vasoconstriction increases total vascular resistance as blood redirects to areas in need. During near-maximal exercise with accompanying dehydration, relatively less blood diverts to peripheral areas for heat dissipation. This reflects the body's attempt to maintain cardiac output despite sweat-induced decreases in plasma volume. *Circulatory regulation and maintenance of muscle blood flow take precedence over temperature regulation, often at the expense of a spiraling core temperature and accompanying health risk.*

Core Temperature During Exercise

Heat generated by active muscles can increase core temperature to fever levels that incapacitate a person if caused by external heat stress alone. Champion distance runners show no ill effects from rectal temperatures as high as 105.8°F (41°C) recorded at the end of a 3-mile race.

Within limits, increased core temperature with exercise does not reflect heat-dissipation failure. To the contrary, this well-regulated response occurs even during cold-weather exercise. **Figure 15.3** illustrates the relationship between esophageal (core) temperature and oxygen uptake (expressed as a percentage of $\dot{V}O_{2max}$) during exercise of increasing severity for men and women of varying fitness levels. Core temperature increases in proportion to exercise intensity. *More than likely, a modest core temperature increase reflects favorable internal adjustments that create an optimal thermal environment for physiologic and metabolic function.*

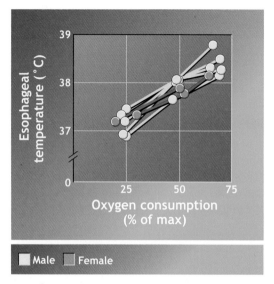

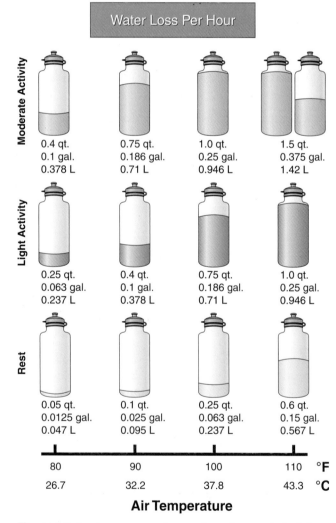

Figure 15.3 Relationship between esophageal temperature and oxygen uptake expressed as a percentage of $\dot{V}O_{2max}$. (Data from Saltin, B., Hermansen, L.: Esophageal, rectal, and muscle temperature during exercise. *J. Appl. Physiol.*, 21:1757, 1966.)

Figure 15.4 Average water loss per hour for a typical adult caused by sweating at various air temperatures during rest and light and moderate physical activity.

Water Loss in the Heat

Dehydration induced by a few hours of intense exercise in the heat often reaches levels that impede heat dissipation and severely compromise cardiovascular function and exercise capacity. **Figure 15.4** shows average water loss per hour from sweating at various air temperatures for a typical adult during rest and light and moderate physical activity.

Magnitude of Exercise Fluid Loss
For an acclimatized person, sweat loss peaks at about 3 $L \cdot h^{-1}$ during intense exercise in the heat and averages nearly 12 L (26 lb) on a daily basis. Intense sweating for several hours can induce sweat gland fatigue that impairs core temperature regulation. Elite marathon runners frequently sweat in excess of 5 L of fluid during competition; this represents 6% to 10% of body mass. For slower paced marathons or ultra-marathons, the average fluid loss rarely exceeds 500 $mL \cdot h^{-1}$. For more intense exercise even in a temperate climate, soccer players lose approximately a 2 L of sweat during a 90-minute game played at about 50°F (10°C).

Hot, humid environments impede the effectiveness of evaporative cooling because of the high vapor pressure of ambient air and promote large fluid losses. **Figure 15.5** illustrates a linear relationship between sweat rate during rest and exercise and the air's moisture content (expressed as wet bulb temperature; see Close Up Box 15.3: *Assessing Heat Quality of the Environment: How Hot is Too Hot?*, page 508). Ironically, excessive sweat output in high humidity contributes little to cooling because minimal evaporation takes place. In this regard, clothing that retards rapid evaporation of sweat creates an extremely humid microclimate at the skin's surface that promotes dehydration and overheating.

Consequences of Dehydration

Any degree of dehydration impairs physiologic function and thermoregulation. When plasma volume decreases as dehydration progresses, peripheral blood flow and sweating rate also decrease to make thermoregulation progressively more difficult. Compared with normal hydration, premature fatigue occurs from reduced plasma volume that increases heart rate, perception of effort, and core temperature. A fluid loss equivalent to only 1% of body mass increases rectal temperature compared with the same exercise performed fully hydrated. Dehydration equivalent to 5% of body mass increases rectal temperature and heart

Questions & Notes

What happens to arterial blood pressure during exercise in the heat?

Give an average peak sweat loss per hour during intense exercise in the heat.

Give the degree of dehydration that can impair physiologic function and thermoregulation.

Name 3 body functions negatively affected by dehydration.

1.

2.

3.

Describe what happens to core body temperature when exercising in the heat.

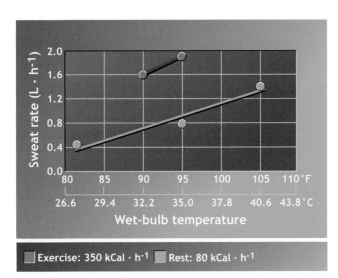

Figure 15.5 Effects of humidity (wet-bulb temperature) on sweat rate during rest and exercise in the heat. Ambient temperature (dry-bulb) equaled 43.3°C (110°F). (Data from Iampietro, P.F.: Exercise in hot environments. In: *Frontiers of Fitness.* Shephard, R.J. (ed.). Springfield, IL: Charles C. Thomas, 1971.)

BOX 15.1 CLOSE UP

Recognizing and Treating Signs and Symptoms of Heat-Related Disorders

Human heat dissipation occurs by:

1. Redistribution of blood from deeper tissues to the periphery
2. Activation of the cooling mechanism provided by evaporation of sweat from the skin's surface and respiratory passages

WHAT HAPPENS DURING HEAT STRESS?

During heat stress at rest, cardiac output increases, vasoconstriction and vasodilation move central blood volume toward the skin, and thousands of previously dormant capillaries threading through the upper skin layer open to accommodate blood flow. Conduction of heat away from warm blood at the skin's cooled surface is accomplished without undue strain on the body's heat-dissipating functions. In contrast, heat production during physical activity often strains heat-dissipating mechanisms, especially in high ambient temperature and high humidity.

SIGNS AND SYMPTOMS OF HEAT-RELATED DISORDERS

Nearly 400 people die each year in the United States from excessive heat stress, and about half of these are men and women age 65 years and older. If the normal signs of heat stress go unheeded—thirst, tiredness, grogginess, and visual disturbances—cardiovascular compensation begins to fail. This initiates a cascade of disabling complications collectively termed **heat illness**. **Heat cramps**, **heat syncope**, **heat exhaustion**, and **heat stroke** constitute the major heat illnesses in order of increasing severity. No clear-cut demarcation exists among these maladies because symptoms often overlap. When symptoms of serious heat illness occur, immediate action must include reducing heat stress and rehydrating the person until medical help arrives. The table lists the causes, signs, and symptoms and preventive methods for the four categories of heat illness.

Heat Illness: Causes, Signs and Symptoms, and Prevention

CONDITION	CAUSES	SIGNS AND SYMPTOMS	PREVENTION
Heat Cramps	Intense, prolonged exercise in the heat	Tightening, cramps, involuntary spasms of active muscles; low serum Na^+	Cease exercise; rehydrate
Heat Syncope	Peripheal vasodilatation and pooling of venous blood; hypotension; hypohydration	Lightheadedness; syncope, mostly in upright position during rest or exercise; pallor; high rectal temperature	Ensure acclimatization and fluid replenishment; reduce exertion on hot days; avoid standing
Heat Exhaustion	Cumulative negative water balance	Exhaustion; hypohydration, flushed skin; reduced sweating in extreme dehydration syncope, high rectal temperature	Proper hydration before exercise and adequate replenishment during exercise; ensure acclimatization
Heat Stroke	Extreme hyperthermia leads to thermoregulatory failure; aggravated by dehydration	Acute medical emergency; includes hyperpyrexia (rectal temperature >41°C, 105.8°F); lack of sweating and neurologic deficit (disorientation, twitching, seizures, coma)	Ensure acclimatization; identify and exclude individuals at risk; adapt activities to climatic constraints

rate while decreasing sweating rate, $\dot{V}O_{2max}$, and exercise capacity compared with the normally hydrated condition.

Blood plasma supplies most of the water lost through sweating; thus, maintaining cardiac output becomes problematic as sweat loss progresses. Loss of plasma volume does the following:

1. Initiates increases in systemic vascular resistance to maintain blood pressure
2. Reduces skin blood flow, which thwarts a major avenue for heat dissipation. *Dehydration reduces circulatory and temperature-regulating capacity to meet the metabolic and thermoregulatory demands of exercise.*

Table 15.2	Water Requirements (L·h⁻¹) for Rest and Varying Intensities of Work in the Heat: Indoors and Outdoors at Diverse Temperatures and Relative Humidity							
AIR TEMP (°F) AND RH[a]	INDOORS (NO SOLAR LOAD)				OUTDOORS (CLEAR SKY)			
	REST	LIGHT	MEDIUM	HEAVY	REST	LIGHT	MEDIUM	HEAVY
85° @ 50%	0.2	0.5	1.0	1.5	0.5	0.9	1.3	1.8
96° @ 30%	0.3	0.9	1.3	1.9	0.8	1.2	1.7	2.0
105° @ 30%	0.6	1.0	1.5	2.0	0.9	1.3	1.9	2.0
115° @ 20%	0.8	1.2	1.7	2.0	1.1	1.5	2.0	2.0
120° @ 20%	0.9	1.3	1.9	2.0	1.3	1.7	2.0	2.0

[a]RH = relative himidity.
From Askew, E.C.: Nutrition and performance in hot, cold, and high altitude environments. In: *Nutrition in Exercise and Sport.* 3rd Ed., Wolinsky, I., (ed.). Boca Raton, FL: CRC Press, 1997.

Seven factors affect sweat-loss dehydration: exercise intensity, exercise duration, environmental temperature, solar load, wind speed, relative humidity, and clothing. **Table 15.2** shows theoretical water requirements at different ambient temperatures and relative humidities with and without a solar load. A 100°F (37.8°C) ambient air temperature increases the resting water requirement by 50% to 60%. Adding physical activity and radiant heat increases the requirement even more. Eight hours of strenuous outdoor physical effort at temperatures of 96°F or higher (relative humidity ≥20%) could increase total fluid requirements to 15 L. Replacing this much fluid requires drinking water at regular intervals throughout the day. First initiated during the 1990 to 1991 Desert War in Iraq and Kuwait and continued currently in Iraq and Afganistan, the U.S. military imposed forced water intake through a planned drinking program before, during, and after job tasks. They also outfitted each soldier with a personal 2.5-L water pack hydration system similar to that illustrated in **Figure 15.6**.

For Your Information

PROFOUND EFFECT ON ENDURANCE PERFORMANCE

Marathon performance decreases progressively as wet bulb–globe temperature (WB-GT) increases. The accompanying figure illustrates the slowing of marathon running performance of men and women as the WB-GT increased from 10° to 25°C (50°–77°F) with performance more negatively affected for slower runners. (From Ely, M.R., et al.: Impact of weather on marathon running performance. *Med. Sci. Sports Exerc.*, 39:487, 2007.)

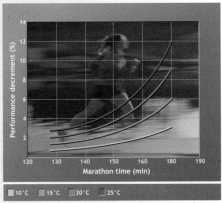

Questions & Notes

Name 4 heat-related illnesses.

1.

2.

3.

4.

Describe the effects of progressive increases in WB-GT on marathon performance. (Hint: Refer to FYI on this page).

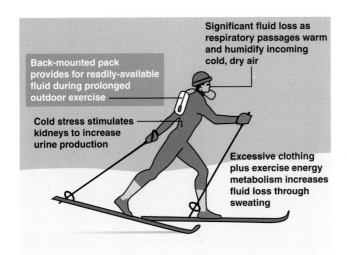

Significant fluid loss as respiratory passages warm and humidify incoming cold, dry air

Back-mounted pack provides for readily-available fluid during prolonged outdoor exercise

Cold stress stimulates kidneys to increase urine production

Excessive clothing plus exercise energy metabolism increases fluid loss through sweating

Figure 15.6 Back-mounted pack provides for readily-available fluid during prolonged outdoor exercise.

Fluid Loss in Winter Environments Dehydration becomes a serious risk during cold-weather exercise. For example, colder air contains less moisture than air at a warmer temperature, particularly at higher altitudes. Fluid volume loss increases from respiratory passages as incoming cold, dry air fully humidifies and warms to body temperature (as much as 1 L of fluid lost daily). In addition, cold stress increases urine production, which also adds to body fluid loss. Ironically, many people overdress for outdoor winter activities. Sweating begins as exercise progresses because body heat production exceeds heat loss. This discrepancy can magnify if individuals consider it unimportant to consume fluids before, during, and after strenuous cold-weather exercise.

Diuretic Use Athletes who take diuretics to rapidly lose body water and body weight reduce their plasma volume; this negatively affects thermoregulation and cardiovascular function. Diuretic drugs can also impair neuromuscular function not noted when comparable fluid loss occurs by exercise. Athletes who vomit and take laxatives to lose weight not only become dehydrated but also lose minerals. These practices weaken muscles and impair motor function.

Water Replacement and Rehydration

Adequate fluid replacement sustains evaporative cooling of acclimatized humans. Properly scheduling fluid replacement maintains plasma volume so that circulation and sweating progress optimally. This, however, may be "easier said than done" because some coaches and athletes cling to the misguided notion that water consumption hinders exercise performance. When left on their own, most athletes voluntarily replace only about half of the water lost during exercise (<500 mL$\cdot$h^{-1}).

Chronic dehydration to lose weight becomes a "way of life" for many athletes, from ballet dancers who strive to maintain a thin appearance to power athletes who try to make weight to compete in a lighter weight category. Enlightened coaches and exercise specialists must remain vigilant about each athlete's hydration status and its impact on exercise performance and safety. *All participants in sports and recreation activities from novice to champion must replenish fluids regularly!*

Cold treatments (e.g., periodic application of cold towels to forehead and abdomen during exercise or taking a cold shower before exercising in a hot environment) at best provide only minimal benefits to facilitate heat transfer at the body's surface compared with the same exercise without skin wetting. Adequate hydration provides the most effective defense against heat stress by balancing water loss with water intake, not by pouring water over the head or body. *A well-hydrated athlete always functions at a higher physiologic and performance level than a dehydrated one.*

Determining the Rate and Quantity of Rehydration Table 15.3 shows sample computations for determining the quantity and rate of fluid loss during exercise. The data under headings A to H show the calculations of sweat rate (column H) for a person who exercises for 90 minutes (column G), with a urine volume (in milliliters; column E) measured before post-exercise body weight measurement (rows A, B, and C). With a sweat rate of 1152 mL$\cdot$h^{-1}, this person needs to consume about 1000 mL (32 oz) during each hour at a rate of 250 mL (8.5 oz) at 15-minute intervals to match total fluid loss during activity.

Partitioning rehydration periods into 10- to 15-minute intervals allows for the maintenance of optimal stomach volume and properly matches fluid loss with fluid intake. Provide for unrestricted access to water during practice and competition. *Athletes must rehydrate on a regular schedule because the thirst mechanism imprecisely gauges water needs.*

Exogenous Glycerol Use Glycerol provides important bodily functions that include:

1. A component of the triacylglycerol molecule
2. A gluconeogenic substrate

Table 15.3	Computing the Magnitude of Sweat Loss and Rate of Sweating in Exercise
A: BW before exercise	61.7 kg
B: BW after exercise	60.3 kg
C: BW difference (A − B)	1400 g
D: Drink volume	420 mL
E: Urine volume output	90 mL[a]
F: Sweat loss (C + D − E)	1730 mL
G: Exercise time	90 min (1.5 h)
H: Sweat rate (F ÷ G)	19.2 ml$\cdot$min^{-1} (1152 ml$\cdot$h^{-1})[b]

BW = body weight in kg.
[a]Weight of urine should be subtracted if urine was excreted before postexercise body weight measurement.
[b]1152 mL$\cdot$h^{-1}; in this example, a person should drink about 1000 mL (32 oz) of fluid during each hour of activity (250 mL [8.5 oz] every 15 min) to remain well hydrated.
Calculations of sweat rate (row H) for a person who exercises for 90 min (row G) and who consumes 420 mL of fluid (row D); BM = body mass; DBM = difference in body mass before and after exercise (row C); urine volume (in mL; row E) measured before postexercise body mass measurement.
Modified from Gatorade Sports Science Institute, Vol. 9, No. 4 (suppl 63), 1996.

BOX 15.2 CLOSE UP

How to Optimally Rehydrate for Exercise

PRE-EXERCISE HYPERHYDRATION

Ingesting "extra" water (hyperhydration) before exercise in the heat offers some protection because it delays hypohydration, increases sweating during exercise, and brings about a smaller increase in core temperature.

Acute hyperhydration results from consuming (1) at least 500 mL of water before sleeping the night before exercising in the heat, (2) another 500 mL upon awakening, and (3) 400 to 600 mL (13–20 oz) of cold water about 20 minutes before exercise. This final pre-exercise intake provides fluid and increases stomach volume to optimize gastric emptying. An extended regimen of pre-exercise hyperhydration (4.5 L fluid per day, starting a few days before heat exposure) also increases body water reserves and improves temperature regulation.

During intense exercise in the heat, matching fluid loss with fluid intake becomes virtually impossible because only 800 to 1000 mL of fluid empty from the stomach each hour. This rate of stomach emptying does not match a water loss that may average nearly 2000 mL per hour. Under these conditions, pre-exercise hyperhydration would prove beneficial.

ADEQUACY OF REHYDRATION

Changes in body weight indicate water loss and the adequacy of rehydration. Voiding small volumes of dark yellow urine with a strong odor also provides a qualitative indication of inadequate hydration. Well-hydrated individuals typically produce urine in large volumes that does not give off a strong smell.

Each pound of weight lost represents 450 mL (15 fluid oz) of dehydration.

Periodic water breaks during activity can deter fluid depletion (see American College of Sports Medicine Clarifies Indicators for Fluid Replacement at *www. acsm-msse.org/*). Alcohol-containing beverages generally impede restoration of fluid balance, particularly if the rehydration fluid contains 4% or more alcohol content.

Optimizing Hydration

Before Exercise
- Drink approximately 17 to 20 oz 2 to 3 hours before activity.
- Consume another 7 to 10 oz after the warm-up (10–15 minutes before exercise).

During Exercise
- Drink approximately 28 to 40 oz every hour of exercise (7–10 oz every 10 to 15 minutes).
- Rapidly replace lost fluids (sweat and urine) within 2 hours after activity to enhance recovery by drinking 20 to 24 oz for every pound of body weight lost through sweating.

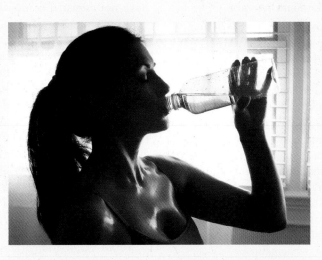

ELECTROLYTE REPLACEMENT

The volume of ingested fluid after exercise must exceed by 25% to 50% of the exercise sweat loss to restore fluid balance because the kidneys continually form urine regardless of hydration status. Unless the beverage contains sufficiently high sodium content, excess fluid intake merely increases urine output without benefit to rehydration. Maintaining a relatively high plasma concentration of sodium by adding sodium to ingested fluid sustains the thirst drive, promotes retention of ingested fluids (less urine output), and more rapidly restores lost plasma volume. The American College of Sports Medicine recommends that sports drinks contain 0.5 to 0.7 g of sodium per liter of fluid consumed during exercise lasting more than 1 hour. A beverage that tastes good to the individual also contributes to voluntary rehydration during exercise and recovery.

With prolonged exercise in the heat, sweat loss can deplete the body of 13 to 17 g of salt (2.3–3.4 g per L of sweat) daily, about 8 g more than typically consumed. With heavy sweating, increasing the intake of potassium-rich foods such as citrus fruits and bananas replaces potassium losses. A glass of orange juice or tomato juice replaces almost all the potassium, calcium, and magnesium excreted in 3 L of sweat.

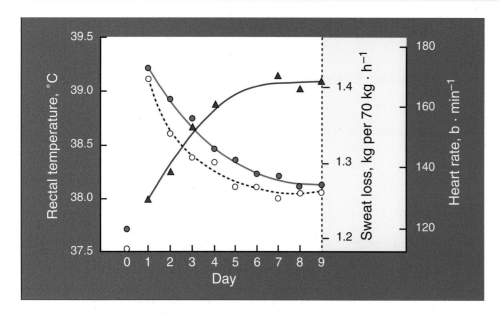

Figure 15.7 Average rectal temperature (○), heart rate (•), and sweat loss (▲) during 100 minutes of daily heat-exercise exposure for 9 consecutive days. On day 0, the men walked on a treadmill at an exercise intensity of 300 kCal·h⁻¹ in a cool climate. Thereafter, they performed the same daily exercise in the heat at 48.9°C (26.7°C wet-bulb). (Data from Lind, A.R., Bass, D.E.: Optimal exposure time for development of acclimatization to heat. *Fed. Proc.*, 22:704, 1963.)

3. An important constituent of the cells' phospholipid plasma membrane
4. An osmotically active natural metabolite

Ingesting a concentrated mixture of glycerol (now permitted by the World Anti-Doping Agency [WADA]) with water increases the body's fluid volume to produce a state of hyperhydration.

The typically recommended pre-exercise glycerol dose of 1 g of glycerol per kg of body mass in 1 to 2 L of water lasts up to 6 hours. This glycerol solution facilitates water absorption from the intestine and causes extracellular fluid retention, mainly in the plasma fluid compartment. Advocates maintain that the hyperhydration effect of glycerol supplementation reduces overall heat stress during exercise as reflected by increased sweating rate; this lowers heart rate and body temperature during exercise and enhances endurance performance under heat stress and increases safety for the exercise participant.

Not all research demonstrates meaningful thermoregulatory or exercise performance benefits of glycerol hyperhydration over pre-exercise hyperhydration with plain water. Its use may be more advantageous during high-intensity endurance exercise. Side effects of exogenous glycerol ingestion include nausea, dizziness, bloating, and lightheadedness. This area requires further research.

FACTORS AFFECTING HEAT TOLERANCE

Factors that interact and affect physiologic adjustments and exercise tolerance during environmental heat stress include acclimatization, exercise training, age, gender, and body composition.

Acclimatization

Relatively light exercise performed easily in cool weather becomes taxing if attempted on the first hot day of spring.

The early stages of spring training often prove hazardous for heat injury because thermoregulatory mechanisms have not adjusted to the dual challenge of exercise and environmental heat. *Repeated exposure to hot environments, when combined with exercise, improves the capacity for exercise with less discomfort during heat stress.*

Heat acclimatization refers to the physiologic adaptive changes that improve heat tolerance. **Figure 15.7** illustrates findings from a classic study in the 1960s of thermoregulatory adjustments over a 9-day heat acclimatization period. Two to 4 hours daily of heat-exercise exposure produce essentially complete acclimatization after 10 days. In practical terms, the first several exercise sessions in a hot environment should be light in intensity and last about 15 to 20 minutes. Thereafter, exercise sessions can increase systematically to reach normal training duration and intensity.

Table 15.4 summarizes the main physiologic adjustments during heat acclimatization. *Optimal acclimatization necessitates adequate hydration.* As acclimatization progresses, proportionately larger quantities of blood transfer to cutaneous vessels, which facilitates heat exchange from the core to the shell. More effective cardiac output distribution maintains blood pressure during exercise; a lowered threshold (earlier onset) for sweating complements this circulatory acclimatization. These responses initiate cooling before internal temperature increases substantially. After 10 days of heat exposure, sweating capacity nearly doubles, and sweat dilutes (less electrolytes lost) and more evenly distributes on the skin surface to facilitate greater cooling. For an acclimatized individual, increased sweat loss increases the need to rehydrate during and after exercise. A heat-acclimatized person exercises with a lower skin and core temperature and heart rate than an unacclimatized individual because of adjustments in circulatory function and evaporative cooling. Unfortunately, major benefits of acclimatization to hot environments dissipate within 2 to 3 weeks after a return to more temperate climates.

Table 15.4	Physiologic Adjustments During Heat Acclimatization	
ACCLIMATIZATION RESPONSE	**EFFECT**
Improved cutaneous blood flow	Transports metabolic heat from deep tissues to the body's shell
Effective distribution of cardiac output	Appropriate circulation to skin and muscles to meet demands of metabolism and thermoregulation; greater stability in blood pressure during exercise
Lowered threshold for start of sweating	Evaporative cooling begins early in exercise
More effective distribution of sweat over skin surface	Optimum use of effective surface for evaporative cooling
Increased sweat output	Maximizes evaporative cooling
Lowered sweat's salt concentration	Dilute sweat preserves electrolytes in extracellular fluid

Exercise Training

The normal exercise-induced "internal" heat stress from strenuous physical activity in a cool environment adjusts peripheral circulation and evaporative cooling in a manner *qualitatively* similar to hot ambient temperature acclimatization. This enables well-conditioned men and women to respond more effectively to severe heat stress than sedentary counterparts.

Exercise training alone increases sweating response sensitivity and capacity so sweating begins at a lower core temperature. It also produces larger volumes of more dilute sweat. These beneficial responses relate to the increase in plasma volume that occurs early in endurance training. Increased plasma volume aids sweat gland function during heat stress and maintains adequate plasma volume to support skin and muscle blood flow demands of exercise. A trained person stores less heat early during exercise and reaches a thermal steady state sooner and at a lower core temperature than an untrained person. The training advantage for thermoregulation occurs *only* if the individual fully hydrates during exercise.

Exercise "heat conditioning" in cool weather proves less effective than acclimatization from similar exercise training in the heat. *Full heat acclimatization does not occur without exposure to environmental heat stress.* Athletes who train and compete in hot weather have a distinct thermoregulatory advantage over those who train in cooler climates but periodically compete in hot weather.

Age

Studies that consider body size and composition, aerobic fitness level, hydration level, and degree of acclimatization show little age-related effects on thermoregulatory capacity or acclimatization to heat stress. For example, in comparing young and middle-aged competitive runners, no age-related decrements emerged in thermoregulatory ability during marathon running. Likewise, temperature regulation was not impaired in physically trained 50-year-old men compared with younger men.

Questions & Notes

Each 1 pound of weight loss represents

_____ mL of dehydration. (Hint: See close-up Box on p. 505).

Give 2 reasons to add a small amount of electrolyte to a rehydration fluid.

1.

2.

Name the component of the triacylglycerol molecule that can increase the body's fluid volume.

Name 5 factors that affect heat tolerance.

1.

2.

3.

4.

5.

 For Your Information

OPTIMAL GOALS FOR FLUID INTAKE WHEN EXERCISING

- **Goal of prehydrating:** Start the activity euhydrated and with normal plasma electrolyte levels. This should be initiated when needed at least several hours before the activity to enable fluid absorption and allow urine output to return to normal levels.
- **Goal of drinking during exercise:** Prevent excessive dehydration (>2% body weight loss from water deficit) and excessive changes in electrolyte balance to avert compromising performance and health. During exercise, consuming beverages containing electrolytes and carbohydrates generally provide benefits over water alone.

American College of Sports Medicine position stand. Exercise and fluid replacement. *Med. Sci. Sports Exerc.*, 39:377, 2007.

BOX 15.3 CLOSE UP

Assessing Heat Quality of the Environment: How Hot Is Too Hot?

Seven important factors determine the physiologic strain imposed by environmental heat:

1. Air temperature and relative humidity
2. Individual differences in body size and fatness
3. State of training
4. Degree of acclimatization
5. Environmental influences such as convective air currents and radiant heat gain
6. Exercise intensity
7. Amount, type, and color of clothing

Several football deaths from heat injury occurred with air temperature below 75°F (23.9°C) but with relative humidity above 95%. *Prevention is the most effective control of heat stress injuries.* Most importantly, acclimatization minimizes the likelihood of heat injury. Another consideration requires evaluating the environment for its potential thermal challenge using the WB-GT index. This index of environmental heat stress developed by the military provides important information to the National Collegiate Athletic Association to establish thresholds for increased risk of heat injury and exercise performance decrements. The WB-GT index depends on ambient temperature, relative humidity, and radiant heat as related in the following equation:

$$WB\text{-}GT = 0.1 \times DBT + 0.7 \times WBT + 0.2 \times GT$$

where DBT represents the dry-bulb temperature (air temperature) recorded by an ordinary mercury thermometer and WBT equals the wet-bulb temperature recorded by a similar thermometer except that a wet wick surrounds the mercury bulb (**Fig. 1**).

With high relative humidity, little evaporative cooling occurs from the wetted bulb, so this thermometer's temperature remains similar to the dry bulb. On a dry day, considerable evaporation occurs from the wetted bulb to maximize the difference between the two thermometer readings. Whereas a small difference between thermometer readings indicates high relative humidity, a large difference indicates little air moisture and rapid evaporation. GT represents the globe temperature recorded by a thermometer with a black metal sphere enclosing its bulb. The black globe absorbs radiant energy from the surroundings to measure this source of heat gain. Most industrial supply companies sell this relatively inexpensive thermometer. **Figure 1** shows an example of a WB-GT measuring devise.

The ACSM proposes the following recommendations concerning risk for heat injury with continuous exercise (e.g., endurance running and cycling) based on the WB-GT:

- **Very high risk:** Above 28°C (82°F)—postpone race
- **High risk:** 23° to 28°C (73°–82°F)—heat-sensitive individuals (e.g., obese, low physical fitness, unacclimatized, dehydrated, history of heat injury) should not compete
- **Moderate risk:** 18° to 23°C (65°–73°F)
- **Low risk:** Below 18°C (65°F)

Without the WBT but knowing relative humidity (local meteorologic stations or media reports), the **heat stress index** (**Fig. 2**) evaluates the relative heat stress. The index should rely on data close to the actual sport site to eliminate potential error from meteorologic data some distance from the event.

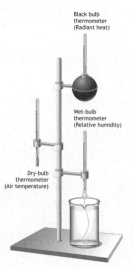

Black bulb thermometer
(Radiant heat)

Wet-bulb thermometer
(Relative humidity)

Dry-bulb thermometer
(Air temperature)

Figure 1 Apparatus to measure wet bulb–globe temperature (WB-GT).

Relative humidity	\multicolumn{11}{c}{Air temperature (°F)}										
	70	75	80	85	90	95	100	105	110	115	120
	\multicolumn{11}{c}{Heat sensation (°F)}										
0%	64	69	73	78	83	87	91	95	99	103	107
10%	65	70	75	80	85	90	95	100	105	111	116
20%	66	72	77	82	87	93	99	105	112	120	130
30%	67	73	78	84	90	96	104	113	123	135	148
40%	68	74	79	86	93	101	110	123	137	151	
50%	69	75	81	88	96	107	120	135	150		
60%	70	76	82	90	100	114	132	149			
70%	70	77	85	93	106	124	144				
80%	71	78	86	97	113	136					
90%	71	79	88	102	122						
100%	72	80	91	108							

90°–105°F	Possibility of heat cramps
105°–130°F	Heat cramps or heat exhaustion likely, heat stroke possible
130°+	Heat stroke a definite risk

Figure 2 The heat stress index.

On the negative side, older adults do not recover from dehydration as readily as younger counterparts owing to a reduced thirst drive. This places elderly individuals in a chronic state of hypohydration (with less than optimal plasma volume) that could impair thermoregulatory dynamics. An altered thirst mechanism and shift in the operating point for control of body fluid volume and composition also decrease total blood volume in older individuals.

Children   Prepubescent children show a lower sweating rate and higher core temperature during heat stress than adolescents and adults despite their larger number of heat-activated sweat glands per unit of skin area. Thermoregulatory differences probably last through puberty without limiting exercise capacity except during extreme environmental heat stress. Sweat composition also differs between children and adults; children show higher concentrations of sodium and chlorine but lower lactate, H^+, and potassium concentrations. Children also take longer to acclimatize to heat compared with adolescents and young adults. *From a practical and health standpoint, children exposed to environmental heat stress should exercise at a reduced intensity and receive additional time to acclimatize than more mature competitors.*

Gender

Women and men equally tolerate the physiologic and thermal stress of exercise when matched for fitness and acclimatization levels. Gender differences occur for the following four thermoregulatory mechanisms:

1. **Sweating:** Women possess more heat-activated sweat glands per unit of skin area than men. Women begin sweating at higher skin and core temperatures; they also produce less sweat for a similar heat-exercise load, even when acclimatized comparably to men.
2. **Evaporative versus circulatory cooling:** Despite a lower sweat output, women show heat tolerance similar to men of equal aerobic fitness at the same exercise level. Whereas women rely more on circulatory mechanisms for heat dissipation, men exhibit greater evaporative cooling. Women who sweat less to maintain thermal balance have less chance of experiencing dehydration during exercise at high ambient temperatures.
3. **Body surface area-to-mass ratio:** Women possess a larger body surface area-to-mass ratio, a favorable dimensional characteristic to dissipate heat. Under identical conditions of heat exposure, women cool at a rate faster than men through a smaller body mass across a relatively large surface area. In this regard, children also possess a "geometric" advantage during heat stress because boys and girls have larger surface areas per unit of body mass compared with adults.
4. **Menstruation:** Initiation of sweating requires a higher core temperature threshold during the menstrual luteal phase. This change in thermoregulatory sensitivity does not affect the ability to exercise or perform strenuous physical work in a hot environment.

Questions & Notes

Prepubescent children show a _____ sweating rate and _____ core temperature during heat stress compared to adolescents and adults.

List 3 gender differences in thermoregulatory mechanisms.

1.

2.

3.

Wet bulb–globe temperature (WB-GT) depends on what 3 factors.

1.

2.

3.

ℹ️ **For Your Information**

AGE-RELATED THERMOREGULATORY DIFFERENCES DO EXIST

Several age-related factors affect thermoregulatory dynamics despite equivalence between young and older adults in capacity to regulate core temperature during heat stress. Aging delays the onset of sweating and blunts the magnitude of the sweating response in one of three ways:

1. Modified sensitivity of thermoreceptors
2. Limited sweat gland output
3. Dehydration-limited sweat output with insufficient fluid replacement

Aging also alters the intrinsic structure and function of the skin and its vasculature to impair mechanisms that mediate cutaneous vasodilation, which attenuates the vasodilation response.

Age-related vascular changes include depressed peripheral sensitivity that impairs cutaneous vasodilation from two factors:

1. Smaller release of vasomotor tone
2. Less active vasodilation when sweating begins

Excess Body Fat

Excess body fat negatively impacts exercise performance in hot environments. Fat's specific heat exceeds that of muscle tissue and subsequently insulates the body's shell to retard heat conduction to the periphery. Large, overfat persons also possess a smaller body surface area-to-mass ratio for sweat evaporation compared with leaner, smaller persons. Excess body fat also directly adds to energy expended in weight-bearing activities. When these effects are compounded by evaporation-retarding characteristics; the added weight of sports equipment (e.g., football uniforms and pads); intense competition; and a hot, humid environment, overfat athletes experience considerable difficulty regulating their body temperature. Fatal heat stroke occurs 3.5 times more frequently in obese young adults than nonobese counterparts.

EXERCISE IN THE COLD

Human exposure to extreme cold produces considerable physiologic and psychological challenges. Cold ranks high among the differing terrestrial environmental stressors for its potentially lethal consequences. Core temperature regulation during cold stress becomes further compromised during chronic exertional fatigue and sleep loss, inadequate nourishment, reduced tissue insulation, and a depressed shivering heat production. Table 15.5 presents the physiologic changes associated with hypothermia that range from mild to severe.

Water represents an excellent medium to study physiologic adjustment to cold; the body loses heat about two to four times faster in cool water compared with air at the same temperature. Metabolic heat generated by muscular activity contributes to thermoregulation during cold stress. Shivering frequently results if people remain inactive in a pool or ocean environment because of a large conductive heat loss. Swimming at a submaximal pace in 18°C (64°F) water requires about 500 mL more oxygen each minute than similar swimming in 26°C (79°F) water. The extra oxygen directly relates to the added energy cost of shivering as the body attempts to combat heat loss. At this point, core temperature declines because additional metabolic heat from shivering and exercise cannot counter the large thermal drain.

Individual differences in body fat content exert a considerable effect on physiologic function in a cold environment during rest and exercise. Successful ocean swimmers have more subcutaneous fat than other endurance athletes. While swimming in cold water, the additional fat greatly increases effective insulation because blood in the periphery moves centrally to the body's core in cold water. These athletes often swim in icy cold ocean waters many hours with almost no decrease in core temperature compared with leaner swimmers, who cannot counter the heat drain to the water. In one of the most amazing endurance ocean swimming feats ever, Benoit Lecomte swam 6 to 8 hours a day at 2-hour intervals in 40° to 50°F water and relentless waves for 3736 nautical miles, crossing the Atlantic ocean from Cape Cod, MA, to Quiberon, France, 72 days later!

Acclimatization to Cold

Humans adapt more successfully to chronic heat exposure than regular cold exposure. Avoiding the cold or minimizing

Table 15.5	Core Temperature and Associated Psychological Changes That Occur as Core Temperature Falls; Individuals Respond Differently at Each Level of Core Temperature		
	CORE TEMPERATURE		
STAGE	**°F**	**°C**	**PHYSIOLOGICAL CHANGES**
Normothermia	98.6	37.0	
Mild Hypothermia	95.0	35.0	Maximal shivering, increased blood pressure
	93.2	34.0	Amnesia; dysarthria; poor judgment; behavior change
	91.4	33.0	Ataxia; apathy
Moderate Hypothermia	89.6	32.0	Stupor
	87.8	31.0	Shivering ceases; pupils dilate
	85.2	30.0	Cardiac arrhythmias; decreased cardiac output
	85.2	29.0	Unconsciousness
Severe Hypothermia	82.4	28.0	Ventricular fibrillation likely; hypoventilation
	80.6	27.0	Loss of reflexes and voluntary motion
	78.8	26.0	Acid–base disturbances; no response to pain
	77.0	25.0	Reduced cerebral blood flow
	75.2	24.0	Hypotension; bradycardia; pulmonary edema
	73.4	23.0	No corneal reflexes; areflexia
	66.2	19.0	Electroencephalographic silence
	64.4	18.0	Asystole
	59.2	15.2	Lowest infant survival from accidental hypothermia
	56.7	13.7	Lowest adult survival from accidental hypothermia

From American College of Sports Medicine position stand. Prevention of cold injuries during exercise. *Med. Sci. Sports Exerc.*, 38:2012, 2007.

its effects represents the basic response of Eskimos and those who inhabit Siberia and Greenland. The clothing of these cold-weather inhabitants provides a near-tropical microclimate.

Some indication of cold adaptation comes from studies of the Ama (AmaSan), the women breath-hold divers of Korea and southern Japan who often dive throughout their pregnancies, even up to the moment of delivery. They tolerate daily prolonged exposure to diving for shellfish, seaweed, and other food in water as cold as 50°F (10°C). In addition to an apparent psychological toughness, a 25% increase in resting metabolism contributes to their cold tolerance. Interestingly, the Ama divers possess similar body fat levels as their nondiving counterparts.

A type of general cold adaptation occurs after prolonged cold-air exposure. Increased heat production does not accompany body heat loss, and individuals regulate at a lower core temperature in the cold. Some peripheral adaptations also reflect a form of acclimation with severe localized cold stress. Repeated cold exposure of the hands or feet brings about blood flow increases through these areas during cold stress as occurs in fishers who handle nets and fish in the cold. Such local adaptations actually facilitate regional heat loss because they provide a form of self-defense because vigorous circulation in exposed areas defends against tissue damage from localized hypothermia known as *congelatio* or frostbite. Frostbite occurs in body parts farthest from the heart (fingers, toes, nose, ears) and areas with larger exposed areas.

EVALUATING ENVIRONMENTAL COLD STRESS

Heightened participation in outdoor winter activities increases cold injuries from overexposure. Pronounced peripheral vasoconstriction during severe cold exposure causes skin temperature in the extremities to decline to dangerous levels. *Early warning signs of cold injury include a tingling and numbness in the fingers and toes or a burning sensation in the nose and ears.* Disregarding these signs of overexposure leads to frostbite; when irreversible damage occurs, the tissue must be removed surgically.

Wind-Chill Index

The **wind chill temperature index** presented in **Figure 15.8** has been used by the National Weather Service (*www.nws.noaa.gov*) since 1973 and modified in 2001. Based on advances in science, technology, and computer modeling, the 2001 revised formula offers a more accurate and useful way to understand the dangers from winter winds and freezing temperatures and provides frostbite threshold values. For example, a 30°F ambient air reading is equivalent to 9°F with a wind speed of 25 mph, and a 10°F reading equals −11°F at the same wind velocity. If a person runs, skis, or skates into the wind, the effective cooling increases directly with forward velocity. Running at 8 mph into a 12-mph headwind creates the equivalent of a 20-mph wind speed. Conversely, running at 8 mph with a 12-mph wind at one's back creates a relative wind speed of only 4 mph. The *white zone* in the left of the figure denotes relatively little danger from cold injury for a properly clothed person. In contrast, the

Questions & Notes

List 2 early warning signs of cold injury.

1.

2.

List 3 reasons excess body fat negatively impacts exercise performance.

1.

2.

3.

Do successful ocean swimmers have more or less body fat than other endurance athletes?

ⓘ For Your Information

THREE STAGES OF FROSTBITE

1. **Stage 1:** Skin appears yellow or white, often with slight burning sensations. This relatively mild stage can be reversed by gradual warming of the affected area.
2. **Stage 2:** Characterized by disappearance of pain with skin reddening and swelling. Treatment may produce blisters and peel the skin.
3. **Stage 3:** The skin becomes waxy and hard. The skin dies, and edema may occur from lack of blood.

Without immediate treatment at stage 3, damage usually becomes permanent, with nerve damage from oxygen deprivation. Frostbitten areas turn discolored—purplish at first, and they soon turn black. Nerve damage produces a loss of feeling in the frostbitten areas. Without feeling in the damaged area, checking it for cuts and breaks in the skin is vital. Infected open skin can lead to gangrene and need for amputation.

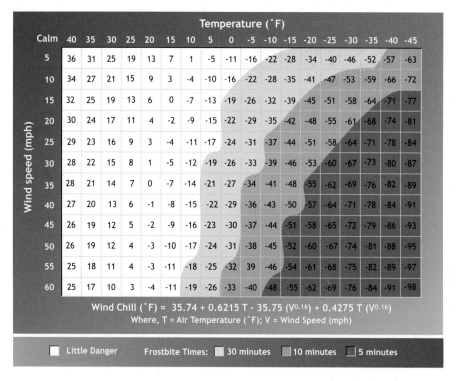

Figure 15.8 The wind chill temperature index, the proper way to evaluate the "coldness" of an environment. Figure shows the wind-chill temperatures for the relative risk of frostbite and the predicted times to freezing of exposed facial skin. Wet skin exposed to wind cools even faster and if the skin is wet *and* exposed to wind, the ambient temperature used for the wind-chill table should be 10°C lower than the actual ambient temperature. (From American College of Sports Medicine position stand. Prevention of cold injuries during exercise. *Med. Sci. Sports Exerc.*, 38:2012, 2006.)

yellow-, orange, and red-shaded zones indicate frostbite threshold values; the danger to exposed flesh increases, especially for the ears, nose, and fingers, when moving to the right of the chart. In the *red-shaded zone,* the equivalent wind-chill temperatures pose serious risk of exposed flesh freezing within minutes.

Respiratory Tract During Cold-Weather Exercise

Cold ambient air does not damage respiratory passages. Even in extreme cold, incoming air warms to between 80°F (27°C) and 90°F (32°C) as it reaches the bronchi. Warming an incoming breath of cold air greatly increases its capacity to hold moisture. Thus, humidification of inspired cold air produces water and heat loss from the respiratory tract, particularly with large ventilatory volumes during intense exercise. This contributes to dryness of the mouth, a burning sensation in the throat, irritation of the respiratory passages, and general dehydration. Wearing a scarf or mask-type "baklava" that covers the nose and mouth and traps the water in exhaled air (and warms and moistens the next incoming breath) reduces uncomfortable respiratory symptoms.

SUMMARY

1. Whereas cutaneous and muscle blood flow increase during exercise in the heat, other tissues temporally compromise their blood supply.

2. Core temperature normally increases during exercise; the relative stress of exercise determines the magnitude of the increase.

3. Excessive sweating strains fluid reserves and creates a relative state of dehydration. Sweating without fluid replacement decreases plasma volume and causes a precipitous, dangerous increase in core temperature.

4. Exercise in a hot, humid environment poses a thermoregulatory challenge because the large sweat loss in high humidity contributes little to evaporative cooling.

5. A small degree of dehydration thwarts heat dissipation, compromises cardiovascular function, and diminishes exercise capacity.

6. Adequate fluid replacement preserves plasma volume to maintain circulation and sweating at optimal levels. The ideal fluid replacement schedule during exercise matches fluid intake to fluid loss.

7. Electrolytes added to a rehydration beverage replenish fluid more effectively than plain water.

8. Repeated heat stress initiates thermoregulatory adjustments that improve exercise capacity and

reduce discomfort on subsequent heat exposure (redistribution of cardiac output while increasing sweating capacity). Full acclimatization generally requires about 10 days of heat exposure.

9. Studies that consider body size and composition, aerobic fitness, level of hydration, and degree of acclimatization show little age-related decrement in thermoregulatory capacity during moderate heat-exercise stress or ability to acclimatize to heat stress.

10. When equated for level of fitness and acclimatization, women and men show equivalent efficiency in thermoregulation during exercise, but women sweat less than men at the same core temperature.

11. The heat stress index uses ambient temperature and relative humidity to evaluate the environment's potential heat challenge to an exercising person.

12. Water conducts heat about 25 times greater than air; thus, immersion in water of only 28° to 30°C provides considerable cold stress. This initiates rapid

thermoregulatory adjustments to conserve body heat.

13. Subcutaneous fat provides excellent insulation against cold stress. It enhances the effectiveness of vasomotor adjustments to maintain a large percentage of metabolic heat.

14. Enhanced insulation from body fat becomes apparent in cold water, where fatter individuals exhibit less thermal and cardiovascular strain and greater exercise tolerance than leaner counterparts.

15. Appropriate clothing enables humans to tolerate the coldest climates on earth.

16. Ambient temperature and wind speed determine the environment's "coldness." The wind-chill index determines the interacting effects of ambient temperature and wind speed on exposed flesh.

17. Inspired ambient air temperature does not pose a danger to the respiratory tract. Considerable water evaporation from the respiratory passages during cold-weather exercise magnifies fluid loss.

THOUGHT QUESTIONS

1. What information contributes to predicting an individual's survival time during extreme cold exposure?

2. In deciding on the starting time for an upcoming summer marathon in Florida, indicate what past meteorologic information would be most valuable and why.

3. Explain whether marathoners should splash water over their body as they run.

4. Suppose you had to jog across a desert for 8 hours (sea level, 115°F [46.1°C], 20% relative humidity) while carrying only a backpack. What items would you take? Why?

Part 3	Exercise at Altitude

Questions & Notes

Define hypoxia.

High-altitude natives live in permanent settlements in the Andes and Himalayan mountains as high as 5486 m (18,000 ft). Prolonged exposure of an unacclimatized person to this altitude can cause death from ambient air's subnormal oxygen pressure, termed **hypoxia**, even if the person remains inactive. The physiologic challenge of even medium altitude becomes apparent during physical activity for unacclimatized newcomers to oxygen's decreased partial pressure.

STRESS OF ALTITUDE

Figure 15.9 illustrates the barometric pressure, pressures of the respired gases, and percentage saturation of hemoglobin at various terrestrial elevations. The density of air decreases progressively with ascents above sea level. For example,

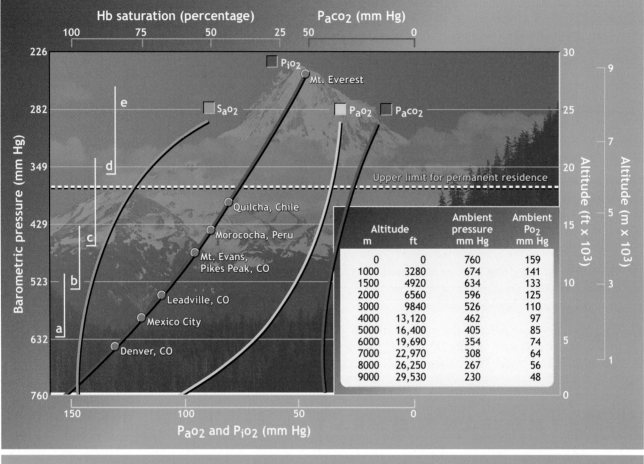

a) Lightheadedness, headache b) Insomnia, nausea, vomiting, pulmonary discomfort
c) Dyspnea, anorexia, GI disturbances d) Lethargy, general weakness e) Impending collapse

Figure 15.9 Changes in environmental and physiologic variables with progressive elevations in altitude. P_aO_2, partial pressure of arterial oxygen; P_aCO_2, partial pressure of arterial carbon dioxide; P_iO_2, partial pressure of oxygen in inspired air; S_aO_2, oxygen saturation of hemoglobin.

whereas the barometric pressure at sea level averages 760 mm Hg, at 3048 m, the barometer reads 510 mm Hg; at an elevation of 5486 m, the pressure of a column of air at the earth's surface represents about half of its pressure at sea level. Dry ambient air, whether at sea level or altitude, contains 20.9% oxygen. The PO_2 (density of oxygen molecules) decreases proportionately to the decrease in barometric pressure upon ascending to higher elevations ($PO_2 = 0.209 \times$ barometric pressure). Ambient PO_2 at sea level averages 150 mm Hg but averages only 107 mm Hg at 3048 m. *Reduced PO_2 and accompanying arterial hypoxia precipitate the immediate physiologic adjustments to altitude and longer term process of acclimatization.*

Oxygen Loading at Altitude

The inherent nature of the oxyhemoglobin dissociation curve (see Chapter 9) dictates only a small change in hemoglobin's percentage saturation with decreasing PO_2 until about 3048 m (10,000 ft). At 1981 m (6500 ft), for example, alveolar PO_2 lowers from its sea level value of

100 mm Hg to 78 mm Hg, yet hemoglobin still remains 90% saturated with oxygen. This relatively small decrease in oxygen carried by blood has little effect on a resting or mildly active individual but exerts a major effect on more intense endurance performance.

In the transition from moderate to higher elevations, values for alveolar (arterial) oxygen partial pressure exist on the steep part of the oxyhemoglobin dissociation curve. This reduces hemoglobin oxygenation dramatically and negatively impacts even moderate aerobic activities. An acute exposure to 4300 m (14,107 ft), for example, reduces aerobic capacity 32% compared with the sea level value. Above 5182 m (17,000 ft), permanent living becomes nearly impossible, and mountain climbing usually progresses with the aid of oxygen equipment. However, acclimatized mountaineers have lived for weeks at 6706 m (22,002 ft) breathing only ambient air. Members of two Swiss expeditions to Mt. Everest remained at the summit for 2 hours without using oxygen equipment (an impressive feat considering arterial PO_2 equals 28 mm Hg with a corresponding 58% oxygen saturation of arterial blood).

An unacclimatized person under these conditions becomes unconscious within 30 seconds. Although such performances clearly represent an exception, they demonstrate the enormous adaptive capability of humans to work and survive without external support at extreme terrestrial elevations.

ACCLIMATIZATION

Altitude acclimatization broadly describes the adaptive responses in physiology and metabolism that improve tolerance to altitude hypoxia. Acclimatization adjustments occur progressively to each higher elevation, and full acclimatization requires time. As a general guideline, it takes about 2 weeks to adapt to 2300 m (7545 ft). Thereafter, each 610-m (2000 ft) altitude increase requires an additional week for full adaptation up to 4572 m (15,000 ft). As summarized in Table 15.6, some compensatory responses to altitude occur almost immediately, but others take weeks or even months.

Immediate Adjustments

At elevations above 2300 m (7546 ft), rapid physiologic adjustments compensate for the thinner air and reduced alveolar oxygen pressure. The most important of these responses include:

1. **Hyperventilation triggered by increased respiratory drive:** *Hyperventilation represents the immediate first line of defense to altitude exposure.* Chemoreceptors located in the aortic arch and branching of the carotid arteries in the neck detect reductions in arterial P_{O_2}. Chemoreceptor stimulation increases ventilation, raising alveolar oxygen concentration toward the level in ambient air. Any increase in alveolar P_{O_2} with hyperventilation facilitates oxygen loading in the lungs.

2. **Increased blood flow (cardiac output) during rest and submaximal exercise:** Submaximal heart rate and cardiac output increase 50% above sea level values in the early stages of altitude acclimatization, but the heart's stroke volume remains essentially unchanged. Sea level and altitude exercise oxygen uptake remain similar, but increased submaximal

Questions & Notes

About how long does it take to fully acclimatize to an altitude of 7500 ft?

List 2 long-term physiological adjustments to altitude hypoxia.

1.

2.

ⓘ For Your Information

NOT MUCH OXYGEN AT THE TOP

At the summit of Mt. Everest (8848 m; 28,028 ft), the pressure of ambient air averages 250 mm Hg with a concomitant alveolar oxygen pressure of 25 mm Hg or about 30% of the oxygen available at sea level. At this altitude, $\dot{V}O_{2max}$ decreases to the sea level value of an average 80-year-old man. Concerning the importance of conserving oxygen in the assault on Mt. Everest, one experienced mountaineer commented: "This is a place where people will cut their toothbrushes in half to reduce weight carried."

Table 15.6	Immediate and Longer Term Adjustments to Altitude Hypoxia	
SYSTEM	**IMMEDIATE**	**LONGER-TERM**
Pulmonary Acid–Base	Hyperventilation Body fluids become more alkaline due to reduced CO_2 (H_2CO_3) with hyperventilation	Hyperventilation Excretion of base (HCO_3^-) via the kidneys with reduced alkaline reserve
Cardiovascular	Increased submaximal heart rate Increased submaximal cardiac output Stroke volume remains the same or lowers slightly Maximum cardiac output remains the same or lowers slightly	Submaximal heart rate remains elevated Submaximal cardiac output falls to or below sea-level values Stroke volume lowers Maximum cardiac output lowers
Hematologic		Decreased plasma volume Increased hematocrit Increased hemoglobin concentration Increased total number of red blood cells Possible increased capillarization of skeletal muscle
Local		Increased red-blood-cell 2,3-DPG Increased mitochondria Increased aerobic enzymes

exercise blood flow at altitude compensates for the reduced arterial oxygen content. In contrast, the circulatory adjustments to acute altitude exposure with *maximal exercise* cannot compensate for the lower oxygen content of arterial blood dramatically decreasing $\dot{V}O_{2max}$ and exercise capacity.

Fluid Loss A depressed thirst sensation at altitude negatively affects body fluid balance. The cool, dry air in mountainous regions also causes considerable body water to evaporate as air warms and moistens the respiratory passages. Respiratory fluid loss often leads to moderate dehydration and accompanying symptoms of dryness of the lips, mouth, and throat, particularly for physically active people with relatively large daily pulmonary ventilations and exercise-related sweat loss. For these active people, body weight should be checked frequently augmented with unlimited fluid availability to ensure against dehydration.

Longer Term Adjustments

Hyperventilation and increased submaximal cardiac output provide a rapid, effective counter to the acute altitude challenge. Other *slower acting* physiologic adjustments commence during a prolonged altitude stay. The three most important longer term adjustments include:

1. **Acid–base adjustment:** Hyperventilation at altitude favorably increases alveolar oxygen concentration, while carbon dioxide concentration decreases. The ambient air contains essentially no carbon dioxide, so increased alveolar ventilation at altitude washes out (dilutes) carbon dioxide in the alveoli. This creates a larger than normal gradient for carbon dioxide diffusion from blood into the lungs, reducing arterial carbon dioxide considerably. During prolonged high-altitude exposure, alveolar carbon dioxide pressure can decrease to 10 mm Hg compared with the sea level value of 40 mm Hg. Carbon dioxide loss from body fluids causes pH to increase as the blood becomes more alkaline. Recall from Chapter 10 that carbonic acid transports the largest amount of the body's carbon dioxide. Control of respiratory alkalosis produced by hyperventilation occurs in the kidneys, which slowly excrete base (HCO_3^-) through the renal tubules. The establishment of acid–base equilibrium with acclimatization occurs with a loss of alkaline reserve. Altitude does not affect anaerobic metabolic pathways per se, but blood's buffering capacity for acids gradually decreases, reducing the critical level for accumulation of acid metabolites such as lactic acid.

2. **Hematologic changes:** *An increase in the blood's oxygen-carrying capacity provides the most important long-term adaptation to altitude.* Two factors account for this adaptation:
   a. Initial decrease in plasma volume
   b. Increase in erythrocytes and hemoglobin synthesis

A rapid decrease in plasma volume increases red blood cell (RBC) concentration during the first few days at altitude. This response causes arterial blood's oxygen *concentration* to increase above values observed on immediate ascent to altitude. The reduced arterial Po_2 stimulates a concurrent increase in RBC mass, a response termed **polycythemia** that directly increases the blood's *capacity* to transport oxygen. The kidneys release the erythrocyte-stimulating hormone **erythropoietin** within 15 hours after altitude ascent. In the weeks that follow, RBC production in the marrow of the long bones increases and remains elevated. For example, the oxygen-carrying capacity of blood for high-altitude residents of Peru averages 28% above sea-level natives. For well-acclimatized mountaineers, oxygen transport capacity for each dL (100 mL) of blood (at sea level Po_2) ranges between 25 and 31 mL compared with about 20 mL for lowland residents. Even with hemoglobin's reduced oxygen saturation

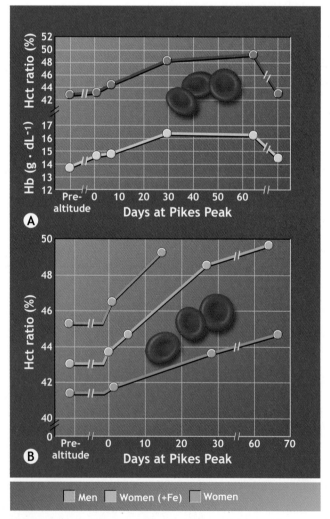

Figure 15.10 Effects of altitude on hemoglobin and hematocrit levels of eight young women before, during, and 2 weeks after exposure to 4267 m. (From Hannon, J.P., et al.: Effects of altitude acclimatization on blood composition of women. *J. Appl. Physiol*, 26:540, 1969.)

at altitude, the actual *quantity* of oxygen in arterial blood of elite mountaineers at altitude nearly equals sea-level values. **Figure 15.10** illustrates the general trend for increased hemoglobin and hematocrit during altitude acclimatization for eight young women at the University of Missouri (altitude, 213 m) who lived and worked for 10 weeks at the 4267-m summit of Pikes Peak. Upon reaching Pikes Peak, their RBC concentrations increased rapidly because of a reduced plasma volume during the first 24 hours. Over the following month, hemoglobin concentration and hematocrit continued to increase and then stabilized for the remainder of the stay. Two weeks after the women returned to Missouri, their hemoglobin and hematocrit levels returned to pre-altitude values.

3. **Cellular adaptations:** Long-term acclimatization initiates peripheral changes that facilitate aerobic metabolism. Three important adaptive changes are as follows:

   a. Increased capillary concentration in skeletal muscle, thus reducing the distance for oxygen diffusion between blood and tissues

   b. Formation of additional mitochondria and an increase in aerobic enzyme concentration

   c. Expanded oxygen storage within specific muscle fibers via increased myoglobin, which facilitates intracellular oxygen delivery and utilization, particularly at low tissue P_{O_2}

HIGH-ALTITUDE–RELATED MEDICAL PROBLEMS

Natives who live and work at high altitudes and newcomers to high altitudes encounter medical problems associated with reduced ambient P_{O_2}. Some mild problems dissipate within hours or several days, depending on the rapidity of ascent and degree of exposure, but other medical complications become severe and compromise overall health and safety. Four medical conditions are associated with high-altitude exposure:

1. **Acute mountain sickness (AMS)** is a relatively benign condition that becomes exacerbated by exercise in the first few hours of exposure. It occurs most often in people who ascend rapidly to high altitude (>10,000 ft; 3000 m) without benefitting from gradual and progressive acclimatization to lower altitudes. Symptoms begin within 4 to 12 hours after exposure and dissipate within 1 week. Treatment usually involves rest and gradual acclimatization.

2. **High-altitude pulmonary edema (HAPE)** is a life-threatening condition that includes fluid accumulation in the brain and lungs. Predisposing factors include high altitude, rate of ascent, and individual susceptibility. Symptoms usually manifest within 24 to 96 hours after a rapid ascent. Preventing severe disability or death requires immediate descent to a lower altitude on a stretcher or being flown to safety. Any physical activity potentiates complications. Supplemental oxygen is helpful during descent.

Questions & Notes

List the 3 most important long-term physiologic adjustment to altitude.

1.

2.

3.

List the 4 medical conditions associated with high altitude exposure.

1.

2.

3.

4.

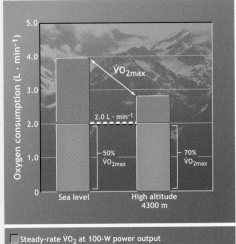

ⓘ For Your Information

SAME COST BUT GREATER STRESS AT ALTITUDE

The oxygen cost of submaximal exercise at 100 watts on a bicycle ergometer at sea level and high altitude remains unchanged at about $2.0 \text{ L} \cdot \text{min}^{-1}$, but the relative strenuousness of effort increases dramatically at altitude. In this example, submaximal exercise representing 50% of sea-level $\dot{V}O_{2max}$ equals 70% of $\dot{V}O_{2max}$ at 4300 m.

☐ Steady-rate $\dot{V}O_2$ at 100-W power output

Comparison of oxygen cost and relative strenuousness of submaximal exercise at sea level and high altitude.

3. **High-altitude cerebral edema (HACE)** is a potentially fatal neurologic syndrome that develops within hours or days in people with AMS. It usually occurs in people exposed to altitudes above 9000 ft (2700 m). Cerebral edema results from cerebral vasodilation and elevation in capillary hydrostatic pressures, causing movement of fluid and protein from the vascular compartment across the blood–brain barrier. Early symptoms similar to those of AMS and HAPE include headache, severe fatigue, and altered mental state. Immediate descent to a lower altitude is required along with supplemental oxygen adminstration.

4. **High-altitude retinal hemorrhage (HARH)** includes hemorrhage in the macula of the eye that produces irreversible visual defects. Retinal bleeding probably results from surges in blood pressure with exercise that cause blood vessels in the eye to dilate and rupture from increased cerebral blood flow. Immediate descent to a lower elevation with supplemental oxygen or use of a hyperbaric chamber is the mandatory treatment.

EXERCISE CAPACITY AT HIGH ALTITUDES

The stress of high altitudes imposes meaningful limitations on exercise capacity and physiologic function. Even at lower altitudes, the body's acclimation adjustments do not fully compensate for reduced oxygen pressure and diminishing exercise performance.

Aerobic Capacity

Figure 15.11 depicts the relationship between decreases in $\dot{V}O_{2max}$ (% of sea-level value) and increasing altitude or simulated exposures reported in diverse civilian and military studies. Small declines in $\dot{V}O_{2max}$ become noticeable at an altitude of 589 m. *Thereafter, arterial desaturation decreases $\dot{V}O_{2max}$ by 7% to 9% per 1000-m altitude increase to 6300 m, where aerobic capacity declines at a more rapid, nonlinear rate.* For example, aerobic capacity at 4000 m averages 75% of the sea-level value. At 7000 m, $\dot{V}O_{2max}$ averages half that at sea level. The $\dot{V}O_{2max}$ of relatively fit men atop Mt. Everest averages about 1000 mL·min^{-1}; this corresponds to a maximal exercise power output of only 50 watts on a bicycle ergometer.

Circulatory Factors

Aerobic capacity remains below sea-level values despite several months of acclimatization. A reduced circulatory efficiency in moderate and strenuous exercise offsets the benefits of acclimatization. The immediate altitude response increases submaximal exercise blood flow; cardiac output decreases in the days that follow and does not improve with longer altitude exposure. A decrease in stroke volume as the altitude stay progresses accounts for diminished cardiac output. At maximal exercise, a decrease in maximum cardiac output occurs after about 1 week above 3048 m (10,000 ft) and persists throughout the altitude stay. *Reduced maximum exercise blood flow results from the combined effect of decreased maximum heart rate and maximum stroke volume.*

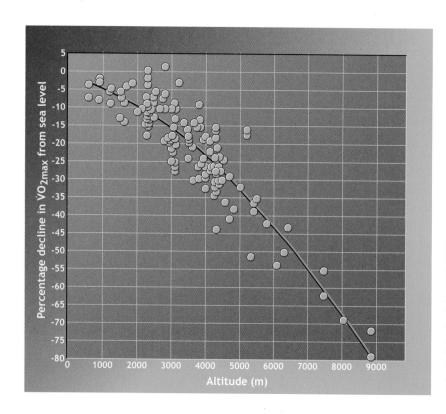

Figure 15.11   Reduction in $\dot{V}O_{2max}$ as a percentage of the sea-level value related to altitude exposure derived from 146 average data points from 67 different civilian and military investigations conducted at altitudes from 580 m (1902 ft) to 8848 m (29,021 ft). "Altitude" represents data from actual terrestrial elevations or simulated elevations with hypoxic chambers or hypoxic gas breathing. (Modified from Fulco, C.S., et al.: Maximal and submaximal exercise performance at altitude. *Aviat. Space Environ. Med.*, 69:793, 1998.)

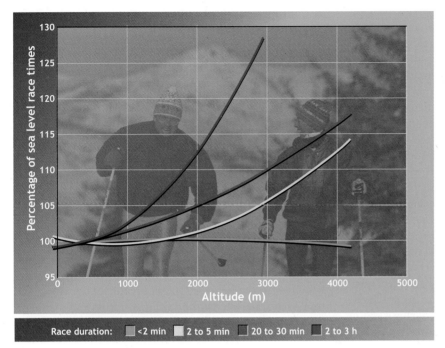

Race duration: ▢ <2 min ▢ 2 to 5 min ▢ 20 to 30 min ▢ 2 to 3 h

Figure 15.12 Generalized trend in exercise performance decrements related to altitude exposure and race duration for runners and swimmers, primarily during competition. (Modified from Fulco, C.S., et al.: Maximal and submaximal exercise performance at altitude. *Aviat. Space Environ. Med.*, 69:793, 1998.)

Exercise Performance

Figure 15.12 illustrates the generalized trend in exercise performance decrements, primarily during competition for athletes at different altitude exposures. *Altitude exerts no adverse effect on events lasting less than 2 minutes.* The threshold for decrements in longer duration events appears at about 1600 m for events of 2 to 5 minutes duration but only a 600- to 700-m (2000–2300 ft) altitude induces poorer performance in events longer than 20 minutes. For the 1- and 3-mile runs, medium altitude (2300 m; 7500 ft) decreases performance by 2% to 13%. This coincides with the 7.2% increase in 2-mile run times for highly trained middle-distance runners. After 29 days of acclimatization, high-altitude exposure still increases 3-mile run time compared with sea-level runs. The small improvements in endurance at high altitude during acclimatization probably relate to:

1. Increases in minute pulmonary ventilation (ventilatory acclimatization)
2. Increases in arterial oxygen saturation
3. A blunted lactate response in exercise

HIGH-ALTITUDE TRAINING AND SEA-LEVEL PERFORMANCE

Altitude acclimatization improves one's capacity to exercise at high altitudes. However, the effect of high-altitude exposure and altitude training on $\dot{V}O_{2max}$ and endurance performance immediately on return to sea level remains equivocal. Altitude adaptations in local circulation and cellular function and compensatory increases in the blood's oxygen-carrying capacity theoretically should enhance sea-level exercise performance. Unfortunately, altitude-exercise research has not adequately evaluated this possibility. Often, poor control exists over subjects' physical activity level, making it difficult to determine whether any improved sea-level $\dot{V}O_{2max}$ or performance score on return from altitude represents a training effect, an altitude effect, or synergism between altitude and training.

Questions & Notes

Describe the relationship between percentage decline in $\dot{V}O_{2max}$ to increased altitude exposure.

List the 2 factors responsible for reduced maximum exercise blood flow.

1.

2.

 For Your Information

DIFFICULT TO MAINTAIN BODY WEIGHT AT HIGH ALTITUDE

Prolonged high-altitude exposure reduces lean body mass (muscle fibers atrophy by 20%) and body fat, with the magnitude of weight loss directly related to terrestrial elevation. This loss results from a reduced energy intake at altitude. In addition to depressed appetite and food intake during high-altitude exposure, efficiency of intestinal absorption decreases, compounding the difficulty in maintaining body weight.

$\dot{V}O_{2max}$ on Return to Sea Level

Sea-level aerobic capacity generally does *not* improve after living at a high altitude. Compared with pre-altitude measures, no change in $\dot{V}O_{2max}$ occurred for young runners on return to sea level after 18 days at 3100 m. Training in chambers designed to simulate high altitude provided no additional benefit to sea-level performance compared with similar training at sea level. As expected, the high-altitude–trained group showed superior physical performance in the altitude experiments compared with sea-level counterparts.

Some physiologic changes produced during prolonged altitude exposure actually *negate* adaptations that could improve exercise performance upon return to sea level. The residual effects of muscle mass loss and reduced maximum heart rate and stroke volume observed with prolonged high-altitude exposure would not enhance immediate exercise performance on return to sea level. Any reduction in maximum cardiac output during a stay at a high altitude offsets benefits derived from the blood's greater oxygen-carrying capacity.

Can Sea-Level Training Be Maintained at a High Altitude?

Exposure to 2300 m (7500 ft) and higher makes it nearly impossible for athletes to train at the same intensity as sea level. At 4000 m (13,123 ft), for example, runners can only train at 40% of their sea-level $\dot{V}O_{2max}$ compared with 80% of this value at sea-level. This high-altitude–related reduction in absolute training intensity makes it difficult for athletes to maintain peak condition for sea-level competition.

High-Altitude Training versus Sea-Level Training

To evaluate the effectiveness of exercise training at a high altitude, middle-distance runners trained at sea level for 3 weeks at 75% of sea-level $\dot{V}O_{2max}$. Another group of six runners trained an equivalent distance at the same percentage $\dot{V}O_{2max}$ measured at 2300 m. The groups then exchanged training sites and continued 3 weeks of similar training. Initially, 2-mile run times decreased by 7.2% at altitude compared with sea-level times. The times improved about 2.0% for both groups after altitude training, but post-altitude performance on return to sea level remained unchanged compared to pre-altitude sea-level runs. The $\dot{V}O_{2max}$ for both groups at altitude decreased initially by about 17% and improved only slightly after 20 days of high-altitude training. When the runners returned to sea level, aerobic capacity averaged 2.8% *below* pre-altitude sea-level values! Clearly, for these highly conditioned runners, no synergistic effect occurred with relatively intense aerobic training at medium altitude compared with equally severe training at sea level.

"Live High, Train Low" *Failure to maintain absolute power outputs of sea-level training at high altitude may initiate a detraining effect.* For these reasons, elite endurance athletes have resorted to the banned and dangerous practices of blood doping or erythropoietin injections to increase hematocrit and hemoglobin concentration without the bother and negative effects of a high-altitude stay.

Strategies that combine altitude acclimatization and maintenance of sea-level training intensity provide *synergistic benefits* to sea-level endurance performance. Regular training exposure to a near–sea-level environment prevents the impaired systolic function (i.e., reduced maximum stroke volume and cardiac output) typically observed during altitude training. Athletes who lived at 2500 m (8200 ft) but returned regularly to 1250 m (4100) ft to train; i.e., "live high, train low", showed greater performance increases in the 5000-m (16,400-ft) run than athletes who lived and trained at 2500 m or athletes who lived and trained at sea level. Altitude acclimatization and maintaining sea-level training intensity provide important additive benefits to endurance at sea level.

At-Home Acclimatization In the absence of a hypobaric chamber used in medical rescue operations at high altitude (see next section), a new approach creates a sea-level "altitude" environment where an athlete, mountaineer, cyclist, endurance runner, or hot-air balloonist living at sea level spends a large enough portion of the day to stimulate a high-altitude acclimatization response. To eliminate the necessity of constructing an enclosure to withstand differentials between ambient sea-level air and reduced pressure within a hypobaric chamber, high altitude has been simulated at sea level by increasing the nitrogen percentage of the air within an enclosure. Increased nitrogen percentage reduces the air's oxygen percentage, thus decreasing the P_{O_2} of inspired air. Nordic skiers have applied this technique by living for 3 to 4 weeks in a specially constructed house that provides air with only 15.3% oxygen compared with the normal concentration of 20.9%. This system does require nitrogen gas and careful monitoring of the breathing mixture.

A relatively new, practical device accomplishes the goals of "living high, training low." The **Hypoxico Altitude Tent**, a suitcase-sized unit initially developed by former British Olympic cyclist Shaun Wallace, continuously supplies air with an oxygen content that eventually equilibrates at 15% to simulate an altitude of 2500 m (8200 ft). The 70-lb unit consists of a portable tent that fits over a normal bed; a hypoxic generator housed in an airline suitcase continually feeds altitude-simulating hypoxic air into the tent. The porosity of the tent's material limits the diffusion rate of outside oxygen into the tent to maintain the 15% value for oxygen within the tent. Equilibration of the tent's environment at the 15% oxygen level requires about 90 minutes.

The method of at-home acclimatization makes use of the observation that altitude's beneficial effects on erythropoiesis and aerobic capacity require relatively short-term exposures to hypoxia. Daily intermittent exposures of 3 to

5 hours for 9 days to simulated altitudes of 4000 to 5500 m in a hypobaric chamber increased the RBC count, hemoglobin concentration, and endurance performance in elite mountain climbers.

Medical Treatment of Altitude Sickness   Another form of hypobaric chamber creates a high-altitude environment for the medical treatment of people with severe forms of altitude illness. The **Gamow Bag Hypobaric Chamber** (named after its inventor, Rustem Igor Gamow from the University of Colorado, and son of famed physicist George Gamow [1904–1968]), is a portable chamber used to treat altitude sickness. The bag has saved the lives of scores of mountain climbers by simulating lower altitudes. Other portable systems also have been developed for medical rescue efforts (*www.high-altitude-medicine.com/ hyperbaric.html*). A person rests and sleeps in the small chamber; reducing the chamber total air pressure simulates the barometric pressure of a given altitude. Increases in barometric pressure bring about proportionate increases in inspired air's P_{O_2}.

Questions & Notes

Explain the statement "Live high, train low".

S U M M A R Y

1. Reduction in ambient P_{O_2} upon high-altitude ascent causes inadequate oxygenation of hemoglobin. This produces noticeable performance decrements in aerobic physical activities at 2000 m and higher.

2. Reduced arterial P_{O_2} and accompanying tissue hypoxia at high altitudes stimulate immediate physiologic responses that improve high-altitude tolerance during rest and exercise. These include hyperventilation and increased submaximal cardiac output via an elevated heart rate.

3. Longer term acclimatization involves physiologic adjustments that greatly improve tolerance to altitude hypoxia. The three main adjustments involve (a) reestablishing the acid–base balance of body fluids, (b) increased hemoglobin and RBC synthesis, and (c) enhanced local circulation and cellular metabolic functions. Adjustments (b) and (c) facilitate oxygen transport, delivery, and utilization.

4. High-altitude level dictates the rate and magnitude of acclimatization. Noticeable improvements occur within several days, but major adjustments require about 2 weeks. Near-full acclimatization to high altitude takes 4 to 6 weeks.

5. For individuals at a simulated altitude that approaches the summit of Mt. Everest, alveolar P_{O_2} equals 25 mm Hg. This reduces $\dot{V}_{O_{2max}}$ by 70%. Unacclimatized individuals at this altitude become unconscious within 30 seconds.

6. Acclimatization does not fully compensate for altitude stress. Even after acclimatization, $\dot{V}_{O_{2max}}$ decreases about 2% for every 300 m above 1500 m. Impaired endurance performance generally parallels the reduced aerobic capacity.

7. Altitude-related decrements in maximum heart rate and stroke volume offset the beneficial effects of acclimatization. This partially explains the inability to achieve sea-level $\dot{V}_{O_{2max}}$ values at altitude.

8. Sea-level $\dot{V}_{O_{2max}}$ and endurance performance do not improve after altitude acclimatization. More than likely, reduced circulatory efficiency in exercise and possibly detraining and a decreased muscle mass offset acclimatization benefits.

9. High-altitude training provides no additional benefit to sea-level exercise performance compared with equivalent training only at sea level.

10. Specialized chambers can simulate an altitude environment by increasing the nitrogen percentage of the air within an enclosure. Increased nitrogen percentage reduces the air's oxygen percentage, thus decreasing the P_{O_2} of inspired air.

11. A portable altitude "bag" has saved the lives of scores of mountain climbers during medical emergencies by simulating lower altitudes as the victim is transported to lower altitudes.

T H O U G H T   Q U E S T I O N S

1. To climb Mt. Everest, elite mountaineers take 3 months to establish base camps at 16,600 ft (4216 m), 19,500 ft (4953 m), 21,300 ft (5410 m), 24,000 ft (6096 m), and 26,000 ft (6604 m) before the final ascent. Explain the physiologic rationale for this "stage ascent" approach to mountaineering.

2. If altitude acclimatization improves endurance exercise performance at high altitude, why doesn't it improve similar performance immediately upon return to sea level?

3. Explain whether periodic breath-holding while exercising at sea level brings about similar physiologic adaptations as training at a high altitude.

4. What advice would you give to an athlete who plans to train for an endurance race at a high altitude in 2 months?

Part 4   Use of Physiologic Agents to Enhance Exercise Performance

Four common nonnutritional, nonpharmacologic procedures to enhance physiologic response to exercise and increase performance include:

1. RBC reinfusion
2. Exogenous use of the hormone erythropoietin
3. Pre-exercise warm-up
4. Breathing hyperoxic gas mixtures

RED BLOOD CELL REINFUSION

RBC reinfusion, often called *induced erythrocythemia*, *blood boosting*, or *blood doping*, came into public prominence as a possible ergogenic technique during the 1972 Munich Olympics—a double gold medallist reported he had used the procedure to prepare for his 5000- and 10,000-m endurance runs.

How It Works

RBC reinfusion requires withdrawal of between 1 and 4 units (1 unit = 450 mL) of a person's blood. Plasma is removed and immediately reinfused, and the packed RBCs are frozen for storage. To prevent reductions in blood cell concentration, removal of each unit of blood occurs over 3 to 8 weeks because it takes this duration to reestablish normal RBC levels. Reinfusion of stored RBCs (referred to as **autologous transfusion**) occurs up to 7 days before endurance competition. (**Homologous transfusion** infuses type-matched donor's blood.) This increases hematocrit and hemoglobin levels by 8% to 20% and increases average hemoglobin concentration for men from a normal of 15 g per dL of blood to 19 g per dL. Theoretically, the added blood volume increases maximal cardiac output, and the increased hematocrit augments the blood's oxygen-carrying capacity to increase the oxygen available to working muscles. This effect benefits endurance athletes, especially long-distance runners, for whom oxygen transport often limits exercise capacity.

Infusing 900 to 1800 mL of freeze-preserved autologous blood usually provides ergogenic benefits. Each 500-mL infusion of whole blood, or its equivalent of 275 mL of RBCs, adds about 100 mL of oxygen to the blood's total oxygen-carrying capacity. This occurs because each deciliter of whole blood normally carries about 20 mL of oxygen. An endurance athlete's total blood volume circulates five times each minute in intense exercise. The potential "extra" oxygen available to the tissues from each unit of reinfused blood (or its RBC component) equals 500 mL (5×100 mL extra O_2).

Blood doping can also create opposite effects to those intended. A large infusion of RBCs (and resulting inordinately large increase in cellular concentration) could increase blood viscosity (thickness) and decrease cardiac output; this effect would reduce aerobic capacity. Any large increase in blood viscosity would compromise blood flow through diseased, narrowed coronary vessels.

Does It Work?

Research generally confirms physiologic and performance improvements with RBC reinfusion. Differences in results among various research studies originate largely from blood storage methods. Frozen RBCs store in excess of 6 weeks without loss of cells compared with conventional storage at 4°C (used in earlier studies); substantial hemolysis (destruction) occurs at 4°C after only 3 weeks. This is important because it usually takes a person about 6 weeks to replenish blood cells after withdrawal of 2 units of whole blood (**Fig. 15.13**).

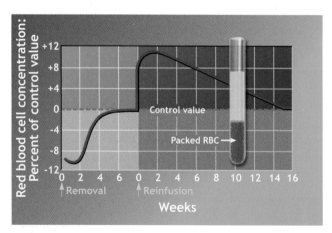

Figure 15.13 Time course of hematologic changes after removal and reinfusion of 900 mL of freeze-preserved blood. (Data from Gledhill, N.: Blood doping and related issues: a brief review. *Med. Sci. Sports Exerc.*, 14:183, 1982.)

RBC reinfusion elevates hematologic characteristics in men and women. This effect translates to a 5% to 13% increase in aerobic capacity, reduced submaximal heart rate and blood lactate for a standard exercise task, and improved endurance at sea level and high altitude. Table 15.7 illustrates hematologic, physiologic, and performance responses for adult men during submaximal and maximal exercise before and 24 hours after a comparatively large 750-mL infusion of RBCs. These response patterns generally reflect the results of the more recent research in this area.

Hormonal Blood Boosting

To eliminate the somewhat cumbersome and lengthy process of blood doping, some endurance athletes now use **erythropoietin**, a hormone normally produced by the kidneys. This hormone stimulates bone marrow to increase production of RBCs. From a medical standpoint, erythropoietin combats anemia in patients with severe kidney disease. Normally, with low hematocrit or when arterial oxygen pressure decreases as in severe lung disease or ascent to a high altitude, erythropoietin release stimulates RBC production. Unfortunately, if administered exogenously in an unregulated and unmonitored fashion (simply injecting the hormone requires much less sophistication than blood doping procedures), hematocrit can dangerously exceed levels in excess of 60%. Excessive hemoconcentration increases blood viscosity and greatly augments the exercise-induced increase in systolic blood pressure. This potentiates the likelihood for stroke, heart attack, heart failure, pulmonary embolism, and even death.

The International Cycling Union (*www.uci.ch*) established a hematocrit threshold of 50% for men and 47% for women; the International Skiing Federation (*www.fis-ski.com*) uses a hemoglobin concentration of 18.5 g · dL^{-1} as the threshold for disqualification. Hematocrit cutoff values of 52% for men and 48% for women (~3 standard deviations above the mean) represent "abnormally high" or extreme values.

WARM-UP

Coaches, trainers, and athletes at all levels of competition believe in the benefit of some type of mild physical activity (**warm-up**) before vigorous exercise. They accept that preliminary exercise enables the performer to (1) prepare either physiologically or psychologically for an event and (2) reduce likelihood of

Questions & Notes

Give another name for red blood cell reinfusion.

Briefly explain why blood boosting works.

Give 2 possible negative effects of blood doping.

1.

2.

Give the average increase in V̇O$_{2max}$ generally achieved with blood doping.

Table 15.7	Physiologic, Performance, and Hematologic Characteristics Before and 24 Hours After the Reinfusion of 750 mL of Packed Red Blood Cells			
VARIABLE	**PRE-INFUSION**	**POST-INFUSION**	**DIFFERENCE**	**DIFFERENCE, %**
Hemoglobin, g · 100 mL blood^{-1}	13.8	17.6	3.8[b]	+27.5[b]
Hematocrit, %[a]	43.3	54.8	11.5[b]	+26.5[b]
Submaximal V̇O$_2$, L · min^{-1}	1.6	1.5	−0.01	−0.6
Submaximal HR, b · min^{-1}	127.4	109.2	18.2	−14.3[b]
V̇O$_{2max}$, L · min^{-1}	3.3	3.7	0.4[b]	+12.8[b]
HR$_{max}$, b · min^{-1}	181.6	180.0	−1.6	−0.9
Treadmill run time, s	793.0	918.0	125.0[b]	+15.8

[a]Hematocrit presented as the percent (%) of 100 mL of whole blood occupied by red blood cells.
[b]Statistically significant difference.
From Robertson, R.J., et al.: Effect of induced erythrocytemia on hypoxia tolerance during physical exercise. *J. Appl. Physiol.*, 53:490, 1982.

joint and muscle injury. For animals, it requires greater forces and increases in muscle length to injure a "warmed-up" muscle compared with a muscle in a "cold" condition. The explanation maintains that warming up stretches the muscle–tendon unit to allow for greater length and less tension at any given load.

Two categories classify warm-up, although considerable overlap exists:

1. **General warm-up** involves calisthenics, stretching, and general body movements or "loosening-up" exercises usually *unrelated* to the specific neuromuscular actions of the anticipated performance.
2. **Specific warm-up** provides *skill rehearsal* for the actual activity. Swinging a golf club, throwing a baseball or football, practicing tennis or basketball, and preliminary lead-up in the high jump or pole vault are examples.

Psychological Considerations

Competitors at all levels believe that some prior activity prepares them mentally for their event so they can concentrate on the upcoming performance. *Evidence supports that a specific warm-up related to the activity improves required skill and coordination patterns.* Athletes participating in sports requiring accuracy, timing, and precise movements benefit from specific or formal preliminary practice.

Competitors also believe that prior exercise, particularly before strenuous effort, gradually prepares them to go "all out" with less fear of injury. The ritual warm-up of baseball pitchers provides a case in point. A starting or relief pitcher would never enter a game throwing at competitive speeds without previously warming up. Would any elite athlete begin competition without first engaging in a particular form, intensity, or duration of warm-up? Because topflight athletes believe in warming up, it becomes nearly impossible to design an experiment with these individuals to resolve whether or not warm-up actually improves subsequent performance and reduces injury potential.

In certain situations, peak performance occurs when play begins, without time for warming up. When a reserve player enters a game in the last few minutes, no time exists for preliminary stretching, vigorous calisthenics, or taking practice shots. The player must go all out with no warm-up except for that done before the game or at intermission.

Effects on Exercise Performance

Little evidence exists that warm-ups per se directly improve subsequent exercise performance. Lack of scientific justification does not mean that warm-ups should be disregarded. Because of the strong psychological component and "possible" physical benefits of warming up, whether passive (massage, heat applications, and diathermy), general (calisthenics and jogging), or specific (practice of the actual movements), we recommend that such procedures

continue. Until substantial evidence justifies elimination, a brief warm-up provides a comfortable way to lead into more vigorous exercise. A gradual warm-up should increase muscle and core temperature without inducing fatigue or reducing immediate energy stores. This consideration makes the warm-ups highly individualized. For example, the duration and intensity of an Olympic swimmer's warm-up would exhaust a recreational swimmer. The competitive event or activity should begin within several minutes from the end of the warm-up. Specific muscles should be engaged in a way that mimics the anticipated activity and brings about a full range of joint motion.

Warm-up and Sudden Strenuous Exercise

Several studies have evaluated the effects of preliminary exercise on cardiovascular responses to sudden, strenuous exercise. The findings provide a different physiologic framework for justifying warm-up for individuals in adult fitness and cardiac rehabilitation programs and occupations and sports requiring a sudden burst of intense exercise.

In one study, 44 men free from overt symptoms of coronary heart disease performed intense, uphill running on a treadmill for 10 to 15 seconds without prior warm-up. Evaluation of post-exercise electrocardiograms (ECGs) revealed that 70% of subjects displayed abnormal ECG changes attributed to inadequate myocardial oxygen supply. These changes did not relate to age or fitness level. To evaluate warm-ups, 22 of the men jogged in place at moderate intensity with a heart rate of 145 b·min^{-1} for 2 minutes before the treadmill run. With warm-ups, 10 men with previously abnormal ECG responses to the treadmill run showed normal tracings, and 10 men improved their ECG results; only two subjects showed ischemic changes (poor oxygen supply) after the warm-up. Warm-ups also improved the blood pressure response. For seven subjects with no warm-up, systolic blood pressure averaged 168 mm Hg immediately after the treadmill run. This decreased to 140 mm Hg with the 2-minute warm-up.

Coronary blood flow adjustments to sudden, intense exercise do not occur instantaneously, and transient myocardial ischemia can occur in apparently healthy and fit individuals. The positive effect of prior warm-up (≥ 2 min of easy jogging) on the ECG and blood pressure indicates a more favorable relationship between myocardial oxygen supply and demand.

Warm-up preceding strenuous exercise probably benefits all people, yet the greatest effect occurs for those with compromised myocardial oxygen supply. A brief pre-exercise warm-up optimizes blood pressure and hormonal adjustments at the onset of subsequent strenuous exercise and serves two important purposes:

1. Reduces myocardial workload and thus myocardial oxygen requirements
2. Enhances coronary blood flow to augment myocardial oxygen supply

BREATHING HYPEROXIC GAS

Athletes often breathe oxygen-enriched or **hyperoxic gas mixtures** during time out, at half-time, or after strenuous exercise at sea-level. They believe this procedure enhances the blood's oxygen-carrying capacity, thus facilitating recovery from exercise. When healthy people breathe ambient air at sea level, hemoglobin in arterial blood leaving the lungs contains nearly 98% of its full oxygen complement. This means the following in physiologic terms:

1. Breathing higher than normal concentrations of oxygen (hyperoxic mixtures) at sea-level increases hemoglobin's oxygen transport by only 10 mL of extra oxygen for every 1000 mL of blood.
2. Oxygen dissolved in plasma when breathing a hyperoxic mixture at sea-level increases only slightly from its normal quantity of 3 mL to about 7 mL per 1000 mL of blood.

Breathing hyperoxic gas at sea-level increases the oxygen-carrying capacity by 14 mL of oxygen for every 1000 mL of blood; 10 mL extra is attached to hemoglobin, and 4 mL extra is dissolved in plasma.

Before Exercise

The blood volume of a 70-kg person equals approximately 5000 mL. Therefore, a hyperoxic breathing mixture potentially adds about 70 mL of oxygen in the total blood volume (5000 mL blood × 14.0 mL extra O_2 per 1000 mL blood = 70 mL O_2). Despite any potential psychological benefit to the athlete who believes that pre-exercise oxygen breathing helps performance, only a slight performance advantage exists from the small amount of extra oxygen (70 mL). Any advantage occurs only if subsequent exercise took place *immediately* after hyperoxic breathing. This means the athlete cannot breathe ambient air in the interval between hyperoxic breathing and exercise. Breathing ambient air (considerably lower P_{O_2} than the previously inspired hyperoxic mixture) facilitates oxygen's movement from the body back into the environment. A halfback who breathes oxygen on the sideline before returning to the game or a swimmer who takes a few deep breaths of oxygen before moving to the blocks for starting instructions (while breathing ambient air) gains no competitive edge from physiologic benefits. This is particularly ironic in American football because the energy to power each play is generated almost completely from metabolic reactions that do *not* require oxygen!

During Exercise

Breathing hyperoxic gas during submaximal and maximal aerobic exercise enhances endurance performance. Oxygen breathing *during* submaximal aerobic exercise reduces blood lactate, heart rate, and ventilation volume and increases maximal oxygen uptake.

In one study, subjects performed a 6.5-minute endurance ride on a bicycle ergometer at an exercise level equivalent to 115% of $\dot{V}O_{2max}$ while breathing either room air or 100% oxygen. Subjects breathed both air and oxygen from identical tanks of compressed gas to mask knowledge of the breathing mixture.

Questions & Notes

Give the 2 effects of breathing 100% oxygen at sea-level.

1.

2.

List 2 important purposes of warm-up prior to strenuous exercise.

1.

2.

Explain if the athlete who breathes 100% oxygen on the sidelines or between plays gains a competitive edge because of physiologic benefits.

Explain if breathing 100% oxygen during intense exercise provides an ergogenic benefit.

 For Your Information

WARM-UP: PHYSIOLOGIC CONSIDERATIONS

The following five physiologic mechanisms suggest how warm-up may improve performance:

1. Increased speed of contraction and relaxation of warmed muscles
2. Greater economy of movement because of lowered viscous resistance within warmed muscles
3. Facilitated oxygen utilization by warmed muscles because hemoglobin releases oxygen more readily at higher muscle temperatures
4. Facilitated nerve transmission and muscle metabolism at higher temperatures; a specific warm-up facilitates motor unit recruitment required in subsequent all-out physical activity
5. Increased blood flow through active tissues as local vascular beds dilate increases metabolism and muscle temperatures

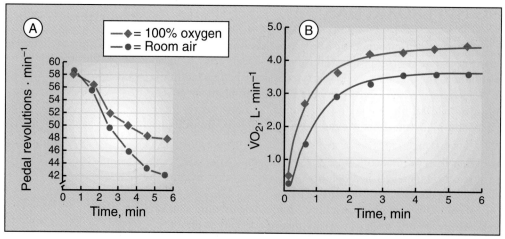

Figure 15.14 (A) Superiority of endurance (measured by pedal revolutions each minute) breathing pure oxygen versus breathing ambient air at sea level. (B) Oxygen uptake curves during the endurance rides show enhanced oxygen uptake while breathing pure oxygen. (Data from Weltman, A., et al.: Effects of increasing oxygen availability on bicycle ergometer endurance performance. *Ergonomics*, 21:427, 1978.)

Figure 15.14A gives the details of the ride, showing superiority in endurance with less drop-off in pedal revolutions during the hyperoxic trials. **Figure 15.14B** shows oxygen uptake curves while participants cycled while breathing either oxygen or room air. A higher oxygen uptake occurred when participants breathed 100% oxygen, with a correspondingly faster increase in oxygen uptake early in exercise. The small increase in hemoglobin saturation with hyperoxic breathing and the additional oxygen dissolved in plasma increase oxygen availability during maximal exercise during which total blood volume circulates up to seven times each minute in an elite endurance athlete. Quantitatively, the 70 mL of extra oxygen in the total blood volume with hyperoxic breathing (circulated seven times each minute) provides an additional 490 mL of oxygen each minute during intense aerobic exercise. Also, increased partial pressure of oxygen in solution while breathing hyperoxic gas facilitates oxygen diffusion across the capillary–tissue membrane to the mitochondria. This accounts for more rapid oxygen utilization early in exercise. Breathing hyperoxic mixtures provides physiologic benefits during some forms of exercise but the sports application of mixtures seems limited. The added weight of an appropriate breathing system would negate any ergogenic benefit. Also, the legality of the system's use during competition seems unlikely.

In Recovery

Figure 15.15 illustrates the effects of breathing hyperoxic gas during recovery from strenuous exercise on subsequent cycle performance. After 1 minute of all-out bicycle ergometer exercise, subjects recovered either passively (quiet sitting) or actively (light pedaling) while breathing room air or 100% oxygen for either 10 or 20 minutes. They then repeated the all-out bicycle ride. No differences emerged in the 6-second revolutions and cumulative revolutions (*top graph*) for the 1-minute ride after breathing

either room air or pure oxygen in recovery. Also, no difference resulted between trials when comparing blood lactate levels at 10 and 20 minutes of recovery. This indicated that oxygen inhalation did not preferentially alter lactate removal.

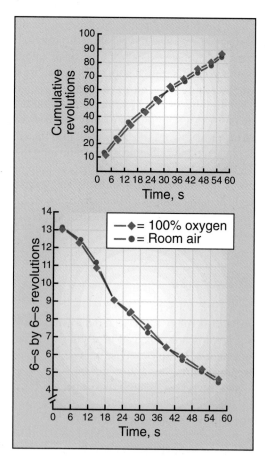

Figure 15.15 Cumulative (*top*) and absolute (*bottom*) pedal revolutions on a bicycle ergometer during 1 minute of maximal exercise subsequent to breathing either oxygen or ambient air during recovery from a previous maximal exercise bout. (Data from Weltman, A., et al.: Exercise recovery, lactate removal, and subsequent high intensity exercise performance. *Res. Q.*, 48:786, 1977.)

Subsequent research supports these findings; breathing hyperoxic mixtures after short intervals of submaximal or maximal exercise does not alter the kinetics for minute ventilation, heart rate, serum lactate, or the level of continued exercise performance.

SUMMARY

1. RBC reinfusion (blood doping) involves drawing, storing, and reinfusing concentrated RBCs for use several weeks later. The added blood volume and RBC concentration theoretically create a larger maximum cardiac output and increase the blood's oxygen-carrying capacity; both factors increase $\dot{V}O_{2max}$.

2. Research supports the ergogenic benefits of RBC reinfusion for aerobic exercise performance and thermoregulation.

3. Diverse physiologic rationales justify warm-up for ergogenic purposes and injury prevention. These include potential benefits for muscular contraction speed and efficiency, tissue compliance, enhanced oxygen delivery and utilization, and facilitated nerve

impulse transmission. Limited research supports the performance benefits of warm-up other than its potential positive effect on psychological factors.

4. A moderate cardiovascular warm-up before sudden strenuous exercise reduces cardiac workload and enhances coronary blood flow by depressing transient myocardial ischemia at the onset of intense physical activity.

5. Breathing 100% oxygen during exercise at sea level extends endurance by increasing oxygen uptake, reducing blood lactate, and lowering pulmonary ventilation. Breathing hyperoxic mixtures before or after sea-level exercise provides no ergogenic benefit.

THOUGHT QUESTIONS

1. As a basketball coach, what warm-up procedures would you recommend before a game?

2. Explain the rationale for oxygen inhalation at the sidelines during a football game played at the moderately high altitude of Denver, Colorado.

SELECTED REFERENCES

American College of Sports Medicine Position Stand. Exertional heat illness during training and competition. *Med. Sci. Sports Exerc.*, 39:556; 2007.

Ashenden, M.J., et al.: "Live high, train low" does not change the total haemoglobin mass of male endurance athletes sleeping at a simulated altitude of 3000 m for 23 nights. *Eur. J. Appl. Physiol.*, 80:479, 1999.

Audran, M., et al.: Effects of erythropoietin administration in training athletes and possible indirect detection in doping control. *Med. Sci. Sports Exerc.*, 31:639, 1999.

Baker, L.B., et al.: Dehydration impairs vigilance-related attention in male basketball players. *Med. Sci. Sports Exerc.*, 39:976, 2007.

Barnard, R.J., et al.: Ischemic response to sudden strenuous exercise in healthy men. *Circulation*, 48:936, 1973.

Bärtsh, P.: High altitude pulmonary edema. *Med. Sci. Sports Exerc.*, 31(Suppl):S23, 1999.

Beidleman, B.A., et al.: Seven intermittent exposures to altitude improves exercise performance at 4300m. *Med. Sci. Sports Exerc.*, 40:141, 2008.

Booth, F.W., Laye M. J.: The future: genes, physical activity and health. *Acta. Physiol. (Oxf).*, 199:549, 2010.

Braun, B.: Effects of high altitude on substrate use and metabolic economy: cause and effect? *Med. Sci. Sports Exerc.*, 40:1495, 2008.

Brothers, M.D., et al.: GXT responses to altitude-acclimatized cyclists during sea-level simulation. *Med. Sci. Sports Exerc.*, 39:1727, 2007.

Brothers, R.M., et al.: Cardiac systolic and diastolic function during whole body heat stress. *Am. J. Physiol. Heart Circ. Physiol.*, 296:H1150, 2009.

Burnley, M., et al.: Effects of prior warm-up regime on severe-intensity cycling performance. *Med. Sci. Sports Exerc.*, 37:838, 2005.

Carter, R. III.: Exertional heat illness and hyponatremia: an epidemiological prospective. *Curr. Sports. Med. Rep.*, 7(Suppl):S20, 2008.

Casa, D.J., et al.: Cold water immersion: the gold standard for exertional heatstroke treatment. *Exerc. Sport Sci. Rev.*, 35:141, 2007.

Cheung, S.S., Sleivert, G.G.: Multiple triggers for hyperthermic fatigue and exhaustion. *Exerc. Sport Sci. Rev.*, 32:100, 2004.

Cheuvront, S.N., et al.: No effect of moderate hypohydration or hyperthermia on anaerobic exercise performance. *Med. Sci. Sports Exerc.*, 38:1093, 2006.

Chinevere, T.D., et al.: Effect of heat acclimation on sweat minerals. *Med. Sci. Sports Exerc.*, 40:886, 2008.

Clark, S.A., et al.: Effects of live high, train low hypoxic exposure on lactate metabolism in trained humans. *J. Appl. Physiol.*, 96:517, 2004.

DeLorey, D.S., et al.: Prior exercise speeds pulmonary O_2 uptake kinetics by increases in both local muscle O_2 availability and O_2 utilization. *J. Appl. Physiol.*, 103:771, 2007.

Dougherty, K.A., et al.: Two percent dehydration impairs and six percent carbohydrate drink improves boys basketball skills. *Med. Sci. Sports Exerc.*, 38:1650, 2006.

Ebert, T.R., et al.: Influence of hydration status on thermo-regulation and cycling hill climbing. *Med. Sci. Sports Exerc.*, 39:323, 2007.

Eichner, E.R.: Heat cramps in sports. *Curr. Sports Med. Rep.*, 7:178; 2008.

Evans, R.K., et al.: Effects of warm-up before eccentric exercise on indirect markers on muscle damage. *Med. Sci. Sports Exerc.*, 34:1892, 2002.

Faigenbaum, A.D., et al.: Acute effects of different warm-up protocols on fitness performance in children. *J. Strength Cond. Res.*, 19:376, 2005.

Gore, C.J., et al.: Nonhematological mechanisms of improved sea-level performance after hypoxic exposure. *Med. Sci. Sports Exerc.*, 39:1600, 2007.

Hajoglou, A., et al.: Effect of warm-up on cycle time trial performance. *Med. Sci. Sports Exerc.*, 37:1608, 2005.

Holowatz, L.A., et al.: Altered mechanisms of vasodilation in aged human skin. *Exerc. Sport Sci. Rev.*, 35:119, 2007.

Hsu, A.R., et al.: Effects of heat removal through the hand on metabolism and performance during cycling exercise in the heat. *Can. J. Appl. Physiol.*, 30:87, 2005.

Judelson, D.A., et al.: Effect of hydration state on strength, power, and resistance exercise performance. *Med. Sci. Sports Exerc.*, 39:1817, 2007.

Katayama, K., et al.: Effect of intermittent hypoxia on oxygen uptake during submaximal exercise in endurance athletes. *Eur. J. Appl. Physiol.*, 92:75, 2004.

Kenney, W.L.: Thermoregulation at rest and during exercise in healthy older adults. *Exerc. Sport Sci. Rev.*, 25:41, 1997.

Kodesh, E., Horowitz, M.: Soleus adaptation to combined exercise and heat acclimation: physio-genomic aspects. *Med. Sci. Sports Exerc.*, 42:943, 2010.

Kuwahara, T., et al.: Effects of menstrual cycle and physical training on heat loss responses during dynamic exercise at moderate intensity in a temperate environment. *Am. J. Physiol. Regul. Integr. Comp. Physiol.*, 288:R1347, 2005.

Lee, J.K., et al.: Cold drink ingestion improves exercise endurance capacity in the heat. *Med. Sci. Sports Exerc.*, 40:1637, 2008.

Leiper, J.B., et al.: The effect of intermittent high-intensity running on gastric emptying of fluids in man. *Med. Sci. Sports Exerc.*, 37:240, 2005.

Levine, B.D., Stray-Gunderson, J.: "Living high-training low": effect of moderate-altitude acclimatization with low-altitude training on performance. *J. Appl. Physiol.*, 83:102, 1997.

Liu, Y., et al.: Effect of "living high-training low" on the cardiac functions at sea level. *Int. J. Sports Med.*, 19:380, 1998.

Mazzeo, R., Reeves J.T.: Adrenergic contribution during acclimatization to high altitude: perspectives from Pikes Peak. *Exerc. Sport Sci. Rev.*, 31:13, 2003.

McArdle, W.D., et al.: Thermal adjustment to cold-water exposure in exercising men and women. *J. Appl. Physiol.*, 56:1572, 1984.

McArdle, W.D., et al.: Thermal responses of men and women during cold-water immersion: influences of exercise intensity. *Eur. J. Appl. Physiol.*, 65:265, 1992.

McCullough, E.A., Kenney, W.L.: Thermal insulation and evaporative resistance of football uniforms. *Med. Sci. Sports Exerc.*, 35:832, 2003.

Mendel, R.W., et al.: Effects of creatine on thermoregulatory responses while exercising in the heat. *Nutrition*, 21:301, 2005.

Montain, S.J.: Hydration recommendations for sport 2008. *Curr. Sports Med. Rec.*, 7:187, 2008.

Mora-Rodriguez, R., et al.: Separate and combined effects of airflow and rehydration during exercise in the heat. *Med. Sci. Sports Exerc.*, 39:1720, 2007.

Mustafa, S., et al.: Hyperthermia-induced vasoconstriction of the carotid artery, a possible causative factor in heatstroke. *J. Appl. Physiol.*, 96:1875, 2004.

Noonan, B., et al.: The effects of hockey protective equipment on high-intensity intermittent exercise. *Med. Sci. Sports Exerc.*, 39:1327, 2006.

Paraskevaidis, I.A., et al.: Repeated exercise stress testing identifies early and late preconditioning. *Int. J. Cardiol.*, 98:221, 2005.

Perry, C.G.R., et al.: Effects of hyperoxic training on performance and cardiorespiratory response to exercise. *Med. Sci. Sports Exerc.*, 37:1175, 2005.

Pugh, L.C.G.E.: Physiological and medical aspects of the Himalayan Scientific and Mountaineering Expedition, 1960–61. *Br. Med. J.*, 2:621, 1962.

Pugh, L.C.G.E.: Athletes at altitude. *J. Physiol. (London)*, 192:619, 1967.

Rae, D.E., et al.: Heatstroke during endurance exercise: is there evidence for excessive endothermy? *Med. Sci. Sports Exerc.*, 40:1193, 2008.

Reisman, S., et al.: Warm-up stretches reduce sensations of stiffness and soreness after eccentric exercise. *Med. Sci. Sports Exerc.*, 37:929, 2005.

Roberts, W.O.: Exertional heat stroke during a cool weather marathon: a case study. *Med. Sci. Sports Exerc.*, 38:1197, 2006.

Robbins, M.K., et al.: Effect of oxygen breathing following submaximal and maximal exercise on recovery and performance. *Med. Sci. Sports Exerc.*, 24:270, 1992.

Roels, B., et al.: Effects of hypoxic interval training on cycling performance. *Med. Sci. Sports Exerc.*, 37:138, 2005.

Rowland, T., et al.: Exercise tolerance and thermoregulation responses during cycling in boys and men. *Med. Sci. Sports Exerc.*, 40:282, 2008.

Saunders, A.G., et al.: The effects of different air velocities on heat storage and body temperature in humans cycling in a hot, humid environment. *Acta. Physiol. Scand.*, 183:241, 2005.

Sawka, M.N., Noakes, T.D.: Does dehydration impair exercise performance? *Med. Sci. Sports Exerc.*, 37:1209, 2006.

Sawka, M.N., et al.: American College of Sports Medicine position stand. Exercise and fluid replacement. *Med. Sci. Sports Exerc.*, 39:377, 2008.

Schneider, M., et al.: Acute mountain sickness: influence of susceptibility, preexposure, and ascent rate. *Med. Sci. Sports Exerc.*, 34:1886, 2002.

Sharwood, K.A., et al.: Weight changes, medical complications, and performance during an Ironman triathlon. *Br. J. Sports Med.*, 38:718, 2004.

Shirreffs, S.M., et al.: Fluid and electrolyte needs for preparation and recovery from training and competition. *J. Sports Sci.*, 22:57, 2004.

Shirreffs, S.M., et al.: The sweating response of elite professional soccer players to training in the heat. *Int. J. Sports Med.*, 26:90, 2005.

Sims, S.T., et al.: Sodium loading aids fluid balance and reduces physiological strain of trained men exercising in the heat. *Med. Sci. Sports Exerc.*, 39:123, 2007.

Smekal, G., et al.: Menstrual cycle: no effect on exercise cardiorespiratory variables or blood lactate concentration. *Med. Sci. Sports Exerc.*, 39:1098, 2007.

Truijens, M.J., et al.: The effect of intermittent hypobaric hypoxic exposure and sea level training on submaximal economy in well-trained swimmers and runners. *J. Appl. Physiol.*, 104:328, 2008.

van Nieuwenhoven, M.A., et al.: The effect of two sports drinks and water on GI complaints and performance during an 18-km run. *Int. J. Sports Med.*, 26:281, 2005.

Wagner, P.D. Lundby, C.: The lactate paradox: does acclimatization to high altitude affect blood lactate during exercise. *Med. Sci. Sports Exerc.*, 39:747, 2007.

Watson, G, et al.: Influence of diuretic-induced dehydration on competitive sprint and power performance. *Med. Sci. Sports Exerc.*, 37:1168, 2005.

Watson, P., et al.: Blood–brain barrier integrity may be threatened by exercise in a warm environment. *Am. J. Physiol. Regul. Integr. Comp. Physiol.*, 288:R1689, 2005.

Wehrlin, J.P., et al.: Live high-train low for 24 days increases hemoglobin mass and red cell volume in elite endurance athletes. *J. Appl. Physiol.*, 101:1938, 2006.

West, J.B.: *High Life: A History of High Altitude Physiology and Medicine.* Oxford, England: Oxford University Press, 1998.

West, J.B.: Point: the lactate paradox does/does not occur during exercise at high altitude. *J Appl. Physiol.*, 102:2398, 2007.

Optimizing Body Composition, Successful Aging, and Health-Related Exercise Benefits

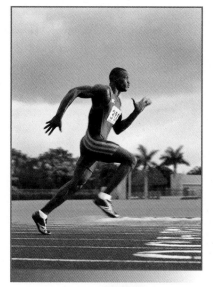

Estimates indicate that one-third of all deaths globally occur from ailments linked to excess body weight and body fat, lack of or decreased physical activity, and smoking—and this trend knows no economic, racial, or cultural borders.

Thirty years ago, age 65 represented the onset of "old" age. Now gerontologists consider 85 as a demarcation of "oldest-old" and age 75 as "young old." Demographers estimate that nearly one-half of the children born in 1996 will survive to age 95 or 100 years. Within this framework, the new gerontology addresses areas beyond age-related diseases and recognizes that *successful aging* requires enhanced physiologic function through improved physical fitness.

The physiologic and exercise capacities of older people generally rate below those of younger counterparts, yet one can question whether such differences reflect true biologic aging or simply the effect of disuse (brought on by negative alterations in lifestyle as people age). A meaningful upswing has occurred in participation of senior citizens in a broad range of physical activities. An active lifestyle retains a relatively high level of functional capacity, thus enabling older men and women to safely engage in leisure sports and more strenuous activities of daily living. Moreover, maintaining this lifestyle offers considerable protection against obesity and other diseases related to musculoskeletal and cardiovascular health.

From the glaciers of the Arctic to the palm-fringed beaches of the South Pacific, there are now more fat people in the world than hungry people! Obesity has become one of the world's leading causes of morbidity and mortality.

— Anonymous

Clinical exercise physiologists have become part of a team approach to health care. The exercise physiologist primarily focuses on restoring the patient's mobility and functional capacity while working closely with the physical therapist, occupational therapist, and physician. To this end, exercise physiologists assume an increasingly important clinical role in sports medicine to evaluate and recondition individuals with diverse diseases and physical limitations.

In this section, Chapter 16 focuses on body composition—its components and assessment, differences between men and women and trained and untrained individuals, topics relevant to the staggering revelations about the obesity epidemic, and basic information about obesity, including the role of diet and increased physical activity for effective weight loss and weight maintenance. In Chapters 17 and 18, we explore aspects of the aging process and the role played by the exercise physiologist as a healthcare professional in the clinical setting.

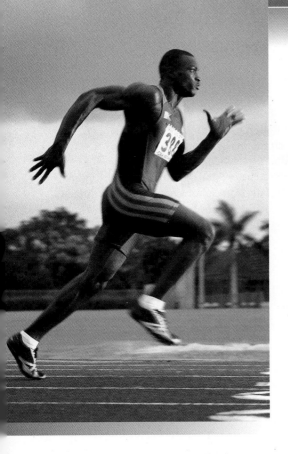

Chapter

16

Chapter

Body Composition, Obesity, and Weight Control

CHAPTER OBJECTIVES

- Outline body composition characteristics of the "reference man" and "reference woman."

- Define *lean body mass*, *fat-free body mass*, and *minimal body mass*.

- Describe Archimedes' principle applied to human body volume measurement.

- List assumptions for computing percentage body fat from body density.

- Explain how population-specific skinfold and girth equations predict body fat.

- Give strengths and weaknesses of the body mass index to assess excess weight, excess fat, and disease risk.

- Describe the current status of overweight and obesity among American adults and children.

- List eight significant health risks of obesity.

- Describe the criterion for obesity.

- Define fat cell hypertrophy and fat cell hyperplasia and explain how each contributes to obesity and how changes in body weight can modify these factors.

- Outline how "unbalancing" the energy balance equation can impact body weight.

- Explain the rationale for including regular physical activity in a prudent weight loss program.

- Explain how a moderate increase in physical activity for a previously sedentary, overweight person affects daily food intake and overall energy expenditure.

- Explain the rationale for and effectiveness of specific exercise for localized fat loss.

- Give diet and exercise advice to a person who wants to gain weight to enhance sports performance.

This chapter describes the gross composition of the human body, including direct and indirect methods to partition the body into two basic compartments—body fat mass and fat-free body mass (FFM). We also present simple, noninvasive methods to analyze an individual's body composition and discuss the important role exercise and diet play to achieve optimal body composition and improve overall health status.

Part 1	Gross Composition of the Human Body

Over the past 75 years, numerous studies have evaluated body composition and how best to measure its various components. Most methodologies partition the body into two distinct compartments: body fat mass and FFM. The density of homogenized snippets of fat-free body tissues in small mammals equals 1.100 g·cm^{-3} at 37°C. Fat stored in adipose tissue has a density of 0.900 g·cm^{-3} at 37°C. Subsequent body composition studies expanded the two-component model to account for biologic variability in three (water, protein, fat) or four (water, protein, bone mineral, fat) distinct components. Not surprisingly, men and women differ in their relative quantities of specific body composition components. Consequently, gender-specific reference standards provide a framework for evaluating "normal" body composition.

MULTICOMPONENT MODEL OF BODY COMPOSITION

Figure 16.1 shows a proposed five-level model for examining the human body. Each level of the model becomes more elaborate (atoms, molecules, cells, tissue systems, and whole body) as the body's complexity of biologic organization increases in accord with advances in physics and chemical assessment techniques. Note that subdivisions exist within each of the five levels. The model primarily attempts to identify and then quantify each level's various components. An essential feature provides separate and distinct levels, each with directly or indirectly measurable characteristics.

Body composition analyses often focuses on tissue and whole-body levels, primarily from methodologic and practical limitations. Gender differences in several of the body's compositional components provide a convenient framework to understand body composition from the framework of a **reference man** and **reference woman** developed in the 1960s by Dr. Albert Behnke (1898–1993; American College of Sports Medicine [ACSM] Honor Award; Navy physician and pioneer body composition research scientist).

BEHNKE'S REFERENCE MAN AND WOMAN MODEL

Figure 16.2 illustrates the body composition of Behnke's reference man and reference woman. The schema partitions body mass into lean body mass (LBM), muscle, and bone, with total body fat subdivided into storage and essential fat components. This model integrates the average physical dimensions from thousands of individuals measured in large-scale civilian and military anthropometric surveys with data from laboratory studies of detailed tissue composition and structure.

The reference man is taller and heavier, his skeleton weighs more, and he possesses a larger muscle mass and lower body fat content than the reference woman. These differences exist even when one expresses fat, muscle, and bone as a percentage of body mass. Just how much of the gender difference in body fat relates to biologic and behavioral factors, perhaps from lifestyle differences, remains unclear. More than likely, hormonal differences play an important role. The reference model still proves useful today for statistical comparisons and interpretations of diverse data from individuals and groups.

Essential and Storage Fat

In the reference model, total body fat exists in two storage sites or depots—**essential fat** and **storage fat**. Essential fat consists of fat in the heart, lungs, liver, spleen, kidneys, intestines, muscles, and lipid-rich tissues of the central nervous system and bone marrow. Normal physiologic functioning requires this fat. In the heart, for example, dissectible fat from cadavers represents approximately 18.4 g or 5.3% of an average heart that weighs 349 g in men and 22.7 g or 8.6% of a 256 g heart in women. In women, essential fat also includes additional **sex-specific fat.**

The storage fat depot includes fat (triacylglycerol) packed primarily in adipose tissue. The adipose tissue energy reserve contains approximately 83% pure fat, 2% protein, and 15% water within its supporting structures. Storage fat includes the visceral fatty tissues that protect the various internal organs within the thoracic and abdominal cavities from trauma and the larger adipose tissue volume deposited beneath the skin's surface called **subcutaneous fat.** A similar proportional distribution of storage fat exists in men and women (12% of body mass in men and 15% in women), but the total percentage of essential fat in women, which includes sex-specific fat, averages four times that in men. More than likely, the additional essential fat in women serves biologically important functions for childbearing and other hormone-related functions. Considering the reference body's total quantity of approximately 8.5 kg of storage fat, this depot theoretically represents 63,500 kCal of available energy, or the energy equivalent of running nonstop at a 9-minute-per-mile pace for 114 hours or approximately 29 consecutive marathons!

Figure 16.3 partitions the distribution of body fat for the reference woman. As part of the 5% to 9% sex-specific fat reserves, breast fat probably contributes no more than 4% of body mass for women whose total fat content ranges between 14% and 35%. We interpret this to mean that other substantial sex-specific fat depots exist (e.g., pelvic, buttock, and thigh regions) that contribute to the female's body fat stores.

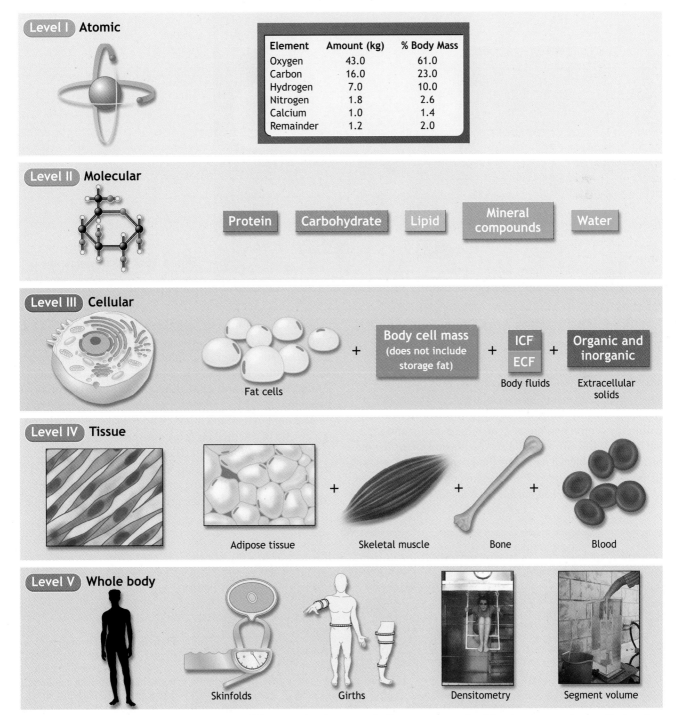

Figure 16.1 Five-level, multicomponent model to assess and interpret body composition. Each level progresses in complexity of biologic organization. ECF = extracellular fluid; ICF = intracellular fluid. (Modified from Wang, Z.M., et al.: The five-component model. A new approach to organizing body composition research. *Am. J. Clin. Nutr.*, 56:19, 1992.)

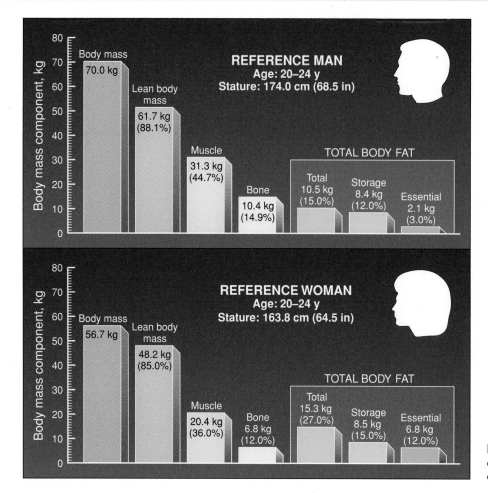

Figure 16.2 Body composition of Behnke's reference man and reference woman.

Fat-Free Body Mass and Lean Body Mass

The terms FFM and LBM refer to specific entities. Although these terms often are used interchangeably, the differences are subtle but real. LBM (a theoretical entity) contains the small percentage of non–sex-specific essential fat equivalent to approximately 4% to 7% of body mass (located chiefly within the central nervous system, bone marrow, and internal organs). In contrast, FFM represents body mass devoid of all extractable fat (FFM = Body mass − Fat mass). Behnke points out that FFM refers to an in vitro entity (*in an artificial environment outside the living organism*) appro-

priate to carcass analysis. Behnke considered the LBM an in vivo (*within a living organism*) entity relatively constant in water, organic matter, and mineral content throughout an active adult's life span. In normally hydrated, healthy adults, the FFM and LBM differ only in the essential fat component.

The LBM in men and **minimal body mass** in women consist chiefly of essential fat (plus sex-specific fat for women), muscle, water, and bone (**Fig. 16.2**). The whole-body density of the reference man with 12% storage fat and 3% essential fat equals 1.070 g·cm^{-3}; the density of his FFM equals 1.094 g·cm^{-3}. If the reference man's total body fat

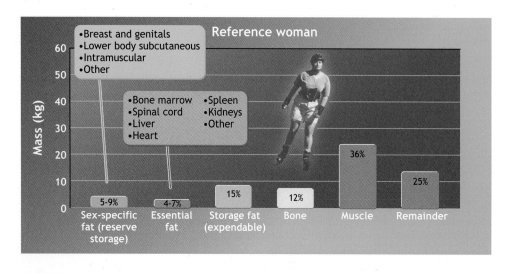

Figure 16.3 Theoretical model for body fat distribution for the reference woman with body mass of 56.7 kg, stature of 163.8 cm, and 27% body fat. (From Katch, V.L., et al.: Contribution of breast volume and weight to body fat distribution in females. *Am. J. Phys. Anthropol.*, 53:93, 1980.)

Table 16.1 Percentage Body Fat of Male and Female Athletes

	PERCENTAGE BODY FAT	
SPORT	MALE	FEMALE
Ballet dancing	8–14	13–20
Baseball/softball	12–15	12–18
Basketball	6–12	20–27
Body building	5–8	10–15
Canoe/Kayak	6–12	10–16
Cycling	5–15	15–20
Football		
Backs	9–12	
Linebackers	13–14	
Lineman	15–19	
Quarterbacks	12–14	
Gymnastics	5–12	10–16
Horse racing	8–12	10–16
Ice/Field hockey	8–15	12–18
Orienteering	5–12	12–24
Racquetball	8–13	15–22
Rock climbing	5–10	13–18
Rowing	6–14	12–18
Rugby		10–17
Skiing		
Alpine	7–14	18–24
Cross-country	7–12	16–22
Jumping	10–15	12–18
Speed skating	10–14	15–24
Synchronized swimming		12–24
Swimming	9–12	14–24
Tennis	12–16	16–24
Track and field		
Discus throwers	14–18	22–27
Jumpers	7–12	10–18
Long distance	6–13	12–20
Shot putters	16–20	20–28
Sprinters	8–10	12–20
Decathletes	8–10	
Triathlon	5–12	10–15
Volleyball	11–14	16–25
Weightlifters	9–16	
Wrestling	5–16	

Data compiled from the research literature.

percentage equals 15.0% (storage fat plus essential fat), the density of a hypothetical fat-free body attains the upper limit of 1.100 g·cm^{-3}.

For the reference woman, the average whole-body density of 1.040 g·cm^{-3} represents a body fat percentage of 27%; of this, approximately 12% consists of essential body fat. A density of 1.072 g·cm^{-3} represents the minimal body mass of 48.5 kg. In actual practice, density values exceeding 1.068 for women (14.8% body fat) and 1.088 g·cm^{-3} for men (5% body fat) rarely occur except in young, lean athletes.

Table 16.1 presents data for percentage body fat for selected groups of male and female athletes. Striking differences exist among these groups, including variability within each athletic group.

Minimal Leanness Standards

A biologic lower limit probably exists beyond which a person's body mass cannot decrease further without lowering the FFM to a degree that impairs health status or alters normal physiologic functions. Wasting diseases of malnutrition in men and women fall into this category, notably the complex eating disorder anorexia nervosa.

Questions & Notes

Describe differences between essential and storage fat.

List 3 essential fat sites.

1.

2.

3.

Describe the primary role of storage fat.

Complete the equation:

FFM =

What is the assumed density of the FFM?

What is the whole-body density for the reference male and female.

Male:

Female:

Men To estimate minimal weight (i.e., LBM), subtract storage fat from body mass. For the reference man, LBM (61.7 kg) includes approximately 3% (2.1 kg) of essential body fat. Encroachment into this reserve may impair optimal health and capacity for exercise.

Low body fat values exist for male world-class endurance athletes and were present in conscientious objectors to military service who voluntarily reduced their body fat stores during a year-long classic nutritional experiment in the 1950s with semistarvation (*en.wikipedia.org/wiki/ Minnesota_Starvation_Experiment*). The low body fat levels of marathon runners, ranging from 1% to 8% of body mass, probably reflect an adaptation to long-term training for distance running and reduced caloric intake. A relatively low body fat level reduces the energy cost of weight-bearing exercise; it also provides an effective gradient to dissipate metabolic heat generated during prolonged, intense exercise.

Women In contrast to the lower limit of body mass for the reference man (with 3% essential fat), the lower limit for the reference woman equals approximately 12% essential fat. This theoretical limit represents 48.5 kg for the reference woman. Generally, the leanest women in the population do not fall below 10% to 12% body fat, which represents a narrow range probably at the lower limit for most women in good health. Behnke's theoretical concept of minimal body mass in women, incorporating approximately 12% essential fat, corresponds to the LBM in men that includes 3% essential fat.

Underweight and Thin

The terms *underweight* and *thin* describe considerably different physical conditions. Measurements in our laboratories have focused on the structural characteristics of "apparently" thin women. We initially screened subjects subjectively as thin or "skinny." Twenty-six women were measured for skinfolds, circumferences, bone diameters, and percentage body fat and FFM by hydrodensitometry (see page 540).

Unexpectedly, the women's percentage of body fat averaged 18.2%, only 7 to 9 percentage points below the values of 25% to 27% body fat typically reported for young adult women. Another striking finding included equivalence in four trunk and four extremity bone diameter measurements for the thin-appearing women compared with 174 women who averaged 25.6% fat and 31 women who averaged 31.4% body fat. Thus, appearing thin or skinny did not necessarily correspond to a diminutive frame size or critically low body fat percentage proposed in the Behnke model for the lower limits of minimal body mass and essential body fat.

Three criteria identify an underweight woman:

1. Body mass lower than minimal body mass calculated from skeletal measurements
2. Body mass lower than the 20th percentile by stature
3. Percentage body fat lower than 17% assessed by a criterion method

LEANNESS, REGULAR EXERCISE, AND MENSTRUAL IRREGULARITY

Physically active women, particularly participants in the "low weight" or "body appearance" sports (e.g., distance running, body building, figure skating, diving, ballet, and gymnastics), increase their likelihood for one of three medical maladies:

1. Delayed onset of menstruation
2. Irregular menstrual cycle (**oligomenorrhea**)
3. Complete cessation of menses (**amenorrhea**)

Menstrual dysfunction results largely from changes in the pituitary gland's normal pulsatile secretion of luteinizing hormone, which is regulated by gonadotropin-releasing hormone from the hypothalamus.

Amenorrhea occurs in 2% to 5% of women of reproductive age in the general population, but it reaches 40% in some athletic groups. As a group, ballet dancers remain lean and exhibit a greater incidence of menstrual dysfunction and eating disorders and a higher mean age at menarche than age-matched, nondance counterparts. One-third to one-half of female endurance athletes exhibit some menstrual irregularity. In premenopausal women, irregularity or absence of menses accelerates bone loss and increases the risk of musculoskeletal injury (e.g., stress fractures), which thus interrupts the normal training process.

A high level of chronic physical stress may disrupt the hypothalamic–pituitary–adrenal axis and modify the output of gonadotropin-releasing hormone to cause irregular menstruation referred to as the **exercise stress hypothesis**. A concurrent hypothesis maintains that an energy reserve inadequate to sustain pregnancy induces cessation of ovulation (**energy availability hypothesis**). Proponents of this "energy deficit" explanation maintain that exercise per se exerts no deleterious effect on the reproductive system other than the potential impact of its additional energy cost on creating a negative energy balance.

Some researchers argue that 17% body fat represents a critical level for onset of menstruation, with 22% fat needed to sustain a normal cycle. They reason that body fat below these levels triggers hormonal and metabolic disturbances that impact the menses. Research with animals has identified **leptin**, a hormone intimately linked to body fat levels and appetite control, as a principal chemical that initiates puberty. Thus, a link exists between hormonal regulation of sexual maturity onset (and perhaps continued optimal sexual function) and the level of stored energy reflected by accumulated body fat.

The LBM-to-body fat ratio may play a key role in normal menstrual function. This could occur through peripheral fat's role in converting androgens to estrogens or through leptin production in adipose tissue. Other factors may also be operative. Many physically active women below the supposedly critical 17% body fat level have normal menstrual cycles without sacrificing a high level of physiologic and exercise capacity. Conversely, some amenorrheic athletes maintain body fat levels considered average for the population.

Potential causes of menstrual dysfunction include a complex interplay of physical, nutritional, genetic, hormonal, regional fat distribution, psychological, and environmental factors. An intense exercise bout triggers release of an array of hormones, some of which can disrupt normal reproductive function.

In all likelihood, 13% to 17% body fat probably represents a minimum range associated with regular menstrual function. The effects and risks of sustained amenorrhea on the reproductive system remain unknown. A gynecologist or endocrinologist should evaluate failure to menstruate or cessation of the normal cycle. Such disrupted function may signal a significant medical condition such as pituitary or thyroid gland malfunction or premature menopause.

 For Your Information

WHEN A MODEL IS NOT IDEAL

In 1967, only an 8% difference existed in body weight between professional fashion models and the average American woman. Today, a model's body weight averages 23% lower than the national average. Twenty years ago, gymnasts weighed about 20 pounds more than their present-day counterparts. Thus, it should come as little surprise that disordered eating patterns and unrealistic weight goals (and general dissatisfaction with one's body) remain so common among girls and women of *all* ages.

 S U M M A R Y

1. Total body fat consists of essential fat and storage fat. Essential fat contains fat in bone marrow, nerve tissue, and organs; it does not represent an energy reserve but is an important component for normal biologic function. Storage fat, the energy reserve, accumulates mainly as adipose tissue beneath the skin and in the deeper visceral depots.

2. Storage fat averages 12% of body mass for young adult men and 15% of body mass for women.

3. True gender differences exist for essential fat. It averages 3% body mass for men and 12% body mass for women. The greater percentage of essential fat for women probably relates to childbearing and hormonal functions (i.e., sex-specific essential fat).

4. A person probably cannot reduce body fat below the essential fat level and still maintain good health and optimal exercise capacity.

5. Menstrual dysfunction occurs among female athletes who train hard, incur an energy deficit, and maintain low levels of body fat. The precise interaction among menstrual dysfunction and the physiologic and psychological stress of regular training and competition, hormonal balance, energy and nutrient intake, and body fat requires further study.

T H O U G H T   Q U E S T I O N

What arguments counter the position that no true sex difference exists in body fat, but only a difference caused by gender-related patterns of regular physical activity and caloric intake?

Part 2 — **Methods to Assess Body Size and Composition**

*Q*uestions & Notes

Discuss differences between the terms underweight and thin.

Two general approaches determine the fat and fat-free components of the human body:

1. Direct measurement by chemical analysis or dissection
2. Indirect estimation by hydrostatic weighing; anthropometric measurements; and other simple procedures, including body stature and mass

DIRECT ASSESSMENT

Two methods directly assess body composition. In one technique, a chemical solution literally dissolves the body into its fat and nonfat (fat-free) components.

The other direct assessment approach involves physical dissection of fat, fat-free adipose tissue, muscle, and bone. Such analyses require extensive time, meticulous attention to detail, and specialized laboratory equipment and pose ethical questions and legal problems in obtaining cadavers for research purposes. The most complete physical dissection study was published in 1984. **Figure 16.4** presents results from 25 cadavers ranging in age from 55 to 94 years. The sample included 12 embalmed (six men and six women) and 13 nonembalmed (six men and seven women) whites. Analyses for each cadaver included removing skeletal muscle and other major organs (brain, heart, lungs, liver, kidneys, and spleen). Bones were then separated at their articulations and scraped to leave surfaces free of muscle and adipose tissue. Muscle included the ligaments, and bone retained the cartilage of any articular surface. Airtight plastic buckets stored all dissected tissues, including scrapings. The tissues were weighed to within 0.1 g and their densities determined as the ratio of mass to volume. Complete dissection took approximately 15 hours and required a team of 10 to 12 anatomists and kinesiologists. The average adipose tissue mass in women equates to 40.5% of total body mass and 28.1% in men (**Fig. 16.4**). The researchers introduced the concept of adipose tissue-free weight (ATFW)—the whole-body mass minus the mass of all dissectible adipose tissue that contains about 83% pure fat. Muscle accounted for 52% of the ATFW in men and 48.1% in women, and bone constituted 19.9% of ATFW in men and 21.3% in women. Combining the data for men and women, the average proportion of the ATFW included 8.5% skin, 50.0% muscle, and 20.6% bone.

INDIRECT ASSESSMENT

Many indirect procedures assess body composition. Archimedes' principle applied to **hydrostatic weighing**, also known as **underwater weighing** and **hydrodensitometry**, computes percentage body fat from **body density**. Other indirect procedures to predict body fat use skinfold thickness and girth measurements, x-ray, total-body electrical conductivity or impedance, near-infrared interactance (NIR), ultrasonography, computed tomography (CT), air plethysmography, magnetic resonance imaging (MRI), and dual-energy x-ray absorptiometry (DXA).

Hydrostatic Weighing (Archimedes' Principle)

The Greek mathematician and inventor Archimedes (287–212 BC; *en.wikipedia.org/wiki/Archimedes*) discovered a fundamental principle renowned in antiquity and still applied to indirectly evaluate human body composition. An itinerant scholar of that period described the interesting circumstances surrounding the event:

> King Hieron of Syracuse suspected that his pure gold crown had been altered by substitution of silver for gold. The King directed Archimedes to devise a method for testing the crown for its gold content without dismantling it. Archimedes pondered over this problem for many weeks without succeeding, until one day, he stepped into a bath filled to the top with water and observed the overflow. He thought about this for a moment, and then, wild with joy, jumped from the bath and ran naked through the streets of Syracuse shouting, "Eureka! Eureka!" I have discovered a way to solve the mystery of the King's crown.

Archimedes reasoned that gold must have a volume in proportion to its mass and to measure the volume of an irregularly shaped object required submersion in water with collection of the overflow. Archimedes took lumps of gold and silver, each having the same mass as the crown, and submerged each in a container full of water. To his delight, he discovered the crown displaced more water than the lump of gold and less than the lump of silver. This could only mean the crown consisted of *both* silver and gold as the King suspected.

Essentially, Archimedes evaluated the **specific gravity** of the crown (i.e., the ratio of the crown's mass to the mass of an equal volume of water) compared with the specific gravities of gold and silver. Archimedes also reasoned that an object submerged or floating in water becomes buoyed up by a counterforce that equals the weight of the volume of water it displaces. This buoyant force supports an immersed object against the downward pull of gravity.

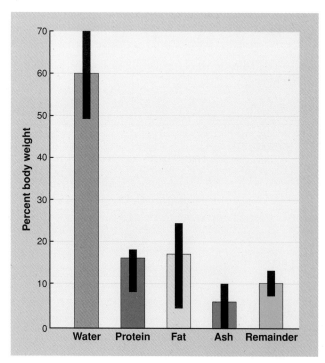

Figure 16.4 Various tissues in the adult male and female body based on cadaver analysis expressed as a percentage of total body mass (in kg). (From Clarys, J.P., et al.: Gross tissue weights in the human body by cadaver dissection. *Hum. Biol.*, 56:459, 1984.)

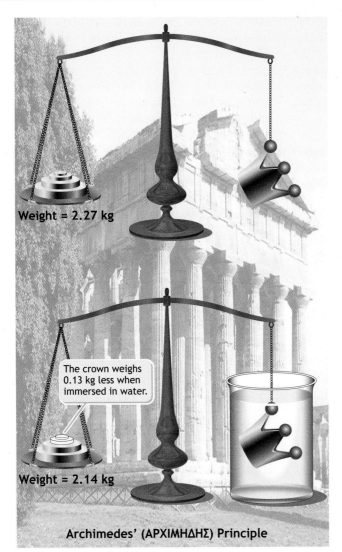

Figure 16.5 Archimedes' principle for determining the volume and specific gravity of the King's crown.

Questions & Notes

List 4 different indirect methods to assess body composition.

1.

2.

3.

4.

Give another name for underwater weighing.

Explain the difference between density and specific gravity?

State Archimedes principle.

Thus, an object "loses weight in water." *The object's loss of weight in water equals the weight of the volume of water it displaces, thus making the specific gravity the ratio of the weight of an object in air divided by its loss of weight in water.* The loss of weight in water equals the weight in air minus the weight in water.

Specific gravity = Weight in air ÷ Loss of weight in water

In practical terms, suppose a crown weighed 2.27 kg in air and 0.13 kg less (2.14 kg) when weighed underwater (**Fig. 16.5**). Dividing the weight of the crown (2.27 kg) by its loss of weight in water (0.13 kg) yields a specific gravity of 17.5. Because this ratio differs considerably from the specific gravity of gold (19.3), we too can conclude: "Eureka, the crown must be fraudulent!"

Archimedes' principle allows the application of hydrodensitometry to indirectly determine the body's volume and from this to compute body density and percentage body fat.

Determining Body Density   For illustrative purposes, suppose a 50-kg woman weighs 2 kg when submerged in water. According to Archimedes' principle, a 48-kg *loss* of weight in water equals the weight of the displaced water. The volume of water displaced is computed easily because chemists have determined the density of water at any temperature. In this example, 48 kg of water equals 48 L or 48,000 cm^3 (1 g of water = 1 cm^3 by volume at 39.2°F). If the woman were measured at the cold-water temperature of 39.2°F, no density correction for water would be necessary. In practice, researchers use warmer water and apply the density value for water at the particular weighing temperature. The whole-body density of this person, computed as Mass ÷ Volume, equals 50,000 g (50 kg) ÷ 48,000 cm^3, or 1.0417 g·cm^{-3}.

Computing Percentage Body Fat, Fat Mass, and Fat-Free Body Mass

The equation that incorporates whole-body density from underwater weighing to estimate the body's fat percentage is derived from the following three premises:

1. Densities of fat mass (all extractable lipid from adipose and other body tissues) and FFM (remaining lipid-free tissues and chemicals, including water) remain relatively constant (fat tissue = 0.90 g·cm^{-3}; fat-free tissue = 1.10 g·cm^{-3}), even with variations in total body fat and FFM components of bone and muscle.
2. Densities for the components of the FFM at a body temperature of 37°C remain constant within and among individuals: water, 0.9937 g·cm^{-3} (73.8% of FFM); mineral, 3.038 g·cm^{-3} (6.8% of FFM); and protein, 1.340 g·cm^{-3} (19.4% of FFM).
3. The person measured differs from the reference body only in fat content (reference body assumed to possess 73.8% water, 19.4% protein, and 6.8% mineral).

The following equation, derived by Berkeley physicist Dr. William Siri (1926–2004), computes percentage body fat from whole-body density:

Siri Equation

Percentage body fat = 495 ÷ Body density − 450

Based on the previous three assumptions, the following example incorporates the body density value of 1.0417 g·cm^{-3} (determined for the woman in the previous example) in the **Siri equation** to estimate percentage body fat:

$$\text{Percentage body fat} = 495 \div \text{Body density} - 450$$
$$= 495 \div 1.0417 - 450$$
$$= 25.2\%$$

The mass of body fat is calculated by multiplying body mass by percentage fat:

$$\text{Fat mass (kg)} = \text{Body mass (kg)}$$
$$\times (\text{Percentage fat} \div 100)$$
$$= 50 \text{ kg} \times 0.252$$
$$= 12.6 \text{ kg}$$

Subtracting mass of fat from body mass yields FFM:

$$\text{FFM (kg)} = \text{Body mass (kg)} - \text{Fat mass (kg)}$$
$$= 50 \text{ kg} - 12.6 \text{ kg}$$
$$= 37.4 \text{ kg}$$

In this example, 25.2% or 12.6 kg of the 50-kg body mass consists of fat, with the remaining 37.4 kg representing the FFM component.

Limitations and Errors in Hydrostatic Weighing The generalized density values for fat-free tissue (1.10 g·cm^{-3}) and fat tissue (0.90 g·cm^{-3}) represent average values for young and middle-aged adults. These constants vary among individuals and groups, particularly the density and chemical composition of the FFM. This variation impacts the accuracy of predicting percentage body fat from whole-body density. For example, African Americans and Hispanics have larger FFM densities than whites (1.113 g·cm^{-3} for African Americans, 1.105 g·cm^{-3} for Hispanics, and 1.100 g·cm^{-3} for whites). Consequently, using existing density-to-fat equations (based on assumptions for whites) to calculate body composition for African Americans or Hispanics *overestimates* FFM and *underestimates* percentage body fat. The following modification of the Siri equation computes percentage body fat from body density for African Americans:

Modification for African Americans

Percentage body fat = 437.4 ÷ Body density − 392.8

Applying constant density values for the various tissues for children (who are growing) or for aging adults (who are concurrently losing muscle and bone mass) also introduces errors in determining body composition from whole-body density values. For example, the water and mineral contents of the FFM continually change during the growth period, and demineralization from osteoporosis occurs with aging. Lower bone density makes density of the fat-free tissues of young children and elderly people lower than the assumed constant of 1.10 g·cm^{-3}, thus overestimating percentage body fat. For this reason, many researchers do not convert body density to percentage body fat in children and aging adults. Others apply a multicompartment model to adjust for such factors in computing percentage body fat from body density in prepubertal children. **Table 16.2** presents equations adjusted to maturation level to determine body fat percentage from whole-body density of boys and girls ages 7 to 17 years.

Table 16.3 presents density estimates of FFM for different adult male and female population subgroups and equations to predict percentage body fat. These were derived from whole-body density based on assumptions regarding the densities and proportions of the body's protein, mineral, and water content. Obviously, different equations to convert body density to percentage body fat yield different values depending on their underlying assumptions. This variation does not reflect an inherent error in the underwater weighing method; rather, hydrostatic weighing to assess body volume generates a technical error for this variable of less than 1%.

Body Volume Measurement

Figure 16.6 illustrates three examples of body volume measurements by hydrostatic weighing. First, the subject's body mass in air

Table 16.2	Percentage Body Fat Estimated From Body Density (Db) Using Age- and Gender-Specific Conversion Constants to Account for Changes in the Density of the Fat-Free Body Mass as a Child Matures	
AGE (y)	BOYS	GIRLS
7–9	%Fat = (5.38/Db – 4.97) × 100	%Fat = (5.43/Db – 5.03) × 100
9–11	%Fat = (5.30/Db – 4.86) × 100	%Fat = (5.35/Db – 4.95) × 100
11–13	%Fat = (5.23/Db – 4.81) × 100	%Fat = (5.25/Db – 4.84) × 100
13–15	%Fat = (5.08/Db – 4.64) × 100	%Fat = (5.12/Db – 4.69) × 100
15–17	%Fat = (5.03/Db – 4.59) × 100	%Fat = (5.07/Db – 4.64) × 100

From Lohman, T. Applicability of body composition techniques and constants for children and youth. *Exerc. Sports Sci., Rev.*, 14:325, 1986.

is assessed usually to the nearest ±50 g. A diver's belt secured around the waist prevents less dense (more fat) subjects from floating to the surface during submersion. Seated with the head out of water, the subject then makes a forced maximal exhalation while lowering the head beneath the water. The breath is held for several seconds while the underwater weight is recorded. The subject repeats this procedure 8 to 12 times to obtain a dependable or "true" underwater weight score. Even when achieving a full exhalation, a small volume of air,

Table 16.3	Equations to Predict Percentage Body Fat From Body Density (Db) Based on Different Estimates of the Fat-Free Body Density (FFDB)	
AGE, y	EQUATION	FFDB[a]
Male		
White		
7–12	%Fat = 5.08/Db − 4.89	1.084
13–16	%Fat = 5.07/Db − 4.64	1.094
17–19	%Fat = 4.99/Db − 4.55	1.098
20–80	%Fat = 4.95/Db − 4.50	1.100
African American		
18–22	%Fat = 4.37/Db − 3.93	1.113
Japanese		
18–48	%Fat = 4.97/Db − 4.52	1.099
61–78	%Fat = 4.87/Db − 4.41	1.105
Female		
White		
7–12	%Fat = 5.35/Db − 4.95	1.082
13–16	%Fat = 5.10/Db − 4.66	1.093
17–19	%Fat = 5.05/Db − 4.62	1.095
20–80	%Fat = 5.01/Db − 4.57	1.097
Native American		
18–60	%Fat = 4.81/Db − 4.34	1.108
African American		
24–79	%Fat = 4.85/Db − 4.39	1.106
Hispanic		
20–40	%Fat = 4.87/Db − 4.41	1.105
Japanese		
18–48	%Fat = 4.76/Db − 4.28	1.111
61–78	%Fat = 4.95/Db − 4.50	1.100
Anorexic		
15–30	%Fat = 5.26/Db − 4.83	1.087
Obese		
17–62	%Fat = 5.00/Db − 4.56	1.098

Equations from the research literature.
[a]Each estimate of the fat-free body density (FFDB) uses slightly different values for the proportions of the body's protein, mineral, and water content.

Questions & Notes

Write the Siri equation for estimating percentage body fat.

Compute the percentage body fat for a person with a body density of 1.0399 g·mL⁻¹.

Compute the percentage fat for a Hispanic female with a body density of 1.0417 g·mL⁻¹.

Compute the percentage fat for an African American male with a body density of 1.0611 g·mL⁻¹.

Compute the percentage fat for a 15-year-old boy with a body density of 1.0444 g·mL⁻¹.

Explain why there are different FFDB for different populations.

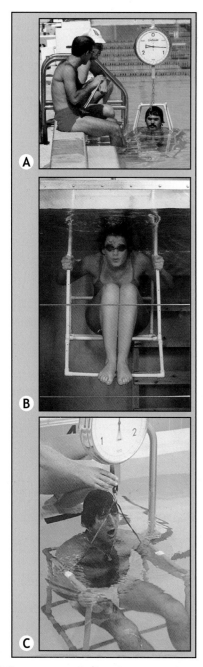

Figure 16.6 Measuring body volume using three methods. Underwater weighing in (**A**) swimming pool, (**B**) stainless steel tank in the laboratory, (**C**) therapy pool at a pro football training facility.

the **residual lung volume (RLV)**, remains in the lungs. Thus, the calculation of body volume requires subtraction of the buoyant effect of the RLV. This can be measured immediately before, during, or following underwater weighing.

A Word About Residual Volume   The greatest source of error in calculating body volume by hydrostatic weighing results from errors in measuring RLV. Its measurement requires specialized equipment and trained personnel. In situations that do not demand research-level accuracy (general screening, fitness assessments, teaching laboratories), RLV

prediction equations based on age, stature, body mass, or vital capacity provide an appropriate estimate (see Close Up, Box 16.1: *Predicting Residual Lung Volume* on page 545).

Body Volume Measurement by Air Displacement   Techniques other than hydrodensitometry can reliably assess body volume. **Figure 16.7** illustrates the **BOD POD**, a plethysmographic device used to assess body volume. Essentially, body volume equals the chamber's reduced air volume when the subject enters the chamber. The subject sits in a structure composed of two chambers, each of known volume. A molded fiberglass seat forms a common wall separating the front (test) and rear (reference) chambers. A volume-perturbing element (a moving diaphragm) connects the two chambers. Changes in pressure between two chambers oscillate the diaphragm, which directly reflects any change in chamber volume. The subject makes several breaths into an air circuit to assess thoracic gas volume (which when subtracted from measured body

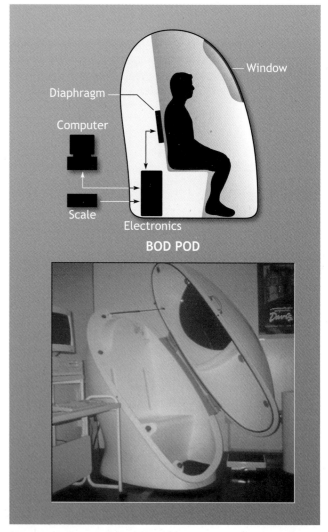

Figure 16.7 (Top) Major system components of the BOD POD, the air displacement chamber used to measure total body volume by air displacement (Bottom). (Photo courtesy of Life Sciences Instruments, Concord, CA.)

BOX 16.1 CLOSE UP

Predicting Residual Lung Volume

Hydrostatic weighing represents a valid and reliable laboratory technique to assess body composition. The procedure accurately assesses body volume in the course of determining whole-body density (body mass ÷ body volume). Body volume equals the difference between body mass measured in air minus body weight measured underwater (subtracting RLV and air in the gastrointestinal [GI] tract) and corrected for water density at the weighing temperature. The small volume of air trapped in the GI tract (<100 mL) can be disregarded. In contrast, RLV represents a large and variable gas volume that must be subtracted to accurately determine body volume.

Laboratory techniques of helium dilution, nitrogen washout, or oxygen dilution routinely measure RLV. Each procedure requires complicated and expensive laboratory equipment. An alternate, although less valid, approach estimates RLV with gender-specific prediction equations based on age, stature, and body mass. The standard error of estimate to predict RLV ranges between ±325 and 500 mL; this can correspond to errors in predicting percentage body fat of up to ±2.5% or more body fat units.

RESIDUAL LUNG VOLUME PREDICTION EQUATIONS

Variables: Age, y; stature (St), cm; body mass (BM), kg
Normal-weight men:

$$RLV, L = (0.022 \times Age) + (0.0198 \times St) - (0.015 \times BM) - 1.54$$

Normal-weight women (uses only age and stature):

$$RLV, L = (0.007 \times Age) + (0.0268 \times St) - 3.42$$

Overfat men (%Fat ≥25) and women (%Fat ≥30):

$$RLV, L = (0.0167 \times Age) + (0.0130 \times BM) + (0.0185 \times St) - 3.3413$$

Examples

1. Man: Age, 21 y; body mass; 80 kg (176.4 lb); stature, 182.9 cm (72 in)

$$RLV (L) = (0.022 \times 21) + (0.0198 \times 182.9) - (0.015 \times 80) - 1.54$$
$$= 0.462 + 3.621 - 1.2 - 1.54$$
$$= 1.34 \text{ L}$$

2. Woman: Age, 19 y; stature, 160.0 cm (63 in)

$$RLV (L) = (0.007 \times 19) + (0.0268 \times 160.0) - 3.42$$
$$= 0.133 + 4.288 - 3.42$$
$$= 1.00 \text{ L}$$

3. Overfat man: Age, 35 y; body mass, 104 kg (229.3 lb); stature, 179.5 cm (70.7 in)

$$RLV (L) = (0.0167 \times 35) + (0.0130 \times 104) + (0.0185 \times 179.5) - 3.3413$$
$$= 0.5845 + 1.352 + 3.321 - 3.3413$$
$$= 1.39 \text{ L}$$

REFERENCES

Grimby, G., Söderholm, B.: Spirometric studies in normal subjects. III: Static lung volumes and maximum ventilatory ventilation in adults with a note on physical fitness. *Acta. Med. Scand.*, 2:199, 1963.

Miller, W.C.T., et al.: Derivation of prediction equations for RV in overweight men and women. *Med. Sci. Sports Exerc.*, 30:322, 1998.

volume yields true body volume). Body density computes as body mass (measured in air) ÷ body volume (measured by BOD POD). The Siri equation converts body density to percentage body fat.

Skinfold Measurements

Simple anthropometric procedures successfully predict body fatness. The most common of these procedures uses **skinfolds**. The rationale for using skinfolds to estimate the body's fat composition results from the close relationships among three factors: (1) subcutaneous fat in adipose tissue deposits directly beneath the skin, (2) the body's internal fat stores, and (3) body density of the intact human body.

Questions & Notes

Compute the residual lung volume for a 22-year-old male with a body mass of 79 kg and a stature of 185.4 cm.

BOX 16.2 CLOSE UP

When Should Skinfold Readings Be Taken?

A frequently asked question about taking skinfold measurements concerns when to read the caliper value. Should you leave the caliper on the site for 1, 3, or 5 seconds or until the pointer stops moving?

Research-quality skinfold calipers exert an average compression force of 10 g per mm² at all jaw openings. This means that the caliper always exerts the same pressure regardless of skin-plus-fat thickness. After it is applied to the skinfold site, the caliper continues to displace subcutaneous interstitial water, connective tissue, and fat throughout the measurement period until the skinfold's rebound force counteracts the caliper pressure.

The *inset* shows the compression data for triceps skinfold for 18 men and 18 women. Modification of the caliper provided for an instantaneous record of skinfold thickness throughout the measurement period. More than 70% of the total compression of skin and underlying fat takes place within the first 4 seconds after applying the caliper. Thus, to

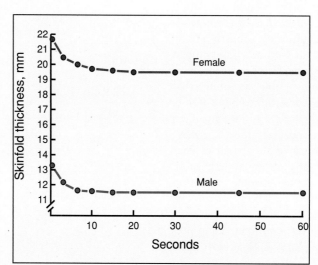

record the uncompressed skin-plus-fat measurement, the reading should be made when applying the caliper to the skin as it exerts its full pressure and certainly within 1 or 2 seconds. Any prolonged delay in reading the caliper *underestimates* the actual skinfold value.

The absolute change in skinfold thickness among subjects over 60 seconds ranged between 0.3 mm and 4.5 mm. Although not a dramatic absolute change, this error can affect the accuracy of percentage body fat when using skinfold prediction equations. For example, using the initial uncompressed versus the final compressed skinfold value (after 60 s) produced differences in predicted percentage body fat that ranged between 2 and 8 fat percentage units (a 10%–50% error). This large error cannot be ignored. Almost all of the research studies using skinfolds have not specified when they recorded their readings. One can only surmise that it occurred immediately after placing the calipers on the skin to obtain an uncompressed value.

REFERENCE

Becque, D.M., et al.: Time course of skin-plus-fat compression in males and females. *Hum. Biol.*, 58:33, 1986.

The Caliper By 1930, a special pincer-type caliper accurately measured subcutaneous fat at selected body sites. The **skinfold calipers** work on the same principle as a micrometer to measure the distance between two points. The pincer jaws exert a constant tension of 10 g·mm⁻² at the point of contact with the double layer of skin plus subcutaneous tissue. The caliper dial indicates skinfold thickness in millimeters.

Figure 16.8 shows three different types of skinfold calipers. Compared with the most costly calipers (Harpenden and Lange), the less expensive models are less precise, exert nonconstant jaw tension throughout the range of measurement, usually have a smaller measurement scale (<60 mm), and produce less consistent scores at the same skinfold site when used by inexperienced testers.

Measuring skinfold thickness requires grasping a fold of skin and subcutaneous fat firmly with the thumb and forefingers and pulling it away from the underlying muscle tis-

sue following the skinfold's natural contour. The skinfold is recorded within 2 seconds after applying the full force of the caliper. This time limitation avoids skinfold compression (see Close Up, Box 16.2, *When Should Skinfold Readings Be Taken?*). For research purposes, the investigator should attain considerable experience in taking measurements and demonstrate consistency in duplicating skinfold values at multiple sites for the same subject made on the same day, consecutive days, or even weeks apart. A good rule of thumb to achieve consistency requires taking duplicate or triplicate practice measurements at all skinfold sites on approximately 50 individuals who range in body fat from "thin" to "obese." Careful attention to details before making "real" meaurements helps to ensure greater measurement reproducibility.

Skinfold Sites The most common skinfold sites include the triceps, subscapular, suprailiac, abdominal, and upper thigh. An average of two or three measurements at each

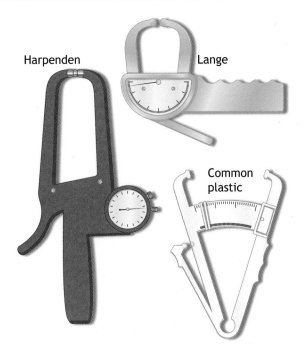

Harpenden

Lange

Common plastic

Figure 16.8 Common calipers to measure subcutaneous fat.

site on the right side of the body with the subject standing represents the skinfold score. Except for the subscapular and suprailiac sites, which are measured diagonally, measurements are taken in the vertical plane. The *lower right schematic* in **Figure 16.9** shows a skinfold caliper and the compression of a double layer of skin and underlying tissue during the measurement along with the anatomic location for five of the most frequently measured skinfold sites:

1. **Triceps:** Vertical fold at the posterior midline of the upper arm, halfway between the tip of the shoulder and tip of the elbow; elbow remains in an extended, relaxed position
2. **Subscapular:** Oblique fold just below the bottom tip of the scapula
3. **Suprailiac (iliac crest):** Slightly oblique fold just above the hip bone (crest of ileum); the fold follows the natural diagonal line
4. **Abdomen:** Vertical fold 1 inch to the right of the umbilicus
5. **Thigh:** Vertical fold at the midline of the thigh, two-thirds of the distance from the middle of the patella (knee cap) to the hip

Two other sites include:

Chest (males): Diagonal fold (with its long axis directed toward the nipple) on the anterior axillary fold as high as possible

Biceps: Vertical fold at the posterior midline of the upper arm

Using Skinfold Data Skinfolds provide meaningful information about body fat and its distribution. Based on research, two practical ways exist to use skinfolds:

1. Sum the individual skinfold values. This "sum of skinfolds" (Σ skf) indicates relative fatness among individuals; it also reflects absolute or percentage changes in fatness before and after a physical conditioning or dietary regimen.
2. Apply mathematical equations to predict body density or percentage body fat from the individual skinfold values or the Σ skf. These equations apply to specific populations because they predict fatness fairly accurately for subjects similar in age, gender, training state, fatness, and race to those used to derive the equations.

Questions & Notes

How long after taking a skinfold should you wait before you read the caliper dial?

List the 5 most common skinfold sites.

1.

2.

3.

4.

5.

List 2 practical ways skinfold data can be used.

1.

2.

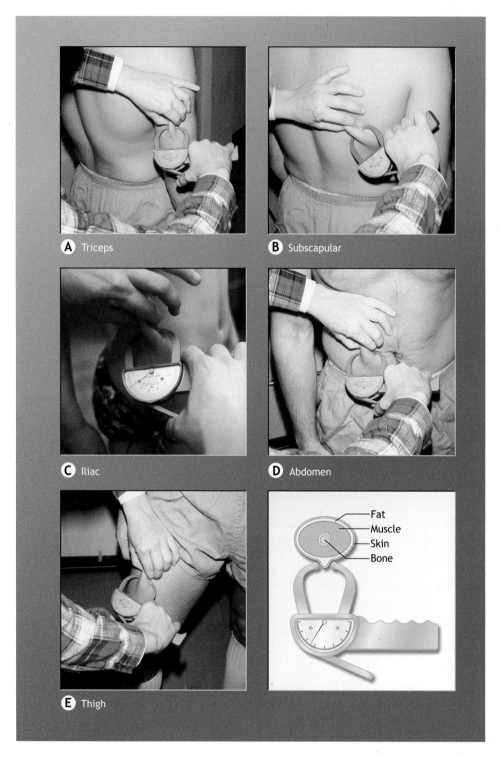

Figure 16.9 Anatomic location of five common skinfold sites: triceps (**A**), subscapular (**B**), suprailiac (**C**), abdomen (**D**), and thigh (**E**).

In young adults, approximately half of the body's total fat consists of subcutaneous fat, with the remainder visceral and organ fat. With advancing age, a proportionately greater quantity of fat deposits internally compared with subcutaneous fat. Thus, the same skinfold score reflects a *greater* percentage body fat as a person grows older. *For this reason, age-adjusted, **generalized equations** should be used to predict body fat from skinfolds that apply to a broad age range of adult men and women* (see Close Up, Box 16.3, *Choosing Appropriate Skinfold Equations to Predict Body Fat in Diverse Populations*, on page 549). We recommend Σ skf

and specific equations as the best alternative to more accurately estimate the body's amount and distribution of fat.

A person can become a skilled skinfold technician by adhering to the following nine guidelines:

1. Be precise in locating and marking anatomical landmarks for each site *before* measurement.
2. Read the caliper dial to the nearest half marking (e.g., 0.5 mm) within 1 to 2 seconds of application of the caliper to the skin.
3. Take a minimum of two measurements at each site and use the average as the skinfold score.

BOX 16.3 CLOSE UP

Choosing Appropriate Skinfold Equations to Predict Body Fat of Diverse Populations

More than 100 different equations exist to predict body density and percentage body fat from skinfolds. The equations, often formulated from homogeneous groups, incorporate between two and seven measurement sites to predict body density, which then converts to percentage body fat using an appropriate equation for the specific population. The different equations yield predicted values that (at best) usually fall within ±3% to 5% body fat units assessed by hydrostatic weighing.

DIFFERENT EQUATIONS

The table presents examples of skinfold equations for different populations. The following abbreviations apply (all skinfolds in mm): Σ Skf = skinfolds; tri = tricep; calf = calf; scap = subscapular; midax = midaxillary; iliac = suprailiac; abdo = abdomen; thigh = thigh; Db = whole body density, g·cm^{-3}; BF = body fat; age in years (y).

Equations to Predict Percentage Body Fat From Skinfolds

POPULATION	AGE, y	VARIABLES	EQUATION	COMMENTS
Children				
Boys	6–10	tri + calf	%BF = 0.735 (Σ2Skf) + 1.0	
		tri + scap	%BF = 0.783 (Σ2Skf) + 1.6	Use when ΣSkf > 35 mm
Girls	6–10	tri + calf	%BF = 0.610 (Σ2Skf) + 5.1	
		tri + scap	%BF = 0.546 (Σ2Skf) + 9.7	Use when ΣSkf > 35 mm
Native Americans				
Women	18–60	tri + midax + iliac	Db = 1.061 − 0.000385 (Σ3Skf) − 0.000204 (age)	%BF = [(4.81 ÷ Db) − 4.34]100
African Americans				
Women	18–55	chest + abdo + thigh + tri + scap + iliac + midax	Db = 1.0970 − 0.00046971 (Σ7Skf) + 0.00000056 (Σ7Skf)^2 − 0.00012828 (age)	%BF = [(4.85 ÷ Db) − 4.39]100
Men	8–61	chest + abdo + thigh + tri + scap + iliac + midax	Db = 1.1120 − 0.00043499 (Σ7Skf) + 0.00000055 (Σ7Skf)^2 − 0.00028826 (age)	%BF = [(4.37 ÷ Db) − 3.93]100
Hispanics				
Women	20–40	chest + abdo + thigh + tri + scap + iliac + midax	Db = 1.10970 − 0.00046971 (Σ7Skf) + 0.00000056 (Σ7Skf)^2 − 0.00012828 (age)	%BF = [(4.87 ÷ Db) − 4.41]100
Native Japanese				
Women	18–23	tri + scap	Db = 1.0897 − 0.00133 (Σ2Skf)	%BF = [(4.76 ÷ Db) − 4.28]100
Men	18–27	tri + scap	Db = 1.0913 − 0.00116 (Σ2Skf)	%BF = [(4.97 ÷ Db) − 4.52]100
White Americans				
Women	18–55	tri + iliac + thigh	Db = 1.0994921 − 0.0009929 (Σ3Skf) + 0.00000023 (Σ3Skf)^2 − 0.0001392 (age)	%BF = [(5.01 ÷ Db) − 4.57]100
Men	18–55	chest + abdo + thigh	Db = 1.109380 − 0.0008267 (Σ3Skf) + 0.00000016 (Σ3Skf)^2 − 0.0002574 (age)	%BF = [(4.95 ÷ Db) − 4.50]100
Athletes (all sports)				
Men	18–29	tri + iliac + abdo + thigh	Db = 1.112 − 0.00043499 (Σ7Skf) + 0.00000055 (Σ7Skf)^2 − 0.00028826 (age)	%BF = [(5.01 ÷ Db) − 4.57]100
Women	18–29	chest + midax + tri + scap + abdo + iliac + thigh	Db = 1.096095 − 0.0006952 (Σ4Skf) + 0.0000011 (Σ4Skf)^2 − 0.0000714 (age)	%BF = [(4.95 ÷ Db) − 4.50]100

4. Take duplicate or triplicate measurements in rotational order rather than consecutive readings at each site to avoid a compression skin plus subcutaneous fat effect.

5. Do not take measurements immediately after the individual stops exercise; the shift in body fluid to the skin spuriously increases the reading.

6. Practice on at least 50 subjects, making multiple measurements at the different skinfold sites, to gain experience.

7. Obtain training from previously skilled technicians in how to take skinfolds; this allows you to compare your results with the results of an "expert."

8. Take measurements on dry, lotion-free skin.

9. If possible, enroll in a course that deals with body composition assessment; some continuing education providers offer courses that award certifications of completion in body composition assessment procedures (*www.sportsnutritionsociety.org/certificates.aspx*).

Girth Measurements

Figure 16.10 shows the six most common sites for girth measurements. Girths offer an easily administered and valid alternative to skinfolds. Apply a linen or plastic measuring tape lightly to the skin surface so the tape remains taut but not tight. This avoids skin compression. Take duplicate measurements at each site and average the scores.

Usefulness of Girth Measurements The equations and constants presented in Appendix C for young and older men and women predict an individual's percentage body fat within ±2.5% to ±4.0% body fat units of the actual value. This applies when the individual's physical characteristics resemble those of the original validation group. Relatively small prediction errors make population-specific girth equations useful to those without access to laboratory facilities. These equations should **not** predict fatness in individuals who appear excessively thin or fat or who participate regularly in strenuous sports or resistance training that can increase girth without altering subcutaneous fat. Girths also can analyze patterns of body fat distribution (**fat patterning**), including changes in fat distribution during weight loss and gain.

Predicting Body Fat from Girths From the appropriate tables in Appendix C, substitute the corresponding constants A, B, and C in the formula shown at

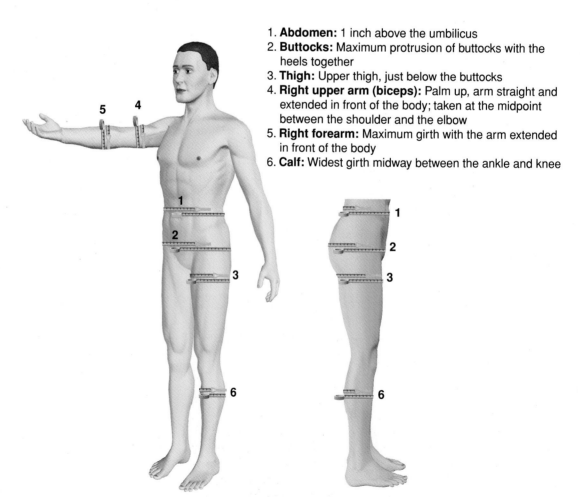

1. **Abdomen:** 1 inch above the umbilicus
2. **Buttocks:** Maximum protrusion of buttocks with the heels together
3. **Thigh:** Upper thigh, just below the buttocks
4. **Right upper arm (biceps):** Palm up, arm straight and extended in front of the body; taken at the midpoint between the shoulder and the elbow
5. **Right forearm:** Maximum girth with the arm extended in front of the body
6. **Calf:** Widest girth midway between the ankle and knee

Figure 16.10 Landmarks for measuring various girths at six common anatomic sites (see text for description).

the bottom of each table. This requires one addition and two subtraction steps. The following five-step example shows how to compute percentage fat, fat mass, and FFM for a 21-year-old man who weighs 79.1 kg:

Step 1. Measure the upper arm, abdomen, and right forearm girths with a cloth tape to the nearest 0.25 in (0.6 cm): Upper arm = 11.5 in (29.21 cm); abdomen = 31.0 in (78.74 cm); right forearm = 10.75 in (27.30 cm).

Step 2. Determine the three constants A, B, and C corresponding to the three girths from Appendix C: Constant A corresponding to 11.5 in = 42.56; constant B corresponding to 31.0 in = 40.68; and constant C corresponding to 10.75 in = 58.37.

Step 3. Compute percentage body fat by substituting the appropriate constants in the formula for young men shown at the bottom of Chart 1 in Appendix C as:

$$\textbf{Percentage Fat} = \textbf{Constant A} + \textbf{Constant B} - \textbf{Constant C} - 10.2$$
$$= 42.56 + 40.68 - 58.37 - 10.2$$
$$= 83.24 - 58.37 - 10.2$$
$$= 24.87 - 10.2$$
$$= 14.7\%$$

Step 4. Calculate the mass of body fat as:

$$\textbf{Fat mass} = \textbf{Body mass} \times (\% \textbf{ Fat} \div 100)$$
$$= 79.1 \text{ kg} \times (14.7 \div 100)$$
$$= 79.1 \text{ kg} \times 0.147$$
$$= 11.6 \text{ kg}$$

Step 5. Determine FFM as:

$$\textbf{FFM} = \textbf{Body mass} - \textbf{Fat mass}$$
$$= 79.1 \text{ kg} - 11.63 \text{ kg}$$
$$= 67.5 \text{ kg}$$

Bioelectrical Impedance Analysis (BIA)

A small, alternating current flowing between two electrodes passes more rapidly through hydrated fat-free body tissues and extracellular water compared with fat or bone tissue because of the greater electrolyte content or lower electrical resistance of the fat-free component. Consequently, impedance to electric current flow relates to the quantity of total body water, which in turn relates to FFM, body density, and percentage body fat.

Bioelectrical impedance analysis requires measurement by trained personnel under strictly standardized conditions, particularly electrode placement and the subject's body position, hydration status, previous food and beverage intake, skin temperature, and recent physical activity. As **Figure 16.11** illustrates, the person lies on a flat, nonconducting surface. Injector (source) electrodes attach on the dorsal surfaces of the foot and wrist, and detector (sink) electrodes attach between the radius and ulna (styloid process) and at the ankle between the medial and lateral malleoli. The *lower illustration* depicts the flow of current and voltage for the right arm, trunk, and right leg.

The person receives a painless, localized electrical current, with impedance (resistance) to current flow between the source and detector electrodes determined. Conversion of the impedance value to body density—adding body mass and stature, gender, age, and sometimes race, level of fatness, and several girths to the equation—computes percentage body fat from the Siri equation or other similar density conversion equation.

Questions & Notes

List 3 most important guidelines that one should follow to become a skilled skinfold technician.

1.

2.

3.

Predict percentage body fat for a 10-year-old female with a tricep skinfold of 20 mm and a subscapular skinfold of 18 mm.

Calculate percentage body fat for an athletic female with a body density of 1.04225 g·mL^{-1}.

List the 6 most common girth measurement sites.

1.

2.

3.

4.

5.

6.

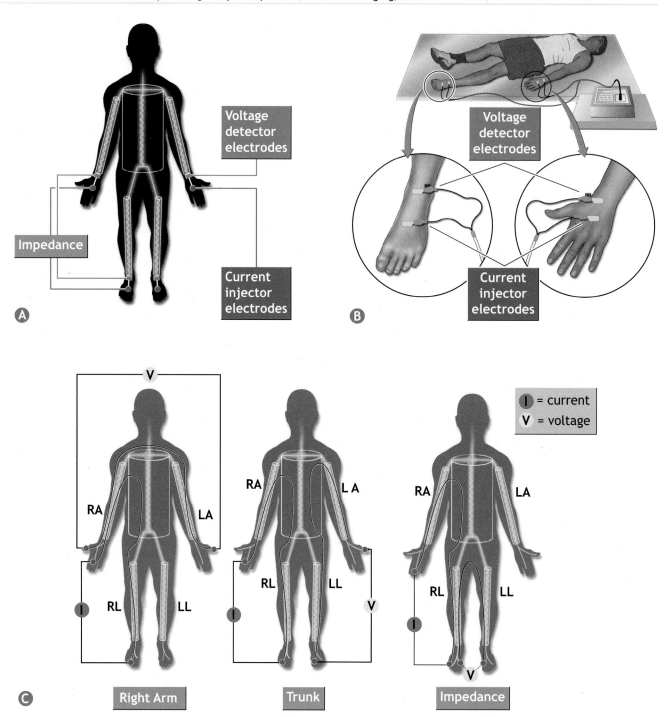

Figure 16.11 Method to assess body composition by bioelectrical impedance analysis. (**A**) Whereas the four-surface electrode technique (whole-body impedance) applies current via one pair of distal (injector) electrodes, the proximal (detector) electrode pair measures electrical potential across the conducting segment. (**B**) Standard placement of electrodes and body position during whole-body impedance measurement. (**C**) Segmental measurement illustrating assessment of current (I) and voltage (V) for the right arm, trunk, and right leg.

Hydration Level Affects BIA Accuracy Either hypohydration or hyperhydration alters the body's normal electrolyte concentrations; this modifies current flow independent of a real change in body composition. For example, impedance decreases from body water loss through sweating in prior exercise or voluntary fluid restriction. This produces a *lower* percentage body fat estimate; hyper-hydration produces the opposite effect (*higher* fat estimate).

Skin temperature (influenced by ambient conditions) also affects whole-body resistance and subsequently the BIA prediction of body fat. A lower predicted body fat occurs in a warm environment (less impedance to electrical flow) compared with a cold environment.

Even under normal hydration and environmental temperature, body fat predictions may be questionable compared with hydrostatic weighing. BIA tends to overpredict body fat in lean and athletic subjects and underpredict fat in obese subjects. Also, conflicting evidence exists whether BIA can detect small changes in body composition during weight loss or other experimental conditions.

Dual-Energy X-Ray Absorptiometry

Dual-energy x-ray absorptiometry (DXA), a high-technology procedure shown in **Figure 16.12** to assess bone mineral density in osteoporosis screening can also quantifies fat and muscle around bony areas of the body, including regions

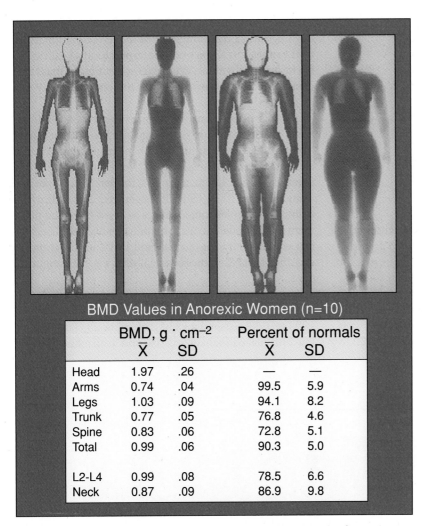

BMD Values in Anorexic Women (n=10)

| | BMD, g · cm⁻² | | Percent of normals | |
	$\overline{X}$	SD	$\overline{X}$	SD
Head	1.97	.26	—	—
Arms	0.74	.04	99.5	5.9
Legs	1.03	.09	94.1	8.2
Trunk	0.77	.05	76.8	4.6
Spine	0.83	.06	72.8	5.1
Total	0.99	.06	90.3	5.0
L2-L4	0.99	.08	78.5	6.6
Neck	0.87	.09	86.9	9.8

Figure 16.12 Dual-energy X-ray absorptiometry (DXA). Example of an anorexic woman (*two left images*) and a typical woman (*two right images*) whose body fat percentage averages 25% of her total body mass of 56.7 kg (125 lb). The average anorexic subject weighed 44.4 kg (97.9 lb) with DXA-estimated 7.5% body fat from the fat percentages at the arms, legs, and trunk regions. The values in the *right column* of the *inset table* present the average percentage values for bone mineral density (BMD) for different regional body areas in the anorexic group compared with a group of 287 normal-weight women ages 20 to 40 years. (Photo courtesy of R.B. Mazess, Department of Medical Physics, University of Wisconsin, Madison, WI, and the Lunar Radiation Corporation, Madison, WI. Data from Mazess, R.B., et al.: *Skeletal and Body Composition Effects of Anorexia Nervosa.* Paper presented at the International Symposium on In Vivo Body Composition Studies, June 20–23, 1989, Toronto, Ontario, Canada.)

Questions & Notes

List 2 factors that affect BIA results.

1.

2.

How many electrodes are used in the BIA method?

What is the most common use for DXA analysis?

without bone present. When used for body composition assessment, DXA does not require assumptions about the biologic constancy of the fat and fat-free components as does hydrostatic weighing.

Two distinct x-ray energies with short exposure with low-radiation dosage penetrate into bone and soft tissue areas to a depth of about 30 cm. Specialized computer software reconstructs an image of the underlying tissues. The computer-generated report quantifies bone mineral content, total fat mass, and FFM. DXA also can target selected body regions for more in-depth analysis.

Body Mass Index

Clinicians and researchers frequently use the **body mass index (BMI)**, derived from body mass related to stature, to assess the "normalcy" of one's body mass.

$$BMI = Body\ mass,\ kg \div Stature,\ m^2$$

Example:
Man: Stature = 175.3 cm, 1.753 m (69 in); body mass = 97.1 kg (214.1 lb)

$$BMI = 97.1\ kg \div (1.753\ m \times 1.753\ m)$$
$$= 97.1 \div 3.073$$
$$= 31.6$$

The importance of this easy-to-obtain index relies on its curvilinear relationship shown in **Figure 16.13** to all-cause mortality; as BMI becomes larger, risk increases for cardiovascular complications including hypertension, diabetes, certain cancers, and renal disease. The level of disease risk along the bottom of the figure represents the degree of risk with each 5-unit change in BMI. The lowest health risk category occurs for BMIs in the range of 20 to

25, with the highest risk for BMIs that exceed 40. For women, 21.3 to 22.1 represents the desirable BMI range; the corresponding range for men equals 21.9 to 22.4. An increased disease incidence occurs when BMI exceeds 27.8 for men and 27.3 for women.

Classifications established by experts convened by the National Heart, Lung and Blood Institute (NHLBI) defined "**overweight**" as a BMI of 25 to 29.9, and "**obesity**" as a BMI of 30 or above (see Part 3 of this chapter).

Limitations of Body Mass Index for Athletes

As with height and weight tables, BMI does not consider the body's fat and nonfat components. Specifically, factors other than excess body fat (i.e., bone and muscle mass and even the increased plasma volume induced by exercise training) affect the numerator of the BMI equation. A high BMI can lead to an incorrect interpretation of excess body fat in lean individuals with excessive muscle mass when genetic makeup or exercise training could actually cause an elevated BMI.

Misclassifying someone as overweight using BMI standards applies particularly to large-size, field-event athletes, body builders, weight lifters, upper–weight class wrestlers, and professional football players. For example, the BMI for seven defensive linemen from a former NFL Super Bowl team averaged 31.9 (team BMI averaged 28.7), clearly signaling these professional athletes as overweight and placing them in the moderate category for mortality risk. Their body fat content, 18.0% for lineman and 12.1% for the team, misclassified them for fatness using BMI as the overweight standard.

In contrast to the professional football players, the average player in the National Basketball Association for the 1993 to 1994 season had a BMI of below 25. This relatively low BMI placed them at low risk and keeps them out of the

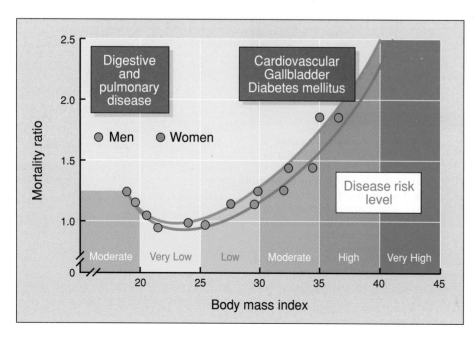

Figure 16.13 Curvilinear relationship based on American Cancer Society data between all-cause mortality and BMI. At extremely low BMIs, the risk for digestive and pulmonary diseases increases; cardiovascular, gallbladder, and type 2 diabetes risk increases with higher BMIs. (Modified from Bray, G.A.: Pathophysiology of obesity. *Am. J. Clin. Nutr.*, 55(Suppl): 488S, 1992).

overweight category, although they would be classified as overweight by height–weight standards.

OTHER INDIRECT PROCEDURES TO ESTIMATE BODY COMPOSITION

Near-Infrared Interactance

Near-infrared interactance (NIR) applies technology developed by the U.S. Department of Agriculture to assess the body composition of livestock and the lipid content of various grains. The commercial versions to assess body composition in humans use a safe, portable, lightweight monitor; require minimal training; and necessitate little physical contact with the subject during measurement. These test administration aspects make NIR popular for body composition assessment in health clubs, hospitals, and weight loss centers. Unfortunately, research with humans has not confirmed NIR's validity compared with hydrostatic weighing and skinfold measurements. NIR does not accurately predict body fat across a broad range of body fat levels, and NIR provides less accuracy than skinfolds. NIR overestimates body fat in lean men and women and underestimates it in fatter subjects.

Ultrasonography

Ultrasound technology can (1) assess the thickness of different tissues (fat and muscle) and (2) obtain an image of muscle's cross-sectional area. The method converts electrical energy through a probe into high-frequency, pulsed sound waves that penetrate the skin surface into the underlying tissues. The sound waves pass through adipose tissue and penetrate the muscle layer. They then reflect from the fat–muscle interface after reflection from a bony surface to produce an echo, which returns to a receiver within the probe. The time required for sound wave transmission through the tissues and back to the transducer converts to a distance score to indicate fat or muscle thickness. Ultrasonography exhibits high reliability for repeat measurements of subcutaneous fat thickness at multiple sites in the lying and standing positions on the same day and different days. The technique has application for determining total and segmental subcutaneous adipose tissue (SCAT) volume. Ultrasonography to map muscle and fat thickness at different body regions quantifies changes in the topographic fat pattern and serves as a valuable adjunct to whole-body composition assessment. In hospitalized patients, ultrasonic fat and muscle thickness determinations aid in nutritional assessment during weight loss and gain.

Computed Tomography and Magnetic Resonance Imaging

Computed Tomography Computed tomography (CT) generates detailed cross-sectional, two-dimensional radiographic images of different body segments when an x-ray beam consisting of ionizing radiation passes through tissues of different densities. The CT scan produces pictorial and quantitative information about total tissue area, total fat and muscle area, and thickness and volume of tissues within an organ.

   Figure 16.14 A and B shows CT scans of the upper legs and a cross-section at the midthigh of a professional walker who walked 11,200 miles through the 50 United States in 50 weeks. Total cross-section and muscle cross section increased, and subcutaneous fat decreased correspondingly in the midthigh region in the "after" scans (not shown). CT scans have established the relationship between simple skinfolds and girths at the abdomen and total adipose tissue

Questions & Notes

Compute your BMI.

HT =

BW =

BMI =

Calculate the BMI for a male who weighs 75 kg, and is 176.5 cm tall.

Classify the body weight of a person with a BMI of 32.

At what BMI does mortality risk due to cardiovascular disease begin to rise?

In terms of body composition analysis, what does ultrasound measure?

In terms of body composition analysis, what do CT scans measure?

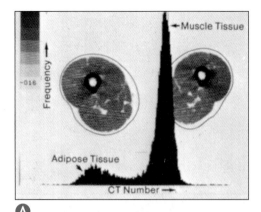

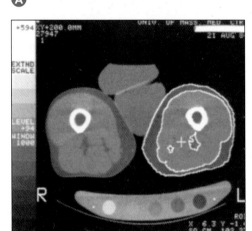

Figure 16.14 CT scans. (**A**) Plot of pixel elements illustrating the extent of adipose and muscle tissue in a cross-section of the thigh. (**B**) A cross-section of the midthigh. (Computed tomography scans courtesy of Dr. Steven Heymsfeld, Obesity Research Center, St. Luke's-Roosevelt Hospital, Columbia University, College of Physicians and Surgeons, New York.)

volume measured from single or multiple pictorial "slices" through this region. The single cut through the L4–L5 region minimizes the radiation dose and provides the best view of visceral and subcutaneous fat.

Magnetic Resonance Imaging Magnetic resonance imaging (**MRI**) offers a valuable, noninvasive assessment of the body's tissue compartments. **Figure 16.15** shows a color-enhanced MRI transaxial image of the midthigh of a 30-year-old male middle-distance runner. Computer software subtracts fat and bony tissues (*lighter-colored areas*) to compute the thigh muscle cross-sectional area (*red area*). With MRI, electromagnetic radiation (not ionizing radiation as in CT scans) in a strong magnetic field excites the hydrogen nuclei of the body's water and lipid molecules. The nuclei then emit a detectable signal that rearranges under computer control to visually represent the various body tissues. MRI effectively quantifies total and SCAT in individuals with varying degrees of body fatness.

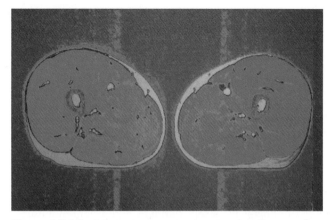

Figure 16.15 Magnetic resonance imaging (MRI) scans of the midthigh of a 30-year-old male middle-distance runner. (MRI scans courtesy of J. Staab, Department of the Army, USARIEM, Natick, MA.)

AVERAGE VALUES FOR BODY COMPOSITION

Table 16.4 presents average values for percentage body fat in men and women from different areas of the United States. The column headed "68% Variation Limits" indicates the range for percentage body fat that includes ±1 standard deviation, or about 68 of every 100 persons measured. As an example, the average percentage body fat of 15.0% for young men from the New York sample includes the ±68% variation limits from 8.9% to 21.1% body fat. Interpreting this statistically, for 68 of every 100 young men measured, percentage fat ranges between 8.9% and 21.1%. Of the remaining 32 young men, 16 possess more than 21.1% body fat, and the 16 other men have a body fat percentage of less than 8.9%. *Percentage body fat for young adult men averages between 12% and 15%; the average fat value for women ranges between 25% and 28%.*

DETERMINING GOAL BODY WEIGHT

No one really knows the optimum body fat or body weight for a particular individual. Inherited genetic factors greatly influence body fat distribution and play an important role in programming body size and its link to disease risk with aging. Values for percentage body fat for young adults average approximately 15% for men and 25% for women. Women and men who exercise regularly or train for athletic competition typically have lower body fat levels than age-matched sedentary counterparts. In contact sports and activities requiring muscular power, successful performance usually requires a large body mass with average to low body fat. In contrast, elite performance in weight-bearing endurance activities requires a lighter body mass and a minimal level of body fat.

Proper assessment of body composition, not body weight, should determine an individual's ideal body weight.

Table 16.4	Average Percentage Body Fat for Younger and Older Women and Men From Selected Studies				
STUDY	AGE RANGE, y	STATURE, cm	BODY MASS, kg	%FAT	68% VARIATION LIMITS
Younger Women					
North Carolina, 1962	17–25	165.0	55.5	22.9	17.5–28.5
New York, 1962	16–30	167.5	59.0	28.7	24.6–32.9
California, 1968	19–23	165.9	58.4	21.9	17.0–26.9
California, 1970	17–29	164.9	58.6	25.5	21.0–30.1
Air Force, 1972	17–22	164.1	55.8	28.7	22.3–35.3
New York, 1973	17–26	160.4	59.0	26.2	23.4–33.3
North Carolina, 1975		166.1	57.5	24.6	—
Army recruits, 1986	17–25	162.0	58.6	28.4	23.9–32.9
Massachusetts, 1994	17–30	165.3	57.7	21.8	16.7–27.8
Older Women					
Minnesota, 1953	31–45	163.3	60.7	28.9	25.1–32.8
	43–68	160.0	60.9	34.2	28.0–40.5
New York, 1963	30–40	164.9	59.6	28.6	22.1–35.3
	40–50	163.1	56.4	34.4	29.5–39.5
North Carolina, 1975	33–50	—	—	29.7	23.1–36.5
Massachusetts, 1993	31–50	165.2	58.9	25.2	19.2–31.2
Younger Men					
Minnesota, 1951	17–26	177.8	69.1	11.8	5.9–11.8
Colorado, 1956	17–25	172.4	68.3	13.5	8.2–18.8
Indiana, 1966	18–23	180.1	75.5	12.6	8.7–16.5
California, 1968	16–31	175.7	74.1	15.2	6.3–24.2
New York, 1973	17–26	176.4	71.4	15.0	8.9–21.1
Texas, 1977	18–24	179.9	74.6	13.4	7.4–19.4
Army recruits, 1986	17–25	174.7	70.5	15.6	10.0–21.2
Massachusetts, 1994	17–30	178.2	76.3	12.9	7.8–18.9
Older Men					
Indiana, 1966	24–38	179.0	76.6	17.8	11.3–24.3
	40–48	177.0	80.5	22.3	16.3–28.3
North Carolina, 1976	27–50	—	—	23.7	17.9–30.1
Texas, 1977	27–59	180.0	85.3	27.1	23.7–30.5
Massachusetts, 1993	31–50	177.1	77.5	19.9	13.2–26.5

Compute a "goal" body weight target that uses a desired (and prudent) percentage of body fat as follows:

$$\text{Goal body weight} = \text{FFM} \div (1.00 - \% \text{ fat desired})$$

Suppose a 23-year-old, 120-kg (265 lb) large man currently with 24% body fat wants to know how much fat weight to lose to attain a body fat composition of 15% (average value for young men). The following computations provide this information:

$$\begin{aligned}
\text{Fat mass} &= \text{Body mass, kg} \times \text{Decimal \% body fat} \\
&= 120 \text{ kg} \times 0.24 \\
&= 28.8 \text{ kg}
\end{aligned}$$

$$\begin{aligned}
\text{FFM} &= \text{Body mass, kg} - \text{Fat mass, kg} \\
&= 120 \text{ kg} - 28.8 \text{ kg} \\
&= 91.2 \text{ kg}
\end{aligned}$$

$$\begin{aligned}
\text{Goal body weight} &= \text{FFM, kg} \div (1.00 - \text{Decimal \% fat desired}) \\
&= 91.2 \text{ kg} \div (1.00 - 0.15) \\
&= 91.2 \text{ kg} \div 0.85 \\
&= 107.3 \text{ kg} (236.6 \text{ lb})
\end{aligned}$$

🛈 For Your Information

A DESIRABLE RANGE FOR GOAL BODY WEIGHT

For practical purposes, recommend a "desirable body weight range" rather than a single goal weight. This range should range within ±2 pounds of the computed "goal body weight." For example, if goal body weight equals 135 pounds, the person should strive for a weight between 133 and 137 pounds.

Desirable fat loss = Present body weight, kg
− Goal body weight, kg
= 120 kg − 107.3 k
= 12.7 kg (28.0 lb)

If this person lost 12.7 kg of body fat, his new body mass of 91.2 kg would have a fat content equal to 15% of body mass. These calculations assume no change in FFM during weight loss. Moderate caloric restriction plus increased daily energy expenditure reduces body fat (and conserves lean tissue). Part 4 of this chapter discusses prudent yet effective approaches to reducing body fat.

SUMMARY

1. Two approaches directly assess body composition. In one technique, a chemical solution literally dissolves the body into its fat and nonfat (fat-free) components. The other approach involves physical dissection of fat, fat-free adipose tissue, muscle, and bone.

2. Hydrostatic weighing determines body volume with subsequent calculation of body density and percentage body fat. The computation assumes a constant density for the body's components of fat and fat-free tissues. Subtracting fat mass from body mass yields FFM.

3. Part of the error inherent in predicting body fat from whole-body density lies in assumptions concerning the densities of the body's fat and fat-free components. These densities, principally FFM, differ from assumed constants because of race, age, and athletic experience.

4. Air displacement (BOD POD) offers an alternative means to quantify body composition because of ease of administration, high reproducibility of body volume scores, and generally high validity compared with hydrostatic weighing.

5. Common field methods to assess body composition use population-specific prediction equations from relationships among selected skinfolds and girths and body density and percentage body fat. These equations predict most accurately with subjects similar to those who participated in the equations' original derivation.

6. BMI relates more closely to body fat and health risk than simply body mass and stature; as with height–weight tables, BMI does not consider the body's proportional composition.

7. The concept of BIA states that hydrated, fat-free body tissues and extracellular water facilitate electrical flow better compared with fat tissue because of the greater electrolyte content of the fat-free component. Impedance to electric current flow relates directly to the body's fat content.

8. NIR should be used with caution when assessing body composition; this methodology currently lacks verification of adequate validity.

9. Ultrasonography, CT, MRI, and DXA indirectly assess body composition. Each has a unique application and inherent limitations for expanding knowledge of the compositional components of the live human body.

10. The average healthy young man possesses 15% body fat, and the average woman possesses 25% body fat. These values can serve as a common yardstick to evaluate deviations from "average" for the body fat of individual athletes and specific athletic groups.

11. Goal body weight computes as FFM ÷ 1.00 − Desired %fat.

12. Top male and female endurance runners represent the lower end of the fat-to-lean continuum.

THOUGHT QUESTIONS

1. How would you use anthropometric data to estimate optimal body composition?

2. Discuss whether the established differences in body composition between men and women justify gender-specific normative standards to evaluate diverse components of physical fitness and motor performance.

3. A friend complains that three fitness centers determined her percentage body fat from skinfolds as 19%, 25%, and 31%. How can you reconcile these discrepancies?

Part 3	Overfatness and Obesity

Questions & Notes

Calculate the desired body weight for a 24-year-old female who weighs 75 kg with a body fat percentage of 32.

Calculate the desirable fat loss in pounds for a 22-year-old female who weighs 70.5 kg with 29% body fat.

To gain insights into the magnitude of the obesity epidemic, a random-digit telephone survey of nearly 110,000 adults in the United States found that nearly 70% struggle to lose weight or just maintain their current body weight. Fifty-eight percent of Americans would like to lose weight and 36% are following a particular diet plan, yet less than 19% of those following such plans closely track their intake of fats, carbohydrates, proteins, and calories. Only 20% of the 50 to 65 million Americans trying to lose weight use the recommended combination of eating fewer calories and engaging in at least 150 minutes of weekly leisure-time physical activity. Those attempting to lose weight spend nearly $60 billion annually on weight-reduction products and services, often using potentially harmful dietary practices and drugs while ignoring sensible weight loss programs. Approximately 2 million Americans pay more than $140 million on appetite-suppressing, over-the-counter diet pills that line drugstore, health food, fitness center, and supermarket shelves, not to mention TV and radio direct marketing and mail order and Internet sales. Despite the upswing in attempts to lose weight, Americans are considerably more overweight than a generation ago, and the trend is for further increases in all regions of the United States.

The latest 2008 data from the Centers for Disease Control and Prevention (CDC) Behavioral Risk Factor Surveillance Survey (*www.cdc.gov/nccdphp/dnpa/obesity/trend/maps/*) provide state-by-state prevalence rates for obesity in the United States (**Fig. 16.16**). The data were collected through the CDC's Behavioral Risk Factor Surveillance System (BRFSS). Each year, state health departments use standard procedures to collect data through a series of monthly telephone interviews with U.S. adults. Mississippi has the highest prevalence of obesity (32.8%) than any other state followed by Alabama at 31.4%, West Virginia at 31.2%, and Tennessee at 30.6%. The rate of obese adults in Mississippi increased for the third year in a row. Adult obesity rates increased in 23 states and did not decrease in a single state during 2008. Eight of the 10 states with the highest percentage of obese adults are in the South. Only one state, Colorado, was lower than 20%, but that percentage will soon exceed 20% if yearly trends continue. The states with the highest adult obesity rates also have the highest prevalence of type 2 diabetes in adults.

A 2009 report, "How Obesity Policies Are Failing in America" from the Trust for Americans Health (*healthyamericans.org/reports/obesity2009/*), provides further alarming data and trends about current strategies (including school nutrition and physical activity policies) regarding the obesity epidemic. By the year 2018, 108 million American adults will classify as obese, and weight gain could drive up health care costs by $344 billion. The *right side* of **Figure 16.16** adds the prevalence of childhood obesity to the accumulating data on adults with Mississippi ranking first in the rate of overweight children (ages 10–17 y) at 44.4% with the percentage of obese and overweight children at or above 30% in 30 states! The crisis is not just confined to children but also minorities. The 2008 data show that blacks have the highest rates of obesity at a 51% higher prevalence than whites, and Hispanics have a 21% higher obesity prevalence.

DEFINITIONS: OVERWEIGHT, OVERFATNESS, AND OBESITY

Confusion surrounds the precise meaning of the terms *overweight*, *overfat*, and *obesity* as applied to body composition. Each term often takes on a different

For Your Information

THE SUPERSIZING OF AMERICA

Substantial changes in genetic makeup cannot account for the rapid increase in obesity among Americans over the past 20 years. More than 60% of the United States population is now overweight, and 25% classify as obese. More than likely, the culprits in the fattening of America are a sedentary lifestyle and the ready availability of tasty, lipid- and calorie-rich foods that are currently served in increasingly larger portions.

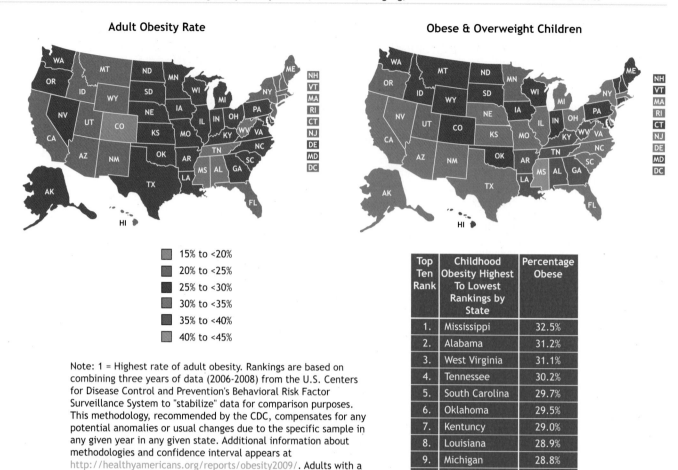

Figure 16.16 Prevalence of adult and childhood obesity in the United States, 2006 to 2008. Top 10 ranking by percentage is for adults (*left*) and children (*right*). (Adapted from Trust for America's Health, F as in Fat 2009: *How Obesity Policies Are Failing America.* Available at *http://healthyamericans.org/reports/obesity2009/.*)

meaning depending on the situation and context of use. The medical literature indicates that the term *overweight* refers to an overfat condition relative to other individuals of the same age or height despite the absence of accompanying body fat measures. Within this context, *obesity* refers to individuals at the extreme of the overfat continuum. This frame of reference delineates the body fat range by BMI (see page 554).

Research and contemporary discussion among diverse disciplines reinforces the need to distinguish between overweight, overfat, and obesity to ensure consistency in use and interpretation. In proper context, the overweight condition refers to a body weight that exceeds some average for stature, and perhaps age, usually by some standard deviation unit or percentage. The overweight condition frequently accompanies an increase in body fat, but not always (e.g., male power athletes), and it may or may not coincide with the comorbidities glucose intolerance, insulin resistance, dyslipidemia, and hypertension.

When body fat measures are available, it becomes possible to accurately place an individual's body fat level on a continuum from low to high, independent of body weight. *Overfatness* then would refer to a condition in which body fat exceeds an age- or gender-appropriate average by a predeter-

mined amount. In most situations, *overfatness* represents the correct term to assess individual and group body fat levels.

The term *obesity* refers to the overfat condition that accompanies a constellation of comorbidities that include one or all of the following components of the **obese syndrome:** glucose intolerance, insulin resistance, dyslipidemia, type 2 diabetes, hypertension, elevated plasma leptin concentrations, increased visceral adipose tissue, and increased risk of coronary heart disease and some cancers. Men and women may be overweight or overfat and yet do not exhibit components of the "obese syndrome." We urge caution in using the term *obesity* in all cases of excessive body weight. We acknowledge that the terms *overweight, overfat,* and *obese* are often used interchangeably to designate the same condition.

OBESITY: A GLOBAL EPIDEMIC

According to the World Health Organization (WHO; *www.who.int*), obesity represents a complex condition with serious social and psychological dimensions that impact all age and socioeconomic groups and threaten to overwhelm both developed and developing countries.

The WHO latest global data from 2005 indicated the following grim statistics:

1. Approximately 1.6 billion adults age 15+ years were overweight.
2. At least 400 million adults were obese.
3. By 2015, approximately 2.3 billion adults will be overweight, and more than 700 million will be obese.
4. At least 20 million children younger than 5 years of age were overweight.

The WHO posits that increased consumption of more energy-dense, nutrient-poor foods with high levels of sugar and saturated fats, combined with reduced physical activity, have led to obesity rates that have risen threefold or more since 1980 in some areas besides North America, including the United Kingdom, Eastern Europe, the Middle East, the Pacific Islands, Australia, and especially China (about one-fifth of the 1 billion overweight or obese people in the world are Chinese; *www.bmj.com/cgi/content/full/333/7564/362*). Taken in total, this makes every fourth person on the planet overfat! It is now estimated that there are more overfat than underweight individuals despite the hunger in many parts of the world.

Table 16.5 presents classification of overweight and obesity by BMI, waist circumference, and associated disease risk. This classification system of obesity by BMI was developed initially by the WHO Obesity Task Force and has been adopted by the U.S. NHLBI of the National Institutes of Health.

The prevalence of overweight and obesity in adults in the United States represents about 134 million Americans (66% of adults age 20 years or older, including 35% of college students). Currently, more than 4 million individuals exceed 300 pounds, and more than 500,000 people (mostly men) exceed 400 pounds—with the average woman now weighing an unprecedented 165 pounds!

Researchers maintain that if this worldwide trend continues, then 70% to 75% of the U.S. adult population may reach overweight or obesity status by the year 2020, with essentially the entire adult population becoming overweight within three generations!

CAUSES OF OBESITY

Obesity frequently begins in childhood. For these children, the chances of becoming obese adults increase threefold compared with children of normal body weight. Simply stated, a child usually does not grow out of obesity. Tracking body weight through generations indicates that obese parents likely give

Questions & Notes

Explain the differences between overweight, obesity, and overfatness.

 For Your Information

ONE IN FIVE AMERICAN CHILDREN ARE OBESE

New research appearing in the *Archives of Pediatrics & Adolescent Medicine* on a nationally representative sample of preschoolers born in 2001 indicates that nearly one in five (more than half a million) American 4-year-old children are obese with an alarmingly high one in three rate among American Indian children. Obesity is also more prevalent among Hispanic and black children but the disparity becomes most startling among American Indians whose obesity doubles that of whites. The alarming statistics are that 13% of Asian children, 16% of whites, 21% of blacks, 22% of Hispanics, and 31% of American Indians are obese.

| Table 16.5 | Classification of Overweight and Obesity by BMI, Waist Circumference, and Associated Disease Risk |

| | | | DISEASE RISK[a] (RELATIVE TO NORMAL WEIGHT AND WAIST CIRCUMFERENCE[b]) | |
CATEGORY	BMI (kg/m^2)	OBESITY CLASS	MEN: ≤40 in (102 cm) WOMEN: ≤35 in (88 cm)	MEN: >40 in (102 cm) WOMEN: >35 in (88 cm)
Underweight	<18.5			
Normal[c]	18.5–24.9			
Overweight	25.0–29.9		Increased	High
Obesity	30.0–34.9	I	High	Very high
	35.0–39.9	II	Very high	Very high
	≥40.0	III	Extremely high	Extremely high

[a]Disease risk for type 2 diabetes, hypertension, and coronary heart disease.
[b]Waist girth measured at the level of the top of the right iliac crest; the tape should be snug but not compressing the skin and held parallel to floor; make at normal respiration.
[c]Increased waist circumference can also be a marker for increased risk even in persons of normal weight.
From Aronne, L.J.: Classification of obesity and assessment of obesity-related health risks. *Obesity Res.*, 10:105, 2002.

BOX 16.4 CLOSE UP

Predicting Percentage Body Fat From Body Mass Index

Many clinicians now view a BMI in excess of 25 to represent overweight and a BMI in excess of 30 to represent the obese state. A lower healthy BMI limit of 18.5 has also been recognized. The basic assumption underlying BMI guidelines lies in its supposed close association with body fatness and consequent morbidity and mortality. This measure exhibits a somewhat higher yet still moderate association with body fat and disease risk than estimates based simply on stature and body mass. Several formulae predict percentage body fat (%BF) from BMI and provide a better indication of health risk than BMI alone.

INDEPENDENT VARIABLES

The following independent variables predict %BF:

1. BMI
2. Age in years
3. Gender: Male or female
4. Race: White, African American, Asian

Calculate Body Mass Index

Use the following formula to calculate BMI using metric or nonmetric data.

Metric Data

$$\text{BMI (kg·m}^{-2}) = \text{Body mass (kg)} \div \text{Stature (m)} \times \text{Stature (m)}$$

Nonmetric Data

$$\text{BMI (lb·in}^{-2}) = \text{Body weight (lb)} \times 703 \div \text{Height (in)} \times \text{Height (in)}$$

EQUATION TO PREDICT PERCENTAGE OF BODY FAT

$$\%BF = 63.7 - 864 \times (1 \div \text{BMI}) - 12.1 \times \text{Sex} + 0.12 \times \text{Age} + 129 \times \text{Asian} \times (1 \div \text{BMI}) - 0.091 \times \text{Asian} \times \text{Age} - 0.030 \times \text{African American} \times \text{Age}$$

where gender = 1 for male and 0 for female; Asian = 1 and 0 for other races; African American = 1 and 0 for other races; age in years; BMI = body weight in kg ÷ stature^2 in m^2.

EXAMPLES

Example 1: African American man; age, 30 y; BMI, 25

$$
\begin{aligned}
\%BF ={}& 63.7 - [864 \times (1 \div \text{BMI})] \\
& - (12.1 \times \text{sex}) + (0.12 \times \text{Age}) \\
& + [129 \times \text{Asian} \times (1 \div \text{BMI})] \\
& - (0.091 \times \text{Asian} \times \text{Age}) \\
& - (0.030 \times \text{African American} \times \text{Age}) \\
={}& 63.7 - (864 \times 0.04) - (12.1 \times 1) \\
& + (0.12 \times 30) + (129 \times 0 \times 0.04) \\
& - (0.091 \times 0 \times 30) \\
& - (0.030 \times 1 \times 30) \\
={}& 63.7 - (34.56) - (12.1) + (3.6) \\
& + (0) - (0) - (0.9) \\
={}& 19.7\%
\end{aligned}
$$

Example 2: Asian woman; age, 50 y; BMI, 30

$$
\begin{aligned}
\%BF ={}& 63.7 - [864 \times (1 \div \text{BMI})] \\
& - (12.1 \times \text{Sex}) + (0.12) \times \text{Age} \\
& + [129 \times \text{Asian} \times (1 \div \text{BMI})] \\
& - (0.091 \times \text{Asian} \times \text{Age}) \\
& - (0.030 \times \text{African American} \times \text{Age}) \\
={}& 63.7 - (864 \times 0.0333) - (12.1 \times 0) \\
& + (0.12 \times 50) + (129 \times 1 \times 0.0333) \\
& - (0.091 \times 1 \times 50) \\
& - (0.030 \times 0 \times 50) \\
={}& 63.7 - (28.80) - (0) + (6.0) \\
& + (4.295) - (4.55) - (0) \\
={}& 40.7\%
\end{aligned}
$$

Example 3: Asian man; age, 70 y; BMI, 28

$$
\begin{aligned}
\%BF ={}& 63.7 - [864 \times (1 \div \text{BMI})] \\
& - (12.1 \times \text{Sex}) + (0.12 \times \text{Age}) \\
& + [129 \times \text{Asian} \times (1 \div \text{BMI})] \\
& - (0.091 \times \text{Asian} \times \text{Age}) \\
& - (0.030 \times \text{African American} \times \text{Age}) \\
={}& 63.7 - (864 \times 0.03571) - (12.1 \times 1) \\
& + (0.12 \times 70) + (129 \times 1 \times 0.03571) \\
& - (0.091 \times 1 \times 70) \\
& - (0.030 \times 0 \times 70) \\
={}& 63.7 - (30.853) - (12.1) + (8.4) \\
& + (4.61) - (6.37) - (0) \\
={}& 25.4\%
\end{aligned}
$$

Example 4: White man; age, 55 y; BMI, 24.5

$$\%BF = 63.7 - [864 \times (1 \div BMI)]$$
$$- (12.1 \times sex) + (0.12 \times Age)$$
$$+ [129 \times Asian \times (1 \div BMI)]$$
$$- (0.091 \times Asian \times Age)$$
$$- (0.030 \times African\ American \times Age)$$
$$= 63.7 - (864 \times 0.0408) - (12.1 \times 1)$$
$$+ (0.12 \times 55) + (129 \times 0 \times 0.0408)$$
$$- (0.091 \times 0 \times 55)$$
$$- (0.030 \times 0 \times 55)$$
$$= 63.7 - (35.25) - (12.1) + (6.6)$$
$$+ (0) - (0) - (0)$$
$$= 22.9\%$$

ACCURACY

The correlation between predicted %BF using the above formulae and measured %BF using a four-compartment model to estimate body fat is r = 0.89 with a standard error for estimating an individual's %BF equal to ±3.9% body fat units. This compares favorably with other prediction methods that use skinfolds and girths.

PREDICTED PERCENTAGE FAT AT GIVEN CRITICAL BODY MASS INDEX VALUES

The table below presents predicted %BF values for different threshold BMI values for men and women of different ethnicities. These data provide a research-based approach for developing healthy percentage body fat ranges from guidelines based on BMI.

Predicted Percentage Body Fat by Sex and Ethnicity Related to BMI Healthy Weight Guidelines

AGE AND BMI	FEMALES			MALES		
	AFRICAN AMERICANS	ASIANS	WHITES	AFRICAN AMERICANS	ASIANS	WHITES
20–39 y						
BMI <18.5	20%	25%	21%	8%	13%	8%
BMI ≥25	32%	35%	33%	20%	23%	21%
BMI ≥30	38%	40%	39%	26%	28%	26%
40–59 y						
BMI <18.5	21%	25%	23%	23%	13%	11%
BMI ≥25	34%	36%	35%	35%	24%	23%
BMI ≥30	39%	41%	42%	41%	29%	29%
60–79 y						
BMI <18.5	23%	26%	25%	11%	14%	13%
BMI ≥25	35%	36%	38%	23%	24%	25%
BMI ≥30	41%	41%	43%	29%	29%	31%

REFERENCE

Gallagher, D., et al.: Healthy percentage body fat ranges: an approach for developing guidelines based on body mass index. *Am. J. Clin. Nutr.*, 72:694, 2000.

birth to children who become overweight and whose offspring also often become overweight. This pattern continues from generation to generation.

Excessive fatness also develops slowly through adulthood, with most of the weight gain occurring between ages 25 and 44 years. The typical American man beginning at age 30 years and woman beginning at age 27 years gains between 0.2 to 0.8 kg (0.5 to 1.8 lb) of body weight each year until age 60 years. For most college students at age 20 years, this means they will weigh, on average, an additional 40 pounds at age 60 years. The degree to which this creeping obesity during adulthood reflects a normal biologic pattern of aging remains unclear.

Questions & Notes

Predict percentage fat for a 29-year-old white female who is 162.5 cm tall and has a BMI of 30.

Overeating and Other Causative Factors

Human obesity results from a complex interaction of factors, including genetic, environmental, metabolic, physiologic, behavioral, social, and perhaps racial influences. Individual differences in specific factors that predispose humans to excessive weight gain include eating patterns and eating environment; food packaging, body image, and variations related to resting metabolic rate; diet-induced thermogenesis; level of spontaneous activity or "fidgeting"; basal body temperature; susceptibility to specific viral infections; levels of cellular adenosine triphosphatase, lipoprotein lipase, and other enzymes; and levels of metabolically active brown adipose tissue.

Regardless of the specific causes of obesity and their interactions, common treatment procedures—diets, surgery, drugs, psychological methods, and exercise, either alone or in combination—have failed miserably on a long-term basis. Nonetheless, researchers continue to devise strategies to prevent and treat this health catastrophe.

Effect of Global Changing of Dietary Patterns

Changes in diet and reduced energy expenditure via patterns of work and leisure, often referred to as the **nutrition transition**, contribute greatly to the increase in obesity worldwide. Moreover, the pace of these changes continues to accelerate, especially in low- and middle-income countries. Dietary changes that characterize the nutrition transition include quantitative and qualitative changes. The adverse changes include shifts in dietary structure toward higher energy density with greater fat and added sugars, greater saturated fat mostly from animal sources, reduced complex carbohydrates and dietary fiber, and reduced fruit and vegetable intakes. These trends in food consumption suggest a causal link to increasing obesity rates.

Food consumption, expressed in kCal per capita per day, provides a key variable to measure and evaluate energy storage. Analysis of worldwide data shows steadily increasing daily kCal per capita from the mid-1960s to the late 1990s, increasing globally by approximately 450 kCal and by more than 600 kCal in developing countries (Table 16.6). These data, coupled with decreased energy expenditure for all populations of the world, help to explain the worldwide creeping obesity epidemic.

Fast Food and Obesity Link in Adolescents An estimated 75% of all U.S. adolescents (ages 12 to 18 years) eat fast food one or more times per week. This increase in fast-food consumption parallels the escalating obesity epidemic, increasing the possibility of a causal relationship. Characteristics of fast food linked to excess energy intake and subsequent adiposity include enormous portion sizes, high-energy density, palatability, excessive amounts of refined starch and added sugars, high fat content, and low levels of dietary fiber. Research demonstrates that fast-food consumption directly relates to total energy intake and inversely relates to diet quality; moreover, a direct and positive association exits between fast food and body weight in adolescents (primarily those who are overweight and obese).

Genetics Play a Role

In our modern scientific era, molecular geneticists are committed to unravel intimate secrets of subcellular function related to obesity, trying to answer a seemingly simple question: "Why have so many people become so fat, and what can be done to ameliorate the problem?" British researchers in December 2009 provided clear evidence of a biological mechanism that helps to explain why some people are more susceptible to gaining weight in a world dominated by high-calorie food and a sedentary lifestyle. The experiment turned the spotlight on the protein-coding gene *FTO* that affects a person's risk of becoming obese or overweight. The *FTO* gene exists in two varieties, and all individuals inherit two copies of the gene. Children who inherit two copies of one variant were 70% more likely to be obese than those who inherited two copies of the other variant. Fifty percent of the children who inherited one copy of each *FTO* variant had a 30% higher risk of obesity. The groundbreaking part of the study involved a subgroup of 76 children whose metabolisms were monitored for 10 days and ate special test meals at the school. The available food was measured before and after consumption to see how much was eaten. Those tests showed the *FTO* variant

Table 16.6	Global and Regional Per Capita Food Consumption (kCal per capita per day)					
REGION	1964–1966	1974–1976	1984–1986	1997–1999	2015	2030
World	2358	2435	2655	2803	2940	3050
Developing countries	2054	2152	2450	2681	2850	2980
Near East and North Africa	2290	2591	2953	3006	3090	3170
Sub-Saharan Africa (excluding South Africa)	2058	2079	2057	2195	2360	2540
Latin America + Caribbean	2393	2546	2689	2824	2980	3140
East Asia	1957	2105	2559	2992	3060	3190
South Asia	2017	1986	2205	2403	2700	2900
Industrialized countries	2947	3065	3206	3380	3440	3500

From Diet, Nutrition and The Prevention of Chronic Diseases. WHO Technical Report Series #916. Report of a Joint WHO/FAO Expert Consultation. Geneva, Switzerland: World Health Organization, 2003.

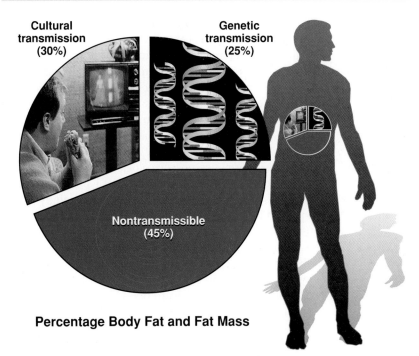

Percentage Body Fat and Fat Mass

Figure 16.17 Total transmissible variance for body fat. Total body fat and percentage body fat determined by hydrostatic weighing. (Data from Bouchard, C., et al.: Inheritance of the amount and distribution of human body fat. *Int. J. Obes.*, 12:205, 1988.)

Questions & Notes

List 5 variables believed to cause human obesity.

1.

2.

3.

4.

5.

Describe the "nutrition transition."

Describe the trend of daily kCal per capita from the mid-1960s to the late 1990s. (Refer to Table 16.6).

did not depress metabolism but instead increased the tendency to eat more high-calorie foods in the test meals. In each case, the extra weight was explained entirely by more body fat, not increased muscle mass or structural differences such as being taller.

Genetic makeup does not necessarily cause obesity, but it does lower the threshold for its development. In fact, it contributes to differences in weight gain for individuals fed identical daily caloric excess. **Figure 16.17** summarizes findings from a large number of individuals representing nine different types of backgrounds. Genetic factors determined about 25% of the transmissible variation among people in percentage body fat and total fat mass, and the largest transmissible variation related to a cultural effect. *In an obesity-producing environment characterized as sedentary and stressful with easy access to calorie-dense food, the genetically susceptible individuals gain weight.*

A Mutant Gene and Leptin

Researchers now link human obesity to a mutant gene. Studies at the University of Cambridge in England identified a specific defect in two genes that control body weight. Two cousins from a Pakistani family in England inherited a defect in the gene that synthesizes leptin, a crucial hormonal body weight–regulating substance produced by fat and released into the bloodstream that acts on the hypothalamus. Congenital absence of leptin produced continual hunger and marked obesity in these children. The second genetic defect observed in an English patient affected the body's response to leptin's "signal." This

For Your Information

THE GOOD AND THE BAD OF BODY FAT

Three studies from researchers in Boston, Finland, and the Netherlands published in the *New England Journal of Medicine* show that some brown fat—the "good fat," which spurs the body to burn calories to generate body heat—remains in adults. This energy-generating fat form stores mostly around the neck and under the collarbone; its energy-storing white (yellow) fat counterpart concentrates around the waistline to store energy and release chemicals that control metabolism and the use of insulin. Three general findings of the research indicate:

1. Lean individuals have more brown fat than overweight counterparts.
2. Brown fat accelerates its energy release in cooler environments.
3. Women tend to have more brown fat than men, with larger and more active deposits.

Devising a means to fully activate the body's brown fat might serve as the Holy Grail in treating the obese condition.

triggering signal largely determines how much one eats, how much energy one expends, and ultimately how much one weighs.

The genetic model in **Figure 16.18** proposes that the *ob* gene normally becomes activated in adipose tissue and perhaps muscle tissue, where it encodes and stimulates production of a body fat–signaling, hormonelike protein called *ob* **protein** or **leptin**, which then enters the bloodstream. This satiety signal molecule travels to the arcuate nucleus, a collection of specialized neurons in the mediobasal hypothalamus that controls appetite and metabolism and develops soon after birth. Normally, leptin blunts the urge to eat when caloric intake maintains ideal fat stores. Leptin may

affect certain neurons in the hypothalamic region that stimulates the production of chemicals that suppress appetite or reduce the levels of neurochemicals that stimulate appetite. Such mechanisms would explain how body fat remains intimately "connected" via a physiologic pathway to the brain to regulate energy balance. In essence, leptin availability, or its lack, affects the neurochemistry of appetite and the brain's dynamic "wiring" to possibly impact appetite and obesity in adulthood.

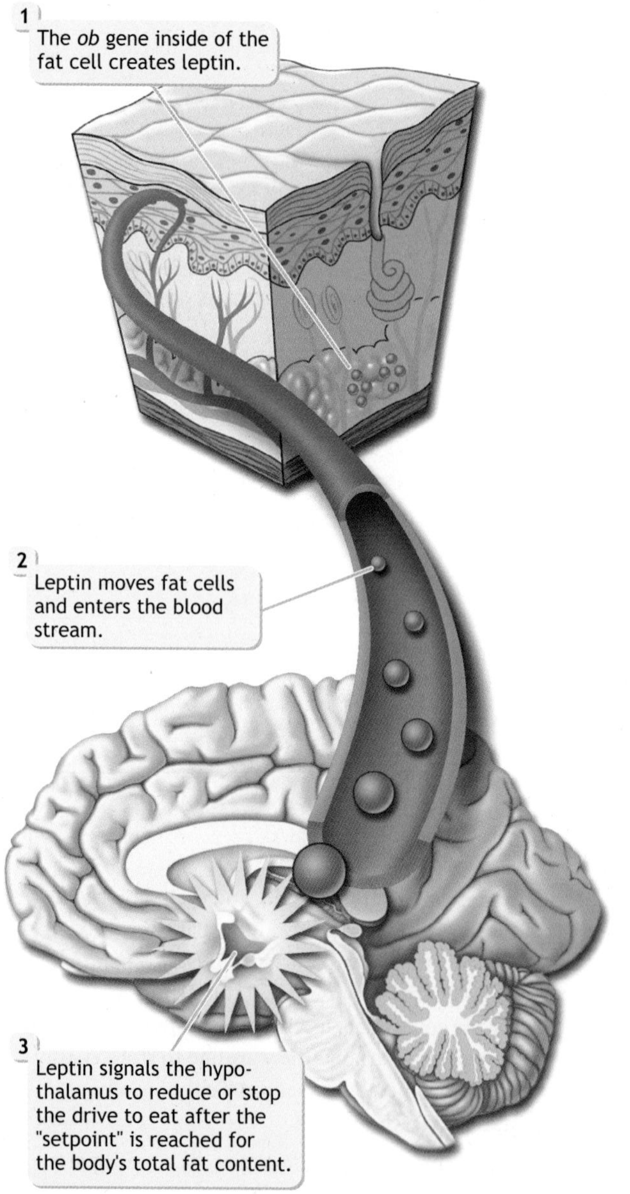

Gender, hormones, pharmacologic agents, and the body's current energy requirements also affect leptin production. Neither short- nor long-term exercise meaningfully affects leptin, independent of the effects of exercise on total adipose tissue mass.

The linkage of genetic and molecular abnormalities to obesity allows researchers to view overfatness as a disease instead of a psychological flaw. Early identification of one's genetic predisposition toward obesity makes it possible to begin diet and exercise intervention before obesity sets in and fat loss becomes exceedingly difficult. Pharmaceutical companies may eventually synthesize compounds that produce satiety or affect the resting rate of fat catabolism. These chemicals would produce weight control with a smaller caloric intake and fewer feelings of hunger and deprivation that often accompany conventional diet plans. Leptin alone does not determine obesity or explain why some people eat whatever they want and gain little weight while others become overfat with the same caloric intake.

Influence of Racial Factors

Racial differences in food and exercise habits, including cultural attitudes toward body weight help to explain the greater prevalence of obesity among black women (nearly 50%) than white women (33%). Research with obese women shows that small differences in resting energy expenditure (REE), related to racial differences in LBM, contribute to the racial differences in obesity. This "racial" effect, which also exists among children and adolescents, predisposes that black women more readily gain weight and regain it after weight loss. On average, black women burn nearly 100 fewer kCal each day during rest than white counterparts. The slower rate of caloric expenditure persists even after adjusting for differences in body mass and body composition. A 100-kCal reduction in daily metabolism translates to nearly 1 pound of body fat gained each month. Total daily energy expenditure (TDEE) of black women averages 10% lower than whites, owing to a 5% lower REE and 19% lower physical activity energy expenditure. Additionally, obese black women showed greater decreases in REE than white women after energy restriction and weight loss. The combination of a lower initial REE and more profound depression of REE with weight loss suggests that black women including athletes experience greater difficulty achieving and maintaining goal body weight than overweight white women.

When evaluating purported racial differences in body composition characteristics and their implications on

1. The *ob* gene inside of the fat cell creates leptin.

2. Leptin moves fat cells and enters the blood stream.

3. Leptin signals the hypothalamus to reduce or stop the drive to eat after the "setpoint" is reached for the body's total fat content.

Figure 16.18 Genetic model of obesity. A malfunction of the satiety gene affects production of the satiety hormone leptin. Underproduction of leptin disrupts proper function of the hypothalamus (step 3), the center that regulates the body's fat level. (Model based on research conducted at Rockefeller University, New York.)

health and physical performance, one must carefully evaluate methods to explore such differences. For example, interethnic and interracial differences in body size, structure, and total body fat and its distribution can mask true differences in body fat at a given BMI. A single generalized BMI–health risk model obscures the potential to document chronic disease risks among different population groups.

Physical Inactivity: An Important Component for Fat Accumulation

Regular physical activity, through either recreation or occupation, effectively impedes weight gain and the adverse changes in body composition. Individuals who maintain weight loss over time show greater muscle strength and engage in more physical activity than counterparts who regained lost weight. Variations in physical activity alone accounted for more than 75% of regained body weight. Such findings point to the need to identify and promote strategies that increase regular exercise. Published 2008 national guidelines by the U.S. Governments Health and Human Services (*www.health.gov/paguidelines/ guidelines/default.aspx*) recommend 60 or more minutes of daily moderate physical activity. We endorse an increase to 80 to 90 minutes of exercise daily, 6 to 7 days a week over and above regular routines, to combat the obesity epidemic in the U.S. population.

Physically active lifestyles lessen the "normal" pattern of fat gain in adulthood. For young and middle-aged men who exercise regularly, time spent in physical activity relates inversely to body fat level. Middle-aged long-distance runners remain leaner than sedentary counterparts. Surprisingly, no relationship emerges between the runners' body fat level and caloric intake. Perhaps the relatively greater body fat among middle-aged runners results from less-vigorous training, *not* greater food intake.

From age 3 months to 1 year, the total energy expenditure of infants who later became overweight averaged 21% lower than infants with normal weight gain. For children ages 6 to 9 years, percentage body fat inversely related to physical activity level in boys but not girls. Obese preadolescent and adolescent children generally spend less time engaging in physical activity or engage in lower intensity physical activity than normal-weight peers. By the time young girls attain adolescence, many do not engage in physical activity. For girls, the decline in time spent in physical activity averaged nearly 100% among blacks and 64% among whites between ages 9 or 10 years and 15 or 16 years. By age 16 years, 56% of the black girls and 31% of the white girls reported no leisure-time physical activity.

Benefits of Increased Energy Output with Aging

Maintaining a lifestyle that includes a regular, consistent level of endurance exercise attenuates but does not fully forestall the tendency to add extra weight through middle age. Sedentary men and women who begin an exercise regimen lose weight and body fat compared with those who remain sedentary; those who stop exercising gain body weight relative to those who remain active. Moreover, the amount of weight change relates proportionally the change in exercise dose. **Figure 16.19** displays the inverse association among distance run and BMI and waist circumference in all age categories. Active men typically remained leaner than sedentary counterparts for each age group; men who ran longer distances each week weighed less than those who ran shorter distances. The typical man who maintained a constant weekly running distance through middle age gained 3.3 pounds, and waist size increased about three-fourths of an inch, regardless of

Questions & Notes

Describe how fast food consumption relates directly to total energy intake and inversely to diet quality.

Discuss genetic factors in determining percentage body fat and total fat mass.

Describe the 2 ways leptin affects body fat levels.

1.

2.

For Your Information

BEWARE OF UNIVERSAL OVERWEIGHT AND OBESITY BODY MASS INDEX CUT-SCORES: A RACIAL OR ETHNIC BIAS DOES EXIST

For the same age and BMI, the percentage body fat of African American men and women, Asian Indian men and women, Hispanic women, and Asian women significantly differed from non-Hispanic white men and women. BMI cut-scores to define overweight and obesity systematically overestimated overweight and obesity prevalence of African American men and women and underestimated prevalence of Asian Indian men and women, Asian women, and Hispanic women.

Reference

Jackson AJ, et al.: Body mass index bias in defining obesity of diverse young adults. The Training Intervention and Genetics of Exercise Response (TIGER) Study. *Br. J. Nutr.*, 102:1084, 2009.

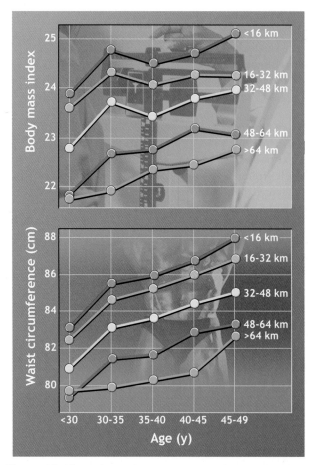

Figure 16.19 Relationship among average body mass index (*top*) and waist circumference (*bottom*) and age for men who maintained constant weekly running for varying distances (<16 to >64 km·wk^{-1}). Men who annually increase their running distance by 1.39 miles (2.24 km) per week compensate for the anticipated weight gain during middle age. (From Williams, P.T.: Evidence for the incompatibility of age-neutral overweight and age-neutral physical activity standards from runners. *Am. J. Clin. Nutr.*, 65:1391, 1997.)

distance run. Such findings suggest that by age 50 years a physically active man can expect to weigh about 10 pounds or more with a 2-in larger waist than he weighed several decades before despite maintaining a constant level of increased physical activity. To counter weight gain in middle age, one should gradually increase the amount of weekly exercise the equivalent of running 1.4 miles for each year of age starting at about age 30 years.

HEALTH RISKS OF OBESITY

Obesity has joined cigarette smoking, hypertension, elevated serum cholesterol, and physical inactivity in the American Heart Association's list of primary coronary heart disease risk factors (*www.americanheart.org/presenter. jhtml?identifier=4639*). Clear associations exist among obesity and hypertension; type 2 diabetes; and various lipid abnormalities (dyslipidemia), including increased risk of cerebrovascular disease, alterations in fatty acid metabo-

lism, and atherosclerosis. The 10 major health consequences of obesity include:

1. Cardiovascular disease
2. Type 2 diabetes
3. Hypertension
4. Dyslipidemia
5. Ischemic stroke
6. Sleep apnea
7. Degenerative joint disease
8. Some types of cancer
9. Gallstones
10. Fertility problems

The costs associated with adult obesity are estimated at more than $147 billion per year, or close to 10% of the U.S. national healthcare budget. If the size of Americans continues to increase at the current rate, one in five health care dollars spent on middle-aged Americans by 2020 will result from obesity.

CRITERIA FOR EXCESSIVE BODY FAT: HOW FAT IS TOO FAT?

Three appropriate approaches measure a person's fat content:

1. Percentage of body mass composed of fat
2. Distribution or patterning of fat at different anatomic regions
3. Size and number of individual fat cells

Percentage Body Fat

The demarcation often becomes arbitrary between what is considered a "normal" body fat level and when obesity begins. Part 1 of this chapter identified "the normal" range of body fat in adult men and women as plus or minus 1 unit of variation (standard deviation) from the average population value. That variation unit equals 5% body fat for men and women between ages 17 and 50 years. Within this statistical boundary, overfatness corresponds to any percentage body fat value above the average value for age and gender, plus 5 percentage points. For young men, whose fat mass averages 15% of body mass, borderline obesity equals 20% body fat. For older men, the average percentage of fat approximates 25%. Consequently, a body fat content in excess of 30% represents overfatness for this group. For young women, obesity corresponds to a body fat content above 30%, but for older women, borderline obesity begins at 37% body fat.

Age-specific demarcations for obesity assumes that men and women *normally* become fatter with age. However, this does not necessarily occur for physically active older men and women. If lifestyle accounts for the greatest portion of body fat increase during adulthood, then the criterion for overfatness could justifiably represent the standard for younger men and women.

We consider that obesity exists along a continuum from the upper limit of average (20% body fat for men and 30% for women) to as high as 50% and a theoretical maximum of nearly 70% of body mass in massively obese individuals. This latter group's weight ranges from 170 to 250 kg or higher. This can create a life-threatening situation in such extreme cases because the body's total fat content would exceed their LBM!

Regional Fat Distribution

The patterning of the body's adipose tissue, independent of total body fat, alters health risks in children, adolescents, and adults. **Figure 16.20** shows two types of regional fat distribution. Increased health risk from fat deposition in the abdominal area (**central** or **android-type obesity**; see Close Up Box 16.5: *Calculating and Interpreting the Waist-to-Hip Girth Ratio* on page 570), particularly internal visceral deposits, may result from this tissue's active lipolysis with catecholamine stimulation. Fat stored in this region shows greater metabolic

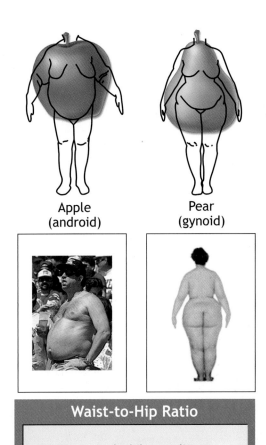

Apple
(android)

Pear
(gynoid)

Waist-to-Hip Ratio

- Waist at navel while standing relaxed, not pulling in stomach

- Hips, over the buttocks where girth is largest

- Divide waist girth by hip girth measure

  Ratio for significant health risk
  Males: ≥0.95
  Females: ≥0.80

Figure 16.20 Male (android pattern) and female (gynoid pattern) fat patterning, including waist-to-hip girth ratio threshold for significant health risk.

Questions & Notes

List 5 major health risks of obesity.

1.

2.

3.

4.

5.

List 3 criteria to evaluate body fat status.

1.

2.

3.

Give the cut-off percentage fat values for adult males and females for defining over-fatness.

Males:

Females:

For Your Information

OBESITY-RELATED ILLNESS

Obesity causes more than 100,000 deaths in the United States each year, according to the latest statistics released by the American Institute of Cancer Research (*www.aich.org*). Excessive body fat causes nearly one-half of endometrial cancers and one-third of esophageal cancers. If Americans maintained normal body weights (BMI ≤25.0), endometrial cancer would decrease by 49%, esophageal cancer by 35%, pancreatic cancer by 28%, kidney cancer by 24%, gallbladder cancer by 21%, breast cancer by 17%, and colon cancer by 9%. Obesity-related illness accounts for nearly 10% of all medical costs in the United States—estimated at greater than $147 billion yearly.

BOX 16.5 CLOSE UP

Calculating and Interpreting the Waist-to-Hip Girth Ratio

Waist-to-hip girth ratio (WHR) indicates relative fat distribution in adults and risk of disease (see table). A higher ratio reflects a greater proportion of abdominal fat with a greater risk for hyperinsulinemia, insulin resistance, type 2 diabetes, endometrial cancer, hypercholesterolemia, hypertension, and atherosclerosis.

WHR computes as Abdominal girth (cm or in) ÷ Hip girth (cm or in); waist girth represents the smallest girth around the abdomen (the natural waist), and hip girth reflects the largest girth measured around the buttocks (see figure).

Waist-to-Hip Girth Ratio and Disease Risk

	AGE, y	LOW	MODERATE	RISK LEVEL HIGH	VERY HIGH
Men	20–29	<0.83	0.83–0.88	0.89–0.94	>0.94
	30–39	<0.84	0.84–0.91	0.92–0.96	>0.96
	40–49	<0.88	0.88–0.95	0.96–1.00	>1.00
	50–59	<0.90	0.90–0.96	0.97–1.02	>1.02
	60–69	<0.91	0.91–0.98	0.99–1.03	>1.03
Women	20–29	<0.71	0.71–0.77	0.78–0.82	>0.82
	30–39	<0.72	0.72–0.78	0.79–0.84	>0.84
	40–49	<0.73	0.73–0.79	0.80–0.87	>0.87
	50–59	<0.74	0.74–0.81	0.82–0.88	>0.88
	60–69	<0.76	0.76–0.83	0.84–0.90	>0.90

CALCULATING WHR

Example 1
Man: Age, 21 y; abdominal girth, 101.6 cm; hip girth, 93.5 cm

$$\text{WHR} = \text{Abdominal girth (cm)} \div \text{Hip girth (cm)}$$
$$= 101.6 \div 93.5$$
$$= 1.08 \text{ (very high disease risk)}$$

Example 2
Woman: Age, 41 y; abdominal girth, 83.2 cm; hip girth, 101 cm

$$\text{WHR} = \text{Abdomen girth (cm)} \div \text{Hip girth (cm)}$$
$$= 83.2 \div 101$$
$$= 0.82 \text{ (high disease risk)}$$

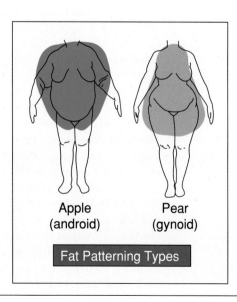

Apple (android)   Pear (gynoid)

Fat Patterning Types

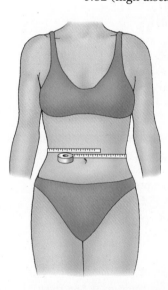

Abdomen: Minimum girth; standing, feet together

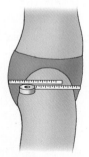

Hips: Maximum girth around buttocks; standing, feet together

responsiveness than fat in the gluteal and femoral regions (**peripheral** or **gynoid-type obesity**). Increases in central fat more readily support processes that cause heart disease. In men, the amount of fat located inside the abdominal cavity called intraabdominal or visceral adipose tissue is twice as large compared with women. For men, the percentage of visceral fat increases progressively with age; this fat deposition in women begins to increase at the onset of menopause.

Central fat deposition, independent of fat storage in other anatomic areas, reflects an altered metabolic profile that increases at least eight of the following medical conditions:

1. Hyperinsulinemia (insulin resistance)
2. Glucose intolerance
3. Type 2 diabetes
4. Endometrial cancer
5. Hypertriglyceridemia
6. Hypercholesterolemia and negatively altered lipoprotein profile
7. Hypertension
8. Atherosclerosis

As a general guideline, waist-to-hip girth ratios that exceed 0.80 for women and 0.95 for men increase the risk of death even after adjusting for BMI. One limitation of the ratio is that it poorly captures the specific effects of each girth measure. Waist and hip circumferences reflect different aspects of body composition and fat distribution. Each has an independent and often opposite effect on cardiovascular disease risk. An increased waist girth is the so-called malignant form of obesity characterized by central fat deposition. This region of fat deposition provides a reasonable indication of the accumulation of intraabdominal visceral adipose tissue. This makes waist girth the trunk measure of clinical choice as a practical measure to evaluate the metabolic and health risks and accelerated mortality with obesity.

Over a broad range of BMI values, men and women with the high waist circumference values possess greater relative risk for cardiovascular disease, type 2 diabetes, cancer, dementia, and cataracts (the leading cause of blindness worldwide) than individuals with small waist circumferences or peripheral obesity. A waist girth that exceeds 91 cm (36 in) in men and 82 cm (32 in) in women and correspondingly high blood insulin levels nearly doubles the risk of colorectal cancer. **Figure 16.21** shows how to apply three BMI categories and waist girth measurements above and below 40 inches for men and 34.6 inches for women to assess a person's risk of health problems ranked from least risk to very high risk.

Fat Cell Size and Number

The size and number of fat cells provide a view of the structure, form, and dimensions of normal and abnormal levels of body fatness. Increases in adipose tissue mass occurs in two ways:

1. Enlarging (filling) of existing fat cells with more fat called **fat cell hypertrophy**
2. Increasing the total number of fat cells called **fat cell hyperplasia**

The technique to assess adipocyte size and number involves sucking small

Questions & Notes

List the waist:hip ratio (WHR) cut-off values that indicate excessive visceral fat accumulation for males and females.

  Males:

  Females:

List 2 medical conditions exacerbated by increased central fat.
  1.

  2.

List the 2 ways that adipose tissue increases.
  1.

  2.

 For Your Information

HIGH BMI AND LARGE WAIST ACCURATELY PREDICT HEART DISEASE RISK

A recent study by Dutch researchers measured BMI and waist size in 20,500 men and women ages 20 to 65 years and correlated these age- and gender-adjusted measurements with nonfatal and fatal cardiovascular disease risk over 10 years. More than 50% of all fatal heart disease cases and 25% of nonfatal heart disease were predicted from having a high BMI or large waist in subjects defined as overweight or obese, with the cardiovascular disease risk equally strong for BMI and waist circumference. Overweight people had BMIs of between 25 and 30 and obese people of 30 or more. Waist circumference in men was defined as 37.0 to 40.1 inches for overweight and more than 40.2 inches for obese. In women, these measurements were 31.5 to 34.6 inches for overweight and more than 34.6 inches for obese.

Reference

Van Dis I, et al.: Body mass index and waist circumference predict both 10-year nonfatal and fatal cardiovascular disease risk: study conducted in 20,000 Dutch men and women aged 20–65 years. *Eur. J. Cardiovasc. Prev. Rehabil.* 16:729, 2009.

BMI category

Waist girth	Normal 18.5 - 24.9 kg · m⁻²	Overweight 25 - 29.9 kg · m⁻²	Obese class I 30 - 34.9 kg · m⁻²
Men: < 102 cm Women: < 88 cm	Least risk	Increased risk	High risk
Men: ≥ 102 cm Women: ≥ 88 cm	Inceased risk	High risk	Very high risk

Figure 16.21 Applying BMI and waist girth measurements in adult men and women from least risk to very high risk for health and longevity and medical problems. For men, high risk = 102 cm (40 in); for women, high risk = 88 cm (34.6 in). (Data from the world literature, including Douketis, J.D.: Body weight classification. *CMAJ.*, 172:995, 2005.)

fragments of subcutaneous tissue by needle biopsy aspiration, usually from the upper back, buttocks, abdomen, and back of the upper arm, directly into the fat depot (**Fig. 16.22**). Chemical treatment of the biopsy sample enables the researcher to separate and count the fat cells. One can estimate the total adipocyte number by determining total body fat by a criterion method such as hydrostatic weighing. For example, an individual who weighs 88 kg with 13% body fat has a total fat mass of 11.4 kg (0.13 × 88 kg). Dividing 11.4 kg by the average fat content per cell estimates

total adipocyte number. If the average adipocyte contains 0.60 μg of fat, then this person's body contains 19 billion adipocytes (11.4 kg ÷ 0.60 μg).

Total adipocyte number = Mass of body fat
÷ Fat content per cell

Cellularity Differences Between Nonobese and Obese Persons
The data in the *left side* of **Figure 16.23** illustrate the strong association between total fat mass

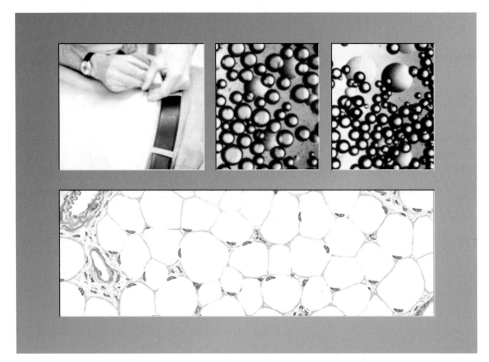

Figure 16.22 *Upper panel.* Needle biopsy procedure to extract fat cells of the upper buttocks region. The area is sterilized and anesthetized, and the biopsy needle is placed beneath the skin surface. The syringe sucks small tissue fragments from the site. The two photomicrographs indicate fat cells biopsied from the buttocks of a physically active professor before (*center*) and after (*right*) 6 months of marathon training. The average fat cell diameter averaged 8.6% smaller after training. The volume of fat in each cell decreased by 18.2%. The large spherical structures in the background represent intracellular lipid droplets. (Photomicrographs courtesy of P.M. Clarkson, Muscle Biology and Imaging Laboratory, University of Massachusetts, Amherst, MA.) *Lower panel.* Cross-section of human fat cells magnified ×440. (From Geneser, F.: *Color Atlas of Histology.* Philadelphia: Lea & Febiger, 1985.)

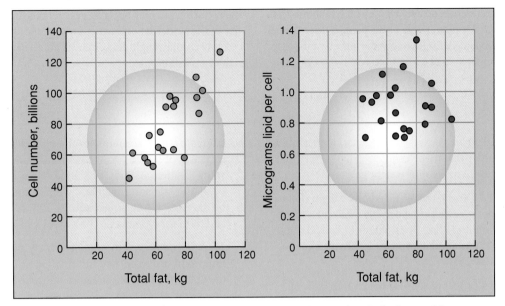

Figure 16.23 Adipose cell number (*left*) and size (*right*) related to the body's total fat mass.

in obese individuals and their number of fat cells. The person with the lowest body fat content had the fewest number of fat cells, whereas the fattest subject had considerably more adipocytes. In contrast, the data displayed in the *right panel* of the figure show little relationship between total body fat and average fat cell size in obese individuals. This suggests that a biologic upper limit exists for fat cell size. After reaching this size, cell number probably becomes the key factor that determines the extent of extreme obesity. Even doubling the size of normal fat cells would not account for the tremendous difference in the fat content between obese and nonobese people. It seems reasonable to conclude, therefore, that the excessive adipose tissue mass in severe obesity occurs by fat cell hyperplasia.

The results from a related early study regarding fat cell size and number displayed in **Figure 16.24** compared body mass, total fat, and adipose tissue cellularity in 25 subjects, 20 of whom classified as clinically obese (BMI ~40.0). The body mass of the obese averaged more than twice that of the nonobese, and they had nearly three times more body fat. In cellularity, adipocytes in the obese averaged 50% larger with nearly three times more cells (75 vs. 27 billion). *Cell number represents the major structural difference in adipose tissue mass between the severely obese and nonobese persons.*

Questions & Notes

Describe the relationship between fat cell number and total body fat.

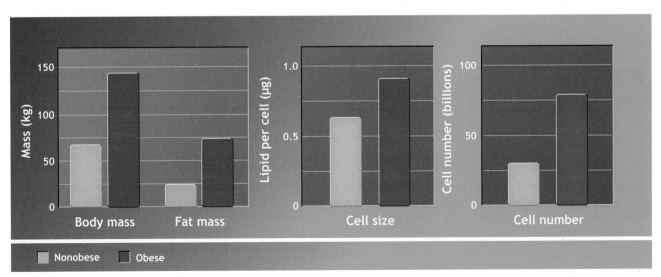

Figure 16.24 Comparison of body mass, total fat mass, and adipocyte size and number in obese and nonobese subjects. (Modified from Hirsch, J., Knittle, J.: Cellularity of obese and non-obese human adipose tissue. *Fed. Proc.*, 29:1518, 1970.)

As a frame of reference, an average person has about 25 to 30 billion fat cells. For moderately obese people, this number ranges between 60 and 100 billion, but the fat cell number for massively obese people may increase to 360 billion or more.

Even during surgery such as gastric banding to reduce the size of the stomach and restrict food intake at any given meal, the substantial weight loss months after surgery still did not reduce fat cell number.

SUMMARY

1. Overfatness, defined as excessive body fat, represents a complex disorder that involves interrelated factors that tip energy balance in favor of weight gain.

2. Over the past 25 years, the average body weight of adult Americans has increased considerably. Currently, 30% of adults (59 million) classify as obese (BMI ≥30), and nearly 65% (130 million adults) are either overweight or obese (BMI ≥25).

3. Genetic factors probably account for 25% to 30% of excessive body fat accumulation. Genetic predisposition does not necessarily cause obesity, but given the right environment, genetically susceptible individuals gain body fat.

4. About 15% to 20% of American children and 12% of adolescents (up from 7.6% in 1976 to 1980) classify as overweight. Excessive body fatness, childhood's most common chronic disorder, is particularly prevalent among poor and minority children.

5. Obesity represents a medical condition that includes overfatness and other conditions such as dyslipidemia, hypertension, insulin resistance, and glucose intolerance.

6. No reason fully accounts for the typical body fat increases observed for American men and women with aging. Therefore, body fat standards for borderline overfatness in adult men and women could justifiably be the values for younger adults: 20% body fat for men and 30% for women.

7. Adipose tissue patterning on the body provides important health-related information. Fat distributed in the abdominal–visceral region (android-type obesity) poses a greater health risk compared with fat deposited at the thigh, hips, and buttocks (gynoid-type obesity).

8. Waist girth provides a second dimension of obesity when assessing the health-risk profile. Men and women with large waist circumferences possess greater relative risk for cardiovascular disease, type 2 diabetes, cancer, and cataracts than individuals with small waist circumferences.

9. Size and the number of adipocytes provides another obesity classification. Before adulthood, body fat increases by enlargement of individual fat cells (fat cell hypertrophy) and increases in total number of fat cells (fat cell hyperplasia).

THOUGHT QUESTIONS

1. Discuss the possibility that excessive food intake does not cause excessive body fat accumulation in children and adults.

2. What possible explanation(s) accounts for the rapid increase in body fat observed worldwide?

3. In your opinion, what are the leading causes of childhood obesity?

4. Explain if and why different body fat standards should apply to people of different ages.

| Part 4 | Achieving Optimal Body Composition Through Diet and Exercise |

The following statement by University of Pennsylvania obesity specialist Dr. Albert Stunkard (1922–) presents a realistic view about the possibility of long-term weight loss for obese individuals:

> Most obese persons will not stay in treatment. Of those who stay in treatment, most will not lose weight, and of those who do lose weight, most will regain it.

This bleak outlook delivered 4 decades ago buttresses the majority of subsequent research showing that initial modifications in body weight have little relation to long-term success. Participants who remain in supervised weight loss programs reduce about 10% of their original body weight.

The potential for successful long-term weight loss maintenance generally varies inversely with the initial degree of fatness (**Fig. 16.25**). For most individuals, initial success in weight loss relates poorly to long-term success. Participants in supervised weight loss programs (pharmacologic or behavioral interventions) generally lose about 8% to 12% of their original body mass. Unfortunately, typically one- to two-thirds of the lost weight returns within 1 year, and almost all of it within 5 years.

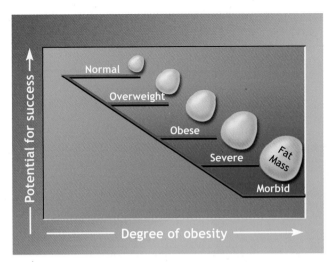

Figure 16.25 Likelihood of success in long-term maintenance of weight loss inversely relates to the level of obesity at the start of intervention.

Is fat cell number or cell size the major structural difference in adipose tissue mass between the obese and nonobese?

Describe the relationship between potential for successful long-term weight loss and initial degree of fatness.

About what percentage of those who start a weight loss program will be successful?

List 3 ways to unbalance the energy balance equation.

1.

2.

3.

Figure 16.26 illustrates that over a 7.3-year follow-up of 121 patients, 50% of the dieters returned to their original weight within 2 to 3 years, and only seven patients remained at their reduced body weights. These discouraging but typical statistics highlight the extreme difficulty of long-term maintenance of a low-calorie diet; it becomes particularly difficult in the relaxed atmosphere of one's home with ready access to food and often little emotional support.

THE ENERGY BALANCE EQUATION: THE KEY TO WEIGHT CONTROL

The first law of thermodynamics often called the *law of conservation of energy* posits that energy can be transferred from one system to another in many forms but cannot be created or destroyed. In human terms, this means that the energy balance equation dictates that body mass remains constant when caloric intake equals caloric expenditure. **Figure 16.27** illustrates that a chronic imbalance on the energy output or input side of the equation changes body weight.

Three ways unbalance the energy balance equation to produce weight loss include:

1. Reducing caloric intake below daily energy requirements
2. Maintaining caloric intake and increase energy expenditure through additional physical activity above daily energy requirements

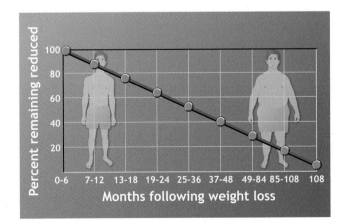

Figure 16.26 General trend for percentage of patients remaining at reduced weights at various time intervals after accomplished weight loss.

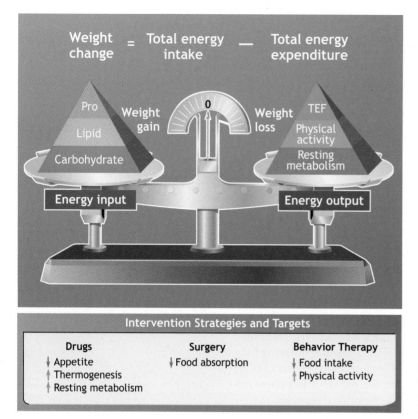

Figure 16.27 The energy balance equation plus intervention strategies and specific targets to alter energy balance in the direction of weight loss. Pro = protein; TEF = thermic effect of food.

3. Decreasing daily caloric intake and increase daily energy expenditure

When considering the sensitivity of the energy balance equation, if caloric intake exceeds output by "only" 100 kCal per day, the surplus calories consumed in a year equal 36,500 kCal (365 days × 100 kCal). Every 0.45 kg (1.0 lb) of body fat contains 3500 kCal (each 1 lb [454 g] of adipose tissue contains about 86% fat, or 390 g × 9 kCal·g^{-1} = 3514 kCal per lb), so this caloric excess causes a yearly gain of about 4.7 kg (10.3 lb) of body fat. In contrast, if daily food intake decreases by just 100 kCal and energy expenditure increases by 100 kCal (e.g., by walking or jogging 1 extra mile each day), then the yearly deficit equals the energy in 9.5 kg (21 lb) of body fat.

Unbalancing the Energy Balance Equation

An objective assessment of energy intake from food and energy expenditure provides the frame of reference for unbalancing the energy balance equation to favorably modify body mass and body composition.

Energy Intake Estimates of caloric intake from daily food intake records usually fall within ±10% of the number of calories consumed. For example, suppose the actual energy value of a person's daily food intake averaged 2130 kCal. Based on a careful 3-day dietary history to estimate caloric intake, the daily value would fall between 1920 and 2350 kCal.

Careful record keeping of food intake also provides the dieter with an objective list of foods consumed rather than a "guesstimate" and triggers an important behavioral aspect of the weight control process—awareness of current food habits and preferences.

Energy Output A physically active lifestyle becomes crucial to long-term success at weight loss. This does not mean playing a token game of tennis twice a year, going for a swim on weekends during the summer, or walking to the store when the car needs repair. Rather, modifying personal exercise habits entails a serious commitment to changing daily routines to include regular periods of moderate to vigorous physical activity. The accompanying Close Up Box 16.6: *Computing Daily Energy (Caloric) Requirement (Including Exercise) for Weight Management and for Weight Loss* on page 578 illustrates how to compute daily energy (kCal) requirement (including exercise) for weight maintenance and for weight loss.

ALTERING THE ENERGY BALANCE EQUATION

The objective of weight loss programs has changed dramatically over the past decade. The previous approach assigned a goal body weight that coincided with an "ideal" weight based on body mass and stature. Achievement of goal body weight heralded the weight loss program's success. Currently, the WHO (*www.who.int*), Institute of

Medicine of the National Academy of Sciences (*www.iom.edu*), and NHLBI (*www.nhlbi.nih.gov/*) recommend that the obese reduce their initial body weight by 5% to 15%. *This more realistic weight loss diminishes weight-related comorbidities and complications from hypertension, type 2 diabetes, and abnormal blood lipids and often exerts a positive effect on social and psychological complications.* Setting the initial weight loss goal beyond the 5% to 15% recommendation often gives patients an unrealistic and potentially unattainable target in light of current treatment methods.

Many people believe that only calories from dietary lipids increase body fat. Individuals reduce fat intake to achieve body fat loss (generally a good idea), but they often disproportionately increase carbohydrate and protein intakes, so total caloric intake remains unchanged or even increases. The prudent dietary approach to weight loss unbalances the energy balance equation by reducing daily energy intake 500 to 1000 kCal *below* the daily energy expenditure while consuming well-balanced meals. Compared with more severe energy restriction, which augments lean tissue loss, a moderate reduction in food intake produces a greater fat loss relative to energy deficit.

Most people do not tolerate prolonged daily caloric restriction of more than 1000 kCal; more extreme semistarvation also increases the likelihood for malnourishment, depletion of glycogen reserves, and loss of lean tissue. **One immutable truth about dieting to achieve success in altering the energy balance equation—the first law of thermodynamics—affirms conclusively that weight loss by dieting occurs whenever energy output *exceeds* energy intake, regardless of the diet's macronutrient mixture.**

Practical Illustration

Suppose an overfat college woman who normally consumes 2800 kCal daily and maintains a body mass of 79.4 kg wishes to lose weight by caloric restriction (dieting). She maintains her regular physical activity but reduces her food intake to 1800 kCal to create a 1000-kCal daily deficit. In 7 days, the accumulated deficit equals 7000 kCal, or the energy equivalent of 0.9 kg of body fat. Actually, she would lose considerably more than 0.9 kg during the first week because initially the body's glycogen stores make up a large portion of the energy deficit. Stored glycogen contains fewer calories per gram and considerably more water than stored fat. For this reason, short periods of caloric restriction often encourage the dieter yet produce a large percentage of water and carbohydrate loss per unit weight loss with only a small decrease in body fat. As weight loss continues, a larger proportion of body fat supports the energy deficit created by food restriction. To reduce body fat by an additional 1.4 kg, the dieter must maintain the reduced caloric intake of 1800 kCal for another 10.5 days; at this point, body fat theoretically decreases at a rate of 0.45 kg every 3.5 days.

Results Are Not Always Predictable

The mathematics of weight loss through caloric restriction seems straightforward, but results do not always follow. First, one assumes that daily energy expenditure remains relatively unchanged throughout the dieting period. Some people experience lethargy because caloric restriction depletes the body's glycogen stores, which actually decreases daily energy expenditure. Second, the energy cost of physical activity decreases in proportion to the weight lost. This also shrinks the energy output side of the energy balance equation. If weight loss progressed proportionately to caloric restriction, a progressive decrease in body weight would depend solely on the extent of caloric deprivation. Metabolic changes also take place during caloric restriction, further blunting the weight loss effort.

Resting Metabolism Lowered A reduction in resting metabolism often occurs when dieting produces weight loss. The decrease in resting metabolism

Describe the energy balance equation.

List the 3 components of total energy expenditure.

1.

2.

3.

One pound of stored body fat contains how many kCal of energy?

What would be a reasonable weight loss recommendation for obese individuals?

Compute the amount of weight loss for a person who expends 100 kCal per day greater than their energy intake for 1 year.

BOX 16.6 CLOSE UP

Computing Daily Energy (Caloric) Requirement (Including Exercise) for Weight Management and for Weight Loss

Successful weight loss requires a negative energy balance, in which total calorie (kCal) expenditure exceeds total intake. Foods consumed in the diet provide the energy the body requires to carry out its metabolic functions. The TDEE, often referred to as the body's "energy requirement," includes:

1. Normal daily energy expenditure (including sleeping and "normal" daily living conditions), excluding energy expenditure during physical activity
2. Energy expenditure during physical activity (including energy expenditure above "normal" daily living activities)

Weight maintenance occurs when intake equals TDEE. Determining TDEE allows one to compute the change in food consumption and physical activity necessary for weight maintenance *or* weight loss.

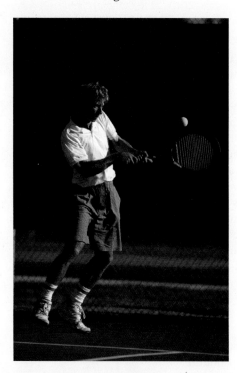

COMPUTING TOTAL DAILY ENERGY EXPENDITURE TO MAINTAIN BODY WEIGHT

Table 1 on the next page presents the computational steps to determine TDEE, including kCal expenditure of physical activity and target number of calories, to achieve a given weight loss.

Example Computations

The following example illustrates the computations for a 24-year-old man who weighs 72.6 kg (160 lb) and who participates in moderate daily physical activity (refer to Table 1).

1. Record body weight (BW): . . . . .160 lb
2. Record caloric requirement per pound BW (see Table 2): 15.0
3. Compute daily caloric requirement without physical activity to maintain current BW (multiply step 1 by step 2): . . . . .2400 kCal
4. Select physical activity (see Table 3; *if selecting more than one physical activity, estimate the average daily calories burned from each additional activity [steps 4 through 11] and add all of these totals to step 12*): . . . . **jogging**
5. Record the number of exercise sessions completed weekly: 4
6. Record the duration of each exercise session in minutes: . . . . 60 min
7. Compute the total *weekly* exercise time in minutes (*multiply step 5 by step 6*): . . . . 240 min
8. Compute the average *daily* exercise time in minutes (*divide step 7 by 7 [round to nearest whole min]*): . . . . 34 min
9. Record the caloric expenditure per pound per minute (kCal·lb⁻¹·min⁻¹) for your physical activity (see Table 3): 0.090
10. Compute total calories burned per minute (kCal·min⁻¹) during physical activity (*Multiply step 1 by step 9*): . . . . 14.4 kCal·min⁻¹
11. Compute average daily calorie expenditure (kCal) during physical activity (*multiply step 8 by step 10 [round to nearest whole number]*): . . . . 490 kCal
12. Compute the daily caloric requirement, including exercise kCal, to maintain current body weight (TDEE) (*add step 3 plus step 11*) . . . . 2890 kCal

COMPUTATIONS OF TARGET ENERGY INTAKE REQUIRED TO REDUCE BODY WEIGHT

In the above example, the TDEE to maintain body weight equals 2890 kCal. Therefore, the total kCal intake must decrease below this value to induce a negative caloric balance for weight loss. The energy deficit should never cause the total daily caloric intake to fall below 1200 kCal for women and 1500 kCal for men. This level of energy intake represents a safe level to ensure adequate intake of protein, vitamins, and minerals. Prudent recommendations include subtracting 500 kCal per day if the TDEE is below 3000 kCal and 1000 kCal for daily TDEE above 3000 kCal.

To compute the target number of calories for weight loss:

1. Compute number of calories to subtract from requirement to achieve a negative calorie balance (*subtract 500 kCal if the total daily kCal expenditure [step 12] is below 3000 kCal or 1000 kCal for daily expenditures above 3000 kCal*): . . . . **500 kCal**
2. Compute the target total caloric intake to reduce weight (*subtract step 13 from step 12*): . . . . . **2390 kCal**

Table 1   Computation of Daily Total Caloric Requirement and Target Caloric Intake to Lose Weight

1. Record body weight (BW) . . . . —
2. Record caloric requirement per pound BW (See **Table 2**) . . . . —
3. Compute daily caloric requirement without physical activity to maintain current BW (*Multiply Step #1 × Step #2*) . . . . —
4. Select physical activity (See **Table 3**) *If more than one physical activity is selected, estimate the average daily calories burned as a result of each additional activity (Steps #4 through #11) and add all of these totals to Step #12* . . . . —
5. Record the number of exercise sessions you do per week . . . . —
6. Record the duration of each exercise session in minutes . . . . —
7. Compute the total weekly exercise time in minutes (*Multiply Step #5 by Step #6*) . . . . —
8. Compute the average daily exercise time in minutes (*Divide Step #7 by 7 [round to nearest whole min]*) . . . . . —

9. Record the caloric expenditure per pound per minute ($kCal \cdot lb^{-1} \cdot min^{-1}$) for your physical activity (See **Table 3**) . . . . —
10. Compute total calories burned per minute ($kCal \cdot min^{-1}$) during physical activity (*Multiply Step #1 by Step #9*) . . . . —
11. Compute average daily calorie expenditure (kCal) during physical activity (*Add Step #3 and Step #11*) . . . . —
12. Compute daily caloric requirement, including exercise kCal, to maintain current BW (TDEE) . . . . . —
13. Compute number of calories to subtract from requirement to achieve a negative calorie balance (*Subtract 500 kCal if the total daily kCal expenditure [Step #12] is below 3000 kCal, 1000 kCal for daily expenditures above 3000 kCal*) . . . . —
14. Compute target caloric intake required to lose weight (*Subtract Step #13 from Step #12*) . . . . —

Table 2   Average 24-h Energy Expenditure Estimated From Body Weight (lb) Based on Different Physical Activity Levels for Men and Women[a]

ACTIVITY LEVEL	kCal PER lb[b]	
	MALES	FEMALES
Sedentary (limited) physical activity [No regular physical activity outside of work]	13.0	12.0
Moderate physical activity [Planned, systematic light to moderate physical activity 2–3 days per week, outside of work]	15.0	13.5
Strenuous physical activity [Planned, systematic heavy physical activity 4–6 days per week, outside of work]	17.0	15.0

[a]Pregnant or lactating women add 3.0 kCal per lb.
[b]For example, the 24-h energy expenditure for a sedentary male weighing 160 lbs equals 2080 kCal (13 kCal per pound × 160 lbs = 2080).

(continued)

BOX 16.6 CLOSE UP

Computing Daily Energy (Caloric) Requirement (Including Exercise) for Weight Management and for Weight Loss (Continued)

Table 3 Sample Caloric Expenditures in kCal Per Pound of Body Weight Per Minute (kCal·lb^{-1}·min^{-1})

ACTIVITY	kCal·lb^{-1}·min^{-1}	ACTIVITY	kCal·lb^{-1}·min^{-1}	ACTIVITY	kCal·lb^{-1}·min^{-1}
Basketball	0.062	Jumping rope		Volleyball	0.023
Circuit weight training		70 jumps/min	0.075	Walking	
Nautilus	0.042	80 jumps/min	0.080	4.5 mph	0.045
Climbing hills	0.055	Racquetball	0.080	grass track	0.037
Cycling		Running		shallow pool	0.090
5.5 mph	0.032	11 min: 30 s/mile	0.062	Swimming	
10 mph	0.050	9 min/mile	0.087	crawl, slow	0.058
13 mph	0.070	8 min/mile	0.097	crawl, fast	0.071
Aerobic dance		7 min/mile	0.1085	back stroke	0.077
medium	0.047	6 min/mile	0.1231	breast stroke	0.074
intense	0.061	Skiing, soft snow, leisure	0.044	side stroke	0.056
Golf	0.038	Skiing, hard snow,		Canoeing	
Gymnastics	0.030	moderate speed	0.054	leisure	0.019
				racing	0.047

REFERENCE

American College of Sports Medicine: Position statement on proper and improper weight loss programs. *Med. Sci. Sports Exerc.*, 15:9, 1993.

exceeds the decrease attributable to loss of either body mass or FFM; severe caloric restriction can depress resting metabolic rate up to 45%! A blunted metabolism characterizes individuals who attempt to lose weight, regardless if they dieted previously or were fat or lean. Reduced metabolism conserves energy, causing the diet to become progressively less effective despite a low caloric intake. Weight loss plateaus and further weight loss slows relative to that predicted from the mathematics of restricted energy intake.

Setpoint Theory: A Case Against Dieting

One can crash off large amounts of weight in a relatively brief time by simply stopping eating. Unfortunately, success is short-lived; eventually, the urge to eat wins out and the lost weight returns. Some argue that the reason for this failure lies in a genetically determined "setpoint" for body weight or body fat that differs from what the dieter would like. The proponents of a **setpoint theory** maintain that all persons fat or thin have a well-regulated internal control mechanism similar to a thermostat located deep within the brain's lateral hypothalamus that maintains with relative ease a preset level of body weight, body fat, or both within a tight range. In a practical sense,

this represents a person's body weight when not counting calories. Regular exercise and Food and Drug Administration–approved antiobesity drugs may lower a person's setpoint, but dieting supposedly exerts no effect. Each time the body weight decreases below one's preestablished setpoint, internal adjustments that affect food intake and regulatory thermogenesis resist the change and conserve or replenish body fat. For example, resting metabolism slows and the individual becomes obsessed with food, unable to control the urge to eat. Even when persons overeat and gain body fat above their normal level, the body resists this change by increasing resting metabolism causing the person to lose interest in food.

The setpoint theory delivers unwelcome news for those with a setpoint "tuned" too high; encouragingly, regular exercise may lower the setpoint level. Concurrently, regular exercise conserves and even increases FFM, increases resting metabolism if FFM increases, and induces metabolic changes that facilitate fat catabolism. These healthful adaptations all augment weight loss efforts. If a physically active lifestyle becomes a reality and body fat decreases, caloric intake balances daily energy requirements to stabilize body mass at a new *lower* level.

Fat Cell Size and Number After Weight Loss

Figure 16.28 highlights the results of a classic study of weight loss effects on changes in adipose tissue cellularity of obese adults during two stages of weight loss. Nineteen obese subjects who initially weighed 149 kg reduced their body mass by 45.8 kg, weighing 103 kg at the end of the first part of the experiment. Before weight reduction, the number of fat cells averaged 75 billion. This number remained essentially unchanged with weight reduction. The average size of the fat cells, in contrast, decreased by 33% from 0.9 µg to a normal value of 0.6 µg of fat per cell. Subjects attained a normal body mass when they lost an additional 28 kg. Cell number again remained unchanged, but cell size continued to shrink to about one-third the size of the fat cells in normal, nonobese subjects. Other experiments have confirmed these findings in young children and adults.

A formerly obese person who reduces body mass and body fat to near average values still does not become "cured" of obesity, at least for adipocyte number. The large number of relatively small fat cells in the reduced obese may somehow relate to appetite control, and the person craves food, overeats, and regains lost weight (fat). This certainly makes sense within the framework of the body fat hormone (leptin)–satiety interaction discussed previously.

Fat cell number increases during three general time periods:

1. Last trimester of pregnancy
2. First year of life
3. Adolescent growth spurt

The total number of fat cells probably cannot be altered to any significant degree during adulthood. Removing large amounts of fat by surgically excising fat

Questions & Notes

Give the calorie expenditure per min for a 160-pound person for each of the following activities: (Hint: see Close-up Box 16.6).

Intense aerobic dance:

Golf:

Running (7 min per mile pace):

Swimming (slow crawl stroke):

Does resting metabolism increase or decrease with dieting?

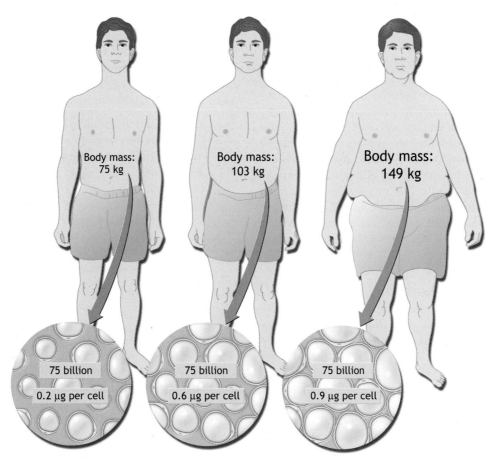

Figure 16.28 Changes in adipose cellularity with weight reduction in obese subjects. (Data from Hirsch, J.: Adipose cellularity in relation to human obesity. In: Stollerman GH, ed. *Advances in Internal Medicine*, Vol 17. Chicago: Year-Book, 1971.)

deposits at selected body sites (liposuction), according to the American Society of Plastic Surgeons (*www.plastic-surgery.org*), has become the third most popular cosmetic procedure in the United States (245,000 procedures in 2008; 30% decline since 2000). Liposuction does not change the person's metabolic profile (i.e., concentration of the hormone leptin, blood cholesterol, triacylglycerols, and blood pressure and insulin levels). Even removing 20 lb of fat from the abdomen in severely obese women did not improve important risk factors for heart disease. Future research needs to determine if removal of deep visceral or storage fat gives more promising health results than liposuction, which primarily removes "pinchable" subcutaneous fat.

New Fat Cells Can Develop

In adult-onset severe obesity, new adipocytes develop in addition to the hypertrophy of existing cells as the person becomes even fatter. This probably occurs because fat cells have an upper-size limit of about 1.0 μg of lipid per cell. In massively obese individuals with 60% body fat (170% of normal weight), almost all adipocytes achieve a hypertrophic limit; for the person to add fat, new cells must proliferate from a preadipocyte cell pool.

How to Select a Diet Plan

The most difficult aspect of dieting involves deciding exactly what foods to include in the daily menu. One can choose from literally hundreds of diet plans—water diets, drinker's diets, zone diets, fruit or vegetable diets, fast-food diets, eat-to-win diets, and diets named after cities (e.g., South Beach, Scarsdale, Hollywood, Beverly Hills) and people (Atkins, Jenny Craig, Ornish, Pritikin, Richard Simmons, Perricone, Suzanne Somers), including the potentially dangerous varieties of high-fat, low-carbohydrate, and liquid-protein diets. Some zealots even state that total caloric intake should *not* be considered but rather the order of eating foods! For individuals desperate to shed excess weight, the tremendous amount of misinformation available in the mainstream media (Internet and TV infomercials) encourages and then reinforces negative eating behaviors, unfortunately causing another repeat cycle of failure.

Low-Carbohydrate Ketogenic Diets *Ketogenic diets emphasize carbohydrate restriction while generally ignoring total calories and the diet's cholesterol and saturated fat content.* Billed as a "diet revolution" and championed by the late Dr. Robert C. Atkins (1930–2003), the diet was first promoted in the late 1800s and has appeared in various forms since then. Long disparaged by the medical establishment, advocates maintain that restricting daily carbohydrate intake to 20 g or less for the initial 2 weeks, with some liberalization afterward, causes the body to mobilize considerable fat for energy. This generates excess plasma ketone bodies—byproducts of incomplete fat

breakdown from inadequate carbohydrate catabolism; ketones supposedly suppress appetite. Theoretically, the ketones lost in the urine represent unused energy that should further facilitate weight loss. Some advocates claim that urinary energy loss becomes so great that dieters can eat all they want as long as they restrict carbohydrates.

The singular focus of the low-carbohydrate diet craze may eventually reduce caloric intake despite claims that dieters need not consider calorie intake as long as lipid represents the excess. Initial weight loss may also result largely from dehydration caused by an extra solute load on the kidneys that increases water excretion. Water loss does *not* reduce body fat. Low-carbohydrate intake also sets the stage for lean tissue loss because the body recruits amino acids from muscle to maintain blood glucose via gluconeogenesis—an undesirable side effect for a diet designed to induce body fat loss.

Three clinical trials compared the Atkins-type, low-carbohydrate diet with traditional low-fat diets for weight loss. The low-carbohydrate diet was more effective in achieving a modest weight loss for severely overweight persons. Some measures of heart health also improved as reflected by a more favorable lipid profile and glycemic control in those who followed the low-carbohydrate diet for up to 1 year. Such findings add a measure of credibility to low-carbohydrate diets and challenge conventional wisdom concerning the potential dangers from consuming a high-fat diet.

Importantly, Atkins-type, high-fat, low-carbohydrate diets require systematic long-term evaluation (≥5 years) for safety and effectiveness, particularly related to the blood lipid profile. The diet, which places no limit on the amount of meat, fat, eggs, and cheese a person consumes, poses nine potential health hazards:

1. Raises serum uric acid levels
2. Potentiates development of kidney stones
3. Alters electrolyte concentrations to initiate cardiac arrhythmias
4. Causes acidosis
5. Aggravates existing kidney problems from the extra solute burden in the renal filtrate
6. Depletes glycogen reserves, contributing to a fatigued state
7. Decreases calcium balance and increases risk for bone loss
8. Causes dehydration
9. Retards fetal development during pregnancy from inadequate carbohydrate intake

For high-performance endurance athletes who train at or above 70% of maximum effort, switching to a high-fat diet remains ill advised because the body needs to maintain adequate blood glucose and glycogen packed in the active muscles and liver storage depots. Fatigue during intense exercise for more than 60 minutes occurs more rapidly when athletes consume high-fat meals than with carbohydrate-rich meals.

High-Protein Diets Low-carbohydrate, high-protein diets may shed pounds in the short term, but their long-term success remains questionable and may even pose health risks. These diets have been promoted to obese individuals as "last-chance diets." Earlier versions consisted of protein in liquid form advertised as a "miracle liquid." Unknown to the consumer, the liquid protein mixture often contained a blend of ground-up animal hooves and horns, with pigskin mixed in a broth with enzymes and tenderizers to "predigest" it. Collagen-based blends produced from gelatin hydrolysis supplemented with small amounts of essential amino acids did not contain the highest quality amino acid mixture and lacked required vitamins and minerals particularly copper. A negative copper balance coincides with electrocardiographic abnormalities and a rapid heart rate. Protein-rich foods often contain high levels of saturated fat, which increase the risk for heart disease and type 2 diabetes. Diets excessively high in animal protein increase urinary excretion of oxalate, a compound that combines primarily with calcium to form kidney stones. The diet's safety improves if it contains high-quality protein with ample carbohydrate, essential fatty acids, and micronutrients.

Some argue that an extremely high protein intake suppresses appetite through reliance on fat mobilization and subsequent ketone formation. The elevated thermic effect of dietary protein, with its relatively low coefficient of digestibility particularly for plant protein, reduces the net calories available from ingested protein compared with a well-balanced meal of equivalent caloric value. This point has some validity, but one must consider other factors when formulating a sound weight loss program, particularly for physically active individuals. A high-protein diet has the potential to promote these four deleterious outcomes:

1. Strain on liver and kidney function and accompanying dehydration
2. Electrolyte imbalance
3. Glycogen depletion
4. Lean tissue loss

Semistarvation Diets A therapeutic fast or **very low-calorie diet** (VLCD) may benefit severe clinical obesity when body fat exceeds 40% to 50% of body mass. The diet provides between 400 and 800 kCal daily as high-quality protein foods or liquid meal replacements. Dietary prescriptions usually last up to 3 months but only as a "last resort" before undertaking more extreme medical approaches for morbid obesity that include various surgical treatments collectively called bariatric surgery. Surgical treatments that considerably reduce the stomach size and reconfigure the small intestine induce a sustained weight loss, but they are generally prescribed for patients with a BMI of at least 40 or a BMI of 35 when accompanied by other obesity-related medical conditions.

Dieting with VLCD requires close supervision, usually in a hospital setting. Proponents maintain that severe food restriction breaks established dietary habits, which in turn improves the long-term prospects for success. These diets may also depress the appetite to help compliance. Daily medications that accompany a VLCD diet include calcium carbonate for nausea, bicarbonate of soda and potassium chloride to maintain consistency of body fluids, mouthwash and sugar-free chewing gum for bad breath (from a high level of ketones from fatty acid catabolism), and bath oils for dry skin. *For most individuals, semistarvation does not compose an "ultimate diet" or proper approach to weight control.* Because a VLCD diet provides inadequate carbohydrate, the glycogen storage depots in the liver and muscles deplete rapidly. This impairs physical tasks that require either intense aerobic effort or shorter duration anaerobic power output. The continuous nitrogen loss with fasting and weight loss reflects an exacerbated lean tissue loss, which may occur disproportionately from critical organs such as the heart. The success rate remains poor for prolonged fasting.

Questions & Notes

List the 3 time periods generally associated with fat cell hyperplasia.

1.

2.

3.

Describe the condition under which new fat cells can develop in adults.

Describe the basis of ketogenic diets.

List 3 possible health risks from consuming a high protein low carb diet.

1.

2.

3.

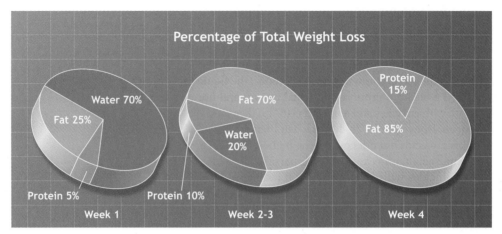

Figure 16.29 General trend for the percentage composition of the weight lost during 4 weeks of caloric restriction.

STRATEGIES TO EFFECT WEIGHT LOSS

Hydration level and duration of the energy deficit affect the amount and composition of weight lost.

Early Weight Loss Is Largely Water

Figure 16.29 presents the general trend for the percentage composition of daily weight loss during 4 weeks of dieting. Approximately 70% of weight lost over the first week of energy deficit consists of water loss. Thereafter, water loss progressively lessens, representing only about 20% of the weight lost in the second and third weeks; concurrently, body fat loss accelerates from 25% to 70%. During the fourth week of dieting, reductions in body fat produce about 85% of the weight loss without further increase in water loss. Protein's contribution to weight loss increases from 5% initially to about 15% after the fourth week. In practical terms, counseling efforts should emphasize that the weight lost during the initial attempts to reduce weight, when successful, consists chiefly of water and not fat; it takes approximately 4 weeks to establish the desired pattern of fat loss for each pound of weight loss.

Hydration Level

Restricting water during the first several days of a caloric deficit increases the proportion of body water lost and decreases the proportion of fat lost. More total weight loss occurs with restricted daily water intake, with the additional weight lost solely from water as dehydration progresses. Dieters lose the same quantity of body fat regardless of fluid intake level.

Longer Term Deficit Promotes Fat Loss

Figure 16.30 reinforces the important general concept that the caloric equivalent of the weight lost increases as

duration of caloric restriction progresses. After 2 months on a diet, the caloric equivalent of weight loss exceeds twice that in the first week. This points out the importance of maintaining a caloric deficit for an extended duration. Shorter periods of caloric restriction produce a larger percentage of water and carbohydrate loss per unit weight reduction with only a minimal decrease in body fat.

EXERCISE CREATES A TIPPING POINT IN THE ENERGY BALANCE EQUATION

Despite debates about contributions of physical inactivity and excessive caloric intake to body fat accretion, a sedentary lifestyle consistently emerges as an important factor in weight gain by children, adolescents, and adults.

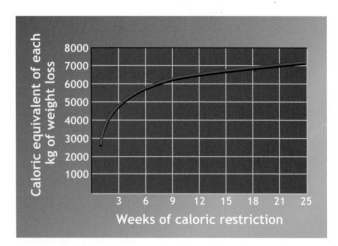

Figure 16.30 General trend for the energy equivalent of the weight lost in relation to duration of caloric restriction. As caloric restriction progresses the energy equivalent per unit of weight lost increases to about 7000 kCal per kilogram after 20 weeks. This occurs because of the large initial body water loss (no calorie value) early in weight loss.

Physically active men and women usually maintain a desirable body composition. An increased level of regular physical activity combined with dietary restraint maintains weight loss more effectively than long-term caloric restriction alone. A negative energy balance induced by increased caloric expenditure, through either lifestyle activities or formal exercise programs, unbalances the energy balance equation for weight loss, improves physical fitness and the health risk profile, and favorably alters body composition and body fat distribution for children and adults. Regular exercise produces less accumulation of central adipose tissue associated with aging. Overweight women show a dose–response relationship between amount of exercise and long-term weight loss. Obese adolescents and adults improve body composition and visceral fat distribution from both moderate physical activity or more vigorous exercise that improves cardiovascular fitness, with more intense physical activity being most effective. Additional benefits of regular exercise includes slowing of the age-related loss in muscle mass, possible prevention of adult-onset obesity, improvement in obesity-related comorbidities, decreased mortality, and beneficial effects on existing chronic diseases.

Two Misconceptions About Exercise

Two arguments attempt to counter the increased physical activity approach to weight loss. One maintains that exercise inevitably increases appetite to produce a proportionate increase in food intake that negates the caloric deficit that increased physical activity produces. The second argument claims that the relatively small calorie-burning effect of a normal exercise workout does not "dent" the body's fat reserves as effectively as food restriction.

Misconception 1: Increased Physical Activity and Food Intake
Sedentary persons often do not balance their energy intake and energy expenditure. Failure to accurately regulate energy balance at the lower end of the physical activity spectrum contributes to the "creeping obesity" observed in highly mechanized and technically advanced societies. In contrast, regular exercisers maintain appetite control within a reactive zone where food intake more readily matches daily energy expenditure.

In considering the effects of exercise on appetite and food intake, one must distinguish between exercise type and duration and the participant's body fat status. Lumberjacks, farm laborers, and endurance athletes consume about twice as many daily calories as sedentary individuals. More specifically, marathon runners, cross-country skiers, and cyclists consume about 4000 to 5000 kCal daily, yet they are the leanest people in the population. Obviously, their large caloric intake meets the energy requirements of training while maintaining a relatively lean body composition.

For overweight or obese individuals, extra energy required for increased physical activity more than offsets moderate physical activity's small compensatory appetite-stimulating effect. To some extent, the large energy reserve of an overfat person makes it easier to tolerate weight loss and exercise without the obligatory increase in caloric intake typically observed for leaner counterparts. No difference emerged in fat, carbohydrate, or protein intake or total calories consumed for overweight men and women during 16 months of supervised, moderate-intensity exercise training compared with a sedentary control group. *In essence, a weak coupling exists between the short-term energy deficit induced by exercise and energy intake. Increased physical activity by overweight, sedentary individuals does not necessarily alter physiologic needs and automatically produce compensatory increases in food intake to balance additional energy expenditure.*

Misconception 2: Low Caloric Stress of Physical Activity   A second misconception concerns the negligible contribution to weight loss of the

Questions & Notes

Describe conditions under which you would recommend a VLCD eating plan.

Which determines the effectiveness of weight loss with low-energy diets: total energy intake or the mixture of macronutrients consumed?

During the first week of weight loss, does the body lose more water or fat per unit of weight lost?

What is one benefit factor determine an increase in the caloric equivalent of weight.

Discuss whether exercise effects appetite.

calories burned in typical exercise. Some argue correctly that it requires an inordinate amount of short-term exercise to lose just 0.45 kg of body fat examples include chopping wood for 10 hours, playing golf for 20 hours, performing mild calisthenics for 22 hours, or playing ping pong for 28 hours or volleyball for 32 hours. Consequently, a 2- or 3-month exercise regimen produces only a small fat loss in an overfat person. From a different perspective, if one played golf without a golf cart for 2 hours daily (350 kCal) 2 days per week (700 kCal), it would take about 5 weeks to lose 0.45 kg of body fat. Assuming the person plays year-round, golfing 2 days a week produces a 4.5-kg yearly fat loss provided food intake remains constant. Even an activity as innocuous as chewing gum burns an extra 11 kCal each hour, a 20% increase over normal resting metabolism. *Simply stated, the calorie-expending effects of increased physical activity add up. A caloric deficit of 3500 kCal equals a 0.45-kg body fat loss, whether the deficit occurs rapidly or systematically over time.*

Effectiveness of Regular Exercise

Adding physical activity to a weight loss program favorably modifies the composition of the weight lost in the direction of greater fat loss and maintains or even enhances physical performance capacity. This muscle-sparing effect of regular exercise is clearly illustrated in **Figure 16.31**, which compares the effect of about 10 pounds of weight loss over

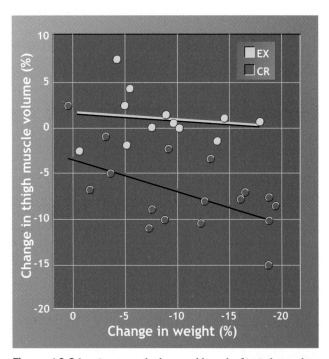

Figure 16.31 Conserve the lean and lose the fat. Relationship between the magnitude of weight loss and the magnitude of change in thigh muscle volume (sum of right and left thighs) in a group losing weight by only caloric restriction (CR) and a group losing weight by only exercise (EX) (From Weiss, E.P., et al.: Lower extremity muscle size and strength and aerobic capacity decrease with caloric restriction but not with exercise-induced weight loss. *J. Appl. Physiol.,* 102:534, 2007.)

12 months induced by either *only* caloric restriction or *only* exercise on MRI-assessed thigh muscle volume of 50- to 60-year-old men and women. Decreases in thigh muscle volume of 6.8% and composite knee flexion strength (–7.2%), and $\dot{V}O_{2max}$ (–6.8%) occurred only in the caloric restriction group, but $\dot{V}O_{2max}$ increased 15.5% in the group losing weight via exercise. Clearly, muscle mass, muscle strength, and aerobic capacity decline in response to 12 months of weight loss by caloric restriction but not in response to similar weight loss by exercise.

The effectiveness of regular physical activity for weight loss relates closely to the degree of excess body fat. Obese persons generally lose weight and fat more readily with increased physical activity than normal-weight persons. In addition, aerobic exercise and resistance training even without dietary restriction provide positive spin-off to the weight loss effort. They alter body composition favorably (reduced body fat with a small increase in FFM) for otherwise healthy overweight children, adolescents, and adults; postmenopausal women; cardiac patients; and physically challenged individuals. Regular exercise and improved aerobic fitness also target excess fat accumulation in the abdominal–visceral area to a greater extent than peripheral fat deposits. This response diminishes a tendency toward insulin resistance and predisposition to type 2 diabetes. **Table 16.7** shows the effects of regular exercise for weight loss by six sedentary, overfat young men who exercised 5 days a week for 16 weeks by walking 90 minutes each session. The men lost nearly 6 kg of body fat, a decrease in percentage body fat from 23.5% to 18.6%. Exercise capacity also improved as did high-density lipoprotein (HDL) cholesterol (15.6%) and the HDL-to-LDL (low-density lipoprotein) cholesterol ratio (25.9%).

Most of the health-related metabolic improvements with regular exercise in obese individuals relate to total exercise volume and quantity of fat loss rather than enhanced cardiorespiratory fitness. Ideal exercise consists of continuous, large-muscle activities with moderate to high caloric cost such as circuit resistance training, walking, running, rope skipping, stair stepping, cycling, and swimming. An expenditure of an extra 300 kCal daily (e.g., jogging for 30 minutes) should produce a 0.45-kg fat loss in about 12 days. This represents a yearly caloric deficit equivalent to the energy in 13.6 kg of body fat.

Figure 16.32 shows body composition changes for 40 obese women placed into one of four groups: (1) control group, no exercise and no diet; (2) diet-only, no exercise (DO) group; (3) diet plus resistance exercise (D+E); and (4) resistance exercise only, no diet (EO) group. The women trained 3 days a week for 8 weeks. They performed 10 repetitions each of three sets of eight strength exercises. Body mass decreased for the DO (–4.5 kg) and D+E groups (–3.9 kg) compared with the EO group (+0.5 kg) and control group (–0.4 kg). Importantly, whereas FFM increased in the EO group (+1 kg), the DO group lost 0.9 kg of FFM. The authors concluded that augmenting a calorie restriction program with resistance exercise training preserved FFM compared with dietary restriction alone.

Table 16.7	Effectiveness of a 16-Week Walking Program on Body Composition and Blood Lipid Changes in Six Overfat Young Men		
VARIABLE	**PRE-TRAINING**[a]	**POST-TRAINING**[a]	**DIFFERENCE**
Body mass (kg)	99.1	93.4	−5.7[b]
Body density, $g \cdot mL^{-1}$	1.044	1.056	+0.012[b]
Body fat (%)	23.5	18.6	−4.9[b]
Fat mass (kg)	23.3	17.4	−5.9[b]
Fat-free body mass (kg)	75.8	76.0	+0.2
Sum of skinfolds (mm)	142.9	104.8	−38.1[b]
HDL cholesterol, $mg \cdot dL^{-1}$	32.0	37.0	5.0[b]
HDL/LDL cholesterol	0.27	0.34	+0.07[b]

[a]Values are means.
[b]Statistically significant.
From Leon A.S. et al.: Effects of a vigorous walking program on body composition, and carbohydrate and lipid metabolism of obese young men. *Am. J. Clin. Nutr.* 33:1776, 1979.

Dose–Response Relationship *The total energy expended in physical activity relates in a dose–response manner to the effectiveness of exercise for weight loss. A reasonable goal progressively increases moderate exercise to between 60 and 90 minutes daily or a level that burns 2100 to 2800 kCal weekly.*

An overfat person who starts out with light exercise such as slow walking accrues a considerable caloric expenditure simply by extending exercise duration. The focus on exercise duration offsets the inadvisability of having a sedentary, obese individual begin a program with more strenuous exercise. The energy cost of weight-bearing exercise relates directly to body mass, allowing the overweight person to expend considerably more calories in such exercise than someone of average weight.

Exercise Frequency To determine the optimal exercise frequency for weight loss, subjects exercised for 30 to 47 minutes for 20 weeks by either running or walking, with exercise intensity maintained between 80% and 95% of maximum heart rate. Training twice weekly produced no changes in body mass,

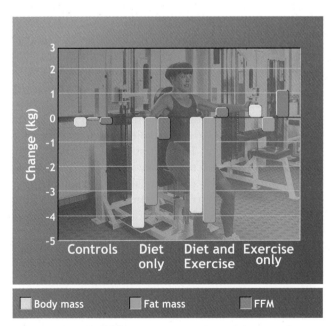

Figure 16.32 Changes in body composition with combinations of resistance exercise, diet, or both in obese women. (From Ballor, D.L., et al.: Resistance weight training during caloric restriction enhances lean body weight. *Am. J. Clin. Nutr.*, 47:19, 1988.)

Questions & Notes

For weight loss, is exercise volume or intensity more important?

Which component of body composition, is most affected by regular physical activity?

List 2 examples of the cumulative effects of regular physical activity designed for weight loss.

1.

2.

Explain why it is desirable to add resistance exercises to aerobic training to enhance body composition changes during weight loss.

What effect does regular exercise have on insulin resistance, independent of weight loss?

What is the optimal exercise frequency to promote weight loss?

skinfolds, or percentage body fat, but training 3 and 4 days weekly did. Subjects who trained 4 days a week reduced their body weight and skinfolds more than subjects who trained 3 days a week. The percentage body fat decreased similarly in both groups. These findings support a recommendation to exercise a *minimum* of 3 days per week to favorably alter body composition; the additional caloric expenditure with more frequent exercise produces even greater results. The threshold exercise energy expenditure for weight loss probably remains highly individualized. The calorie-burning effect of each exercise session should eventually reach *at least* 300 kCal whenever possible. This generally occurs with 30 minutes of moderate to vigorous running, swimming, bicycling, or circuit resistance training or 60 minutes of brisk walking.

Self-Selected Energy Expenditures: Mode of Exercise

No selective effect exists among diverse modes of large-muscle aerobic exercise to favorably reduce body weight, body fat, skinfold thickness, and girths, yet other differences may emerge. For individuals without physical activity limitations, running usually provides the most suitable exercise mode for maximizing energy expenditure during self-selected intensities of continuous exercise.

THE IDEAL COMBINATION FOR SUCCESS: CALORIC RESTRAINT PLUS EXERCISE

Combinations of increased physical activity and caloric restraint offer considerably more flexibility for achieving a negative caloric imbalance than either exercise alone or diet alone. Dietary restraint plus increased physical activity through lifestyle changes offers health and weight loss benefits similar to those from combining dietary restraint and a vigorous program of structured exercise. Adding exercise to a weight control program facilitates longer term maintenance of fat loss than total reliance on either food restriction alone or increased exercise alone. Table 16.8 summarizes eight benefits of exercise in a weight loss program.

MAINTENANCE OF GOAL BODY WEIGHT

The popular and scientific literature, including TV reality shows, is replete with success stories of individuals who have lost considerable amounts of weight using different interventions that include nutritional, exercise, and behavioral approaches.

Success of the National Weight Control Registry

A project in the National Weight Control Registry (NWCR; *www.nwcr.ws*) recruited 784 individuals (629 women;

Table 16.8	Eight Benefits of Adding Exercise to Dietary Restriction for Weight Loss

1. Increases overall size of the energy deficit
2. Facilitates lipid mobilization and oxidation, especially from visceral adipose tissue deposits
3. Increases relative body fat loss by preserving fat-free body mass
4. Blunts the decrease in resting metabolism that accompanies weight loss by conserving and even increasing fat-free body mass
5. Requires less reliance on caloric restriction to create an energy deficit
6. Contributes to long-term success of the weight loss effort
7. Provides significant health-related benefits
8. Offsets the deterioration in immune system function that often accompanies weight loss

155 men), the largest database of individuals who successfully achieved prolonged weight loss. Criteria for NWCR membership included age 18 years or older and maintenance of weight loss of at least 30 pounds (13.6 kg) for 1 year or longer. Participants averaged 66 pounds (30 kg) of weight loss, and 14% lost more than 100 pounds (45.4 kg). Members maintained the required minimum 30-pound weight loss for a 5.5-year average, and 16% maintained the loss for 10 years or longer. Most participants had been overweight since childhood; nearly 50% had one overweight parent, and more than 25% had both parents overweight. *Genetic background may have predisposed these persons to obesity, but an impressive weight loss and its maintenance proves that heredity alone need not predestine a person to the obese condition.*

About 55% of the NWCR members used either a formal program or professional assistance to reduce weight; the rest succeeded on their own. Regarding weight loss methods, 89% modified their food intake and maintained relatively high physical activity levels (2800 kCal weekly on average) to achieve goal weight loss. Many walked briskly for at least 1 hour daily. About 92% exercised at home, and one-third exercised regularly with friends. Whereas women primarily walked and did aerobic dancing, men chose competitive sports and resistance training. Only 10% relied solely on diet, and 1% used exercise exclusively. The diet strategy of nearly 90% of participants restricted intake of certain types or amounts of foods—44% counted calories, 33% limited lipid intake, and 25% restricted grams of lipid. Forty-four percent ate the same foods they normally ate but in reduced amounts (Table 16.9).

A follow-up study in 2008 provides additional details about the weekly energy expenditure patterns among the men and women enrolled in the NWCR between 1993 and 2004. Interestingly, participants expended an average of 2621 kCal·wk^{-1} in physical activity, but the range of expenditure (2252 kCal·wk^{-1}) was almost as large as the average. Approximately 25.3% reported less than 1000 kCal·wk^{-1} in physical activity, and 34.9% reported

Table 16.9	Dietary Strategies to Achieve Weight Loss of Participants of the National Weight Control Registry (*top*) and Effects of Weight Loss on Various Dimensions of Life as Reported by Participants (*bottom*)

| | PERCENTAGE | | |
STRATEGY	WOMEN	MEN	TOTAL
Restricted intake of certain types or classes of food	87.8	86.7	87.6
Ate all foods but limited the quantity	47.2	32.0	44.2
Counted calories	44.8	39.3	43.7
Limited % lipid intake	31.1	36.7	33.1
Counted lipid grams	25.7	21.3	25.2
Followed exchange diet	25.2	11.3	22.5
Used liquid formula	19.1	26.0	20.4
Ate only 1 or 2 food types	5.1	6.7	5.5

| | PERCENTAGE | | |
AREA OF LIFE	IMPROVED	NO DIFFERENCE	WORSENED
Quality of life	95.3	4.3	0.4
Level of energy	92.4	6.7	0.9
Mobility	92.3	7.1	0.6
General mood	91.4	6.9	1.6
Self-confidence	90.9	9.0	0.1
Physical health	85.8	12.9	1.3
Interactions with:			
Opposite sex	65.2	32.9	0.9
Same sex	5.0	46.8	0.4
Strangers	69.5	30.4	0.1
Job performance	54.5	45.0	0.6
Hobbies	49.1	36.7	0.4
Spouse interactions	56.3	37.3	5.9

From Klem MI, et al.: A descriptive study of individuals successful at longterm maintenance of substantial weight loss. *Am. J. Clin. Nutr.* 66:239, 1997.

Questions & Notes

Is it possible to gain muscle and lose fat during weight loss? Explain.

List 4 benefits of adding exercise to dietary restriction for weight loss.

1.

2.

3.

4.

Discuss the effectiveness of specific exercises to achieve a spot-reducing effect.

When gaining weight, what type of exercises are most beneficial?

less than 3000 kCal·wk^{-1}. The amount of activity reported by men decreased over time, but no change was observed in women. The large amount of individual variability in energy expenditure of successful "weight losers" makes it extremely difficult to pinpoint what amount of activity would constitute optimum to maintain weight loss.

Can Targeted Exercise Selectively Reduce Local Fat Deposits?

The notion of spot reduction stems from the belief that an increase in a muscle's metabolic activity stimulates relatively greater fat mobilization from the adipose tissue in proximity to the active muscle. As such, exercising a specific body area region to "sculpt" it should selectively reduce more fat from that area than exercising a different muscle group at the same metabolic intensity. Advocates of spot reduction recommend performing large numbers of sit-ups or side-bends to reduce excessive abdominal and hip fat. The promise of spot reduction with exercise seems attractive from an aesthetic and health risk standpoint—unfortunately, critical evaluation of the research evidence does not support its use.

To examine claims for spot reduction, researchers compared the girths and subcutaneous fat stores of the right and left forearms of high-caliber tennis

i For Your Information

EXCESS CALORIES ACCUMULATE FAT

Each 0.45 kg (1 lb) of adipose tissue contains about 87% pure lipid or 3500 kcal (395 g × 9 kcal·g^{-1}). An excess intake of 3500 kCal accumulates 0.45 kg of extra fat. Magic potions, trick diets, or special formula foods cannot undo this strategic ratio.

players. As expected, the girths of the dominant or playing arms exceeded the girths of nondominant arms because of a modest muscular hypertrophy from the exercise overload of tennis. Measurements of skinfold thickness, however, clearly showed that regular and prolonged tennis exercise did not reduce subcutaneous fat in the playing arm. Another study evaluated fat biopsy specimens from abdominal, subscapular, and buttock sites before and after 27 days of sit-up exercise training. The number of sit-ups increased from 140 at the end of the first week to 336 on day 27. Despite the considerable amount of localized exercise, adipocytes in the abdominal region were no smaller than adipocytes in the unexercised buttocks or subscapular control regions.

Undoubtedly, the negative energy balance created through regular exercise contributes to reducing total body fat. Conventional wisdom maintains that exercise stimulates mobilization of fatty acids via hormones and enzymes that act on fat depots throughout the body, not simply from areas closest to the active muscle mass. In this connection, recent advances in microinvasive measurements of subcutaneous adipose tissue (SCAT) make it possible to study if localized lipolysis is possible with localized exercise. One study estimated blood flow and lipolysis in femoral SCAT adjacent to contracting and resting skeletal muscle during one-legged knee extension exercise at 25% of maximum. Blood flow and SCAT lipolysis were higher adjacent to contracting muscle versus adjacent to resting muscle independent of exercise intensity. Whether this translates to sustained fat loss at a particular site remains unknown, and additional experiments certainly seem warranted.

GAINING WEIGHT

For most people, weight loss to reduce body fat and improve overall health and aesthetic appearance becomes the primary focus of any attempt to alter body composition. Many individuals desire to gain weight to improve the body composition profile or performance in sports or exercises that require muscular strength and power. This goal poses a unique dilemma that is not easily resolved. Gaining weight per se occurs all too easily by tilting the body's energy balance to favor greater caloric intake. In a sedentary person, an accumulated excess intake of 3500 kCal produces a body fat gain of 1 pound because adipocytes store the excess calories. Weight gain for athletes should ideally occur in the form of lean tissue, specifically muscle mass and accompanying connective tissue. Generally, this form of weight gain takes place if an increased caloric intake (adequate carbohydrate for energy and protein sparing and enough protein for tissue synthesis) accompanies the proper exercise regimen. Athletes attempting to increase muscle mass often fall easy prey to health food and diet supplement manufacturers who market "high-potency, tissue-building" substances, including chromium, boron, vanadyl sulfate, β-hydroxy-methyl butyrate, and various protein and amino acid mixture, none of which reliably increases muscle mass.

Increase Lean, Not Body Fat Mass

Endurance exercise training usually increases FFM only slightly, but the overall effect reduces body weight because of fat loss from the calorie-burning and possible appetite-depressing effects of this exercise mode. In contrast, muscular overload through resistance training, supported by adequate energy and protein intake (with sufficient recovery), increases muscle mass and strength. Adequate energy intake ensures that no catabolism of protein available for muscle growth occurs from an energy deficit. *Thus, intense aerobic training should not coincide with resistance training to increase muscle mass.* More than likely, the added energy (and perhaps protein) demands of concurrent resistance and aerobic exercise training impose a limit on muscle growth and responsiveness to resistance training. In addition, on the molecular level, aerobic exercise training may inhibit signaling to the protein synthesis machinery of skeletal muscle to negatively impact the muscle's adaptive response to resistance training. A prudent recommendation increases daily protein intake to about 1.6 g per kg of body mass during the resistance-training period. The individual should consume a variety of plant and animal proteins; relying solely on animal protein which is high in saturated fatty acids and cholesterol potentially increases heart disease risk.

If all calories consumed in excess of the energy requirement during resistance training sustained muscle growth, then 2000 to 2500 extra kCal could supply each 0.5-kg increase in lean tissue. In practical terms, 700 to 1000 kCal added to a well-balanced daily meal plan supports a weekly 0.5- to 1.0-kg gain in lean tissue and additional energy needs for training.

HOW MUCH GAIN TO EXPECT

A 1-year program of intense resistance training for young, athletic men increases body mass by about 20%, mostly from lean tissue accrual. The rate of lean tissue gain rapidly plateaus as training progresses beyond the first year. For athletic women, first-year gains in lean tissue mass average 50% to 75% of the absolute values for men, probably from women's smaller initial LBM. Individual differences in the daily quantity of nitrogen incorporated into body protein and protein incorporated into muscle also limit and explain differences among persons in muscle mass increases with resistance training.

Individuals with relatively high androgen-to-estrogen ratios and greater percentages of fast-twitch muscle fibers probably increase their lean tissue to the greatest extent. Muscle mass increases most at the start of training in individuals with the largest relative FFM corrected for stature and body fat. Regularly monitoring body mass and body fat verifies whether the combination of training and additional food intake increases lean tissue and not body fat. This requires a valid appraisal of body composition at regular intervals throughout the training period.

SUMMARY

1. Three methods can unbalance the energy balance equation to create weight loss: (1) reduce energy intake below daily energy expenditure, (2) maintain normal energy intake and increase energy output, and (3) combine both methods and decrease food intake and increase energy expenditure.

2. Long-term maintenance of weight loss through dietary restriction has a success rate of less than 20%. Typically, one- to two-thirds of the lost weight returns within 1 year, and almost all of it returns within 5 years.

3. A caloric deficit of 3500 kCal created through either diet or exercise equals the calories in 1 pound (0.45 kg) of body fat.

4. Disadvantages of extreme semistarvation include loss of lean body tissue, lethargy, possible malnutrition and metabolic disorders, and decrease in the basal energy expenditure.

5. Adipocyte number stabilizes sometime before adulthood; any weight gain or loss thereafter usually relates to a change in fat cell size. In extreme obesity, cell number can increase after adipocytes reach their hypertrophic limit.

6. Increases in adipocyte number involve three general time periods: the last trimester of pregnancy, the first year of life, and the adolescent growth spurt before adulthood.

7. The calories expended in exercise accumulate; a modest amount of extra exercise performed routinely creates a dramatic calorie-burning effect over time.

8. For previously sedentary, overfat men and women, moderate increases in physical activity do not necessarily increase food intake proportionately. Most individuals consume adequate calories to counterbalance caloric expenditure.

9. Combining exercise and caloric restriction offers a flexible yet effective means to weight control. Exercise enhances fat mobilization and utilization for energy, improves insulin sensitivity, and retards lean tissue loss.

10. Rapid weight loss during the first few days of caloric deficit comes mainly from body water loss and glycogen depletion. Continued weight reduction occurs at the expense of greater fat loss per unit weight loss.

11. Successful weight losers generally rely on both food intake and physical activity to achieve their goal weight. Increased physical activity for weight maintenance represents a significant component for these individuals.

12. A triggering event or incident (medical, emotional, lifestyle, weight incident, inspirational) usually precedes successful weight loss. For weight loss success, intervention strategies must couple with "readiness criteria."

13. Selective fat reduction of specific body areas by targeted or "spot exercise" does not occur.

14. The areas of greatest body fat concentration or lipid-mobilizing enzyme activity supply the greatest amount of energy.

15. Athletes should gain weight as lean body tissue. This occurs with a modest increase in caloric intake plus systematic resistance training.

THOUGHT QUESTIONS

1. What strategy, advice, and words of encouragement can you offer to a person who has attempted several diets yet never achieved long-term weight loss?

2. Respond to this comment: "The only way to lose weight is to stop eating. It's that simple!"

3. Outline a prudent yet effective plan for losing weight for a middle-age woman whose physician advises her to shed 20 pounds of excess weight. Provide the rationale for each of your recommendations.

SELECTED REFERENCES

Allen, T.W.: Body size, body composition, and cardiovascular disease risk factors in NFL players. *Phys. Sportsmed.*, 38:21, 2010.

Ansari, R.M.: Effect of physical activity and obesity on type 2 diabetes in a middle-aged population. *J. Environ. Public Health*, 195:285, 2009.

Arner, E., et al.: Adipocyte turnover: relevance to human adipose tissue morphology. *Diabetes.* 59:105, 2010.

Arsenault, B.J., et al.: Body composition, cardiorespiratory fitness, and low-grade inflammation in middle-aged men and women. *Am. J. Cardiol.*, 104:240, 2009.

Ballard, T.P., et al.: Comparison of Bod Pod and DXA in female collegiate athletes. *Med. Sci. Sports Exerc.*, 36:731, 2004.

Behnke, A.R., Wilmore, J.H.: *Evaluation and Regulation of Body Build and Composition.* Englewood Cliffs, NJ: Prentice Hall, 1974.

Behnke, A.R., et al.: The specific gravity of healthy men. *JAMA.*, 118:495, 1942.

Booth, F.W., et al.: Waging war on modern chronic diseases: primary prevention through exercise biology. *J. Appl. Physiol.*, 88:774, 2000.

Bouchard, C.: Defining the genetic architecture of the predisposition to obesity: a challenging but not insurmountable task. *Am. J. Clin. Nutr.*, 91:5, 2010.

Bouchard, C.: Human variation in body mass: evidence for a role of the genes. *Nutr. Rev.*, 55(Suppl):S21, 1997.

Brandon, L.J.: Comparison of existing skinfold equations for estimating body fat in African American and white women. *Am. J. Clin. Nutr.*, 67:1115, 1998.

Brozek, J., et al.: Densitometric analysis of body composition: revision of some quantitative assumptions. *Ann. N.Y. Acad. Sci.*, 110:113, 1963.

Buchan, D.S., et al.: The influence of a high intensity physical activity intervention on a selection of health related outcomes: an ecological approach. *B.M.C. Public Health.*, 10:8, 2010.

Burton, R.F., Cameron, N.: Body fat and skinfold thicknesses: a dimensional analytic approach. *Ann. Hum. Biol.*, 36:717, 2009.

Cameron, N., et al.: Regression equations to estimate percentage body fat in African prepubertal children aged 9 y. *Am. J. Clin. Nutr.*, 80:70, 2004.

Carbuhn, A.F.: Sport and training influence bone and body composition in women collegiate athletes. *J. Strength Cond. Res.*, 24:1710, 2010.

Cartier, A., et al.: Sex differences in inflammatory markers: what is the contribution of visceral adiposity? *Am. J. Clin. Nutr.* 89:1307, 2009.

Chakravarthy, M.V., Booth, F.W.: Eating, exercise, and "thrifty" genotypes: connecting the dots toward an evolutionary understanding of modern chronic diseases. *J. Appl. Physiol.*, 96:10, 2004.

Chaput J.P., et al.: Risk factors for adult overweight and obesity in the Quebec Family Study: have we been barking up the wrong tree? *Obesity (Silver Spring)*, 17:1964, 2009.

Chaput J.P., Tremblay A.: Obesity and physical inactivity: the relevance of reconsidering the notion of sedentariness. *Obes. Facts*, 2:249, 2009.

Clark, R.R., et al.: Minimum weight prediction methods cross-validated by the four-component model. *Med. Sci. Sports Exerc.*, 36:639, 2004.

Clarys, J.P., et al.: Gross tissue weights in the human body by cadaver dissection. *Hum. Biol.*, 56:459, 1984.

Collins, A.L., et al.: Within- and between-laboratory precision in the measurement of body volume using air displacement plethysmography and its effect on body composition assessment. *Int. J. Obes. Relat. Metab. Disord.*, 28:80, 2004.

Coppini, L.Z., et al.: Limitations and validation of bioelectrical impedance analysis in morbidly obese patients. *Curr. Opin. Clin. Nutr. Metab. Care.*, 8:329, 2005.

Dietz, W.H.: Health consequences of obesity in youth: childhood predictors of adult disease. *Pediatrics*, 101:518, 1998.

Diliberti, N., et al.: Increased portion size leads to increased energy intake in a restaurant meal. *Obes. Res.*, 12:562, 2004.

Donnelly, J.E., et al.: Physical activity across the curriculum (PAAC): a randomized controlled trial to promote physical activity and diminish overweight and obesity in elementary school children. *Prev. Med.*, 49:336, 2009.

Dorsey, K.B., et al.: Diagnosis, evaluation, and treatment of childhood obesity in pediatric practice. *Arch. Pediatr. Adolesc. Med.*, 159:632, 2005.

Ebbeling, C.B., et al.: Compensation for energy intake from fast food among overweight and lean adolescents. *JAMA.*, 291:2828, 2004.

Elsawy, B., Higgins, K.E.: Physical activity guidelines for older adults. *Am. Fam. Physician*, 81:55, 2010.

Farpour-Lambert N.J., et al.: Physical activity reduces systemic blood pressure and improves early markers of atherosclerosis in pre-pubertal obese children. *J. Am. Coll. Cardiol.*, 54:2396, 2009.

Fernández, J.R., et al.: Is percentage body fat differentially related to body mass index in Hispanic Americans, African Americans, and European Americans? *Am. J. Clin. Nutr.*, 77:71, 2003.

Fields, D.A., et al.: Assessment of body composition by air-displacement plethysmography: influence of body temperature and moisture. *Dyn. Med.*, 3:3, 2004.

Flegal, K.M., et al.: Excess deaths associated with underweight, overweight, and obesity. *JAMA.*, 293:1861, 2005.

Frank, L.L., et al.: Effects of exercise on metabolic risk variables in overweight postmenopausal women: a randomized clinical trial. *Obes. Res.*, 13:615, 2005.

Freedson, P.A., et al.: Physique, body composition, and psychological characteristics of competitive female body builders. *Phys. Sports Med.*, 11:85, 1983.

Frisch, R.E., et al.: Lower lifetime occurrence of breast cancer and cancers of the reproductive system among former college athletes. *Am. J. Clin. Nutr.*, 45:328, 1987.

Garcia, A.L., et al.: Improved prediction of body fat by measuring skinfold thickness, circumferences, and bone breadths. *Obes. Res.*, 13:626, 2005.

Giannopoulou, I., et al.: Exercise is required for visceral fat loss in postmenopausal women with type 2 diabetes. *J. Clin. Endocrinol. Metab.*, 90:1511, 2005.

Gregg, E.W., et al.: Secular trends in cardiovascular disease risk factors according to body mass index in US adults. *JAMA.*, 293:1868, 2005.

Haroun, D., et al.: Composition of the fat-free mass in obese and nonobese children: matched case-control analyses. *Int. J. Obes. Relat. Metab. Disord.*, 29:29, 2005.

Hedley, A., et al.: Prevalence of overweight and obesity among US children, adolescents, and adults, 1999–2002. *JAMA.*, 291:2847, 2004.

Hirsch, J., Batchelor, B.R.: Adipose tissue cellularity in human obesity. *Clin. Endocrinol. Metab.*, 5:299, 1976.

Hirsch, J., et al.: Diet composition and energy balance in humans. *Am. J. Clin. Nutr.*, 67(Suppl):551S, 1998.

Jackson, A.J., et al.: Body mass index bias in defining obesity of diverse young adults. The Training Intervention and Genetics of Exercise Response (TIGER) Study. *Br. J. Nutr.*, 102:1084, 2009.

Jackson, A.S., Pollock, M.L.: Generalized equations for predicting body density of men. *Br. J. Nutr.*, 40:497, 1978.

Jakicic, J.M., Gallagher, K.I.: Exercise considerations for the sedentary, overweight adult. *Exerc. Sport Sci. Rev.*, 31:91, 2003.

Janssen, I., et al.: Body mass index and waist circumference independently contribute to prediction of nonabdominal, abdominal subcutaneous, and visceral fat. *Am. J. Clin. Nutr.*, 75:683, 2002.

Johnson W.D., et al.: Prevalence of risk factors for metabolic syndrome in adolescents: National Health and Nutrition Examination Survey (NHANES), 2001–2006. *Arch. Pediatr. Adolesc Med.*, 163:371, 2009.

Kah-Banerjee, P., et al.: Prospective study of the association of changes in dietary intake, physical activity, alcohol consumption, and smoking with 9-y gain in waist circumference among 16587 US men. *Am. J. Clin. Nutr.*, 78:719, 2003.

Kahn, H.S., Valdez, R.: Metabolic risks identified by the combination of enlarged waist and elevated triacylglycerol concentration. *Am. J. Clin. Nutr.*, 78:928, 2003.

Katch, F.I., Katch, V.L.: Measurement and prediction errors in body composition assessment and the search for the perfect prediction equation. *Res. Q. Exerc. Sport*, 51:249, 1980.

Katch, F.I., McArdle, W.D.: Prediction of body density from simple anthropometric measurements in college-age men and women. *Hum. Biol.*, 45:445, 1973.

Katch, F.I., McArdle, W.D.: Validity of body composition prediction equations for college men and women. *Am. J. Clin. Nutr.*, 28:105, 1975.

Katch, F.I., et al.: Effects of situp exercise training on adipose cell size and adiposity. *Res. Q. Exerc. Sport*, 55:242, 1984.

Katch, F.I., et al.: Validity of bioelectrical impedance to estimate body composition in cardiac and pulmonary patients. *Am. J. Clin. Nutr.*, 43:972, 1986.

Katch, V.L., et al.: Contribution of breast volume and weight to body fat distribution in females. *Am. J. Phys. Anthropol.*, 53:93, 1980.

Katch, V.L., et al.: The underweight female. *Phys. Sports Med.*, 8:55, 1980.

Katzmarzyk, P.T., et al.: Racial differences in abdominal depot-specific adiposity in white and African American adults. *Am. J. Clin. Nutr.*, 91:7, 2010.

Katzmarzyk, P.T., et al.: Sitting time and mortality from all causes, cardiovascular disease, and cancer. *Med. Sci. Sports Exerc.*, 41:998, 2009.

Keys, A., Brozek, J.: Body fat in adult men. *Physiol. Rev.*, 33:245, 1960.

Kim, J., et al.: Intramuscular adipose tissue-free skeletal muscle mass: estimation by dual-energy X-ray absorptiometry in adults. *J. Appl. Physiol.*, 97:655, 2004.

Kondo, M., et al.: Upper limit of fat-free mass in humans: a study of Japanese sumo wrestlers. *Am. J. Hum. Biol.*, 6:613, 1994.

Kullberg, J.: Adipose tissue distribution in children: automated quantification using water and fat MRI. *J. Magn. Reson. Imaging.*, 32:204, 2010.

Lang, T.: Computed tomographic measurements of thigh muscle cross-sectional area and attenuation coefficient predict hip fracture: the health, aging, and body composition study. *J. Bone Miner. Res.*, 25:513, 2010.

Lazzer, S., et al.: Assessment of energy expenditure associated with physical activities in free-living obese and nonobese adolescents. *Am. J. Clin. Nutr.*, 78:471, 2003.

Liu A, et al.: Differential intra-abdominal adipose tissue profiling in obese, insulin-resistant women. *Obes. Surg.*, 19:1564, 2009.

Loucks, A.B.: Energy availability, not body fatness, regulates reproductive function in women. *Exerc. Sport Sci. Rev.*, 31:144, 2003.

Maddalozzo, G.F., et al.: Concurrent validity of the BOD POD and dual energy x-ray absorptiometry techniques for assessing body composition in young women. *J. Am. Diet Assoc.*, 102:1677, 2002.

Mayo, M.J., et al.: Exercise-induced weight loss preferentially reduces abdominal fat. *Med. Sci. Sports Exerc.*, 35:207, 2003.

Mota, J.: Television viewing and changes in body mass index and cardiorespiratory fitness over a two-year period in schoolchildren. *Pediatr. Exerc. Sci.*, 22:245, 2010.

National Task Force on the Prevention and Treatment of Obesity: Obesity, overweight and health risk. *Arch. Intern Med.*, 160:898, 2000.

Oda, E., Kawai R.: Comparison among Body Mass Index (BM), Waist Circumference (WC), and Percent Body Fat (%BF) as Anthropometric Markers for the Clustering of Metabolic Risk Factors in Japanese. *Intern. Med.*, 49:1477, 2010.

Ostojic, S.M.: Adiposity, physical activity and blood lipid profile in 13-year-old adolescents. *J. Pediatr. Endocrinol. Metab.*, 23:333, 2010.

Pérusse, L., et al.: Familial aggregation of abdominal visceral fat level: results from the Quebec family. *Metabolism*, 45:378, 1996.

Peterson, M.J., et al.: Development and validation of skinfold-thickness prediction equations with a 4-compartment model. *Am. J. Clin. Nutr.*, 77:1186, 2003.

Pollock, M.L., et al.: Twenty-year follow-up of aerobic power and body composition of older track athletes. *J. Appl. Physiol.*, 82:1508, 1997.

Portal, S.: Body fat measurements in elite adolescent volleyball players: correlation between skinfold thickness, bioelectrical impedance analysis, air-displacement plethysmography, and body mass index percentiles. *J. Pediatr. Endocrinol. Metab.*, 23:395, 2010.

Rhéaume, C., et al.: Low cardiorespiratory fitness levels and elevated blood pressure: What is the contribution of visceral adiposity? *Hypertension*, 54:91, 2009.

Rolls B.J., et al.: The relationship between energy density and energy intake. *Physiol. Behav.*, 97:609, 2009.

Romaguera, D.: Dietary determinants of changes in waist circumference adjusted for body mass index—a proxy measure of visceral adiposity. *PLoS. One.*, 14: 5:e11588, 2010.

Sacks F.M., et al.: Comparison of weight-loss diets with different compositions of fat, protein, and carbohydrates. *N. Engl. J. Med.*, 360:859, 2009.

Schoeller, D.A.: Balancing energy expenditure and body weight. *Am. J. Clin. Nutr.*, 68(Suppl):956S, 1998.

Schutte, J.E., et al.: Density of lean body mass is greater in blacks than whites. *J. Appl. Physiol.*, 56:1647, 1984.

Sisson, S.B., et al.: Ethnic differences in subcutaneous adiposity and waist girth in children and adolescents. *Obesity (Silver Spring)*, 17:2075, 2009.

Sisson, S.B., et al.: Profiles of sedentary behavior in children and adolescents: the US National Health and Nutrition Examination Survey, 2001–2006. *Int. J. Pediatr. Obes.*, 4:353, 2009.

St.-Onge, M.P., et al.: Changes in childhood food consumption patterns: a cause for concern in light of increasing body weights. *Am. J. Clin. Nutr.*, 78:1068, 2003.

Stern, L., et al.: The effects of low-carbohydrate versus conventional weight loss diets in severely obese adults: one-year follow-up of a randomized trial. *Ann. Intern. Med.*, 140:778, 2004.

Stommel, M., Schoenborn, C.A.: Variations in BMI and prevalence of health risks in diverse racial and ethnic populations. *Obesity (Silver Spring)*, 2010, Epub ahead of print.

Sun, G., et al.: Comparison of multifrequency bioelectrical impedance analysis with dual-energy X-ray absorptiometry for assessment of percentage body fat in a large, healthy population. *Am. J. Clin. Nutr.*, 81:74, 2005.

Torstveit, M.K., Sundgot-Borgen, J.: Participation in leanness sports but not training volume is associated with menstrual dysfunction: a national survey of 1276 elite athletes and controls. *Br. J. Sports Med.*, 39:14, 2005.

Tran, Z.V., Weltman, A.: Generalized equation for predicting body density of women from girth measurements. *Med. Sci. Sports Exerc.*, 21:101, 1989.

Utter, A.C., et al.: Evaluation of air displacement for assessing body composition of collegiate wrestlers. *Med. Sci. Sports Exerc.*, 35:500, 2003.

van Marken Lichtenbelt, et al.: Body composition changes in bodybuilders: a method comparison. Med. *Sci. Sports Exerc.*, 36:490, 2004.

Wagner, D.R., Heyward, V.H.: Measures of body composition in blacks and whites: a comparative review. *Am. J. Clin. Nutr.*, 71:1392, 2000.

Weltman, A., et al.: Accurate assessment of body composition in obese females. *Am. J. Clin. Nutr.*, 48:1179, 1988.

Whitlock, E.P., et al.: Screening and interventions for childhood overweight: A summary of evidence for the US Preventive Services Task Force. *Pediatrics*, 116:e125, 2005.

Wijndaele, K., et al.: Increased cardiometabolic risk is associated with increased TV viewing time. *Med. Sci. Sports Exerc.*, 42:1511, 2010.

Witham, M.D., Avenell A.: Interventions to achieve long-term weight loss in obese older people: a systematic review and meta-analysis. *Age Ageing*, 39:172, 2010.

Wyshak, G.: Percent body fat, fractures and risk of osteoporosis in women. *J. Nutr. Health Aging*, 14:428, 2010.

Yu, OK.: Comparisons of obesity assessments in over-weight elementary students using anthropometry, BIA, CT and DEXA. *Nutr. Res. Pract.*, 4:128, 2010.

Zoladz, J.A., et al.: Effect of moderate incremental exercise, performed in fed and fasted state on cardio-respiratory variables and leptin and ghrelin concentrations in young healthy men. *J. Physiol. Pharmacol.*, 56:63, 2005.

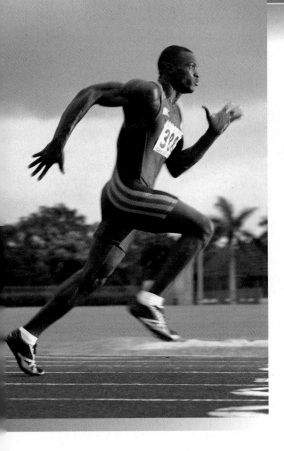

17

Physical Activity, Exercise, Successful Aging, and Disease Prevention

At least half of all babies born in America in 2007 will live to the age of 104!

— *Lancet* 374, October 2009

CHAPTER OBJECTIVES

- Describe the meaning of the the term *healthspan*.

- Explain the concept of successful aging compared with traditional views of the aging process.

- Distinguish between the terms *exercise* and *physical activity*.

- Explain the basis of the Physical Activity Pyramid.

- Answer the question, "How safe is exercise?"

- Describe the goals of Healthy People 2010.

- What is SeDS, and why is it so important?

- List important age-related changes in muscular strength, joint flexibility, nervous system function, cardiovascular function, pulmonary function, endocrine function, and body composition.

- Describe five field tests to assess the flexibility of major body areas.

- Describe research showing that regular physical activity protects against disease and may even extend life.

- List the three major causes of death in the United States.

- List and describe the four major coronary heart disease (CHD) risk factors.

- List secondary and novel risk factors for CHD.

- List specific components of the blood lipid profile and give values considered desirable for each.

- Discuss factors that affect cholesterol lipoprotein levels.

- Explain how regular physical activity reduces the risk of CHD.

- Describe the occurrence of CHD risk factors in children.

- Explain interactions between CHD risk factors.

THE GRAYING OF AMERICA

Elderly persons make up the fastest growing segment of American society. Forty years ago, age 65 years indicated the onset of "old age" and represented the average retirement age of most men in the workforce. Gerontologists now consider age 85 years the demarcation of "**oldest-old**" and age 75 years "**young-old**." Currently, nearly 12%, or approximately 35 million Americans, exceed age 65 years. By the year 2030, 70 million Americans will exceed age 85 years. Some demographers project that half of the girls and one-third of the boys born in developed countries near the end of the 20th century will live in three centuries. Based on the latest research, at least half of all babies born in America in 2007 will live to the age of 104 years. Most babies born since the year 2000 in countries with long-lived residents will celebrate their 100th birthday if the present yearly growth in life expectancy continues through the 21st century (**Table 17.1**).

In the short term, disease prevention, improved health care, and more effective treatment of age-related heart disease and osteoporosis help people live longer. Far fewer people now die from infectious childhood diseases, and those with the genetic potential actualize their proclivity for longevity. On a different but parallel front, anticipated breakthroughs in genetic therapies may slow the aging of individual cells. Cellular damage results from (1) accumulated mutations in mitochondrial DNA, perhaps induced by injury and deterioration from oxidative stress and (2) gene alterations that depress telomerase synthesis enzyme that protects the protective caps (telomers) at the ends of chromosomes that allow cells to divide properly. Gene therapies could boost human life spans to a much greater extent than improved medical treatment or even eradication of deadly diseases.

Figure 17.1A shows that proportionately, centenarians currently represent the fastest growing age group in the United States. Numbers range from 30,000 to 50,000, up from the estimated 15,000 in 1980 and almost none at the beginning of the 20th century. No longer viewed as a quirk of nature, one in 10,000 Americans now lives to the age of 100 years. Demographers project that by the middle of this century, more than 800,000 Americans will exceed age 100 years, with many in relatively good health. Old-age mortality appears to be on the decline because the death rate (number of people per 100 in a specific age group) levels off in the 90-year-old age category (approximately 11 per 100) and decreases to eight per 100 after age 100 years.

Figure 17.1B indicates the percentage of individuals age 65 years who survive to specified ages. Among current 65-year-old people, 95.5% will live to age 70 years, 63.3% will live to age 85 years, and nearly 10% will live to be 100 years old. A child born in 2007 should survive to age 100 years or more. Life expectancy in the United States has been on the rise for the past decade, increasing 1.4 years—from 76.5 years in 1997 to 77.9 in 2007, according to the latest statistics from the Centers for Disease Control and Prevention (CDC; *www.cdc.gov/nchs*).

Cigarette smoking, elevated body mass index (BMI), excess body fatness, and reduced physical activity provide potent predictors of subsequent morbidity and mortality. Changing to a more physically active lifestyle reduces mortality from common ailments and greatly improves cardiovascular and muscular functional capacities, quality of life, and capacity for independent living. At any age, behavioral changes such as becoming more physically active, quitting cigarette smoking, and controlling body weight and blood pressure act independently to delay all-cause mortality and extend life. Persons with more healthful lifestyles survive longer with a reduced risk of disability as life progresses.

THE NEW GERONTOLOGY: SUCCESSFUL AGING

Many gerontologists maintain that research on aging should not focus on increasing life span but rather on improving **healthspan**, the total number of years a person remains in excellent health. The **new gerontology** addresses areas beyond age-related diseases and their prevention to recognize that successful aging requires maintenance of enhanced physiologic function and physical fitness. Much of the physiologic deterioration previously

| Table 17.1 | Oldest Age in Years at Which at Least 50% of a Birth Cohort Is Still Alive in Eight of the World's Industrialized Countries |||||||||

	BIRTH YEAR							
COUNTRY	**2000**	**2001**	**2002**	**2003**	**2004**	**2005**	**2006**	**2007**
Canada	102	102	103	103	103	104	104	104
Denmark	99	99	100	100	101	101	101	101
France	102	102	103	103	103	104	104	104
Germany	99	100	100	100	101	101	101	102
Italy	102	102	102	103	103	103	104	104
Japan	104	105	105	105	106	106	106	107
UK	100	101	101	101	102	102	103	103
USA	101	102	102	103	103	103	104	104

From Human Mortality Database. Available at *http://www.mortality.org/cgi-bin/hmd/hmd_download.php*.

considered "normal aging" included deleterious changes in blood pressure, bone mass, body composition, body fat distribution, insulin sensitivity, and homocysteine levels. These maladies convey increased health risk, dysfunction, or actual disease, and depend on lifestyle and environmental influences subject to considerable modification with proper diet and exercise. For those achieving older age, low muscular strength, diminished cardiovascular function, poor range of joint motion, and sleep disturbances relate directly to functional limitations regardless of disease status. Gerontologists consider that successful aging includes four components:

1. Physical health
2. Spirituality
3. Emotional and educational health
4. Social satisfaction

Healthy Life Expectancy: A New Concept

Life expectancy estimates consider the overall length of life based on mortality data without considering the quality of life during aging. At some point during the life span, some level of disability detracts from life's quality. For example, the CDC (*www.cdc.gov/nchs/fastats/lifexpec.htm*) reports that nearly 1 in 10 Americans older than age 70 years requires help with daily activities such as bathing, and 4 in 10 use assistive devices such as walkers or hearing aids. Approximately one-half of men and two-thirds of women older than age 70 years have arthritis; more than one-third of all Americans in this age group also have high blood pressure, and 11% have diabetes. Of all seniors, women older than age 85 years are the most likely to need everyday help, and 23% require assistance with at least one basic activity (e.g., dressing or going to the toilet).

Questions & Notes

What is the prognosis for how long "you" will live?

Explain the term "new gerontology."

ⓘ For Your Information

PHYSICAL ACTIVITY MODIFICATIONS FOR ELDERLY INDIVIDUALS

Physical activity recommendations for elderly people are similar to those of the updated American College of Sports Medicine/American Heart Association (AHA) recommendations for healthy adults but with several important differences. For example, the level of exercise intensity takes into account the older adult's relatively lower level of aerobic fitness. Recommended activities also focus on joint flexibiltiy and balance to reduce risks of falls. Physical activity in this population emphasizes moderate-intensity aerobic activity, muscle-strengthening exercises, reduction of sedentary behavior, and lifestyle risk management. (From Nelson M.E., et al.: Physical activity and public health in older adults: recommendation from the American College of Sports Medicine and the American Heart Association. *Med. Sci. Sports Exerc.*, 39:1435, 2006.)

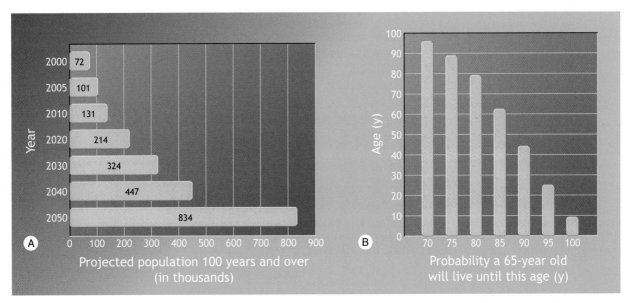

Figure 17.1 The graying of America. (**A**) Growth in number of centenarians in the United States. (**B**) Probability that a current 65-year-old person will live to a certain age. (Data from U.S. Bureau of the Census, National Center for Health Statistics, Centers for Disease Control and Prevention: Washington, DC, and actuarial tables from insurance companies.)

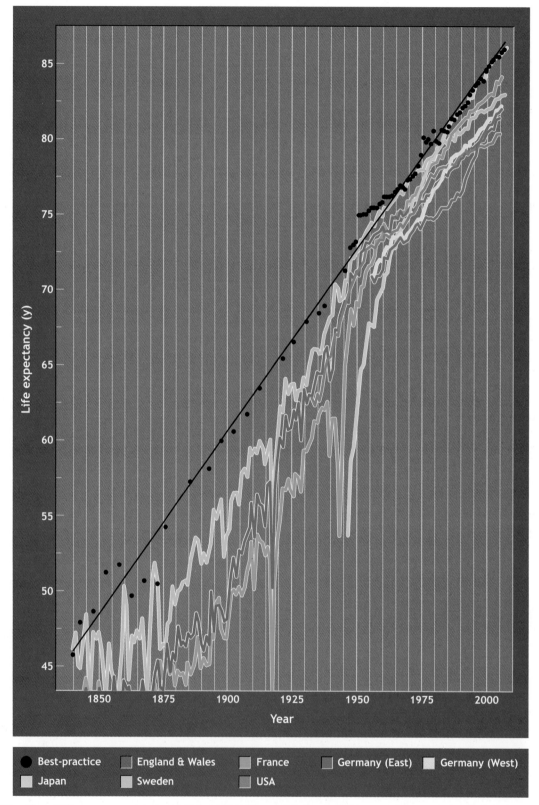

Figure 17.2 Plot of life expectancy (y) since 1850 to 2010. The *straight line* and *data points* represent the "best-practice life expectancy," the highest values recorded in a national population. Life expectancy has risen by 3 months per year since 1840. The *colored lines* represent individual country average life expectancy.

To estimate healthful longevity, the World Health Organization (*www.who.int/whr*) introduced the concept of **healthy life expectancy (HALE)**, the expected number of years a person might live in the equivalent of full health. HALE considers the years of ill health weighted according to severity and subtracted from expected overall life expectancy to compute the equivalent years of healthy life. Of the 191 countries evaluated, HALE estimates reached 70 years in 24 countries and 60 years in more than half. Thirty-two countries were at the lower extreme of less than 40 years. Many of these countries bear the burden of the major epidemics of HIV/AIDS and other causes of death and disability.

Figure 17.2 shows that life expectancy increases almost linearly in most developed countries, with no sign of deceleration. In fact, best-practice life expectancy—the highest value recorded in a national population—has risen by 3 months per year since 1840 and continues unabated. In the record-holding country, Japan, female life expectancy achieved 86.0 years in 2007, surpassing 85 years considered the upper-limit life expectancy for any one population. Although with lower life expectancies than Japan's, most developed countries show similar yearly life expectancy increases since 1950. The linear increase in the record life expectancy for more than 170 years does not suggest a looming limit to the human life span. If life expectancy were approaching its limit, some deceleration of progress would probably occur. Continued increases in life expectancy in the longest living populations suggests that we are not close to a limit and a further rise seems likely.

The six most prominent factors in order of importance responsible for decreased life expectancy in non-Western countries include those related most to disease occurrence and environmental insults:

1. Low birth weight
2. Vitamin and mineral deficiency (particularly vitamin A and iron)
3. Unsafe water and sanitation procedures
4. Unsafe sex, including HIV
5. Introduction of carcinogens
6. Work-related risk

In the Americas and Europe, the six major factors contributing to a decrease in healthy life span relate to lifestyle choices:

1. Tobacco use
2. High blood pressure
3. Increased blood cholesterol
4. Obesity
5. Low levels of physical activity
6. Limited fruit and vegetable consumption

PHYSICAL ACTIVITY EPIDEMIOLOGY

Epidemiology involves quantifying factors that influence the occurrence of illness to better understand, modify, or control a disease pattern in the general population. The specific field of **physical activity epidemiology** applies the general research strategies of epidemiology to study physical activity as a health-related behavior linked to disease and other outcomes.

Terminology

Physical activity epidemiology applies specific definitions to characterize behavioral patterns and outcomes of the groups under investigation. Relevant terminology includes the following:

- **Physical activity:** Body movement produced by muscle action that increases energy expenditure
- **Exercise:** Planned, structured, repetitive, and purposeful physical activity

Questions & Notes

Explain the concept of healthy life expectancy.

List 3 factors responsible for decreased life expectancy in non-Western countries.

1.

2.

3.

List 3 factors responsible for decreased life expectancy in the Americas and European countries.

1.

2.

3.

Explain differences between the terms physical activity and exercise.

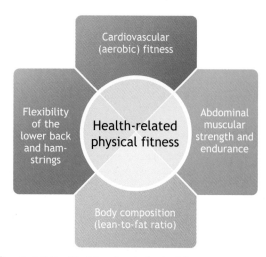

Figure 17.3 Health-related physical fitness components.

- **Physical fitness:** Attributes related to how well one performs physical activity
- **Health:** Physical, mental, and social well-being, not simply absence of disease
- **Health-related physical fitness:** Components of physical fitness associated with some aspect of good health or disease prevention (**Fig. 17.3**)
- **Longevity:** Length of life

Within this framework, *physical activity* becomes a generic term with exercise its major component. Similarly, the definition of *health* focuses on the broad spectrum of well-being that ranges from complete absence of health (near death) to the highest levels of physiologic function. Such definitions often challenge our ability to measure and quantify health and physical activity objectively. They do, however, provide a broad perspective to study the role of physical activity in health and disease.

The trend in physical fitness assessment during the past 40 years deemphasizes tests of motor performance and athletic fitness (i.e., speed, power, balance, agility). Current assessment focuses on functional capacities related to overall good health and disease prevention. The four most common components of **health-related physical fitness** include aerobic or cardiovascular fitness, body composition, abdominal muscular strength and endurance, and lower back and hamstring flexibility (see Close Up Box 17.1: *How to Assess Joint Flexibility in Common Body Areas*, on page 602).

Physical Activity Participation

More than 30 different methods can assess physical activity. They include direct and indirect calorimetry, self-reports and questionnaires, job classifications, physiologic markers, behavioral observations, mechanical or electronic monitors, and activity surveys. Each approach offers both unique advantages and disadvantages depending on the situation and population studied. Obtaining valid estimates of physical activity of large groups remains difficult because such studies by necessity apply self-reports of daily activity and exercise participation rather than direct monitoring or

objective measurement. Despite limitations in assessment, a discouraging picture of physical activity participation worldwide consistently emerges. In the United States, adult participation in any physical activity remains quite low as revealed by these statistics:

- Only about 15% engage in regular, vigorous physical activity during leisure time, three times a week for at least 30 minutes.
- More than 60% do not engage in any regularly physical activity.
- About 25% lead sedentary lives (i.e., do not exercise).
- Walking, gardening, and yard work are the most popular leisure-time activities.
- About 22% engage in light-to-moderate physical activity regularly during leisure time (five times a week for at least 30 min).
- Physical inactivity occurs more frequently among women than men, blacks and Hispanics than whites, older than younger adults, and less-affluent than wealthier persons.
- Participation in fitness activities declines with age; older citizens typically have such poor functional capacity that they cannot rise from a chair or bed, walk to the bathroom, or climb a single stair without assistance.

Equally discouraging data emerge for children and teenagers:

- Nearly half of those between ages 12 and 21 do not exercise vigorously on a regular basis regardless of gender.
- About 14% report no recent physical activity; this is more prevalent among females, particularly black females.
- About 25% engage in light to moderate physical activity (e.g., walk or bicycle) nearly every day.
- Participation in all types of physical activity declines strikingly as age and school grade increase.
- More boys than girls participate in vigorous physical activity, strengthening activities, and walking or bicycling.

Getting America More Physically Active

On July 11, 1996, in a landmark announcement, the Surgeon General of the United States acknowledged the importance of physical activity to the nation with the release of the **First Surgeon General's Report on Physical Activity and Health** (*www.cdc.gov/NCCDPHP/sgr/ataglan.htm*). This encompassing report summarized the benefits of regular physical activity in disease prevention. The Surgeon General proposed a national agenda that urged the nation to adopt and maintain a physically active lifestyle to combat ailments associated with the country's generally low level of energy expenditure. The report stated that men and women of all ages benefit from regular physical activity. It became a stated goal of the government to encourage all citizens to

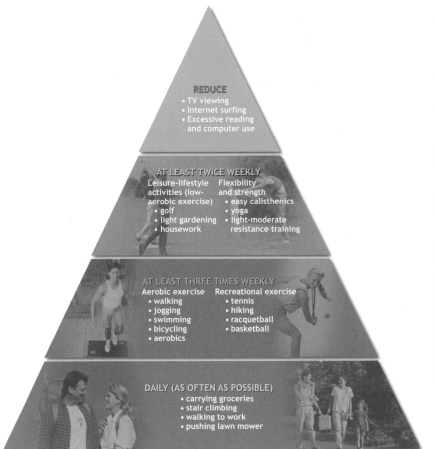

Physical Activity Pyramid

Figure 17.4 The Physical Activity Pyramid: prudent goals for increasing daily physical activity.

Questions & Notes

List the 4 components of health-related physical fitness.

1.

2.

3.

4.

List 4 methods to assess physical activity.

1.

2.

3.

4.

List 2 major goals of the Healthy People 2010 initiative.

1.

2.

include moderate physical activity such as 30 minutes of brisk walking or raking leaves, 15 minutes of running, or 45 minutes of playing volleyball on most, if not all, days of the week.

The **Physical Activity Pyramid (Fig. 17.4)** summarizes major goals for increasing the level of regular physical activity in the general population; the pyramid emphasizes diverse forms of behavioral and lifestyle options.

Healthy People 2010

The **Healthy People 2010** initiative (*www.healthypeople.gov*) launched on January 25, 2000, builds on the initiatives of the previous two decades as an instrument to improve national health for the first decade of the 21st century. Healthy People 2010 outlines a comprehensive, nationwide health promotion and disease prevention agenda as a roadmap to promote health and prevent illness, disability, and premature death among all people in the United States.

ⓘ For Your Information

LET'S MOVE – THE NEW INITIATIVE TO COMBAT CHILDHOOD OBESITY

In February 2010 First Lady Michelle Obama with support from the U.S. government rolled out a national initiative against childhood obesity, dubbed "Let's Move." Along with the First Lady's influential leadership, the project received a commitment of $1 billion a year in federal funds for 10 years, and the first national task force on solving the childhood obesity epidemic with members from the departments of the Interior, Health and Human Services, Agriculture and Education.

The initiative has four core pillars: better nutrition information, increased physical activity, easier access to healthy foods and personal responsibility. Specific actions revolve around food labeling, school food quality, and encouraging kids to exercise each day and doctors to monitor body mass index.

This campaign is comprehensive in nature that builds on effective strategies, and mobilizes public and private sector resources. Let's Move will engage every sector that impact the health of children and will provide schools, families and communities simple tools to help kids be more active, eat better, and get healthy. To support Let's Move the nation's leading children's health foundations have come together to create a new independent foundation - the *Partnership for a Healthier America* - to accelerate existing efforts towards the national goal of solving childhood obesity within a generation.

BOX 17.1 CLOSE UP

How to Assess Joint Flexibility in Common Body Areas

Two types of flexibility include (1) **static**, which is full range of motion (ROM) of a specific joint, and (2) **dynamic**, which is torque or resistance encountered as the joint moves through its ROM. Improper alignment of the vertebral column accounts for more than 80% of all lower back and pelvic girdle ailments; this often results from poor flexibility in regions of the lower back, trunk, hip, and posterior thigh (common in runners) and weak abdominal and erector spinae muscles.

SPECIFICITY AND FLEXIBILITY

Considerable specificity exists for joint ROM depending on joint structure. Triaxial joints (ball and socket) of the hip and shoulder afford a greater degree of movement than either uniaxial or biaxial joints (wrist, knee, elbow, and ankle). "Tightness" of the soft tissue structures of the joint capsule and muscle and its fascia, tendons, ligaments, and skin constitute major factors that influence static and dynamic flexibility. Other influences include a well-developed musculature and excess fatty tissue of adjacent body segments. Flexibility progressively decreases with advancing age, mainly because of decreased soft-tissue extensibility. How decrements in flexibility reflect true aging or result from a "disuse" effect of an increasingly sedentary lifestyle remains unclear. On average, women remain more flexible than men at any age.

FIVE COMMON FIELD TESTS OF STATIC FLEXIBILITY

Field tests assess static flexibility indirectly through linear measurement of ROM. A minimum of three trials should be administered after a warm-up.

Test 1: Hip and Trunk Flexibility (Modified Sit-and-Reach Test)

Starting position: Sit on the floor with the back and head against a wall with the legs fully extended with the bottom of the feet against the sit-and-reach box. Place the hands on top of each other, stretching the arms forward while keeping the head and back against the wall (**A**). Measure the distance from the fingertips to the box edge with a yardstick. This becomes the zero or starting point.

Movement: Slowly bend and reach forward as far as possible (the head and back move away from the wall), sliding the fingers along the yardstick; hold the final position for 2 seconds (**B**).

Score: The total distance reached to the nearest one-tenth inch

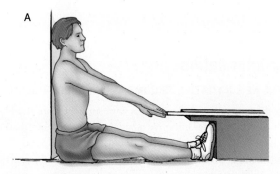
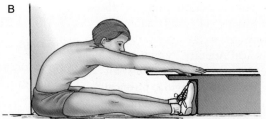

Modified Sit and Reach, Age Range				
PERFORMANCE RATING	**MEN**		**WOMEN**	
	AGE <35 YEARS	**AGE 36–49 YEARS**	**AGE <35 YEARS**	**AGE 36–49 YEARS**
Excellent	>17.9	>16.1	>17.9	>17.4
Good	17.0–17.9	14.6–16.1	16.7–17.9	16.2–17.4
Average	15.8–17.0	13.9–14.6	16.2–16.7	15.2–16.2
Fair	15.0–15.8	13.4–13.9	15.8-16.2	14.5–15.2
Poor	<15.0	<13.4	<15.4	<14.5

Adapted from Johnson, B.L., Nelson, J.K.: *Practical Measurements for Evaluation in Physical Education*, 4th ed. New York: Macmillan Publishing, 1986.

Test 2: Shoulder–Wrist Flexibility (Shoulder and Wrist Elevation Test)

Starting position: Lie prone on the floor with the arms fully extended overhead; grasp a yardstick with the hands shoulder width apart.

Movement: Raise the stick at high as possible.

1. Measure the vertical distance (nearest 1/2 in) the yardstick rises from the floor.
2. Measure arm length from the acromial process to the tip of longest finger.
3. Subtract the best vertical score from arm length.

Score: Arm length − Best vertical score (nearest 1/4 in)

Shoulder and Wrist Elevation		
PERFORMANCE RATING	**MEN**	**WOMEN**
Excellent	≥12.75	≥12.00
Good	12.50–11.75	11.75–11.0
Average	11.50–8.50	10.75–7.75
Fair	8.25–6.25	7.50–5.75
Poor	≤6.00	≤5.50

Adapted from Johnson, B.L., Nelson, J.K.: *Practical Measurements for Evaluation in Physical Education*, 4th ed. New York: Macmillan Publishing, 1986.

Test 3: Trunk and Neck Flexibility (Trunk and Neck Extension Test)

Starting position: Lie prone on the floor with the hands clasped together behind the head.

Movement: Raise the trunk as high as possible while keeping the hips in contact with the floor. An assistant can hold down the legs.

Score: Vertical distance (nearest 1/4 in) from the tip of the nose to the floor

Trunk and Neck Extension		
PERFORMANCE RATING	**MEN**	**WOMEN**
Excellent	≥10.25	≥10.00
Good	10.00–8.25	9.75–8.00
Average	8.00–6.25	7.75–6.00
Fair	6.00–3.25	5.75–2.25
Poor	≤3.00	≤2.00

Adapted from Johnson, B.L., Nelson, J.K.: *Practical Measurements for Evaluation in Physical Education*, 4th ed. New York: Macmillan Publishing, 1986.

Test 4: Shoulder Flexibility (Shoulder Rotation Test)

Starting position: Grasp one end of a rope with the left hand; 4 inches away, grasp the rope with the right hand.

Movement: Extend both arms in front of the chest and rotate the arms overhead and behind the back; as resistance occurs, slide the right hand farther from the left hand along the rope until the rope touches against the back.

1. Measure the distance on the rope between the thumb of each hand after successfully rotating overhead with the rope against the back.
2. Measure shoulder width from deltoid to deltoid. Subtract the rope distance from the shoulder width distance.

Score: Shoulder-width distance − Rope distance (nearest 1/4 in)

Shoulder Rotation		
PERFORMANCE RATING	**MEN**	**WOMEN**
Excellent	≥20.00	≥18.00
Good	19.75–14.75	17.75–13.25
Average	14.50–11.75	13.00–10.00
Fair	11.50–7.25	9.75–5.25
Poor	≤7.00	≤5.00

Adapted from Johnson, B.L., Nelson, J.K.: *Practical Measurements for Evaluation in Physical Education*, 4th ed. New York: Macmillan Publishing, 1986.

Test 5: Ankle Flexibility (Ankle Flexion Test)

Starting position: Stand facing a wall. With the feet flat on the floor, lean into the wall.

Movement: Slowly slide back from the wall as far as possible while keeping the feet flat on the floor, body and knees fully extended, and chest in contact with the wall.

Score: Distance between the toe line and the wall (nearest 1/4 in)

Ankle Flexion		
PERFORMANCE RATING	**MEN**	**WOMEN**
Excellent	≥35.50	≥32.00
Good	35.25–32.75	31.75–30.50
Average	32.50–29.75	30.25–26.75
Fair	29.50–26.75	26.50–24.50
Poor	≤26.50	≤24.25

Adapted from Johnson, B.L., Nelson, J.K.: *Practical Measurements for Evaluation in Physical Education*, 4th ed. New York: Macmillan Publishing, 1986.

Healthy People 2010 attempts to achieve two primary goals:

1. Increase the quality and years of healthy life
2. Eliminate health disparities among the nation's citizens

Progress will be monitored through achievements within 467 objectives in 28 focus areas. Many goals and objectives, several of which either directly or indirectly involve upgrading the national level of regular physical activity, converge on interventions designed to reduce or eliminate illness, disability, and premature death among individuals and communities. Other objectives focus on broader issues such as improving access to quality health care, strengthening public health services, and improving availability and dissemination of health-related information. Each objective has a target for specific improvements and explicit guidelines on how to achieve the stated goal by the year 2010.

Safety of Exercising

Several well-publicized reports of sudden death during exercise raise the question of exercise safety. It may surprise some that the death rate during exercise has declined over the past 25 years despite an overall increase in exercise participation. In one report of cardiovascular episodes over a 65-month period, 2935 exercisers recorded 374,798 hours of exercise that included 2,726,272 km of running and walking. No deaths occurred during this time, and only two nonfatal cardiovascular complications occurred. This amounts to two complications per 100,000 hours of exercise for women and three complications for men.

The relative risk of sudden death among athletes versus nonathletes was 1.95 for men and 2.00 for women. The higher risk of sudden death in athletes strongly related to underlying cardiovascular diseases such as congenital coronary artery anomaly, arrhythmogenic right ventricular cardiomyopathy, premature coronary artery disease. Interestingly, athletic participation did not cause the enhanced mortality, but instead triggered sudden death in athletes affected by cardiovascular conditions predisposing them to life-threatening ventricular arrhythmias during physical exercise.

Intense physical exertion poses a small risk of sudden death (e.g., one sudden death per 1.51 million episodes of exertion) during the activity compared with resting an equivalent time, particularly for sedentary people with a genetic predisposition to sudden death. Prospective epidemiologic research evaluated clinically significant medical incidents and emergencies for 7725 low-risk, apparently healthy corporate fitness enrollees in a supervised facility at a major medical center. Over 2.5 years, 15 medically significant events (0.048 per 1000 participant-hours) and two medical emergencies (both recovered; 0.0063 per 1000 participant-hours). This extremely low rate of medical incidents in a supervised health-fitness facility shows that the health-related fitness benefits far outweigh the small risk of participation.

The most recent report in 2007 from the National Electronic Injury Surveillance System All Injury Program (*www.cpsc.gov/LIBRARY/neiss.html*) that characterizes sports- and recreation-related injuries in the U.S. population revealed an overall rate of 11.2 injuries per 100,000 population participants. For persons 15 to 24 years of age the injury rate equalled 30 injuries per 100,000 population, the highest recorded for any age group. Basketball reported 159 injuries per 100,000 participants, and bicycle-related injuries were 171 per 100,00 participants. With 150 injuries per 100,000 participants, football ranked close behind. The most frequent injury diagnosis included strains or sprains, fractures, contusions or abrasions, and lacerations. The body parts injured most commonly were the ankles, fingers, face, head, and knees.

SEDENTARY DEATH SYNDROME

A review of the world literature over the past 60 years has led to the conclusion that physical *inactivity* produces a constellation of problems and conditions that eventually lead to premature death. **Sedentary death syndrome** (**SeDS**; *hac.missouri.edu*) describes this condition that denotes a collection of disorders directly caused by or worsened by physical inactivity that ends in death. SeDS will contribute to 1 in 10 premature deaths, or 2.5 million deaths in the United States alone, at a projected cost of $1.5 trillion over the next 10 years. In summary:

- SeDS will cause 2.5 million Americans to die prematurely over the next decade.
- SeDS will cost $1.5 trillion in health care expenses in the United States in the next decade.
- Chronic diseases have increased because of physical inactivity. In the United States, type 2 diabetes has increased ninefold since 1958, obesity has doubled since 1980, and heart disease remains a leading cause of death.
- Children are now experiencing SeDS-related diseases. American children have become increasingly overweight, showing fatty streaks in their arteries and developing type 2 diabetes at an alarming rate.
- SeDS relates to 26 medically related conditions that include angina, heart attack, coronary artery disease, arthritis pain, arrhythmias, breast cancer, colon cancer, congestive heart failure, depression, digestive problems, gallstone disease, gastroesophageal disease, high blood triglyceride level, high blood cholesterol level, hypertension, less cognitive function, low blood high-density lipoprotein cholesterol (HDL-C) level, lower quality of life, menopausal symptoms, osteoporosis, pancreatic cancer, peripheral vascular disease, physical frailty, premature mortality, prostate cancer, respiratory problems, sleep apnea, stroke, and type-2 diabetes.

More medical-based evidence must convince the world population that *physical inactivity* promotes unhealthy gene expression. We wholeheartedly endorse that regular, vigorous physical activity should play an increasingly more important role in the lives of all individuals.

AGING AND BODILY FUNCTION

Figure 17.5 shows that bodily functions improve rapidly during childhood and reach a maximum at about age 30 years; thereafter, a decline in functional capacity occurs. A similar age trend exists for physically active persons; physiologic function averages about 25% higher compared with sedentary counterparts at each age category (e.g., an active 50-year-old man or woman often maintains the functional level of a 30-year-old man or woman). All physiologic measures eventually decline with age, but not all decrease at the same rate.

Nerve conduction velocity, for example, declines only 10% to 15% from age 30 to 80 years, but resting cardiac index (ratio of cardiac output to body surface area) and joint flexibility decline 20% to 30%; maximum breathing capacity at age 80 years averages 40% of values for a 30-year-old person. Brain cells die at a fairly constant rate until age 60 years, but the liver and kidneys lose 40% to 50% of their function between ages 30 and 70 years. By the seventh decade of life, the average woman has lost 30% of her bone mass, while men lose only 15%.

Aging and Muscular Strength

Men and women achieve maximum strength between ages 20 to 30 years, when muscle cross-sectional area often achieves maximum size. Thereafter, strength progressively declines for most muscle groups; by age 70 years, overall "general" strength has decreased by 30%.

Decrease in Muscle Mass *Strength decreases with age because of reduced fat-free body mass (FFM), a condition termed* **sarcopenia.** *The smaller muscle mass in older adults reflects a loss of total muscle protein induced by physical inactivity, aging, or the combined effects. Some loss in muscle fiber number also takes place with aging. For example, whereas the biceps of a newborn contains about 500,000 individual fibers, the same muscle for an 80-year-old man contains 300,000 fibers, or 40% less.*

Muscle Trainability Among Middle Aged and Elderly Persons
Regular exercise retains body protein and blunts the loss of muscle mass and strength with aging. Healthy men between age 60 and 72 years participated in a 12-week

Questions & Notes

Identify the most prevalent medical complication from exercising.

What do the initials SeDS stand for?

List 10 medical conditions related to SeDS.

1.

2.

3.

4.

5.

6.

7.

8.

9.

10.

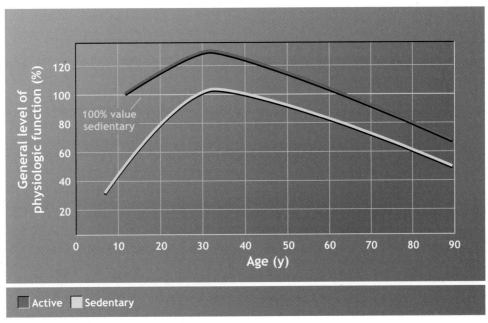

Figure 17.5 Generalized curve for age-related changes in physiologic function. All comparisons were made against the 100% value achieved by the 20- to 30-year-old sedentary person.

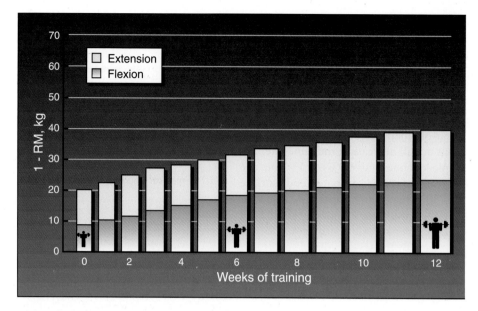

Figure 17.6 Weekly measurement of dynamic muscle strength (1-RM) in left knee extension (*yellow*) and flexion (*red*) during a 12-week period of resistance training in men age 60 to 72 years. (Data from Frontera, W.R., et al.: Strength conditioning in older men: Skeletal muscle hypertrophy and improved function. *J. Appl. Physiol.*, 64:1038, 1988.)

standard resistance-training program. **Figure 17.6** shows that the men's muscle strength increased progressively throughout the program, averaging about 5% each exercise session (a training response similar to young adults). Exercise specialists who work with elderly people argue that improving strength effectively maintains muscle mass, increases mobility, and reduces injury incidence for this age group.

Aging and Joint Flexibility

With advancing age, connective tissue (cartilage, ligaments, and tendons) becomes stiffer and more rigid, which reduces joint flexibility. It is unclear whether these changes result from biologic aging or reflect the impact of chronic disuse through sedentary living or degenerative tissue diseases of specific joints. Regardless of the cause, appropriate exercises that regularly move the joints through their full ROM increase flexibility 20% to 50% in men and women at all ages.

Endocrine Changes with Aging

Endocrine function changes with age, particularly the pituitary, pancreas, adrenal, and thyroid glands. About 40% of individuals between ages 65 and 75 years and 50% of individuals older than age 80 years have impaired glucose tolerance that leads to type 2 diabetes, the most common diabetes form. Impaired glucose metabolism leading to high blood glucose levels in type 2 diabetes results from three factors:

1. Decreased effect of insulin on peripheral tissue (**insulin resistance**)
2. Inadequate pancreatic insulin production to control blood sugar (**relative insulin deficiency**)
3. Combined effect of insulin resistance and relative insulin deficiency

With the exception of a genetic predisposition, increased prevalence of type 2 diabetes largely relates to "controllable" factors such as poor diet, inadequate physical activity, and increased body fat (particularly in the visceral–abdominal fat).

Thyroid dysfunction from lowered pituitary gland release of the thyroid-stimulating hormone thyrotropin (and reduced output of thyroxine from the thyroid gland) commonly occurs among elderly people. This affects metabolic function that includes decreased glucose metabolism and protein synthesis.

Figure 17.7 depicts changes in three additional hormonal systems associated with aging: the hypothalamic–pituitary–gonadal axis, adrenal cortex, and growth hormone (GH) and insulin-like growth factor-1 (IGF-1) axis.

Hypothalamic–Pituitary–Gonadal Axis Alterations in the interaction among stimulating hormones from the hypothalamus and anterior pituitary gland and gonads decrease ovarian output of estradiol. This effect probably initiates permanent cessation of menses (**menopause**) in aging women. Changes in hypothalamic–pituitary–gonadal axis activity in men occur more slowly and subtly. For example, serum total and free testosterone decline with aging in men. Age-related decreases in gonadotropic secretions from the anterior pituitary gland characterize male **andropause**.

Adrenal Cortex **Adrenopause** refers to the decrease in adrenal cortext output of dehydroepiandrosterone (DHEA) and its sulfated ester (DHEAS). In contrast to the glucocorticoid and mineralocorticoid adrenal steroids whose plasma levels remain relatively high with aging, a long, progressive, but slow decline in DHEA occurs after about age 30 years. This has led to speculation concerning DHEA's role in aging, prompting a dramatic increase in unregulated supplementation of this hormone.

Growth Hormone and Insulin-Like Growth Factor-1 Axis Mean pulse amplitude, duration, and fraction of secreted GH gradually decrease with aging, a condition termed **somatopause**. A parallel decrease in circulating levels of IGF-1 also occurs. IGF-1, produced by the liver and other cells, stimulates tissue growth and protein synthesis. The trigger for the age-related GH decrease

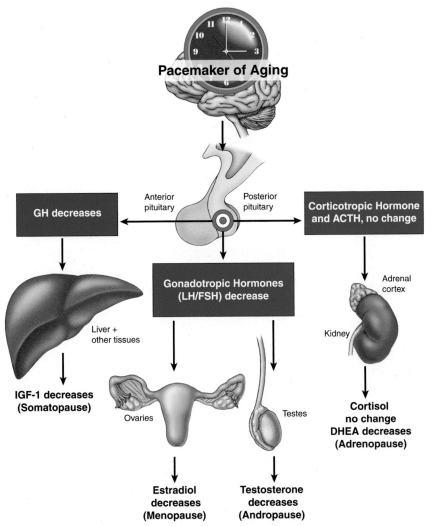

Pacemaker of Aging

GH decreases

Anterior pituitary

Posterior pituitary

Corticotropic Hormone and ACTH, no change

Gonadotropic Hormones (LH/FSH) decrease

Adrenal cortex

Liver + other tissues

Kidney

IGF-1 decreases (Somatopause)

Ovaries

Testes

Cortisol no change DHEA decreases (Adrenopause)

Estradiol decreases (Menopause)

Testosterone decreases (Andropause)

Figure 17.7   Age-related decline in three hormone systems that affect the rate of biological aging. **Left**. Decreased growth hormone (GH; released by the anterior pituitary) depresses production of insulin-like growth factor-1 (IGF-1) to inhibit cellular growth (a condition of aging termed *somatopause*). **Middle**. Decreased output of luteinizing hormone (LH) and follicle-stimulating hormone (FSH) by the anterior pituitary, coupled with reduced estradiol secretion from ovaries and testosterone from testes, causes menopause (in women) and andropause (in men). **Right**. Adrenocortical cells responsible for dehydroepiandrosterone (DHEA) production decrease their activity (termed *adrenopause*) without clinically evident changes in this gland's corticotropin (adrenocorticotropic hormone [ACTH]) and cortisol secretion. A central "pacemaker" in the hypothalamus or higher brain areas probably mediates these processes to produce aging-related changes in the ovaries, testicles, and adrenal cortex.

Questions & Notes

Give 2 reasons older individuals develop impaired glucose tolerance leading to type 2 diabetes.

  1.

  2.

Define the term menopause.

Define the term andropause.

Define the term adrenopause.

Define the term somatopause.

probably lies in the interaction between the hypothalamus and anterior pituitary gland.

To what extent changes in gonadal function (menopause and andropause) contribute to adrenopause and somatopause in both genders remains unknown. A growing body of evidence indicates that functional correlates, such as muscle size and strength, body composition, bone mass alterations, and progression of atherosclerosis, directly relate to hormonal changes with aging. Hormone replacement therapy, nutritional supplementation, and regular exercise may suppress aspects of hormone-related aging dysfunction.

Aging and Nervous System Function

A 37% decline in the number of spinal cord axons and 10% decline in nerve conduction velocity reflect cumulative effects of aging on central nervous system (CNS) function. Such changes partially explain age-related decrements in neuromuscular performance. Partitioning reaction time into central processing time and muscle contraction time indicates that aging exerts the greatest effect on stimulus detection and information processing to produce a response. For example, the knee-jerk reflex does not require CNS processing; it becomes less affected by aging than voluntary responses and movement patterns.

Despite the real effects of aging on reaction and movement time, physically active young or old groups move faster than a corresponding less active age group. These observations fuel speculation that regular participation in physical activity thwarts biologic aging of certain neuromuscular functions.

Aging and Pulmonary Function

Cross-sectional studies indicate that dynamic pulmonary capacity of older endurance-trained athletes exceeds that of sedentary peers. Although longitudinal studies will provide a definitive answer, available data suggest that regular physical activity retards pulmonary function deterioration associated with aging. Regular, more vigorous exercise promotes the maintenance of ventilatory musculature power and endurance.

Aging and Cardiovascular Function

Regular physical activity exerts a profound influence on age-related decrements in cardiovascular function and exercise endurance.

Maximal Oxygen Uptake
Beyond age 35, $\dot{V}O_{2max}$ declines at a nonlinear rate that accelerates after age 45 years so that by age 60 years, it averages 11% below values for

35-year-old men and 15% below values for women (see **Fig. 7.14**). A slower rate of decline occurs for individuals who maintain an active lifestyle that includes regular aerobic training. *Physical activity does not entirely offset aging's effect on $\dot{V}O_{2max}$ even when adjusting for a person's quantity of muscle mass.*

Figure 17.8 shows the relationship between $\dot{V}O_{2max}$ and active appendicular muscle mass for younger (average age, 25 y) and older (average age, 63 y) aerobically trained men and women. Younger subjects had trained for 9 consecutive years, and older subjects had trained for 20 consecutive years. Older men and women exhibited a 14% lower $\dot{V}O_{2max}$ than younger counterparts throughout the broad range of variation in muscle mass among subjects. In other words, despite an equivalence in appendicular muscle mass between a young and older person, the younger person exhibited a *higher* $\dot{V}O_{2max}$.

Three factors partially account for the deterioration in $\dot{V}O_{2max}$ with aging:

1. Age-associated loss of muscle mass
2. Increase in body fat
3. Altered cardiovascular and pulmonary functions

The reductions in aerobic power per kilogram of active muscle mass with aging displayed in **Figure 17.8** can reflect only age-associated reduced oxygen delivery, reduced oxygen extraction at the active muscle, or both. Skeletal muscle oxidative capacity and capillarization, both important components of oxygen extraction, remain similar in older and younger individuals with comparable physiologic characteristics and training histories. Consequently, the well-documented reduction in cardiac output (decreases in maximum heart rate and stroke volume) represents the most likely explanation for the decrease in $\dot{V}O_{2max}$ per kilogram of active muscle that accompanies aging.

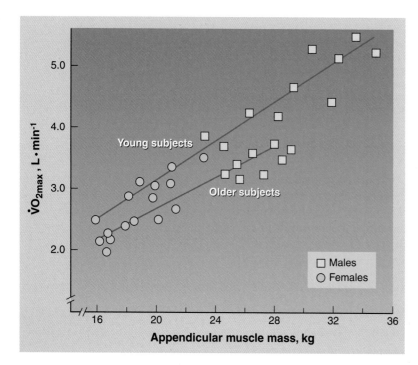

Figure 17.8 Maximal oxygen uptake ($\dot{V}O_{2max}$) related to appendicular muscle mass in young and older endurance-trained men and women. $\dot{V}O_{2max}$ per kg of active muscle mass decreases with age, independent of training status. (Modified from Proctor, D.N., Joyner, J.: Skeletal muscle mass and the reduction of $\dot{V}O_{2max}$ in trained older subjects. *J. Appl. Physiol.*, 82:1411, 1997.)

Aging Response to Exercise Training *For the healthy elderly, exercise training enhances the heart's capacity to pump blood and increases aerobic capacity to the same relative degree as in younger adults.* Nine to 12 months of endurance training in healthy older adults increased $\dot{V}O_{2max}$ 19% in men and 22% in women. These values represent the high end of the typical training response for young adults. Middle-aged men who regularly engaged in aerobic training for more than 20 years delayed the expected 10% to 15% decline in exercise capacity and aerobic fitness. At age 55 years, these active men maintained nearly the same values for blood pressure, body mass, and $\dot{V}O_{2max}$ as at age 35 years; by age 70 years, their $\dot{V}O_{2max}$ equaled values for individuals 25 years younger. These remarkable findings attest to the adaptability of the aerobic system to successful training at any age.

Cardiovascular and Body Composition Age-Related Changes

Figure 17.9 shows longitudinal changes for maximum heart rate, minute pulmonary ventilation, and different body composition variables of 21 men tested at ages 50 (T1), 60 (T2), and 70 years (T3). The men trained continuously throughout the 20-year period; each had placed either first, second, or third in regional, national, or international competition in running events during a 10-year measurement interval.

With the exception of pulmonary ventilation (small increase at T2), each shows definitive "aging effects." Maximum heart rate decreased by 5 to 7 beats per min at each measurement over the 20 years (a smaller decrease than

$\mathcal{Q}$uestions & Notes

Give the percentage rate decline in $\dot{V}O_{2max}$ between ages 20 and 60.

Describe the general relationship between $\dot{V}O_{2max}$, $L \cdot min^{-1}$ and appendicular muscle mass, kg.

Can the healthy elderly enhance cardiovascular capacity with exercise training to the same relative extent as younger counterparts.

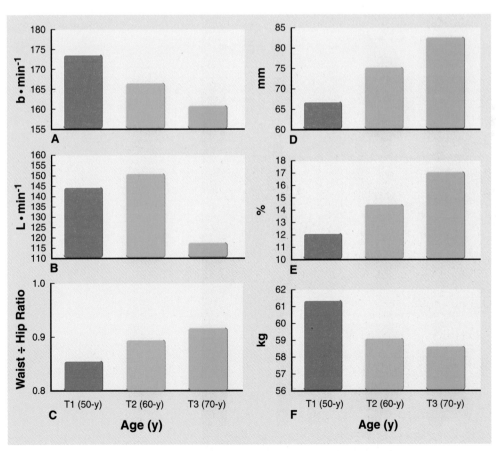

Figure 17.9   Changes in maximum heart rate (**A**), minute ventilation (**B**), waist-to-hip girth ratio (**C**), sum of skinfolds (**D**), percentage body fat (**E**), and fat-free body mass (**F**) for 21 endurance athletes who continued to train over a 20-year period, starting at age 50 years. (Modified from Pollock, M.L., et al.: Twenty-year follow-up of aerobic power and body composition of older track athletes. *J. Appl. Physiol.*, 82:1508, 1997.)

generally reported for nonathletes). Age-related decrements in maximum heart rate have been attributed to three factors:

1. Alterations in sinoatrial (SA) node activity
2. Reduced sympathetic activity output from the medulla
3. Reluctance of researchers to encourage older, nonathletic individuals to train "all out" to achieve a maximal effort during testing

Other age-related cardiovascular changes include reduced blood flow capacity to peripheral tissues, narrowing of the coronary arteries (30% obstruction by middle age), and decreased elasticity or compliance of major blood vessels.

Despite the almost 30 years of continuous training without changes in body mass (T1, 70.1 kg; T2, 69.4 kg; T3, 70.8 kg), gains occurred in body fat while FFM declined. The roughly 3% body fat unit increase per decade paralleled similar increases in waist girth. These data support an argument that some alterations in body composition and body fat distribution represent a normal aging response.

Other studies of physically active older individuals suggest that the typical individual grows fatter with age, but those who remain physically active counter the "normal" age-related loss in FFM while depressing the typical increase in body fat percentage.

In addition to weight-bearing exercise's positive role in preserving FFM, the lack of weight-bearing (mechanical loading) exercise deserves concern because such exercise helps to counter the deleterious effects of osteoporosis with aging. Longitudinal research of bone mineral content assessed every 6 months in children from age 6 to 12 years showed that 26% of adult total body bone mineral accrued during just 2 years of peak bone mineral deposition. Such direct evidence seems self-evident for its long-range implications in helping to preserve lean tissue mass. Perhaps the eventual "cure" for osteoporosis and its attendant medical and societal costs really should be viewed as a problem of young age (pediatric medicine) and not older age (geriatric medicine). We strongly endorse the position that vigorous physical activity should play an increasingly more important role in the home and schools as children grow into adolescence and adulthood.

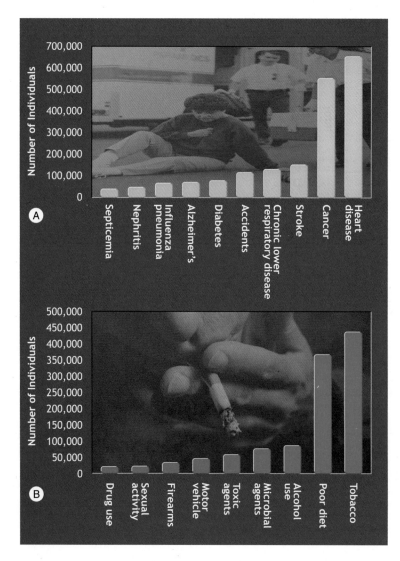

Figure 17.10 (A) Leading causes of deaths in the United States in 2006. (B) Actual causes of preventable deaths in the United States in 2006. (From the National Heart Lung and Blood Institute. Available at *http://www.nhlbi.nih.gov.*)

REGULAR EXERCISE: A FOUNTAIN OF YOUTH?

Exercise may not necessarily represent a "fountain of youth," yet the preponderance of evidence shows that regular physical activity retards the decline in functional capacity associated with aging and disuse. Exercise participation can reverse the loss of function regardless of when a person becomes more physically active.

Causes of Death in the United States

During the past 2 decades, changes in lifestyle have resulted in variations in causes of death in the United States. Whereas mortality rates from heart disease, stroke, and cancer have declined, prevalence of obesity and type 2 diabetes increased **Figure 17.10A** summarizes the latest research detailing causes of death in the United States for the year 2006 (reported in late 2009). Clearly, diseases of the heart, malignant neoplasms and cancers, and cerebrovascular disease account for the majority of deaths.

Figure 17.10B shows causes of preventable deaths during the same time period. The most striking finding is the substantial increase in the number of deaths attributable to poor diet and physical inactivity. The gap between deaths caused by poor diet and physical inactivity and those caused by cigarette smoking has narrowed substantially. *Clearly, most preventable deaths can be attributed to a small number of largely preventable behaviors and exposures that relate directly to physical inactivity, dietary exccess, and overfatness.* Unless curtailed, the increasing trend of overfatness, poor diet, and physical inactivity will overtake cigarette smoking as the leading preventable cause of mortality.

Does Exercise Improve Health and Extend Life?

Medical experts have debated whether a lifetime of regular exercise contributes to good health and perhaps longevity compared with a sedentary "good life." Because older, fit individuals exhibit many functional characteristics of younger people, one could argue that improved physical fitness and a vigorous lifestyle in older age retard biologic aging and confer health benefits later in life.

Research concerning lifestyles and exercise habits of 17,000 Harvard alumni who entered college between 1916 and 1950 showed that only moderate aerobic exercise, equivalent to jogging 3 miles a day, promotes good health and adds time to life. Men who expended 2000 kCal in weekly exercise had up to one-third lower death rates than classmates who did little or no exercise. To achieve a 2000-kCal energy output weekly requires moderate additional physical activity such as a daily 30- to 45-minute brisk walk or a moderate run, cycle, swim, cross-country ski, or aerobic dance participation. The following summarizes the results of the long-term study of alumni:

1. Regular exercise counters the life-shortening effects of cigarette smoking and excess body weight.
2. Even for people with high blood pressure (a primary heart disease risk), those who exercised regularly reduced their death rate by half.
3. Regular exercise countered genetic tendencies toward early death. Individuals with one or both parents who died before age 65 years (another significant but nonmodifiable risk) reduced their death risk by 25% with a lifestyle of regular exercise.

Questions & Notes

Give 2 reasons for age-related decrements in maximum heart rate.

1.

2.

Describe what happens to waist girth, percentage body fat, and FFM with aging, independent of physical activity level.

List the 3 leading causes of death in the United States in the year 2006.

1.

2.

3.

Give 2 major findings of the Harvard Alumni Study of physical activity and health.

1.

2.

(i) For Your Information

LARGE ARTERY COMPLIANCE

Compliance of large arteries declines with age from changes in the arterial wall's structural and nonstructural properties. The inability of the internal diameter of an artery to expand and recoil in response to fluctuations in intravascular pressure during the cardiac cycle associates with impaired cardiovascular function and elevated heart disease risk factors, including hypertension, stroke, atherosclerosis, thrombosis, myocardial infarction, and congestive heart failure. Regular endurance exercise slows or prevents the "stiffening" of the large arteries with advancing age and slows the decline in limb vasodilator capacity with healthy aging.

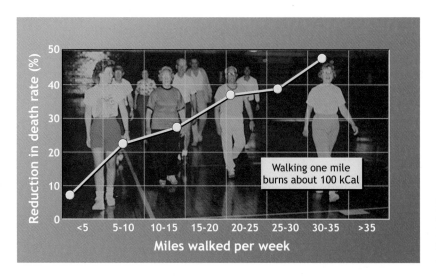

Figure 17.11 Reduced risk of death with regular exercise. (Data from Paffenbarger, R.S. Jr., et al.: Physical activity, all-cause mortality, and longevity of college alumni. *N. Engl. J. Med.*, 314:605, 1986.)

4. A 50% reduction in mortality rate occurred for active men whose parents lived beyond 65 years.

Figure 17.11 shows that among physically active people, the more a person exercises, the more risk of death declines. For example, men who walked 9 or more miles a week had a 21% lower mortality rate than men who walked 3 miles or less. Exercising in light sports activities increased life expectancy 24% over men who remained sedentary. From a perspective of energy expenditure, the life expectancy of Harvard alumni increased steadily from a weekly exercise energy output of 500 to 3500 kCal, the equivalent of 6 to 8 hours of strenuous weekly exercise. In addition, active men lived an average of 1 to 2 years longer than sedentary classmates. Additional research confirms that regular exercise confers an expected increase in life expectancy of about 10 months.

No additional health or longevity benefits accrued beyond weekly exercise of 3500 kCal. Men who performed extreme exercise had higher death rates than less active colleagues, an example of why *more* does not necessarily produce *greater* exercise benefits.

Improved Fitness: A Little Goes a Long Way

A study of more than 13,000 men and women over an 8-year interval indicates that even modest amounts of exercise substantially reduce the risk of death from heart disease, cancer, and other causes. The study evaluated fitness performance directly rather than relying on verbal or written reports of physical activity habits. To isolate the effect of physical fitness per se, the researchers accounted for factors of smoking, cholesterol and blood sugar levels, blood pressure, and family history of coronary heart disease. Based on age-adjusted death rates per 10,000 person-years, **Figure 17.12** illustrates that the least fit group died at a three times greater rate than the most fit subjects.

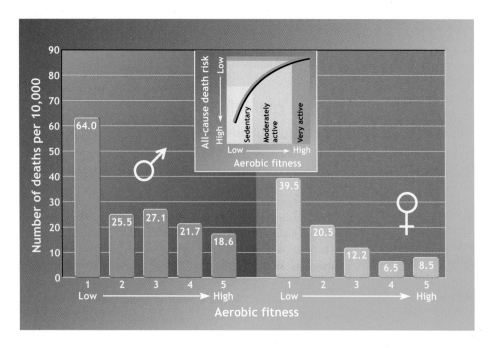

Figure 17.12 Physical fitness and risk of death. The greatest reduction in death rate risk occurs when going from the most sedentary category to a moderate fitness level. (Data from Blair, S.N., et al.: Physical fitness and all-cause mortality: a prospective study of healthy men and women. *JAMA.*, 262:2395, 1989.)

Importantly, the group rated just above the most sedentary category derived the greatest change in health benefits. Whereas the decrease in death rate for men from the least fit to the next category equaled 38 (64.0 vs. 25.5 deaths per 10,000 person-years), the decline from the second group to the most fit category equaled only seven deaths per 10,000 person-years. Women obtained similar benefits as men. The amount of exercise required moving from the most sedentary category to the next more fit category (the jump showing the greatest increase in health benefits) was moderate-intensity exercise such as walking briskly for 30 minutes several times weekly. *If life-extending benefits of exercise exist, they associated more with preventing early mortality than improving overall life span.* Only moderate exercise enables individuals to live more productive and healthy lives.

Questions & Notes

Describe the relationship between reduced risk of death with increases in regular exercise.

Changes in Physical Activity and Mortality Among Older Women

Studies of changes in physical activity and mortality have mostly examined middle-aged male populations. It remains unclear whether adoption of a physically active lifestyle by previously sedentary older women, particularly those with chronic cardiovascular disease, diabetes, and physical frailty, produces similar benefits typically observed for men. **Figure 17.13** summarizes a unique study of 9704 mostly white, 65-year-old women followed for 12.5 years. They were classified at baseline and 4.0 to 7.7 years later into one of four groups (quintiles, from highest to lowest) based on physical activity level (amount of walking per day and frequency and duration of other leisure time activities such as dancing, gardening, aerobics, or swimming). The four groups were (1) active at baseline and stayed active during follow-up, (2) active at baseline but became sedentary during the follow-up, (3) sedentary at baseline and remained sedentary at follow-up, and (4) sedentary at baseline but became active at follow-up. All-cause mortality data

 For Your Information

STRUCTURED PHYSICAL ACTIVITY NOT NECESSARY

Researchers monitored two groups of sedentary middle-aged men and women ages 35 to 60 years during a 2-year clinical trial. One group exercised vigorously for 20 to 60 minutes by swimming, stair stepping, walking, or biking at a fitness center up to 5 days a week. The other group incorporated 30 minutes a day of "lifestyle" exercises such as extra walking, raking leaves, stair climbing, walking around the airport while waiting for a plane, and participating in a walking club most days of the week. The lifestyle participants also learned cognitive and behavioral strategies to increase daily physical activity. For each of the programs, the intervention consisted of 6 months of intensive exercise followed by 18 months of maintenance. At the end of 24 months, *both* groups showed similar improvements in physical activity, cardiorespiratory fitness, systolic and diastolic blood pressure, and body fat percentage. These findings reinforce the conclusion that the health-derived benefits from regular exercise do not require highly structured or vigorous exercise.

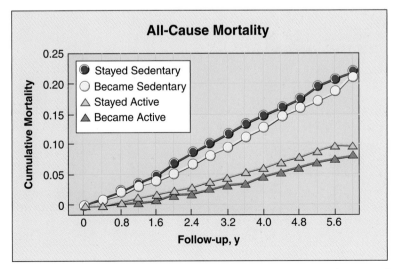

Figure 17.13 All-cause mortality by change in total physical activity by years of follow-up in older women. (From Gregg, E.W., et al.: Relationship of changes in physical activity and mortality among older women. *JAMA.*, 289:2379, 2003.)

For Your Information

MOST POPULAR EXERCISES FOR AMERICANS

Activity	Men (%)	Women (%)
Walking	30	48
Resistance training	20	9
Cycling	16	15
Running	12	6
Stair climbing	10	12
Aerobics	3	10

were compared between groups up to 12.5 years after baseline (6.7 y after the follow-up visit).

Compared with continually sedentary women, those who were active or who became active had lower all-cause mortality. Notably, sedentary women who increased daily physical activity to the equivalent of 1 mile of walking between baseline and follow-up had 40% to 50% lower all-cause mortality rates than chronically sedentary women. These findings take on added importance because the population of older women in the United States will double in the next 30 years, and more than one-third are now sedentary.

CORONARY HEART DISEASE

The main graph of **Figure 17.14** shows the prevalence of cardiovascular diseases in U.S. adults age 20 and older by age and gender for 2005 to 2006. The *inset pie chart* illustrates the percentage breakdown of deaths from the diverse diseases of the heart and blood vessels.

Deaths from CHD have declined more than 35% since 1970, yet heart disease remains the leading cause of death in the Western world. For every American who dies of cancer, almost two die of heart-related diseases. Death rates for women lag about 10 years behind men, but the gap has rapidly closed for women who smoke; for them, heart disease is now the leading cause of death. Available evidence indicates that disease symptoms, progression, and outcome differ in women and men. Four gender-related heart disease differences include:

1. Women usually die sooner after a heart attack.
2. Women who survive a heart attack frequently experience a second episode.
3. Women become more incapacitated by heart disease-related pain and disability.
4. Women are less likely to survive coronary artery bypass surgery.

Changes on the Cellular Level

Apparent Breakthrough Predisposing factors to CHD involve degenerative changes in the intima or inner lining of the larger arteries that supply the myocardium. Damage to the arterial walls begins as a low-grade chronic inflammatory response to injury. Eight contributing factors include hypertension, cigarette smoking, infection, homocysteine, elevated cholesterol, free radicals, reaction to obesity-related substances, and immunologically mediated factors. Discovering the cause(s) of CHD had escaped researchers until a recent breakthrough by a team of English researchers identified the trigger for inflammation and tissue breakdown in arterial plaque. The specialized molecule, toll-like receptor 2 (TLR-2), resides on the surface of an immune cell. When TLR-2 recognizes harmful molecules and cells its role switches the immune cell into attack mode

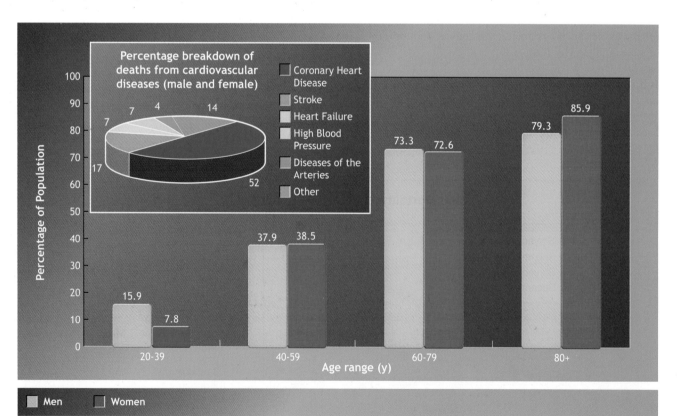

Figure 17.14 Prevalence of cardiovascular diseases in adults age 20 and older by age and gender in the United States for 2005 to 2006. The *inset pie chart* illustrates the percentage breakdown of deaths from the diverse diseases of the heart and blood vessels. (From *Heart Disease and Stroke Statistics: 2009 Update at a Glance. American Heart Association.* Available at *www.americanheart.org/downloadable/heart/1240250946756LS-1982%20Heart%20and%20Stroke%20Update.042009.pdf.*)

to protect the body. TLR-2 also can switch on immune cells when the body encounters stress. In addition, bacteria may switch on the TLR-2 molecules, increasing the risk of plaques bursting and causing strokes and heart attacks. The scientists demonstrated for the first time that antibodies could block the TLR-2 trigger mechanism. In their experiment, sections of the atherosclerotic carotid arteries were taken from 58 patients after they had a stroke. The arterial tissues were decomposed with enzymes until they formed a suspension of single cells in liquid. They analyzed the liquid after 4 days and found that the cells had produced an unusually large amount of inflammatory molecules and enzymes known to damage the arteries. The cells were then grown with several different antibodies designed to block different receptors and other molecules involved in the inflammation process. Blocking TLR-2 using an antibody dramatically reduced the production of inflammation molecules and enzymes. The next step in future research would be to pinpoint specific parts of molecules that switch on TLR-2 and trigger inflammation.

Other Considerations   One response in the degenerative changes in the coronary arterial wall triggers the chemical modification of various compounds, including oxidation of low-density lipoprotein cholesterol (LDL-C). LDL-C oxidation represents a crucial step in a complex series of changes that produce lesions that sometimes bulge into the vessel lumen or protrude into the arterial wall. The first signs of atherosclerosis involve lesions that take the form of fatty streaks, With further inflammatory damage from continued lipid deposition and proliferation of smooth muscle and connective tissue, the vessels congest with lipid-filled plaques, fibrous scar tissue, or both. Progressive occlusion gradually reduces blood flow capacity, causing the myocardium to become ischemic or poorly supplied with oxygen.

Vulnerable Plaque: Difficult to Detect Yet Lethal   Vulnerable plaque, a soft type of metabolically active, unstable plaque, does not necessarily produce significant coronary artery narrowing but tends to fissure and burst. The rupture of unstable plaque—the sudden breakdown of fatty plaques in the lining of the coronary arteries—exposes the blood to thrombogenic compounds. This triggers a cascade of chemical events that culminates in clot formation (thrombus) and leads to a myocardial infarction (MI) and possible death. The sudden, complete obstruction of a coronary artery frequently occurs in blood vessels with only mild to moderate obstructions (~70% blockage). Arterial blockage often occurs before the coronary vessel has narrowed enough to produce angina symptoms or ECG abnormalities or to indicate the need for revascularization procedures (e.g., coronary bypass surgery or balloon angioplasty). Acute disruption and rupture of arterial plaque provides a plausible explanation for sudden death from acute physical exertion or emotional stress in middle-aged men with coronary artery disease compared with sudden death under resting conditions. The beneficial effects of cholesterol-lowering strategies on heart disease risk do not always improve coronary blood flow. A reduction in overall blood cholesterol, however, may improve the stability of vulnerable plaque, which would reduce the likelihood of future rupture of existing arterial plaque.

A Lifelong Process

Landmark studies of atherosclerosis in 22-year-old American soldiers killed in Korea in 1950–1953 showed advanced lesions. These findings surprised the medical community and focused attention on the possible childhood origins of atherosclerosis. Researchers now know that fatty streaks and clinically significant fibrous plaques develop rapidly during adolescence through the third decade of life.

BMI, systolic and diastolic blood pressure, and total serum cholesterol, triacylglycerols, and LDL-C strongly and positively related (HDL-C related negatively)

*Q*uestions & Notes

Health benefits from regular exercise are about the same for men and women.

Name the leading cause of death in the Western world.

Give 2 gender-specific differences related to heart disease.

1.

2.

Describe the function of the TLR-2 molecule.

i **For Your Information**

DIABETES RISK LOWERED WITH REGULAR EXERCISE

Men who exercise five or more times a week show a 42% lower risk of type 2 diabetes than men who exercise less than once a week. The exercise benefits become most pronounced among obese participants. The risk of diabetes decreases approximately 6% for every 500 kCal of additional weekly exercise.

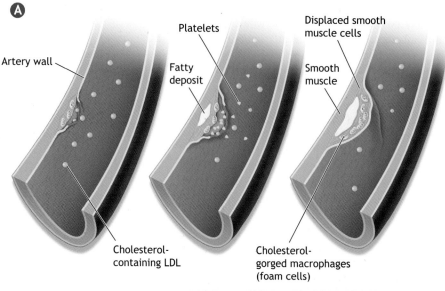

Platelets

Displaced smooth
muscle cells

Artery wall

Fatty
deposit

Smooth
muscle

Cholesterol-
containing LDL

Cholesterol-
gorged macrophages
(foam cells)

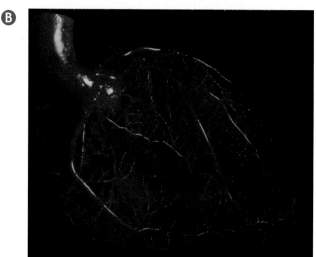

Figure 17.15 **A.** Deterioration of a coronary artery in atherosclerosis; deposits of fatty substances roughen the vessel's center. **B.** Cast of coronary artery vasculature.

to the extent of vascular lesions in the deceased young people. History of cigarette smoking magnified the vascular damage. As the number of risk factors increased, so did the severity of atherosclerosis. Analyses of microscopic qualities of coronary atherosclerosis in teenagers and young adults who died as a result of accidents, suicide, and murder indicated that many had arteries so clogged that they could experience an MI. Two percent of those ages 15 to 19 years and 20% of those ages 30 to 34 years had advanced plaque formation, the blockages considered most likely to separate from the arterial walls and trigger a heart attack or stroke. Collectively, these and other data support the wisdom of primary prevention through risk factor identification and intervention of artherosclerosis early in childhood or adolescence.

Figure 17.15 shows the progressive occlusion of an artery from a buildup of calcified fatty substances in atherosclerosis. The first overt sign of atherosclerotic change occurs when lipid-laden macrophage cells cluster under the endothelial lining to form a bulge (fatty streak) in the artery. Over time, proliferating smooth muscle cells accumulate to narrow the artery's lumen (center). Typically, a

thrombus (clot) forms and plugs the artery, depriving the myocardium of normal blood flow with its oxygen supply. When the thrombus blocks one of the smaller coronary vessels, a portion of the heart muscle dies (called *necrosis*), and the person has a heart attack or MI.

If coronary artery narrowing leads to brief periods of inadequate myocardial perfusion, the person may experience temporary chest pains termed **angina pectoris** (see Chapter 18). These pains usually emerge during exertion because increased physical activity creates a greater demand for myocardial blood flow. Anginal attacks provide painful, dramatic evidence of the importance of adequate myocardial oxygen supply.

Seven Heart Attack Warning Signs The AHA (*www.aha.org*) and other medical experts claim that one or more of these seven warning signs help identify an impending heart attack:

1. Uncomfortable pressure, fullness, squeezing, or pain in the center of the chest lasting more than a few minutes

2. Pain spreading to the shoulders, neck, or arms. The pain ranges from mild to intense. It may feel like pressure, tightness, burning, or heavy weight. It may be located in the chest, upper abdomen, neck, jaw, or inside the arms or shoulders

3. Chest discomfort with lightheadedness, fainting, sweating, nausea, or shortness of breath

4. Anxiety; nervousness; or cold, sweaty skin

5. Paleness or pallor

6. Increased or irregular heart rate

7. Feeling of impending doom

Cardiovascular Disease Epidemic

Each year, cardiovascular diseases top the list of the country's most serious health problems. CHD remains the leading health problem and the primary cause of death. It represents the most expensive condition to treat as it exemplifies a resource-intensive chronic condition. Consider recent (2005–2006) statistics for the United States released by the AHA shown in the accompanying box:

- At least 80 million people (one person in three) has some form of cardiovascular disease.
- Cardiovascular disease is the primary killer of women and men. Diseases of the cardiovascular system claim the lives of more than half a million women every year, about one death per minute.
- Cardiovascular disease accounts for almost 1 of every 2.4 deaths.
- Since 1900, cardiovascular disease was the leading cause of death every year but 1918, and it caused more deaths than the next seven causes combined.
- Every 37 seconds, a person has a coronary event, and each minute, someone dies from one.
- Among whites, only 11.4% have heart disease, 6.1% have CHD, and 2.2% have had a stroke.
- Among African Americans, 10.2% have heart disease, 6.0% have CHD, 31.7% have hypertension, and 3.7% have had a stroke.
- Among Asian Americans, 6.9% have heart disease, 4.3% have CHD, 19.5% have hypertension, and 2.6% have had a stroke.

Cigarette Smoking

Cigarette smoking, either active or passive through environmental exposure, directly increases the risk of CHD. Smokers experience twice the risk of death from heart disease as nonsmokers. The risk increases further for smokers with diabetes and hypertension. The CDC estimates that every cigarette smoked steals 7 minutes from a smoker's life. This adds up to 5 million years of potential life Americans lose to cigarettes yearly. CHD risk increases the more one smokes or receives passive exposure, the deeper one inhales, and the stronger the cigarette (for tars and noxious by-products). The increasing death rate from heart disease among women in the United States almost parallels their increased cigarette use. British researchers estimate that smokers between ages 30 and 40 years have five times as many heart attacks as nonsmokers in the same age range. When these relatively young smokers have a heart attack, an 80% chance exists that smoking caused it; this percentage averages nearly 70% for smokers in their 50s and 50% for smokers in their 60s and 70s. Also, smokers run a five times greater risk for stroke than nonsmokers, and those who smoke one pack or more each day are 11 times more likely to have a specific type of a sudden, deadly stroke most common in younger men and women. Surprisingly, the CHD risk from smoking correlates with a greater number of deaths than excess mortality of cigarette smokers from lung cancer.

Smoking risk usually remains independent of other risk factors. If additional risk factors exist, then smoking accentuates their influence. Cigarette smoking

Questions & Notes

List 4 variables that positively relate to vascular lesions.

1.

2.

3.

4.

List 3 heart attack warning signs.

1.

2.

3.

For Your Information

HEART ATTACK VERSUS CARDIAC ARREST

- **Heart attack:** Caused by (1) blockage in one or more arteries supplying the heart, thus cutting off myocardial blood supply, or (2) sudden spasms (constrictions) of a coronary vessel, causing part of the heart muscle to die (necrosis) from lack of oxygen (anoxia).

- **Cardiac arrest:** Caused by irregular neural–electrical transmission within the myocardium. This produces chaotic, unregulated beating in the heart's lower chambers (ventricular fibrillation).

For Your Information

EXERCISE IS GOOD MEDICINE FOR THE COLON

Research based on the health and exercise habits of Harvard alumni indicates that physically active men had about half the risk of colon cancer as inactive classmates. The protection disappeared if the men stopped exercising. One mechanism proposes that exercise protects against this major killer by speeding the passage of food residues through the digestive tract that reduces the colon's exposure to potential food carcinogens.

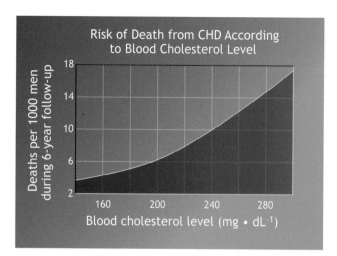

Figure 17.16 Generalized risk for death from coronary heart disease (CHD) in relation to total serum cholesterol level. (Adapted from Martin, M.J., et al.: Serum cholesterol, blood pressure and mortality: implications from a cohort of 361,662 men. *Lancet*, 2:933, 1986.)

facilitates heart disease through its potentiating effect on serum lipoproteins; individuals who smoke have lower levels of HDL-C than nonsmokers. When smokers quit, the HDL-C and heart disease risk return to levels of nonsmokers. A frightening statistic predicts that by the year 2030, smoking will become the world's single leading cause of death and disability (unless obesity continues its meteoric increases with unprecedented effects on disease processes).

Blood Lipid Abnormalities

An abnormal blood lipid level, or hyperlipidemia, provides a crucial component in the genesis of atherosclerosis. **Figure 17.16** shows the increasing rate of death from CHD related to total serum cholesterol. Current guidelines focus less on total cholesterol and more on its lipoprotein components (see Close Up Box 17.2: *How to Classify Cholesterol, Lipoproteins, and Triacylglycerol Values*, on page 619). Early treatment becomes crucial because of a strong association between high serum cholesterol as a young adult and cardiovascular disease in middle age. A cholesterol level of 200 mg·dL^{-1} or lower is usually desirable, although risk for a fatal heart attack begins to increase at

150 mg·dL^{-1}. A cholesterol level of 230 mg·dL^{-1} increases heart attack risk to about twice that of 180 mg·dL^{-1}, and 300 mg·dL^{-1} increases the risk fourfold. For triacylglycerols, the National Cholesterol Education Program (*www.nhlbi.nih.gov/about/ncep/index.htm*) considers 200 mg·dL^{-1} an upper limit of normal triacylglycerol level, with 200 to 400 mg·dL^{-1} as borderline, requiring changes in exercise, diet, and possibly drug treatment if accompanied by other CHD risk factors. More than likely, triacylglycerol levels above 100 mg·dL^{-1} pose a cardiac risk. Individuals with triacylglycerol levels above 100 mg·dL^{-1} (after a 12-h fast) show a 50% greater CHD risk than those with triacylglycerols below 100 mg·dL^{-1}, even after controlling for HDL-C.

Major clinical drug trials show conclusively that reducing cholesterol lowers death rates and attenuates heart attacks. Medications that affect blood lipids include (1) bile acid sequestrants (e.g., cholestyramine resin and colestipol hydrochloride), which bind (sequester) cholesterol-rich bile in the gastrointestinal tract and prevent its reabsorption from the gut; (2) fibric acid derivatives (e.g., gemfibrozil, probucol, clofibrate), which lower triacylglycerols and LDL-C (5% to 20%) and elevate HDL-C (average 6% per year); and (3) the remarkably effective statins (e.g., lovastatin, pravastatin, simvastatin, atorvastatin), which inhibit an enzyme that controls cholesterol synthesis by the cells, increase LDL-C receptors in the liver, and facilitate LDL-C removal from serum (18% to 55% reduction). Raising HDL-C by 34 mg·dL^{-1} via a 5-year gemfibrozil therapy trial reduced heart attacks, strokes, and death by 24% in patients with initially low HDL-C levels.

Lipids do not circulate freely in blood plasma; rather, they combine with a carrier protein to form lipoproteins composed of a hydrophobic cholesterol core and coat of free cholesterol, phospholipid, and a regulatory protein (apolipoprotein [Apo]). **Table 17.2** lists the four different lipoproteins, their approximate gravitational densities, and their percentage composition in the blood. *Serum cholesterol reflects a composite of the total cholesterol contained in each of the different lipoproteins.* Although discussions commonly refer to hyperlipidemia, the more meaningful focus addresses the different types of hyperlipoproteinemias.

Cholesterol distribution among the various lipoproteins provides a more powerful predictor of heart disease

Table 17.2	Approximate Composition of Lipoproteins in the Blood			
	CHYLOMICRONS	**VERY LOW-DENSITY LIPOPROTEINS (VLDL: PREBETA)**	**LOW-DENSITY LIPOPROTEINS (LDL:BETA)**	**HIGH-DENSITY LIPOPROTEINS (HDL: ALPHA)**
Density, g·cm^{-3}	0.95	0.95–1.006	1.006–1.019	1.063–1.210
Protein, %	0.5–1.0	5–15	25	45–55
Lipid, %	99	95	75	50
Cholesterol, %	2–5	10–20	40–45	18
Triacylglycerol, %	85	50–70	5–10	2
Phospholipid, %	3–6	10–20	20–25	30

BOX 17.2 CLOSE UP

How to Classify Cholesterol, Lipoproteins, and Triacylglycerol Values

Important risk factors for the development of atherosclerosis include high levels of serum cholesterol, triacylglycerol, and LDL-C and a low level of HDL-C. The primary sites for artery-narrowing plaque formation (i.e., incorporation of connective tissue, smooth muscle, cellular debris, minerals, and cholesterol) include the aorta and carotid, coronary, femoral, and iliac arteries. Specific cutoff values for the diverse blood lipid forms relate to increased CHD risk. The following tables present current guidelines for the various blood lipids and lipoproteins.

Table 1 Classification of Serum Total Cholesterol, Low-Density Lipoprotein Cholesterol, and High-Density Lipoprotein Cholesterol Levels

CHOLESTEROL ($mg \cdot dL^{-1}$)	CLASSIFICATION
Total	
<200	Desirable cholesterol
200–239	Borderline high cholesterol
>240	High cholesterol
LDL	
<70	Optimal (recommended for people with CHD or diabetes)
<130	Desirable
130–159	Borderline high cholesterol
160–189	High cholesterol
>190	Very high cholesterol
HDL	
<35	Low cholesterol
>60	High cholesterol

From Diabetes Education Research Center and American Heart Association, 2004.

Table 2 Classification of Triacylglycerol Levels

SERUM TRIACYLGLYEROLS ($mg \cdot dL^{-1}$)	CLASSIFICATION	COMMENTS
<150	Normal	
150–199	Borderline high	Check for accompanying primary or secondary dyslipidemias
200–499	High	Check for accompanying primary or secondary dyslipidemias
>500	Very high	Increased risk for acute pancreatitis

From Diabetes Education Research Center and American Heart Association, 2004.

risk than total blood cholesterol. Specifically, elevated HDL-C levels relate causally with a *lower* heart disease risk, even among individuals with total cholesterol below 200 $mg \cdot dL^{-1}$. Overwhelming evidence links high LDL-C and Apo B levels with *increased* CHD risk. A more effective evaluation of heart disease risk than either total cholesterol or LDL-C levels divides total cholesterol by HDL-C. A ratio greater than 4.5 indicates a high heart disease risk; a ratio of 3.5 or lower represents a more desirable risk level.

 ## For Your Information

SHOULD CHOLESTEROL BE MEASURED IN CHILDREN?

Guidelines issued by the National Cholesterol Education Program (*www.americanheart.org*) conclude "yes" if a family history of high cholesterol or heart disease exists particularly if a parent had a heart attack before age 50 years. Shockingly, this parental "cardiac proneness" includes up to 25% of the United States adult population! Research with children ages 10 to 15 years indicates that lifestyle habits of regular exercise, improved cardiovascular fitness, and a prudent nutritional profile contribute to favorable lipid profiles similar to effects with adults.

LDL-C (synthesized in the liver) and very low–density lipoprotein cholesterol (VLDL-C) provide the transport medium for fats to cells, including the smooth muscle walls of arteries. Upon oxidation, LDL-C participates in artery-clogging, plaque-forming atherosclerosis by stimulating monocyte–macrophage infiltration and lipoprotein deposition. LDL-C's surface coat contains the specific apolipoprotein (Apo B) that facilitates cholesterol removal from the LDL-C molecule by binding to LDL-C receptors of specific cells. Prevention of LDL-C oxidation slows the progression of CHD. The potential benefit of the dietary antioxidants vitamins C and E and β-carotene on heart disease risk reflect how well they blunt LDL-C oxidation.

LDL-C targets peripheral tissue and contributes to arterial damage, and HDL-C (also produced in the liver and whose levels relate to genetic factors) facilitates reverse cholesterol transport. HDL-C promotes surplus cholesterol removal from peripheral tissues including arterial walls for transport to the liver for bile synthesis and subsequent excretion via the digestive tract. The apolipoprotein A-1 (Apo A-1) in HDL-C activates the enzyme lecithin acetyl transferase (LCAT) that converts free cholesterol into cholesterol esters. This facilitates removal of cholesterol from lipoproteins and other tissues.

Factors that Affect Blood Lipids

Six behaviors favorably impact the blood lipid profile:

1. Weight loss
2. Regular aerobic exercise (independent of weight loss)
3. Increased intake of water-soluble fibers (fibers in beans, legumes, and oat bran)
4. Increased intake of polyunsaturated to saturated fatty acid ratio and monounsaturated fatty acids and elimination of trans fatty acids
5. Increased intake of the polyunsaturated fatty acids in fish oils (omega-3 fatty acids)
6. Moderate alcohol consumption

Four variables adversely affect cholesterol and lipoprotein levels:

1. Cigarette smoking
2. Diet high in saturated fatty acids, trans fatty acids, and preformed cholesterol
3. Emotionally stressful situations
4. Oral contraceptives

Hypertension: A Prevalent Disorder

About 73.6 million people in the United States age 20 years and older have high blood pressure that exceeds 140 mm Hg (systolic hypertension) or diastolic pressure that exceeds 90 mm Hg (diastolic hypertension; *www.americanheart.org/ presenter.jhtml?identifier=4621*). These values form the lower limit for the classification of *borderline* high blood pressure. One of every four or five people experiences chronic, abnormally high blood pressure sometime during life. Uncorrected hypertension can precipitate heart failure, heart attack, stroke, and kidney failure. From 1995 to 2005, the death rate from hypertension increased 25.2%, and the number of deaths rose 56.4%.

Modification of lifestyle behaviors can lower high blood pressure, often called the "silent killer"; important modifications include weight loss, regular physical activity, cessation of smoking (nicotine constricts peripheral blood vessels that elevates blood pressure), and reducing salt intake (excess sodium retains fluid that elevates blood pressure in susceptible individuals). Unfortunately, the cause(s) of hypertension remains unknown in more than 90% of individuals. Men and women ages 30 to 54 years with mild hypertension modestly lowered their systolic by 2.9 mm Hg and diastolic blood pressure by 2.3 mm Hg when they reduced their body weight and salt intake over an 18-month period. No blood pressure changes occurred for subjects who undertook only stress reduction and relaxation techniques or consumed calcium, magnesium, phosphorus, and fish oil dietary supplements. Prescription drugs that either reduce fluid volume or decrease peripheral resistance to blood flow effectively treat high blood pressure. Lowering systolic blood pressure just 2 mm Hg reduces deaths from stroke by 6% and heart disease by 4%.

Diabetes

Diabetics are up to four times more likely to develop cardiovascular disease from multiple risk factors usually coincident with the diabetic condition. These four factors include:

1. **Obesity** represents a major risk factor for cardiovascular disease that strongly associates with insulin resistance. Insulin resistance may provide the mechanism by which obesity leads to cardiovascular disease. Weight loss improves cardiovascular risk, decreases blood insulin concentrations, and increases insulin sensitivity.
2. **Physical inactivity** is a modifiable risk factor for insulin resistance and cardiovascular disease. Exercising more while reducing excess body weight (and fat) prevents or delays the onset of type 2 diabetes, reduces blood pressure, and reduces heart attack and stroke risk.
3. **Hypertension** positively correlates with insulin resistance in diabetes. For a person with both hypertension and diabetes, a common combination, the risk for cardiovascular disease doubles.
4. **Atherogenic dyslipidemia**, often called *diabetic dyslipidemia* in people with diabetes, relates to insulin resistance characterized by high levels of triacylglycerols (hypertriglyceridemia) and high levels of small LDL particles and low levels of HDL. The components of this *lipid triad* contribute to atherosclerotic risk.

According to the latest statistics from the 2007 National Diabetes Fact Sheet (the most recent year for which data are available; *www.diabetes.org/diabetes-basics/diabetes-statistics*), 3.6 million children and adults in the United States—7.8% of the population—have diabetes. Roughly 17.9 million people have been diagnosed, 5.7 million people remain undiagnosed, and 57 million people are prediabetic. Unfortunately, 1.6 million new cases of diabetes will be diagnosed in people age 20 years and older each year, and the numbers continue to increase yearly at an alarming rate.

Other Coronary Heart Disease Risk Factor Candidates

The following factors represent potentially potent CHD risk predictors.

Age, Gender, and Heredity   Age represents a CHD risk factor as it associates with other risk factors—hypertension, elevated blood lipid levels, and glucose intolerance. After age 35 years in men and age 45 years in women, the chances of dying from CHD increase progressively and dramatically. Heredity also represents a risk factor in that heart attacks that strike at an early age tend to run in families. Such familial predisposition probably relates to a genetic role in determining the risk of heart disease.

Immunologic Factors   An immune response may trigger plaque development within arterial walls. During this process, mononuclear immune cells produce proteins called *cytokines,* some of which stimulate plaque buildup; others inhibit plaque formation. Within this framework, regular exercise may stimulate the immune system to inhibit agents that facilitate arterial disease. For example, 2.5 hours of weekly exercise for 6 months *decreased* cytokine production that facilitates plaque development by 58%; cytokines that inhibit plaque formation *increased* by 36%.

Homocysteine   Homocysteine, a highly reactive, sulfur-containing amino acid, forms as a by-product of methionine metabolism. Researchers in the 1960s and 1970s described three different inborn errors of homocysteine metabolism involving B-vitamin enzymes. High levels of homocysteine in the blood and urine were common to all three disorders of the affected individuals, and half of these individuals developed arterial or venous thrombosis by age 30 years. It was postulated that moderate elevation of homocysteine in the general population predisposes individuals to atherosclerosis similarly to elevated cholesterol concentration.

Numerous studies have shown a nearly lockstep association between plasma homocysteine levels and heart attack and mortality in men and women similar to that of smoking and hyperlipidemia. This metabolic abnormality is present in nearly 30% of CHD patients and 40% of patients with cerebrovascular disease. Excessive homocysteine causes blood platelets to clump, fostering blood clots and deterioration of smooth muscle cells that line the arterial wall. Chronic homocysteine exposure eventually scars and thickens arteries and provides a fertile medium for circulating LDL-C to initiate damage. In the presence of other conventional CHD risks (e.g., smoking and hypertension), synergistic

Questions & Notes

List the 4 major risk factors for diabetes.

1.

2.

3.

4.

ⓘ For Your Information

FIBER INTAKE AND CORONARY HEART DISEASE IN THE ELDERLY

An inverse association exists between fiber consumption from cereal sources (including whole grains and bran) and coronary heart disease risk in elderly men and women (average age, 72+ y). Compared with medical or surgical interventions, increasing fiber intake by the equivalent of two slices of whole grain bread per day is easy to incorporate into the daily routine, is low cost, and is widely available.

ⓘ For Your Information

PHYSICAL ACTIVITY AND WOMEN: HOW MUCH IS GOOD ENOUGH?

Modest levels of physical activity (30 minutes per day on most days) decrease the risk of chronic diseases, including breast cancer. Appropriate dietary restraint, coupled with increased physical activity, can help overweight women reduce their weight. When prescribing physical activity, set a goal of 30 minutes per day of moderate-intensity activity. This can be accumulated in bouts of at least 10 minutes daily. For those willing to do more and for whom no contraindications exist, greater duration and increased intensity of activity confers additional benefits. (Jakicic, J.M.: Effect of exercise duration and intensity on weight loss in overweight, sedentary women: a randomized trial. *JAMA.,* 290:1323, 2003; Lee, I.-M. Physical Activity and Women: How Much Is Good Enough? *JAMA.,* 290:1377, 2003; and Manson, J.E.: Walking compared with vigorous exercise for the prevention of cardiovascular events in women. *N. Engl. J. Med.,* 347:716, 2002.)

effects magnify the negative impact of homocysteine on cardiovascular health. In general, people in the highest quartile for homocysteine levels have nearly twice the risk of heart attack or stroke compared with those in the lowest quartile. Why some people accumulate homocysteine is uncertain, but the evidence points to a deficiency of B vitamins (B_6, B_{12}, and particularly folic acid); cigarette smoking, frequent coffee intake, and high meat consumption are also associated with elevated homocysteine concentrations.

Excessive Body Fat Excess body fat has received attention as a CHD risk factor, but its relationship frequently coexists with hypertension, elevated cholesterol, type 2 diabetes, and cigarette smoking. The number of annual deaths attributable to overfatness in the United States adult population easily exceeds 350,000. Weight loss and accompanying body fat reduction, whether through diet or exercise, usually normalize cholesterol and triacylglycerol levels and exert beneficial effects on blood pressure and type 2 diabetes.

Physical Inactivity Regular physical activity offers protection against heart disease. Sedentary men and women are twice as likely to suffer a fatal heart attack as more physically active counterparts. Maintenance of aerobic fitness throughout life also provides protection against CHD risk factors and disease occurrence. One could argue that genetic factors contribute more to fitness level than to daily exercise patterns. However, fitness level relates closely to individual differences in physical activity level among most individuals, making regular exercise assume greater importance than simply genetics in determining physical fitness and related health benefits. **Table 17.3** summarizes possible biologic mechanisms for how regular aerobic exercise confers protection against CHD progression.

C-Reactive Protein Mounting evidence indicates that painless chronic low-grade arterial inflammation, including that of the coronary arteries remains central to every stage of atherosclerotic disease and a major trigger for heart attack—more substantial even than high cholesterol. The inflammation produces heart attacks by weakening blood vessels walls, making plaque burst, and interfering with substances that increase myocardial circulation. **C-reactive protein (CRP)** is a protein found in the blood that increases during the inflammatory response to tissue injury or infection. The liver primarily synthesizes CRP with its release stimulated by interleukin 6 (IL-6) and other proinflammatory cytokines. Small increases in CRP within the normal range predict future vascular events in apparently healthy, asymptomatic individuals. Such predictive accuracy of CRP extends to patients with preexisting vascular disease. Higher CRP levels are associated with abdominal obesity, and increased levels predict the risk of developing type 2 diabetes. Strategies to lower CRP include weight loss, abstinence from cigarette smoking, consuming a healthful diet, and regular exercise (e.g., combined aerobic/resistance training).

Lipoprotein(a) Liporotein(a) [Lp(a)] is an LDL-like particle largely under genetic control that varies substantially between individuals depending on the size of the apo(a) isoform present. Lp(a) levels vary little with diet or exercise, unlike the other lipoproteins LDL and HDL. The biological function of Lp(a) remains unclear, but strong evidence suggests its role in responding to tissue injury and vascular lesions, to prevent infectious pathogens from invading cells, and to promote wound healing. High Lp(a) in blood is a risk factor for coronary artery disease, cerebrovascular disease, atherosclerosis, thrombosis, and stroke. Lp(a)'s most important role may be to inhibit the breakdown of clots (fibrinolysis) at the site of tissue injury. These properties make Lp(a) a highly atherothrombotic lipoprotein.

Table 17.3	**Possible Mechanisms for Eight Beneficial Effects of Regular Aerobic Exercise on Risk of Coronary Heart Disease and Mortality**

1. Improves myocardial circulation and metabolism to protect the heart from hypoxic stress. Improvements include enhanced vascularization and increased coronary blood flow capacity via altered control of coronary vascular smooth muscle and increased reactivity of coronary resistance vessels. Modest increases in cardiac glycogen stores and glycolytic capacity also prove beneficial if the heart's oxygen supply suddenly becomes compromised.
2. Enhances the mechanical properties of the myocardium to enable the exercise-trained heart to maintain or increase contractility during a specific challenge.
3. Establishes more favorable blood-clotting characteristics and other hemostatic mechanisms, including increased fibrinolysis and production of endothelial prostacyclin.
4. Normalizes the blood lipid profile to slow or reverse atherosclerosis.
5. Favorably alters heart rate and blood pressure so myocardial work decreases during rest and exercise.
6. Suppresses age-related body weight gain and promotes a more desirable body composition and body fat distribution (particularly a reduced level of intraabdominal adipose tissue).
7. Establishes a more favorable neural–hormonal balance to conserve oxygen for the myocardium; improves the mixture of carbohydrate and fat metabolized by the body.
8. Provides a favorable outlet for psychological stress and tension.

Fibrinogen Fibrinogen, a circulating glycoprotein synthesized by the liver, acts at the final step in the coagulation response to vascular tissue injury. Fibrinogen, similar to CRP, is an acute-phase reactant, with other characteristics that make it biologically plausible as a possible participant in vascular disease: (1) regulation of cell adhesion, chemotaxis (movements of cells in response to substances exhibiting chemical properties), and cell proliferation; (2) vasoconstriction at sites of vessel wall injury; (3) stimulation of platelet aggregation; and (4) determinants of blood viscosity.

Epidemiologic data support an independent association between elevated fibrinogen levels and cardiovascular morbidity and mortality. Elevated blood fibrinogen, independent of classic CHD risk factors, correlates with ischemic stroke and peripheral vascular disease. Several factors other than inflammation modulate fibrinogen levels. A dose–response relationship exists between number of cigarettes smoked and fibrinogen level. Fibrinogen tends to be higher in patients with diabetes, hypertension, obesity, and a sedentary lifestyle.

CORONARY HEART DISEASE RISK FACTOR INTERACTIONS

Smoking generally acts independently of other risk factors to increase CHD risk. The other risk factors interact with each other and CHD itself to accentuate disease risk. **Figure 17.17** quantifies the interaction of three primary CHD risk factors in the same person. With one risk factor, a 45-year-old man's chance for CHD symptoms during the year averages about twice that of a man without risks. The chance for chest pain, heart attack, or sudden death with three risk factors increases five times compared with no risk factors.

CORONARY HEART DISEASE RISK FACTORS IN CHILDREN

The frequent occurrence of multiple CHD risk factors in young children emphasizes the need for early CHD initiatives to reduce atherosclerosis risk later in life. Obesity and a family history of heart disease represent the two most common risk factors in physically active and apparently healthy boys and girls. A relatively large percentage of these children also show abnormally high blood lipid concentrations.

As with adults, the association between body fat and serum lipid levels becomes apparent in overfat children. The fattest children usually have the highest levels of serum cholesterol and triacylglycerols. For them, general adiposity and visceral adipose tissue relate to unfavorable hemostatic factors that increase CHD morbidity and mortality in adulthood. Of 62 overfat children ages 10 to 15 years, only 1 child had just one CHD risk factor. Of the remaining children, 14% had two risk factors, 30% had three risk factors, 29% had four risk factors, 18% had five risk factors, and the remaining five children (8%) had six risk factors. A subsample of these children was then enrolled in a 20-week program to evaluate the effects on the risk profile of either (1) diet plus behavior therapy (DB) or (2) regular exercise plus diet and behavior therapy (EDB). No changes resulted in multiple-risk reduction in the control group (CON) or in those receiving diet with behavior treatment. In contrast, children who exercised, dieted, and underwent behavior therapy

$\mathcal{Q}$*uestions & Notes*

List 6 factors not causally linked that are nevertheless potent CHD risk factors.

1.

2.

3.

4.

5.

6.

List 3 possible exercise-induced mechanisms for reducing CHD risk.

1.

2.

3.

Briefly explain the role of C-reactive protein as a CHD risk factor.

$\textit{i}$ For Your Information

APOPROTEIN

Apoproteins represent a class of specific proteins embedded in the outer shell of a lipoprotein particle that (1) increase the solubility of the lipoprotein's cholesterol and triacylglycerol components, (2) act as ligands for specific lipoprotein receptors in cell membranes, and (3) serve as important cofactors to activate enzymes in lipoprotein metabolism. Specific apoproteins may more reliably predict heart disease proneness than total cholesterol level.

BOX 17.3 CLOSE UP

Calculate Your Coronary Heart Disease Risk

CHD risk inventories provide a qualitative means to assess an individual's susceptibility to CHD. The table below presents the Framingham 10-year CHD risk estimate. This is the most widely used "traditional" risk analysis system.

To determine risk profile, review each risk factor and accompanying numerical "point" value. Insert the respective points into the applicable box at the top of the table. The total number of points represents the 10-year risk for developing CHD expressed as a percentage.

Framingham 10-Year CHD Risk Estimate Worksheet

□	+	□	+	□	+	□	+	□	+	□	=	□
AGE		HDL-C		SBP		TC		SMOKING		TOTAL POINTS		10-y RISK (%)

Age (y)				Systolic Blood Pressure (SBP), mm Hg					

Women	Points	Men	Points	Women	Points		Men	Points	
				mm Hg	Treated	Untreated	mm Hg	Treated	Untreated
20–34	−7	20–34	−9	<120	0	0	<120	0	0
35–39	−3	35–39	−4	120–129	1	3	120–129	0	1
40–44	0	40–44	0	130–139	2	4	130–139	1	2
45–49	3	45–49	3	140–159	3	5	140–159	1	2
50–54	6	50–54	6	>160	4	6	>160	2	3
55–59	8	55–59	8						
60–64	10	60–64	10						
65–69	12	65–69	11						
70–74	14	70–74	12						
75–79	16	75–79	13						

Points for Total Cholesterol (TC) at Each Age Category (y) Women						Points for Total Cholesterol (TC) at Each Age Category (y) Men					

TC $(mg \cdot dL^{-1})$	20–39	40–49	50–59	60–69	70–79	TC $(mg \cdot dL^{-1})$	20–39	40–49	50–59	60–69	70–79
<160	0	0	0	0	0	<160	0	0	0	0	0
160–199	4	3	2	1	1	160–199	4	3	2	1	0
200–239	8	6	4	2	1	200–239	7	5	3	1	0
240–279	11	8	5	3	2	240–279	9	6	4	2	1
>280	13	10	7	4	2	>280	11	8	5	3	1

Points for Smoking at Each Age Category (y) Women						Points for Smoking at Each Age Category (y) Men					

	20–39	40–49	50–59	60–69	70–79		20–39	40–49	50–59	60–69	70–79
Nonsmoker	0	0	0	0	0	Nonsmoker	0	0	0	0	0
Smoker	9	7	4	2	1	Smoker	8	5	3	1	1

Predicated 10-Year CHD Risk From Point Total

Women		Men	
Point Total	10-Year Risk (%)	Point Total	10-Year Risk (%)
<9	<1	0	<1
9–12	1	1–4	1
13–14	2	5–6	2
15	3	7	3
16	4	8	4
17	5	9	5
18	6	10	6
19	8	11	8
20	11	12	10
21	14	13	12
22	17	14	16
23	22	15	20
24	27	16	25
≥25	≥30	≥17	≥30

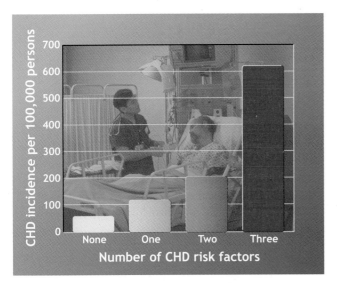

Figure 17.17   Relationship between a combination of abnormal CHD risk factors (cholesterol >250 mg·dL^{-1}; systolic blood pressure >160 mm Hg; smoking >1 pack a day) and incidence of CHD.

dramatically reduced multiple risks (**Fig. 17.18**). These encouraging findings demonstrate that supervised programs of moderate food restriction and exercise with behavior modification reduces CHD risk factors in obese adolescents. Adding regular exercise augmented the effectiveness of risk factor intervention.

If regular physical activity upgrades or at least stabilizes a poor risk factor profile, then school curricula at all grade levels particularly at the kindergarten and elementary grades, should strongly encourage more physically active lifestyles. In this regard, not implementing daily, required physical education seems counterproductive from a public health policy standpoint.

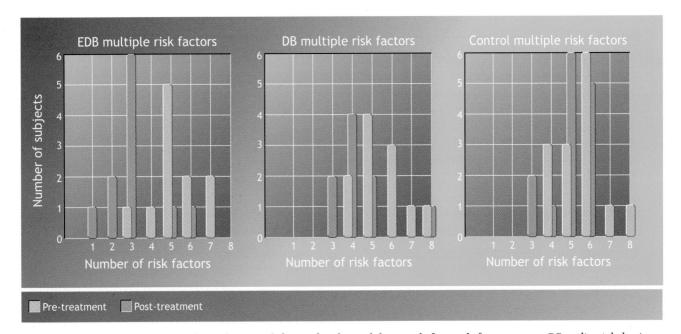

Figure 17.18   Multiple coronary heart disease risk factors for obese adolescents before and after treatment. DB = diet + behavior change group; EDB = exercise + diet + behavior change group. (From Becque, M.D., et al.: Coronary risk incidence of obese adolescents: reduction by exercise plus diet intervention. *Pediatrics*, 81:605, 1988.)

SUMMARY

1. Elderly persons make up the fastest growing segment of American society. Thirty years ago, age 65 years represented the onset of old age. Gerontologists now consider 85 years the demarcation of "oldest-old" and age 75 years "young-old."

2. Nearly 12% or approximately 35 million Americans exceed age 65 years; by the year 2030, 70 million Americans will exceed age 85 years.

3. "Healthspan" refers to the total number of years a person remains in excellent health.

4. The "new gerontology" addresses areas beyond age-related diseases and their prevention to recognize that successful aging maintains enhanced physiologic function and physical fitness.

5. "Healthy life expectancy" refers to the expected number of years a person might live in the equivalent of full health.

6. The specific field of physical activity epidemiology applies the general research strategies of epidemiology to study physical activity as a health-related behavior linked to disease and other outcomes.

7. The Physical Activity Pyramid summarizes major goals to increase the level of regular physical activity in the general population; it emphasizes many forms of behavioral and lifestyle options.

8. Healthy People 2010 describes a comprehensive, nationwide health promotion and disease prevention agenda as a roadmap for promoting health and preventing illness, disability, and premature death among all people in the United States.

9. Inactivity alone produces a constellation of conditions eventually leading to premature death. The term *SeDS* identifies this condition.

10. Physiologic and performance capabilities generally decline after age 30 years. The decline rates of various functions differ within and among individuals. Regular exercise enables older persons to retain higher levels of functional capacity, particularly cardiovascular and muscular functions.

11. Aging alters endocrine function, particularly for the pituitary, pancreas, adrenal, and thyroid glands.

12. A physically active lifestyle throughout life confers considerable health-related benefits.

13. Approximately one-half of all deaths in the United States reflect a limited number of largely preventable behaviors and exposures, most of which relate directly to physical inactivity and overweight and obesity.

14. Life-extending benefits of exercise correlate more with preventing early mortality than improving overall life span. Although the maximum life span may not extend greatly, only moderate exercise enables many men and women to live more productive and healthy lives.

15. Sedentary white women who increase their physical activity to the equivalent of about 1 mile/day of walking exhibit approximately 40% to 50% lower all-cause mortality rates than chronically sedentary counterparts.

16. CHD represents the single largest cause of death in the Western world. The pathogenesis of CHD involves degenerative changes in the inner lining of the arterial wall that leads to progressive occlusion.

17. Four major modifiable cardiovascular risk factors (smoking, diabetes mellitus, hypertension, and hypercholesterolemia) account for 80% to 90% of CHD cases. Physical inactivity and excessive body weight also contribute to disease risk.

18. Cigarette smoking, either active or passive through environmental exposure, directly relates to CHD risk. Smokers experience twice the risk of death from heart disease as nonsmokers.

19. The receptor molecule TLR-2 represents the trigger for inflammation and tissue breakdown in arterial plaque that leads to CHD.

20. A cholesterol level of 200 mg·dL^{-1} or lower is usually desirable, although risk for a fatal heart attack begins to increase at 150 mg·dL^{-1}. A cholesterol level of 230 mg·dL^{-1} increases heart attack risk to about twice that of 180 mg·dL^{-1}, and 300 mg·dL^{-1} increases the risk fourfold.

21. For triacylglycerol level, less than 150 mg·dL^{-1} is considered a nominal level, with 200 to 499 mg·dL^{-1} considered high.

22. Behaviors that favorably affect cholesterol and lipoprotein levels include weight loss; regular aerobic exercise; increased intake of water-soluble fibers; moderate alcohol consumption; increased intake of fatty acids in fish oils (omega-3 fats); elimination of trans fatty acids; and adjusting the intake of polyunsaturated, monounsaturated, and saturated fatty acids.

23. Variables that adversely affect cholesterol and lipoprotein levels include cigarette smoking, a diet high in saturated fatty acids and preformed cholesterol, emotionally stressful situations, and oral contraceptives.

24. A systolic blood pressure that exceeds 140 mm Hg or diastolic pressure that exceeds 90 mm Hg form the

lower limit for the classification of borderline high blood pressure (hypertension).

25. People with diabetes are two to four times more likely to develop cardiovascular disease from obesity, physical inactivity, hypertension, and atherogenic dyslipidemia, maladies usually coincident with the diabetic condition.

26. The following ten variables represent positive CHD predictors: age, gender, heredity, immunologic factors, homocysteine, excessive body fat, physical inactivity, C-reactive protein, lipoprotein(a), and fibrinogen.

27. CHD risk factors interact with each other and CHD itself to accentuate disease risk.

28. The frequent occurrence of multiple CHD risk factors in young children emphasizes the need for early initiatives to reduce atherosclerotic risk later in life

29. Implementing daily, required physical education to reduce childhood CHD risk should become a prioritized public health policy imperative.

 THOUGHT QUESTIONS

1. Does risk factor modification always change disease risk?

2. If regular physical activity contributes little to overall life span, what other reasons exist for maintaining a physically active lifestyle throughout middle and old age?

3. Respond to the question: "Overwhelming epidemiologic evidence links physical activity on the job or in leisure time to reduced CHD risk, but does this prove that exercise benefits cardiovascular health?"

 SELECTED REFERENCES

Aagaard P, et al.: Mechanical muscle function, morphology, and fibert type in lifelong trained elderly. *Med. Sci. Sports Exerc.*, 39:1989, 2007.

ADA/ACSM: ADA/ACSM diabetes mellitus and exercise joint position paper. *Med. Sci. Sports Exerc.*, 29:I, 1997.

Albert, C.M., et al.: Triggering of sudden death from cardiac causes by vigorous exertion. *N. Engl. J. Med.*, 9:343, 2000.

Always, S.E., Siu, P.M.: Nuclear apoptosis contributes to sarcopenia. *Exerc. Sport Sci. Rev.*, 36:51, 2008.

American College of Sports Medicine: ACSM position stand on exercise and type 2 diabetes. *Med. Sci. Sports Exerc.*, 32:1345, 2000.

American College of Sports Medicine: ACSM position stand on physical activity and bone health. *Med. Sci. Sports Exerc.*, 36:1985, 2004.

American College of Sports Medicine and American Heart Association: Joint position statement. Exercise and acute cardiovascular events: placing the risks into perspective. *Med. Sci. Sports Exerc.*, 9:886, 2007.

Andrews, N.P., et al.: Telomeres and immunological diseases of aging. *Gerontology*, 56:390, 2010.

Baker, J., et al.: Physical activity and successful aging in Canadian older adults. *J. Aging Phys. Act.*, 17:223, 2009.

Banda, J.A., et al.: Protective health factors and incident hypertension in men. *Am. J. Hypertens.*, 23:599, 2010.

Barnes, D.E., et al.: Physical activity and dementia: the need for prevention trials. *Exerc. Sport Sci. Rev.*, 35:24, 2007.

Blair, S.N.: Physical activity, physical fitness, and health. *Res. Q. Exerc. Sport*, 64:365, 1993.

Blair, S.N., Connelly, J.C.: How much physical activity should we do? The case for moderate amounts and intensities of physical activity. *Res. Q. Exerc. Sport*, 67:193, 1996.

Blair, S.N., et al.: Changes in physical fitness and all cause mortality: a prospective study of healthy and unhealthy men. *JAMA.*, 273:1093, 1995.

Blair, S.N., et al.: Influences of cardiorespiratory fitness and other precursors on cardiovascular disease and all-cause mortality in men and women. *JAMA.*, 276:205, 1996.

Blair, S.N., et al.: Physical activity, nutrition, and chronic disease. *Med. Sci. Sports Exerc.*, 28:335, 1997.

Bodegard, J., et al.: Reasons for terminating an exercise test provide independent prognostic information: 2014 apparently healthy men followed for 26 years. *Eur. Heart J.*, 26:1394, 2005.

Booth, F.W., et al.: Waging war on modern chronic diseases: primary prevention through exercise biology. *J. Appl. Physiol.*, 88:774, 2000.

Booth, F.W., Laye M.J.: The future: genes, physical activity and health. *Acta. Physiol. (Oxf).*, 199:549, 2010.

Carnethon, M.R., et al.: A longitudinal study of physical activity and heart rate recovery: CARDIA, 1987–1993. *Med. Sci. Sports Exerc.*, 37:606, 2005.

Caspersen, C.J., Fulton, J.E.: Epidemiology of walking and type 2 diabetes. *Med. Sci. Sports Exerc.*, 40(Suppl):S519, 2008.

Chen, F.Y., et al.: Effects of a lifestyle program on risks for cardiovascular disease in women. *Taiwan J. Obstet. Gynecol.*, 48:49, 2009.

Church, T.S., et al.: Metabolic syndrome and diabetes, alone and in combination, as predictors of cardiovascular disease mortality among men. *Diabetes Care*, 32:1289, 2009.

Corrado, D., et al.: Does sport activity enhance the risk of sudden death in adolescent and young adults? *J. Am. Coll. Cardiol.*, 42:1959, 2003.

Davi, G., et al.: Nutraceuticals in diabetes and metabolic syndrome. *Cardiovasc. Ther.*, 28:216, 2010.

Djousse, L., et al.: Dietary linolenic acid is associated with a lower prevalence of hypertension in the NHLBI Family Heart Study. *Hypertension*, 45:368, 2005.

Di Angelantonio, E., et al.: Major lipids, apolipoproteins, and risk of vascular disease. Emerging Risk Factors Collaboration. *JAMA.*, 302:1993, 2009.

Esfahani, A., et al.: Session 4: CVD, diabetes and cancer: a dietary portfolio for management and prevention of heart disease. *Proc. Nutr. Soc.*, 8:1, 2009.

Fleg, J.L., et al.: Accelerated longitudinal decline of aerobic capacity in healthy older adults. *Circulation*, 112:674, 2005.

Fries, J.F., Aging, natural death and the compression of morbidity. *N. Engl. J. Med.*, 303:130, 1980.

Frimel, T.N., et al.: Exercise attenuates the weight-loss-induced reduction in muscle mass in frail obese older adults. *Med. Sci. Sports Exerc.*, 40:1213, 2008.

Frontera, W.R., et al.: Aging of skeletal muscle: a 12-yr longitudinal study. *J. Appl. Physiol.*, 88:1321, 2000.

Gotsch, K., et al.: Nonfatal sports- and recreation-related injuries treated in emergency departments—United States, July 2000–June 2001. *Morbid. Mortal. Wkly. Rep. M.M.W.R.*, 51:736, 2002.

Graham, M.R., et al.: Arterial pulse wave velocity, inflammatory markers, pathological GH and IGF states, cardiovascular and cerebrovascular disease. *Vasc. Health Risk. Manag.*, 4:1361, 2008.

Greenland, P.: Improving risk of coronary heart disease: can a picture make the difference. *JAMA*, 289:2270, 2003.

Haskell, W.L., et al.: Physical activity and public health: updated recommendation for adults from the American College of Sports Medicine and the American Heart Association. *Med. Sci. Sports Exerc.*, 39:1423, 2006.

Héroux, M., et al.: Dietary patterns and the risk of mortality: impact of cardiorespiratory fitness. *Int. J. Epidemiol.*, 39:197, 2010.

Holmes, J.S., et al.: Heart disease and prevention: race and age differences in heart disease prevention, treatment, and mortality. *Med. Care*, 43:133, 2005.

Hu, F.B., et al.: Trends in the incidence of coronary heart disease and changes in diet and lifestyle in women. *N. Engl. J. Med.*, 343:530, 2000.

Jackson, A., et al.: Role of lifestyle and aging on the longitudinal changes in cardiorespiratory fitness. *Arch. Intern. Med.*, 169:1781, 2009.

Jahangir, A., Aging and cardioprotection. *J. Appl. Physiol.*, 103:2128, 2007.

Janssen, I., Jolliffe, C.J.: Influence of physical activity on mortality in elderly with coronary artery disease. *Med. Sci. Sports Exerc.*, 38:418, 2006.

Jouven, X., et al.: Heart-rate profile during exercise as a predictor of sudden death. *N. Engl. J. Med.*, 352:1951, 2005.

Kesäniemi, A., et al.: Advancing the future of physical activity guidelines in Canada: an independent expert panel interpretation of the evidence. *Int. J. Behav. Nutr. Phys. Act.*, 11;7:41, 2010.

Kurl, S., et al.: Cardiac power during exercise and the risk of stroke in men. *Stroke*, 36:820, 2005.

Kurozawa, Y., et al.: JACC Study Group. Levels of physical activity among participants in the JACC study. *J. Epidemiol.*, 15(Suppl):S43, 2005.

Larose, J., et al.: Effect of exercise training on physical fitness in type II diabetes mellitus. *Med. Sci. Sports Exerc.*, 42:1439, 2010.

Lavie, C.J., et al.: Impact of cardiac rehabilitation on coronary risk factors, inflammation, and the metabolic syndrome in obese coronary patients. *J. Cardiometab. Syndr.*, 3:136, 2008.

Lee, I.-M., Buchner, D.M.: The importance of walking to public health. *Med. Sci. Sports Exerc.*, 40(Suppl):S512, 2008.

Lee, S., et al.: Cardiorespiratory fitness attenuates metabolic risk independent of abdominal subcutaneous and visceral fat in men. *Diabetes Care*, 28:895, 2005.

Lyerly, G.W., et al.: Maximal exercise electrocardiographic responses and coronary heart disease mortality among men with metabolic syndrome. *Mayo Clin. Proc.*, 85:239, 2010.

Martinez, M.E.: Primary prevention of colorectal cancer: lifestyle, nutrition, exercise. *Recent Results Cancer Res.*, 166:177, 2005.

McGill, H.C., et al.: Starting earlier to prevent heart disease. *JAMA.*, 290:2320, 2003.

Metzger, J.S., et al.: Patterns of objectively measured physical activity in the United States. *Med. Sci. Sports Exerc.*, 40:630, 2008.

Miller, M.G., et al.: Aspirin under fire: aspirin use in the primary prevention of coronary heart disease. *Pharmacotherapy*, 25:847, 2005.

Mitchell, J.A., et al.: The impact of combined health factors on cardiovascular disease mortality. *Am. Heart J.*, 160:102, 2010.

Moholdt, T., et al.: Physical activity and mortality in men and women with coronary heart disease: a prospective population-based cohort study in Norway (the HUNT study). *Eur. J. Cardiovasc. Prev. Rehabil.*, 15:639, 2008.

Monaco, C., et al.: Toll-like receptor-2 mediates inflammation and matrix degradation in human atherosclerosis. *Circulation*, 120:2462, 2009.

Morris, J.N.: Exercise in the prevention of coronary heart disease: today's best bet in public health. *Med. Sci. Sports Exerc.*, 26:807, 1994.

Morris, J.N., et al.: Coronary heart disease and physical activity of work. *Lancet*, 265:1053, 1953.

Mujica, V., et al.: Intervention with education and exercise reverses the metabolic syndrome in adults. *J. Am. Soc. Hypertens.*, 4:148, 2010.

Nader, P.R., et al.: Moderate-to-vigorous physical activity from ages 9 to 15 years. *JAMA.*, 30:295, 2008.

Nelson, R.: Exercise could prevent cerebral changes associated with AD. *Lancet Neurol.*, 4:275, 2005.

Oeppen, J., Vaupel, J.W.: Broken limits to life expectancy. *Science*, 296:1029, 2002.

Olshansky, S.J., et al.: Prospects for longevity. *Science*, 291:1491, 2001.

Ornish, D., et al.: Intensive lifestyle changes for reversal of coronary heart disease. *JAMA.*, 280:2001, 1998.

Panagiotakos, D.B., et al.: The association between lifestyle-related factors and plasma homocysteine levels in healthy individuals from the "ATTICA" Study. *J. Cardiol.*, 98:471, 2005.

Panagiotakos, D.B., Polychronopoulos, E.: The role of Mediterranean diet in the epidemiology of metabolic syndrome; converting epidemiology to clinical practice. *Lipids Health Dis.*, 4:7, 2005.

Parker, B.A., et al., Sex-specific influence of aging on exercising leg blood flow. *J. Appl. Physiol.*, 104:655, 2008.

Pessana, F., et al.: Subclinical atherosclerosis modeling: integration of coronary artery calcium score to Framingham equation. *Conf. Proc. IEEE Eng. Med. Biol. Soc.*, 1:5348, 2009.

Phillips, A.C., et al.: Stress and exercise: getting the balance right for aging immunity. *Exerc. Sport Sci. Rev.*, 35:35, 2007.

Pollock, M.L., et al.: Twenty-year follow-up of aerobic power and body composition of older track athletes. *J. Appl. Physiol.*, 82:1508, 1997.

Ramsey, F., et al. Prevalence of selected risk behaviors and chronic diseases—Behavioral Risk Factor Surveillance System (BRFSS), 39 steps communities, United States, 2005. *Morbid. Mortal. Wkly. Rep. M.M.W.R.*, 57:1, 2008.

Ridker, P.M., et al.: C-reactive protein levels and outcomes after statin therapy. *N. Engl. J. Med.*, 352:20, 2005.

Rimm, E.B., Stampfer, M.J.: Diet, lifestyle, and longevity—the next step. *JAMA.*, 292:1490, 2004.

Robinson, J.G., Maheshwari, N.: A "poly-portfolio" for secondary prevention: a strategy to reduce subsequent events by up to 97% over five years. *Am. J. Cardiol.*, 95:373, 2005.

Salem, G.J., et al.: ACSM position stand on exercise and physical activity for older adults. *Med. Sci. Sports Exerc.*, 41:1510, 2009.

Schweiger, B., et al.: Physical activity in adolescent females with type 1 diabetes. *Int. J. Pediatr.*, 328318, 2010.

Shephard, R.J.: Maximal oxygen intake and independence in old age. *Br. J. Sports Med.*, 40:1058, 2008.

Simon, A., et al.: Differences between markers of atherogenic lipoproteins in predicting high cardiovascular risk and subclinical atherosclerosis in asymptomatic men. *Atherosclerosis*, 179:339, 2005.

Slentz, C.A., et al.: Modest exercise prevents the progressive disease associated with physical inactivity. *Exerc. Sport Sci. Rev.*, 35:18, 2007.

Smith, D.A., et al.: Abdominal diameter index: a more powerful anthropometric measure for prevalent coronary heart disease risk in adult males. *Diabetes Obes. Metab.*, 7:370, 2005.

Spirduso, W.W., Clifford, P.: Replication of age and physical activity effects on reaction and movement time. *J. Gerontol.*, 33:26, 1978.

Stanner, S.: Diet and lifestyle measures to protect the ageing heart. *Br. J. Community Nurs.*, 14:210, 2009.

Stefan, M.A., et al.: Effect of activity restriction owing to heart disease on obesity. *Arch. Pediatr. Adolesc. Med.*, 159:477, 2005.

Talbot, L.A., et al.: Army Physical Fitness Test scores predict coronary heart disease risk in Army National Guard soldiers. *Mil. Med.*, 174:245, 2009.

Tanaka, H.: Swimming exercise: impact of aquatic exercise on cardiovascular health. *Sports Med.*, 39:377, 2009.

Thomas, N.E., et al.: Relationship of fitness, fatness, and coronary-heart-disease risk factors in 12- to 13-year-olds. *Pediatr. Exerc. Sci.*, 19:93, 2007.

Tota-Maharaj, R., et al.: A practical approach to the metabolic syndrome: review of current concepts and management. *Curr. Opin. Cardiol.*, 22:502, 2010.

Tully, M.A., et al.: Brisk walking, fitness, and cardiovascular risk: A randomized controlled trial in primary care. *Prev. Med.*, 41:622, 2005.

Van den Hoogen, P.C., et al.: Blood pressure and long-term coronary heart disease mortality in the Seven Countries study: implications for clinical practice and public health. *Eur. Heart J.*, 21:1639, 2000.

Visser, M., et al.: Muscle mass, muscle strength, and muscle fat infiltration as predictors of incident mobility limitations in well-functioning older persons. *J. Gerontol. A. Biol. Sci. Med. Sci.*, 60:324, 2005.

Weiss, E.P., et al.: Gender differences in the decline in aerobic capacity and its physiological determinants during the later decades of life. *J. Appl. Physiol.*, 101:938, 2006.

Williams, P.T.: Physical fitness and activity as separate heart disease risk factors: a meta-analysis. *Exerc. Sport Sci. Rev.*, 33:754, 2001.

Williams, P.T.: Reduced diabetic, hypertensive, and cholesterol medication use with walking. *Med. Sci. Sports Exerc.*, 40:433, 2008.

Williams, P.T.: Vigorous exercise, fitness and incident hypertension, high cholesterol, and diabetes. *Med. Sci. Sport Exerc.*, 40:998, 2008.

Yanez, N.D., et al.: CHS Collaborative Research Group; Sibling history of myocardial infarction or stroke and risk of cardiovascular disease in the elderly: the Cardiovascular Health Study. *Ann. Epidemiol.*, 19:858, 2009.

Young, D.R., et al.: Physical activity, cardiorespiratory fitness, and their relationship to cardiovascular risk factors in African Americans and non-African Americans with above-optimal blood pressure. *J. Community Health*, 30:107, 2005.

NOTES

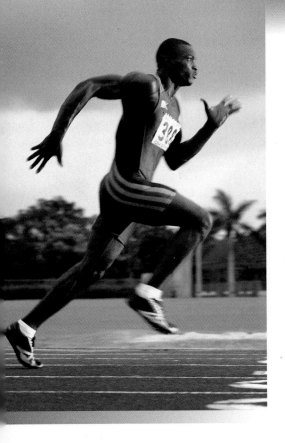

Chapter

18

Clinical Aspects of Exercise Physiology

CHAPTER OBJECTIVES

- List six clinical areas and corresponding diseases and disorders in which physical activity (exercise) as therapy exerts positive influence.

- List three different diseases of the heart muscle.

- Categorize two diseases that affect heart valves and the cardiac nervous system.

- Describe the major steps in cardiac disease assessment.

- List different laboratory-based coronary heart disease (CHD) screening tools.

- List three reasons for including stress testing to evaluate CHD.

- List several indicators of CHD during an exercise stress test.

- Give two advantages and limitations of different modes of exercise for graded exercise stress testing.

- Define the following terms for stress test results: *true-positive*, *false-negative*, *true-negative*, and *false-positive*.

- List four reasons for stopping an exercise stress test.

- Outline the approach for individualizing an "exercise prescription."

- Give advantages and disadvantages of submaximal versus maximal exercise stress testing.

- Give the pros and cons of the different stress test protocols.

- Discuss of the role of physical activity and exercise prescription in pulmonary rehabilitation.

- Describe the role of exercise in the diagnosis and treatment for diseases and disorders of the cardiovascular system.

- Describe the role of exercise in the diagnosis and treatment for diseases and disorders of the neuromuscular system.

- Describe the role of exercise in the diagnosis and treatment for cancer.

- Describe the role of exercise in the diagnosis and treatment for depression.

The promotion of regular exercise is widespread and increasing in the global prevention of disease, in the rehabilitation from injury, and as adjunctive therapy for diverse medically related disorders. This chapter focuses on understanding the mechanisms by which exercise improves health, physical fitness, and the rehabilitation potential of patients challenged by chronic disease and disability. This chapter highlights several clinical applications of exercise interventions for some of the medical and health conditions that exercise positively influences listed in **Table 18.1**.

CARDIOVASCULAR DISEASES AND DISORDERS

As detailed in Chapter 17, diseases of the cardiovascular system account for the greatest number of deaths in industrialized nations. Because increased physical activity represents the prudent first line of defense to combat cardiovascular diseases, exercise physiologists need to become familiar with all aspects of this category of disease. **Table 18.2** lists three categories of heart disease that lead to functional disability:

1. Diseases affecting the heart muscle
2. Diseases affecting heart valves
3. Diseases affecting the cardiac nervous system

Diseases of the Myocardium

Diseases of the myocardium become prevalent with advancing age. The following terms frequently describe these diseases: degenerative heart disease (DHD), atherosclerotic cardiovascular disease, arteriosclerotic cardiovascular disease, coronary artery disease (CAD), and coronary heart disease (CHD).

Advances in molecular biology have isolated possible genetic links to CHD. One of these genes (on chromosome 19 near the gene related to low-density lipoprotein [LDL] cholesterol receptor functioning), called the **atherosclerosis susceptibility gene (*ATHS*)**, accounts for about 50% of all CHD cases. The *ATHS* gene causes a set of characteristics that triples a person's risk of **myocardial infarction (MI)**. These include abdominal obesity

Table 18.1	Clinical Areas and Corresponding Diseases and Disorders Where Exercise Therapy Applies
Cardiovascular diseases and disorders	Ischemia, chronic heart failure, dyslipidemias, cardiomyopathies, cardiac valvular disease, heart transplantation, congenital abnormalities
Pulmonary diseases and disorders	Chronic obstructive pulmonary disease, cystic fibrosis, asthma and exercise-induced asthma
Neuromuscular diseases and disorders	Stroke, multiple sclerosis, Parkinson's disease, Alzheimer's disease, polio, cerebral palsy
Metabolic diseases and disorders	Obesity (adult and pediatric), diabetes, renal disease, menstrual dysfunction
Immunologic and hematologic diseases and disorders	Cancer, breast cancer, immune deficiency, allergies, sickle cell disease, HIV and AIDS
Orthopedic diseases and disorders	Osteoporosis, osteoarthritis and rheumatoid arthritis, back pain, sports injuries
Aging	Sarcopenia
Cognitive and emotional disorders	Anxiety and stress disorders, mental retardation, depression

and low HDL (high-density lipoprotein) and high LDL cholesterol levels.

CHD pathogenesis progresses as follows:

1. Injury to the coronary artery's endothelial cell wall
2. Fibroblastic proliferation of the artery's inner lining or intima
3. Accumulation of lipids at the junction of the arterial intima and middle lining, further obstructing blood flow
4. Deterioration and formation of hyaline (a clear, homogeneous substance formed in degeneration) in the vessel's intima
5. Calcium deposition at the edges of the hyalinated area

The major disorders from reduced myocardial blood supply include angina pectoris, MI, and congestive heart failure (CHF).

Table 18.2	Three Categories of Heart Disease That Lead to Functional Disability	
DISEASES AFFECTING THE HEART MUSCLE	**DISEASES AFFECTING THE HEART VALVES**	**DISEASES AFFECTING THE CARDIAC NERVOUS SYSTEM**
Congestive heart disease	Rheumatic fever	Arrhythmias
Angina	Endocarditis	Tachycardia
Myocardial infarction	Mitral valve prolapse	Bradycardia
Pericarditis	Congenital malformations	
Congestive heart failure		
Aneurysms		

Table 18.3	Similarity of Symptoms of Angina and Heartburn
ANGINA	**HEARTBURN**
Gripping, viselike feelings of pain or pressure	Frequent feeling of heartburn
Pain that radiates to the neck, jaw, back, shoulders, or arms (usually left)	Frequent use of antacids to relieve pain
Toothache	Waking up at night
Burning indigestion	Acidic or bitter taste in mouth
Shortness of breath	Burning sensation in chest
Nausea	Discomfort after eating spicy food
Frequent belching	Difficulty swallowing

Angina Pectoris

Angina pectoris, characterized by acute chest pain, occurs from an imbalance between the oxygen demands of the heart and its oxygen supply. The pain results from metabolite accumulation within an ischemic segment of heart muscle. The sensation of angina pectoris, often confused with simple heartburn, includes squeezing, burning, and pressing or "choking" in the chest region (Table 18.3). The pain usually lasts up to 3 minutes but can continue for longer intervals. One-third of all individuals who have angina will die suddenly from MI. Several types of angina exist, including **chronic stable angina,** often referred to as "walk-through" angina; it occurs at a predictable level of physical exertion (e.g., metabolic equivalent [MET] level or exercise heart rate). Vasodilators (e.g., fast-acting nitroglycerin, commonly used since the 19th century, and longer acting isosorbide dinitrate and mononitrate) reduce cardiac workload and thus oxygen requirements to effectively control this uncomfortable and potentially debilitating condition.

Figure 18.1 shows the usual pain pattern associated with acute angina pectoris. Pain frequently occurs in the left shoulder or along the arm to the elbow. Occasionally, angina pain emanates in the back area of the left scapula along the spinal cord.

Myocardial Infarction

MI (heart attack or coronary occlusion) results from a severely inadequate perfusion of blood in the coronary arteries or a

Questions & Notes

Diseases of which organ become most prevalent with advancing age?

Name 3 terms to describe diseases of the myocardium.

1.

2.

3.

List 3 characteristics of the ATHS gene.

1.

2.

3.

Name the 3 disorders resulting from reduced myocardial blood supply.

1.

2.

3.

Name 2 diseases that affect the myocardium.

1.

2.

List 3 common symptoms of angina pectoris.

1.

2.

3.

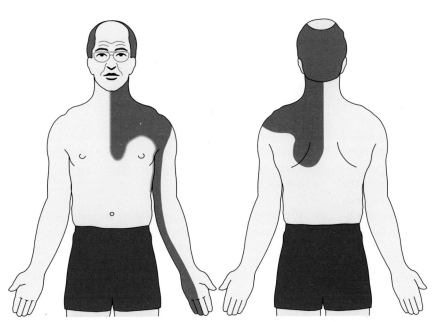

Figure 18.1 Location of pain generally associated with angina pectoris.

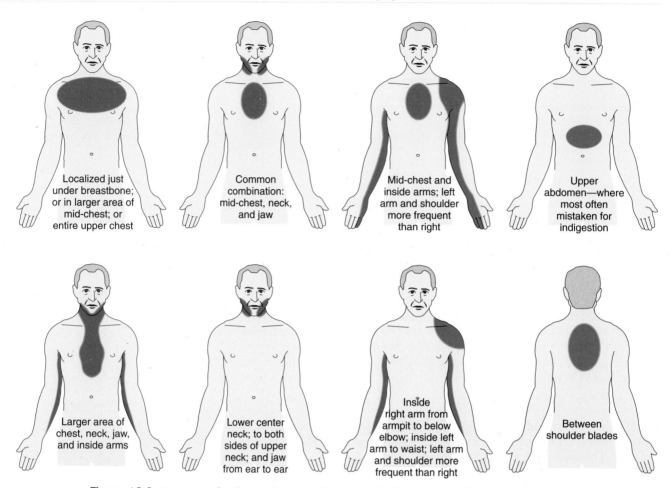

Figure 18.2 Location of early warning signs of myocardial infarction. Note diverse locations of pain.

dramatic imbalance in myocardial oxygen demand and supply from occlusion of a portion of the coronary vasculature. Sudden occlusion results from prior clot formation initiated by plaque accumulation in one or more coronary arteries. Severe fatigue for several days without specific pain often precedes the onset of an MI.

Figure 18.2 displays the locations of early warning signs of an MI. Severe, unrelenting chest pain can last up to 1 hour during an MI.

Pericarditis Pericarditis, an inflammation of the heart's outer pericardial lining, classifies as either acute or chronic (recurring or constrictive). Acute pericarditis symptoms vary but usually include chest pain, shortness of breath (dyspnea), and elevated resting heart rate and body temperature. In chronic pericarditis, inflammation creates extreme chest pain caused by fluid accumulation in the pericardial sac, which prevents the heart from fully expanding during diastole. The prognosis for acute viral pericarditis remains excellent, but chronic pericarditis from bacterial origin presents a persistent serious pathology.

Heart Failure Heart failure (HF; CHF or chronic decompensation) occurs when cardiac output cannot keep pace with venous return. This common incurable condition varies widely in severity and often can be effectively

counteracted by lifestyle changes that include diet, exercise, and medications. The heart can fail from intrinsic myocardial disease, chronic hypertension, or structural defects that impair pump performance. In HF, the amount of blood pumped from the left ventricle relative to the total amount of blood received, called the **ejection fraction**, decreases. With diminished left ventricular output (ejection fraction usually well below 50%), blood accumulates in the pulmonary vasculature. This causes dyspnea and eventual flooding of the pulmonary alveoli with plasma filtrate, a condition termed **pulmonary congestion**. Common HF symptoms include dyspnea, coughing with large amounts of frothy blood-tinged sputum, pulmonary edema, general fatigue, and overall muscle weakness. HF can occur from the right or left side of the heart, each with different symptoms and prognosis depending on initiation of treatment.

Aneurysm Aneurysm represents an abnormal dilatation in the walls of arteries or veins or within the myocardium itself. Vascular aneurysms occur when a vessel's wall weakens from trauma, congenital vascular disease, infection, or atherosclerosis. Aneurysms are identified as either "arterial" or "venous" and classified according to the specific vasculature area affected (e.g., thoracic aneurysm). Routine chest radiography uncovers most aneurysms. Common symptoms include chest pain with a specific, palpable, pulsating mass in the chest, abdomen, or lower back.

Heart Valve Diseases

Diseases and abnormalities that affect heart valve structure and function include:

- **Stenosis:** Valve narrowing or constriction that prevents the valve from opening fully; caused by growths, scars, or abnormal mineral deposits.
- **Insufficiency** (also called *regurgitation*): Valves do not close properly, causing blood to flow back into the heart's chambers during diastole.
- **Prolapse** (only affects mitral valve): Enlarged valve leaflets bulge backward into the left atrium during the cardiac cycle.

Valvular abnormalities increase myocardial workload, requiring the heart to generate greater force to pump blood through a constricted valve or to maintain cardiac output if blood seeps back into a chamber. **Rheumatic fever**, a potentially fatal infection by streptococcal bacteria that can lead to rheumatic heart disease causing valvular scarring and heart valve deformity, usually causes heart valve stenosis. The two most common symptoms of this heart valve pathology include fever and joint pain.

Endocarditis
Endocarditis, an inflammation of the innermost layer of the heart (endocardium) usually of bacterial origin, damages the tricuspid, aortic, or mitral valves from direct invasion of bacteria into the tissue. Patients initially have musculoskeletal symptoms, including arthritis, low-back pain, and general weakness in one or more joints. Many antibiotic drugs effectively treat this disease before it becomes fatal.

Congenital Malformations
Congenital heart defects appear in one of every 100 births; they include defects of the heart valves, such as ventricular or atrial septal defects (a hole between the ventricles and atria) and patent ductus arteriosus (a shunt caused by an opening between the aorta and pulmonary artery). These defects require surgical repair.

Mitral Valve Prolapse
Mitral valve prolapse (MVP) occurs in about 10% of Americans and involves variations in either the mitral valve's shape or structure. This defect has been called "floppy valve syndrome," "Barlow's syndrome," and the "click-murmur syndrome." MVP usually remains benign, but the frequency of diagnosis has increased over the past decade because of MVP's association with endocarditis, atherosclerosis, and muscular dystrophy. MVP probably results from connective tissue abnormalities in mitral valve leaflets. Sixty percent of patients with MVP have no symptoms; the remainder experience profound fatigue during exercise.

Cardiac Nervous System Diseases

Diseases that affect the heart's electrical conduction system include **dysrhythmias (arrhythmias)** that cause the heart to beat too quickly (tachycardia), beat too slowly (bradycardia), generate extra beats (ectopic, extrasystole, or **premature ventricular contractions [PVCs]**), or fibrillate (fine, rapid contractions or twitching of myocardial fibers).

Dysrhythmias usually change circulatory dynamics and result in low blood pressure, HF, and shock. They often occur after a stroke induced by physical exertion or other stressor.

In adults, **sinus tachycardia** represents a resting heart rate greater than 100 b·min^{-1}, and **sinus bradycardia** represents a resting heart rate below 60 b·min^{-1}. Asymptomatic sinus bradycardia often occurs in endurance

Questions & Notes

Name 3 locations generally associated with early warning signs of myocardial infarction.

1.

2.

3.

Name a symptom of acute pericarditis.

Name a symptom of chronic pericarditis.

Give 2 reasons for heart failure.

1.

2.

List 2 diseases that affect heart valves.

1.

2.

List 2 diseases that affect the cardiac nervous system.

1.

2.

List 2 types of dysrhythmias.

1.

2.

athletes. This benign dysrhythmia may reflect a beneficial training adaptation because it provides a longer diastole for ventricular filling during the cardiac cycle and hence the possibility for a greater stroke volume.

CARDIAC DISEASE ASSESSMENT

A thorough cardiac disease assessment typically includes the following:

1. Patient medical history
2. Physical examination
3. Laboratory tests
4. Physiologic tests

Patient Medical History

A proper patient history documents the most common complaints and establishes a basis for CHD risk profiling. Because CHD symptoms frequently include chest pain, making this pain's differential diagnosis is a primary focus. Table 18.4 lists a limited differential diagnosis of chest pain, including possible causes and pathogenesis.

Physical Examination   A physician, nurse, or physician's assistant usually conducts the physical examination that includes the patient's vital signs (body temperature, heart rate, breathing rate, and blood pressure; see accompanying Close Up Box 18.1: *How to Recognize Vital Signs*, on page 637).

For purposes of prescribing exercise and identifying early warning signs of CHD, the clinical exercise physiologist must know the patient's heart rate and blood pressure response to incremental exercise. For example, an increase in systolic blood pressure of 20 mm Hg or more in low-level physical activity of 2 to 4 METs (**hypertensive exercise response**) indicates overall cardiovascular impairment and warns of increased myocardial oxygen demand suggestive of

potential coronary ischemia. In contrast, failure of systolic blood pressure to increase during moderate physical activity (**hypotensive exercise response**) indicates left ventricular dysfunction; a hypotensive response in intense exercise signals a serious mortality risk. Individuals unable to elevate systolic blood pressure above 140 mm Hg during maximal exercise often have serious but dormant cardiac disease.

Heart Auscultation   Listening to heart sounds, termed **auscultation**, provides important information about cardiac function. Exercise physiologists should become familiar with abnormal heart sounds, including how to identify those related to heart murmurs. Auscultation can readily diagnose valvular diseases (e.g., MVP diagnosed by the classic click-murmur sounds) and congenital abnormalities (e.g., regurgitation sounds in ventricular septal defects).

Laboratory-Based Screening and Assessment

The following laboratory-based screenings provide considerable information for confirming and documenting the extent of CHD:

- **Chest radiography:** Chest radiographs reveal the size and shape of the heart and lungs.
- **Electrocardiogram (ECG):** Resting and exercise ECG provide essential information to assess myocardial electrical conductivity and oxygenation. Correctly reading and interpreting an ECG requires specialized training and considerable practice. Table 18.5 lists the six different categories of ECG interpretations. Later in this chapter, various ECG abnormalities and abnormal physiologic responses to exercise are described; we also detail how to count heart rate from ECG tracings. Careful monitoring of ECG changes during exercise targets individuals with potential CHD for further evaluation. Table 18.6 lists common ECG changes associated with CHD.

Table 18.4	Chest Pain Diagnosis		
PAIN/COMPLAINT/FINDINGS	**POSSIBLE CAUSES**	**STIMULI**	**POSSIBLE PATHOLOGY**
Pressure, ache, tightness, or burning in midsternum, left shoulder, arm; diaphoresis; nausea; vomiting; S-T segment changes	MI	Exertion; cold; smoking; heavy meal; fluid overload	CHD
Sharp pain worsens with inspiration, improves with sitting	Inflammation	Acute MI	Pericarditis
Chest tightness with breathlessness; low-grade fever	Infection	IV drug use; microbes	Myocarditis; endocarditis
Sharp, stabbing pain; breathlessness; cough; loss of consciousness	Pulmonary	Recent surgery	Pulmonary embolism
Burning pain in stomach; indigestion relieved by antacids	Referred pain	Heavy meal; spicy food	Esophageal reflux
Angina pain; breathlessness; wide pulse pressure; ventricular hypertrophy on ECG	Ventricular outflow tract obstruction	Exertion; CHD	Aortic stenosis; mitral valve prolapse

BOX 18.1 CLOSE UP

How to Recognize Vital Signs

Proper handling of potentially critical situations requires recognition of the following nine **vital signs**:

1. Heart (pulse) rate
2. Breathing rate
3. Blood pressure
4. Body temperature
5. Skin color
6. Pupils of the eye
7. State of consciousness
8. Body movements
9. Pain or abnormal nerve response

HEART (PULSE) RATE

A normal pulse rate for adults ranges between 60 and 80 b·min^{-1} and 80 to 100 b·min^{-1} for children. Any long-term alteration from normal may indicate the presence of a pathologic condition. For example, a rapid but weak pulse could indicate shock, diabetic coma, or heat exhaustion. A rapid and strong pulse may indicate heatstroke or severe fright, and a strong but abnormally slow pulse could indicate a stroke.

BREATHING RATE

The normal breathing rate approximates 12 breaths/min in adults and 20 to 25 breaths/min in children. Breathing can be shallow, irregular, or gasping. Frothy blood from the mouth indicates a chest (lung) injury. *Look, listen, and feel*: look to ascertain whether the chest is rising or falling; listen for air passing in and out of the mouth, nose, or both; and feel how the chest is moving.

BLOOD PRESSURE

Normal systolic blood pressure for 15- to 20-year-old young men ranges from 115 to 120 mm Hg, and diastolic pressure ranges from 75 to 80 mm Hg. Blood pressure for young women is usually 8 to 10 mm Hg lower for both systolic and diastolic pressures. Between the ages of 15 and 20 years, a systolic pressure of 135 mm Hg and above may be excessive, and a pressure of 110 mm Hg or lower may be considered too low. Diastolic pressure should not exceed 60 mm Hg for young women and 85 mm Hg for young men. A dramatically lowered blood pressure can indicate hemorrhage, shock, heart attack, or internal organ injury.

BODY TEMPERATURE

Normal resting body temperature averages 98.6°F (37°C). Temperature can be measured under the tongue, in the armpit, or in the rectum. Changes in body temperature can also be palpated. Hot, dry skin indicates disease, infection, or heat overexposure. Cool, clammy skin indicates trauma, shock, or heat exhaustion. Cool, dry skin can indicate overexposure to cold.

SKIN COLOR

For lightly pigmented individuals, skin color can be a good indicator of health. Three skin colors are commonly identified in medical emergencies:

1. **Red:** Heat stroke, high blood pressure, or carbon monoxide poisoning
2. **White** (pale, ashen, or white): Insufficient circulation, shock, fright, hemorrhage, heat exhaustion, or insulin shock
3. **Blue:** Circulating blood is poorly oxygenated, indicating an airway obstruction or respiratory insufficiency

Assessing dark-skinned individuals is complicated. They normally have pink coloration of the nail beds and inside the lips, mouth, and tongue. Changes in these areas strongly indicate a medical emergency.

PUPILS OF THE EYE

The pupils are extremely sensitive to situations affecting the nervous system. Most persons have pupils of regular outline and equal size. A constricted pupil can indicate a central nervous system (CNS) response to a depressant drug. If one or both pupils are dilated, the individual may have sustained a head injury; may be experiencing shock, heat stroke, or hemorrhage; or may have ingested a stimulant drug. The pupils' response to light should also be noted. If one or both pupils fail to accommodate to light, there may be brain injury or alcohol or drug poisoning. Pupil response is more critical in evaluation than pupil size.

STATE OF CONSCIOUSNESS

Normally, individuals are alert, aware of their environment, and respond quickly to vocal stimulation. Head injury, heat stroke, and diabetic coma can vary an individual's level of conscious awareness.

BODY MOVEMENTS

Inability to move a body part can indicate a serious CNS injury. Inability to move one side of the body can result from a head injury or cerebrovascular accident. Paralysis of the upper limb can indicate a spinal injury; inability to move the lower extremities could mean an injury below the neck; and pressure on the spinal cord could lead to limited use of the limbs.

PAIN OR ABNORMAL NERVE RESPONSE

Numbness or tingling in a limb with or without movement can indicate nerve or cold damage. Blocking of a main artery can produce severe pain, loss of sensation, or lack of a limb pulse. A complete lack of pain or of awareness of serious but obvious injury can be caused by shock, hysteria, drug usage, or spinal cord injury. Generalized or localized pain in an injured region probably indicates no spinal cord injury.

Table 18.5	Six Categories for ECG Interpretation
1. Measurements	• Heart rate (atrial and ventricular) • PR interval (0.12–0.20 s) • QRS duration (0.03–0.10 s) • QT interval (HR dependent) • Frontal plane QRS axis (–30° to +90°)
2. Rhythm diagnosis	
3. Conduction diagnosis	
4. Waveform description	• P wave (atrial enlargement) • QRS complex (ventricular hypertrophy, infarction) • S-T segment (elevated or depressed) • T wave (flattened or inverted) • U wave (prominent or inverted)
5. ECG diagnosis	• Within normal limits • Borderline abnormal • Abnormal
6. Comparison with previous ECG	

ECG = electrocardiographic.
From Fardy, P., Yanowitz, F.G.: *Cardiac Rehabilitation, Adult Fitness and Exercise Testing.* Baltimore, MD: Williams & Wilkins, 1996.

- **Blood lipid and lipoproteins:** Routine laboratory testing for CHD risk includes analysis of the blood lipid and lipoprotein profiles. Individuals with heart disease often have elevated cholesterol and LDL cholesterol.
- **Serum enzymes:** Alterations in serum enzymes can diagnose or rule out an acute MI. When myocardial cell death (**necrosis**) or prolonged lack of blood flow (**ischemia**) occur, enzymes from the damaged muscle leak into the blood because of the plasma membrane's increased permeability. This leakage increases serum levels of three enzymes: (1) **creatine phosphokinase (CPK)**, which reflects either skeletal or cardiac muscle necrosis depending on one of three isoenzymes that form; (2) **lactate dehydrogenase (LDH)**, which also fractionates into different isoenzyme markers, one of which increases during an MI; and (3) **serum glutamic oxaloacetic transaminase (SGOT)**, which elevates during an MI.

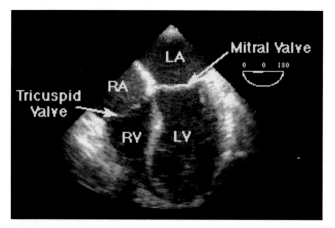

Figure 18.3 Still picture of an echocardiogram that shows the right and left ventricles, right and left atria, and mitral and tricuspid valves.

Noninvasive Physiologic Screening and Assessment

Noninvasive physiologic tests identify specific cardiovascular/cardiac dysfunction with minimal patient discomfort and risk.

Echocardiography
Echocardiography uses pulses of reflected ultrasound to evaluate heart function and morphology; it identifies the heart's structural components and measures distances within the myocardial chambers. This allows estimation of various chamber sizes (volumes) in addition to blood vessel dimensions and thickness of various myocardial components. The echocardiogram has surpassed the ECG in recognizing chamber enlargement, myocardial hypertrophy, and other structural abnormalities. Echocardiograms can diagnose heart murmurs, evaluate valvular lesions, and determine the extent of congenital heart diseases and cardiomyopathies.

Figure 18.3 presents a typical still echocardiographic image showing the left and right atrium and left and right ventricle, the tricuspid valves and the mitral valves. The echocardiogram provides the ability to measure different parameters of size and function of the heart's chambers for diagnostic purposes. The advent of new

Table 18.6	Normal and Abnormal ECG Changes Commonly Observed During Exercise
NORMAL ECG CHANGES IN HEALTHY INDIVIDUALS	**ABNORMAL ECG CHANGES WITH CHD**
1. Slight increase in P wave amplitude	1. Appearance of bundle branch block at a critical HR
2. Shortening of PR interval	2. Recurrent or multifocal PVCs during exercise and recovery
3. Shift to the right of QRS axis	3. Ventricular tachycardia
4. S-T segment depression <1.0 mm	4. Appearance of bradyarrhythmias and tachyarrhythmias
5. Decreased T wave amplitude	5. S-T segment depression/elevation of >1.0 mm 0.08 s after J point
6. Single or rare PVC during exercise and recovery	6. Exercise bradycardia
7. Single or rare PVC or PAC	7. Submaximal exercise tachycardia
	8. Increase in frequency or severity of any known arrhythmia

PVC - , premature ventricular contraction; PAC - , premature atrial contraction.

three-dimensional echocardiogram has enhanced echocardiography as a valuable diagnostic tool (*depts.washington.edu/cvrtc/ocarinas.html*).

Graded Exercise Stress Test

A **graded exercise stress test (GXT)** describes the systematic use of exercise for two purposes:

1. Observe cardiac rhythm abnormalities during exercise
2. Assess overall physiologic adjustments to increased metabolic demands

The most common modes for exercise stress testing include multistage bicycle and treadmill tests. The test, "graded" for exercise intensity, includes submaximal exercise levels of 3 to 5 minutes in duration, each level progressing up to self-imposed fatigue or a specific target heart rate. The graded nature of testing allows detection of ischemic manifestations and rhythm disorders with small increments in exercise intensity. The GXT provides a reliable, quantitative index of the person's level of functional impairment. *For most screening purposes, the test does not require maximal effort; instead, the person exercises to at least 85% of age-predicted maximum heart rate.* Laboratory-based GXTs remain preferable to field tests (walking or running tests) because of closer control over the test environment and exercise intensity.

A resting ECG precedes the GXT to establish whether the person can engage safely in subsequent graded exercise. The resting ECG also provides an important baseline measure for subsequent comparisons.

Why Stress Test? Stress testing serves six important roles in an overall CHD evaluation:

1. **Detect heart disease:** An exercise ECG can diagnose overt heart disease and screen for possible "silent" coronary disease in seemingly healthy individuals. Between 25% and 40% of people with confirmed CHD have normal resting ECGs. ECG analysis during exercise uncovers about 80% of these abnormalities.

2. **Reproduce and assess exercise-related chest symptoms:** Individuals older than age 40 years often experience angina symptoms with physical exertion. ECG analysis during graded exercise provides a more objective and valid diagnosis of exercise-induced chest discomfort.

3. **Screen candidates for preventive and rehabilitative exercise programs:** Stress test results help design an exercise program within the person's functional capacity and health status. Repeated testing evaluates training progress and safely modifies the initial exercise prescription.

Questions & Notes

Give a typical heart rate for sinus tachycardia.

Give a typical heart rate for sinus bradycardia.

List 5 vital signs.

1.

2.

3.

4.

5.

For Your Information

MAJOR SIGNS AND SYMPTOMS OF CARDIOPULMONARY DISEASE

Individuals with undiagnosed cardiopulmonary diseases exhibit specific signs and symptoms during rest and exercise:

- Pain or discomfort (or other angina equivalent) in the chest, neck, or arms
- Shortness of breath at rest or with mild exertion
- Dizziness or syncope (feeling of lightheadedness or faintness)
- Dyspnea (shortness of breath or labored breathing) on rising from a supine position or at night during sleep
- Palpitations or tachycardia (unexplained increased heart rate) during rest or mild exercise
- Ankle edema (swelling)
- Intermittent claudication (ischemic pain described as an aching, weakness, tightness, or cramping sensation during physical activity) in the calf of the leg
- Known heart murmur
- Unusual fatigue accompanied by moderate to extreme dyspnea during usual activities

For Your Information

CHRONIC FATIGUE SYNDROME AND EXERCISE

Chronic fatigue syndrome (CFS) involves continual and severe fatigue. Its prevalence has been estimated at between 1 and 4 million Americans. The cause(s) of CFS remains unknown but may represent a common end point from multiple causes that include infectious agents (similar to Epstein-Barr virus), immunologic variables (perhaps inappropriate production of cytokines such as interleukin-1), hypothalamic–pituitary–adrenal (HPA) axis stimulation leading to increased release of cortisol and other hormones that influence the immune system and other body systems, diabetes, neurally mediated hypotension, substance abuse, and possible nutritional deficiencies. Modest regular exercise to avoid deconditioning is important for all CFS patients (*www.ncpad.org*).

4. **Detect abnormal blood pressure responses:** Exercise hypertension often signifies underlying cardiovascular complications.

5. **Monitor responses to various therapeutic interventions designed to improve cardiovascular health and function:** Periodic stress testing objectifies the degree of benefit derived from pharmacologic, surgical, or dietary treatment of heart disease.

6. **Quantify functional aerobic capacity and evaluate its degree of deviation from established standards:** Metabolic measurements during the GXT allow determination of the $\dot{V}O_{2max}$ or $\dot{V}O_{2peak}$.

Who Should Be Stress Tested? **Table 18.7** shows a classification system by age and health status for screening and supervisory procedures for both stress testing and participation in a regular exercise program. These guidelines apply for healthy individuals and those at higher risk. Healthy young adults can begin moderate intensity exercise at 40% to 60% $\dot{V}O_{2max}$ without an exercise stress test or medical examination. Men older than age 40 years and women older than age 50 years should have a medical examination that includes a stress test before starting an exercise program. A GXT that precedes exercise training takes on added importance for high-risk individuals of any age. *This pertains to people with two or more major CHD risk factors or symptoms suggestive of cardiopulmonary or metabolic disease.*

Informed Consent "Informed volunteers" must be the participants in all exercise testing and training. *Informed consent raises awareness about potential risks of participa-tion.* This consent must include a written statement that the person has had an opportunity to ask questions about the procedures with sufficient information clearly provided so consent occurs from a knowledgeable (informed) perspective. A minor requires prior legal consent from a legal guardian or parent. Individuals need assurance that test results remain confidential. Minors must clearly understand that they may terminate the exercise testing or training program at any time and for any reason. **Table 18.8** presents a sample informed consent statement.

Contraindications to Stress Testing Certain conditions preclude administering a stress test (*absolute contraindications*) and other conditions require the GXT be administered under more closely monitored conditions (*relative contraindications*).

Absolute Contraindications to Stress Testing Under no circumstances should a stress test be administered without direct medical supervision if any of the following 12 conditions exist:

1. Resting ECG suggestive of acute cardiac disease
2. Recent complicated MI
3. Unstable angina pectoris
4. Uncontrolled ventricular arrhythmia
5. Uncontrolled atrial arrhythmia that compromises cardiac function
6. Third-degree atrioventricular heart block without a pacemaker
7. Acute congestive heart failure
8. Severe aortic stenosis
9. Active or suspected myocarditis or pericarditis
10. Recent systemic or pulmonary embolism

Table 18.7	Recommendations for Medical Examination, Graded Exercise Stress Testing (GXT), and Physician Supervision of GXT Before Participation in an Exercise Program	
RISK CATEGORY	**MEDICAL EXAMINATION AND GXT**	**M.D. SUPERVISION**
Low risk Men <45 years Women <55 years; asymptomatic with ≤1 risk factor[a,b]	Moderate exercise; not necessary Vigorous exercise, not necessary	Moderate exercise; not necessary Vigorous exercise; not necessary
Moderate risk Men ≥45 years Women ≥55 years, with ≥2 risk factors[a,b]	Moderate exercise; not necessary Vigorous exercise; recommended	Moderate exercise; not necessary Vigorous exercise; recommended

High risk
Individuals with ≥1 sign/symptom of
  cardiovascular or pulmonary disease[c] or
  known cardiovascular (cardiac, peripheral
  vascular, or cerebrovascular), pulmonary
  (obstructive pulmonary disease, asthma,
  cystic fibrosis), or metabolic (diabetes,
  thyroid disorder, renal or liver) disease
	Moderate exercise; recommended
	Vigorous exercise; recommended
		Moderate exercise; recommended
		Vigorous exercise; recommended

[a]Risk factors: family history of heart disease, cigarette smoking, hypertension, hypercholesterolemia, impaired fasting glucose, obesity, and sedentary lifestyle.
[b]HDL > 60 mg·dL^{-1} (subtract 1 risk factor from the sum of other risk factors because high HDL decreases CHD risk).
[c]Signs and symptoms of cardiovascular and pulmonary disease: pain, discomfort in chest, neck, jaw, left arm; shortness of breath at rest or with mild exertion; dizziness or syncope; orthopnea or paroxysmal nocturnal dyspnea; ankle edema; tachycardia; intermittent claudication; heart murmur; and unusual fatigue or shortness of breath with mild activity.

Table 18.8	Example of Informed Consent for a Graded Exercise Stress Test

Name _____

1. **Explanation of the Exercise Test**
   You will perform an exercise test on a cycle ergometer or a motor-driven treadmill. The exercise intensity begins at a level you can easily accomplish and will advance in stages of difficulty depending on your fitness level. We may stop the test at any time because of signs of fatigue, or you may stop the test when you wish because of fatigue or discomfort that you feel, particularly at the higher exercise levels.
2. **Risks and Discomforts**
   The possibility exists that certain abnormal changes can occur during the test. These include abnormal blood pressure, fainting, disorder of heart beat, and in rare instances, heart attack, stroke, or death. Every effort will be made to minimize these risks by evaluating preliminary information related to your health and fitness, and by observations during testing. Emergency equipment and available trained personnel can deal with unusual situations that may arise.
3. **Responsibilities of the Participant**
   Information you possess about your health status or previous experiences of unusual feelings with physical effort may affect the safety and value of your exercise test and you should report this information now. Your prompt reporting of how you feel during the exercise test also is important. You are responsible for fully disclosing such information when requested to do so by the testing staff.
4. **Expected Benefits From the Test**
   The results obtained from the exercise test may assist in diagnosing your illness, or evaluating what type of physical activities you might do with low risk.
5. **Inquires**
   We encourage you to ask any questions about the procedures used in the exercise test or in the estimation of your functional capacity. If you have doubts or questions, please ask us for further explanations.
6. **Freedom of Consent**
   Your permission to perform this exercise test is voluntary. You are free to deny consent or stop the test at any point.
   I have read this form and understand the test procedures. I voluntarily consent to participate in this test.

Date: _____
Signature of Patient: _____
Signature of Witness: _____
Questions: _____

Responses: _____
Signature of Physician or Delegate: _____

11. Acute infections
12. Acute emotional distress

Relative Contraindications to Stress Testing Administer a GXT with caution and with medical personnel in close proximity to the test area if any of the following 10 conditions exist:

1. Resting diastolic blood pressure above 115 mm Hg or systolic blood pressure above 200 mm Hg
2. Moderate valvular disease
3. Electrolyte abnormalities
4. Frequent or complex ventricular ectopic beats
5. Ventricular aneurysm
6. Uncontrolled metabolic disease (diabetes, thyrotoxicosis)
7. Chronic infectious disease (hepatitis, mononucleosis, AIDS)
8. Neuromuscular or musculoskeletal disorders
9. Pregnancy (complicated or in the last trimester)
10. Psychological distress or apprehension about taking the test

Maximal Versus Submaximal Stress Testing A maximal GXT (GXT_{max}) *represents the most common noninvasive method to screen for CHD and determine* $\dot{V}O_{2max}$ *or* $\dot{V}O_{2peak}$. Individuals exercise until they decide to stop or develop

Questions & Notes

List 3 common laboratory-based screening tests for CHD.

1.

2.

3.

Define the term ischemia.

Name 2 common noninvasive physiologic CHD screening tests.

1.

2.

List 2 purposes for administering a GXT.

1.

2.

List 4 absolute contraindications to stress testing.

1.

2.

3.

4.

List 4 relative contraindications to stress testing.

1.

2.

3.

4.

Table 18.9	Criteria for Stopping a GXT in Apparently Healthy Adults

1. Onset of angina or angina-like symptoms
2. Ventricular tachycardia
3. Significant decrease in systolic blood pressure of ≥ 20 mm Hg
4. Failure of systolic blood pressure or heart rate to increase with an increase in exercise load
5. Lightheadedness, confusion, ataxia, pallor, cyanosis, nausea, or signs of severe peripheral circulatory insufficiency
6. Early onset horizontal or downsloping S-T segment depression or elevation (>4 mm)
7. Increasing ventricular ectopy, multiform PVCs
8. Excessive increase in blood pressure: systolic >260 mm Hg; diastolic >115 mm Hg
9. Increase in heart rate <25 b$\cdot$min^{-1} of predicted normal value (in the absence of β-blockade medication)
10. Sustained supraventricular tachycardia
11. Subject requests to stop test for whatever reason
12. Equipment failure

PVC = premature ventricular contraction.
From *ACSM's Guidelines for Exercise Testing and Prescription*, 7th ed. Baltimore: Lippincott Williams & Wilkins, 2006.

abnormal symptoms that signal test termination (Table 18.9). The term *symptom limited* describes such stress tests.

GXT$_{max}$ normally progress through several stages (multistage): the duration, starting point, and increments between stages vary with the person (e.g., young active, healthy sedentary, and questionable health status). Advantages of a GXT$_{max}$ include direct determination of $\dot{V}O_{2max}$ and maximal cardiovascular responses, screening for abnormal ECG patterns not revealed during rest or low-intensity exercise, and establishing more precise exercise training levels. Disadvantages include the considerable stress placed on the person; although GXT$_{max}$ exhibits low risk, the discomfort of being pushed to maximum without prior physical conditioning may deter some persons from participating in a subsequent fitness program. For most healthy people, about the same physiologic information can be obtained from a submaximal test (80%–90% HR$_{max}$ [maximal safe heart rate]) as from a test requiring all-out effort.

The criteria for stopping a test distinguish one GXT protocol from another; otherwise, any of the protocols are effective. In all instances, an abnormal response should terminate the test.

Nine important factors influence physiologic responses to submaximal or maximal exercise:

1. Ambient temperature and relative humidity
2. Subject's sleep state (number of sleep hours prior to testing)
3. Emotional state
4. Medication
5. Time of day
6. Caffeine intake
7. Time since last meal
8. Time since last exercise
9. Testing environment (type and appearance of testing room, physical appearance and behavior of test personnel)

Stress Test Protocols Test duration, initial exercise intensity level, and increments of intensity between stages for GXT protocols dictate the test to administer. In a national survey of 1400 exercise stress test centers, 71% used treadmills, 17% used bicycle ergometers, and only 12% used step tests. No statistics exist for arm-crank or swim stress tests.

Treadmill Tests Treadmill tests accommodate individuals through a broad spectrum of fitness using the "natural" activities of walking and running. (See Chapter 7, page 225, for a discussion of different treadmill protocols.) Table 18.10 presents some of the more common exercise test protocols and the predicted $\dot{V}O_2$ (mL $\cdot$ kg^{-1} $\cdot$ min^{-1}) for each exercise level for each test.

Each protocol has advantages and disadvantages. The Bruce test, one of the more common protocols, uses large increments every 3 minutes, resulting in less uniform responses compared with tests with smaller increments (e.g., Bruce test) and is better suited for screening of younger and or physically active invidiuals. Protocols with smaller increments, such as Naughton test or the modified Balke test, are preferable for older or deconditioned individuals and patients with chronic diseases. The ramp test is an attractive alternative approcah to incremental exercise testing in which the work rate increases in a constant and continuous manner.

All stress tests begin at a relatively low level, with 2- to 3-minute increments in exercise intensity. A warm-up should be used either separately or incorporated into the initial phase of the test. The total test duration should last at least 8 to 12 minutes. A test longer than 20 minutes provides no additional useful ECG or physiologic data but can establish more precise end points for estimating performance capacity.

Bicycle Ergometer Tests Bicycle ergometers have distinct advantages over other exercise devices. In contrast to treadmills, power output easily calculated and regulated on the ergometer remains independent of body mass. Most ergometers are portable, safe, and relatively inexpensive. Electrically braked and weight-loaded, friction-type devices represent the two most common cycle ergometers. For electrically braked ergometers, preselected power output remains fixed within a range of pedaling frequencies. Power output with weight-loaded ergometers relates directly to frictional resistance and pedaling rate.

The same general guidelines for treadmill testing apply to the bicycle ergometer and arm-crank ergometer. Power output on a bicycle ergometer is expressed in kg-m$\cdot$min^{-1} or watts (1 W = 6.12 kg-m$\cdot$min^{-1}). Bicycle ergometer tests generally use 2- to 4-minute stages of graded exercise. Initial resistance ranges between 0 and 30 W; power output generally increases 15 to 30 W per stage. Pedaling at 50 or 60 revolutions per minute (rpm) represents the typical rpm for weight-loaded ergometers.

| Table 18.10 | Modified Treadmill Protocols for Different Populations |

STAGE	TREADMILL MPH	TREADMILL % GRADE	TIME (min)	O₂ COST (mL · kg⁻¹ · min⁻¹)	METs
Bruce Test (Normally Used for Young Active Adults)					
1	1.7	10	3	14.0–17.5	4–5
2	2.5	12	3	24.5–28.0	7
3	3.4	14	3	31.5–35.0	9.5
4	4.2	16	3	45.5–49.0	13.5
5	5.0	18	3	59.5–63.0	17
6	5.5	20	3	70.0–73.5	20.5
Modified Balke Test (Normally Used for Normal Sedentary Adults)					
1	2	0	2	8.75	2.5
2	3	0	2	12.25	3.5
3	3	2.5	2	15.75	4.5
4	3	5	2	19.25	5.5
5	3	7.5	2	22.75	6.5
6	3	10	2	26.26	7.5
7	3	12.5	2	29.75	8.5
8	3	15	2	33.25	9.5
9	3	17.5	2	36.75	10.5
10	3	20	2	40.25	11.5
11	3	22.5	2	43.75	12.5
12	3	25	2	47.25	13.5
Modified Naughton Test (Normally Used for Very Sedentary Adults)					
1	1	0	3	3.5	1
2	1.5	0	3	7.0	2
3	2	3.5	3	12.25	3.5
4	2	7	3	15.75	4.5
5	2	10.5	3	19.25	5.5
6	3	7.5	3	22.75	6.5
7	3	10	3	26.26	7.5
8	3	12.5	3	29.75	8.5
9	3	15	3	33.25	9.5
10	3	17.5	3	36.75	10.5
11	3	20	3	40.25	11.5
12	3	22.5	3	43.75	12.5
13	3	25	3	47.25	13.5

MET = metabolic equivalent; MPH = miles per hour.
Adapted from Figure 5.3 in Thompson, W.R., et al.: *ACSM's Guidelines for Exercise Testing and Prescription*, 8th ed. Baltimore: Lippincott Williams & Wilkins, 2010:114–115.

Arm-Crank Ergometer Tests Stress testing uses arm cranking (**Fig. 18.4**) as the exercise stressor when formulating the prescription for upper-body exercise. Arm-crank exercise generally produces up to 30% lower $\dot{V}O_{2max}$ values and a 10 to 15 b · min⁻¹ lower maximum heart rate compared with treadmill or bicycle exercise. Unfortunately, arm-crank exercise interferes with conventional blood pressure measurement during exercise. Blood pressure, heart rate, and oxygen uptake values remain higher during submaximal arm cranking compared with the same power output in leg exercise. Protocols developed for leg cycling tests can evaluate the response to upper-body exercise with a lower starting frictional resistance and incremental power outputs adjusted accordingly.

 For Your Information

FIBROMYALGIA AND EXERCISE

Fibromyalgia (FM) represents a complex condition experienced by 3.4% of women and 0.5% of men in the United States. FM causes persistent pain in muscles, ligaments, tendons, and joints. Other symptoms include disturbed sleep and headaches. Symptoms can worsen with anxiety, cold environments, depression, hormonal changes, physical overexertion, and increased stress. FM can exist by itself but usually accompanies rheumatoid arthritis, hypothyroidism, and chronic fatigue syndrome.

Individuals with FM benefit from tailored exercise programs that condition muscles and decrease symptoms by countering the effects of prolonged deconditioning. Primary exercises combine slow stretching, light resistance exercise for all major muscle groups, and low-intensity aerobic activity. Low-impact walking, stair climbing, or swimming is particularly well suited for FM patients. Avoid exercises that include high-impact or high-loading, jogging, aerobic dancing, weight training, racquet sports, basketball, or other activities that involve repetitive jumping (*www.ncpad.org/*).

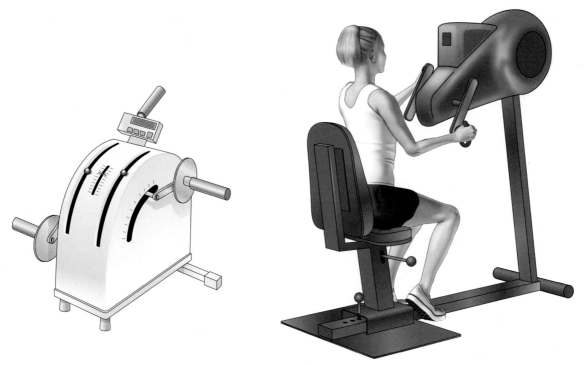

Figure 18.4 Examples of 2 arm-crank ergometers for testing physiologic and metabolic responses to upper-body exercise.

Safety of Stress Testing The yearly death rate from stress testing ranges between 2% and 12% for men with clinical evidence of heart disease. Such broad variation in expected mortality directly relates to the number and severity of diseased coronary arteries.

In approximately 170,000 submaximal and maximal stress tests, only 16 high-risk but apparently healthy patients experienced coronary episodes. This represents about 1 person per 10,000 or approximately 0.01% of the total group. In more than 9000 stress tests, no cardiovascular episodes occurred for subjects with increased heart disease risk. In other reports, the risk of coronary episodes for healthy, middle-aged adults during a maximum stress test equaled about 1 in 3000. In most middle-aged individuals, test risk generally increases about 6 to 12 times higher than for young adults. For patients with documented CHD (including previous MI or episodes of angina), the risk of cardiovascular incident in stress testing increases 30 to 60 times above normal. Based on total risk analyses, many experts believe that a *lower* "overall risk" exists for those who take a GXT and then initiate a regular exercise program than for those who refrain from testing and remain sedentary.

Stress Test Outcomes The clinical value of a stress test depends on how well it detects heart disease or its degree of **sensitivity**. *Sensitivity of a stress test refers to the percentage of people with actual disease who have an abnormal test result (true-positive test result)*. Four possible outcomes from a graded exercise stress test include:

- **True-positive:** Test results correctly diagnose heart disease (test is successful).
- **False-negative:** Normal test results but heart disease is present (test is unsuccessful; heart disease is undiagnosed).
- **True-negative:** Test results are normal; no heart disease is present (test is successful).
- **False-positive:** Test results are abnormal but the person does not have heart disease (test is unsuccessful; healthy person diagnosed with heart disease).

False-negative results occur 25% of the time, and false-positives 15%. False-negative and false-positive test results have dramatic ramifications, particularly a false-negative result when an individual's heart disease goes undiagnosed. Whenever a stress test indicates the presence of heart disease, subsequent thallium imaging or angiocardiography (see p. 648) must confirm the diagnosis. Despite these limitations, the predictive value of an abnormal stress test result exceeds the predictive value of a normal test result.

Exercise-Induced Indicators of Coronary Heart Disease

The prognostic value of exercise testing in asymptomatic individuals comes from exercise-induced observations of ECG ischemia and other abnormalities and fitness-related variables obtained during the GXT.

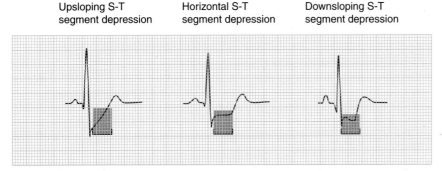

Upsloping S-T segment depression   Horizontal S-T segment depression   Downsloping S-T segment depression

Figure 18.5 Three types of S-T segment depression: upsloping, horizontal, and downsloping.

Exercise-Induced Electrocardiographic Indicators of Coronary Heart Disease

Angina Pectoris Approximately 30% of initial manifestations of CHD during exercise are revealed from chest-related pain, termed angina pectoris. This condition indicates insufficiency of coronary blood flow, where oxygen supply momentarily reaches critically low levels. Myocardial ischemia (insufficient oxygen supply caused by coronary atherosclerosis) stimulates sensory nerves in the walls of coronary arteries and myocardium. (Refer to **Fig. 18.3** for locations of angina pain.) After resting a few minutes the pain usually subsides without permanent damage to the heart muscle.

Electrocardiographic Disorders Alterations in the heart's normal pattern of electrical activity rarely present until the heart's metabolic and blood flow requirements increase above rest. The most common ECG abnormalities during exercise indicate myocardial ischemia from coronary artery obstruction. This obstruction generally relates to more than 50% diameter reduction from occlusion. A significantly obstructed coronary artery can still maintain adequate blood flow at rest but cannot deliver sufficient blood (and oxygen) to meet increased myocardial needs with exercise. Ischemia does not always produce angina pectoris; its diagnosis most readily occurs through depressions of the S-T segment of the ECG. **Figure 18.5** shows three types of **S-T segment depressions**: upsloping, horizontal, and downsloping.

Alterations in cardiac rhythm (arrhythmia) with exercise frequently appear as PVCs (**Fig. 18.6**). In this case, the ventricles demonstrate disorganized electrical activity. The ECG shows this as an "extra" ventricular beat (QRS complex) that occurs without a P wave normally preceding it.

Exercise PVCs generally herald the presence of severe ischemic atherosclerotic heart disease, often involving two or more major coronary vessels. Individuals who experience frequent PVCs have a high risk of sudden death from ventricular fibrillation, an electrical instability when ventricles fail to contract synchronously. This

*Q*uestions & Notes

List 3 factors that influence a person's physiologic response to submaximal or maximal exercise.

1.

2.

3.

Describe the Bruce GXT protocol.

Describe the Balke GXT protocol.

Give the units of measurement for power on a bicycle ergometer.

Define PVC.

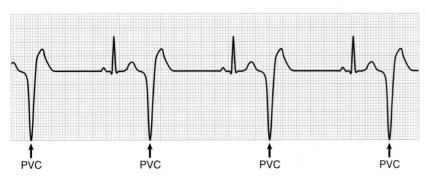

PVC   PVC   PVC   PVC

Figure 18.6 Electrocardiographic tracing illustrating premature ventricular contractions (PVCs).

BOX 18.2 CLOSE UP

Determining Heart Rate From an Electrocardiographic Tracing

The ECG depicts the pattern of electrical activity across the myocardium recorded by an **electrocardiograph**. As the wave of depolarization travels throughout the heart, electrical currents spread through the highly conductive body fluids for monitoring by electrodes placed on the skin's surface. Standard markings on the ECG paper allow time interval and voltage measurements during ECG propagation.

STANDARD ELECTROCARDIOGRAPH TRACING

Figure 1 shows a standard ECG tracing with time recorded on the horizontal axis. The paper normally moves at 25 mm per second. A repeating grid marks the ECG paper; major grid lines occur 5 mm apart (at 25 mm·s^{-1} paper speed, 5 mm = 0.20 s), minor grid

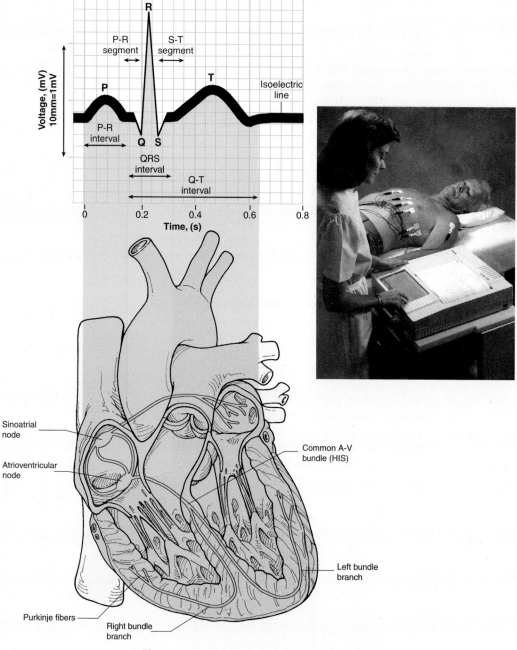

Figure 1 Normal electrocardiographic tracing.

lines occur 1 mm apart (at 25 mm · s^{-1} paper speed, 1 mm = 0.04 s). The graph's vertical axis indicates electrical voltage. The standard calibration factor equals 0.1 mV (millivolt) per mm of vertical deflection.

DETERMINING HEART RATE

Three methods determine heart rate from the standard ECG tracing.

Method 1

Figure 2A shows the standard **R-R method**. The R-R interval indicates the time between successive R waves. An approximate heart rate in beats per minute (b·min^{-1}) can be determined by dividing 1500 (60 s × 25 mm·s^{-1}) by the number of mm between adjacent R waves. In the example, heart rate equals 125 b·min^{-1} because 12 mm occurs between two successive R waves.

Method 2

This method begins with an R wave that falls on a thick blue line of the tracing (**Fig. 2B**). Moving to the right, the next six thick lines represent heart rates of 300, 150, 100, 75, 60, and 50 mm·s^{-1} (these numbers need to be memorized). If the next R wave (after the first one falling on the thick line) falls on either the first through sixth subsequent thick lines, the corresponding number (300 to 50) indicates heart rate in mm·s^{-1}. Interpolation becomes necessary if the next R wave falls between two thick lines. In this instance, the first R wave falls between points 60 and 75 at 70 mm·s^{-1}.

Method 3

This method (**Fig. 2C**), often used with irregular heart rates, counts the number of complete R-R intervals in a 6-s ECG strip multiplied by 10. In this example, six complete R-to-R intervals occur in 6 s; this equals a heart rate of 60 b·min^{-1} (6 × 10 = 60).

A

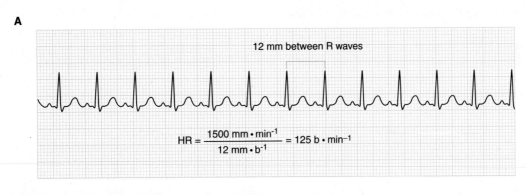

12 mm between R waves

$$HR = \frac{1500 \text{ mm} \cdot \text{min}^{-1}}{12 \text{ mm} \cdot \text{b}^{-1}} = 125 \text{ b} \cdot \text{min}^{-1}$$

B

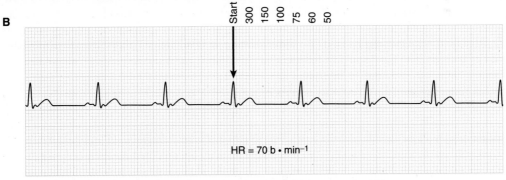

Start 300 150 100 75 60 50

HR = 70 b · min^{-1}

C

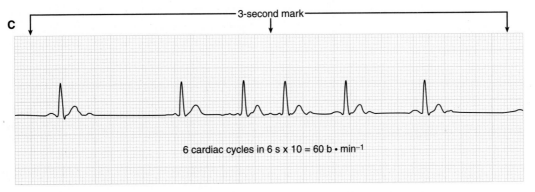

3-second mark

6 cardiac cycles in 6 s x 10 = 60 b · min^{-1}

Figure 2   Three methods for determining heart rate from electrocardiographic tracings.

disrupts myocardial function, causing cardiac output to decrease dramatically.

Exercise-Induced Nonelectrocardiographic Indicators of Coronary Heart Disease

Two useful nonelectrocardiographic indicators of possible CHD include blood pressure and heart rate response to exercise.

Hypertensive or Hypotensive Response During a graded exercise test, a normal, progressive transition in systolic blood pressure occurs from about 120 mm Hg at rest to 160 to 190 mm Hg during peak exercise. Diastolic blood pressure generally changes less than 10 mm Hg. A hypertensive response in strenuous exercise can elevate systolic blood pressure to 250 mm Hg or higher, and diastolic blood pressure can approach 150 mm Hg. Abnormal blood pressure responses to exercise often provide an important clue to cardiovascular disease.

Failure of blood pressure to increase with graded exercise called a hypotensive response indicates cardiovascular malfunction. For example, diminished cardiac reserve may exist if systolic blood pressure does not increase by at least 20 or 30 mm Hg during graded exercise.

Heart Rate Response An abnormally rapid heart rate (tachycardia) early in submaximal exercise often foretells cardiac problems. Likewise, abnormally low exercise heart rate (bradycardia) usually reflects sinus node malfunction (**sick sinus node syndrome**). An inability of the heart rate to increase during exercise, especially when accompanied by extreme fatigue, indicates cardiac strain and underlying heart disease.

In asymptomatic women, heart rate recovery provides a more sensitive predictor of cardiovascular disease and all-cause mortality than S-T segment depression. Because nearly two-thirds of women who die suddenly from cardiovascular disease have no previous symptoms, the important potential role of treadmill testing this population should be recognized.

Invasive Physiologic Tests

Invasive physiologic tests provide diagnostic information unavailable through noninvasive procedures. This information includes the extent, severity, and location of coronary atherosclerosis, degree of ventricular dysfunction, and specific cardiac abnormalities. The three most common invasive physiologic tests are:

1. **Radionucleotide studies** include two types: (1) **thallium imaging**, which evaluates areas of myocardial blood flow and tissue perfusion to differentiate between a true- and a false-positive S-T segment depression (by ECG evaluation), and (2) **ventriculography**, an imaging procedure that provides information about left ventricular functional dynamics.
2. **Cardiac catheterization** involves threading a small-diameter, flexible tube (catheter), guided by x-ray, directly into an arm or leg vein or artery into the right or left side of the heart. Sensors on the catheter tip accurately measure pressure gradients at various locations within the heart's chambers or large vessels and also assess the heart's electrical patterns to determine coronary artery blockage. The oxygen content of arterial and mixed-venous blood comes from blood sampled from the ventricles or atria. Cardiac catheterization takes place under local anesthesia, depending on the point of catheter entry into the arm or leg. The patient remains awake during the procedure, and test results usually become available on the day of testing.
3. **Coronary angiography** provides an intracardiac radiograph after a radiopaque contrast medium enters the coronary blood vessels, and its passage viewed during a cardiac cycle. This technique accurately assesses the extent of atherosclerosis and serves as the criterion "gold standard" for viewing coronary blood flow. It also creates a baseline for other test comparisons and validations. Angiography does not show how readily blood flows within local portions of the myocardium (not a measure of capillary blood flow) and cannot be used during exercise.

Functional Classification of Heart Disease

Table 18.11 shows a system for classifying the functional and therapeutic characteristics of various stages of heart disease. Substantial individual differences exist in symptoms, functional capacities, and appropriate rehabilitation requirements. Whenever patients undertake rehabilitation, their classification should include available medical screening information and a recent GXT.

Exercise Prescription for Cardiac Patients

Heart rate and oxygen uptake obtained during the GXT form the basis for an individualized exercise prescription. Many people who start exercising do not recognize their limitations and exercise above a prudent level. Even group exercise programs that require medical clearance may not be appropriate because all members often exercise at about the *same* work level (walk, jog, or swim at a similar pace) without much attention paid to individual differences in fitness status.

Figure 18.7 illustrates a practical approach for functional translation of treadmill or cycle ergometer exercise test responses to an exercise prescription. Heart rate (**A**) during the Bruce test is plotted as a function of time. Line **B** depicts a mathematical line of "best fit" drawn through the data points. A target zone for heart rate equals 60% to 75% of maximum heart rate (167 b·min⁻¹; *shaded portion* represented as **C**). The individualized prescription includes pace (14.0–15.4 min per mile, **D**) or METs (3.9 to 5.9, **E**). The acceptable range of exercise intensity in area C, based

Functional Capacity Classification

Class I   No limitation of physical activity. Ordinary physical activity does not cause undue fatigue, palpitation, dyspnea, or anginal pain.

Class II   Slight limitation of physical activity. Comfortable at rest, but ordinary physical activity results in fatigue, palpitation, dyspnea, or anginal pain.

Class III   Marked limitation of physical activity. Comfortable at rest, but less than ordinary activity causes fatigue, palpitation, dyspnea, or anginal pain.

Class IV   Unable to carry on any physical activity without discomfort. Symptoms of cardiac insufficiency or angina may be present even at rest. If any physical activity is undertaken, discomfort increases.

Therapeutic Classification

Class A   Physical activity need not be restricted.

Class B   Ordinary physical activity need not be restricted, but unusually severe or competitive efforts should be avoided.

Class C   Ordinary physical activity should be moderately restricted, and more strenuous efforts should be discontinued.

Class D   Ordinary physical activity should be markedly restricted.

Class E   Patient should be at complete rest and confined to bed or a chair.

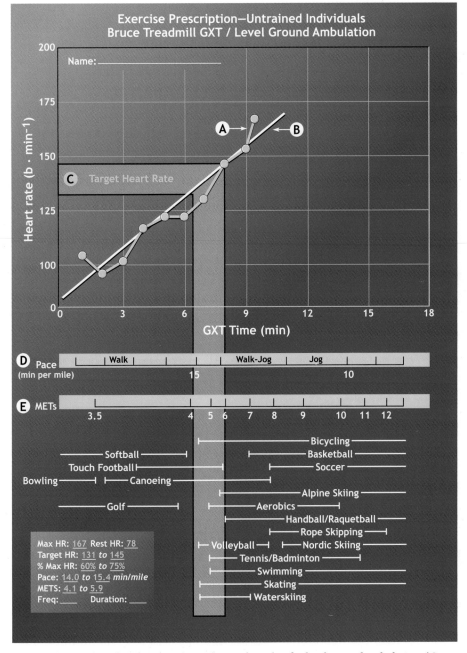

Figure 18.7   Exercise prescription based on functional translation algorithm for level ground ambulation. (Courtesy of Dr. C. Foster, Professor, Department of Exercise and Sport Science; Director, Department of Exercise and Sport Science, University of Wisconsin-La Crosse.)

BOX 18.3 CLOSE UP

The Revised rPAR-Q to Assess Readiness for Physical Activity

Physical Activity Readiness
Questionnaire - PAR-Q
(revised 2002)

PAR-Q & YOU

(A Questionnaire for People Aged 15 to 69)

Regular physical activity is fun and healthy, and increasingly more people are starting to become more active every day. Being more active is very safe for most people. However, some people should check with their doctor before they start becoming much more physically active.

If you are planning to become much more physically active than you are now, start by answering the seven questions in the box below. If you are between the ages of 15 and 69, the PAR-Q will tell you if you should check with your doctor before you start. If you are over 69 years of age, and you are not used to being very active, check with your doctor.

Common sense is your best guide when you answer these questions. Please read the questions carefully and answer each one honestly: check YES or NO.

YES	NO		
☐	☐	1.	Has your doctor ever said that you have a heart condition <u>and</u> that you should only do physical activity recommended by a doctor?
☐	☐	2.	Do you feel pain in your chest when you do physical activity?
☐	☐	3.	In the past month, have you had chest pain when you were not doing physical activity?
☐	☐	4.	Do you lose your balance because of dizziness or do you ever lose consciousness?
☐	☐	5.	Do you have a bone or joint problem (for example, back, knee or hip) that could be made worse by a change in your physical activity?
☐	☐	6.	Is your doctor currently prescribing drugs (for example, water pills) for your blood pressure or heart condition?
☐	☐	7.	Do you know of <u>any other reason</u> why you should not do physical activity?

If

you

answered

YES to one or more questions

Talk with your doctor by phone or in person BEFORE you start becoming much more physically active or BEFORE you have a fitness appraisal. Tell your doctor about the PAR-Q and which questions you answered YES.

• You may be able to do any activity you want — as long as you start slowly and build up gradually. Or, you may need to restrict your activities to those which are safe for you. Talk with your doctor about the kinds of activities you wish to participate in and follow his/her advice.

• Find out which community programs are safe and helpful for you.

NO to all questions

If you answered NO honestly to all PAR-Q questions, you can be reasonably sure that you can:

• start becoming much more physically active — begin slowly and build up gradually. This is the safest and easiest way to go.

• take part in a fitness appraisal — this is an excellent way to determine your basic fitness so that you can plan the best way for you to live actively. It is also highly recommended that you have your blood pressure evaluated. If your reading is over 144/94, talk with your doctor before you start becoming much more physically active.

→

DELAY BECOMING MUCH MORE ACTIVE:
• if you are not feeling well because of a temporary illness such as a cold or a fever — wait until you feel better; or
• if you are or may be pregnant — talk to your doctor before you start becoming more active.

PLEASE NOTE: If your health changes so that you then answer YES to any of the above questions, tell your fitness or health professional. Ask whether you should change your physical activity plan.

Informed Use of the PAR-Q: The Canadian Society for Exercise Physiology, Health Canada, and their agents assume no liability for persons who undertake physical activity, and if in doubt after completing this questionnaire, consult your doctor prior to physical activity.

No changes permitted. You are encouraged to photocopy the PAR-Q but only if you use the entire form.

NOTE: If the PAR-Q is being given to a person before he or she participates in a physical activity program or a fitness appraisal, this section may be used for legal or administrative purposes.

"I have read, understood and completed this questionnaire. Any questions I had were answered to my full satisfaction."

NAME _____

SIGNATURE _____ DATE _____

SIGNATURE OF PARENT _____ WITNESS _____
or GUARDIAN (for participants under the age of majority)

Note: This physical activity clearance is valid for a maximum of 12 months from the date it is completed and becomes invalid if your condition changes so that you would answer YES to any of the seven questions.

CSEP
SCPE © Canadian Society for Exercise Physiology   Supported by: 🍁 Health   Santé
                                                                    Canada Canada

continued on other side...

REFERENCE

Canadian Society for Exercise Physiology: *Par-Q and You*. Gloucester, Ontario, Canada: Canadian Society for Exercise Physiology, 1994.

on heart rate response during the graded exercise test, includes the following recreational activities: bicycling, canoeing, alpine skiing, aerobics, volleyball, tennis and badminton, swimming, skating, and waterskiing. This quantitative method of assigning exercise improves exercise prescription specificity and precision for previously sedentary, healthy individuals and patients with diagnosed cardiovascular diseases.

Guidelines Any exercise prescription should begin with 5 to 10 minutes of light stretching and range of motion (ROM) activities followed by several minutes of light to moderate rhythmic "warm-up" movements. The aerobic conditioning phase should progress in duration so individuals eventually perform 30 to 45 minutes of continuous activity at the prescribed intensity followed by 5 to 15 minutes of low-intensity walking or other rhythmic "cool-down" activities.

Most cardiac rehabilitation patients easily tolerate exercising 3 days per week with no more than a 2-day lapse between exercise sessions. For elderly patients or those with poor functional capacity (<5 METs), low-intensity exercise should be performed daily or twice daily. As a patient's functional capacity improves, exercise intensity and duration can increase progressively with little fear of complications. The most recent GXT serves as the basis for updating the exercise prescription.

Three other important components of cardiac rehabilitation include (1) patient education, (2) appropriate pharmacologic intervention, and (3) family support counseling. A trained social worker often coordinates these aspects of the rehabilitative process.

Beneficial Effects of Resistance Exercise Resistance exercise helps restore and maintain muscular strength, preserve fat-free body mass (FFM), improve psychological status and quality of life, and increase glucose tolerance and insulin sensitivity. Combining resistance training and aerobic training yields more pronounced physiologic adaptations (improved aerobic capacity, muscle strength, and lean body mass) in patients with CAD than aerobic training alone. The following six conditions preclude cardiac patients from participating in resistance training:

1. Unstable angina
2. Uncontrolled arrhythmias
3. Left ventricular outflow obstruction (e.g., hypertrophic cardiomyopathy with obstruction)
4. Recent history of CHF without follow-up and treatment
5. Severe valvular disease, hypertension (systolic blood pressure >160 mm Hg or diastolic blood pressure >105 mm Hg)
6. Poor left ventricular function and exercise capacity below 5 METs with anginal symptoms or ischemic S-T segment depression

Resistance Training Prescription Cardiac patients should exercise with light resistance (range of 30%–50% of 1-RM) because of exaggerated blood pressure responses with straining-type exercise. In the absence of contraindications, elastic bands, light (1–5 lb) cuff and hand weights, light free weights, and wall pulleys can be applied at entrance to an outpatient program. Low-level resistance training should not be started until 2 to 3 weeks after MI. Barbells or weight machines should be introduced after 4 to 6 weeks of convalescence.

Most cardiac patients begin ROM exercises using relatively light weights for the lower and upper extremities. In accordance with recommendations of the American Heart Association (AHA; *www.americanheart.org*), they should perform one set of 10 to 15 repetitions to moderate fatigue using 8 to 10 different exercises (e.g., chest press, shoulder press, triceps extension, biceps curl, lat pull-down, lower back extension, abdominal crunch or curl-up, quadriceps extension or leg press, leg curl, calf raise). Exercises performed 2 to 3 days a week produce favorable adaptations. The rating of perceived exertion (RPE)

Questions & Notes

List 2 common noninvasive physiologic tests for CHD.

1.

2.

List 2 variables used to formulate an exercise Rx for cardiac patients.

1.

2.

List 2 nonelectrocardiographic indicators of CHD.

1.

2.

Under what conditions would you use the PAR-Q questionance?

List 2 benefits of including resistance exercise as part of the exercise Rx for patients with CAD.

1.

2.

should range from 11 to 14 on the Borg scale ("fairly light" to "somewhat hard"). To minimize dramatic blood pressure fluctuations during lifting, patients should be warned to avoid straining, performing the Valsalva maneuver, and gripping weight handles or bars tightly.

For heart transplant patients, a carefully supervised total body resistance training program 3 days weekly for 6 months increases functional strength and muscle mass to counter the generally debilitating effects of immunosuppressive medication.

PULMONARY DISEASES AND DISORDERS

The exercise physiologist's involvement in treating patients with pulmonary disease focuses on improving ventilation, decreasing the work of breathing, and increasing the overall level of functional capacity. The exercise physiologist applies clinical information from the patient's personal history, physical examination, pertinent laboratory data, and imaging studies. Disorders of the cardiovascular system usually impair pulmonary function. Conversely, cardiovascular complications often occur after the onset of pulmonary disease.

Restrictive (reduced lung volume dimensions) and obstructive (impeded air flow) lung diseases represent two common classifications for pulmonary dysfunction. Several pulmonary disorders combine *both* restrictive and obstructive impairments.

Restrictive Lung Dysfunction

Restrictive lung dysfunction (RLD), characterized by abnormal reduction in pulmonary ventilation, includes diminished lung expansion and decreased tidal volume. The chest and lung tissues in RLD tend to stiffen and offer considerable resistance to expansion under normal pulmonary pressure differentials. This represents a reduction in **lung compliance**, that is, the change in lung volume per unit change in intra-alveolar pressure. Decreased pulmonary compliance increases the energy cost of ventilation even at rest. Eventually, RLD progresses to a point where considerable decreases occur in all lung volumes and capacities.

Table 18.12 lists major RLDs along with causes, signs and symptoms, and treatments. Other known causes of RLD include rheumatoid arthritis, immunologic impairment, massive obesity, diabetes mellitus, trauma from impact injuries, penetrating wounds, burns and other inhalation injuries, radiation trauma, poisoning, and complications from drug therapy (including negative reactions to antibiotics and anti-inflammatory drugs).

Chronic Obstructive Pulmonary Disease

Chronic obstructive pulmonary disease (COPD), also termed *chronic airflow limitations* (CAL), includes respiratory diseases that produce airflow obstruction. This ulti-

mately affects the lung's mechanical function and compromises alveolar gas exchange. In the United States, COPD ranks as the fourth leading cause of death and the second leading cause of morbidity; its economic burden averages about $43 billion annually. The natural history of COPD spans 20 to 50 years and closely links to chronic cigarette smoking.

COPD is usually diagnosed from changes in pulmonary function, most notably a decrease in expiratory flow rate and increase in residual lung volume. Classic symptoms include spontaneous spasms of bronchial smooth muscle that produce chronic coughing, inflammation and thickening of the mucosal lining of the bronchi and bronchioles, increased mucus production, wheezing, and dyspnea upon physical exertion. Table 18.13 summarizes the differences among major COPD conditions.

In all forms of COPD, the airways narrow to obstruct airflow. Airway narrowing hinders alveolar ventilation by trapping air in the bronchi and alveoli; in essence, COPD increases physiologic dead space. Obstruction principally increases resistance to airflow during expiration, impairs normal alveolar gas exchange, diminishes exercise capacity, and reduces ventilatory capacity.

The following brief discussion centers on three major COPD diseases: chronic bronchitis, emphysema, and cystic fibrosis. Chapter 11 discussed the obstructive conditions of asthma and exercise-induced bronchospasm.

Chronic Bronchitis **Acute bronchitis** refers to self-limiting and short-duration inflammation of the trachea and bronchi. In contrast, **chronic bronchitis** mostly occurs with long-term exposure to nonspecific irritants. Increases in mucus secretion accompany prolonged respiratory tract inflammation. Over time, the swollen mucous membranes and thick sputum obstruct airways, causing wheezing and persistent coughing. Partial or complete airway blockage from mucus secretion causes insufficient arterial oxygen saturation and edema, which produces the characteristic look of the "blue bloater" (**Fig. 18.8**). Chronic bronchitis develops slowly and worsens over time. Patients usually have been long-term smokers. Functional exercise capacity remains low, and fatigue occurs readily with only moderate effort. If left untreated, the disease can lead to death.

Emphysema Abnormal, permanent enlargement of air spaces distal to the terminal bronchi characterizes **emphysema**. This disease often develops from chronic bronchitis and occurs frequently in long-term cigarette smokers. Symptoms include extreme dyspnea, abnormally increased arterial carbon dioxide tension (hypercapnia), persistent cough, cyanosis, and digital clubbing (evidence of chronic hypoxemia; **Fig. 18.9**). Patients frequently appear thin; they lean forward with their arms braced on their knees to support their shoulders and chest for easier breathing. The effects of trapped air and alveolar distention change the size and shape of the chest, causing the characteristic emphysemic "barrel chest" appearance (**Fig. 18.10**).

Table 18.12 Major Restrictive Lung Diseases and Their Causes, Signs and Symptoms, and Treatment

CAUSES/TYPE	ETIOLOGY	SIGNS AND SYMPTOMS	TREATMENT
I. Maturational			
a. *Abnormal fetal lung development*	Premature birth (hypoplasia-reduced lung tissue)	Asymptomatic; pulmonary insufficiency	No specific treatment
b. *Respiratory distress syndrome* (hyaline membrane disease)	Insufficient maturation of lungs due to premature birth	↑ respiration rate; ↓ lung volumes; ↓ PaO_2; acidemia; rapid and labored respiration pressure	Treat mother prior to birth (corticosteroids); hyperalimentation; continuous positive airway
c. *Aging*	Aging and cumulative effects of pollution, noxious gas, inhaled drug use, and cigarette smoking	↑ residual volume; ↓ vital capacity; repetitive periodic apnea	No specific treatment; increase physical activity
II. Pulmonary			
a. *Idiopathic pulmonary fibrosis* (IPF)	Unknown orign (perhaps viral or genetic)	↓ lung volumes; pulmonary hypertension; dyspnea; cough; weight loss, fatigue	Corticosteriods; maintain adequate nutrition and ventilation
b. *Coal workers' pneumoconiosis*	Repeated inhalation of coal dust over 10–12 y	↓ TLC, VC, FRC; ↓ lung compliance; dyspnea; ↓ PaO_2; pulmonary hypertension; cough	Nonreversible, no known cure
c. *Asbestosis*	Chronic exposure to asbestos	↓ lung volumes; abnormal x-ray; ↓ PaO_2; dyspnea on exertion; shortness of breath	Nonreversible, no known cure
d. *Pneumonia*	Inflammatory process caused by various bacteria, microbes, viruses	↓ lung volumes; abnormal x-ray; tachypneic dyspnea; high fever, chills, cough; pleuritic pain	Drug therapy (antibiotic)
e. *Adult respiratory distress syndrome*	Acute lung injury (fat emboli, drowning, drug induced, shock, blood transfusion, pneumonia)	Abnormal lung function tests; $PaO_2 < 60$ mm Hg; extreme dyspnea; cyanotic; headache; anxiety	Intubation and mechanical ventilation
f. *Bronchogenic carcinoma*	Tobacco use	Variable depending on type and location of growth	Surgery; radiation; chemotherapy
g. *Pleural effusions*	Accumulation of fluid within pleural space; heart failure; cirrhosis	Shortness of breath; pleuritic chest pain; ↓ PaO_2	Specific drainage
III. Cardiovascular			
a. *Pulmonary edema*	↑ pulmonary capillary hydrostatic pressure secondary to left ventricular failure	↑ respiration rate; ↓ lung volumes; ↓ PaO_2; arrhythmias; feeling of suffocation, shortness of breath, cyanotic, cough	Drug therapy; diuretics; supplemental O_2
b. *Pulmonary emboli*	Complications of venous thrombosis	↓ lung volumes, ↓ PaO_2; tachycardia; acute dyspnea, shortness of breath; syncope	Heparin therapy; mechanical ventilation

Table 18.13 Differences Among Major Chronic Obstructive Pulmonary Diseases

NAME	AREA AFFECTED	RESULT
Bronchitis	Membrane lining bronchial tubes	Inflammation of bronchial lining
Bronchiectasis	Bronchial tubes (bronchi or air passages)	Bronchial dilation with inflammation
Emphysema	Air spaces beyond terminal bronchioles (aleveoli)	Breakdown of alveolar walls; air spaces enlarged
Asthma	Bronchioles (small airways)	Bronchioles obstructed by muscle spasm; swelling of mucosa; thick secretions
Cystic fibrosis	Bronchioles	Bronchioles become obstructed and obliterated; plugs of mucus cling to airway walls leading to bronchitis, atelectasis, pneumonia, or pulmonary abscess

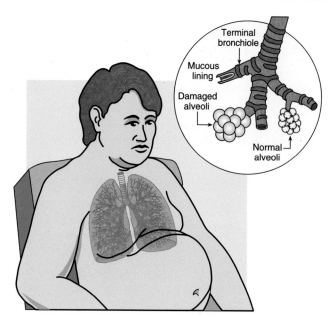

Figure 18.8   Individuals with chronic bronchitis usually develop cyanosis and pulmonary edema with the characteristic appearance known as "blue bloater." The effects of chronic bronchitis displayed in the *inset* illustrate misshapen or large alveolar sacs with reduced surface for oxygen and carbon dioxide exchange.

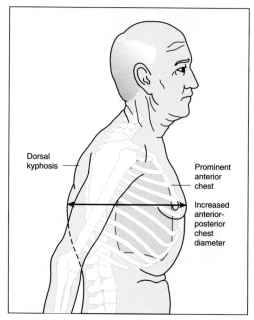

Figure 18.10   Emphysema traps air in the lungs, making exhalation difficult. With time, changes in the patient's physical features include a "barrel chest" appearance.

Exercise cannot "cure" emphysema, but it does enhance cardiovascular fitness and strengthen the respiratory musculature. Regular exercise also improves patients' psychological state.

Cystic Fibrosis

The term **cystic fibrosis** (**CF**; *www.cff.org*) originated from observing cysts and scar tissue on the pancreas of autopsied patients. These, however, are not primary characteristics of the disease (although the term *cystic fibrosis* remains in use). Table 18.14 lists clinical signs and symptoms of CF. This disease, characterized by thickened secretions of all exocrine glands (e.g., pancreatic, pulmonic, and gastrointestinal), eventually obstructs pulmonary airflow. The most common inherited genetic disease in whites, CF affects approximately 1 in about 3500 white newborn infants in the United States (1 in 15,000 African Americans and 1 in 32,000 Asian Americans). The disease, inherited as a recessive trait because both parents are carriers, has no current cure and remains fatal.

Pulmonary system involvement represents the most common and severe manifestation of CF. Airway obstruction leads to a chronic state of hyperinflation. Over time, RLD superimposes on the obstructive disorder, leading to chronic hypoxia, hypercapnia, and acidosis. Pneumothorax and pulmonary hypertension eventually follow and cause death.

Treatment of CF includes antibiotics, enzyme supplements, nutritional intervention, and frequent secretion removal. Regular physical activity can provide beneficial

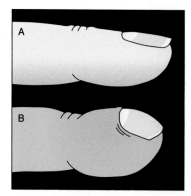

Figure 18.9   Normal digit configuration (**A**) and example of digital clubbing (**B**), indicating chronic tissue hypoxia, a common physical symptom of emphysema.

Table 18.14	Clinical Signs and Symptoms of Cystic Fibrosis and Related Pulmonary Involvement
Early stages	• Persistent cough and wheezing • Recurrent pneumonia • Excessive appetite but poor weight gain • Salty skin or sweat • Bulky, foul-smelling stools (undigested lipids)
Latter stages (with significant pulmonary involvement)	• Tachypnea (rapid breathing) • Sustained chronic cough with mucus production on vomiting • Barrel chest • Cyanosis and digital clubbing • Exertional dyspnea with decreased exercise capacity • Pneumothorax • Right heart failure secondary to pulmonary hypertension

outcomes. Twenty minutes of aerobic exercise replaces one session of secretion removal in some children. Increased minute ventilation with aerobic exercise helps clear excessive secretions from the airways. Improved physical fitness may also play a role in delaying the severe effects of CF.

Pulmonary Assessments

Chest and lung imaging provide the most common pulmonary assessment techniques. These include conventional radiography and computed tomography (CT) scanning to (1) screen for abnormalities, (2) provide a baseline for subsequent assessments, and (3) monitor disease progression. Magnetic resonance imaging (MRI) plays a limited role because the density of large portions of the lungs cannot generate clear magnetic signals. Static and dynamic tests of lung function, pulmonary diffusing capacity, and flow–volume loops also provide important diagnostic information.

Pulmonary Rehabilitation and Exercise Prescription

Pulmonary rehabilitation receives considerably less attention than rehabilitative programs for cardiovascular and musculoskeletal diseases. Perhaps deemphasis results from rehabilitation's failure to markedly improve pulmonary function or reverse the natural progression of these debilitating and often deadly diseases. Pulmonary rehabilitation can have marked, positive effects on exercise capacity, respiratory muscle function, psychological status, quality of life variables (e.g., self-esteem and self-efficacy), frequency of hospitalization, and disease progression. Nine major goals for pulmonary rehabilitation include the following:

1. Improve health status
2. Improve respiratory symptoms (shortness of breath and cough)
3. Recognize early signs requiring medical intervention
4. Decrease the frequency and severity of respiratory problems
5. Obtain maximal arterial oxygen saturation
6. Improve daily functional capacity through enhanced muscular strength, joint flexibility, and cardiorespiratory endurance
7. Improve strength and power of the ventilatory musculature
8. Improve body composition
9. Improve nutritional status

Pulmonary rehabilitation programs include the following five components:

1. General care
2. Pulmonary respiratory care
3. Exercise and functional training
4. Education
5. Psychosocial management

The exercise and functional training aspects of rehabilitation are particularly important to individuals with end-stage disease because the effects of weakness, fatigue, and severe dyspnea profoundly limit physical activity. Physiologic monitoring during exercise rehabilitation should assess heart rate, blood pressure, respiratory rate, arterial oxygen saturation by pulse oximetry (indicates arterial oxygen desaturation), and dyspnea.

Dyspnea monitoring involves a perceived dyspnea "Likert-type" scale (**Fig. 18.11**), similar to psychometric scales for RPE. Extreme shortness of breath, fatigue, palpitations, chest discomfort, or a decrease of 3% to 5% on pulse oximetry indicates the need to terminate the exercise test.

The pretraining GXT and spirometric analyses govern the exercise prescription. Exercise stress test interpretation includes the following:

1. Whether the test terminated for cardiovascular or ventilatory end points

Questions & Notes

List 3 symptoms of cystic fibrosis.

1.

2.

3.

List 3 goals for pulmonary rehabilitation.

1.

2.

3.

List 3 components of a pulmonary rehabilitation program.

1.

2.

3.

For Your Information

EIGHT FACTORS PREDISPOSING TO CHRONIC OBSTRUCTIVE PULMONARY DISEASE

1. Chronic cigarette smoking
2. Air pollution
3. Occupational exposure to irritating dusts or gases
4. Heredity
5. Infection
6. Allergies
7. Aging
8. Drugs

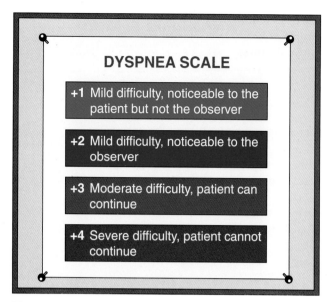

Figure 18.11 Dyspnea scale. Grading of subjective ratings of dyspnea intensity during exercise testing occurs on a scale of 1 to 4. Dyspnea usually accompanies poor exercise capacity and impaired ability to increase systolic blood pressure during graded exercise testing.

2. Difference between pre- and postexercise pulmonary function (e.g., a decrease of 10% in forced expiratory volume in 1 second [$FEV_{1.0}$] indicates the need for bronchodilator therapy before exercise)
3. Need for supplemental oxygen from arterial oxygen desaturation during exercise with a decrease in PaO_2 of >20 mm Hg or a PaO_2 of <55 mm Hg

The exercise prescription for a patient with mild pulmonary disease (shortness of breath with intense exercise) mirrors that for a healthy individual. For patients with moderate disease (shortness of breath with normal daily activities or clinical symptoms of RLD or COPD), exercise training can proceed as follows:

1. An intensity no greater than 75% of ventilatory reserve
2. The middle of the calculated training heart rate range (50% to 70% of age-predicted HR_{max})
3. The point where the patient becomes noticeably dyspneic between 40% to 85% of maximum MET level on a GXT.

Under these circumstances, exercise duration usually lasts 20 minutes and is performed three times a week. If 5- to 15-minute exercise durations are more desirable, exercise frequency should increase to 5 to 7 days weekly.

Patients with severe pulmonary disease (shortness of breath during most daily activities, and forced vital capacity [FVC] and $FEV_{1.0}$ below 55% of predicted values) require a modified approach to exercise testing and prescription. Usually low-level, discontinuous testing can begin at 2 to 3 METs with increments every several minutes. Symptom-limited walking speeds and distances provide helpful guidelines for formulating an exercise prescription. Brief bouts of interval exercise often benefit this population. Patients should exercise a minimum of once daily because of the relatively low initial training prescription. Even small gains in exercise tolerance improve an individual's functional capacity and quality of life indices.

For all patients with pulmonary disease, regular exercise contributes to improved respiratory muscle function. Two approaches achieve this goal:

1. Resistance training of the ventilatory muscles by use of a **continuous positive airway pressure (CPAP)** device improves their strength and power. Overload takes place in a manner similar to progressive resistance exercise for other skeletal muscles.
2. Increases in endurance performance capacity of respiratory muscles through a general program of regular and progressive aerobic exercise training.

NEUROMUSCULAR DISEASES AND DISORDERS

Neuromuscular diseases represent conditions affecting the brain in specific ways. Progressive nerve degeneration or trauma to specific brain neurons result in impairment that ranges from simple to complex. *More Americans are hospitalized with neurologic and mental disorders than any other major disease group, including heart disease and cancer!* The economic costs of brain dysfunction are enormous, but they pale in comparison with the staggering emotional toll on victims and families.

Stroke

Stroke, sometimes called *acute cerebrovascular attack,* refers to a potentially fatal reduction in oxygen supply to part of the brain from restricted blood supply (ischemia) or bleeding (hemorrhage). The resulting brain injury affects multiple systems depending on the injury site and the amount of damage sustained. Effects include motor and sensory impairment and language, perception, and affective and cognitive dysfunction. Strokes can cause severe limitations in mobility and cognition or can be mild with only short-term, nonpermanent consequences.

Clinical Features Clinical features of stroke depend on the location and severity of the injury. Signs of a hemorrhagic stroke include altered levels of consciousness, severe headache, and elevated blood pressure. Cerebellar hemorrhage usually occurs unilaterally and associates with disequilibrium, nausea, and vomiting. **Table 18.15** presents the typical physical and psychological traits and comorbidities associated with stroke.

Cerebral blood flow (CBF) represents the primary marker for assessing ischemic strokes. When CBF decreases below 10 mL·100 g^{-1}·min^{-1} (reference range,

$50–55 \ mL \cdot 100 \ g^{-1} \cdot min^{-1}$), synaptic transmission failure occurs, and a CBF of $8 \ mL \cdot 100 g^{-1} \cdot min^{-1}$ or below results in cell death.

Strokes cause physical and cognitive damage. Left-hemisphere lesions typically accompany expressive and receptive language deficits compared with right-hemisphere lesions. Motor impairment usually results in hemiplegia (paralysis) or hemiparesis (weakness). Damage to descending neural pathways produces an abnormal regulation of spinal motoneurons, resulting in adverse changes in postural and stretch reflexes and difficulty with voluntary movement. Deficits in motor control may involve muscle weakness, abnormal synergistic organization of movement, impaired regulation of force, decreased reaction times, abnormal muscle tone, and loss of active range of joint motion.

Exercise Prescription   The emphasis for stroke survivors centers on rehabilitation of movement during the first 6 months of recovery (increase flexibility [passive and active-assisted], strength development). The few exercise-training studies with stroke patients support the use of exercise to improve mobility and functional independence and to prevent or further reduce disease and functional impairment. Stroke survivors vary widely in age; degree of disability; motivational level; and number and severity of comorbidities, secondary conditions, and associated circumstances. The specific exercise prescription intervention should focus on reducing these conditions and improving functional capacity.

Multiple Sclerosis

Multiple sclerosis (MS) represents a chronic, often disabling disease characterized by destruction of the myelin sheath (demyelination) that surrounds nerve fibers of the CNS (see Chapter 11.) Lesions of inflammatory demyelination can be present in any part of the brain and spinal cord.

Clinical Features   Two or more areas of demyelination confirm the diagnosis of MS. MS usually develops between the ages of 20 and 40 years. Frequently, a history emerges of transient neurologic deficits such as numbness or weakness of an extremity, weakness, blurring of vision, and diplopia (double vision) in childhood or adolescence before development of more persistent neurologic deficits that lead to the definitive diagnosis. MS occurs worldwide at a higher frequency in latitudes farther from the equator. The prevalence of MS in the United States below the 37th parallel occurs at a rate of 57 to 78 cases per 100,000, but the prevalence rate above the 37th parallel averages 140 cases per 100,000. Reasons for these differences remain unknown. Patients with a definite MS diagnosis more likely have a variety of the autoimmune illnesses such as systemic lupus erythematosus, rheumatoid arthritis, polymyositis, and myasthenia gravis. A person with a first-degree relative with MS has a 12- to 20-fold increased chance of developing MS.

*Q*uestions & Notes

List 2 variables that require monitoring during exercise rehabilitation.

1.

2.

Briefly describe the dyspnea grading scale.

Describe the major clinical feature of a stroke.

Describe the most common clinical symptom of multiple sclerosis.

Table 18.15	**Physical and Psychological Conditions and Comorbidities Associated With Stroke Patients**	
PHYSICAL CONDITIONS	**PSYCHOLOGICAL CONDITIONS**	**COMORBIDITIES**
Aphasia	Cognitive impairment	Coronary heart disease
Balance problems	Emotional instability	Diabetes mellitus
Falls	Depression	Hypertension
Fatigue	Memory loss	Hyperlipidemia
Muscle weakness	Low self-esteem	Obesity
Obesity	Social isolation	Peripheral vascular disease
Paralysis		
Paresis		
Spasticity		
Visual impairments		

Fatigue manifests as the most common early MS symptom. Other symptoms include one or all of the following: painful blurring or loss of vision in one eye, muscle weakness in the extremities, clumsiness, numbness and tingling, bowel and bladder dysfunction, sexual dysfunction, joint contractures, urinary tract infection, osteoporosis, and spasticity.

Exercise Prescription   Patients with MS benefit from a comprehensive health prescription that involves aerobic, strength, balance, and flexibility exercises. One important factor that hinders endurance training in about 80% of MS patients relates to adverse effects to heat, whether generated environmentally by outside climatic changes or internally via fever or exercise-induced thermogenesis. This effect makes continuous exercise training difficult and poorly tolerated. Nevertheless, MS patients still can improve cardiovascular function. Stationary cycling, walking, and low-impact chair or water aerobics provide excellent training choices, depending on personal interest and level and nature of physical impairment. Ideal exercise consists of walking in a climate-controlled area that provides stable temperatures, a level surface, and the opportunity to rest frequently. Controlling body temperature represents a primary consideration in the exercise prescription. A realistic and achievable goal for structured exercise provides training three times per week for a minimum of 30 minutes each session divided into three 10-minute sessions.

Parkinson's Disease

Parkinson's disease (PD), a common neurodegenerative disease of the CNS that often impairs motor skills, speech, and other functions, has a prevalence of 60 to 187 per 100,000 people worldwide (no population is immune to PD). The risk of developing this movement disorder increases with age; 10% of patients become symptomatic before age 40 years, 30% become symptomatic before age 50 years, and 40% become symptomatic between 50 and 60 years.

Clinical Features   Clinical symptoms of PD include varying degrees of tremor, a decrease in spontaneity and movement (bradykinesia), rigidity, and impaired postural reflexes. These conditions produce extreme gait and postural instability, resulting in increased episodes of falling or freezing and great difficulty walking. Some patients exhibit a complete lack of movement (**akinesia**). Functional problems also include difficulty getting out of bed or a car and rising from a chair. Other problems include difficulties dressing, writing, talking, and swallowing. Persons with PD generally experience difficulty with performing more than one task simultaneously. As the disease progresses, such problems become more pronounced as the person eventually loses the ability to perform even the most common activities of daily living. In the last stage of the disease, the person must begin to use a wheelchair for mobility and may become bed bound.

Exercise Prescription   Most exercise prescriptions for PD patients are individualized and directed toward interventions that impact associated motor control problems. The rehabilitation exercises emphasize slow, controlled movements for specific tasks through various ranges of motion while lying, sitting, standing, and walking. Treatment protocols include ROM exercises that use slow, static stretches for all major muscle and joint areas, balance and gait training, mobility, and muscle coordination exercises. Little research has assessed the effects of training on aerobic capacity, and no guidelines exist. Anecdotal reports indicate that swimming provides a well-tolerated exercise mode.

RENAL DISEASE AND DISORDERS

Treatment modalities for the major metabolic diseases of obesity, diabetes, and renal disease use regular exercise as adjunctive therapy. Obesity and diabetes have been discussed in different chapters of this text. This section reviews aspects of renal disease associated with kidney function as they relate to exercise physiology.

Chronic kidney disease occurs when the kidneys no longer adequately filter toxins and waste products from blood. Acute renal failure occurs from a toxin (e.g., drug allergy or poison) or severe blood loss or trauma. Diabetes is the number one cause of kidney disease and remains responsible for about 40% of all kidney failures; high blood pressure is the second cause, responsible for about 25% of all kidney failures. Genetic diseases, autoimmune diseases, and birth defects also cause kidney disorders.

Clinical Features   Common symptoms of chronic kidney disease, sometimes referred to as **uremia** (retention in the blood of waste products normally excreted in urine), include the following:

1. **Changes in urination:** Making more or less urine than usual, feeling pressure when urinating, changes in the color of urine, foamy or bubbly urine, or having to get up at night to urinate.
2. **Swelling of the feet, ankles, hands, or face:** Fluid retention in the tissues from failure of kidney filtration.
3. **Fatigue or weakness:** A buildup of wastes or a shortage of red blood cells (anemia) causes these problems as the kidneys begin to fail.
4. **Shortness of breath:** Kidney failure is sometimes confused with asthma or HF because fluid builds up in the lungs.
5. **Ammonia breath or an ammonia or metal taste in the mouth:** Waste buildup can cause bad breath, changes in taste, or an aversion to high-protein foods.
6. **Back or flank pain:** The kidneys are located on either side of the spine in the back.
7. **Itching:** Waste accumulation can cause severe itching, especially of the legs.

8. Loss of appetite.
9. Nausea and vomiting.
10. **Increased hypoglycemic episodes, if the person has diabetes.**

Chronic uremia eventually progresses to **end-stage renal disease (ESRD)** that requires lifelong dialysis or a kidney transplant. The number of renal transplants has increased steadily in the past decade worldwide and generally offers a more normal lifestyle and full rehabilitation. More kidney transpants are performed in the United States (16,517 in 2008, about two-thirds from cadavers) than any other country in the world (almost by a factor of 9). Nearly 80% of transplant patients function at near normal levels compared with 40% to 60% of those treated with various forms of dialysis. Almost 75% of transplant patients resume a normal work schedule compared with about 50% to 60% for dialysis patients.

Exercise Prescription   Regular exercise serves an important role in rehabilitating dialysis and kidney transplant patients to better adapt to their illness. The rehabilitation program should begin before the start of dialysis to optimize beneficial effects. Normal low-level endurance training (following American College of Sports Medicine [ACSM] guidelines) reduces muscle protein degradation in moderate renal insufficiency, reduces resting blood pressure in some hemodialysis patients, and modestly improves aerobic capacity in patients undergoing hemodialysis.

No longitudinal data exist on the effects of aerobic training or a more physically active lifestyle on the survival of patients with chronic uremia or kidney transplants. However, patients with uremia who maintain a lifetime of diverse physical activity do report an enhanced quality of life, including participation in competitive athletics (*www.kidney.org/news/tgames/index.cfm*).

CANCERS

Cancer represents a group of diseases collectively characterized by uncontrolled growth of abnormal cells. More than 100 different types of cancers exist, most occurring in adults. **Carcinomas** refer to cancers that develop from epithelial cells that line the surface of the body, glands, and internal organs. They account for 80% to 90% of all cancers, including prostate, colon, lung, cervical, and breast cancer. Cancers also can arise from cells of the blood (**leukemias**); the immune system (**lymphomas**); and connective tissues such as bones, tendons, cartilage, fat, and muscle (**sarcomas**).

Figure 18.12 presents estimated U.S. cancer deaths for 2009. Lung and bronchus cancers for men and lung and bronchus and breast cancer for women account for the majority of cancer deaths in the adult U.S. population. Although lung and bronchus cancer relate to smoking and environmental smoke exposure, much less is known about the causes of breast cancer.

Cancer has currently replaced heart disease as the top killer of Americans younger than age 85 years, and approximately one-third of the population has some type of cancer (*www.cancer.gov/statistics*). Minorities (with different cultural backgrounds and health and nutrition beliefs) consistently have higher cancer rates, although the reasons remain unknown. Cancer represents the leading cause of death in women between age 25 and 44 years.

The current population of more than 8 million cancer survivors (many initially diagnosed in the 1970s and 1980s) illustrates the ongoing need for rehabilitative and maintenance options in this important area of medicine. The most serious outcomes for most cancer patients and survivors include loss of muscle mass and functional status. Reduced functional status encompasses difficulty walking (even short distances) and serious fatigue that limits completion of simple household chores. Approximately 75% of cancer survivors report extreme fatigue during and after radiotherapy or chemotherapy, accompanied

$\mathcal{Q}$uestions & Notes

Give 2 clinical symptoms of Parkinson's disease.

1.

2.

_____ *is the number one cause of kidney disease.*

List 3 common symptoms of kidney disease.

1.

2.

3.

List 3 primary breast cancer risk factors.

1.

2.

3.

ⓘ **For Your Information**

DECREASED CANCER PREVALENCE ASSOCIATED WITH INCREASED PHYSICAL ACTIVITY

Evidence from more than 25 human research studies from different continents with different diets, ways of life, environmental circumstances, race, ethnicity, and socioeconomic backgrounds and laboratory animals undergoing voluntary or forced exercise show that a reduced risk of cancer development associates with higher levels of regular physical activity.

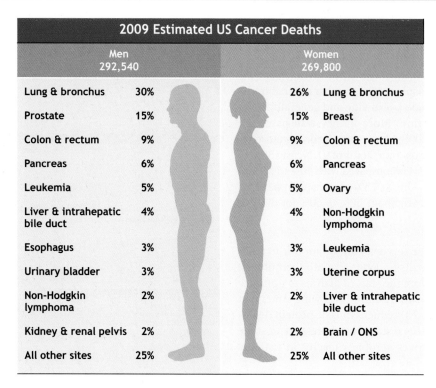

Figure 18.12 2009 estimated U.S. cancer deaths. (American Cancer Society, 2009.)

by weight loss and decreased muscular strength and cardiovascular endurance. Maintaining and restoring functional capacity challenges cancer survivors, even patients considered "cured." Sufficient rationale now justifies exercise intervention for cancer patients during and after different treatment modalities.

Clinical Features

Cancer's clinical features relate to the effects of the three primary cancer treatment modalities: surgery, radiation, and systemic pharmacologic therapy.

Surgery represents the oldest and most common modality. Surgeries include operations to remove high-risk tissues to prevent cancer development, biopsies of abnormal tissue to diagnose cancer, excision of tumors with curative intent, insertion of central venous catheters to support chemotherapy infusions, reconstruction after definitive surgery, and palliative or symptom relief for incurable disease (i.e., partial bowel removal).

Radiation treatment occurs in more than 50% of all cancer survivors. It involves photon penetration into specific tissue, which produces an ionized electrically charged particle that damages DNA to inhibit cell replication and produce cell death. Radiation treatment is typically given daily for between 5 and 8 weeks.

Pharmacologic therapy is prescribed for patients with many advanced solid tumors if cancer cells are suspected of metastasizing beyond the primary site and regional lymph nodes. Chemotherapy, endocrine therapy, and biologic therapy represent the three major types of systemic therapy.

Table 18.16 presents common clinical symptoms resulting from surgery, radiation therapy, and systemic therapy interventions.

Exercise Prescription

Regular physical activity helps cancer patients recuperate and return to a normal lifestyle with greater independence and functional capacity. Health and fitness professionals generally recommend a symptom-limited, progressive, and individualized exercise prescription. Prudent ambulation of any kind proves beneficial for the most sedentary and deconditioned patient.

The benefits of regular exercise include decreased fatigue symptoms, improved functional capacity, decreased neutropenia (abnormally small numbers of neutrophils in circulating blood), reduced severity of pain and diarrhea, and shortened hospital stays. Exercise intervention also decreases psychological distress (improves mood state) and enhances immune function. Current research focuses on psychosocial outcomes such as general fatigue, satisfaction with life, level of depression, self-concept, and quality of life. Such studies report positive associations between regular exercise and improvement in psychosocial outcomes.

Cancer patients can participate in exercise stress tests, which also serve as a basis for exercise prescriptions. Similar testing procedures apply as with healthy individuals, but feelings of fatigue require greater attention. Table 18.17 presents special precautions to consider when testing the functional capacity of cancer patients. Generally, patients should not exercise to maximum.

Table 18.16	Cancer Therapies and Their Complications

TYPE OF TREATMENT	DESCRIPTION AND EFFECTS/OUTCOME
Surgery	**Lung**—reduced lung capacity, dyspnea, deconditioning **Neck**—reduced range of motion, muscle weakness, occasional cranial nerve palsy **Pelvic region**—urinary incontinence, erectile dysfunction, deconditioning **Abdomen**—deconditioning, diarrhea **Limb amputation**—chronic pain, deconditioning
Radiation Therapy	**Skin**—redness, pain, dryness, peeling, sloughing, reduced elasticity **Brain**—nausea, vomiting, fatigue, memory loss **Thorax**—some degree of irreversible lung fibrosis, heart may receive radiation causing pericardial inflammation or fibrosis, premature atherosclerosis, cardiomyopathy **Abdomen**—vomiting, diarrhea **Pelvis**—diarrhea, pelvic pain, bladder scarring, occasional incontinence, sexual dysfunction **Joints**—connective tissue and joint capsule fibrosis, possible decreased range of motion
Systemic Therapy	**Chemotherapies** [depending on type and amount]—extreme fatigue, anorexia, nausea, anemia, neutropenia, muscle pain, sensory and motor peripheral neuropathy, ataxia, anemia, vomiting, loss of muscle mass, deconditioning, infection **Endocrine Therapies** [depending on type and amount]—fat redistribution (truncal and facial obesity), proximal muscle weakness, osteoporosis, edema, infection, weight gain, extreme fatigue, hot flashes, loss of muscle mass **Biologic Therapies** [depending on type and amount]—fevers or allergic reactions, chills, fever, headache, extreme fatigue, low blood pressure, skin rash, anemia

From Courneya, K.S., et al.: *ACSM's Resource Manual for Clinical Exercise Physiology for Special Populations*. In: Myers, J. (ed.). Baltimore: Lippincott Williams & Wilkins, 2002.

Table 18.17	Special Precautions for Testing the Functional Capacity of Cancer Patients

COMPLICATION	PRECAUTION
Ataxia, dizziness, or peripheral sensory neuropathy	Avoid tests that require balance and coordination (treadmill, weights).
Bone pain	Avoid high-impact tests that increase risk of fracture (treadmill, weights).
Low blood count (hemoglobin ≤ 8.0 g·dL^{-1}; neutrophil count $\leq 0.5 \times 10^9 \cdot$ L^{-1})	Avoid tests that require high oxygen uptake or high impact (risk of bleeding); ensure proper sterilization of equipment.
Dyspnea	Avoid maximal tests.
Fever $\geq 38°$C (100.4°F)	May indicate systemic infection; avoid exercise testing.
Mouth sores or ulcerations	Avoid mouthpieces; use face masks.
Low functional status	Avoid exercise testing.
Surgical wounds or tenderness	Avoid pressure or trauma to surgical site.
Severe nausea or vomiting	Avoid or postpone exercise testing.

Modified from Courneya, K.S., et al.: Coping with cancer: can exercise help? *Phys. Sports Med.*, 28:49, 2000.

Questions & Notes

List the 3 primary cancer treatment modalities.

1.

2.

3.

List 3 benefits of regular exercise for cancer patients.

1.

2.

3.

i For Your Information

LIFE EXPECTANCY INCREASED BY 73 DAYS

According to preliminary data from the National Center for Health Statistics (*www.cdc.gov/nchs*), life expectancy in the United States rose 10.4 weeks to a record 77.9 years, from 77.7 in 2006. A continuing decline in mortality rates for the top two killers—heart disease and cancer and a 10% decrease in deaths from the AIDS virus contributed to the change. Heart disease and cancer accounted for 48.5% of all deaths, and HIV, the sixth leading cause of death among Americans age 25 to 44 years, accounted for 11,061 deaths. Applied to both genders, life expectancy averaged 75.3 years for men and 80.4 years for women. Life expectancy for black men increased to 70.2 years in 2007 from 69.7 years in 2006.

| Table 18.18 | General Aerobic Exercise Guidelines for Otherwise Healthy Cancer Survivors |

PRESCRIPTION VARIABLE	GUIDELINES
Frequency	At least three to five times per week; daily activity may be optimal for deconditioned patients
Intensity	Depends on fitness status and GXT results; usually 50%–70% $\dot{V}O_{2peak}$; or 60%–80% HR_{max}; or RPE 11–14
Type (mode)	Large muscle group activity, particularly walking and cycling in some cases
Time (duration)	20 to 30 continuous minutes per session; this goal can be achieved through multiple intermittent shorter sessions with adequate rest intervals
Progression	May not always be linear; rather, it may be cyclical with periods of regression, depending on treatments

GXT = graded exercise stress test; HR_{max} = maximal safe heart rate; RPE = rating of perceived exertion; $\dot{V}O_{2peak}$ = peak oxygen consumption.
Modified from Courneya, K.S., et al.: Coping with cancer: can exercise help? *Phys. Sports Med.,* 28:49, 2000.

The exercise prescription should encourage ambulation if the patient has no specific exercise contraindications. Also encouraged are ROM and flexibility exercises and exercises to improve muscular strength, augment FFM, and improve overall mobility (e.g., submaximal static exercises for antigravity muscles, deep breathing exercises, and dynamic trunk rotation movements). In most cases, preference goes to low-level exercise for short periods performed several times daily. Exercise progression and intensity are individualized, with initial work to rest ratios of 1:1 progressing to 2:1. Eventually, continuous exercise for up to 15 minutes can replace intermittent exeercise bouts. Table 18.18 presents general aerobic exercise guidelines for otherwise healthy cancer survivors.

Breast Cancer

Carcinoma of the breast, one of the most common forms of cancer in white women age 40 years and older, represents the leading cause of death in women between ages 40 and 60 years. In 2009, nearly 192,370 new cases of breast cancer for women and 1910 cases for men were reported, with 40,170 deaths for women. Only lung cancer accounts for more cancer deaths in women. About one in eight women develops breast cancer at some time during life with a high rate of recurrence. The National Cancer Institute estimates that approximately 2.5 million women with a history of breast cancer were alive in January 2006. Most of these individuals were cancer free, but others still had evidence of cancer and may have been undergoing treatment.

Primary breast cancer risk factors include a family history of breast cancer, a personal history of cancer, first menstrual period at an early age, menopause at a late age, first childbirth after age 30 years or no childbirth, and a high-fat diet.

Daily low- to moderate-intensity aerobic exercise reduces fatigue in women with breast cancer undergoing chemotherapy and improves a wide range of quality of life outcomes from breast cancer treatment. Regular exercise produces positive improvements in functional capacity, body composition, side effects of treatment, mood, and self-image.

A study from one of our laboratories illustrates the benefits of regular exercise in breast cancer survivors. The program, conducted 4 days per week, consisted of self-paced hydraulic resistance exercises performed in a 14-station aerobic exercise circuit by 28 patients recovering from breast cancer surgery. **Figure 18.13** illustrates that exercisers decreased depression by 38% compared with a 13%

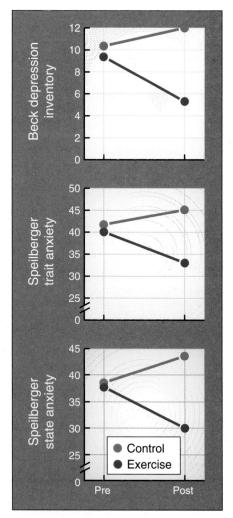

Figure 18.13 Effects of 10 weeks of moderate aerobic circuit resistance exercise on depression (*top*) and trait (*middle*) and state (*lower*) anxiety in women recovering from breast cancer surgery. (Data courtesy of M. Segar, Applied Physiology Laboratory, University of Michigan, Ann Arbor, MI, 1996.)

increase for nonexercising counterparts also recovering from breast cancer surgery. Exercisers decreased trait anxiety by 16% and state anxiety by 20% compared with increases in both variables for nonexercisers. These results demonstrate that a planned, moderate aerobic resistance exercise program exerts positive effects on psychosocial variables during breast cancer rehabilitation.

COGNITIVE AND EMOTIONAL DISEASES AND DISORDERS

The National Institutes of Mental Health (*www.nimh.nih.gov/index.shtml*) estimates that nearly 19 million Americans older than 18 years of age experience major depression. Suicide linked to depression, represents the third leading cause of death among 10- to 24-year old individuals. Also, 6% to 8% of all outpatients in primary care settings have major depression. Despite the large numbers of depressed patients, mental disorders remain underdiagnosed; only about one-third of people diagnosed receive treatment.

The five major classifications of cognitive/emotional diseases include:

1. **Major depressive disorder:** Commonly referred to as "depression"
2. **Dysthymia:** Mildly depressed on most days over a period of at least 2 years; symptoms resemble major depression but less severe
3. **Seasonal affective disorder:** Recurrence of the depressive symptoms during certain seasons (e.g., winter)
4. **Postpartum depression:** Occurs after birth; typically in the first few months after delivery but can happen within the first year after birth
5. **Bipolar disorder** (previously known as manic-depressive illness) characterized by extremes in mood and behavior lasting for at least 2 weeks

Clinical Features Depression has no single cause but often results from a combination of factors or events. Whatever its cause, depression is not just a state of mind. Rather, it relates to physical changes in the brain and a chemical imbalance of neurotransmitters.

Women are roughly twice as likely to experience depression as men, partly from hormonal changes from puberty, menstruation, menopause, and pregnancy. Men are more likely go undiagnosed and less likely to seek help. Men may show the typical symptoms of depression; they tend to be angry and hostile and mask their condition with alcohol or drug abuse. Suicide becomes a serious risk for depressed men, who are four times more likely than women to kill themselves. Depression among the elderly poses a unique situation. Older people often lose loved ones and have to adjust to living alone. Physical illness decreases normal levels of physical activity. Such changes all contribute to depression. Loved ones may attribute the signs of depression to normal aging, and many older people are reluctant to talk about their symptoms. As such,

 For Your Information

KEEP YOUR BRAIN YOUNG

Five behavioral changes that preserve brain functions with age:

1. Exercise 30 to 60 minutes daily. Regular exercise reverses age-related shrinkage of memory regions in the brain.
2. Lose (or at least do not gain) excess body weight. Excess body fat can increase insulin that interferes with enzymes that break down plaque in cerebral blood vessels.
3. Control blood pressure. Hypertension may precipitate silent strokes that diminish brain reserve.
4. Stay socially and mentally active. People who stay mentally and socially engaged throughout life show less decline in mental functions in later years.
5. Consume enough vitamin D by eating more leafy green vegetables, and increase seafood intake.

 For Your Information

RESISTANCE TRAINING HELPS BREAST CANCER SURVIVORS

For decades, physicians have advised breast cancer survivors (currently 2.4 million Americans) that lifting weights or carrying heavy objects may cause harmful arm swelling. New research shows that a program of resistance training (90-minute weightlifting classes twice a week for 13 weeks continued on their own for 39 more weeks) actually helps alleviate the problem of radiation treatment–related buildup of fluids that causes painful and unsightly swelling of arms and hands.

Questions & Notes

Using the FITT principle, outline an exercise Rx for cancer survivors.

Table 18.19	Twelve Common Signs and Symptoms of Depression

1. Loss of enjoyment from things that were once pleasurable
2. Loss of energy
3. Feelings of hopelessness or worthlessness
4. Difficulty concentrating
5. Difficulty making decisions
6. Insomnia or excessive sleep
7. Stomach ache and digestive problems
8. Sexual problems (e.g., decreased sex drive)
9. Aches and pains (e.g., recurrent headaches)
10. A change in appetite causing weight loss or gain
11. Thoughts of death or suicide
12. Attempting suicide

older people may not receive proper treatment for their depression.

Four common factors in depression include:

1. **Family situation:** Trauma and stress from financial problems, breakup of a relationship, death of a loved one, or other major life changes
2. **Pessimistic personality:** Higher risk for individuals who have low self-esteem and a negative outlook
3. **Health status:** Medical conditions such as heart disease, cancer, and HIV contribute to depression
4. **Other psychological disorders:** Anxiety disorders, eating disorders, schizophrenia, and substance abuse often appear with depression

Table 18.19 presents common signs and symptoms of depression.

Exercise Prescription

Exercise studies in clinically depressed populations include hospitalized and ambulatory patients. Overall, the data support the positive effects of exercise on depressive symptoms. In most cases, exercising patients decreased their depression scores.

No mode of exercise has a greater impact on depression than other types of exercise, yet most studies have focused on running or other aerobic-type activities. Interestingly, positive psychological outcomes do not depend on achieving physical fitness, although fitness-related indicators of lower blood pressure and increased aerobic capacity frequently do improve.

Different psychological and physiologic mechanisms may explain the beneficial effects of exercise on depression. Psychologically, exercise enhances one's sense of mastery and self-esteem important for depressed individuals who feel a loss of control over their lives. Exercise also provides a therapeutic distraction that diverts attention from areas of worry, concern, and guilt. Improving one's health, flexibility, and physique status can also enhance mood. Large-muscle activity in exercise may help to discharge feelings of pent-up frustration, anger, and hostility. Exercise may exert its beneficial effect on mood by influencing the metabolism and availability of central neurotransmitters with mood-improving capability.

Researchers continue to study exercise effects on the neurochemistry of mood regulation, specifically turnover of monoamines and other central neurotransmitters at presynaptic and postsynaptic sites. Antidepressant medications, including the selective serotonin reuptake inhibitors (SSRIs), exert their effect by increasing neurotransmitters availability at receptor sites. Exercise may exert its beneficial effect on mood by influencing the metabolism and availability of these central medications.

The role of β-endorphins in mood regulation has received considerable attention. These endogenous chemicals that reduce pain and can induce euphoria have been linked to the "runner's high" experienced by intensive exercisers. The ability of exercise to produce enough β-endorphins to affect depression remains questionable, but the possibility still exists for depressed patients.

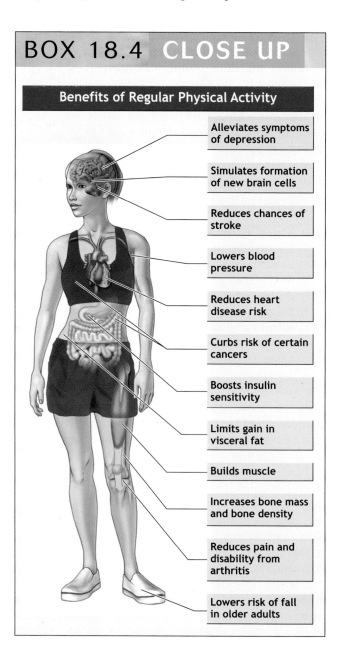

BOX 18.4 CLOSE UP

Benefits of Regular Physical Activity

- Alleviates symptoms of depression
- Simulates formation of new brain cells
- Reduces chances of stroke
- Lowers blood pressure
- Reduces heart disease risk
- Curbs risk of certain cancers
- Boosts insulin sensitivity
- Limits gain in visceral fat
- Builds muscle
- Increases bone mass and bone density
- Reduces pain and disability from arthritis
- Lowers risk of fall in older adults

Disturbed sleep represents both a symptom and an aggravating factor of depression making beneficial effects of exercise on sleep take on added importance. Depressed individuals demonstrate improved subjective sleep quality and a corresponding improvement in depression measures.

The exercise prescription for patients with depression considers the following eight factors:

1. **Anticipate barriers.** Common symptoms of depression, such as fatigue, lack of energy, and psychomotor retardation, pose formidable barriers to physical activity. Feelings of hopelessness and worthlessness also interfere with motivation to exercise.
2. **Keep expectations realistic.** Make exercise recommendations with caution. Depressed patients often self-blame and may view exercise as another occasion for failure. Do not raise false expectations that can arouse anxiety and guilt. Explain that exercise provides an adjunct to, not a substitute for, primary treatment.
3. **Design a feasible plan.** Make the exercise prescription realistic and practical, not an additional burden to compound the patient's sense of futility. Consider the individual's background and history. For severely depressed patients, postpone exercise until medication and psychotherapy alleviate symptoms. Previously sedentary patients should start with a light exercise schedule such as just a few minutes of daily walking.
4. **Accentuate pleasurable aspects.** Guide the choice of exercise by the patient's preferences and circumstances. Use pleasurable activities that can easily add to the patient's schedule.
5. **Include group activities.** Depressed, isolated, and withdrawn patients are most likely to benefit from increased social involvement. The stimulation of being outdoors in a pleasant setting can enhance mood; exposure to light exerts therapeutic effects for seasonal depression.
6. **State specifics.** Walking is almost universally acceptable, carries minimal injury risk, and benefits mood enhancement. In keeping with ACSM recommendations for healthy adults, a goal of 20 to 60 minutes of walking or other aerobic exercise three to five times a week remains reasonable. The ACSM also recommends resistance and flexibility training 2 to 3 days per week.
7. **Encourage compliance.** Improved fitness serves as a valuable consequence of exercise participation without an antidepressant effect. Compliance increases with less physically demanding exercise programs.
8. **Integrate exercise with other treatments.** The primary treatments for depression should not present exercise obstacles. Antidepressant medication can impair a patient's ability to function.

Combatting depression relies on a spectrum of brief and longer term psychotherapies, either alone or with antidepressant medication. An exercise prescription complements psychotherapy when the goal increases the patient's overall activity level and adds pleasurable, satisfying experiences. The patient's difficulties with exercise (e.g., motivational problems, fear of interpersonal situations, a tendency to transform exercise into a burdensome chore), may shed light on dysfunctional attitudes that psychotherapy adequately explores.

Questions & Notes

List 5 major classifications of cognitive and emotional diseases.

1.

2.

3.

4.

5.

Name the neurochemical substance usually associated with the "runners high."

For Your Information

JUST A LITTLE EXERCISE ADDS LIFE TO SENIORS 85+ YEARS

Little is known about the potential benefits of regular physical activity for the oldest-old, those in their 80s. Recent finding suggest that even the oldest-old benefit from regular physical activity. Even previously sedentary 85-year-olds who participated in 4 hours per week of physical activity (this level of activity classifies as "active" for this age group) reaped the benefits. Even if the walks were broken up into 15-minue strolls, the benefits equaled those who participated for longer durations. The physically active octogenarians also experienced less depression and loneliness and showed greater ability to perform tasks of daily living more easily. (*Arch. Intern. Med.* 169:1476, 2009)

SUMMARY

1. An exercise physiologist health and fitness professional becomes part of a team approach in the clinical setting for comprehensive patient health care. The exercise physiologist focuses on restoring the patient's mobility and functional capacity.

2. The major cardiovascular diseases affect the heart muscle directly, the heart valves, or neural regulation of cardiac function.

3. A gene (*ATHS*) on chromosome 19 near the gene related to LDL-cholesterol receptor functioning accounts for almost 50% of CHD cases.

4. An imbalance between the oxygen demands of the heart and its oxygen supply causes angina pectoris.

5. MI results from inadequate perfusion of blood in the coronary arteries or imbalance in myocardial oxygen demand and supply during physical activity.

6. Pericarditis, an inflammation of the heart's outer pericardial lining, is classified as either acute (recurring) or chronic (constrictive).

7. CHF occurs when cardiac output cannot keep pace with venous return. The heart fails from intrinsic myocardial disease, chronic hypertension, or structural defects that impair pump performance.

8. Aneurysm represents an abnormal dilatation in the wall of an artery or vein or the myocardium. Vascular aneurysms occur when a vessel's wall weakens from trauma, congenital vascular disease, infection, or atherosclerosis.

9. Aerobic exercise programs implemented for cardiac patients should consider specific disease pathophysiology, mechanisms that limit exercise capacity, and individual differences in functional capacity.

10. Heart valve diseases include stenosis, regurgitation, and prolapse.

11. The dysrhythmias bradycardia, tachycardia, and PVCs represent diseases of the heart's nervous system.

12. A thorough cardiac disease assessment includes medical history, physical examination, laboratory assessments (chest radiography, ECG, blood lipid analyses, serum enzyme testing), and physiologic tests.

13. The "stress test" describes systematic exercise for two purposes: (1) ECG observations and (2) evaluation of physiologic adjustments to metabolic demands that exceed resting requirements.

14. Multistage bicycle and treadmill tests represent the most common modes for exercise stress testing. These tests, graded for exercise intensity, include several levels of 3 to 5 minutes of exercise that bring the person to self-imposed, symptom-limited fatigue.

15. Graded exercise stress testing provides a low-risk screening for CHD preventive and rehabilitative exercise programs.

16. Four possible outcomes from a stress test include true-positive (test a success), false-negative (heart disease not diagnosed when present), true-negative (test a success), and false-positive (healthy person diagnosed with heart disease) results.

17. Exercise-induced indicators of CHD include angina pectoris, ECG disorders, cardiac rhythm abnormalities, and abnormal blood pressure and heart rate responses.

18. Invasive physiologic tests that include radionucleotide studies, cardiac catheterization, and coronary angiography provide diagnostic information unavailable through noninvasive procedures.

19. Cardiac patients improve their functional capacity similar to healthy people of the same age.

20. Cardiac patients enter different cardiac rehabilitation phases depending on disease severity and degree of risk.

21. RLD and COPD represent two major pulmonary disease categories.

22. RLD increases chest-lung resistance to lung inflation. COPD (including bronchitis, emphysema, asthma, exercise-induced bronchospasm, and CF) affects expiratory flow capacity and ultimately impedes aeration of alveolar blood.

23. Pulmonary disease assessment requires different diagnostic tools that include chest radiography, CT scanning, MRI, and standard spirometric lung volume testing.

24. Exercise contributes to pulmonary disease management if close attention focuses on exercise intensity, patient monitoring, and exercise progression.

25. The most prominent neuromuscular diseases impacting the brain include stroke, multiple sclerosis, and Parkinson's disease.

26. Patients with chronic kidney disease benefit from individualized and structured exercise programs.

27. More than 100 different types of cancers affect adults, including carcinomas, leukemias, lymphomas, and sarcomas.

28. The exercise prescription for cancer patients is symptom limited, progressive, and individualized, with improved ambulation the primary goal.

29. For women recovering from breast cancer surgery, a carefully planned, aerobic circuit resistance exercise program decreases depression and state and trait anxieties.

30. Depression relates to physical changes in the brain produced by neurotransmitter imbalance. No one kind of exercise has a greater impact on depression than others.

31. Exercise-related positive psychological outcomes do not depend on achieving physical fitness, yet fitness-related indicators such as lower blood pressure and increased aerobic capacity improve with regular exercise in depressed individuals.

THOUGHT QUESTIONS

1. Give two recommendations to a middle-aged man who wants to begin an aerobic training program because he feels breathless and experiences chest discomfort while walking the golf course.

2. What type of aerobic training prescription would prove most beneficial for a CHD patient who experiences angina during upper-body work as a plasterer and paper hanger?

3. List two possible mechanisms that might account for the experience of a mildly depressed person who states: "Whenever I begin to feel 'down,' I take a brisk walk, and my mental attitude perks right back up."

SELECTED REFERENCES

Ahluwalia, I.B., et al.: Report from the CDC. Changes in selected chronic disease-related risks and health conditions for nonpregnant women 18-44 years old BRFSS. *J. Womens Health (Larchmt.)*, 14:382, 2005.

American Psychiatric Association: *Diagnostic and Statistical Manual of Mental Disorders: DSM-IV*, 4th ed. Washington, DC: American Psychiatric Association, 1994.

Angermayr, L., et al.: Multifactorial lifestyle interventions in the primary and secondary prevention of cardiovascular disease and type 2 diabetes mellitus—a systematic review of randomized controlled trials. *Ann. Behav. Med.*, 40:49, 2010.

ASCM's Guidelines to Exercise Testing and Prescription, 10th ed. Baltimore, MD: Lippincott Williams & Wilkins, 2010.

Bartholomew, J.B., et al.: Effects of acute exercise on mood and well-being in patients with major depressive disorder. *Med. Sci. Sports Exerc.*, 37:2032, 2005.

Bauman, A.E.: Updating the evidence that physical activity is good for health: an epidemiological review, 2000–2003. *J. Sci. Med. Sport*, 7(1 Suppl):6, 2004.

Blain, G., et al.: Assessment of ventilatory thresholds during graded and maximal exercise test using time varying analysis of respiratory sinus arrhythmia. *Br. J. Sports Med.*, 39:448, 2005.

Blair, S.N., et al: Physical activity, nutrition, and chronic disease. *Med. Sci. Sports Exerc.*, 28:335, 1996.

Bodegard, J., et al.: Reasons for terminating an exercise test provide independent prognostic information: 2014 apparently healthy men followed for 26 years. *Eur. Heart J.*, 26:1394, 2005.

Braith, R.W., et al.: Exercise training in patients with CHF and heart transplant recipients. *Med. Sci. Sports Exerc.*, 30(Suppl):S367, 1998.

Brown, T.R., Kraft, G.H.: Exercise and rehabilitation for individuals with multiple sclerosis. *Phys. Med. Rehabil. Clin. N. Am.*, 16:513, 2005.

Church T, Blair SN.: When will we treat physical activity as a legitimate medical therapy. . . even though it does not come in a pill? *Br. J. Sports Med.*, 43:80, 2009.

Clark, C.J., et al.: Low intensity peripheral muscle conditioning improves exercise tolerance and breathlessness in COPD. *Eur. J. Respir. J.*, 9:2590, 1996.

Cooper, C.B.: Determining the role of exercise in patients with chronic pulmonary disease. *Med. Sci. Sports Exerc.*, 27:147, 1995.

D'Andrea, A., et al.: Prognostic value of supine bicycle exercise stress echocardiography in patients with known or suspected coronary artery disease. *Eur. J. Echocardiogr.*, 6:271, 2005.

Demark-Wahnefried, W., et al.: Lifestyle intervention development study to improve physical function in older adults with cancer: outcomes from Project LEAD. *J. Clin. Oncol.*, 24:3465, 2006.

Dimeo, F., et al.: Aerobic exercise as therapy for cancer fatigue. *Med. Sci. Sports Exerc.*, 30:475, 1998.

Doyne, E.J., et al.: Running versus weight lifting in the treatment of depression. *J. Consult Clin. Psychol.*, 55:748, 1987.

Emaus, A., et al.: Physical activity, heart rate, metabolic profile, and estradiol in premenopausal women. *Med. Sci. Sports Exerc.*, 40:1022, 2008.

Fairey, A.S., et al.: Randomized controlled trial of exercise and blood immune function in postmenopausal breast cancer survivors. *J. Appl. Physiol.*, 98:1534, 2005.

Feiereisen, P., et al.: Is strength training the more efficient training modality in chronic heart failure? *Med. Sci. Sports Exerc.*, 39:1910, 2007.

Franco, M.J., et al.: Comparison of dyspnea ratings during submaximal constant work exercise with incremental testing. *Med. Sci. Sports Exerc.*, 30:479, 1998.

Frazer, C.J., et al.: Effectiveness of treatments for depression in older people. *Med. J. Aust.*, 182:627, 2005.

Freedman, D.S., et al.: Changes and variability in high levels of low-density lipoprotein cholesterol among children. *Pediatrics.*, 126:266, 2010.

Galvao, D.A., Newton, R.U.: Review of exercise intervention studies in cancer patients. *J. Clin. Oncol.*, 1;23:899, 2005.

Hamer, M., et al.: The impact of physical activity on all-cause mortality in men and women after a cancer diagnosis. *Cancer Causes Control*, 20:225, 2009.

Hebestreit, H., et al.: Oxygen uptake kinetics are slowed in cystic fibrosis. *Med. Sci. Sports Exerc.*, 37:10, 2005.

Holmes, M.D., et al.: Physical activity and survival after breast cancer diagnosis. *JAMA.*, 293:2479, 2005.

Hutnick, N.A., et al.: Exercise and lymphocyte activation following chemotherapy for breast cancer. *Med. Sci. Sports Exerc.*, 37:1827, 2005.

Irwin, M.L.: Randomized controlled trials of phyical activity and breast cancer prevention. *Exerc. Sport Sci. Rev.*, 34:182, 2006.

Irwin, M.L.: Physical activity interventions for cancer survivors. *Br. J. Sports Med.*, 43:32, 2009.

Jarrell, L.A., et al.: Gender differences in functional capacity following myocardial infarction: An exploratory study. *Can. J. Cardiovasc. Nurs.*, 15:28, 2005.

Katzmarzyk, P.T., et al.: Sitting time and mortality from all causes, cardiovascular disease, and cancer. *Med. Sci. Sports Exerc.*, 41:998, 2009.

Klika, R.J., et al.: Exercise capacity of a breast cancer survivor: A case study. *Med. Sci. Sports Exerc.*, 40:1711, 2008.

Kohl, H.W., et al.: Maximal exercise hemodynamics and risk of mortality in apparently healthy men and women. *Med. Sci. Sports Exerc.*, 28:601, 1998.

Lee, I.M.: Physical activity and cardiac protection. *Curr. Sports Med. Rep.*, 9:214, 2010.

Malin, A., et al.: Energy balance and breast cancer risk. *Cancer Epidemiol. Biomarkers Prev.*, 14:1496, 2005.

Marzolini, S., et al.: Aerobic and resistance training in coronary disease: Single versus multiple sets. *Med. Sci. Sports Exerc.*, 40:1557, 2008.

McClure, M.K., et al.: Randomized controlled trial of the Breast Cancer Recovery Program for women with breast cancer-related lymphedema. *Am. J. Occup. Ther.*, 64:59, 2010.

McCartney, N.: Role of resistance training in heart disease. *Med. Sci. Sports Exerc.*, 30(Suppl):S396, 1998.

Minam, D.S., et al.: Physical activity and quality of life after radical prostatectomy. *Can Urol. Assoc. J.*, 4:180, 2010.

Mirza, M.A.: Anginalike pain and normal coronary arteries. Uncovering cardiac syndromes that mimic CAD. *Postgrad. Med.*, 117:41, 2005.

Mock, V., et al.: Exercise manages fatigue during breast cancer treatment: A randomized controlled trial. *Psychooncology*, 14:464, 2005.

Morris, J.N.: Exercise in the prevention of coronary heart disease: Today's best bet in public health. *Med. Sci. Sports Exerc.*, 26:807, 1994.

Mousa, T.M., et al.: Exercise training enhances baroreflex sensitivity by an angiotensin II-dependent mechanism in chronic heart failure. *J. Appl. Physiol.*, 104:616, 2008.

Nilsson, B.B., et al.: Effects of group-based high-intensity aerobic interval training in patients with chronic heart failure. *Am. J. Cardiol.*, 102:1361, 2008.

Ohkawara, K., et al.: Response of coronary heart disease risk factors to changes in body fat during diet-induced weight reduction in Japanese obese men: A pilot study. *Ann. Nutr. Metab.*, 56:1, 2010.

Paffenbarger, R.S. Jr., et al.: Physical activity and personal characteristics associated with depression and suicide in American college men. *Acta. Psychiatr. Scand.*, 377(Suppl):16, 1994.

Pelletier, A.R., et al.: Revisions to chronic disease surveillance indicators, United States, 2004. *Prev. Chronic Dis.*, 2(Suppl A):A15, 2005.

Resnick, B.: Research review: exercise interventions for treatment of depression. *Geriatr. Nurs.*, 26:196, 2005.

Samad, A.K., et al.: A meta-analysis of the association of physical activity with reduced risk of colorectal cancer. *Colorectal Dis.*, 7:204, 2005.

Schwartz, A.L., et al.: Exercise reduces daily fatigue in women with breast cancer receiving chemotherapy. *Med. Sci. Sports Exerc.*, 33:718, 2001.

Sesso, H.D., et al.: Physical activity and breast cancer risk in the College Alumni Health Study (United States). *Cancer Causes Control*, 9:433, 1998.

Shephard, R.J., Baldy, G.J.: Exercise as cardiovascular therapy. *Circulation*, 99:963, 1999.

Singh, N.A., et al.: A randomized controlled trial of the effect of exercise on sleep. *Sleep*, 20:95, 1997.

Spence, J.C., et al.: The effect of physical-activity participation on self-concept: A meta-analysis. *J. Sport Exerc. Psychol.*, 19(Suppl):S109, 1997.

Theisen, V., et al.: Blood pressure Sunday: Introducing genomics to the community through family history. *Prev. Chronic Dis.*, 2(Suppl A):A23, 2005.

Verrill, D.E., Ribisl, P.M.: Resistive exercise training in cardiac rehabilitation (an update). *Sports Med.*, 21:371, 1996.

Visovsky, C., Dvorak, C.: Exercise and cancer recovery. *Online J. Issues Nurs.*, 10:7, 2005.

White, L.J., Dressendorfer, R.H.: Exercise and multiple sclerosis. *Sports Med.*, 34:1077, 2004.

Winzer, B.M., et al.: Exercise and the Prevention of Oesophageal Cancer (EPOC) study protocol: a randomized controlled trial of exercise versus stretching in males with Barrett's oesophagus. *BMC Cancer.*, 10:292, 2010.

Wilson, D.B., et al.: Anthropometric changes using a walking intervention in African American breast cancer survivors: A pilot study. *Prev. Chronic Dis.*, 2(Suppl A):A16, 2005.

Yach, D., et al.: Improving diet and physical activity: 12 lessons from controlling tobacco smoking. *Br. Med. J.*, 330:898, 2005.

Yamazaki, T., et al.: Circadian dynamics of heart rate and physical activity in patients with heart failure. *Clin. Exp. Hypertens.*, 27:241, 2005.

Yang, P.S., Chen, C.H.: Exercise stage and processes of change in patients with chronic obstructive pulmonary disease. *J. Nurs. Res.*, 13:97, 2005.

Youngstedt, S.D.: Effects of exercise on sleep. *Clin. Sports Med.*, 24:355, 2005.

Zhang, Y.: Cardiovascular diseases in American women. *Nutr. Metab. Cardiovasc. Dis.*, 20:386, 2010.

The Metric System and Conversion Constants in Exercise Physiology

Appendix A has two parts. Part 1 deals with the metric system, and Part 2 discusses the Système International d'Unités (SI units).

THE METRIC SYSTEM

Most measurements in science are expressed in terms of the metric system. This system uses units that are related to one another by some power of 10. The prefix *centi* means one-hundredth, *milli* means one-thousandth, and *kilo* is derived from a word that means one thousand. In the following sections, we show the relationship between metric units and English units of measurement that are relevant to the material presented in this book.

Units of Length

METRIC UNIT	EQUIVALENT METRIC UNITS	EQUIVALENT ENGLISH UNITS
meter (m)	100 cm; 1000 mm	39.37 in; 3.28 ft; 1.09 yd
centimeter (cm)	0.01 m; 10 mm	0.3937 in
millimeter (mm)	0.001 m; 0.1 cm	0.03937 in

UNITS OF WEIGHT

Use the following conversions for common units of mass (weight) and volume. For example, 1 oz = 0.06 lb. Therefore, 2 oz equals 2 × 0.06 = 0.12 lb, and 16 oz = 0.96 lb (16 × 0.06).

Units of Weight

METRIC UNIT	EQUIVALENT METRIC UNITS	EQUIVALENT ENGLISH UNITS
kilogram (kg)	1000 g; 1,000,000 mg	35.3 oz; 2.2046 lb
gram (g)	0.001 kg; 1000 mg	0.353 oz
milligram (mg)	0.000001 kg; 0.001 g	0.0000353 oz

Units of Volume

METRIC UNIT	EQUIVALENT METRIC UNITS	EQUIVALENT ENGLISH UNITS
liter (L)	1000 mL	1.057 qt
milliliter (mL) or cubic centimeter (cc)	0.001 L	0.001057 qt

Temperature

To convert Fahrenheit to Celsius: $°C = (°F - 32) \div 1.8$

To convert Celsius to Fahrenheit: $°F = (1.8 \div °C) + 32$

On the Fahrenheit scale, water freezes at 32°F and boils at 212°F. On the Celsius scale, water freezes at 0°C and boils at 100°C.

Units of Speed

mph	$km \cdot h^{-1}$	$m \cdot sec^{-1}$
1	1.6	0.47
2	3.2	0.94
3	4.8	1.41
4	6.4	1.88
5	8.0	2.35
6	9.6	2.82
7	11.2	3.29
8	12.8	3.76
9	14.4	4.23
10	16.0	4.70
11	17.7	5.17
12	19.3	5.64
13	20.9	6.11
14	22.5	6.58
15	24.1	7.05
16	25.8	7.52
17	27.4	7.99
18	29.0	8.46
19	30.6	8.93
20	32.2	9.40

Common Expressions of Work, Energy, and Power

WATTS	KILOCALORIES (kCal)	FOOT-POUNDS (ft-lb)
1 watt = 0.73756 ft-lb·sec^{-1}	1 kCal = 3086 ft-lb	1 ft·lb = 3.2389 × 10^{-3} kCal
1 watt = 0.01433 kCal·min^{-1}	1 kCal = 426.8 kg-m	1 ft·lb = 0.13825 kg-m
1 watt = 1.341 × 10^{-3} hp or 0.0013 hp	1 kCal = 3087.4 ft-lb	1 ft·lb = 5.050 × 10^{-3} hp·h^{-1}
1 watt = 6.12 kg-m·min^{-1}	1 kCal = 1.5593 × 10^{-3} hp·h^{-1}	

TERMINOLOGY AND UNITS OF MEASUREMENT

The American College of Sports Medicine (*www.acsm.org/*) suggests that the following terminology and units of measurement be used in scientific endeavors to promote consistency and clarity of communication and to avoid ambiguity. The following terms are defined using the units of measurement of the Système International d'Unités (SI units).

Exercise: Any and all activity involving generation of force by the activated muscle(s) that results in disruption of a homeostatic state. In dynamic exercise, the muscle may perform shortening (concentric) contractions or be overcome by external resistance and perform lengthening (eccentric) contractions. When muscle force results in no movement, the contraction should be termed *static* or *isometric*.

Exercise intensity: A specific level of maintenance of muscular activity that can be quantified in terms of power (energy expenditure or work performed per unit of time), isometric force sustained, or velocity of progression.

Endurance: The time limit of a person's ability to maintain either a specific isometric force or a specific power level involving combinations of concentric or eccentric muscular contractions.

Mass: A quantity of matter of an object; a direct measure of the object's inertia (note: Mass = Weight ÷ Acceleration due to gravity; unit: gram or kilogram).

Weight: The force with which a quantity of matter is attracted toward Earth by normal acceleration of gravity (traditional unit: kilogram).

Energy: The capability of producing force, performing work, or generating heat (unit: joule or kilojoule).

Force: That which changes or tends to change the state of rest or motion in matter (unit: Newton).

Speed: Total distance traveled per unit of time (unit: meters per second).

Velocity: Displacement per unit of time. A vector quantity requiring that direction be stated or strongly implied (unit: meters per second or kilometers per hour).

Work: Force expressed through a distance but with no limitation on time (unit: joule or kilojoule). Quantities of energy and heat expressed independently of time should also be presented in joules. The term *work* should *not* be used synonymously with *muscular exercise*.

Power: The rate of performing work; the derivative of work with respect to time; the product of force and velocity (unit: watt). Other related processes, such as energy release and heat transfer, should, when expressed per unit of time, be quantified and presented in watts.

Torque: Effectiveness of a force to produce axial rotation (unit: Newton meter).

Volume: A space occupied, for example, by a quantity of fluid or gas (unit: liter or milliliter). Gas volumes should be indicated as ATPS, BTPS, or STPD.

Amount of a substance: The amount of a substance is frequently expressed in moles. A mole is the quantity of a chemical substance that has a weight in mass units (e.g., grams) numerically equal to the molecular weight or that, in the case of a gas, has a volume occupied by such a weight under specified conditions. One mole of a respiratory gas is equal to 22.4 L at STPD.

SI UNITS

The uniform numerical value system is known as the Système International d'Unités (SI units). SI was developed through international cooperation to create a universally acceptable system of measurement. SI ensures that units of measurement are uniform in concept and style. The SI system permits quantities in common use to be more easily compared. Many scientific organizations endorse the concept of the SI, and leading journals in nutrition, health, and exercise science now require that laboratory data be presented in SI units. The information in this appendix has been summarized from a detailed description about the SI published in the following article: Young, D.S.: Implementation of SI units for clinical laboratory data. Style specifications and conversion tables. *Ann. Intern. Med.*, 106:114, 1987.

For SI units in exercise physiology, the term *body weight* is properly referred to as mass (kg), height should be referred to as stature (m), second is sec, minute is min, hour is h, week is wk, month is mo, year is y, day is d, gram is g, liter is L, hertz is Hz, joule is J, kilocalorie is kCal, ohm is V, pascal is Pa, revolutions per minute is rpm, volt is V, and watt is W. These abbreviations or symbols are used for the singular and plural forms.

Definitions of Common SI Units

Degree Celsius (°C)	The degree Celsius (centigrade) is equivalent to K − 273.15.
Radian (rad)	The radian is the plane angle subtended by a circular arc as the length of the arc divided by the radius of the arc.
Joule (J)	The joule is the work done when the point of application of a force of 1 N is displaced through a distance of 1 m in the direction of the force. 1 J = 1 Nm.
Kelvin (K)	The Kelvin is the fraction 1/273.16 of the thermodynamic temperature of the triple point of water.
Kilogram (kg)	The kilogram is a unit of mass equal to the mass of the international prototype of the kilogram.
Meter (m)	The meter is the length equal to 1,650,763.73 wavelengths in vacuum of the radiation that corresponds to the transition between the levels $2p_{10}$ and $5d_5$ of the krypton 86 atom.
Newton (N)	The Newton is the force that, when applied to a mass of 1 kg, gives it an acceleration of $1\ m^{-1}\cdot sec^{-2}$. $1\ N = 1\ kg\cdot m^{-1}\cdot sec^{-2}$.
Pascal (Pa)	The Pascal is the pressure produced by a force of 1 N applied, with uniform distribution, over an area of $1\ m^{-2}$. $1\ Pa = 1\ N\cdot m^{-2}$.
Second (sec)	The second is the duration of 9,192,631,770 periods of the radiation that corresponds to the transition between the two hyperfine levels of the ground state of the cesium 133 atom.
Watt (W)	The Watt is the power that, in 1 sec, gives rise to the energy of 1 joule. $1\ W = 1\ J\cdot sec^{-1}$.

Base Units of SI Nomenclature

PHYSICAL QUANTITY	BASE UNIT	SI SYMBOL
Length	meter	m
Mass	kilogram	kg
Time	second	sec
Amount of substance	mole	mol
Thermodynamic temperature	kelvin	K
Electric current	ampere	A
Luminous intensity	candela	cd

Base Units of SI Style Guidelines

GUIDELINES	EXAMPLE	INCORRECT STYLE	CORRECT STYLE
Lowercase letters are used for symbols or abbreviations	kilogram	Kg	kg
Exceptions:	kelvin	k	K
	ampere	a	A
	liter	l	L
Symbols are not followed by a period	meter	m.	m
Exception: end of sentence	mole	mol.	mol
Symbols are not to be pluralized	kilograms	kgs	kg
	meters	ms	m
Names and symbols are not to be combined	force	$kilogram\cdot meter\cdot sec^{-2}$	$kg\text{-}m\cdot sec^{-2}$ $kg\text{-}m/sec^2$
When numbers are printed, symbols are preferred		100 meters	100 m
		2 moles	2 mol
A space should be placed between the number and the symbol		50 ml	50 mL
The product of units is indicated by a dot above the line		$kg \times m/sec^2$	$kg\text{-}m\cdot sec^{-2}$ $kg\text{-}m/sec^2$
Only one solidus (/) should be used per expression		mmol/L/sec	mmol/(L·sec)
A zero should be placed before the decimal		.01	0.01
Decimal numbers are preferable to fractions		$^3/_4$	0.75
		75%	0.75
Spaces are used to separate long numbers		1,500,000	1 500 000
Exception: optional with four-digit number		1,000	1000 or 1 000

Metabolic Computations in Open-Circuit Spirometry

STANDARDIZING GAS VOLUMES: ENVIRONMENTAL FACTORS

Gas volumes obtained during physiologic measurements are usually expressed in one of three ways: *ATPS*, *STPD*, or *BTPS*.

ATPS refers to the volume of gas at the specific conditions of measurement, which are, therefore, at *a*mbient *t*emperature (273°K + ambient temperature°C), ambient *p*ressure, and *s*aturated with water vapor. Gas volumes collected during open-circuit spirometry and pulmonary function tests are measured initially at ATPS.

The volume of a gas varies depending on its temperature, pressure, and content of water vapor, even though the absolute number of gas molecules remains constant. These environmental influences are summarized as follows:

Temperature: The volume of a gas varies *directly* with temperature. Increasing the temperature causes the molecules to move more rapidly; the gas mixture expands, and the volume increases proportionately (*Charles' law*).

Pressure: The volume of a gas varies *inversely* with pressure. Increasing the pressure on a gas forces the molecules closer together, causing the volume to decrease in proportion to the increase in pressure (*Boyle's law*).

Water vapor: The volume of a gas varies depending on its water vapor content. The volume of a gas is greater when the gas is saturated with water vapor than it is when the same gas is dry (i.e., contains no moisture).

These three factors—temperature, pressure, and the relative degree of saturation of the gas with water vapor—must be considered, especially when gas volumes are to be compared under different environmental conditions and used subsequently in metabolic and physiologic calculations. The standards that provide the frame of reference for expressing a volume of gas are either STPD or BTPS.

STPD refers to the volume of a gas expressed under standard conditions of *t*emperature (273°K or 0°C), *p*ressure (760 mm Hg), and *d*ry (no water vapor). Expressing a gas volume STPD, for example, makes it possible to evaluate and compare the volumes of expired air measured while running in the rain at high altitude, along a beach in the cold of winter, or in a hot desert environment below sea level. *In all metabolic calculations, gas volumes are always expressed at STPD.*

1. To reduce a gas volume to standard temperature (ST), the following formula is applied:

$$\textbf{Gas volume ST} = V_{ATPS} \times \frac{273°K}{273°K + T°C} \quad (1)$$

where $T°C$ = temperature of the gas in the measuring device and 273°K = absolute temperature kelvin, which is equivalent to 0°C.

2. The following equation is used to express a gas volume at standard pressure (SP):

$$\textbf{Gas volume SP} = V_{ATPS} \times \frac{P_B}{760 \text{ mm Hg}} \quad (2)$$

where P_B = ambient barometric pressure in mm Hg and 760 = standard barometric pressure at sea level, mm Hg.

3. To reduce a gas to standard dry (SD) conditions, the effects of water vapor pressure at the particular environmental temperature must be subtracted from the volume of gas. Because expired air is 100% saturated with water vapor, it is not necessary to determine its percent saturation from measures of relative humidity. The vapor pressure in moist or completely humidified air at a particular ambient temperature can be obtained in Table B.1 and expressed in mm Hg. This vapor pressure (P_{H_2O}) is then subtracted from the ambient barometric pressure (P_B) to reduce the gas to standard pressure dry (SPD) as follows:

$$\textbf{Gas volume SPD} = V_{ATPS} \times \frac{P_B - P_{H_2O}}{760} \quad (3)$$

By combining equations (1) and (3), any volume of moist air can be converted to STPD as follows:

Gas volume STPD

$$= V_{ATPS}\left(\frac{273°K}{273 + T°C}\right)\left(\frac{P_B - P_{H_2O}}{760}\right) \quad (4)$$

Table B.1	Vapor Pressure (P_{H_2O}) of Wet Gas at Temperatures Normally Encountered in the Laboratory		
T (°C)	P_{H_2O} (mm Hg)	T (°C)	P_{H_2O} (mm Hg)
20	17.5	31	33.7
21	18.7	32	35.7
22	19.8	33	37.7
23	21.1	34	39.9
24	22.4	35	42.2
25	23.8	36	44.6
26	25.2	37	47.1
27	26.7	38	49.7
28	28.4	39	52.4
29	30.0	40	55.3
30	31.8		

Table B.2 Factors to Reduce Moist Gas to a Dry Gas Volume at 0°C and 760 mm Hg

BAROMETRIC PRESSURE	TEMPERATURE (°C)																	
	15	16	17	18	19	20	21	22	23	24	25	26	27	28	29	30	31	32
700	0.855	851	847	842	838	834	829	825	821	816	812	807	802	797	793	788	783	778
702	857	853	849	845	840	836	832	827	823	818	814	809	805	800	795	790	785	780
704	860	856	852	847	843	839	834	830	825	821	816	812	807	802	797	792	787	783
706	862	858	854	850	845	841	838	832	828	823	819	814	810	804	800	795	790	785
708	865	861	856	852	848	843	839	834	830	825	821	816	812	807	802	797	792	787
710	867	863	859	855	850	846	842	837	833	828	824	819	814	809	804	799	795	790
712	870	866	861	857	853	848	844	839	836	830	826	821	817	812	807	802	797	792
714	872	868	864	859	855	851	846	842	837	833	828	824	819	814	809	804	799	794
716	875	871	866	862	858	853	849	844	840	835	831	826	822	815	812	807	802	797
718	877	873	869	864	860	856	851	847	842	838	833	828	824	819	814	809	804	799
720	880	876	871	867	863	858	854	849	845	840	836	831	826	821	816	812	807	802
722	882	878	874	869	865	861	856	852	847	843	838	833	829	824	819	814	809	804
724	885	880	876	872	867	863	858	854	849	845	840	835	831	826	821	816	811	806
726	887	883	879	874	870	866	861	856	852	847	843	838	833	829	824	818	813	808
728	890	886	881	877	872	868	863	859	854	850	845	840	836	831	826	821	816	811
730	892	888	884	879	875	871	866	861	857	852	847	843	838	833	828	823	818	813
732	895	890	886	882	877	873	868	864	859	854	850	845	840	836	831	825	820	815
734	897	893	889	884	880	875	871	866	862	857	852	847	843	838	833	828	823	818
736	900	895	891	887	882	878	873	869	864	859	855	850	845	840	835	830	825	820
738	902	898	894	889	885	880	876	871	866	862	857	852	848	843	838	833	828	822
740	905	900	896	892	887	883	878	874	869	864	860	855	850	845	840	835	830	825
742	907	903	898	894	890	885	881	876	871	867	862	857	852	847	842	837	832	827
744	910	906	901	897	892	888	873	878	874	869	864	859	855	850	845	840	834	829
746	912	908	903	899	895	890	866	881	876	872	867	862	857	852	847	842	837	832
748	915	910	906	901	897	892	888	883	879	874	869	864	860	854	850	845	839	834
750	917	913	908	904	900	895	890	886	881	876	872	867	862	857	852	847	842	837
752	920	915	911	906	902	897	893	888	883	879	874	869	864	859	854	849	844	839
754	922	918	913	909	904	900	895	891	886	881	876	872	867	862	857	852	846	841
756	925	920	916	911	907	902	898	893	888	883	879	874	869	864	859	854	849	844
758	927	923	918	914	909	905	900	896	891	886	881	876	872	866	861	856	851	846
760	930	925	921	916	912	907	902	898	893	888	883	879	874	869	864	859	854	848
762	932	928	923	919	914	910	905	900	896	891	886	881	876	871	866	861	856	851
764	936	930	926	921	916	912	907	903	898	893	888	884	879	874	869	864	858	853
766	937	933	928	924	919	915	910	905	900	896	891	886	881	876	871	866	861	855
768	940	935	931	926	922	917	912	908	903	898	893	888	883	878	873	868	863	858
770	942	938	933	928	924	919	915	910	905	901	896	891	886	881	876	871	865	860

Table B.3	**BTPS Factors**		
T (°C)	**BTPS[a]**	**T (°C)**	**BTPS**
20	1.102	29	1.051
21	1.096	30	1.045
22	1.091	31	1.039
23	1.085	32	1.032
24	1.080	33	1.026
25	1.075	34	1.020
26	1.068	35	1.014
27	1.063	36	1.007
28	1.057	37	1.000

[a]Body temperature, ambient pressure, and saturated with water vapor.

As was the case with the correction to STPD, appropriate BTPS *correction factors* are available for converting a moist gas volume at ambient conditions to a volume BTPS. These BTPS factors for a broad range of ambient temperatures are presented in Table B.3. These factors have been computed assuming a barometric pressure of 760 mm Hg, and small deviations of ±10 mm Hg from this pressure introduce only a minimal error.

CALCULATION OF OXYGEN UPTAKE

In determining oxygen uptake by open-circuit spirometry, we are interested in knowing how much oxygen has been removed from the *inspired air*. Because the composition of inspired air remains relatively constant (CO_2 = 0.03%; O_2 = 20.93%; N_2 = 79.04%), it is possible to determine how much oxygen has been removed from the inspired air by measuring the amount and composition of the expired air. When this is done, the expired air contains more carbon dioxide (usually 2.5%–5.0%), less oxygen (usually 15.0%–18.5%), and more nitrogen (usually 79.04%–79.60%). It should be noted, however, that nitrogen is inert in terms of metabolism; any change in its concentration in expired air reflects the fact that the number of oxygen molecules removed from the inspired air is not replaced by the same number of carbon dioxide molecules produced in metabolism. This results in the volume of expired air (V_E, STPD) being unequal to the inspired volume (V_I, STPD). For example, if the respiratory quotient is less than 1.00 (i.e., less CO_2 produced in relation to O_2 consumed) and 3 L of air is inspired, *less than* 3 L of air will be expired. In this case, the nitrogen concentration is higher in the expired air than in the inspired air. This is not to say that nitrogen has been produced, only that nitrogen molecules now represent a larger percentage of V_E compared with V_I. In fact, V_E differs from V_I in direct proportion to the change in nitrogen concentration between the inspired and expired volumes. Thus, V_I can be determined from V_E using the relative

change in nitrogen in an equation known as the *Haldane transformation*.

$$V_I, STPD = V_E, STPD \times \frac{\%N_{2E}}{\%N_{2I}} \quad (5)$$

where $\%N_{2I}$ = 79.04 and $\%N_{2E}$ = percent nitrogen in expired air computed from gas analysis as:

$$[(100 - (\%O_{2E} + \%CO_2)]$$

The volume of O_2 in the inspired air ($\dot{V}O_{2I}$) can then be determined as follows:

$$VO_{2I} = V_I \times \%O_{2I} \quad (6)$$

Substituting equation (5) for $\dot{V}_I$,

$$\dot{V}O_{2I} = \dot{V}_E \times \frac{\%N_{2E}}{79.04\% \times \%O_{2I}} \quad (7)$$

where $\%O_{2I}$ = 20.93%

The amount or volume of oxygen in the expired air ($\dot{V}O_{2E}$) is computed as:

$$\dot{V}O_{2E} = \dot{V}_E \times \%O_{2E} \quad (8)$$

where $\%O_{2E}$ is the fractional concentration of oxygen in expired air determined by gas analysis (chemical or electronic methods).

The amount of O_2 removed from the inspired air *each minute* ($\dot{V}O_2$) can then be computed as follows:

$$\dot{V}O_2 = (\dot{V}_I \times \%O_{2I}) - (\dot{V}_E \times \%O_{2E}) \quad (9)$$

By substitution

$$\dot{V}O_2 = \left[\left(\dot{V}_E \times \frac{\%N_{2E}}{79.04\%} \right) \times 20.93\% \right] - (\dot{V}_E \times \%O_{2E}) \quad (10)$$

where $\dot{V}O_2$ = volume of oxygen consumed per minute, expressed in milliliters or liters, and $\dot{V}_E$ = expired air volume per minute expressed in milliliters or liters.

Equation 10 can be simplified to:

$$\dot{V}O_2 = \dot{V}_E \left[\left(\frac{\%N_{2E}}{79.04\%} \times 20.93\% \right) - \%O_{2E} \right] \quad (11)$$

The final form of the equation is:

$$\dot{V}O_2 = \dot{V}_E [(\%N_{2E} \times 0.265) - \%O_{2E}] \quad (12)$$

The value obtained within the brackets in equations 11 and 12 is referred to as the *true O_2*; this represents the "oxygen extraction" or, more precisely, the percentage of oxygen consumed for any volume of air *expired*.

Although equation 12 represents the equation used most widely to compute oxygen uptake from measures of expired air, it is also possible to calculate $\dot{V}O_2$ from direct measurements of both $\dot{V}_I$ and $\dot{V}_E$. In this case, the Haldane transformation is not used, and oxygen uptake is calculated directly as:

$$\dot{V}O_2 = (\dot{V}_I \times 20.93) - (\dot{V}_E \times \%O_{2E}) \quad (13)$$

In situations in which only $\dot{V}_I$ is measured, the $\dot{V}_E$ can be calculated from the Haldane transformation as:

$$\dot{V}_E = \dot{V}_I \frac{\%N_{2I}}{\%N_{2E}}$$

By substitution in equation 13, the computational equation is:

$$\dot{V}O_2 = \dot{V}_I\left[\%O_{2I} - \left(\frac{\%N_{2I}}{\%N_{2E}} \times \%O_{2E}\right)\right] \quad (14)$$

CALCULATION OF CARBON DIOXIDE PRODUCTION

The carbon dioxide production per minute ($\dot{V}CO_2$) is calculated as follows:

$$\dot{V}CO_2 = \dot{V}_E(\%CO_{2E} - \%CO_{2I}) \quad (15)$$

where $\%CO_{2E}$ = percent carbon dioxide in expired air determined by gas analysis and $\%CO_{2I}$ = percent carbon dioxide in inspired air, which is essentially constant at 0.03%.

The final form of the equation is:

$$\dot{V}CO_2 = \dot{V}_E(\%CO_{2E} - 0.03\%) \quad (16)$$

CALCULATION OF RESPIRATORY QUOTIENT

The respiratory quotient (RQ) is calculated in one of two ways:

1.
$$RQ = \dot{V}CO_2/\dot{V}O_2 \quad (17)$$

   or

2.
$$RQ = \frac{(\%CO_{2E} - 0.03\%)}{\text{"True" } O_2} \quad (18)$$

SAMPLE METABOLIC CALCULATIONS

The following data were obtained during the last minute of a steady-rate, 10-minute treadmill run performed at 6 mph at a 5% grade.

$\dot{V}_E$: 62.1 L, ATPS
Barometric pressure: 750 mm Hg
Temperature: 26°C
$\%O_2$ expired: 16.86 (O_2 analyzer)
$\%CO_2$ expired: 3.60 (CO_2 analyzer)
$\%N_2$ expired: $[100 - (16.86 + 3.60)] = 79.54$

Determine the following:
1. $\dot{V}_E$, STPD
2. $\dot{V}O_2$, STPD
3. $\dot{V}CO_2$ STPD
4. RQ
5. kCal·min^{-1}

1. $\dot{V}_E$, STPD (use equation 4 or STPD correction factor in **Table B.2**).

$$\dot{V}_E, STPD = \dot{V}_E, ATPS \left(\frac{273}{273 + T°C}\right)\left(\frac{P_B - P_{H_2O}}{760}\right)$$
$$= 62.1\left(\frac{273}{299}\right)\left(\frac{750 - 25.2}{760}\right)$$
$$= 54.07 \text{ L·min}^{-1}$$

2. $\dot{V}O_2$, STPD (use equation 12)

$$\dot{V}O_2, STPD = \dot{V}_E, STPD[(\%N_{2E} \times 0.265) - \%O_{2E}]$$
$$= 54.07[(0.7954 \times 0.265) - 0.1686]$$
$$= 54.07(0.0422)$$
$$= 2.281 \text{ L·min}^{-1}$$

3. $\dot{V}CO_2$, STPD (use equation 16)

$$\dot{V}CO_2, STPD = \dot{V}_E, STPD(CO_{2E} - 0.03\%)$$
$$= 54.07(0.0360 - 0.0003)$$
$$= 54.07(0.0357)$$
$$= 1.930 \text{ L·min}^{-1}$$

4. RQ (use equation 17 or 18)

$$RQ = \dot{V}CO_2/\dot{V}O_2$$
$$= \frac{1.930}{2.281}$$
$$= 0.846$$

or

$$RQ = \frac{(\%CO_{2E} - 0.03\%)}{\text{"True" } O}$$
$$= \frac{3.60 - 0.03}{4.22}$$
$$= 0.846$$

Because the exercise was performed in a steady-rate of aerobic metabolism, the obtained RQ of 0.846 can be applied in Table 7.2 to obtain the appropriate caloric transformation. In this way, the exercise oxygen uptake can be transposed to kCal of energy expended per minute as follows:

5. Energy expenditure (kCal·min^{-1}) = $\dot{V}O_2$ (L·min^{-1}) × caloric equivalent per liter O_2 at the given steady-rate RQ:

$$\textbf{Energy expenditure} = 2.281 \times 4.862$$
$$= 11.09 \text{ kCal·min}^{-1}$$

Assuming that the RQ value reflects the nonprotein RQ, a reasonable estimate of both the percentage and quantity of lipid and carbohydrate metabolized during each minute of the run can be obtained from Table 7.2.

Percentage kCal derived from lipid = 50.7%
Percentage kCal derived from carbohydrate = 49.3%
Grams of lipid used = 0.267 g per liter of oxygen, or approximately 0.61 g per minute (0.267×2.281 L O_2)
Grams of carbohydrate used = 0.580 g per liter of oxygen, or approximately 1.36 g per minute (0.580×2.281 L O_2)

Evaluation of Body Composition—Girth Method

This appendix contains the age- and gender-specific equations to predict body fat percentage based on three girth measurements. There are four charts, one each for younger and older men and women. In our experience, it is important to calibrate the tape measure before using it. Use a meter stick as the standard and check the markings on the cloth tape at 10-cm increments. A cloth tape is preferred over a metal one because of little skin compression when applying a cloth tape to the skin's surface at a relatively constant tension.

To use the charts, measure the three girths for your age and gender as follows:

AGE (years)	GENDER	SITE A	SITE B	SITE C
18–26	M	Right upper arm	Abdomen	Right forearm
	F	Abdomen	Right thigh	Right forearm
27–50	M	Buttocks	Abdomen	Right forearm
	F	Abdomen	Right thigh	Right calf

Chapter 16 presents the specific measurements sites and a step-by-step explanation of how to compute the relative and absolute values for body fat, lean body mass, and desirable body mass from the Appendix C charts. The bottom of each of the Appendix C charts presents specific equation to predict percentage body fat with its corresponding constant.

Chart C.1	Conversion Constants to Predict Percentage Body Fat for Young Men[a]								

UPPER ARM			ABDOMEN			FOREARM		
in	cm	CONSTANT A	in	cm	CONSTANT B	in	cm	CONSTANT C
7.00	17.78	25.91	21.00	53.34	27.56	7.00	17.78	38.01
7.25	18.41	26.83	21.25	53.97	27.88	7.25	18.41	39.37
7.50	19.05	27.76	21.50	54.61	28.21	7.50	19.05	40.72
7.75	19.68	28.68	21.75	55.24	28.54	7.75	19.68	42.08
8.00	20.32	29.61	22.00	55.88	28.87	8.00	20.32	43.44
8.25	20.95	30.53	22.25	56.51	29.20	8.25	20.95	44.80
8.50	21.59	31.46	22.50	57.15	29.52	8.50	21.59	46.15
8.75	22.22	32.38	22.75	57.78	29.85	8.75	22.22	47.51
9.00	22.86	33.31	23.00	58.42	30.18	9.00	22.86	48.87
9.25	23.49	34.24	23.25	59.05	30.51	9.25	23.49	50.23
9.50	24.13	35.16	23.50	59.69	30.84	9.50	24.13	51.58
9.75	24.76	36.09	23.75	60.32	31.16	9.75	24.76	52.94
10.00	25.40	37.01	24.00	60.96	31.49	10.00	25.40	54.30
10.25	26.03	37.94	24.25	61.59	31.82	10.25	26.03	55.65
10.50	26.67	38.86	24.50	62.23	32.15	10.50	26.67	57.01
10.75	27.30	39.79	24.75	62.86	32.48	10.75	27.30	58.37
11.00	27.94	40.71	25.00	63.50	32.80	11.00	27.94	59.73
11.25	28.57	41.64	25.25	64.13	33.13	11.25	28.57	61.08
11.50	29.21	42.56	25.50	64.77	33.46	11.50	29.21	62.44
11.75	29.84	43.49	25.75	65.40	33.79	11.75	29.84	63.80
12.00	30.48	44.41	26.00	66.04	34.12	12.00	30.48	65.16

Chart C.1	**Conversion Constants to Predict Percentage Body Fat for Young Men[a]** *(Continued)*							

UPPER ARM			ABDOMEN			FOREARM		
in	cm	CONSTANT A	in	cm	CONSTANT B	in	cm	CONSTANT C
12.25	31.11	45.34	26.25	66.67	34.44	12.25	31.11	66.51
12.50	31.75	46.26	26.50	67.31	34.77	12.50	31.75	67.87
12.75	32.38	47.19	26.75	67.94	35.10	12.75	32.38	69.23
13.00	33.02	48.11	27.00	68.58	35.43	13.00	33.02	70.59
13.25	33.65	49.04	27.25	69.21	35.76	13.25	33.65	71.94
13.50	34.29	49.96	27.50	69.85	36.09	13.50	34.29	73.30
13.75	34.92	50.89	27.75	70.48	36.41	13.75	34.92	74.66
14.00	35.56	51.82	28.00	71.12	36.74	14.00	35.56	76.02
14.25	36.19	52.74	28.25	71.75	37.07	14.25	36.19	77.37
14.50	36.83	53.67	28.50	72.39	37.40	14.50	36.83	78.73
14.75	37.46	54.59	28.75	73.02	37.73	14.75	37.46	80.09
15.00	38.10	55.52	29.00	73.66	38.05	15.00	38.10	81.45
15.25	38.73	56.44	29.25	74.29	38.38	15.25	38.73	82.80
15.50	39.37	57.37	29.50	74.93	38.71	15.50	39.37	84.16
15.75	40.00	58.29	29.75	75.56	39.04	15.75	40.00	85.52
16.00	40.64	59.22	30.00	76.20	39.37	16.00	40.64	86.88
16.25	41.27	60.14	30.25	76.83	39.69	16.25	41.27	88.23
16.50	41.91	61.07	30.50	77.47	40.02	16.50	41.91	89.59
16.75	42.54	61.99	30.75	78.10	40.35	16.75	42.54	90.95
17.00	43.18	62.92	31.00	78.74	40.68	17.00	43.18	92.31
17.25	43.81	63.84	31.25	79.37	41.01	17.25	43.81	93.66
17.50	44.45	64.77	31.50	80.01	41.33	17.50	44.45	95.02
17.75	45.08	65.69	31.75	80.64	41.66	17.75	45.08	96.38
18.00	45.72	66.62	32.00	81.28	41.99	18.00	45.72	97.74
18.25	46.35	67.54	32.25	81.91	42.32	18.25	46.35	99.09
18.50	46.99	68.47	32.50	82.55	42.65	18.50	46.99	100.45
18.75	47.62	69.40	32.75	83.18	42.97	18.75	47.62	101.81
19.00	48.26	70.32	33.00	83.82	43.30	19.00	48.26	103.17
19.25	48.89	71.25	33.25	84.45	43.63	19.25	48.89	104.52
19.50	49.53	72.17	33.50	85.09	43.96	19.50	49.53	105.88
19.75	50.16	73.10	33.75	85.72	44.29	19.75	50.16	107.24
20.00	50.80	74.02	34.00	86.36	44.61	20.00	50.80	108.60
20.25	51.43	74.95	34.25	86.99	44.94	20.25	51.43	109.95
20.50	52.07	75.87	34.50	87.63	45.27	20.50	52.07	111.31
20.75	52.70	76.80	34.75	88.26	45.60	20.75	52.70	112.67
21.00	53.34	77.72	35.00	88.90	45.93	21.00	53.34	114.02
21.25	53.97	78.65	35.25	89.53	46.25	21.25	53.97	115.38
21.50	54.61	79.57	35.50	90.17	46.58	21.50	54.61	116.74
21.75	55.24	80.50	35.75	90.80	46.91	21.75	55.24	118.10
22.00	55.88	81.42	36.00	91.44	47.24	22.00	55.88	119.45
			36.25	92.07	47.57			
			36.50	92.71	47.89			
			36.75	93.34	48.22			
			37.00	93.98	48.55			
			37.25	94.61	48.88			
			37.50	95.25	49.21			
			37.75	95.88	49.54			
			38.00	96.52	49.86			
			38.25	97.15	50.19			
			38.50	97.79	50.52			
			38.75	98.42	50.85			
			39.00	99.06	51.18			
			39.25	99.69	51.50			
			39.50	100.33	51.83			
			39.75	100.96	52.16			
			40.00	101.60	52.49			
			40.25	102.23	52.82			
			40.50	102.87	53.14			
			40.75	103.50	53.47			
			41.00	104.14	53.80			
			41.25	104.77	54.13			
			41.50	105.41	54.46			
			41.75	106.04	54.78			
			42.00	106.68	55.11			

Note: Percentage Fat = Constant A + Constant B − Constant C − 10.2.

[a]Copyright © 1986, 1991, 1996, 2000, 2006, 2010 by Frank I. Katch, Victor L. Katch, William D. McArdle, and Fitness Technologies, Inc., 5043 Via Lara Ln. Santa Barbara, CA 93111. No part of this appendix may be reproduced in any manner without written permission from the copyright holders.

Chart C.2	Conversion Constants to Predict Percentage Body Fat for Older Men[a]

BUTTOCKS			ABDOMEN			FOREARM		
in	cm	CONSTANT A	in	cm	CONSTANT B	in	cm	CONSTANT C
28.00	71.12	29.34	25.50	64.77	22.84	7.00	17.78	21.01
28.25	71.75	29.60	25.75	65.40	23.06	7.25	18.41	21.76
28.50	72.39	29.87	26.00	66.04	23.29	7.50	19.05	22.52
28.75	73.02	30.13	26.25	66.67	23.51	7.75	19.68	23.26
29.00	73.66	30.39	26.50	67.31	23.73	8.00	20.32	24.02
29.25	74.29	30.65	26.75	67.94	23.96	8.25	20.95	24.76
29.50	74.93	30.92	27.00	68.58	24.18	8.50	21.59	25.52
29.75	75.56	31.18	27.25	69.21	24.40	8.75	22.22	26.26
30.00	76.20	31.44	27.50	69.85	24.63	9.00	22.86	27.02
30.25	76.83	31.70	27.75	70.48	24.85	9.25	23.49	27.76
30.50	77.47	31.96	28.00	71.12	25.08	9.50	24.13	28.52
30.75	78.10	32.22	28.25	71.75	25.29	9.75	24.76	29.26
31.00	78.74	32.49	28.50	72.39	25.52	10.00	25.40	30.02
31.25	79.37	32.75	28.75	73.02	25.75	10.25	26.03	30.76
31.50	80.01	33.01	29.00	73.66	25.97	10.50	26.67	31.52
31.75	80.64	33.27	29.25	74.29	26.19	10.75	27.30	32.27
32.00	81.28	33.54	29.50	74.93	26.42	11.00	27.94	33.02
32.25	81.91	33.80	29.75	75.56	26.64	11.25	28.57	33.77
32.50	82.55	34.06	30.00	76.20	26.87	11.50	29.21	34.52
32.75	83.18	34.32	30.25	76.83	27.09	11.75	29.84	35.27
33.00	83.82	34.58	30.50	77.47	27.32	12.00	30.48	36.02
33.25	84.45	34.84	30.75	78.10	27.54	12.25	31.11	36.77
33.50	85.09	35.11	31.00	78.74	27.76	12.50	31.75	37.53
33.75	85.72	35.37	31.25	79.37	27.98	12.75	32.38	38.27
34.00	86.36	35.63	31.50	80.01	28.21	13.00	33.02	39.03
34.25	86.99	35.89	31.75	80.64	28.43	13.25	33.65	39.77
34.50	87.63	36.16	32.00	81.28	28.66	13.50	34.29	40.53
34.75	88.26	36.42	32.25	81.91	28.88	13.75	34.92	41.27
35.00	88.90	36.68	32.50	82.55	29.11	14.00	35.56	42.03
35.25	89.53	36.94	32.75	83.18	29.33	14.25	36.19	42.77
35.50	90.17	37.20	33.00	83.82	29.55	14.50	36.83	43.53
35.75	90.80	37.46	33.25	84.45	29.78	14.75	37.46	44.27
36.00	91.44	37.73	33.50	85.09	30.00	15.00	38.10	45.03
36.25	92.07	37.99	33.75	85.72	30.22	15.25	38.73	45.77
36.50	92.71	38.25	34.00	86.36	30.45	15.50	39.37	46.53
36.75	93.34	38.51	34.25	86.99	30.67	15.75	40.00	47.28
37.00	93.98	38.78	34.50	87.63	30.89	16.00	40.64	48.03
37.25	94.61	39.04	34.75	88.26	31.12	16.25	41.27	48.78
37.50	95.25	39.30	35.00	88.90	31.35	16.50	41.91	49.53
37.75	95.88	39.56	35.25	89.53	31.57	16.75	42.54	50.28
38.00	96.52	39.82	35.50	90.17	31.79	17.00	43.18	51.03
38.25	97.15	40.08	35.75	90.80	32.02	17.25	43.81	51.78
38.50	97.79	40.35	36.00	91.44	32.24	17.50	44.45	52.54
38.75	98.42	40.61	36.25	92.07	32.46	17.75	45.08	53.28
39.00	99.06	40.87	36.50	92.71	32.69	18.00	45.72	54.04
39.25	99.69	41.13	36.75	93.34	32.91	18.25	46.35	54.78
39.50	100.33	41.39	37.00	93.98	33.14			
39.75	100.96	41.66	37.25	94.61	33.36			
40.00	101.60	41.92	37.50	95.25	33.58			
40.25	102.23	42.18	37.75	95.88	33.81			
40.50	102.87	42.44	38.00	96.52	34.03			
40.75	103.50	42.70	38.25	97.15	34.26			
41.00	104.14	42.97	38.50	97.79	34.48			
41.25	104.77	43.23	38.75	98.42	34.70			
41.50	105.41	43.49	39.00	99.06	34.93			
41.75	106.04	43.75	39.25	99.69	35.15			
42.00	106.68	44.02	39.50	100.33	35.38			
42.25	107.31	44.28	39.75	100.96	35.59			
42.50	107.95	44.54	40.00	101.60	35.82			
42.75	108.58	44.80	40.25	102.23	36.05			
43.00	109.22	45.06	40.50	102.87	36.27			
43.25	109.85	45.32	40.75	103.50	36.49			

Chart C.2	Conversion Constants to Predict Percentage Body Fat for Older Men[a] *(Continued)*

BUTTOCKS			ABDOMEN			FOREARM		
in	cm	CONSTANT A	in	cm	CONSTANT B	in	cm	CONSTANT C
43.50	110.49	45.59	41.00	104.14	36.72			
43.75	111.12	45.85	41.25	104.77	36.94			
44.00	111.76	46.12	41.50	105.41	37.17			
44.25	112.39	46.37	41.75	106.04	37.39			
44.50	113.03	46.64	42.00	106.68	37.62			
44.75	113.66	46.89	42.25	107.31	37.87			
45.00	114.30	47.16	42.50	107.95	38.06			
45.25	114.93	47.42	42.75	108.58	38.28			
45.50	115.57	47.68	43.00	109.22	38.51			
45.75	116.20	47.94	43.25	109.85	38.73			
46.00	116.84	48.21	43.50	110.49	38.96			
46.25	117.47	48.47	43.75	111.12	39.18			
46.50	118.11	48.73	44.00	111.76	39.41			
46.75	118.74	48.99	44.25	112.39	39.63			
47.00	119.38	49.26	44.50	113.03	39.85			
47.25	120.01	49.52	44.75	113.66	40.08			
47.50	120.65	49.78	45.00	114.30	40.30			
47.75	121.28	50.04						
48.00	121.92	50.30						
48.25	122.55	50.56						
48.50	123.19	50.83						
48.75	123.82	51.09						
49.00	124.46	51.35						

Note: Percentage Fat = Constant A + Constant B − Constant C − 15.0.

[a]Copyright © 1986, 1991, 1996, 2000, 2006 by Frank I. Katch, Victor L. Katch, William D. McArdle, and Fitness Technologies, Inc., 5043 Via Lara Ln. Santa Barbara, CA 93111. No part of this appendix may be reproduced in any manner without written permission from the copyright holders.

Chart C.3	Conversion Constants to Predict Percentage Body Fat for Young Women[a]

ABDOMEN			THIGH			FOREARM		
in	cm	CONSTANT A	in	cm	CONSTANT B	in	cm	CONSTANT C
20.00	50.80	26.74	14.00	35.56	29.13	6.00	15.24	25.86
20.25	51.43	27.07	14.25	36.19	29.65	6.25	15.87	26.94
20.50	52.07	27.41	14.50	36.83	30.17	6.50	16.51	28.02
20.75	52.70	27.74	14.75	37.46	30.69	6.75	17.14	29.10
21.00	53.34	28.07	15.00	38.10	31.21	7.00	17.78	30.17
21.25	53.97	28.41	15.25	38.73	31.73	7.25	18.41	31.25
21.50	54.61	28.74	15.50	39.37	32.25	7.50	19.05	32.33
21.75	55.24	29.08	15.75	40.00	32.77	7.75	19.68	33.41
22.00	55.88	29.41	16.00	40.64	33.29	8.00	20.32	34.48
22.25	56.51	29.74	16.25	41.27	33.81	8.25	20.95	35.56
22.50	57.15	30.08	16.50	41.91	34.33	8.50	21.59	36.64
22.75	57.78	30.41	16.75	42.54	34.85	8.75	22.22	37.72
23.00	58.42	30.75	17.00	43.18	35.37	9.00	22.86	38.79
23.25	59.05	31.08	17.25	43.81	35.89	9.25	23.49	39.87
23.50	59.69	31.42	17.50	44.45	36.41	9.50	24.13	40.95
23.75	60.32	31.75	17.75	45.08	36.93	9.75	24.76	42.03
24.00	60.96	32.08	18.00	45.72	37.45	10.00	25.40	43.10
24.25	61.59	32.42	18.25	46.35	37.97	10.25	26.03	44.18
24.50	62.23	32.75	18.50	46.99	38.49	10.50	26.67	45.26
24.75	62.86	33.09	18.75	47.62	39.01	10.75	27.30	46.34
25.00	63.50	33.42	19.00	48.26	39.53	11.00	27.94	47.41
25.25	64.13	33.76	19.25	48.89	40.05	11.25	28.57	48.49
25.50	64.77	34.09	19.50	49.53	40.57	11.50	29.21	49.57
25.75	65.40	34.42	19.75	50.16	41.09	11.75	29.84	50.65
26.00	66.04	34.76	20.00	50.80	41.61	12.00	30.48	51.73
26.25	66.67	35.09	20.25	51.43	42.13	12.25	31.11	52.80
26.50	67.31	35.43	20.50	52.07	42.65	12.50	31.75	53.88

(continued)

Chart C.3 | **Conversion Constants to Predict Percentage Body Fat for Young Women[a] (Continued)**

ABDOMEN			THIGH			FOREARM		
in	cm	CONSTANT A	in	cm	CONSTANT B	in	cm	CONSTANT C
26.75	67.94	35.76	20.75	52.70	43.17	12.75	32.38	54.96
27.00	68.58	36.10	21.00	53.34	43.69	13.00	33.02	56.04
27.25	69.21	36.43	21.25	53.97	44.21	13.25	33.65	57.11
27.50	69.85	36.76	21.50	54.61	44.73	13.50	34.29	58.19
27.75	70.48	37.10	21.75	55.24	45.25	13.75	34.92	59.27
28.00	71.12	37.43	22.00	55.88	45.77	14.00	35.56	60.35
28.25	71.75	37.77	22.25	56.51	46.29	14.25	36.19	61.42
28.50	72.39	38.10	22.50	57.15	46.81	14.50	36.83	62.50
28.75	73.02	38.43	22.75	57.78	47.33	14.75	37.46	63.58
29.00	73.66	38.77	23.00	58.42	47.85	15.00	38.10	64.66
29.25	74.29	39.10	23.25	59.05	48.37	15.25	38.73	65.73
29.50	74.93	39.44	23.50	59.69	48.89	15.50	39.37	66.81
29.75	75.56	39.77	23.75	60.32	49.41	15.75	40.00	67.89
30.00	76.20	40.11	24.00	60.96	49.93	16.00	40.64	68.97
30.25	76.83	40.44	24.25	61.59	50.45	16.25	41.27	70.04
30.50	77.47	40.77	24.50	62.23	50.97	16.50	41.91	71.12
30.75	78.10	41.11	24.75	62.86	51.49	16.75	42.54	72.20
31.00	78.74	41.44	25.00	63.50	52.01	17.00	43.18	73.28
31.25	79.37	41.78	25.25	64.13	52.53	17.25	43.81	74.36
31.50	80.01	42.11	25.50	64.77	53.05	17.50	44.45	75.43
31.75	80.64	42.45	25.75	65.40	53.57	17.75	45.08	76.51
32.00	81.28	42.78	26.00	66.04	54.09	18.00	45.72	77.59
32.25	81.91	43.11	26.25	66.67	54.61	18.25	46.35	78.67
32.50	82.55	43.45	26.50	67.31	55.13	18.50	46.99	79.74
32.75	83.18	43.78	26.75	67.94	55.65	18.75	47.62	80.82
33.00	83.82	44.12	27.00	68.58	56.17	19.00	48.26	81.90
33.25	84.45	44.45	27.25	69.21	56.69	19.25	48.89	82.98
33.50	85.09	44.78	27.50	69.85	57.21	19.50	49.53	84.05
33.75	85.72	45.12	27.75	70.48	57.73	19.75	50.16	85.13
34.00	86.36	45.45	28.00	71.12	58.26	20.00	50.80	86.21
34.25	86.99	45.79	28.25	71.75	58.78			
34.50	87.63	46.12	28.50	72.39	59.30			
34.75	88.26	46.46	38.75	73.02	59.82			
35.00	88.90	46.79	29.00	73.66	60.34			
35.25	89.53	47.12	29.25	74.29	60.86			
35.50	90.17	47.46	29.50	74.93	61.38			
35.75	90.80	47.79	29.75	75.56	61.90			
36.00	91.44	48.13	30.00	76.20	62.42			
36.25	92.07	48.46	30.25	76.83	62.94			
36.50	92.71	48.80	30.50	77.47	63.46			
36.75	93.34	49.13	30.75	78.10	63.98			
37.00	93.98	49.46	31.00	78.74	64.50			
37.25	94.61	49.80	31.25	79.37	65.02			
37.50	95.25	50.13	31.50	80.01	65.54			
37.75	95.88	50.47	31.75	80.64	66.06			
38.00	96.52	50.80	32.00	81.28	66.58			
38.25	97.15	51.13	32.25	81.91	67.10			
38.50	97.79	51.47	32.50	82.55	67.62			
38.75	98.42	51.80	32.75	83.18	68.14			
39.00	99.06	52.14	33.00	83.82	68.66			
39.25	99.69	52.47	33.25	84.45	69.18			
39.50	100.33	52.81	33.50	85.09	69.70			
39.75	100.96	53.14	33.75	85.72	70.22			
40.00	101.60	53.47	34.00	86.36	70.74			

Note: Percentage Fat = Constant A + Constant B − Constant C − 19.6.

[a]Copyright © 1986, 1991, 1996, 2000, 2006, 2010 by Frank I. Katch, Victor L. Katch, William D. McArdle, and Fitness Technologies, Inc., 5043 Via Lara Ln. Santa Barbara, CA 93111. No part of this appendix may be reproduced in any manner without written permission from the copyright holders.

Chart C.4		Conversion Constants to Predict Percentage Body Fat for Older Women[a]							
ABDOMEN			**THIGH**			**FOREARM**			
in	cm	CONSTANT A	in	cm	CONSTANT B	in	cm	CONSTANT C	
25.00	63.50	29.69	14.00	35.56	17.31	10.00	25.40	14.46	
25.25	64.13	29.98	14.25	36.19	17.62	10.25	26.03	14.82	
25.50	64.77	30.28	14.50	36.83	17.93	10.50	26.67	15.18	
25.75	65.40	30.58	14.75	37.46	18.24	10.75	27.30	15.54	
26.00	66.04	30.87	15.00	38.10	18.55	11.00	27.94	15.91	
26.25	66.67	31.17	15.25	38.73	18.86	11.25	28.57	16.27	
26.50	67.31	31.47	15.50	39.37	19.17	11.50	29.21	16.63	
26.75	67.94	31.76	15.75	40.00	19.47	11.75	29.84	16.99	
27.00	68.58	32.06	16.00	40.64	19.78	12.00	30.48	17.35	
27.25	69.21	32.36	16.25	41.27	20.09	12.25	31.11	17.71	
27.50	69.85	32.65	16.50	41.91	20.40	12.50	31.75	18.08	
27.75	70.48	32.95	16.75	42.54	20.71	12.75	32.38	18.44	
28.00	71.12	33.25	17.00	43.18	21.02	13.00	33.02	18.80	
28.25	71.75	33.55	17.25	43.81	21.33	13.25	33.65	19.16	
28.50	72.39	33.84	17.50	44.45	21.64	13.50	34.29	19.52	
28.75	73.02	34.14	17.75	45.08	21.95	13.75	34.92	19.88	
29.00	73.66	34.44	18.00	45.72	22.26	14.00	35.56	20.24	
29.25	74.29	34.73	18.25	46.35	22.57	14.25	36.19	20.61	
29.50	74.93	35.03	18.50	46.99	22.87	14.50	36.83	20.97	
29.75	75.56	35.33	18.75	47.62	23.18	14.75	37.46	21.33	
30.00	76.20	35.62	19.00	38.26	23.49	15.00	38.10	21.69	
30.25	76.83	35.92	19.25	48.89	23.80	15.25	38.73	22.05	
30.50	77.47	36.22	19.50	49.53	24.11	15.50	39.37	22.41	
30.75	78.10	36.51	19.75	50.16	24.42	15.75	40.00	22.77	
31.00	78.74	36.81	20.00	50.80	24.73	16.00	40.64	23.14	
31.25	79.37	37.11	20.25	51.43	25.04	16.25	41.27	23.50	
31.50	80.01	37.40	20.50	52.07	25.35	16.50	41.91	23.86	
31.75	80.64	37.70	20.75	52.70	25.66	16.75	42.54	24.22	
32.00	81.28	38.00	21.00	53.34	25.97	17.00	43.18	24.58	
32.25	81.91	38.30	21.25	53.97	26.28	17.25	43.81	24.94	
32.50	82.55	38.59	21.50	54.61	26.58	17.50	44.45	25.31	
32.75	83.18	38.89	21.75	55.24	26.89	17.75	45.08	25.67	
33.00	83.82	39.19	22.00	55.88	27.20	18.00	45.72	26.03	
33.25	84.45	39.48	22.25	56.51	27.51	18.25	46.35	26.39	
33.50	85.09	39.78	22.50	57.15	27.82	18.50	46.99	26.75	
33.75	85.72	40.08	22.75	57.78	28.13	18.75	47.62	27.11	
34.00	86.36	40.37	23.00	58.42	28.44	19.00	48.26	27.47	
34.25	86.99	40.67	23.25	59.05	28.75	19.25	48.89	27.84	
34.50	87.63	40.97	23.50	59.69	29.06	19.50	49.53	28.20	
34.75	88.26	41.26	23.75	60.32	29.37	19.75	50.16	28.56	
35.00	88.90	41.56	24.00	60.96	29.68	20.00	50.80	28.92	
35.25	89.53	41.86	24.25	61.59	29.98	20.25	51.43	29.28	
35.50	90.17	42.15	24.50	62.23	30.29	20.50	52.07	29.64	
35.75	90.80	42.45	24.75	62.86	30.60	20.75	52.70	30.00	
36.00	91.44	42.75	25.00	63.50	30.91	21.00	53.34	30.37	
36.25	92.07	43.05	25.25	64.13	31.22	21.25	53.97	30.73	
36.50	92.71	43.34	25.50	64.77	31.53	21.50	54.61	31.09	
36.75	93.35	43.64	25.75	65.40	31.84	21.75	55.24	31.45	
37.00	93.98	43.94	26.00	66.04	32.15	22.00	55.88	31.81	
37.25	94.62	44.23	26.25	66.67	32.46	22.25	56.51	32.17	
37.50	95.25	44.53	26.50	67.31	32.77	22.50	57.15	32.54	
37.75	95.89	44.83	26.75	67.94	33.08	22.75	57.78	32.90	
38.00	96.52	45.12	27.00	68.58	33.38	23.00	58.42	33.26	
38.25	97.16	45.42	27.25	69.21	33.69	23.25	59.05	33.62	
38.50	97.79	45.72	27.50	69.85	34.00	23.50	59.69	33.98	
38.75	98.43	46.01	27.75	70.48	34.31	23.75	60.32	34.34	
39.00	99.06	46.31	28.00	71.12	34.62	24.00	60.96	34.70	
39.25	99.70	46.61	28.25	71.75	34.93	24.25	61.59	35.07	
39.50	100.33	46.90	28.50	72.39	35.24	24.50	62.23	35.43	
39.75	100.97	47.20	28.75	73.02	35.55	24.75	62.86	35.79	
40.00	101.60	47.50	29.00	73.66	35.86	25.00	63.50	36.15	
40.25	101.24	47.79	29.25	74.29	36.17				

(continued)

Chart C.4	Conversion Constants to Predict Percentage Body Fat for Older Women[a] (*Continued*)							
ABDOMEN			**THIGH**			**FOREARM**		
in	cm	CONSTANT A	in	cm	CONSTANT B	in	cm	CONSTANT C
40.50	102.87	48.09	29.50	74.93	36.48			
40.75	103.51	48.39	29.75	75.56	36.79			
41.00	104.14	48.69	30.00	76.20	37.09			
41.25	104.78	48.98	30.25	76.83	37.40			
41.50	105.41	49.28	30.50	77.47	37.71			
41.75	106.05	49.58	30.75	78.10	38.02			
42.00	106.68	49.87	31.00	78.74	38.33			
42.25	107.32	50.17	31.25	79.37	38.64			
42.50	107.95	50.47	31.50	80.01	38.95			
42.75	108.59	50.76	31.75	80.64	39.26			
43.00	109.22	51.06	32.00	81.28	39.57			
43.25	109.86	51.36	32.25	81.91	39.88			
43.50	110.49	51.65	32.50	82.55	40.19			
43.75	111.13	51.95	32.75	83.18	40.49			
44.00	111.76	52.25	33.00	83.82	40.80			
44.25	112.40	52.54	33.25	84.45	41.11			
44.50	113.03	52.84	33.50	85.09	41.42			
44.75	113.67	53.14	33.75	85.72	41.73			
45.00	114.30	53.44	34.00	86.36	42.04			

Note: Percentage Fat = Constant A + Constant B − Constant C − 19.6.

[a]Copyright © 1986, 1991, 1996, 2000, 2006, 2010 by Frank I. Katch, Victor L. Katch, William D. McArdle, and Fitness Technologies, Inc., 5043 Via Lara Ln. Santa Barbara, CA 93111. No part of this appendix may be reproduced in any manner without written permission from the copyright holders.

Evaluation of Body Composition—Skinfold Method

Skinfold equations to predict body density (Db) or percentage body fat (%BF) use regression analyses in which scores obtained on several variables are multiplied by constants to arrive at a predicted Db or %BF. Solving these equations requires extensive computations that are ill suited for field work and are subject to error, particularly when done by hand or with calculators.

A nomogram is a pictorial method that simplifies computations by providing a simple "look-up" method to solve the equation.

THE NOMOGRAM

Figure D.1 presents the nomogram to estimate %BF for college-aged men and women from the sum of three skinfolds plus age using generalized equations.

VARIABLES

- For men, obtain the following variables: skinfolds in millimeters (chest, abdomen, thigh) and age in years.
- For women, obtain the following variables: skinfolds in millimeters (triceps, thigh, suprailiac) and age in years.

USING THE NOMOGRAM

1. Sum the three skinfolds.
2. Locate on the right scale (sum of the three skinfolds in millimeters).
3. Locate on the left scale (age in years).
4. With a ruler, connect the two points (right scale and left scale); read the resulting %BF from the center scale (male or female).

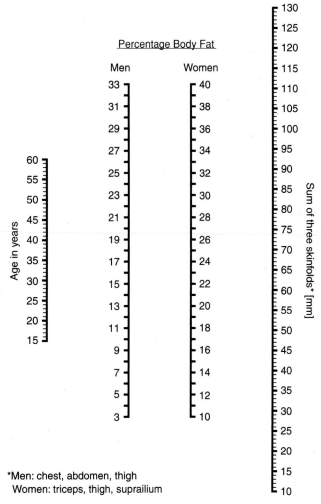

*Men: chest, abdomen, thigh
  Women: triceps, thigh, suprailium

Figure D.1   Nomogram to estimate percentage body fat of college-aged men and women using the Jackson et al. generalized equations. (From Baun, W.B., Baun, M.R.: A nomogram for the estimate of percent body fat from generalized equations. *Res. Q. Exerc. Sport*, 52:382, 1981. Copyright 1981 by AAHPERD. Reprinted by permission.)

EXAMPLE

Data for a woman, age 30 y; triceps skinfold = 15 mm; thigh skinfold = 15 mm; suprailiac skinfold = 25 mm.

1. Sum skinfolds = 55 mm.
2. Place rule on right scale over 55 mm; connect to left scale at age 30 y.
3. Read percentage body fat: 23%.

CAUTION

Although nomograms can save time, they are subject to error, particularly interpolation errors in which precision and accuracy can be compromised. At best, interpolation of the %BF value for men and women in the present nomogram becomes limited to no more than half a whole percentage point. Also, because the nomogram uses the Siri equation to convert Db to %BF, it should not be used with populations in which other density-to-percentage fat conversions are more appropriate.

EQUATIONS

Check the accuracy of using the nomogram by solving the following equations to predict percentage Db.

Convert Db to %BF using the Siri equation (%BF = 495 ÷ Db − 450).

1. Equation for men: Σ3SKF equals sum of chest, abdomen, and thigh skinfolds:

$$Db = 1.10938 - (0.0008267 \times \Sigma 3SKF) \\ + ([0.0000016 \times \Sigma 3SKF]^2) \\ - (0.0002574 \times Age)$$

2. Equation for women: Σ3SKF equals sum of triceps, thigh, and suprailiac skinfolds:

$$Db = 1.0994921 - (0.0009929 \times \Sigma 3SKF) \\ + ([0.0000023 \times \Sigma 3SKF]^2) \\ - (0.0001392 \times Age)$$

REFERENCES

Baun, W.B., Baun M.R.: A nomogram for the estimate of percent body fat from generalized equations. *Res. Quart. Exerc. Sport,* 52:382, 1981.

Jackson, A.S., et al.: Generalized equations for predicting body density of women. *Med. Sci. Sports Exerc.,* 12:175, 1980.

Jackson, A.S., Pollock, M.L.: Generalized equations for predicting body density of men. *Br. J. Nutr.,* 40:497, 1978.

Index

CCS1110